Pediatric Nutrition Handbook

6TH EDITION

Ronald E. Kleinman, MD
Editor

Policy of the American Academy of Pediatrics

American Academy of Pediatrics
141 Northwest Point Blvd
Elk Grove Village, IL 60007-1098

Library of Congress Control Number: 2008922528
ISBN: 978-1-58110-298-7
MA0442

The recommendations in this publication do not indicate an exclusive course of treatment or serve as a standard of medical care. Variations, taking into account individual circumstances, may be appropriate.

Cover photo credits: (t) Getty Images; (ml) Getty Images; (mr) Bananastock/Jupiterimages; (bl) Superstock; (bc) Getty Images; (br) Corbis; (b) Superstock

Committee on Nutrition
2007-2008

Frank R. Greer, MD, Chairperson
Jatinder J. S. Bhatia, MD
Stephen R. Daniels, MD, PhD
Marcie B. Schneider, MD
Janet Silverstein, MD
Dan W. Thomas, MD
Nicolas Stettler, MD, MSCE

Former Committee Members

Nancy F. Krebs, MD, MS, Former Chairperson
Robert D. Baker, Jr, MD, PhD
Melvin B. Heyman, MD
Fima Lifshitz, MD

Liaisons

Laurence Grummer-Strawn, PhD, *Centers for Disease Control and Prevention*
Van S. Hubbard, MD, PhD, *National Institutes of Health*
Donna Blum-Kemelor, MS, RD, *US Department of Food and Agriculture*
Valerie Marchand, MD, *Canadian Paediatric Society*
Benson M. Silverman, MD, *US Food and Drug Administration*

Staff

Debra L. Burrowes, MHA

Preface

The role of nutrition in the well-being of infants and children has expanded beyond determining the quantities of nutrients needed to prevent classic deficiency states such as scurvy. Modern nutritional science now seeks to understand the interaction between nutrition and human physiology at the level of genetics and molecular biology. In addition, a major direction in nutritional research is to examine how those interactions that occur early in life affect health and development not only at different periods during infancy and childhood but also over the life span of the individual. To provide one example, does the provision of specific nutrients such as long-chain fatty acids during pregnancy or during early infancy influence cognition, behavior, and vision of the young infant, and if so, do those benefits persist into later childhood and even adulthood? We also have come to recognize that nutrients, foods, and eating patterns are not synonymous. What and how infants and children are fed and eat have many determinants, including those that are cultural, traditional, behavioral, cognitive, and environmental, and this is another major current focus of investigation.

Thus, this sixth edition of the *Pediatric Nutrition Handbook* attempts to provide the latest information about nutrient metabolism and nutrition to support normal development and health of infants and children who are well, those born with congenital anomalies or disorders of metabolism, and those with acute and chronic illness. It is meant to serve as a useful and ready reference for practicing clinicians. Within the chapters, every attempt has been made to provide the reader with additional resources, including references to printed materials, agencies, and Web sites that may be useful in practice and for patients to access directly. The chapters on specific nutrients are meant to serve as the basis for subsequent chapters that deal with specific health conditions. Breastfeeding is discussed early in this book to emphasize its roles in promoting a healthy infancy and in protecting against chronic disease, for example, obesity. An entire chapter is dedicated to cultural implications of feeding children, and other chapters focus on topics such as how children develop preferences for specific tastes, foods, and meal patterns; how to best support those with chronic illness; and enteral and parenteral nutrition support for those who cannot eat.

From a public health perspective, in all industrialized nations and increasingly in most developing nations, overweight and obesity are among the most important chronic conditions affecting children today. The persistent and accumulating adverse effects of excessive body fat during childhood have been and continue to be documented in well-designed ecologic studies. Overweight in childhood is a consequence of the pernicious effect of environmental influences that encourage eating and the repeated consumption of high-calorie foods and discourage activity, overlaid on a genetic background that is designed to conserve or store excess consumed energy. Thus, the introductory chapter of this edition of the handbook, "Nutrition, Physical Activity, and Health: An Office-Based Approach," speaks to office-based practices that can be directed toward identifying overweight as well as other nutritional disorders, and other chapters focus on in-depth discussions of nutrition assessment, obesity, food labeling, and other issues that affect our understanding and treatment of overweight as well as other nutritional disorders.

This handbook is the result of the work of more than 70 authors, some of whom contributed to the previous edition and all of whom are recognized experts in the topics on which they have written. Several new chapters and appendices have been added, including chapters on nutrition support of patients with liver disease and inflammatory bowel disease and appendices that display and discuss the newest food guide pyramids, now called MyPyramid. The newly developed growth standards from the World Health Organization for healthy breastfed infants and young children are also provided, along with the reference growth charts for infancy through adolescence from the Centers for Disease Control and Prevention. All chapters have been updated to reflect the latest information available, and summaries of the current position statements and guidelines of the American Academy of Pediatrics Committee on Nutrition are included in relevant chapters. Many thanks go to the members of the Committee on Nutrition, who have served as the editorial board and have guided and overseen the content of the handbook under the expert leadership of the chairperson, Frank Greer, MD. It has been a particular privilege to work with Dr. Greer, whose knowledge, experience, and counsel on all "things nutritional" is unsurpassed.

Ronald E. Kleinman, MD, Editor

Contributors

The American Academy of Pediatrics gratefully acknowledges the invaluable assistance provided by the following individuals who contributed to the preparation of this edition of the *Pediatric Nutrition Handbook*. Every attempt has been made to recognize all who have contributed; we regret any omissions that may have occured.

Steven Abrams, MD, *Children's Nutrition Research Center, Baylor College of Medicine,* Houston, TX

Sue Ann Anderson, PhD, RD, *Food and Drug Administration,* College Park, MD

Jean Ashland, PhD, *Massachusetts General Hospital,* Boston, MA

Robert D. Baker, MD, PhD, *Women and Children's Hospital of Buffalo,* Buffalo, NY

Jatinder Bhatia, MD, FAAP, *Medical College of Georgia,* Augusta, GA

Donna Blum-Kemelor, MS, RD, *USDA/FNS/OANE/NSS,* Alexandria, VA

John Bradley, MD, *Children's Hospital San Diego,* San Diego, CA

Caren L. Brown, RD, CDE, *University of Florida,* Gainesville, FL

Nancy Butte, MD, *Children's Nutrition Research Center, Baylor College of Medicine,* Houston, TX

Hilary Creed-Kanashiro, *Instituto de Investigación Nutricional,* Lima, PERU

Stephen R. Daniels, MD, PhD, FAAP, *Denver Children's Hospital,* Denver, CO

Peter R. Durie, MD, *The University of Toronto,* Toronto, Ontario, CANADA

Robert Earl, MPH, RD, *Food Products Association,* Washington, D.C.

Drew Feranchak, MD, *UT Southwestern Medical School,* Dallas, TX

Jerry Z. Finkelstein, MD, *David Geffen School of Medicine at University of California Los Angeles,* Los Angeles, CA

Marta Fiorotto, PhD, *Children's Nutrition Research Center, Baylor College of Medicine,* Houston, TX

Shahin Firouzbakhsh, RD, *Miller Children's Hospital at Long Beach Memorial Medical Center,* Long Beach, CA

Jennifer O. Fisher, PhD, *Baylor College of Medicine,* Houston, TX

Deborah A. Frank, MD, *Boston University School of Medicine,* Brookline, MA

Michael K. Georgieff, MD, *University of Minnesota,* Minneapolis, MN

William Greenhill, DMD, *Children's Hospital Medical Center,* Cincinnati, OH

Frank Greer, MD, *Perinatal Center – Meriter Hospital,* Madison, WI

Carey O. Harding, MD, *Oregon Health & Science University,* Portland, OR

William C. Heird, MD, *Children's Nutrition Research Center, Baylor College of Medicine,* Houston, TX

Melvin B. Heyman, MD, FAAP, *University of California,* San Francisco, CA

Kathleen Huntington, RD, *Oregon Health & Science University,* Portland, OR

Esther Israel, MD, *MassGeneral Hospital for Children, Harvard Medical School,* Boston, MA

W. Daniel Jackson, MD, *University of Utah School of Medicine,* Salt Lake City, UT

Thomas Jaksic, MD, PhD, *Children's Hospital,* Boston, MA

Craig L. Jensen, MD, *Children's Nutrition Research Center, Baylor College of Medicine,* Houston, TX

Susan L. Johnson, PhD, *University of Colorado Health Sciences Center,* Denver, CO

Daina Kalnins, RD, *The Hospital for Sick Children,* Toronto, Ontario, CANADA

William J. Klish, MD, *Texas Children's Hospital,* Houston, TX

Richard Kreipe, MD, *University of Rochester,* Rochester, NY

Michele LaBotz, MD, FAAP, *Intermed PA,* South Portland, ME

Alan M. Lake, MD, Pediatric Consultants, Lutherville, MD

Michael Laposata, *Massachusetts General Hospital,* Boston, MA

Rudolph L. Leibel, MD, *Division of Molecular Genetics and Naomi Berrie Diabetes Center,* New York, NY

Lynne L. Levitsky, MD, *MassGeneral Hospital for Children, Harvard Medical School,* Boston, MA

Bo Lonnerdal, PhD, *University of California,* Davis, CA

Martha Lynch, *MassGeneral Hospital for Children,* Boston, MA

William C. MacLean, Jr, MD, *The Ohio State University College of Medicine,* Columbus, OH

Valerie Marchand, MD, *Hopital Ste Justine,* Montreal, Quebec, CANADA

Martín G. Martín, MD, MPP, *University of California Los Angeles,* Los Angeles, CA

Tracie Miller, MD, *University of Miami School of Medicine,* Miami, FL

Bruce Z. Morgenstern, MD, *Phoenix Children's Hospital,* Phoenix, AZ

Theresa Nicklas, PhD, *Children's Nutrition Research Center, Baylor College of Medicine,* Houston, TX

Carol O'Neil, PhD, MPH, LDN, RD, *Louisiana State University,* Baton Rouge, LA

Lois Parker, RPh, *MassGeneral Hospital for Children,* Boston, MA

Heidi Pfeifer, RD, LDN, *MassGeneral Hospital for Children,* Boston, MA

Mary Frances Picciano, PhD, *National Institutes of Health,* Bethesda, MD

Michael Rosenbaum, MD, *Naomi Berrie Diabetes Center,* New York, NY

Philip Rosenthal, *University of California,* San Francisco, CA

Gary Russell, MD, *MassGeneral Hospital for Children, Harvard Medical School,* Boston, MA

Hugh A. Sampson, MD, *Mount Sinai Medical Center,* New York, NY

Richard J. Schanler, MD, *North Shore University Hospital,* Manhasset, NY

Kathleen B. Schwarz, MD, *Johns Hopkins University School of Medicine,* Baltimore, MD

Robert Shaddy, MD, *Primary Children's Medical Center,* Salt Lake City, UT

Katherine M. Shea, MD, MPH, *Duke University School of Medicine,* Durham, NC

Robert J. Shulman, MD, *Children's Nutrition Research Center, Baylor College of Medicine,* Houston, TX

Benson M. Silverman, MD, *Food and Drug Administration,* College Park, MD

Janet Silverstein, MD, *University of Florida College of Medicine,* Gainesville, FL

John Snyder, MD, *Children's Hospital,* Washington, DC

Ronald J. Sokol, MD, *University of Colorado Health Sciences Center,* Denver, CO

Chad Soupir, MD, *Harvard Medical School,* Boston, MA

Virginia A. Stallings, MD, *The Children's Hospital of Philadelphia,* Philadelphia, PA

Elizabeth Thiele, *MassGeneral Hospital for Children,* Boston, MA

Patti J. Thureen, MD, *University of Colorado School of Medicine,* Denver, CO

Vasundhara Tolia, MD, *Michigan State University College of Human Medicine,* Southfield, MI

John N. Udall, Jr., MD, *West Virginia University–Charleston,* Charleston, WV

Steven J. Wassner, MD, *The Penn State University College of Medicine,* Hershey, PA

William B. Weil, MD, *Michigan State University,* East Lansing, MI

Marc-Alain Widdowson, *Centers for Disease Control,* Atlanta, GA

Table of Contents

Introduction

Nutrition, Physical Activity, and Health: An Office-Based Approach

Background

For those of us in community practice of pediatrics, this sixth edition of the American Academy of Pediatrics (AAP) *Nutrition Handbook* will bring a much-needed updated resource with which to expand our knowledge and practical needs to address issues of child "wellness." Never before have the needs of children required such focus on nutrition, physical activity, and establishing a model for lifestyle change to promote healthy habits that can extend into the adult years. Twenty years ago, the second edition of the AAP *Nutrition Handbook* emphasized evaluation of failure to thrive and included one sentence on exercise. Now, the emphasis is on awareness of the intervals from the prenatal environment to adolescence that contribute to possible "programming" of the child for a life of obesity and its comorbid complications. Although the pendulum has thus swung to concern with excess energy intake for level of activity and growth, it is critical that health care professionals remain focused on health and wellness, emphasizing nutritional health and physical activity for normal growth and development throughout childhood, independent of body weight.

Studies reported by the Institute of Medicine and the Centers for Disease Control and Prevention confirm that the prevalence of obesity has nearly tripled across the spectrum of childhood, from toddler to adolescent.[1-3] Most of the developed world has entered the era of affluent malnutrition, with intakes of energy-rich foods exceeding the intakes of nutrient-rich foods. Complications of obesity, once rare in childhood, are now encountered frequently and mandate monitoring. The basic physics of weight gain are such that when energy or caloric intake exceeds energy use by 3500 kcal, weight gain of 1 pound occurs. An excess of only 100 kcal per day yields weight gain of 10 pounds a year.

Community physicians must devote increased time for early recognition of nutritional and activity concerns and early intervention by increasing parent and family awareness of inadequate or excess weight for height, age, and activity. A consistent theme of the intervention will be the need for the family members to be role models and assume a family-based commitment to a more active lifestyle. Reference will be made to reviews and recommendations from the AAP, the American Heart Association, the American

Dietetic Association, Bright Futures, the Centers for Disease Control and Prevention, and the Institute of Medicine.

Documentation of Growth and Body Mass Index

It is imperative that growth data are generated for every child at the time of physical examinations for preventive health maintenance. Weight, length, and head circumference are measured and plotted in the first 3 years. For children younger than 2 years, one can plot the weight for length on the standard growth chart and confirm whether the percentile is a cause for concern. For children 2 years and older, the body mass index (BMI) can be determined and plotted. The BMI is a weight-for-height index determined by dividing the weight in kg by the height in m². BMI calculators are readily available and can be plotted on the reverse side of most growth charts (see Appendix D) as a percentile for age. The level of weight concern is now defined on the basis of these percentiles for age. If the BMI is less than the 5th percentile, the child is underweight; if between the 5th and 85th percentile, the child is of normal weight; if between the 85th and 95th percentile, the child is considered "at risk" of being overweight, and if above the 95th percentile for age, the child is considered overweight. It is acknowledged that BMI is not a perfect measure, especially if the child is of small or very large frame.

In addition to an elevated BMI percentile, a yearly increase or decrease of 3 units in the BMI is a cause for concern. The waist circumference is the best measure of central adiposity and best predictor of insulin resistance. Nationally representative reference standards for waist circumference have been published for children in the United States.[4] A recent practice-based study of office evaluation and management of childhood obesity underscored the slow acceptance of the BMI calculation; among 600 patients, 39.8% of whom were either at risk of or already overweight, the BMI was calculated in only 0.5% of charts.[5]

In 2003, the AAP endorsed routine yearly screening by BMI documentation in children older than 2 years.[6] In 2005, the Childhood Obesity Working Group of the US Preventive Services Task Force reminded us that, despite expert consensus, the evidence to date does not allow recommendations for or against routine BMI screening for the prevention of adult obesity.[7] This is not an indictment of screening, but a call to monitor for complications of screening and to generate the "practice-based evidence" required to achieve "evidence-based practice."[8] Overweight and obesity are discussed in greater depth in Chapter 33.

Recognition of the Role of the Intrauterine Environment

Evidence is accumulating that some children are "primed" for long-term weight concerns and type 2 diabetes early in gestation.[9] Maternal obesity and the attendant role of intrauterine overnutrition appear to lead to metabolic adaptations that may extend well into early adulthood and beyond. Similarly, Barker and colleagues remind us that early gestational maternal undernutrition leads to small-for-gestational-age neonates with metabolic adaptations predisposing to overweight and early-onset cardiovascular disease and diabetes.[10,11] Thus, children with birth weight less than 5 pounds or greater than 9 pounds need more careful monitoring for excessive early weight gain.

Genetic factors, of course, also play a role, with most research addressing the "survival genes"—those that created a metabolic ability to survive intervals of relative starvation that truly plagued our forefathers. Not surprisingly, both animal and human studies have demonstrated more than 200 genes that predispose to energy conservation or obesity and fewer than 5 genes that predispose to remaining lean. Thus, although the survival gene historically was a benefit, it is prudent that we limit its effect on our current health needs.

Risk Assessment

As patients are followed through the pediatric age group, it is essential to establish a habit of regular review of risk factors in nutrition and physical activity with the goal of early recognition and early intervention. In 1998, Barlow and Dietz established evaluation guidelines for children with nutritional concerns.[12] Assessment of nutritional status is discussed in greater depth in Chapter 24.

Physical Examination

As noted previously, weight and length up to 2 years of age, and weight and height beyond 2 years of age, should be measured and documented, and growth percentiles should be confirmed. BMI should be calculated and percentile for age should be plotted. Progress, or lack thereof, should be reviewed with the family and child, keeping in mind that pace of growth is more important than the percentile. Blood pressure should be documented in all children 3 years and older. Tanner staging of pubertal status should be documented and its significance with regard to nutritional demands should be reviewed.

Patient History
Gestation, birth weight, and rate of gain since infancy should be documented. Contributory roles of acute and chronic illness, medications, and allergies should be documented. The history for underweight children includes patterns of eating, early satiety, reflux or emesis, specific questions about stool pattern, discomfort with meals, and their personal weight goals. The review of systems for overweight children includes glucose intolerance, orthopedic concerns, features of polycystic ovary syndrome, sleep disorders, headache, and dramatic shifts in weight.

Family History
Parental weight, height, and risk of or established features of the metabolic syndrome should be documented. Specifically, predispositions to early cardiovascular disease, hypertension, dyslipidemia, diabetes, sleep apnea, gallbladder or fatty liver disease, other endocrine concerns, and eating disorders should be addressed. The parent's (and grandparent's) ability to be a role model for improved nutrition and physical activity should be reviewed.

Nutrition History
Early feeding practices, tolerance and duration of breastfeeding, use of formulas, and timing of introduction of solids should be documented. Current eating patterns, including meals, snacks, fast food, and beverage choices, should be reviewed. Servings of fruits, vegetables, salads, fiber, and sources of calcium, folic acid, and iron as well as the use of vitamins should be documented. The "habits" of family meals should be reviewed. If concern is high or the reports are inconsistent, a prospective 3-day diet record should be requested.

Physical Activity
Family and child opportunities for daily physical activity should be reviewed. Factors that limit access, such as safety, lack of commitment from child care providers, or lack of recess time or physical education classes in school, should be identified. "Screen-time" with television, personal computers, video games, and hand held games should be documented.

Opportunities for Intervention
The child's and family's acceptance of any concern, which is a critical component to motivate for change, should be documented. Nutritional and activity options should be addressed, and the child's and family's ideas and preferences should be incorporated while setting reasonable goals. Television or "screen-time" should be limited to no more than 2 hours per day

for all children older than 2 years and should be eliminated for children younger than 2 years. Judgmental or threatening comments should be avoided. Health care professionals should appeal to the parent's recognition of the long-term complications of being overweight and the child's need to avoid peer teasing. Health care professionals should appeal to the child's desire for improved appearance, improved exercise tolerance, and improved social opportunities. Regardless of whether calorie supplements or reductions in energy intake are advised, close follow-up and encouragement should be planned to underscore the health care professional's concern. Everyone in the child's environment—from siblings to parents to teachers to physicians—must recognize their potential value as a role model.

Age-Specific Concerns

Although nutritional and activity status and opportunities for intervention are addressed throughout childhood, there are some issues that are more age specific. These concerns are presented as follows within the ranges of infancy and toddlerhood and preschool, primary school, and secondary school ages.

Infancy and Toddlerhood: Birth to 2 Years of Age

Many pediatricians have the first opportunity to discuss a child's nutritional health at the prenatal visit. Parental concerns and expectations can be addressed, and the value of breastfeeding can be underscored. Intrauterine concerns in regard to fetal health can be identified and discussed as well. The goal is for the prospective parents to buy into the need for child wellness.

The value of breastfeeding has been well established and is discussed in Chapter 2. The AAP recently updated its policy statement "Breastfeeding and the Use of Human Milk."[13] The role of the pediatrician in facilitating proper nursing techniques has also been summarized in an article by Lawrence.[14] In addition to the well-documented advantages of human milk, the process of breastfeeding adds the crucial component of the baby's ability to self-regulate intake. Although the studies to date are far from conclusive, there is some demonstrated reduction in risk of childhood obesity with breastfeeding for greater than 4 to 6 months.[15] Breastfeeding is associated with increased mean triglyceride and low-density lipoprotein concentrations in infancy but lower concentrations in adulthood.[16] Furthermore, a recent study suggests that the more rapid initial weight gain seen in formula-fed babies, even in the first week of life, may contribute to adult obesity.[17] Vitamin D supplementation is now recommended for all breastfed newborns.

The schedule of formula feedings should be reviewed with an eye to avoiding overfeeding or use of the bottle as a pacifier. Parents should be encouraged to feed infants and children when they are hungry, not solely on a schedule convenient to the parents. It should be confirmed that the formula is being prepared correctly and that fluoride is available after 6 months of age. After 6 months of age, there is no need for routine feeding between midnight and 6 AM. Cereals and pureed foods should not be introduced until after 4 to 6 months of age, and unless there is a specific need to thicken liquids, cereals should not be added to bottles. Parents should be reminded that a baby's tolerance of initial solids is often based more on texture than on taste. The early introduction of inappropriate solids should be discouraged.

The recent Feeding Infants and Toddlers Study (FITS), undertaken in 3000 children by the American Dietetic Association and Gerber, demonstrated that 4- to 6-month-olds received 10% more calories per day than optimal for growth, that 7- to 11-month-olds received 23% more calories than optimal for growth, and that 1- to 2-year-olds received 31% more calories than optimal for growth.[18] The subset of study participants who were receiving benefits under the Special Supplemental Nutrition Program for Women, Infants, and Children (WIC) had even higher energy intakes; 7- to 11-month-olds received 32% more calories per day than optimal for growth, and 1- to 2-year olds received 40% more calories per day than optimal for growth. Nearly 30% of the infants younger than 4 months were already receiving solid foods daily. By daily diet reporting at 2 years of age, 30% of children were not eating any fruit and 20% were not eating any vegetables on a daily basis.[18] Not surprisingly, the vegetable that was most commonly consumed was potato.

By 9 to 11 months of age, the diets of most children begin to resemble those of their parents, reinforcing the need for the parent to be aware of their influence even before 1 year of age. By 12 to 15 months of age, children ideally should be eating meals with the family. Toddlers should have 3 balanced meals a day and 1 or 2 nutritious snacks. One serving size is approximately the size of the individual's fist.[19]

According to the National Health and Nutrition Examination Survey (NHANES) III data, extended bottle feeding is a concern. For each month after 18 months of age that a toddler continues daily bottle use, there is a 3% increase in risk of having a BMI higher than the 95th percentile by 10 years of age. In the NHANES, 20% of 2-year-olds and 9% of 3-year-olds still drank juice or milk from a bottle daily.[20] Counseling families to minimize sugary juice and to eliminate bottle use by 18 months of age is, thus, encouraged.

Although an increase in BMI percentile is a feature of excessive weight gain, infants developing failure to thrive may not have as dramatic a decline in BMI percentile, because reduced weight gain may be associated with reduced height gain, regardless of whether the infant has maldigestion, malabsorption, or inadequate caloric delivery. When weight gain slows in the infant or toddler, a careful review of caloric delivery should be conducted, including questions about use of dilute formulas or fat-free dairy products, excessive juice intake, and inappropriate early introduction of low–caloric-density solids, and there should be a discussion about opportunities to increase calorie and nutrient delivery. Caregivers are encouraged to provide a 3- to 5-day dietary intake record for review by the pediatrician or consulting dietitian. Before embarking on an expensive, if not invasive, evaluation, a trial of increased caloric delivery can be attempted by enriching the diet with more calorie-dense nutrients while documenting stool frequency, addressing chronic disease issues, and addressing relevant psychosocial issues for the family. See Chapter 26 for a more extensive review of inadequate growth.

In infancy, physical activity is encouraged to promote developmental milestones, such as reaching, transferring, rolling, sitting, creeping, crawling, walking, climbing, and running. Parents are encouraged to allow their infants "tummy time" for several minutes, several times a day. Parents should be reminded of the need to create a safe area for unstructured play on the floor several times a day. From 1 to 3 years of age, parents should seek more than 30 minutes of structured play and more than 60 minutes of free, unstructured play for their children every day. Safe outdoor play, free from the constraints of strollers, is also encouraged once ambulation is achieved. Unfortunately, recent surveys demonstrate that 75% of 3-year-olds and 39% of 4-year-olds are predominately confined to strollers when outdoors, even at parks. Table I.1 summarizes the nutritional and activity goals for infants and toddlers.

Preschool: 2 to 5 Years of Age

During the preschool years, the adiposity of children generally declines with a decline in BMI as the child's length increases and fat cell size declines. A nadir is reached between 4 and 6 years, which is followed by the "adiposity rebound" of the BMI, which increases linearly to puberty. Evidence suggests that children who enter the rebound earlier or have a higher BMI at 4 to 6 years of age as they enter the rebound are at greater risk of adult obesity and glucose intolerance.[21] The Healthy Start Preschool Study suggests that children should gain 1.0 kg of weight per linear increase of 2 cm from 3 to 5 years of age. A weight gain of 1.8 kg per linear increase of 2 cm predicted overweight at elementary school.[22] For children younger than 3 years, the best predictor of adult obesity is parent weight; for children between 3 and 9 years of age, the predictor is combined child and parent weight; and for children older than 9 years, the child's degree of obesity is the best predictor.[23] The preschool years, thus, appear to be important in potentially determining nutritional status in later childhood, if not into adulthood.

Table I.1
Nutrition and Physical Activity in Infants and Toddlers: Guidelines for Parents

Nutrition Goals
Encourage and support breastfeeding through the first year.
Feed the child when hungry, not solely by habits of schedules.
Defer introduction of solid foods until after 4 to 6 months of age.
Monitor for inadequate or excessive weight gain closely.
Expect to offer new foods repeatedly before child accepts the food.
Minimize juice and other sugar-based beverages.
Eat meals as a family; be a good role model.
Activity Goals
Create a safe space for unstructured play.
In infancy, gear activity to developmental progress.
Encourage "tummy time" several times a day until baby can crawl.
Encourage creeping, crawling, and safe crawling up and down stairs.
Use a stroller for safe transportation, but encourage free play when ambulatory.
From 1 to 3 years, seek more than 30 minutes of structured play and more than 60 minutes of free, unstructured play daily.

Parents typically describe frustration in achieving a healthy diet for the preschool-aged child. This tends to be an age group prone to excess sugary foods, limited interest in acceptance of new foods, and sensitivity to portion size. Twenty years ago, Birch and associates demonstrated that preschoolers could self-regulate their own intake.[24] Children should not be encouraged to "clean the plate." Two- and 3-year-olds will not increase intake when given larger portion sizes, but children older than 4 years will increase their intake by more than 30% when offered larger portions.[25] The consensus is, thus, that parents should decide when and what to eat, and children should decide how much and whether to eat. New nutritious foods should be offered on the plate next to accepted food and, on average, will need to be offered 8 to 10 times before they are accepted. Most parents give up after 3 to 4 refusals, so patience is critical. Parents should be encouraged to offer nutrient-dense foods rather than energy-dense foods, using low-fat or nonfat dairy in place of whole milk (which should be used up to 2 years of age).[26]

Parents should be reminded that food should not be used as a reward or punishment for behavior and that "low-fat" food is often not low in calories. Preschool-aged children can help with shopping for appropriate foods and assist in food preparation at meals. They should have 3 nutritious meals and 2 nutritious snacks a day. Meals should be a family event, and routinely feeding the child first should be discouraged. Physicians should be sensitive to ethnic and cultural issues with regard to diet, appropriate activity, and sense of wellness. On the other hand, it is imperative that parents and grandparents accept the reality that a "chubby" child is not the accepted goal.

The role of physical activity in weight control is underscored by the observation that obesity risk in preschoolers and beyond is reduced 10% by every hour of moderate to vigorous activity daily. Regrettably, the average preschool child spends 75% of his or her waking hours inactive and only 12 minutes a day in vigorous activity. Even on the playground, preschool children devote only 11% of their time engaging in vigorous play.

For children 3 to 6 years of age, the best predictors of increased BMI are baseline BMI (at the nadir of the adiposity rebound), decreased physical activity, and increased television viewing.[27] The AAP recommends that "screen time," including television, personal computers, and video games, be limited to 2 hours or less a day for children older than 2 years. Televisions should not be placed in children's bedrooms. Moderate to vigorous activity is encouraged for at least 1 hour per day. An ideal goal in preschool programs is 10 minutes of active play per hour in school. Families should be encouraged to exercise together, go for walks, limit use of strollers, use safe outdoor play areas, and become community advocates for increased opportunities for all. The recommendations for nutritional awareness and physical activity for preschool-aged children are summarized in Table I.2.

Table I.2
Nutrition and Physical Activity in the Preschool-Aged Child: Guidelines for Parents

Nutrition Goals
Choose meal time and content.
Let child self-regulate amount of intake; do not demand a clean plate.
Avoid juices, sugary snacks, and high-fat foods.
Do not use food as a reward or punishment.
Offer new foods 6 to 10 times to expect acceptance.
Avoid large portion sizes; be a role model.
Activity Goals
Create or find a safe area for unstructured play daily.
Seek 1 hour or more of vigorous play daily.
Encourage child care providers to offer 10 minutes of active play per hour.
Reduce television and other screen time to less than 2 hours a day, and avoid television in bedroom.
Limit use of strollers to encourage spontaneous walking, running, and playing.
Establish regular family exercise; be a role model.

Primary School: 5 to 11 Years of Age

The highest rate of increase in obesity from 1980 to 2000 occurred in the age group from 6 to 11 years of age, from 4% with a BMI percentile above the 95th percentile to 15%.[1] This is attributed to many factors, including increased consumption of fast food and super-sized meals, more screen time, less daily exercise, working parents too tired for family exercise, reduction of safe play areas in urban settings, reduced physical education and recess at schools, and increased academic demands. All undoubtedly play a variable role in each child and family. In the prepubertal years, the child gains an average of 7 pounds and grows 2.5 inches per year. The adiposity rebound underscores the steady increase in both the size and number of fat cells that extends into puberty.

The period from 5 to 11 years of age is commonly when many children first begin to eat and snack in the absence of parent supervision. Most primary school-aged children do not eat a nutritious breakfast and get more than 30% of calories from snacks readily available at home, at friends' houses, at after-school care programs, or from neighborhood fast food resources. With multiple caregivers involved, most parents have little idea of their child's actual daily intake. Multiple after-school programs and family obligations often limit family meals at home.

In September 2005, the US Department of Agriculture released MyPyramid for Kids (see Appendix K), an interactive Web-based program designed to improve nutritional and activity awareness targeting 6- to 11-year-olds. The Web site (www.mypyramid.gov/kids) is based on the 2005 Dietary Guidelines for Americans and addresses food choices, portion sizes, and daily physical activity guidelines.[28] It includes a 2-sided parent handout called "Tips for Families," which has nutritional information on one side and physical activity tips on the other. Lesson plans for teachers are also available. Updated dietary recommendations for childhood, with an eye to prevention of the comorbidities of developing overweight in childhood, were published by the American Heart Association and endorsed by the AAP.[26]

During the annual physical examination or other opportunity, questions in regard to nutrition should focus on meal content and acceptance, frequency of fast food meals, volumes of daily juices and sodas, choices at school breakfast and lunch, and willingness to increase use of vegetables and fruits. By 1990, 1 in every 3 meals eaten by school-aged children was fast food—twice the number in the 1950s. On days when fast foods are consumed, the child's caloric intake is 175 calories higher. This alone would contribute to an excess weight gain of more than 6 pounds in a year. One additional 12-ounce can of high-calorie soda per day is related to a 60% increased risk of BMI higher than the 95th percentile.[29]

Chewable vitamins with iron can be incorporated as an "insurance" option. For children older than 9 years, it is recommended to increase calcium intake to 1300 mg per day, a level usually requiring supplementation. Parents should be encouraged to include children at this age to join them when shopping for food, discussing relative nutritional value of different food options, and helping in food preparation for a family meal. As always, parents and other caregivers need to be reminded of the importance of being a role model in food choice and portion size. Parents need to be particularly aware of problems that can develop if they keep a less-than-secret "stash" of their preferred snacks—doing so not only sends the wrong message but also increases the appeal of the "forbidden" food to the observant child.

The role of physical activity remains paramount for the health and wellness of primary school-aged children. On average, an elementary school-aged child spends 75% of his or her waking hours inactive. The average 5- to 12-year-old spends 6 hours per day watching television, sitting at a computer, or playing video games. For every hour they spend on screen time per day, they increase their risk of obesity by up to 10%. Television programming aimed at elementary school-aged children now includes 40 000 ads per year, produced at a cost of $13 billion dollars per year, up 100% since the 1970s, with 70% devoted to food. Not surprisingly, 70% of children 6 to 8 years of age respond that fast food is healthier than home-prepared meals.

Although weekly sports programs, especially for girls, have increased, daily exercise has dramatically decreased. In 1969, nearly 80% of children played sports daily; now only 20% do. Only 17% of primary school-aged students walk to school, including only 30% of those who live within 1 mile. Less than 10% of American elementary schools have daily physical education class. Furthermore, in the average physical education class, the child is aerobically active for only 3 minutes. With the justification of needing more academic class time, many elementary schools have cancelled or reduced recess. Between 1977 and 1997, there was a 40% reduction in walking and bicycling by preadolescents. Table I.3 summarizes the major nutritional and physical activity issues during the primary school years.

Table I.3
Nutrition and Physical Activity in the Elementary School-Aged Child: Guidelines for Parents

Nutrition Goals
Prepare and eat regular meals as a family; be a role model.
Seek 5-a-day intake of fruits and vegetables.
Reduce fast food meals, avoiding super-sized portions.
Increase daily intake of whole grains and fiber.
Use reduced-fat dairy products to help meet calcium needs.
Discuss school breakfast and lunch options and nutritious snacks.
Physical Activity
Seek 1 hour of moderate to vigorous activity daily.
Reduce "screen time" to less than 2 hours a day.
Encourage after-school and weekend physical activity and bike riding.
Advocate for safe parks and school physical education and recess time.
Encourage family physical activity on a regular basis; be a role model.
Plan active parties for birthdays, play dates, and casual get-togethers.

Secondary School: 12 to 18 Years of Age

Adolescence is a particularly difficult interval with the increased nutritional demands of puberty, psychosocial drives for independence, and a reduction in physical activity for most teenagers. Not surprisingly, the gamut of concerns ranges from primary eating disorders of anorexia, bulimia, and binge eating; to increased awareness of sports-performance nutrition; to obesity-related health complications rarely seen by past generations of pediatricians. BMI, of course, is sensitive to simultaneous rapid weight gain and height acceleration. For example, a teenager can gain 15 pounds in a year with a 4-inch height gain and the BMI will not change.

As primary health care professionals, pediatricians often have the benefit of a several-year rapport with adolescent patients. Pediatricians can draw on this mutual respect to develop a plan of evaluation and management for any nutritional concerns. Teenagers should be asked privately how they feel about their weight, their level of physical activity, status of puberty (confirmed by Tanner staging on examination), and social pressures to eat more or less. Actual intakes, including meals, lunches, beverages, snacks, purchases from school vending machines, after-school fast food ("chicken boxes"), and vitamins and minerals such as calcium, iron, and folic acid should be documented. The average teenager now drinks 850 cans of soda per year—double the volume of the 1970s. The average size of a soda at the movies has increased from 6.5 oz in 1970 to 20 oz now. It requires 2.5 miles of walking to burn off the calories from that drink.

The primary eating disorders are discussed in Chapter 38. If suspicious, ask direct questions and inquire about menstrual regularity, cold intolerance, constipation, early satiety, dry skin, fatigue, compulsive exercise, emesis, laxative use, purging, binge eating, palpitations, and syncopal episodes. Teenagers with increasing BMI percentiles should give complete nutritional histories outlined previously as well as a daily and weekly review of physical activity. Health care professionals should be alert for features of depression or loss of self-esteem.

Typically, girls between 9 and 19 years of age have an 83% reduction in regular physical activity. Remind teenagers that for every hour per day of moderate exercise, they reduce their risk of obesity by 10%. For every daily half-mile walked (even at the mall), the risk of obesity is reduced by 5%. Regrettably, only 65% of teenagers engage in any vigorous physical activity more than 3 days a week. Television viewing and video games remain a major concern in adolescence. By 17 years of age, the average child spends 38% more time watching television than in school, averaging more than 20 hours per week of screen time. Reducing screen time alone does not reduce obesity; increased physical activity is required. Adolescents should be encouraged to include a component of physical activity in their parties and social events by going swimming, bowling, or dancing or playing sports. By 12th grade, fewer than one third of students participate in daily physical education programs, and after-school athletic programs are limited to elite athletes. The general advice for nutrition and physical activity for adolescents is noted in Table I.4.

Table I.4
Nutrition and Physical Activity for Secondary School-Aged Children: Guidelines for Parents

Nutrition Goals
Prepare and eat meals as a family; be a role model.
Encourage a daily, healthy breakfast as part of 3 balanced meals a day.
Discourage calorie-dense snacks, high-sugar sodas, and candy.
Avoid having "stash" of unhealthy snack foods in the home.
Encourage 5-a-day intake of fruits and vegetables as well as good sources of whole grains and fiber.
Use a vitamin supplement for iron and folic acid, and confirm calcium intake.
Physical Activity
Encourage at least 1 hour of moderate to vigorous physical activity daily.
Limit "screen time" to less than 2 hours a day.
Avoid having a television in the bedroom.
Encourage individual sports, such as tennis, biking, hiking, and swimming.
Encourage active parties and social events by incorporating dancing, bowling, swimming, etc.
Be a community activist to increase safe opportunities for all to exercise.

Eliciting nutritional information from competitive adolescent athletes is also critical. Many have distorted ideas as to ideal weights and diets for performance. In December 2005, the AAP published a policy statement on healthy weight control practices in young athletes.[30] Most adolescent athletes will do fine on a normal, healthy diet with 60% to 70% of calories from carbohydrates with an emphasis on low– and moderate–glycemic-index complex starches, with higher-energy, high–glycemic-index beverages and food primarily reserved for endurance-demanding exercise. Twenty percent to 30% of calories should come from fat, primarily unsaturated; slightly more fat is acceptable for prolonged low-intensity competition. Protein contributes 5% to 10% of the energy used in prolonged activity. Most athletes require approximately 1.2 g of high-quality protein per kg of body weight daily, increasing to 1.8 g for prolonged, heavy-resistance exercise.[31] When weight training is used to add muscle, to gain 1 pound of muscle in 1 week requires intakes of 2000 to 2500 kcal more than one expends, consumption of 1.5 to 1.75 g of protein per kg per day, and a strength-training program. Muscle hypertrophy is best achieved with a high number of repetitions per set. Weight gain should not exceed more than 1.5% of body weight per week during such training.[30]

Many athletes focus on their percentage of body fat as a specific sport-specific goal. In reality, no specific body composition goals have ever been confirmed. The normal body fat of the "reference adolescent" ranges from 12.7% to 17.2% for males and 21.5% to 25.4% for females.[30] Low body fat is considered 10% to 13% for males and 17% to 20% for females. Very low body fat is 7% to 10% for males and 14% to 17% for females.[30]

For most athletes, adequate hydration during performance is a bigger issue than meal content. Fluid intake normally is 1 qt per 1000 kcal eaten. For exercise lasting an hour or less, 4 to 6 oz of cool water every 15 to 20 minutes will generally meet hydration needs. For longer activity, hydration with carbohydrate-electrolyte sports drinks is appropriate. All adolescent athletes should be asked about their exposure to and understanding of the limited value of and significant risk with performance enhancing drugs.[32]

Salt depletion with exercise is increasingly frequent as a result of both increased sweat losses and low salt intakes in health-conscious diets. The clinical presentation is early fatigue during endurance performances, vasovagal syncopal episodes with extended standing, and orthostatic hypotension on physical examination. Salt repletion with sports beverages or salt tablets will usually suffice.

Monitoring for Complications of Nutritional Concerns

When there are concerns regarding underweight or overweight, historical data must be obtained, the physical examination must be directed at areas of concern, and laboratory monitoring must be initiated. The need for accurate weight and height measurements, waist circumference (as a risk factor for insulin resistance), and determination of BMI percentile has been emphasized repeatedly. Determining Tanner stage to correlate with pubertal demands is important, as is accurate blood pressure measurement with the proper cuff size.

In 2003, the AAP published a policy statement on identifying and treating eating disorders[33] that outlined the need to document physical findings, such as bradycardia, edema, atrophic breasts, emaciation, dry skin, oral ulcers and dental enamel erosions, and calluses on knuckles from self-induced emesis. Laboratory screening could include a complete blood cell count; sedimentation rate; chemistry panel, including electrolytes, amylase, lipase, thyroid profile, follicle-stimulating hormone, luteinizing hormone, prolactin, and human chorionic gonadotropin; stool test for blood; and urinalysis. An electrocardiogram is required if any electrolyte changes, bradycardia, or history of syncope is noted.

The medical consequences of obesity, once limited to adults, are now increasingly encountered in adolescents and occasionally even in preadolescents. Screening for obesity-related problems, mostly by laboratory testing, has been proposed, but results have been inconsistent and cost effectiveness has been limited thus far.[34,35] In adults, a number of health concerns constitute the "metabolic syndrome," including hyperinsulinemia, obesity, hypertension, and hyperlipidemia.[22] Recent studies confirm that more than 30% of overweight adolescents already have 2 or more features of the metabolic syndrome.

Endocrine concerns lead the list of acute comorbid disease associated with overweight and obesity. Insulin resistance progressing to type 2 diabetes is the first concern. The American Diabetes Association has recommended fasting glucose testing for all children older than 10 years with BMI at or higher than the 85th percentile with 2 of the following risk factors: a family history of type 2 diabetes in first- or second-degree relatives, nonwhite race, and conditions associated with insulin resistance, such as acanthosis nigricans, hypertension, dyslipidemia, or polycystic ovary syndrome.[36] A number of other guidelines are under revision, including proposals to document fasting insulin and/or hemoglobin A1C in all adolescents with BMI higher than the 85th percentile. Certainly, any child in a treatment program needs to have baseline insulin concentrations documented. Early-intervention drug trials, mostly with metformin, are now underway. Other endocrine concerns include increased frequency of polycystic ovary syndrome (attributed to hyperinsulinemia and hyperandrogenemia), early puberty, and an acute hyperglycemic, hyperosmolar syndrome with emesis, dizziness, and weakness that can progress to coma.

Cardiovascular concerns, both acute and long-term, are also increasing.[22,26] Hypertension, generally defined as a systolic or diastolic pressure higher than the 95th percentile for age, is now reported in more than 10% of overweight adolescents. Most guidelines include a fasting lipid profile to check for elevated triglyceride, elevated low-density lipoprotein, and low high-density lipoprotein concentrations. Overweight adolescents are also at risk of pulmonary embolism, with contributory factors such as hypoventilation, sleep apnea, and reduced activity.

An acute left ventricular dysfunction, even in the absence of hypertension, has also been seen and attributed to increased blood volume and increased metabolic activity in the excess adipose tissue. Stress tests are advised for adolescents with a BMI greater than 40.

Hypoventilation and sleep apnea are the major respiratory complications of childhood obesity. If suspected, an overnight sleep study will usually clarify the child's ventilatory status. Sleep disruption can also be a feature of the increased gastroesophageal reflux typical in overweight children.

Increased hepatic fat storage in association with overweight is termed nonalcoholic fatty liver disease (NAFLD), and steatosis with inflammation has been labeled nonalcoholic steatohepatitis. Once felt to be relatively benign, if not reversible, it is now recognized that NAFLD may progress to hepatic fibrosis and cirrhosis.[37] Regular liver enzyme determinations, including aspartate transaminase, alanine transaminase, and gamma-glutamyl transpeptidase concentrations, as well as ultrasonography of the liver, aid in monitoring for NAFLD.

Orthopedic complications of overweight and obesity include slipped capital femoral epiphysis, mostly in males, and Blount disease, an overgrowth of the medial proximal tibial metaphysis. Because of weight dynamics with exercise, overuse injuries, in the context of relatively minimal and infrequent use, are also common.

The psychosocial ramifications of being overweight, in children of all ages, are not insignificant. Low self-esteem and depression are most common. Overweight children are more likely to develop bullying behavior while also being more likely to be the victims of bullying. Recent studies also report reduced school performance.

As primary health care professionals, we must maintain a low threshold for documenting these concerns. Early referral for intervention to minimize or reverse comorbidities is the goal.

Treatment Programs

The emphasis of this chapter has been on early recognition with the goal of early intervention to prevent the complications of failure to thrive, weight loss, or excessive weight gain. The specific treatment approaches are summarized in other chapters: Chapter 26 for failure to thrive, Chapter 38 for primary eating disorders, and Chapter 33 for overweight and obesity. Several excellent reviews in 2005 by Daniels and colleagues along with the American Heart Association,[21] Dietz and Robinson,[34] and Schuster and Brill[38] addressed the multifaceted treatment options for obesity.

References for this chapter have been drawn from the published literature; however, there are a large number of Web sites with excellent information for patients, parents, and physicians. Many of these sites are listed in Table I.5. Food exchange lists are provided in Appendix A, and a table for converting conventional units to Systéme International (SI) Units is available in Appendix B.

Table I.5
Web-Based Educational Material for Physicians and Families

American Academy of Pediatrics
    www.aap.org/topics.html
    www.aap.org/parents.html

American Dietetic Association   www.eatright.org
American Heart Association   www.americanheart.org
Bright Futures in Practice: Nutrition and Physical Activity   http://brightfutures.aap.org/web

Centers for Disease Control and Prevention
    Healthy Schools, Healthy Youth: www.cdc.gov/HealthyYouth
    Project VERB: www.cdc.gov/youthcampaign/ and www.verbnow.com

President's Council on Physical Fitness and Sports   www.fitness.gov and www.presidentschallenge.org
Shape Up America   www.shapeup.org

US Department of Agriculture
    Food and Nutrition Information Center: www.nal.usda.gov/fnic
    Healthy School Meals: http://www.fns.usda.gov/cnd/
    Eat Smart, Play Hard: www.fns.usda.gov/eatsmartplayhard/
    MyPyramid: www.mypyramid.gov
    2005 Dietary Guidelines: www.healthierus.gov/dietaryguidelines

National Diabetes Education Program, Tip Sheets for Kids for obesity prevention   www.ndep.nih.gov

References

1. Institute of Medicine, Committee on Prevention of Obesity in Children and Youth. *Preventing Childhood Obesity: Health in the Balance*. Koplan JP, Liverman CT, Kraak VA, eds. Washington, DC: National Academies Press; Washington, DC: 2005. Available at: http://books.nap.edu/catalog.php?record_id=11015. Accessed July 6, 2007

2. Centers for Disease Control and Prevention, National Center for Health Statistics. Prevalence of Overweight Among Children and Adolescents: United States, 1999–2002. Available at: www.cdc.gov/NCHS/products/pubs. Accessed July 6, 2007

3. Hedley A, Ogden CL, Johnson CL, Carrol MD, Curtis LR, Flegal KM. Prevalence of overweight and obesity among US children, adolescents, and adults, 1999–2002. *JAMA*. 2004;291:2847–2850

4. Fernández JR, Redden DT, Pietrobelli A, Allison DB. Waist circumference percentiles in nationally representative samples of African-American, European-American, and Mexican-American children and adolescents. *J Pediatr*. 2004;145:439–444

5. Dorsey KB, Wells C, Krumholz HM, Concato JC. Diagnosis, evaluation and treatment of childhood obesity in pediatric practice. *Arch Pediatr Adolesc Med*. 2005;159:632–638

6. Krebs NF, Jacobson MS, American Academy of Pediatrics, Committee on Nutrition. Prevention of pediatric overweight and obesity. *Pediatrics*. 2003;112:424–430

7. Whitlock EP, Williams SB, Gold R, Smith PR, Shipman SA. Screening and intervention for childhood overweight: a summary of evidence for the US Preventive Services Task Force. *Pediatrics*. 2005;116(1):e125-e144. Available at: http://pediatrics.aappublications.org/cgi/content/full/116/1/e125. Accessed July 6, 2007

8. Krebs NF. Screening for overweight in children and adolescents: a call to action. *Pediatrics*. 2005;116:238–239

9. Whitaker RC, Dietz WH. Role of the prenatal environment in the development of obesity. *J Pediatr*. 1998;132:768–776

10. Hales CN, Barker DJ, Clark PM, et al. Fetal and infant growth and impaired glucose tolerance at age 64. *BMJ*. 1991;303:1019–1022

11. Barker DJ. Early growth and cardiovascular disease. *Arch Dis Child*. 1999;80:305–307

12. Barlow SE, Dietz WH. Obesity evaluation and treatment: expert committee recommendations. The Maternal and Child Health Bureau, Health Resources and Services Administration and the Department of Health and Human Services. *Pediatrics*. 1998;102(3):e29. Available at: http://pediatrics.aappublications.org/cgi/content/full/102/3/e29. Accessed July 6, 2007

13. American Academy of Pediatrics, Section on Breastfeeding. Breastfeeding and the use of human milk. *Pediatrics*. 2005;115:496–506

14. Lawrence R. The clinician's role in teaching proper infant feeding techniques. *J Pediatr*. 1995;126:S112–S117

15. Owen CG, Morton RM, Whincup PH, Smith GD, Cook DG. Effect of infant feeding on the risk of obesity over the life course. A quantitative review of published evidence. *Pediatrics*. 2005;115:1367–1377

16. Owen CG, Whincup PH, Odoki K, Gilg JA, Cook DG. Infant feeding and blood cholesterol: a study in adolescents and systematic review. *Pediatrics*. 2002;110:597–608

17. Stettler N, Stallings VA, Troxel AB, et al. Weight gain in the first week of life and overweight in adulthood. *Circulation.* 2005;111:1897–1903

18. Ryan C, Dwyer J, Ziegler P, Yang E, Moore L, Song WO. What do infants really eat? *Nutr Today.* 2002;37:50–56

19. National Center for Education in Maternal and Child Health. *Bright Futures in Practice: Nutrition.* Story M, Holt K, Sofka D, eds. Washington, DC: National Center for Education in Maternal and Child Health; 2000

20. Centers for Disease Control and Prevention, National Center for Health Statistics. National Health and Nutrition Examination Survey. Available at: www.cdc.gov./nchs/nhanes.htm. Accessed July 6, 2007

21. Daniels SR, Arnett DK, Echel RH, et al. American Heart Association scientific statement. Overweight in children and adolescents: pathophysiology, consequences, prevention, and treatment. *Circulation.* 2005;111:1999–2012

22. Williams CL, Strobino BA, Bollella M, Brotanek J. Cardiovascular risk reduction in preschool children: the "Healthy Start" project. *J Am Coll Nutr.* 2004;23:117–123

23. Whitaker RC, Wright JA, Pepe MS, Seidel KD, Dietz WH. Predicting obesity in young adulthood from childhood and parental obesity. *N Engl J Med.* 1997;337:869–873

24. Birch LL, McPhee L, Shoba BC, Steinberg L. "Clean up your plate": effects of child feeding practices on the conditioning of meal size. *Learn Motiv.* 1987;18:301–317

25. Rolls BJ, Engell D, Birch LL. Serving portion size influences 5-year-old but not 3-year-old children's food intake. *J Am Diet Assoc.* 2000;100:232–234

26. Giddings S, Dennison BA, Birch LL, et al. American Heart Association. Dietary guidelines for children and adolescents: a guide for practitioners. *Pediatrics.* 2006;117:544–559

27. Jago R, Baranowski T, Baranowski JC, Thompson D, Greaves KA. BMI from 3–6 years of age is predicted by television viewing and physical activity, not diet. *Int J Obesity (Lond).* 2005;29:557–564

28. US Department of Agriculture. MyPyramid for Kids. Available at: http://www.mypyramid. gov/kids/index.html. Accessed July 6, 2007

29. Ludwig DS, Peterson KE, Gortmaker SL. Relation between consumption of sugar-sweetened drinks and childhood obesity: a prospective analysis. *Lancet.* 2001;357:505–508

30. American Academy of Pediatrics, Committee on Sports Medicine and Fitness. Promotion of healthy weight-control practices in young athletes. *Pediatrics.* 2005;116:1557–1564

31. Dimeff RJ. Sports nutrition. *Curr Rev Sports Med.* 1994;15:201–221

32. Gomez J, American Academy of Pediatrics, Committee on Sports Medicine and Fitness. Use of performance enhancing substances. *Pediatrics.* 2005;115:1103–1106

33. American Academy of Pediatrics, Committee on Adolescence. Identifying and treating eating disorders. *Pediatrics.* 2003;111:204–211

34. Barlow SE, Dietz WH, Klish WH, Trowbridge FL. Medical evaluation of overweight children and adolescents: reports from pediatricians, pediatric nurse practitioners, and registered dietitians. *Pediatrics.* 2002;110:222–228

35. Dietz WH, Robinson TN. Clinical practice. Overweight children and adolescents. *N Engl J Med.* 2005;352:2100–2109

36. American Diabetes Association. Type 2 diabetes in children and adolescents. *Diabetes Care*. 2000;23:381–389

37. Schwimmer JB, Deutsch R, Rauch JB, Behling C, Newbury R, Lavine JE. Obesity, insulin resistance, and other clinicopathological correlates of pediatric nonalcoholic fatty liver disease. *J Pediatr*. 2003;143:500–505

38. Schuster MB, Brill SR. Obesity in children and adolescents. *Pediatr Rev*. 2005;26:155–162

Feeding the Infant

I

Infant Nutrition and Development of Gastrointestinal Function

Development of Gastrointestinal Function

The design of the gastrointestinal tract allows for the assimilation of environmental nutrients for the purposes of growth, maintenance, and reproduction. The gut has an incredibly intricate physiological and mechanical design with a large, yet limited, capacity for nutrient assimilation.[1] The absorptive capacity of the gut is a function of multiple variables, including surface area, digestion, facilitative and active transport, motility, perfusion, microflora, and metabolism. Ultimately, capacity of the gut is designed to assimilate the dietary load to meet energy requirements for growth and metabolism.[2] Study of the development of gastrointestinal function has revealed strong evolutionary concepts and critical adaptations for the purposes served.[3]

Development of the Gastrointestinal Tract

The embryonic period is the time of organogenesis for the gastrointestinal tract. Development begins in the third week of gestation with gastrulation, the process that establishes the 3 germ layers—ectoderm, mesoderm, and endoderm. The mammalian digestive tract begins to form soon after the embryo begins to undergo cephalocaudal and lateral folding, resulting in the incorporation of a portion of the endoderm-lined yolk sac cavity into the embryo. This forms the primitive gut, which is differentiated into 3 parts: foregut, midgut, and hindgut.[4] Throughout embryogenesis, the gut lumen seals and recanalizes several times for the purpose of elongation. Most of the gut and visceral organs are derived from the endodermal cell layer; however, the interaction of ectodermal and mesodermal tissues is crucial, and several structures contain a mixture of primordial cells.

The lining of the digestive tube and its glands are generated by endodermal cells.[5] Endodermal cells also derive the parenchyma of the liver, gallbladder, and pancreas, and mesodermal tissue surrounds the tube and forms the smooth muscle necessary for intestinal peristalsis. Regional patterning sets the stage for the differential development of primary organs. Anterior (cranial) and posterior (caudal) patterning of the gut tube occurs through the expression of several genes (eg, sonic hedgehog) that regulate gut development.[6,7] As primary organs emerge, endodermal and mesodermal layers coordinate their differentiation via direct signaling between adjacent tissues and cells.[8]

The foregut differentiates into the pharynx, esophagus, and stomach, up to the second part of the duodenum, and gives rise to the liver and pancreas. Organs of the foregut ingest food and initiate digestion. The midgut is largely responsible for nutrient absorption and gives rise to the structures from the third part of the duodenum to the first two thirds of the large intestine. The hindgut gives rise to the structures from the remaining large intestine through to the rectum and is responsible for the resorption of water and ions as well as fermentation and expulsion of digestive waste.

The glandular epithelium of the liver and the biliary drainage system, including the gallbladder, are formed from the hepatic diverticulum, a tube of endoderm that extends out from the foregut into the surrounding mesenchyme. The pancreas develops from the fusion of 2 distinct dorsal and ventral diverticula, both derived of endodermal cells immediately caudal to the stomach. Portions of the gut tube and its derivatives are designated intraperitoneal if they are suspended from the dorsal and ventral body wall by a double layer of peritoneum that enclose and connect them to the body wall. Organs and portions of the intestinal tube that lie up against the posterior body-wall, covered by peritoneum on their anterior surface only, are called retroperitoneal. Most of the gut lies intraperitoneally and is free floating, exceptions being the majority of the duodenum and parts of the colon. The duodenum turns and exits into the retroperitoneal space just past the bulb and re-enters the peritoneum at the location of its fixation to the left crus of the diaphragm by the ligament of Treitz, which also marks the beginning of the jejunum. In most individuals, the left colon and right colon also lay retroperitoneally.[5]

Developmental Disorders

Several well-known complications of embryogenesis constitute a significant portion of the developmental abnormalities seen in neonates and infants.[9] Esophageal abnormalities include esophageal atresia, stenosis, and tracheoesophageal fistula. Esophageal stenosis can be the result of a vascular abnormality. Stomach malformations include duplication and prepyloric septum. Duodenal atresia and stenosis are usually the result of incomplete recanalization of the intestinal lumen. Midgut atresias are often caused by a vascular accident secondary to intestinal malrotation. Normally, the primary intestinal loop rotates 270° counterclockwise during embryogenesis. Failure of the gut to rotate fully, or its reverse rotation, results in malrotation and predisposes the child to abnormal movement of the gut and volvulus.

Gastroschisis (ie, the herniation of abdominal contents through the body wall directly into the amniotic cavity) and omphalocele (ie, the herniation of abdominal contents through an enlarged umbilical ring) can also result in loss of viable intestines, leading to short gut syndrome. Rectoanal atresias and congenital fistulas are caused by abnormalities in formation of the cloaca and ectopic positioning of the anal opening. Imperforate anus occurs because of improper recanalization of the lower portion of the anal canal. Hirschsprung disease is caused by the absence of parasympathetic ganglia in the bowel wall. These ganglia are neural crest derived and normally migrate from the neural folds down to the wall of the bowel.[10]

Variation in liver architecture and lobulation is most often asymptomatic. Extrahepatic ducts can fail to recanalize, resulting in extrahepatic biliary atresia. Intrahepatic biliary duct hypoplasia may be caused by fetal infections (eg, cytomegalovirus) and usually represents a more benign condition. Pancreatic abnormalities are relatively common, are often asymptomatic, and are usually the result of poor migration of the pancreatic buds. The lack of fusion of the 2 pancreatic ducts is called pancreatic divisum and is an important differential diagnosis for pancreatitis in children. The most serious malformation is when the duodenum is surrounded by an annular pancreas. This can constrict the duodenum and present with intestinal obstructive symptoms.

Development of the Intestinal Epithelium

The rapid epithelial cell turnover of the gastrointestinal tract continues throughout life. This process is maintained and regulated by a population of stem cells, which give rise to both absorptive and secretory epithelial cell lineages.[11] These cells form a clonal population called a "niche" toward the base of crypts, and their activity is regulated by paracrine secretion of growth factors and cytokines from surrounding mesenchymal cells. Stem cell division is usually asymmetric, with the identical daughter cell becoming a committed progenitor cell and retaining the ability to continue dividing until terminally differentiating. Symmetric division may result in either 2 daughter cells, with loss of stem cell function, or formation of 2 stem cells and eventual clone dominance. The apparent stochastic extinction of some stem cell lines with eventual dominance of a single cell line is called "niche succession."[12]

The cells of the epithelium become increasingly differentiated along the crypt-villus axis, undergo spontaneous apoptosis within 4 to 5 days, and are shed into the lumen, where they are digested and phagocytosed.[13] Four main epithelial cell lineages are derived from this process: columnar cells are the most abundant and are specialized for absorption by the presence of apical microvilli; goblet cells are named for their swollen shape, a consequence of mucin granule production; neuroendocrine or enteroendocrine cells secrete peptide hormones in an endocrine and paracrine fashion, influencing gastrointestinal function in a variety of ways; and Paneth cells are large cells that migrate down to the crypt base, where they express and secrete several proteins including lysozyme, tumor necrosis factor-alpha, and antibacterial defensins, all of which help keep the crypt sterile.[14,15] M (membranous or microfold) cells are a fifth type of epithelial cell found near Peyer patches and are involved in antigen transportation.[16]

The lamina propria forms the basement membrane, providing a supporting network for the epithelium and regulating epithelial cell function. It contains numerous kinds of cells, including fibroblasts, myofibroblasts, fibrocytes, vascular endothelial, and smooth muscle cells, and various blood lineages. Some of these cells secrete growth factors, such as transforming growth factor beta-2, essential for epithelial cell differentiation and proliferation.[17]

Infant Nutrient Assimilation

The neonatal gut has several major functions. It is obviously an organ of nutrition, with digestive, absorptive, secretory, and motile functions adapted to a milk diet. However, the neonatal gut is also part of the immune system, containing both humoral and cellular elements of the gut-associated lymphoid tissue. The neonatal gut is a large and diffuse endocrine organ that secretes locally acting gut hormones and paracrine factors, which help regulate intestinal and metabolic adaptation to extrauterine life.[18] It plays a role in water conservation and electrolyte homeostasis and maintains a symbiotic relationship with a microbial flora, which assists in the digestion and absorption of certain nutrients. The intestinal microbiota also plays a vital role in health and disease.[19]

The neonatal intestine replaces the role of the placenta quite abruptly at birth, with most intestinal nutrient transport mechanisms intact well before birth. The neonatal intestine is uniquely capable of absorbing intact macromolecules via endocytosis, a process by which various maternal growth factors imperative for intestinal development are transported.[20,21] Yet, the overall absorptive and digestive capacity of the gut is impaired in the neonatal period, and early infant growth requires a special nutrient environment.[22] The degree to which alterations in digestive and absorptive capacity seen during and after infancy are genetically determined has yet to be established. For example, although the decrease in lactase activity seen with weaning occurs despite an ongoing lactose load, the up-regulation of fructose transporters in response to increased fructose consumption is altered by load.[23] Thus, we see evidence of both genetic preprogramming and an adaptation mechanism responsive to nutrient load.

Dietary Fats

Fat, or lipid, is defined as a class of compounds insoluble in water but soluble in organic solvents, such as alcohol. Lipids contain carbon, hydrogen, and oxygen but have far less oxygen, proportionally, than do carbohydrates. Lipids vary considerably in size and polarity, ranging from hydrophobic triglycerides and sterol esters to the more water-soluble phospholipids and cardiolipins. Dietary lipids also include cholesterol and phytosterols. These compounds are distinguished from other dietary macronutrients in that they must undergo specialized processing during digestion, absorption, transport, storage, and utilization.[24]

Triglycerides make up the largest proportion of dietary lipids. Triglycerides are composed of 3 fatty acids esterified onto a glycerol molecule. These fatty acids are generally nonbranched and have an even number of carbons, from 4 to 26, although very long-chain fatty acids are found in the brain and specialized tissue, such as the retina and spermatozoa.[25] Double bonds are identified relative to the methyl end by the designation "n" or "ω" to indicate the distance from the first bond. For example, ω-6 indicates that the initial double bond is situated between the sixth and seventh carbon atom from the methyl group end. Because the biosynthetic process can only insert double bonds at the ω-9 position or higher, essential fatty acids are considered those with double bonds at the ω-6 and ω-3 positions. Most food contains double bonds in the cis configuration, while bonds that are trans result from hydrogenation, an industrial process used to increase the viscosity of oils. Trans fatty acids have reduced internal rotation, which makes them more resistant to electrophilic additions, such as hydration, and increases their melting point. Trans fatty acids may contribute to development of heart disease and atherosclerosis.[26]

Phospholipids are distinct from triglycerides in that they contain polar head groups that makes them amphipathic and, therefore, capable of forming micelles in water. They include glycerol, choline, serine, inositol, and ethanolamine. Sterols, such as cholesterol, are also amphipathic molecules made up of a steroid nucleus and a branched hydrocarbon tail. Although cholesterol is found only in food of animal origin, plants do contain phytosterols, which are chemically related to cholesterol.

Fat Digestion

Digestion of dietary fat requires a series of processes that enable absorption through the water-soluble epithelium of the gut. Digestion begins in the oral cavity as salivation, mastication, and lingual lipase begin to release largely short-chain fatty acids from triglycerides. Lingual lipase is produced by von Ebner serous glands located on the proximal, dorsal tongue,[27] and gastric lipase is produced by stomach chief cells.[28] Both lipases have been shown to remain largely active in the gastric milieu.[29] Both lingual and gastric (ie, preduodenal) lipases preferentially hydrolyze short-chain fatty acids and medium-chain triglycerides, which can be absorbed directly from the stomach.[30–32] Thus, monoglycerides are poorly hydrolyzed in the stomach, and the release of long-chain fatty acids and very long-chain fatty acids requires the presence of bile and pancreatic lipases.

Pancreatic lipase requires the presence of colipase to remove the inhibitory effect of bile salts. It is more active against insoluble, emulsified substrates. A second pancreatic lipase, carboxylase esterase, is more active against micellar (ie, soluble) substrates and is strongly stimulated by bile salts.

Bile is composed of bile salts, phospholipids, and sterols. It emulsifies the hydrophobic groups of dietary lipids and allows pancreatic lipases to hydrolyze the ester bonds of the glycerol moiety. Bile also increases the surface area available to enzymes and protects enzymes from proteolysis themselves. Infant bile has a lower concentration of bile acids than that of older children and adults, with a higher relative ratio of cholic acid to chenodeoxycholic acid.[33] This is believed to be secondary to a slower rate of synthesis of bile acids in neonates than in adults.[34] Moreover, bile acids in neonates are conjugated primarily with taurine, whereas in older infants, they are conjugated primarily with glycine.[35] The ileal mechanism for transport of cholyltaurine (ie, the expression of the apical sodium-dependent bile acid transporter) is not well developed in the neonate, resulting in poor recycling of bile acids.[36,37]

Fat Absorption

The absorption of lipids is through both active transport and passive diffusion of micellar products and free fatty acids across the brush-border membrane (BBM). Fatty acid binding proteins assist in the transmucosal shunting of free fatty acids, monoglycerides, and bile salts.[38] Both increased FA saturation and chain length correlate negatively with absorptive efficiency across the BBM.[39]

Fat Assimilation in the Neonate

Human milk consists of approximately 4% fat, mostly in the form of medium-chain triglycerides and long-chain triglycerides.[40] Because almost half of the total calories in an infant's diet are derived from fat, the digestion and absorption of fat must be very efficient in infancy.[41,42] Both salivary and gastric lipases are produced early in fetal development (gastric lipase is detectable in the developing fetus as early as 10 weeks' gestation and reaches adult levels by early infancy)[43]; yet, neonatal pancreatic and biliary excretion is generally low in early infancy.[44-46] Therefore, it is likely that certain evolutionary measures were preferentially selected, such as the greater capacity for absorption of intact macromolecules by receptor-mediated endocytosis in the neonatal intestine and the production of various lipases and proteolytic inhibitors in the maternal mammary glands. The importance of human milk factors in infant fat digestion is well-documented, as hydrolysis of fat has been shown to be more than twice as efficient in breastfed infants compared with formula-fed infants.[47]

Human milk lipases include bile salt-stimulated lipase (BSSL), which is made in the mammary glands and remains inactive until coming in contact with bile salts in the infant's duodenum.[48,49] BSSL survives the stomach milieu and is activated in the duodenum by bile acids to convert monoglycerides to glycerol and free fatty acids.[50,51] Without BSSL, the monoglyceride load would likely exceed neonatal absorptive capacity, and much would escape unabsorbed. BSSL performs other functions, such as the hydrolysis of retinol esters allowing for retinol absorption,[52] as well as hydrolysis of ceramide, the main sphingomyelin (a phospholipid) in human milk.[53] The importance of BSSL is supported by a study of preterm infants with low birth weight (3 to 6 weeks of age) who were fed raw versus heat-treated (ie, pasteurized or boiled) human milk. Fat absorption was significantly higher in the former group (74%) compared with the latter (54% in the pasteurized group and 46% in the boiled group).[54] Other lipases, such as lipoprotein lipase, are also present in human milk.[55]

Dietary Carbohydrates

Carbohydrates are a class of substances with a molar ratio of carbon to hydrogen to oxygen of 1:2:1 [$C_n(H_2O)_n$] plus oligosaccharides, polysaccharides, and the sugar alcohols (sorbitol, maltitol, mannitol, galactitol, and lactitol). Complex carbohydrates are mainly plant starch and animal glycogen, but include also pectin, cellulose, and gum. Simple carbohydrates include the hexose monosaccharides glucose, galactose, and fructose; the disaccharides maltose (glucose-glucose), sucrose (glucose-fructose), and lactose (glucose-galactose); and sporadic trioses, tetroses, and pentoses. Pentoses (ie, ribose [$C_5H_{10}O_5$]) are important constituents of nucleic acids.[56]

Oligosaccharides are generally defined as yielding 3 to 10 monosaccharides on hydrolysis (eg, maltose, isomaltose, maltotriose, maltodextrin), whereas polysaccharides yield more than 10.[57] Starch, by far the most common dietary polysaccharide, consists of only glucose units and is thus designated a glucosan. It is composed of 2 homopolymers of glucose: amylose (linear 1–4 linkages) and amylopectin (branched 1–6 and 1–4 linkages).

Carbohydrate Digestion

The digestion of carbohydrates requires complete hydrolysis of polysaccharides, oligosaccharides, and disaccharides, because absorption of dietary carbohydrates in the intestine is limited to the monosaccharides glucose, galactose, and fructose. Digestion begins with salivary amylase, which acts only on the interior (1–4) linkages of polysaccharides, not the outer (1–6) linkages, releasing α-disaccharides (eg, maltose) and trisaccharides (eg, maltotriose) and creating large oligosaccharides (eg, dextrins). Dextrins are sugar molecules containing an average of 8 glucose units with 1 or more outer links, requiring further digestion by glucoamylase. Pancreatic amylase, similar to salivary amylase, cleaves only interior links. The disaccharidases (eg, lactase, fructase, and sucrase-isomaltase) are necessary to ultimately yield free monosaccharide molecules.

Carbohydrate Absorption

Glucose is the major source of metabolic energy. As a hydrophilic polar molecule, it relies on transport across the relatively impermeable hydrophobic intestinal BBM. Transport occurs via both a family of facilitative glucose transporters (GLUTs) and active symporters, such as the sodium-glucose cotransporters (SGLTs).[58–60] GLUTs are membrane integral proteins found on the surface of all cells. They transport glucose down its concentration gradient, and the energy for the transfer comes from dissipation of the concentration difference. The SGLTs allow for glucose transport against the concentration gradient and are expressed mostly in enterocytes of the small intestine and epithelial cells of the kidney's proximal tubule.[61] The transport of glucose up its concentration gradient occurs in the presence of sodium and results in the passive resorption of water.[62] This concept explains the rationale behind oral rehydration solutions.

Galactose shares the same transport mechanisms as glucose in the enterocytes, namely, apical SGLT cotransporters and the basolateral GLUT2. Once it enters the portal blood circulation, galactose is practically cleared in its first passage through the liver, where it is converted by galactokinase into galactose-1-phosphate. The latter is then transformed enzymatically into glucose-1-phosphate and converted into glycogen. Lactose is the sole dietary source of galactose in humans, although glucose can be converted into galactose for supply of cellular needs (eg, glycoproteins and mucopolysaccharides).

Fructose is transported across the BBM by the facilitated transporter GLUT5. Fructose malabsorption is well documented in infants and toddlers and is associated with diarrhea and abdominal pain.[63] GLUT5 is believed to undergo up-regulation with increased dietary intake of fructose. Once absorbed, fructose is metabolized by the abundant enzyme fructokinase and then cleaved by aldolase to produce glyceraldehyde and dihydroxyacetone phosphate. The metabolites ultimately enter the glycolytic pathway and produce glycogen. Small amounts of fructose act catalytically to enhance glucose metabolism, perhaps via activation of glucokinase.[64] However, large amounts of fructose may saturate the glycolytic pathway with intermediate metabolites that may be used for triglyceride synthesis.

Carbohydrate Assimilation in the Neonate

The concentrations of salivary and pancreatic amylase, as well as BBM glucoamylase and disaccharidases (eg, lactase), are low in the neonatal period but increase to mature concentrations quite rapidly in the postnatal period.[65–67] Approximately 25% of 1-week-old term infants exhibit some lactose malabsorption, and lactase activity in the neonatal period appears to be inducible by lactose intake.[68–71] Lactose malabsorption in the neonate is generally mild and asymptomatic, with malabsorbed lactose salvaged in the colon with bacterial fermentation and production of SCFAs. Thus, the finite capacity of the neonatal intestine to absorb lactose may serve to promote healthy intestinal microflora and provide colonocytes with an important nutrient (ie, butyric acid).[72]

Starch digestion is limited in newborn infants, and pancreatic secretion of α-amylase may remain insufficient for several months.[73] Thus, carbohydrate needs in infancy are met largely via the digestion of lactose into glucose and galactose, and the need for α-amylase digestion is minimal until weaning. Weaning is also the time at which all studied nonhuman mammals and most humans begin to experience a decline in lactase concentrations.[74] Individuals who are lactase persistent are generally of western European descent, the product of natural selection in areas where animal farming and milking have occurred for centuries. Hypolactasia occurs in most other individuals, as early as 2 years of age in children from Thailand and Bangladesh and 10 years of age for Asian, black, and Hispanic children. For many white children (eg, Finnish, Irish descent), it is a steady and slow decrease.[75,76]

Dietary Protein

Consisting of amino acids, proteins direct and facilitate the biochemical reactions of life. Proteins include enzymes, transporters, signaling peptides, and muscle fiber. The body's requirement for proteins diminishes greatly after infancy as the rate of accretion of new protein is reduced. However, during accelerated growth phases, as seen in early childhood and adolescence, as well as in athletes, protein requirement is increased to near-infant levels. The metabolic rate of conversion and utilization of individual amino acids differs in the body depending on age, gender, nutrient exposure, and level of activity.[77]

Essential amino acids constitute approximately one third of the protein requirement in infancy but only about one fifth later in childhood and one tenth in adulthood.[78] The need for high-quality protein, defined by the protein's ability to support growth, also decreases with age.[79] High-quality proteins characteristically have an abundance of indispensable amino acids, are easily digestible, and lack contaminating molecules, such as inhibitors of digestive enzymes (eg, trypsin inhibitors) or antigens that may trigger allergic stimuli.

Protein differs from carbohydrates and fat in that it contains nitrogen, on average approximately 16% by weight. When amino acids are oxidized in the citric acid (ie, Krebs or tricarboxylic acid) cycle to carbon dioxide and water to produce energy, nitrogen is produced as a waste product and must be expelled from the body. The body can use dietary protein for energy, muscle incorporation, or incorporation into other nitrogen-containing compounds.

Amino acids can be converted to glucose via gluconeogenesis to provide a continuous supply of glucose after glycogen stores are consumed. Similar to carbohydrates, degradation of amino acids by oxidation produces approximately 4 kcal/g of protein. The carbon skeletons may also be used for formation of fat via elongation of acetyl units as well as carbohydrates through the conversion of alanine into pyruvate. Amino acids are also incorporated into various products, such as creatine, nitric oxide, purines and pyrimidines, glutathione, porphyrins (hemoglobin and cytochromes), histamine, serotonin, nicotinic acid, thyroid hormone, catecholamines, and carnitine, among many others.

Protein Digestion

Digestion of protein begins in the stomach with pepsin secretion in gastric juice. Pepsin cleaves the carboxyl terminus of tyrosine, phenylalanine, and tryptophan. Pepsin output and parietal cell activity are believed to be lower in the neonate than in older infants.[80] The buffering of gastric acidity after milk feeds may also result in suboptimal pepsin activity in early infancy.[81,82] Yet, it is important to note that secretion of gastric acid, intrinsic factor, and gastrin is noted as early as the middle of the second gestational trimester,[83] and infants are able to maintain a gastric pH well below 4 from the first day of life.[84,85] Indeed, infants have been shown to be capable of hydrogen ion secretion,[86] with the level of gastric H^+/K^+-adenosine triphosphatase proton pump increasing significantly with advanced gestational age and during the first 3 months of life.[87] Pepsin activity is shown to increase soon after initiating feeding.[88]

Proteolytic enzymes secreted from the pancreas and intestinal mucosa break proteins down into smaller peptides. Their activity is largely dependent on the amino acid residue composition of the protein ingested. Pancreatic excretion begins in utero at approximately the fifth month of gestation.[89] Although trypsin values may be lower in the preterm infant,[90] a substantial difference in trypsin concentration in duodenal fluid between 2 days and 7 weeks of age is not observed,[91] and mature trypsin concentration is reached as early as 1 to 3 months of age.[24,44] Chymotrypsin activity may also be low in the newborn infant but increases rapidly, approaching the levels of older children at about 6 months of age and adult levels by 3 years of age.[92] Nonetheless, adults can digest protein at about a 60% faster rate than children.[93]

Pancreatic digestive enzymes are secreted in the form of zymogens, precursors that are converted into active proteolytic enzymes in the intestinal lumen. Trypsin is activated from trypsinogen by enterokinase, a brush-border enzyme. Trypsin cleaves the carboxyl terminus of positively charged amino acids such as lysine and arginine and activates chymotrypsin from chymotrypsinogen. Chymotrypsin attacks the same bonds cleaved by pepsin, which is inactivated by the increased pH of duodenal content. Carboxypeptidase cleaves the amide bond at the carboxyl terminus of aromatic and branched-chain amino acids, such as tyrosine, tryptophan, and phenylalanine. Elastase preferentially cleaves peptide bonds at the carboxyl terminus of small, hydrophobic amino acids, such as glycine, alanine, serine, and valine. Elastase is highly active against elastin, a component of connective tissue. Nucleases hydrolyze ingested nucleic acids (RNA and DNA) into their component nucleotides.

The oligopeptide products of gastric and pancreatic proteolysis undergo further hydrolysis in the BBM of the small intestine by carboxypeptidase and aminopeptidase. These 2 enzymes hydrolyze the carboxyl and amino terminuses of oligopeptides, respectively, releasing tripeptides, dipeptides, and individual amino acids. Tripeptides and dipeptides can cross the BBM to be hydrolyzed intracellularly by tripeptidases and dipeptidases. Activity of carboxypeptidase, aminopeptidase, tripeptidase, and dipeptidase is detectable in the intestines of fetuses as early as in the second trimester of gestation.[69,94]

Protein Absorption

Free amino acids are absorbed by active and specific transporters into the mucosa. Several transport systems are ubiquitously expressed and exhibit preference for certain amino acids. Systems A and ASC, for example, prefer amino acids with small side chains (eg, glycine, alanine, serine). System L transports amino acids with bulky side chains (eg, tyrosine, arginine, valine, asparagine, glutamine). The B system (eg, B^0, $B^{0,+}$), which has broad specificity for neutral amino acids, is produced largely in the small intestine.[95] Other specific amino acid transport systems in the intestine include IMINO (proline and glycine) and rBAT (cystine and dibasic amino acids). The transport of amino acids across the mucosa of the small intestine has been shown in fetuses as young as 12 weeks' gestational age.[96]

Protein Assimilation in the Neonate

Larger peptides and proteins can enter the gut intact. Although the adult intestine absorbs approximately a quarter of its dietary protein as dipeptides and tripeptides, using intracellular hydrolases to free amino acids into the portal blood, the neonate relies on the transfer of macromolecules to a much greater extent. Macromolecules in human milk include enzymes, growth factors, and immunologlobulins (Igs) that help shape the neonate's digestive, barrier, and immunologic function. Macromolecules can cross the intestinal epithelium either transcellularly (ie, through cells) or paracellularly (ie, between cells). Endocytosis, a transcellular pathway, is the major pathway for macromolecules to cross the mucosal brush border.[97] The paracellular passage of macromolecules across "leaks" between epithelial cell junctions (ie, tight junctions) remains controversial.

The uptake of macromolecules by the neonatal gut may represent the persistence of intrauterine absorptive processes, because the amniotic fluid is known to contain a range of protein macromolecules, including immunoglobulins, hormones, enzymes, and growth factors.[98] The small intestine is noted to be more permeable to intact proteins in the neonatal period, and infant serum often contains higher titers of antibodies to food antigens than does the serum of adults.[99–101] It is not fully understood how protein antigens escape luminal digestion and cross the BBM in sufficient amount to trigger an immune response, but the transport of maternal biological compounds intact may have served an evolutionary advantage.[102] Recent data suggest that the epithelial IgG receptor (FcRn) facilitates the recycling of IgG between the intestinal lumen and systemic circulatory compartments, including antigen-Ig complexes.[103]

Vitamins and Minerals

Fat-soluble micronutrients, such as prostaglandins and vitamins A, D, E, and K, are emulsified within lipid and cross the mucosal BBM as lipophilic molecules. Water-soluble vitamins cross the intestinal BBM by the action of specific carrier-mediated transport. These include the sodium-dependent multivitamin transporter, which is produced by enterocytes and transports vitamins such as B complex and pantothenate.[104] Vitamin C (L-ascorbic acid) transport occurs via the recently identified mammalian family of a sodium-dependent L-ascorbic acid transporter. Thought to be essential in diminishing oxidant injury in rapidly growing tissue, vitamin C serum concentrations decline rapidly postpartum. Thus, sodium-dependent L-ascorbic acid transporter expression in neonates may be of vital importance for vitamin C regulation.[105,106]

Most mineral absorption depends on specific carrier-mediated transport as well. Mineral accretion in the fetus occurs only during the last trimester of gestation, increasing the risk of mineral deficiencies in the preterm infant. The transport of calcium is sensitive to the presence and abundance of other nutrients, such as lactose and fatty acids.[107–109] The effect of calcium on newborn bone mineral content (BMC) depends on several factors, including maternal vitamin D concentrations, gestational age, fetal size, and maternal glucose homeostasis.[110] Infants of mothers with diabetes have low BMC at birth, implying that factors in pregnancy have an effect on fetal BMC or that decreased transplacental mineral transfer may occur, because otherwise, BMC is consistently increased with increased newborn weight and length. Moreover, although race and gender differences in BMC appear early in life, they do not appear to exist at birth.

Young animals absorb iron, lead, calcium, and strontium much better than do adults.[111,112] A divalent cation transporter named DCT1 is the main iron carrier in the small intestine.[113] The specificity of this transporter is limited to the reduced or ferrous form of iron. However, it can transport other divalent cationic minerals, such as zinc, copper, manganese, nickel, lead, cobalt, and cadmium. Its affinity to lead puts infants at greater risk than of lead toxicity than adults.[114]

Human Milk

The relationship between lactating mammary function and neonatal gastrointestinal function is an example of the parallel evolution of 2 organs that, after birth, together undertake functions previously performed by the placenta.[102] Human milk contains both nutrients required by the newborn infant for energy and metabolism and nonnutritional components that promote infant health, growth, and development. Nonnutritional components include antimicrobial factors, digestive enzymes, hormones, trophic factors, and growth modulators. Energy nutrients include metabolic fuel (ie, fat, protein, carbohydrates), free water, and raw material necessary for tissue growth and development, such as long-chain fatty acids, essential amino acids, minerals, vitamins, and trace elements. For most infants, nutrient intake from human milk becomes increasingly insufficient after 4 to 6 months of age, and other foods need to be added to the diet.

More than 98% of the fat in human milk is in the form of triglycerides, made within the mammary glands from medium-chain fatty acids and LCFAs. Oleic acid (18:1) and palmitic acid (16:0) are the most abundant fatty acids, with palmitic acid occupying the central position of the glycerol molecule in most human milk triglycerides, a property that increases its overall digestibility.[115] Similarly high proportions of the essential fatty acids linoleic acid (18:2 ω-6) and linolenic acid (18:3 ω-3) and of other long-chain polyunsaturated fatty acids (LCPUFAs), such as arachidonic acid (20:4 ω-6 [ARA]) and docosahexaenoic acid (22:6 ω-3 [DHA]), are also present.[116] These LCPUFAs are constituents of brain and neural tissue and are needed in early life for mental and visual development.[117] Studies have established that concentrations of LCPUFAs in plasma and red blood cells of infants fed formulas supplemented with both ω-6 and ω-3 LCPUFAs were closer to those of breastfed infants than to those of infants fed formulas containing no LCPUFAs.[118] However, those concentrations in infants fed supplemented formulas did not match those of breastfed infants.[119] Although fewer than half of all studies report beneficial effects of LCPUFAs on visual, mental, and/or psychomotor function, the body of literature suggests that LCPUFAs are important to the growth and development of infants.[120]

Proteins account for approximately 75% of the nitrogen-containing compounds in human milk. Nonprotein nitrogen substances include urea, nucleotides, peptides, free amino acids, and DNA. The proteins of human milk can be divided into 2 categories: micellar caseins and aqueous whey proteins, present in a ratio of approximately 40:60.[121] The predominant casein of human milk is beta-casein, which forms micelles of relatively small volume and produces a soft, flocculent curd in the infant's stomach. Certain human milk proteases, such as plasmin, which is highly active against casein, increase infant capacity for protein digestion.

The major whey proteins found in human milk are α-lactalbumin, lactoferrin, secretory IgA, and serum albumin, with a large number of other proteins present in smaller amounts. Secretory IgA is the principal Ig of human milk, and together with lactoferrin, it represents about 30% of all milk protein.[122] It is synthesized in the mammary epithelial cell when 2 IgA molecules, produced locally by lymphocytes resident in the breast tissue, are coupled with 2 proteins, a J-chain and a secretory component. The specificity of human milk secretory IgA antibodies reflects the mother's exposure to various antigens and is independent of the specificity profile of bloodborne

IgA.[123,124] Lactoferrin, which transports and promotes the absorption of iron, is also a bacteriostatic agent to a range of organisms. Ultimately, once digested into amino acids, it can be absorbed and used by the body for energy requirement.[122]

The principal carbohydrate of human milk is lactose, a β-disaccharide manufactured in the mammary epithelial cell from glucose by a reaction involving α-lactalbumin.[125] In addition, human milk contains significant quantities of oligosaccharides, predominantly lacto-N-tetraose and its mono-fucosylated derivatives, representing approximately 10% of total milk carbohydrate. Oligosaccharides can escape luminal digestion and are believed to serve as growth factors for intestinal microflora (eg, *Bifidobacterium bifidum*).[126] Oligosaccharides are also suspected of altering bacterial adhesion to intestinal epithelial cells.[127]

In addition to energy nutrients, human milk contains a wealth of bioactive components that have beneficial yet nonnutritional functions.[128,129] Nonnutrient factors compensate for the neonate's immature digestive and barrier functions and modulate the transition from intrauterine to extrauterine life. These factors include a wide range of specific and nonspecific antimicrobial factors, cytokines, and anti-inflammatory substances as well as hormones, growth modulators, and digestive enzymes. These components may be of particular importance for young infants, as the digestive system and host defense are still immature and susceptible to infection. The physiological significance of many of these substances is not fully determined, and some may represent merely a "spillover" of excretory products from metabolic processes occurring within the mammary epithelial cell. For those with established significance, the site of action may be within the mother's breast, within the infant's alimentary canal, or within the infant's body.

Of the trophic factors active in the neonate, epidermal growth factor (EGF) is the best studied. A small polypeptide with mitogenic, antisecretory, and cytoprotective properties, EGF is present in amniotic fluid and colostrum, suggesting that it plays an important role in perinatal adaptation to extrauterine nutrition and gut function.[130] Its roles in activating mucosal function, diminishing gastric hydrolysis of potentially useful milk macromolecules, and protecting the gut epithelium from autodigestion are well described.[131,132] EGF has also been implicated in the induction of lactase secretion and the repression of sucrase activity.[133]

Pancreatic lipase secretion in the preterm infant is only approximately 10% of that of an adult, and the bile-salt pool is only about 50% of that found in the mature neonate.[134] The depressed pancreatic function ensures that the immature microvillus membrane is spared digestion by pancreatic proteolytic enzymes and permits prolonged activity of essential brush border enzymes and mammary gland factors. The evolutionary advantage of maintaining certain human milk proteins intact is clear. Breastfed infants are able to maintain the function of Igs and other biologically important peptides, including enzymes such as salivary and human milk amylases and lipases that are able to continue their activity in the neutral environment of the duodenum even after temporary inactivation in gastric pH. A sufficient proportion of antimicrobial proteins is known to escape digestion altogether and emerge in the feces, suggesting that antimicrobial activity continues throughout the length of the infant's gastrointestinal tract.

Some antimicrobial components are active both within the breast, minimizing the risk of breast infection and mastitis,[135] and within the infant's gastrointestinal and respiratory tracts, protecting the mucosal surfaces from infection by bacteria, viruses, and parasites.[121] The site of action of the peptide feedback inhibitor of lactation, for example, is within the breast itself, its function being the autocrine regulation of milk production.[136] Many bioactive substances also become valuable nutrient sources once they are digested and absorbed (see also Chapter 2).

Intestinal Microbiota in the Infant

The gastrointestinal tract is sterile at birth and is subsequently colonized by microbes acquired from the mother and the surrounding environment.[137] Bacteria are predominant, but a variety of protozoa, yeasts, bacteriophages, and anaerobic fungi are present.[138,139] It is estimated that the human colon contains more than 10^{11} bacterial cells/g of mucosa; the bacteria outnumber host cells by a factor of 10 and comprise as many as 400 different species.[140] Anaerobic bacteria predominate, and more than 99% of the bacteria isolated from human fecal specimens will not grow in the presence of atmospheric oxygen.[141] Because of the vital role of gastrointestinal microbiota and its profound influence on immunologic, nutritional, physiological, and protective processes, some consider it the largest metabolically adaptable and rapidly renewable organ of the body.[142]

The gut is initially colonized by lactic acid bacteria (eg, lactobacillus, bifidobacteria), enterobacteria, and streptococci. The gastric content of newborn infants is similar to that of their mothers' cervix,[143] and the content of the nasopharynx of most neonates is consistent with that of their mothers' vagina immediately before delivery.[144] Enterobacteria and streptococci are the first groups to colonize the intestines, and all infants are colonized with *Escherichia coli* within a few days.[145] The intestinal microflora differs between breastfed and formula-fed infants, with the predominant species in breastfed infants being *Lactobacillus* species and *Bifidobacterium* species, whereas formula-fed infants have a large proportion of *Bacteroides* species and *Enterobacter* species.[146,147] Human milk contains up to 10^9 microbes/L, the most common groups being staphylococci, streptococci, corynebacteria, lactobacilli, micrococci, propionibacteria, and bifidobacteria.[148,149] After the introduction of solid foods, obligate anaerobes increase in number and diversity until a pattern similar to that seen in adults is achieved, normally by the age of 2 to 3 years. Lactobacilli and most gram-negative bacteria, such as *E coli* and other members of the Enterobacteriaceae family, can adhere to enterocytes.[150] The study of the molecular basis for bacterial adhesion to enterocytes may help elucidate some of the mechanisms by which indigenous bacteria stimulate the development of host immunity in the intestinal tract. This may lead to insights into a variety of pediatric conditions, including food allergies, inflammatory bowel disease, and autoimmune conditions, including eczema.[151]

References

1. Steyermark AC, Lam MM, Diamond J. Quantitative evolutionary design of nutrient processing: glucose. *Proc Natl Acad Sci U S A.* 2002;99:8754–8759

2. O'Connor TP, Lam MM, Diamond J. Magnitude of functional adaptation after intestinal resection. *Am J Physiol.* 1999;276:R1265–R1275

3. Tracy CR, Diamond J. Regulation of gut function varies with life–history traits in chuckwallas (Sauromalus obesus: Iguanidae). *Physiol Biochem Zool.* 2005;78:469–481

4. Sadler TW. Third to eighth week: the embryonic period. In: *Langman's Medical Embryology.* 9th ed. Philadelphia, PA: Lippincott Williams & Wilkins; 2004:87–115

5. Sadler TW. Digestive system. In: *Langman's Medical Embryology.* 9th ed. Philadelphia, PA: Lippincott Williams & Wilkins; 2004:285–319

6. Apelqvist A, Ahlgren U, Edlund H. Sonic hedgehog directs specialized mesoderm differentiation in the intestine and pancreas. *Curr Biol.* 1997;7:801–804

7. Moore-Scott BA, Manley NR. Differential expression of Sonic hedgehog along the anterior-posterior axis regulates patterning of pharyngeal pouch endoderm and pharyngeal endoderm-derived organs. *Dev Biol.* 2005;278:323–335

8. Kiefer JC. Molecular mechanisms of early gut organogenesis: a primer on development of the digestive tract. *Dev Dyn.* 2003;228:287–291

9. Stevenson RE, Hall JG, Goodman RM. *Human Malformations and Related Anomalies.* New York, NY: Oxford University Press; 1993

10. Amiel J, Lyonnet S. Hirschsprung disease, associated syndromes, and genetics: a review. *J Med Genet.* 2001;38:729–739

11. Bjerknes M, Cheng H. Gastrointestinal stem cells. II. Intestinal stem cells. *Am J Physiol Gastrointest Liver Physiol.* 2005;289:G381–G387

12. Leedham SJ, Brittan M, McDonald SA, Wright NA. Intestinal stem cells. *J Cell Mol Med.* 2005;9:11–24

13. Hall PA, Coates PJ, Ansari B, Hopwood D. Regulation of cell number in the mammalian gastrointestinal tract: the importance of apoptosis. *J Cell Sci.* 1994;107:3569–3577

14. Bjerknes M, Cheng H. The stem-cell zone of the small intestinal epithelium. I. Evidence from Paneth cells in the adult mouse. *Am J Anat.* 1981;160:51–63

15. Ouellette AJ. Defensin-mediated innate immunity in the small intestine. *Best Pract Res Clin Gastroenterol.* 2004;18:405–419

16. Gerbert A. The role of M cells in the protection of mucosal membranes. *Histochem Cell Biol.* 1997;108:455–470

17. Powell DW, Mifflin RC, Valentich JD, Crowe SE, Saada JI, West AB. Myofibroblasts. II. Intestinal subepithelial myofibroblasts. *Am J Physiol.* 1999;277:C183–C201

18. Aynsley-Green A. Metabolic and endocrine interrelations in the human fetus and neonate. *Am J Clin Nutr.* 1985;41:339–417

19. Salminen S, Isolauri E. Intestinal colonization, microbiota, and probiotics. *J Pediatr.* 2006;149(5 Suppl):S115–S120

20. Menard D. Growth-promoting factors and the development of the human gut. In: Lebenthal E, ed. *Human Gastrointestinal Development.* New York, NY: Raven Press; 1989:123–150

21. Weaver LT, Laker MF, Nelson R. Intestinal permeability in the newborn. *Arch Dis Child.* 1984;59:236–241

22. Lebenthal E. Concepts in gastrointestinal development. In: Lebenthal E, ed. *Human Gastrointestinal Development.* New York, NY: Raven Press; 1989:3–18

23. Ferraris RP, Diamond JM. Specific regulation of intestinal nutrient transporters by their dietary substrates. *Annu Rev Physiol.* 1989;51:125–141

24. Jones PJH, Kubow S. Lipids, sterols, and their metabolites. In: Shils ME, Shike M, Ross AC, Caballero B, Cousins RJ, eds. *Modern Nutrition in Health and Disease.* 10th ed. Philadelphia, PA: Lippincott Williams & Wilkins: 92–122

25. Poulos A, Beckman K, Johnson DW, et al. Very long-chain fatty acids in peroxisomal disease. *Adv Exp Med Biol.* 1992;318:331–340

26. Hu FB, van Dam RM, Liu S. Diet and risk of type II diabetes: the role of types of fat and carbohydrate. *Diabetologia.* 2001;44:805–817

27. von Ebner K. Die acinosen drusen der zunge und ihre beziehungen zu den geschmacksorganen. In: Hoelliker V, ed. *Handbook der Geweblehre des Menschen.* Graz, Austria: Leuschner and Lubensky; 1899:18–38

28. Menard D, Monfils S, Tremblay E. Ontogeny of human gastric lipase and pepsin activities. *Gastroenterology.* 1995;108:1650–1656

29. Fink CS, Hamosh P, Hamosh M. Fat digestion in the stomach: stability of lingual lipase in the gastric environment. *Pediatr Res.* 1984;18:248–254

30. Jensen RG, DeJong FA, Clark RM, Palmgren LG, Liao TH, Hamosh M. Stereospecificity of premature human infant lingual lipase. *Lipids.* 1982;17:570–572

31. Gargouri Y, Pieroni G, Riviere C, et al. Kinetic assay of human gastric lipase on short- and long-chain triacylglycerol emulsions. *Gastroenterology.* 1986;91:919–925

32. Faber J, Goldstein R, Blondheim O, et al. Absorption of medium chain triglycerides in the stomach of the human infant. *J Pediatr Gastroenterol Nutr.* 1988;7:189–195

33. Encrantz JC, Sjovall J. On the bile acids in duodenal contents of infants and children. Bile acids and steroids 72. *Clin Chim Acta.* 1959;4:793–799

34. Heubi JE, Balistreri WF, Suchy FJ. Bile salt metabolism in the first year of life. *J Lab Clin Med.* 1982;100:127–136

35. Boehm G, Bierbach U, Senger H, et al. Activities of lipase and trypsin in duodenal juice of infants small for gestational age. *J Pediatr Gastroenterol Nutr.* 1991;12:324–327

36. de Belle RC, Vaupshas V, Vitullo BB, et al. Intestinal absorption of bile salts: immature development in the neonate. *J Pediatr.* 1979;94:472–476

37. Wong MH, Oelkers P, Craddock AL, Dawson PA. Expression cloning and characterization of the hamster ileal sodium-dependent bile acid transporter. *J Biol Chem.* 1994;269:1340–1347

38. Reinhart GA, Mahan DC, Lepine AJ, Simmen FA, Moore BE. Dietary clofibric acid increases intestinal fatty acid binding protein activity and apparent lipid digestibility in weanling swine. *J Anim Sci.* 1993;71:2693–2699

39. Liao TH, Hamosh M, Scanlon JW, Hamosh P. Preduodenal fat digestion in the newborn infant: effect of fatty acid chain length on triglyceride hydrolysis. *Clin Res.* 1980;28:820

40. Bitman J, Wood L, Hamosh M, Hamosh P, Mehta NR. Comparison of the lipid composition of breast milk from mothers of term and preterm infants. *J Clin Nutr.* 1983;38:300–312

41. Roy CC, Ste-Marie M, Chartrand L, Weber A, Bard H, Doray B. Correction of the malabsorption of the preterm infant with a medium-chain triglyceride formula. *J Pediatr.* 1975;86:446–450

42. Tantibhedhyangkul P, Hashim SA. Medium-chain triglyceride feeding in premature infants: effects on fat and nitrogen absorption. *Pediatrics.* 1975;55:359–370

43. Sarles J, Moreau H, Verger R. Human gastric lipase: ontogeny and variations in children. *Acta Paediatr.* 1992;81:511–513

44. Zoppi G, Andreotti G, Pajno-Ferrara F, Njai DM, Gaburro D. Exocrine pancreas function in premature and full term neonates. *Pediatr Res.* 1972;6:880–886

45. Boehm G, Bierbach U, DelSanto A, Moro G, Minoli I. Activities of trypsin and lipase in duodenal aspirates of healthy preterm infants: effects of gestational and postnatal age. *Biol Neonate.* 1995;67:248–253

46. Brueton MJ, Berger HM, Brown GA, Ablitt L, Iyngkaran N, Wharton BA. Duodenal bile acid conjugation patterns and dietary sulphur amino acids in the newborn. *Gut.* 1978;19:95–98

47. Armand M, Hamosh M, Mehta NR, et al. Effect of human milk or formula on gastric function and fat digestion in the premature infant. *Pediatr Res.* 1996;40:429–437

48. Mehta NR, Jones JB, Hamosh M. Lipases in preterm human milk: ontogeny and physiologic significance. *J Pediatr Gastroenterol Nutr.* 1982;1:317–326

49. Blackberg L, Hernell O. The bile-salt stimulated lipase in human milk: purification and characterization. *Eur J Biochem.* 1981;116:221–225

50. Hernell O, Blackberg L. Digestion of human milk lipids: physiologic significance of sn-2 monoglycerol hydrolysis by bile salt-stimulated lipase. *Pediatr Res.* 1982;16:882–885

51. Hernell O. Human milk lipases. III. Physiological implications of the bile salt-stimulated lipase. *Eur J Clin Invest.* 1975;5:267–272

52. Fredrikzon B, Olivecrona T. Decrease of lipase and esterase activities in intestinal contents of newborn infants during test meals. *Pediatr Res.* 1978;12:631–634

53. Nyberg L, Farooqi A, Blackberg L, Duan RD, Nilsson A, Hernell O. Digestion of ceramide by human mild bile salt-stimulated lipase. *J Pediatr Gastroenterol Nutr.* 1998;27:560–567

54. Williamson S, Finucane E, Ellis H, Gamsu HR. Effect of heat treatment of human milk on absorption of nitrogen, fat, sodium, calcium, and phosphorus by preterm infants. *Arch Dis Child.* 1978;53:555–563

55. Wang CS, Kuksis A, Manganaro F. Studies on the substrate specificity of purified human milk lipoprotein lipase. *Lipids.* 1982;17:278–284

56. Keim NL, Levin RJ, Havel PJ. Carbohydrates. In: Shils ME, Shike M, Ross AC, Caballero B, Cousins RJ, eds. *Modern Nutrition in Health and Disease.* 10th ed. Philadelphia, PA: Lippincott Williams & Wilkins; 2006:62–82

57. Eggermont E. The hydrolysis of the naturally occurring alpha-glucosides by the human intestinal mucosa. *Eur J Biochem.* 1969;9:483–487

58. Wright EM, Loo DD. Coupling between Na^+, sugar, and water transport across the intestine. *Ann N Y Acad Sci.* 2000;915:54–66

59. Koldovsky O, Heringova A, Jirsova V, Jirasek JE, Uher J. Transport of glucose against a concentration gradient in everted sacs of jejunum and ileum of human fetuses. *Gastroenterology.* 1965;48:185–187

60. Malo C. Separation of two distinct Na^+/D-glucose cotransport systems in the human fetal jejunum by means of their differential specificity for 3-O-methylglucose. *Biochim Biophys Acta.* 1990;1022:8–16

61. Lee WS, Kanal Y, Wells RG, Hediger MA. The high affinity Na^+/glucose cotransporter. Re-evaluation of function and distribution of expression. *J Biol Chem.* 1994;269:12032–12039

62. Loo DD, Hirayama BA, Meinild AK, Chandy G, Zeuthen T, Wright EM. Passive water and ion transport by cotransporters. *J Physiol.* 1999;518(Pt 1):195–202

63. Hoekstra JH. Fructose breath hydrogen tests in infants with chronic non-specific diarrhoea. *Eur J Pediatr.* 1995;154:362–364

64. Moore MC, Charrington AD, Mann SL, Davis SN. Acute fructose administration decreases the glycemic response to an oral glucose tolerance test in normal adults. *J Clin Endocrinol Metab.* 2000;85:4515–4519

65. Rossiter MA, Barrowman JA, Dand A, Wharton BA. Amylase content of mixed saliva in children. *Acta Paediatr Scand.* 1974;63:389–392

66. Delachaume-Salem E, Sarles H. [Normal human pancreatic secretion in relation to age.] [Article in French.] *Biol Gastroenterol (Paris).* 1970;2:135–146

67. Lebenthal E, Lee PC. Development of functional responses in human exocrine pancreas. *Pediatrics*. 1980;66:556–560

68. Antonowicz I, Chang SK, Grand RJ. Development and distribution of lysosomal enzymes and disaccharides in human fetal intestine. *Gastroenterology*. 1974;67:51–58

69. Raul F, Lacroix B, Aprahamian M. Longitudinal distribution of brush border hydrolases and morphological maturation in the intestine of the preterm infant. *Early Hum Dev*. 1986;13:225–234

70. Shulman RJ, Schanler RJ, Lau C, Heitkemper M, Ou CN, Smith EO. Early feeding, feeding intolerance, and lactase activity in preterm infants. *J Pediatr*. 1998;133:645–649

71. Douwes AC, Oosterkamp RF, Fernandes J, Los T, Jongbloed AA. Sugar malabsorption in healthy neonates estimated by breath hydrogen. *Arch Dis Child*. 1980;55:512–515

72. Topping DL, Clifton PM. Short-chain fatty acids and human colonic function: roles of resistant starch and nonstarch polysaccharides. *Physiol Rev*. 2001;81:1031–1064

73. Gray CM. Starch digestion and absorption in nonruminants. *J Nutr*. 1992;122:172–177

74. Rings EH, Grand RJ, Buller HA. Lactose intolerance and lactase deficiency in children. *Curr Opin Pediatr*. 1994;6:562–567

75. Northrop-Clewes CA, Lunn PG, Downes RM. Lactose maldigestion in breast-feeding Gambian infants. *J Pediatr Gastroenterol Nutr*. 1997;24:257–263

76. Koldovsky O. Digestive-absorptive functions in fetuses, infants, and children. In: Polin RA, Fox WW, eds. *Fetal and Neonatal Physiology*. Vol 2. Philadelphia, PA: WB Saunders Co; 1992:1060–1077

77. Matthews DE. Proteins and amino acids. In: Shils ME, Shike M, Ross AC, Caballero B, Cousins RJ, eds. *Modern Nutrition in Health and Disease*. Philadelphia, PA: Lippincott Williams & Wilkins; 2006:23–61

78. Young VR. Adult amino acid requirements: the case for a major revision in current recommendations. *J Nutr*. 1994;124[8 Suppl]:1517S–1523S

79. Bjelton L, Sandberg G, Wennberg A, et al. Assessment of biological quality of amino acid solutions for intravenous nutrition. In: Kinney JM, Borum PR, eds. *Perspectives in Clinical Nutrition*. Baltimore, MD: Urban & Schwarzenberg; 1989:31–42

80. Mouterde O, Dacher JN, Basuyau JP, Mallet E. Gastric secretion in infants. Application to the study of sudden infant death syndrome and apparently life-threatening events. *Biol Neonate*. 1992;62:15–22

81. Mitchell DJ, McClure BG, Tubman TR. Simultaneous monitoring of gastric and oesophageal pH reveals limitations of conventional oesophageal pH monitoring in milk fed infants. *Arch Dis Child*. 2001;84:273–276

82. Omari TI, Davidson GP. Multipoint measurement of intragastric pH in healthy preterm infants. *Arch Dis Child Fetal Neonatal Ed*. 2003;88:F517–F520

83. Kelly EJ, Brownlee KG. When is the fetus first capable of gastric acid, intrinsic factor and gastrin secretion? *Biol Neonate*. 1993;63:153–156

84. Kelly EJ, Brownlee KG, Newell SJ. Gastric secretory function in the developing human stomach. *Early Hum Dev*. 1992;31:163–166

85. Hyman PE, Clarke DD, Everett SL, et al. Gastric acid secretory function in preterm infants. *J Pediatr.* 1985;106:467–471

86. Kelly EJ, Newell SJ, Brownlee KG, Primrose JN, Dear PR. Gastric acid secretion in preterm infants. *Early Hum Dev.* 1993;35:215–220

87. Grahnquist L, Ruuska T, Finkel Y. Early development of human gastric H,K-adenosine triphosphatase. *J Pediatr Gastroenterol Nutr.* 2000;30:533–537

88. Yahav J, Carrion V, Lee PC, Lebenthal E. Meal-stimulated pepsinogen secretion in premature infants. *J Pediatr.* 1987;110:949–951

89. Lieberman J. Proteolytic enzyme activity in fetal pancreas and meconium: demonstration of plasminogen and trypsinogen activators in pancreatic tissue. *Gastroenterology.* 1966;50:183–190

90. Borgstrom, Lindquist B, Lundh G. Enzyme concentration and absorption of protein and glucose in duodenum of premature infants. *Am J Dis Child.* 1960;99:338–343

91. Madey S, Dancis J. Proteolytic enzymes of the premature infant: with special reference to his ability to digest unsplit protein food. *Pediatrics.* 1949;4:177–182

92. Bujanover Y, Harel A, Geter R, Blau H, Yahav J, Spirer Z. The development of the chymotrypsin activity during postnatal life using the bentiromide test. *Int J Pancreatol.* 1988;3:53–58

93. Lindberg T. Proteolytic activity in duodenal juice in infants, children, and adults. *Acta Paediatr Scand.* 1974;63:805–808

94. Kushak RI, Winter HS. Regulation of intestinal peptidases by nutrients in human fetuses and children. *Comp Biochem Physiol A Mol Integr Physiol.* 1999;124:191–198

95. Palacin M, Estevez R, Bertran J, Zorzano A. Molecular biology of mammalian plasma membrane amino acid transporters. *Physiol Rev.* 1998;78:969–1054

96. Malo C. Multiple pathways for amino acid transport in brush border membrane vesicles isolated from the human fetal small intestine. *Gastroenterology.* 1991;100:1644–1652

97. Weaver LT, Walker WA. Uptake of macromolecules in the neonate. In: Lebenthal E, ed. *Human Gastrointestinal Development.* New York, NY: Raven Press; 1989:731–748

98. Lind T. Amniotic fluid. In: Lentner C, ed. *Geigy Scientific Tables.* Vol 1. 8th rev ed. Basel, Switzerland: Geigy; 1981:197–212

99. Roberton DM, Paganelli R, Dinwiddie R, Levinsky RJ. Milk antigen absorption in the preterm and term neonate. *Arch Dis Child.* 1982;57:369–372

100. Walker WA. Absorption of protein and protein fragments in the developing intestine: role in immunologic/allergic reactions. *Pediatrics.* 1985;75(Suppl):167–171

101. Gruskay FL, Cooke RE. The gastrointestinal absorption of unaltered protein in normal infants and in infants recovering from diarrhea. *Pediatrics.* 1955;16:763–769

102. Weaver LT. Breast and gut: the relationship between lactating mammary function and neonatal gastrointestinal function. *Proc Nutrition Soc.* 1992;51:155–163

103. Yoshida M, Kobayashi K, Kuo TT, et al. Neonatal Fc receptor for IgG regulates mucosal immune responses to luminal bacteria. *J Clin Invest.* 2006;116:2142–2151

104. Prasad PD, Wang H, Huang W, et al. Molecular and functional characterization of the intestinal Na+-dependent multivitamin transporter. *Arch Biochem Biophys.* 1999;366:95–106

105. Bass WT, Malati N, Castle MC, White LE. Evidence for the safety of ascorbic acid administration to the premature infant. *Am J Perinatol.* 1998;15:133–140

106. Tsukaguchi H, Tokui T, Mackenzie B, et al. A family of mammalian Na⁺-dependent L-ascorbic acid transporters. *Nature.* 1999;399:70–75

107. Ziegler EE, Fomon SJ. Lactose enhances mineral absorption in infancy. *J Ped Gastroenterol Nutr.* 1983;2:288–294

108. Ghishan FK, Stroop S, Meneely R. The effect of lactose on the intestinal absorption of calcium and zinc in the rat during maturation. *Pediatr Res.* 1982;16:566–568

109. Barnes LA, Morrow G III, Silverio J, Finnegan LP, Heitman SE. Calcium and fat absorption from infant formulas with different fat blends. *Pediatrics.* 1974;54:217–221

110. Namgung R, Tsang RC. Factors affecting newborn bone mineral content: in utero effects on newborn bone mineralization. *Proc Nutr Soc.* 2000;59:55–63

111. Ghishan FK, Parker P, Nichols S, Hoyumpa A. Kinetics of intestinal calcium transport during maturation in rats. *Pediatr Res.* 1984;18:235–239

112. Forbes GB, Reina JC. Effect of age on gastrointestinal absorption (Fe, Sr, Pb) in the rat. *J Nutr.* 1972;102:647–652

113. Gunshin H, Mackenzie B, Berger UV, et al. Cloning and characterization of a mammalian proton-coupled metal-ion transporter. *Nature.* 1997;388:482–488

114. Ziegler EE, Edwards BB, Jensen RL, Mahaffey KR, Fomon SJ. Absorption and retention of lead by infants. *Pediatr Res.* 1978;12:29–34

115. Carnielli VP, Luijendijk IH, van Goudoever JB, et al. Feeding premature newborn infants palmitic acid in amounts and stereoisomeric position similar to that of human milk: effects on fat and mineral balance. *Am J Clin Nutr.* 1995;61:1037–1042

116. Jensen RG. Lipids in human milk-composition and fat soluble vitamins. In: Lebenthal E, ed. *Textbook of Gastroenterology and Nutrition in Infancy.* New York, NY: Raven Press; 1989:157–208

117. Ballabriga A. Essential fatty acids and human tissue composition. An overview. *Acta Paediatr Suppl.* 1994;402:63–68

118. Clandinin MT. Brain development and assessing the supply of polyunsaturated fatty acid. *Lipids.* 1999;34:131–137

119. Sala-Vila A, Castellote AI, Campoy C, Rivero M, Rodriquez-Palmero M, Lopez-Sabater MC. The source of long-chain PUFA in formula supplements does not affect the fatty acid composition of plasma lipids in full-term infants. *J Nutr.* 2004;134:868–873

120. Fleith M, Clandinin MT. Dietary PUFA for preterm and term infants: review of clinical studies. *Crit Rev Food Sci Nutr.* 2005;45:205–229

121. Lonnerdal B. Biochemistry and physiological function of human milk proteins. *Am J Clin Nutr.* 1985;42:1299–1317

122. Prentice A, Ewing G, Roberts SB, et al. The nutritional role of breast milk IgA and lactoferrin. *Acta Paediatr Scand.* 1987;76:592–598

123. Kleinman RE, Walker WA. The enteromammary immune system: an important new concept in breast milk host defense. *Dig Dis Sci.* 1979;24:876–882

124. Mata L. Breastfeeding and host defense. *Front Gastrointest Res.* 1986;13:119–133

125. Mepham TB. *Physiology of Lactation*. Philadelphia, PA: Open University Press; 1987

126. Kunz C, Rudloff S. Biological functions of oligosaccharides in human milk. *Acta Paediatr.* 1994;82:903–912

127. Gnoth MJ, Rudloff S, Kunz C, Kinne RK. Investigations on the in vitro transport of human milk oligosaccharides by a Caco-2 monolayer using a novel high performance liquid chromatography-mass spectrometry technique. *J Biol Chem.* 2001;276:34363–34370

128. Koldovsky O. Hormonally active peptides in human milk. *Acta Pediatr Suppl.* 1994;402:89–93

129. Goldman AS, Goldblum RM. Defense agents in milk. A. Defense agents in human milk. In: Jensen RG, ed. *Handbook of Milk Composition*. San Diego, CA: Academic Press; 1995:727–745

130. Weaver LT, Walker WA. Epidermal growth factor and the developing human gut. *Gastroenterology.* 1988;94:845–847

131. Weaver LT, Freiberg E, Israel EJ, Walker WA. Epidermal growth factor in human amniotic fluid. *Gastroenterology.* 1989:95:1436

132. Weaver LT, Gonnella PA, Israel EJ, Walker WA. Uptake and transport of epidermal growth factor by the small intestinal epithelium of the fetal rat. *Gastroenterology.* 1990;98:828–837

133. Menard D, Arsenault P, Pothier P. Biologic effects of epidermal growth factor in human fetal jejunum. *Gastroenterology.* 1988;94:656–663

134. Watkins JB, Szczepanik P, Gould JP, Klein P, Lester R. Bile salt metabolism in the human premature infant. Preliminary observations of pool size and synthesis rate following prenatal administration of dexamethasone and phenobarbital. *Gastroenterology.* 1975;69:706–713

135. Prentice A, Prentice AM, Lamb WH. Mastitis in rural Gambian mothers and the protection of the breast by milk antimicrobial factors. *Trans R Soc Trop Med Hyg.* 1985;79:90–95

136. Wilde CJ, Prentice A, Peaker M. Breastfeeding: matching supply with demand in human lactation. *Proc Nutr Soc.* 1995;54:401–406

137. Mackie RI, Sghir A, Gaskins HR. Developmental microbial ecology of the neonatal gastrointestinal tract. *Am J Clin Nutr.* 1999;69(Suppl):1035S–1045S

138. Clarke RTJ. The gut and its micro-organisms. In: Clarke RTJ, Bauchop T, eds. *Microbial Ecology of the Gut.* New York, NY: Academic Press; 1977:36–71

139. Hespell RB, Akin DE, Dehority BA. Bacteria, fungi and protozoa of the rumen. In: Mackie RI, White BA, Isaacson RE, eds. *Gastrointestinal Microbiology.* Vol 2. New York, NY: Chapman and Hall; 1997:59–141

140. Conway PL. Microbial ecology of the human large intestine. In: Gibson GR, Macfarlane GT, eds. *Human Colonic Bacteria: Role in Nutrition, Physiology, and Pathlogy.* Boca Raton, FL: CRC Press; 1995:1–24

141. Savage DC. Microbial ecology of the gastrointestinal tract. *Annu Rev Microbiol.* 1977;31:107–133

142. Berg RD. The indigenous gastrointestinal microflora. *Trends Microbiol.* 1996;4:430–435

143. Brook I, Barrett CT, Brinkman CR, Martin WJ, Finegold SM. Aerobic and anaerobic bacterial flora of the maternal cervix and newborn gastric fluid and conjunctiva: a prospective study. *Pediatrics.* 1979;63:451–455

144. MacGregor RR, Tunnessen WW. The incidence of pathogenic organisms in the normal flora of the neonates external ear and nasopharynx. *Clin Pediatr (Phila)*. 1973;12:697–700

145. Adlerberth I, Carlsson V, de Man P, et al. Intestinal colonization with Enterobacteriaceae in Pakistan and Swedish hospital-delivered infants. *Acta Paediatr Scand*. 1991;80:602–610

146. Parrett AM, Edwards CA. In vitro fermentation of carbohydrate by breast fed and formula fed infants. *Arch Dis Child*. 1997;76:249–253

147. Mata LJ, Urrutia JJ. Intestinal colonization of breast fed children in a rural area of low socioeconomic level. *Ann N Y Acad Sci*. 1971;176:93–108

148. Asquith MT, Harrod JR. Reduction in bacterial contamination in banked human milk. *J Pediatr*. 1979;95:993–994

149. West PA, Hewitt JH, Murphy OM. The influence of methods of collection and storage on the bacteriology of human milk. *J Appl Bacteriol*. 1979;46:269–277

150. Duguid JP, Old DC. Adhesive properties of Enterobacteriaceae. In: Beachey EH, ed. *Bacterial Adherence, Receptors and Recognition*. Series B. Vol 6. London, England: Chapman and Hall; 1980:185–217

151. Kalliomäki M, Salminen S, Arvilommi H, Kero P, Koskinen P, Isolauri E. Probiotics in primary prevention of atopic disease: a randomised placebo-controlled trial. *Lancet*. 2001;357:1076–1079

2 Breastfeeding

Introduction

The American Academy of Pediatrics (AAP) strongly recommends breast-feeding as the preferred feeding for all infants, including preterm newborn infants.[1] The success of adequate lactation depends substantially on a supportive attitude of professional personnel in pediatrics, family practice, and obstetrics services; a hospital climate that is conducive to the initiation and maintenance of breastfeeding; and the realization by health care professionals that although breastfeeding is a natural function, many mothers need instruction and support. Much information must be conveyed to new parents in the short postpartum hospital stay. Caregivers should observe and document breastfeeding, and early follow-up at 3 to 5 days of age should be arranged.[1] Public awareness of the benefits of breastfeeding has increased, which has prompted caregivers to request more formal education in the field.[2] Numerous programs have been developed to enhance the knowledge of pediatricians and support their practices, and the AAP and American College of Obstetricians and Gynecologists together published the *Breastfeeding Handbook for Physicians*.[3]

Rates of Breastfeeding in the United States

Infant feeding practices in the United States have changed substantially over the past several decades. Breastfeeding was the norm in the early part of this century, with a mean duration of more than 4 months in 1931.[4] However, after World War II, the proportion of babies who were breastfed decreased dramatically, probably as a result of the great influx of women into the workforce and the use of the readily available and widely marketed commercial infant formulas.[5] Recognition of the benefits of breastfeeding by the public and health professionals, however, grew during the 1970s, and breastfeeding rates increased from a low of 24.7% in 1971 to 59.7% in 1984.[6] In 1995, 60% of mothers breastfed and 20% continued to 6 months.[7] The Centers for Disease Control and Prevention began monitoring annual breastfeeding rates through the National Immunization Survey in 2003 (http://www.cdc.gov/breastfeeding/data/index.htm) and published the first data in 2003. In 2003 and 2004, 70.9% and 70.3%, respectively, of all US women initiated breastfeeding—close to the *Healthy People 2010* (Table 2.1) objective of 75% breastfeeding initiation.[8] Although this time period had the highest rates in recent years, only approximately 40% were breastfeeding exclusively at 3 months. At 6 months, 36% of infants were receiving any human milk, well below the *Healthy People 2010* goal of 50%, and only 14% were breastfeeding exclusively. When viewed by state, in 2004, 14 states achieved the national *Healthy People 2010* objective of 75% breastfeeding initiation rate, whereas only 3 states achieved the objective of having 50% of mothers report any breastfeeding at 6 months, and 5 states achieved the objective of having 25% of mothers report any breastfeeding at 12 months. However, no US state achieved an exclusive breastfeeding rate of 25% through 6 months.

Table 2.1
***Healthy People 2010* Goals**[8]

Breastfeeding initiation	75%
Breastfeeding duration to 6 months	50%
Breastfeeding duration to 12 months	25%

Unfortunately, the increases in breastfeeding rates have not been distributed equally among all population subgroups. Demographically, formula feeding is more common among less-educated women[9-11] and those who are single[9] or young.[6] Although well below national rates, significant increases in breastfeeding rates have been reported among these subgroups: mothers 20 years or younger (any breastfeeding: 48% initiation and 14% at 6 months of age), primiparous women, mothers of infants with low birth weight, and participants in the Special Supplemental Nutrition Program for Women, Infants, and Children (WIC) (any breastfeeding: 64% initiation and 29% at 6 months). The WIC program has made significant strides in increasing the rates of breastfeeding among its participants, although the rates have still been low.[12,13]

Employment has been associated with lower rates of initiation and duration of breastfeeding in some studies.[5] However, breastfeeding rates have decreased among both unemployed and working women.[6] Nevertheless, women who work outside the home may need assistance and support in balancing breastfeeding with experiences in the workplace. Efforts have been made to develop breastfeeding support programs in many work locations, often with great success.

There also is considerable disparity in breastfeeding rates among racial and ethnic minority groups. Data on breastfeeding from the National Immunization Survey revealed that non-Hispanic black and socioeconomically disadvantaged women had lower breastfeeding rates. Black women are significantly less likely to breastfeed.[6,9,10,14] Although in 2004 and 2003, breastfeeding rates among black women approximated 54% for initiation and 23% at 6 months, this group had the most rapid gains in breastfeeding rates in recent years (30% increase from 1996–2004). Breastfeeding rates in 2003–2004 for Hispanic mothers are greater than those for the total US population (approximately 79% at initiation). Ethnicity also influences attitudes cited in support of feeding decisions, with some feeding beliefs being culturally specific.[15,16] Hispanic mothers sometimes express concern about transmitting dangerous negative emotions to their babies through their milk.[17,18] In contrast, Navajo mothers believe that breastfeeding passes on maternal attributes and models proper behavior, thereby ensuring a good life for the infant.[19] In addition, support for breastfeeding from the baby's father,[20] other relatives, such as the maternal grandmother,[21] or friends,[22] which influences duration of breastfeeding, may also vary by ethnicity.[18]

Data on breastfeeding rates at 1 year of age have only recently been collected. Whereas the *Healthy People 2010* goal for any breastfeeding at 1 year of age is 25%, the rate for the United States in 2004 and 2003 approximated 17%, but the rate among black women was 9.8%. *Healthy People 2010* goals include eliminating health disparities among subgroups of the population, including racial and ethnic disparities.[23] Thus, improvements in breastfeeding rates in many subgroups of the population are needed. Such improvements can be facilitated through knowledgeable health care practitioners.

The Evidence to Support Breastfeeding

The AAP recommends exclusive breastfeeding for a minimum of 4 months but preferably for 6 months. Breastfeeding should be continued, with the addition of complementary foods, at least through the first 12 months of age and thereafter as long as mutually desired by mother and infant.[1,24,25] The recommendation for feeding full-term and preterm infants with human milk arises because of its acknowledged benefits to infant nutrition, gastrointestinal function and host defense, and the potential beneficial influence on neurodevelopment and chronic diseases of childhood. In addition, benefits of breastfeeding to maternal health as well as significant societal benefits have been described.

Nutritional Aspects

The human milk model is used to design the composition of human milk substitutes, because the goal for infant nutrition through the first year is to mimic the body composition of the breastfed infant. A reference tabulation of the composition of human milk, comparing early and more mature milk, is provided in Appendix C.[26] However, because human milk has a dynamic nutrient composition, making a single tabulation of its contents is unrealistic. Nutrient contents may change through lactation, over the course of a day, and within a feeding and differ among women. Components in human milk also exert dual roles, one in nutrition and one involved in immunity and/or development. In the first few weeks after birth, the total nitrogen content of milk from mothers who deliver prematurely (preterm milk) is greater than milk obtained from women delivering at term (term milk).[27] The total nitrogen content in both milks, however, decreases similarly to approach what is called mature milk.[28] The protein quality (proportion of whey [70%] and casein [30%]) of human milk differs from that in bovine milk (82% casein, 18% whey). Caseins are proteins with low solubility in gastric acid. Whey proteins remain in solution after acid precipitation. Generally, the whey fraction of soluble proteins is more easily digested and promotes more rapid gastric emptying. The whey protein fraction provides lower concentrations of phenylalanine, tyrosine, and methionine and higher concentrations of taurine than the casein fraction of milk. The plasma amino acid pattern in the breastfed infant serves as the model on which enteral and parenteral amino acid solutions are based.

The type of proteins contained in the whey fraction differs between human and bovine milks. The major human whey protein is α-lactalbumin. Lactoferrin, lysozyme, and secretory immunoglobulin A (sIgA) are specific human whey proteins involved in host defense.[29] Because these host defense proteins resist proteolytic digestion, they serve as a first line of defense by lining the gastrointestinal tract. The major whey protein in bovine milk is β-lactoglobulin, the particular protein associated with cow milk allergy.

The lipid system in human milk, responsible for providing approximately 50% of the calories in the milk, is structured to facilitate fat digestion and absorption. The system is composed of an organized milk fat globule, bile salt-stimulated lipase, and a pattern of fatty acids (high in palmitic [C16:0], oleic [C16:1 ω-9], linoleic [C18:2 ω-6], and linolenic [C18:3 ω-3] acids) characteristically distributed on the triglyceride molecule (C16:0 at the 2 position of the molecule). Because the lipase is heat-labile, the superior fat absorption from human milk is reported only when unprocessed milk is fed. The mixture of fatty acids in infant formula differs from that in human milk. Manufacturers have modified the fat blends in formula to contain greater medium- and intermediate-chain fatty acids, in part, to match the superior fat absorption from human milk. The pattern of fatty acids in human milk also is unique in its composition of very long-chain polyunsaturated fatty acids. Arachidonic acid (C20:4 ω-6 [ARA]) and docosahexaenoic acid (C22:6 ω-3 [DHA]), derivatives of linoleic and linolenic acids, respectively, are found in human but not bovine milk. ARA and DHA are constituents of retinal and brain phospholipid membranes and functionally have been associated with improved short-term visual function and neurodevelopmental outcomes in some studies (see Chapter 16). Knowledge of their presence in human milk and their beneficial effects influenced their recent addition to many infant formulas.

The carbohydrate composition of human milk is important as a nutritional source of lactose and for the presence of oligosaccharides. Although studies in full-term infants demonstrate a small proportion of unabsorbed lactose in the feces, the presence of lactose is assumed to be a physiological effect of feeding infants with human milk. A softer stool consistency, more nonpathogenic fecal flora, and improved absorption of minerals have been attributed to the presence of small quantities of unabsorbed lactose resulting from feeding infants with human milk. Oligosaccharides are carbohydrate polymers (also including glycoproteins) that, in addition to their role in nutrition, help protect the infant, because their structure mimics specific bacterial antigen receptors and prevents bacterial attachment to the host mucosa.

The concentrations of calcium and phosphorus in human milk are significantly lower than in other milks, because they are present in more bioavailable forms—bound to digestible proteins and in complexed and ionized states.[30] Thus, despite differences in mineral intake, bone mineral content of breastfed infants is similar to that of infants fed formula.[31] The concentrations of iron, zinc, and copper decrease throughout lactation.[32,33] The concentrations of copper and zinc, despite their decrease throughout lactation, appear adequate to meet the infant's nutritional needs until approximately 6 months of age. The concentration of iron may also not meet the infant's needs beyond 6 months of breastfeeding.[34] At that time, most authorities agree that an iron supplement, in the form of iron-containing complementary feedings, is indicated to prevent subsequent iron-deficiency anemia.

Vitamin K deficiency may be a concern in the infant, because bacterial flora are responsible for ensuring vitamin K adequacy. The intestinal flora of the breastfed infant produce less vitamin K, and the content in human milk is low. Therefore, to meet vitamin K needs, a single dose of vitamin K is given at birth.[35] The content of vitamin D in human milk is low; nutrient needs for vitamin D are met by adequate sunlight exposure. Vitamin D deficiency, however, has been reported in breastfed infants who have dark skin pigmentation, inadequate exposure to sunlight, and/or when appropriate sunscreen ointments are prescribed.[36–38] Thus, giving the breastfed infant supplemental vitamin D is indicated.[39]

Gastrointestinal Function

Gastric emptying is faster for infants fed human milk than for infants fed commercial cow milk-based formula. Large gastric residual volumes are reported less frequently in preterm infants fed human milk. Many factors in human milk may stimulate gastrointestinal growth and motility and enhance maturity of the gastrointestinal tract. Bioactive factors, such as lactoferrin, may affect intestinal growth. Glutamine affects intestinal cellular metabolism, and nucleotides affect fecal flora. Enzymes such as acetylhydrolase, which blocks the ischemic injury produced by platelet-activating factor in the pathogenesis of necrotizing enterocolitis, may lower the risk of this condition.[40] In addition, components such as epidermal growth factor provide a surveillance system for the intestinal mucosa to repair any sites of injury, and interleukin-10 exerts anti-inflammatory properties.

Host Defense

Specific factors such as sIgA, lactoferrin, lysozyme, oligosaccharides, growth factors, and cellular components may affect the host defense of the infant (Table 2.2).[41] A description of the enteromammary immune system summarizes an important part of the protective nature of human milk.[42] In the enteromammary immune system, the mother produces sIgA antibody when exposed to foreign antigens and is stimulated to make specific antibodies that are elaborated at mucosal surfaces and in her milk. By ingesting the milk that contains specific sIgA antibody, the infant receives specific passive immunity. The system is active against a variety of antigens in infants.

In Brazil, infants who were completely weaned had 14.2 times the risk of death from diarrhea and 3.6 times the risk of respiratory infection compared with exclusively breastfed infants.[43] Not only in developing countries, but also in affluent US populations, there is a reduction in the incidence of gastrointestinal and respiratory diseases and otitis media that is directly attributed to breastfeeding (Table 2.3).[3] As noted previously, limited data also suggest that human milk protects the preterm infant from infection and necrotizing enterocolitis.[44] Research conducted over the past decade has addressed methodologic issues in older studies, and current studies in the industrialized world have demonstrated that breastfeeding provides clear health benefits.

Table 2.2
Selected Bioactive Factors in Human Milk

Secretory IgA	Specific antigen-targeted anti-infective action
Lactoferrin	Immunomodulation, iron chelation, antimicrobial action, anti-adhesive, trophic for intestinal growth
Lysozyme	Bacterial lysis, immunomodulation
κ-casein	Anti-adhesive, bacterial flora
Oligosaccharides	Bacterial attachment
Cytokines	Anti-inflammatory, epithelial barrier function
Growth factors 　Epidermal growth factor 　Transforming growth factor (TGF) 　Nerve growth factor	 Luminal surveillance, repair of intestine Promotes epithelial cell growth (TGF-α) Suppresses lymphocyte function (TGF-β) Growth
Enzymes 　Platelet-activating factor-acetylhydrolase 　Glutathione peroxidase	 Blocks action of platelet activating factor Prevents lipid oxidation
Nucleotides	Enhance antibody responses, bacterial flora
Vitamins A, E, C	Antioxidants
Amino acids 　Glutamine	 Intestinal cell fuel, immune responses
Lipids	Anti-infective properties

IgA indicates immunoglobulin A.

Adapted from American Academy of Pediatrics and American College of Obstetricians and Gynecologists. The importance of breastfeeding for infants, mothers, and society. In: *Breastfeeding Handbook for Physicians*. Elk Grove Village, IL: American Academy of Pediatrics; 2006:19–36[3]

　　Large, prospective studies of otitis media show a protective effect of breastfeeding.[45–48] Infants exclusively breastfed for at least 4 months may experience as few as half the number of episodes of otitis media as formula-fed infants and also half as many recurrent episodes.[45] Otitis media also is less prevalent among breastfed infants with cleft palate.[49] In many of these studies, not only is the incidence of disease diminished with breastfeeding, but also, the duration of individual episodes is reduced.[50]

Lower respiratory tract illnesses and gastroenteritis also are less common or less severe among breastfed infants. For example, breastfeeding for 1 month or longer has been associated with significantly lower rates of wheezing and lower respiratory tract illness during the first 4 months of life.[51–53] Breastfeeding also confers a strong protective effect against *Haemophilus influenzae* type b infection.[54,55] Infants breastfed for at least 13 weeks had significantly fewer gastrointestinal illnesses during the first year of life as well as lower rates of respiratory illness during several time periods. Additionally, illnesses in infants who were breastfed for at least 13 weeks seemed to be less severe because the infants were significantly less likely to be hospitalized for gastrointestinal illness.[56]

Table 2.3
Pediatric Diseases Against Which Human Milk May Protect

Acute disorders
Diarrhea
Otitis media
Recurrent otitis media
Urinary tract infection
Necrotizing enterocolitis
Septicemia
Infant botulism
Hospitalizations
Infant mortality
Chronic disorders
Insulin-dependent diabetes mellitus
Celiac disease
Crohn disease
Childhood cancer
Lymphoma
Leukemia
Allergy
Obesity and overweight

Adapted from American Academy of Pediatrics and American College of Obstetricians and Gynecologists. The importance of breastfeeding for infants, mothers, and society. In: *Breastfeeding Handbook for Physicians.* Elk Grove Village, IL: American Academy of Pediatrics; 2006:19–36[3]

Urinary tract infections have been reported to be more common among formula-fed infants than among breastfed infants.[57,58] Reduced adhesion to uroepithelial cells by pathogens as mediated by oligosaccharides,[59] sIgA,[60] or lactoferrin[61,62] has been hypothesized as the mechanism for this protective effect in breastfed infants.

In a study of infant botulism and its role in sudden infant death, formula-fed infants tended to be younger than breastfed infants at onset of the disease and were more likely to experience severe illness.[63] Indeed, breastfeeding has been a protective factor in sudden infant death syndrome.[64] Fewer episodes of late-onset sepsis and necrotizing enterocolitis are reported in preterm infants fed human milk.[65–68] Lastly, infant mortality rates in the United States and throughout the world are lower in breastfed infants compared with those fed formula.[69,70]

Chronic Diseases of Childhood

Data from epidemiologic studies suggest that specific chronic disorders have a lower incidence in children who were breastfed as infants. Because of the nature of these studies, causal relationships between breastfeeding and the health outcome of interest cannot be inferred. Among these chronic disorders are Crohn disease,[71] celiac disease,[72] lymphoma and leukemia,[73–76] juvenile-onset diabetes mellitus,[77] and certain allergic conditions. Data are conflicting regarding protection against allergic disease in general afforded by breastfeeding.[53,78] Breastfeeding, however, may be protective against some food allergies,[79,80] and the incidence of atopic dermatitis may be lessened in breastfeeding infants whose mothers follow a restricted diet. A lower incidence of atopic conditions is reported in breastfed infants with a family history of atopy.[53,81]

There may be a relationship between breastfeeding and the development of type 1 diabetes, although this remains very controversial.[77,82,83] In one report, insulin-dependent diabetes mellitus was more likely when breastfeeding occurred for fewer than 3 months and cow milk proteins were introduced before 4 months of age.[77] Increased concentrations of immunoglobulin G antibodies specific to bovine serum albumin that cross-react with β-cell–specific surface proteins have been identified in children with insulin-dependent diabetes mellitus.[84] However, it should be noted that type 1 diabetes mellitus is largely thought to be a T-lymphocyte–mediated disorder. Lactation also is associated with a decreased risk of type 2 diabetes mellitus in mothers.[85]

Several reports suggest a significant inverse relationship between breastfeeding duration and the development of overweight and obesity in adolescents and young adults.[86–88] Most, but not all, studies describe this relationship between breastfeeding and overweight/obesity in preschool children, school-aged children, and/or older adolescents, and in many of the studies, the reported data were adjusted for maternal body mass index. It is speculated that breastfeeding promotes internal self-regulation of energy intake,[89,90] promotes less rapid early weight gain,[91] is associated with lower rates of diabetes, and affects long-term programming of leptin metabolism.[92,93]

Neurobehavioral Aspects
Maternal-infant bonding is enhanced during breastfeeding. In addition, improved long-term cognitive and motor abilities in full-term infants have been directly correlated with duration of breastfeeding.[94,95] Improved long-term cognitive development in preterm infants also has been correlated with the receipt of human milk during hospitalization.[96,97] A meta-analysis of studies in which a multitude of confounding factors were considered concluded that breastfeeding conferred a benefit to cognitive function beyond the period of actual breastfeeding in term infants,[98] although this remains unresolved.

Maternal Benefits
There are positive effects of breastfeeding for the mother. There is a notion that postpartum weight loss and uterine involution are more rapid in breastfeeding women than in nonlactating mothers.[99] Exclusive breastfeeding delays the resumption of normal ovarian cycles and the return of fertility in most mothers.[100] The lowest pregnancy rates are achieved with the lactational amenorrhea method (LAM) of birth control when the following 3 criteria are met: full breastfeeding (round-the-clock), no resumption of menses, and an infant younger than 6 months.[101] The LAM method is a highly effective global program, with efficacy rates of 98.5% to 100%.[101] As such, the contraceptive effect of breastfeeding contributes to global child spacing.

Epidemiologic studies have identified a decreased incidence of premenopausal breast cancer in women who have lactated; the greater the duration of lactation, the lower the odds ratio of developing breast cancer.[102] In addition, similar studies report a decreased incidence of ovarian cancer in women who have lactated.[103,104] There also is speculation that lactation might protect against the development of osteoporosis.[104] This observation is of interest, because during lactation, there is a drain on the maternal skeleton such that maternal bone density decreases. However, maternal bone mineralization in the postweaning period is normal, suggesting a catch-up mineralization.[105,106] The adaptations necessary to remineralize the skeleton possibly have an effect on decreasing the risk of late-onset osteoporosis.

Societal Effects of Breastfeeding

The economic advantages of breastfeeding can be tangibly calculated at both personal and national levels. The obvious personal advantage is in the savings accrued by not buying infant formula. A more meaningful comparison is made by computing health care expenditures. The increased rates of illness in nonbreastfed infants result in more expenses for medical care and, if the child is ill, expenses arising from parental absence from work.

From the perspective of the national economy, it has been estimated that if 50% of infants enrolled in the WIC program were breastfed exclusively for just the first 3 months of life, a savings of approximately $4 million per month would be realized.[107] These savings would come from a combined reduction in household expenditure on formula as well as reductions in expenditures for health care. In addition, it is estimated that significant costs of health care decrease with every additional month of breastfeeding and with each month of delay in a mother's return to work after 3 months.[108] Thus, the societal economic incentives for women to breastfeed are strong and should be promoted.

Contraindications to Breastfeeding

Few true contraindications to breastfeeding exist. Infants with galactosemia cannot ingest lactose-containing milk. Therefore, because the principal carbohydrate in human milk is lactose, infants with galactosemia should not breastfeed. Infants with other inborn errors of metabolism may ingest some human milk, but this recommendation would depend on the desired protein intake and other factors. Women in the United States who are infected with human immunodeficiency virus (HIV) and those with human T-cell lymphotropic virus infection should not breastfeed. Globally, the health risks of not breastfeeding must be balanced with the risk of HIV acquisition. Indeed, some studies suggest that short-term exclusive breastfeeding may decrease maternal-to-child transmission of HIV compared with mixed feedings. When herpetic lesions are localized to the breast, women should not breastfeed. However, women with vaginal herpes should be allowed to breastfeed. Those with varicella lesions on the breast should provide expressed milk to their infant until their lesions are crusted over, and the infant should receive varicella immune globulin. Women with miliary tuberculosis should not breastfeed until they are no longer contagious, approximately 2 weeks. Women with breast cancer should not delay treatment so they can breastfeed. Depending on the therapy, women receiving antimetabolite chemotherapy should not breastfeed.[109] Most other medications are compatible with breastfeeding, or a substitute medication may exist. Women ingesting drugs of abuse need counseling and should not breastfeed until they are free of the abused drugs.[109] Mothers with fever or other minor illness should be permitted to breastfeed.

The Management of Breastfeeding

Prenatal Considerations

The successful management of lactation begins early, before and during pregnancy.[110,111] Prenatal visits provide significant opportunities for the obstetrician to support and encourage breastfeeding. The early breast examination not only serves to identify potential problems that could affect lactation but also is an advantageous time to encourage the new mother and let her know that she should have no problems with breastfeeding. Although only 11% of pediatricians said that prenatal visits were a part of their office practice,[2] prenatal pediatric visits are an ideal time to discuss feeding plans along with issues of infant care. Because these opportunities before delivery are limited, breastfeeding education should not wait for a pregnancy. The function of the mammary gland should be taught in secondary school and should continue throughout the reproductive life cycle. Then, at the appropriate time, prenatal classes should provide further information to facilitate an informed choice on infant feeding method closer to the time of delivery.

Hospital Issues: Getting Started

The early days of lactation are critical to the establishment of a good milk supply and effective letdown reflex. The Baby Friendly Hospital Initiative of the United Nations Children's Fund (UNICEF) and the World Health Organization (WHO) outlines 10 steps to ensure breastfeeding success in the hospital (Table 2.4). Postpartum units must maintain a written policy on breastfeeding that is communicated to the entire staff. All health care professionals should be trained in the implementation of this policy. Pregnant women should be informed of the benefits of breastfeeding. Breastfeeding should commence within 1 hour of birth unless not indicated medically. Health care staff must be able to demonstrate appropriate breastfeeding skills to mothers. Infants should be given nothing but human milk unless otherwise medically indicated. Mother and infant should not be separated; they should remain together through the recovery process unless there is a medical problem requiring separation. Rooming-in for 24 hours per day should be practiced to allow unrestricted breastfeeding. Mother and baby should sleep in close proximity so mother can identify early infant feeding cues and for ease in handling the infant in the postpartum period.

Table 2.4
Ten Steps to Successful Breastfeeding

Step 1	Have a written breastfeeding policy that is routinely communicated to all health care staff.
Step 2	Train all health care professionals in skills necessary to implement this policy.
Step 3	Inform all pregnant women about the benefits and management of breastfeeding.
Step 4	Help mothers initiate breastfeeding within 1 hour of birth.
Step 5	Show mothers how to breastfeed and how to maintain lactation even if they should be separated from their infants.
Step 6	Give newborn infants no food or drink other than human milk, unless medically indicated.
Step 7	Practice rooming-in—allow mothers and infants to remain together 24 hours a day.
Step 8	Encourage breastfeeding on demand.
Step 9	Give no artificial teats or pacifiers to breastfeeding infants.
Step 10	Foster the establishment of breastfeeding support groups and refer mothers to them on discharge from the hospital or clinic, and give each mother a phone number to call for breastfeeding assistance.

Adapted from American Academy of Pediatrics and American College of Obstetricians and Gynecologists. Peripartum care: the transition to lactation. In: *Breastfeeding Handbook for Physicians*. Elk Grove Village, IL: American Academy of Pediatrics; 2006:67–80[3]

Early initiation of breastfeeding within the first hour after birth should be practiced unless the medical condition of the mother or infant indicates otherwise. Although infant identification bands are essential immediately after delivery, eye prophylaxis, vitamin K administration, glucose monitoring, weighing, and other procedures can be postponed until after the first latch-on/breastfeeding has been achieved.

Hospital staff should evaluate breastfeeding formally at least once per nursing shift and document their findings in the medical record. Families should have access to knowledgeable information on breastfeeding. All breastfed infants should be seen by a knowledgeable health care professional at 3 to 5 days of age to avoid potential problems of dehydration and severe jaundice. Each hospital should establish breastfeeding support groups or work with organized community support groups so that families have a resource on leaving the hospital.

Mechanics of Breastfeeding

Positioning
There are many different positions for the nursing mother to use, but regardless of position, she should be comfortable. Pillows and footstools may provide assistance. The baby should be positioned so that the head, shoulders, and hips are in alignment and the infant faces the mother's body. The "football" or "clutch" and "side-lying" positions may provide an advantage for mothers who have undergone cesarean delivery by avoiding contact with the surgical incision. The football or clutch position often is used for preterm infants or those with low birth weight or infants having trouble latching on, because it allows for good control of the infant's head and good visibility of the infant's mouth on the breast. No matter which position is used, it is important to avoid pushing on the back of the infant's head, because doing so may cause the infant to arch away from the breast. To ensure proper latch-on, the infant should be held so that the mouth is opposite the mother's nipple and the neck is slightly extended, with the head, shoulders, and hips in alignment. Proper latch-on is facilitated if the breast is supported with 4 fingers underneath and the thumb on top or by a scissor-hold. The infant must open his or her mouth wide, grasp the entire nipple and as much of the areola as comfortably possible (about 1 to 2 inches from the base of the nipple), and draw it into the mouth. If the infant is well positioned, the nose and chin will touch the breast, and the lips will be flanged outward around the breast tissue. The infant's tongue compresses the lactiferous sinuses beneath the areola against the hard palate. When the infant is latched correctly, the mother will feel a gentle undulating motion but no pain with each suck.

Frequency
Beginning in the first 24 hours after birth, the newborn infant should breast-feed 8 to 12 times or more every 24 hours, usually for 10 to 15 minutes per breast. Frequent breastfeeding in the first few days minimizes postnatal weight loss, decreases bilirubin concentrations, and helps establish a good milk supply. Although every 1.5 to 3 hours is the average, there is a great deal of variation from infant to infant and day to day. Human milk empties from the stomach faster than does formula. Without anticipatory guidance, new mothers often compare their infants to bottle-fed infants and misinterpret the normal frequency of breastfeeding to mean that they have insufficient milk. As infants get older, they breastfeed more efficiently, and the frequency and duration of feedings decrease. Many new parents expect their

baby to cry when hungry, but they need to be informed that crying is a late sign of hunger and can result in an infant who is difficult to calm and latch to the breast.

Supplements

There is no reason to provide supplements for a breastfeeding newborn infant who is otherwise healthy. Supplemental fluids are likely to interfere in the process of successful initiation of breastfeeding by the mother and newborn infant. If the appetite or the sucking response is partially satiated by water or formula, the infant will take less from the breast, causing diminished milk production, which may lead to lactation failure. Water and glucose water supplements may exacerbate hyperbilirubinemia, because they prevent adequate milk (calorie) intake and gastrocolic stimulation. However, if there are medical reasons for supplementation, milk (either as the mother's expressed milk, pasteurized donor human milk, or infant formula) should be used; glucose water or sterile water should not be used. The use of pacifiers in the early breastfeeding period has been shown to be associated with shorter breastfeeding duration and should be avoided until after breastfeeding is well established. As discussed previously, all infants require vitamin K after birth, a supplement of vitamin D beginning in the first few days, and a supplement of iron beginning in the first few months of life.

Assessment of the Breastfeeding Infant

History

The birth history, gestational age assessment, and birth weight should be reviewed. Risk factors that might herald lactation problems should be queried, such as low birth weight, preterm birth (<37 weeks' gestation), multiple gestation, persistently sleepy infant, medical problems (jaundice, hypoglycemia, respiratory distress, infection, neurologic problems, genetic syndromes), difficulty latching on or ineffective/unsustained suckling, oral anatomic abnormalities (cleft lip/palate, micrognathia, macroglossia), or excessive infant weight loss. A history of formula supplementation, effective breastfeeding not established by hospital discharge, early discharge from hospital, and/or early pacifier use also might raise concerns about potential breastfeeding issues.

Hydration Status

The most accurate appraisal of the adequacy of breastfeeding is the serial measurement of the infant's naked weight. Nearly all infants lose weight for the first few days after birth. Infants who are feeding well should not continue to lose weight after the completion of lactogenesis stage 2 (days 2 through 4). When lactogenesis and milk transfer are proceeding normally, a weight loss greater than 7% of birth weight may be excessive, and if present, milk production and transfer must be assessed. Once lactogenesis stage 2 is completed, an infant who did not lose excessive weight and who is nursing effectively should obtain enough milk to begin gaining weight by day 4 or 5 at a rate of approximately 15 to 30 g per day. At this rate, most breastfed infants will exceed their birth weight by 10 to 14 days and gain 150 to 210 g per week for the first 2 months. A breastfed infant who weighs less than his or her birth weight at 2 weeks of age requires evaluation and intervention.

Elimination patterns, such as voiding and stooling, also serve as indicators of the adequacy of milk intake. A journal kept by the mother recording feeding and elimination by the infant in the first few weeks can be helpful. The number of voids increases from 1 in the first 24 hours, to 2 or 3 in the second 24 hours, 4 to 6 during the third and fourth days, to 6 to 8 on day 5 and thereafter. Stool output and character also change and increase. There usually is 1 meconium stool in the first 24 hours and 1 the next day. The normal green-black meconium stool should change to transitional dark green on day 3, then lighter transitional green on day 4. By 5 to 7 days of age, well-nourished breastfed infants usually pass a medium-sized yellow stool at least 3 to 4 times a day. Some infants pass stool after most feedings. Anticipatory guidance is helpful, because stools of the normal breastfed newborn infant may be loose and may be confused with diarrhea if parents are accustomed to seeing the firm brown stools typical of formula-fed infants. After the first month, the volume of each stool increases and the frequency decreases. Insufficient milk intake in an infant older than 5 days of age may be signaled by the presence of meconium stools, green-brown transitional stools, infrequent (less than 3 per day) stools, or scant stools.

Physical Examination

The examination includes vital signs, growth percentiles, and percent weight change from birth and a more detailed oral-motor examination (mandible size, frenulum, rooting, sucking). The presence of congenital anomalies and overall tone should be noted. Breastfeeding should be observed to evaluate infant positioning at the breast, the ability of infant to latch on, quality of latch, milk letdown, presence of audible swallowing, characteristics of the anatomy and physiology of the nipple, maternal responses, and whether the health care professional needs to provide assistance with feeding.

Maternal Breastfeeding Issues

Nipple Pain

Sore nipples are the most common complaint of breastfeeding mothers in the immediate postpartum period. Early, mild nipple discomfort is common among breastfeeding women. Severe nipple pain, the presence of cracks and skin lesions, pain that continues throughout a feeding, or pain that is not improving at the end of the first week should not be considered a normal part of breastfeeding. Improper breastfeeding technique—specifically, poor position and improper latch—is the most common cause of nipple pain in the immediate postpartum period. Limited milk transfer occurs when the infant is attached incorrectly, resulting in poor infant weight gain and impaired milk production. Other potential causes of nipple pain include sources of trauma that produce cracking, such as breast care rituals (eg, overzealous breast cleansing), failing to release suction before removing the infant from the breast, climate variables, and unique skin sensitivity. Treatment for nipple pain depends on the underlying etiology. Skilled help with position and latch-on are primary interventions. If severe trauma exists, it may be necessary either to manually or mechanically express milk until the tissue has healed. Nipple healing might be hastened if a small amount of milk is applied to the area after a feeding. Sore nipples resulting from fungal infections, such as candidiasis, are not uncommon later in the postpartum period.

Engorgement

Physiological breast fullness occurs as a result of vascular congestion during lactogenesis stage 2. Pathologic engorgement is the firm, diffuse, and painful overfilling and edema of breasts, usually caused by infrequent or ineffective milk removal. The best treatment of engorgement is prevention by frequent breastfeeding. If left untreated, engorgement may lead to difficulties in latch-on and to mastitis. Engorgement should not be confused with a plugged milk duct, which can result in a localized lump in one area of the breast.

Mastitis

As a single area of localized warmth, tenderness, edema, and erythema in one breast more than 10 days after delivery, mastitis may present with a sudden onset of breast pain, myalgia, and fever, or with flu-like symptoms such as fatigue, nausea, vomiting, and headache. The infection commonly enters through a break in the skin, usually a cracked nipple. However, milk stasis and congestion from engorgement or obstruction from plugged ducts also can lead to mastitis. The treatment of mastitis includes administration of antimicrobial agents and continuation of breastfeeding with frequent feeding (or pumping) to allow the drainage of the affected breast. Additional therapy includes the encouragement of fluid intake, rest, and pain control.

Neonatal Issues and Breastfeeding

Hypoglycemia

The risk of hypoglycemia may be reduced by immediate and sustained mother-infant skin-to-skin contact and early initiation of breastfeeding. Blood glucose concentrations reach a nadir 1 to 2 hours after birth. An adaptive response to low blood glucose concentrations in breastfed infants is an increased concentration of ketone bodies and other substrates, which act as alternate fuels for the infant until breastfeeding is established. Infants of mothers with diabetes, infants who are small for gestational age, and preterm infants are the common subgroups of infants at risk of hypoglycemia. Thus, routine monitoring of blood glucose concentration in asymptomatic, not-at-risk, term neonates is unnecessary. In general, healthy, term breastfed neonates do not develop symptomatic hypoglycemia. If they develop symptomatic hypoglycemia, an underlying illness must be excluded. Serial monitoring does not preclude routine breastfeeding. The intervention for hypoglycemia in an asymptomatic breastfed infant is to breastfeed and recheck the blood glucose concentration before the next feeding. If breastfeeding alone cannot correct and maintain an appropriate blood glucose concentration, expressed human milk or formula should be offered. Symptomatic hypoglycemia requires treatment with intravenous glucose.

Inadequate Milk Intake

Insufficient milk syndrome refers to failure of mother's milk production, either primary or secondary. Because most infants leave the hospital around 48 hours after birth, insufficient milk intake and dehydration are problems that may be seen in follow-up. Dehydration, hypernatremia, and hyperbilirubinemia result from insufficient milk intake but can be prevented with appropriate interventions. The infant with an insufficient milk intake may have delayed stool output, decreased urinary output, weight loss greater than 7% of birth weight, jaundice, and hunger, crying, or lethargy.

Causes of insufficient milk intake may be related either to failure of the mother to produce milk or failure of the infant to extract milk. Although primary lactation failure is rare (and often heralded by a lack of breast growth during pregnancy), delayed lactogenesis stage 2 may be the result of maternal conditions, such as retained placental fragments, primary pituitary insufficiency, diabetes, or previous breast surgery. Insufficient milk supply more commonly is caused by inappropriate early feeding routines, including infrequent feeding, maternal-infant separation, or use of supplements. Occasionally, an infant with oral-motor abnormalities or neurologic problems may not be able to extract milk effectively, leading to a gradual decrease in milk supply. Preterm infants, especially "late preterm" infants (born between 34 0/7 and 36 6/7 weeks of gestation), particularly are at risk of insufficient milk intake. Any factor that limits milk removal may result in diminished milk synthesis, because local factors in the breast govern milk production.

A review of the perinatal history may identify maternal and/or infant factors that predispose to insufficient milk syndrome. A significant predictor of insufficient milk syndrome is a mother whose breasts did not enlarge during pregnancy or do not become full by 5 days after birth. Direct observation of breastfeeding may reveal anatomical abnormalities, improper latch, improper positioning, or inadequate infant effort. Manual milk expression or mechanical milk expression techniques may be needed to ascertain total milk volume before feeding or residual milk volume in the breast after a feeding. If the residual milk volume is high (greater than 30 mL), it may be a reason for concern. The major goal in management is to increase milk production and milk transfer. The primary management depends on the cause but usually involves increasing the frequency and effectiveness of breastfeeding. Mothers also may need to mechanically express milk after each breastfeeding to increase stimulation and breast drainage. Insufficient milk is a primary reason for supplementation of the breastfed infant.

Jaundice
The association between breastfeeding and jaundice is observed in 2 distinct entities: breastfeeding jaundice and breast milk jaundice.

Breastfeeding Jaundice: Severe jaundice is the most common reason for readmission of near-term and term infants, many of whom are breastfed. Insufficient milk production, discussed previously, often is the major contributing factor to breastfeeding jaundice. Severe jaundice may be part of the clinical picture of the dehydrated, malnourished breastfed infant in the first week after birth. Many infants with severe hyperbilirubinemia and/or kernicterus are near-term breastfed infants.[112,113] In their first week, such infants with breastfeeding jaundice have increasing total serum unconjugated bilirubin (TSB) concentrations and poor intake of breast milk. Usually, the history reveals decreased maternal milk production and/or poor milk intake by the infant. Dehydration, weight loss, failure to gain weight, and/or hypernatremia also may be observed.[114] Late preterm infants (born between 34 0/7 and 36 6/7 weeks of gestation) have been noted to be at particularly high risk of developing kernicterus, especially if breastfeeding.[115] Clinicians cannot assume that these infants feed like term infants. In the hospital, these infants seem to feed adequately, because milk production has not maximized. Once home, as milk production increases, late preterm infants may not be capable of ingesting larger volumes. Thus, they often have more breastfeeding problems and also have less well-developed hepatic mechanisms for disposal of bilirubin. Closer observation is indicated, and slightly lower concentrations of bilirubin may indicate need for intervention.

Breastfed infants with an insufficient milk intake early in their first week may have an increase in TSB concentration as a result of an exaggerated enterohepatic circulation of bilirubin. Lack of milk leads to intestinal milk stasis and intestinal action of glucuronidase enzymes to cleave conjugated bilirubin to unconjugated bilirubin, which readily is reabsorbed. This entity also is known as breast-nonfeeding jaundice, because it is similar to starvation jaundice in adults. The evaluation and treatment of these infants are similar to those for infants with mothers with insufficient milk syndrome. TSB and conjugated bilirubin concentrations should be monitored serially. Other causes of jaundice (hemolytic, infection, metabolic) should be considered to ensure optimal overall management. A good milk supply must be established. Breastfed infants should follow the same criteria for intervention as formula-fed infants as recommended by the AAP.[116] Breastfed infants usually may continue to receive breast milk if phototherapy is initiated. A plot of serum bilirubin concentration on a bilirubin nomogram before hospital discharge is helpful to predict future risk. The follow-up for all breastfed infants on the third to fifth day after birth to assess general health and breastfeeding competency and the presence of jaundice is important to prevent the most serious consequences of breastfeeding jaundice.[1]

Breast Milk Jaundice: In many breastfed infants, TSB concentrations remain high, and in a few infants, this may last for as long as 6 to 12 weeks. In formula-fed infants, serum bilirubin concentration decreases, reaching a value of less than 1.5 mg/dL by the 11th or 12th day after birth. In contrast, by week 3, 65% of normal, thriving breastfed infants have serum bilirubin concentrations above 1.5 mg/dL, and 30% will be clinically jaundiced. It has been suggested that the high serum bilirubin concentration may be protective against oxidative injury, because it has been shown to be an effective antioxidant in vitro. Because this is a normal response to breastfeeding, other than jaundice, the infants appear healthy and are thriving. The results of the physical examination are normal and the infants are growing normally. Mature human milk contains an unidentified factor that enhances the intestinal absorption of bilirubin, resulting in jaundice. As the production of the factor diminishes over time and the liver matures, the serum bilirubin concentration eventually returns to normal. The infant may be evaluated to ensure that no other causes of prolonged unconjugated hyperbilirubinemia (galactosemia, hypothyroidism, urinary tract infection, pyloric stenosis, low-grade hemolysis) are present. These etiologies may be identified on newborn screening or from the hospital records and physical examination. The TSB concentration should be measured if the clinical examination indicates a high concentration. The unconjugated and conjugated bilirubin concentrations should be monitored if jaundice persists for more than 3 weeks.

Breastfeeding should be continued. Parents should be reassured. A persistently high serum bilirubin concentration may necessitate a diagnostic challenge by interrupting breastfeeding for 24 to 48 hours. After interruption of breastfeeding, the serum bilirubin concentration will decrease markedly and not increase to previous concentrations with resumption of breastfeeding. If breastfeeding is interrupted, the mother should be encouraged and helped to maintain her milk supply. The mother may be reluctant to resume breastfeeding because of the association between breastfeeding and jaundice. Positive attitudes of health care professionals and assurance that this will not occur later may avoid termination of breastfeeding.

Growth of the Breastfed Infant

The rate of weight gain of the population of breastfed infants may differ from that of infants fed formula after 3 months of age.[117,118] Several factors might explain these differences; most notably is that the growth charts used in the comparison were derived from infants predominantly fed formula.[119] Several studies have concluded that the pattern of growth of the population of breastfed infants should be considered the norm.[118,120] Indeed, breastfed infants regulate their energy intakes at lower levels than formula-fed infants.[119] Body temperature and minimal observable metabolic rates are lower in breastfed than formula-fed infants.[121] Thus, it is argued that the increased weight gain in formula-fed infants is excessive and that no deleterious outcomes are associated with a slower rate of weight gain in breastfed infants.

The WHO recently published a new international growth reference based on the growth of healthy breastfed infants throughout the first year of life (see Appendix D).[122] The new WHO Child Growth Standards (http://www.who.int/childgrowth/) are the result of an intensive global study initiated by the WHO in 1997 to develop a new international measurement tool for children from birth to 5 years of age. More than 8000 children from 6 countries (Brazil, Ghana, India, Norway, Oman, and the United States) representing all regions of the world were involved. The participating children were selected on the basis of criteria for optimum environments for healthy development, including healthy feeding practices (specifically, breastfeeding and good complementary feeding), good health care (including vaccinations/immunizations), and mothers who did not smoke. The standards are based on the breastfed infant as the normative growth model.

Since the late 1970s, the US National Center for Health Statistics (NCHS)/WHO growth reference has been used. This reference describes how children grow in a particular region and time and is based on data from a limited sample of children from the United States, some of whom were breastfed and others who were fed formula. Since the new WHO standards include only breastfed babies, the shape of the growth curve is slightly different: it shows leaner infants, who grow to be slightly taller in later months than if they had been measured on the old references.

The WHO and UNICEF jointly developed the *Global Strategy for Infant and Young Child Feeding*[24] in 2003 as a guide for countries to develop policies addressing feeding practices and the nutritional status, growth, health, and therefore, the very survival of infants and children. The strategy states that breastfeeding is an unequalled way of providing ideal food for the healthy growth and development of infants. It recommends that infants should be exclusively breastfed for the first 6 months of life to achieve optimal growth, development, and health. Thereafter, to meet their evolving nutritional requirements, they should receive adequate and safe complementary foods while breastfeeding continues up to 2 years or beyond.

For the individual infant, clinicians occasionally are in doubt about when to intervene if a breastfed infant is not gaining adequate weight.[123] A newborn infant younger than 2 weeks whose weight is more than 10% below birth weight should be evaluated. An older infant who fails to regain birth weight by 2 weeks of age or is not gaining a minimum of 20 grams per day should be evaluated. An infant with faltering growth, when the weight-for-age (or weight-for-length) is less than 2 standard deviations below the mean or weight-for-age crosses more than 2 percentile channels downward on the growth chart, should be evaluated. Assessments of milk supply and intake, appropriateness of complementary foods, and the feeding environment all are part of the evaluation of the infant with slow weight gain or faltering growth.

Collection and Storage of Human Milk

There are many instances when mothers will be separated from their infants, and prior knowledge of this separation allows them to select methods to express and store their milk for future use. Return to work or school, illness, and hospitalization are some of the common reasons encountered by mothers who wish to learn about the methods for milk collection and storage. General techniques for ensuring cleanliness during milk expression begin with good hand washing with soap and water. Electric breast pumps generally are more effective than mechanical pumps or manual expression. Bicycle horn-type hand pumps may cause breast trauma and contamination of milk and should not be used. Many mothers find the double-collecting kits that enable simultaneous breast pumping from both breasts more efficient for milk expression. Collection kits should be rinsed, cleaned with hot soapy water, and dried in the air. Dishwasher cleaning is also adequate. Glass or hard plastic containers should be used for milk storage. Bacteriologic testing may not be necessary for milk collected for feeding to a mother's own infant unless caregivers suspect that the technique for milk collection is not optimal. Milk to be fed within 3 days of collection can be refrigerated without significant bacterial proliferation.

Freezing is the preferred method of storing milk that will not be fed within 72 hours. Single-milk expressions should be packaged separately for freezing and labeled with the date (and name of the infant if the infant is cared for in a child care center or hospital). Unlike heat treatment, freezing preserves many of the nutritional and immunologic benefits of human milk. When frozen appropriately, milk can be stored for as long as 3 to 6 months. Milk should be thawed rapidly, usually by holding the container under running tepid (not hot) water. Milk should never be thawed in a microwave oven. After milk is thawed, it should not be refrozen. Thawed milk should be used completely within 24 hours.

Preterm Infants

Electric breast pumps enable optimal milk production for mothers separated from their hospitalized infants. Mothers should maintain a milk pumping frequency of 6 to 8 times per day to achieve and maintain their milk production. Preterm infants weighing less than 1500 g at birth should be given a human milk fortifier, a multinutrient supplement designed to meet their nutritional needs. This fortifier can be added once the preterm infant is tolerating tube feeding of approximately 100 mL/kg per day. The fortifier should be continued until the infant has achieved all oral feedings or a body weight of 1800 g or is near the time of discharge from the hospital. Subsequently, the infant may be fed unfortified breast milk. Because human milk is not homogenized, the fat will separate from the milk on standing. Efforts should be made to ensure that the separated fat is not left behind when the milk is fed. To ensure the best delivery of fat when continuous tube-feeding methods are used, the feeding syringe should be oriented with the tip upright, the syringe emptied completely after each use, and the shortest amount of tubing used.

Donor Human Milk

A variety of bacteria, bacterial toxins, and viruses, such as rubella, cytomegalovirus, and hepatitis B and C, may be transmitted by breastfeeding, but generally, mothers also pass along antibodies to their infant through milk and via the placenta. However, in some situations, such as with HIV, the milk may infect the infant directly. The transmission of disease, therefore, is even more of a concern if milk is given to another mother's infant, namely, as donor human milk. The possibility that maternal T-lymphocytes may be absorbed intact through the gastrointestinal tract of newborn infants also raises theoretic questions about the safety of feeding fresh (unfrozen or unheated) human milk from a mother other than the infant's own. Standards have been published by the Human Milk Banking Association of North America.[124] For these reasons, human milk banks processing pooled milk from multiple donors use pasteurization methods to avoid disease transmission.

Conclusion

Strong evidence now demonstrates that breastfeeding is associated with lower rates of infectious illness during infancy in developing and industrialized countries. Of particular importance, exclusive breastfeeding for 6 months is associated with one third the risk of developing otitis media and half the risk of having a wheezing illness during the first 6 months of life. Indications exist that breastfeeding may have some long-term effects on infant health and development, although the mechanisms behind these effects are unknown. Research continues to identify components of human milk to which these findings could be attributed, including bioactive factors with immunologic and/or growth-promoting properties. Unfortunately, substantial improvements must occur in breastfeeding rates, particularly among the groups that suffer most from infant morbidity.

Health care professionals are uniquely situated to influence women in their decision to breastfeed. Discussing the benefits of breastfeeding permits the mother to make an informed choice. In addition, health care professionals should be prepared to assist in the management of breastfeeding problems and in the logistics of breastfeeding. For many women, physician support of breastfeeding is critical to their success in providing the best possible means of nourishing and nurturing their infants.

References

1. American Academy of Pediatrics, Section on Breastfeeding. Breastfeeding and the use of human milk. *Pediatrics.* 2005;115:496–506

2. Schanler RJ, O'Connor KG, Lawrence RA. Pediatricians' practices and attitudes regarding breastfeeding promotion. *Pediatrics.* 1999;103(3):e35. Available at: http://pediatrics.aappublications.org/cgi/content/full/103/3/e35. Accessed July 3, 2007

3. American Academy of Pediatrics, American College of Obstetricians and Gynecologists. *Breastfeeding Handbook for Physicians.* Elk Grove Village, IL: American Academy of Pediatrics; 2006

4. Hirschman C, Butler M. Trends and differentials in breast feeding: an update. *Demography.* 1981;18:39–54

5. Wright AL. The rise of breastfeeding in the United States. *Pediatr Clin North Am.* 2001;48:1–12

6. Ryan AS, Rush D, Kreiger FW, Lewandowski GE. Recent declines in breast-feeding in the United States, 1984 through 1989. *Pediatrics.* 1991;88:719–27

7. Ryan AS. The resurgence of breastfeeding in the United States. *Pediatrics.* 1997;99(4):e12. Available at: http://pediatrics.aappublications.org/cgi/content/full/99/4/e12. Accessed July 3, 2007

8. Department of Health and Human Services, Office on Women's Health. *Breastfeeding: HHS Blueprint for Action on Breastfeeding.* Washington, DC: US Department of Health and Human Services; 2000

9. Rassin DK, Richardson CJ, Baranowski T, et al. Incidence of breastfeeding in a low socioeconomic group of mothers in the United States: ethnic patterns. *Pediatrics.* 1984;73:132–137

10. Wright AL, Holberg C, Taussig LM. Infant feeding practices among middle-class Anglos and Hispanics. *Pediatrics.* 1988;82:496–503

11. Hirschman C, Butler M. Trends and differentials in breastfeeding. *Demography.* 1975;64:686–692

12. Provisional Section on Breastfeeding, American Academy of Pediatrics. WIC Program. *Pediatrics.* 2001;108:1216–1217

13. Ryan AS, Zhou W. Lower breastfeeding rates persist among the Special Supplemental Nutrition Program for Women, Infants, and Children participants, 1978–2003. *Pediatrics.* 2006;117:1136–46

14. Bee DE, Baranowski T, Rassin DK, Richardson CJ, Mikrut W. Breast-feeding initiation in a triethnic population. *Am J Dis Child.* 1991;145:306–309

15. Scrimshaw SCM. The cultural context of breastfeeding in the United States. In: *Report of the Surgeon General's Workshop on Breastfeeding & Human Lactation*. Rockville, MD: US Department of Health and Human Services; 1984:23–29

16. Baranowski T, Rassin DK, Richardson CJ, Brown JP, Bee DE. Attitudes toward breastfeeding among Mexican-American women. *Dev Behav Pediatr*. 1986;7:367–377

17. Shapiro J, Saltzer EB. Attitudes toward breastfeeding among Mexican-American women. *J Trop Pediatr*. 1985;31:13–16

18. Weller SC, Dungy CI. Personal preferences and ethnic variations among Anglo and Hispanic breast and bottle feeders. *Soc Sci Med*. 1986;23:539–548

19. Wright AL, Bauer M, Clark C, Morgan F, Begishe K. Cultural interpretations and individual beliefs about breastfeeding among the Navajo. *Am Ethnologist*. 1993;20:781–796

20. Freed GL, Fraley JK, Schanler RJ. Attitudes of expectant fathers regarding breast-feeding. *Pediatrics*. 1992;90:224–227

21. Mackey S, Fried PA. Infant breast and bottle feeding practices: some related factors and attitudes. *Can J Public Health*. 1981;72:312–318

22. Ekwo EE, Dusdieker LB, Booth BM. Factors influencing initiation of breastfeeding. *Am J Dis Child*. 1983;137:375–377

23. US Department of Health and Human Services. *Healthy People 2010. With Understanding and Improving Health and Objectives for Improving Health*. 2 vols. 2nd ed. Washington, DC: US Government Printing Office; 2000

24. World Health Organization. *Global Strategy for Infant and Young Child Feeding*. Geneva, Switzerland: World Health Organization; 2003

25. World Health Organization. *Expert Consultation. Global Strategy for Infant and Young Child Feeding: The Optimal Duration of Exclusive Breastfeeding*. WHO/54th World Health Assembly. Geneva, Switzerland: World Health Organization; 2001. WHO Publication No. A54/INF.DOC./4. 5-1-2001. Available at: http://ftp.who.int/gb/archive/pdf_files/WHA54/ea54id4.pdf. Accessed November 2, 2007

26. Picciano MF. Representative values for constituents of human milk. *Pediatr Clin North Am*. 2001;48:263–264

27. Schanler RJ. Suitability of human milk for the low-birthweight infant. *Clin Perinatol*. 1995;22:207–222

28. Blanc B. Biochemical aspects of human milk: comparison with bovine milk. *World Rev Nutr Diet*. 1981;36:1–89

29. Goldman AS, Chheda S, Keeney SE, Schmalsteig FC, Schanler RJ. Immunologic protection of the premature newborn by human milk. *Semin Perinatol*. 1994;18:495–501

30. Neville MC, Watters CD. Secretion of calcium into milk: a review. *J Dairy Sci*. 1983;66:371–380

31. Venkataraman PS, Luhar H, Neylan MJ. Bone mineral metabolism in full-term infants fed human milk, cow milk-based, and soy-based formulas. *Am J Dis Child*. 1992;146:1302–1305

32. Casey CE, Hambidge KM, Neville MC. Studies in human lactation: zinc, copper, manganese, and chromium in human milk in the first month of lactation. *Am J Clin Nutr*. 1985;41:1193–1200

33. Dallman PR, Siimes MA, Stekel A. Iron deficiency in infancy and childhood. *Am J Clin Nutr.* 1980;33:86–118

34. Lonnerdal B, Hernell O. Iron, zinc, copper and selenium status of breast-fed infants and infants fed trace element fortified milk-based infant formula. *Acta Paediatr.* 1994;83:367–373

35. Greer FR, Suttie JW. Vitamin K and the newborn. In: Tsang RC, Nichols BL, eds. *Nutrition During Infancy.* Philadelphia, PA: Hanley & Belfus; 1988:289–297

36. Martinez GA, Krieger FW. 1984 milk-feeding patterns in the United States. *Pediatrics.* 1985;76:1004–1008

37. Bates CJ, Prentice AM, Prentice A, Lamb WH, Whitehead RG. The effect of vitamin C supplementation on lactating women in Keneba, a West African rural community. *Int J Vitam Nutr Res.* 1983;53:68–76

38. Kreiter SR, Schwartz RP, Kirkman HN, Charlton PA, Calikoglu AS, Davenport ML. Nutritional rickets in African American breast-fed infants. *J Pediatr.* 2000;137:153–157

39. Gartner LM, Greer F, American Academy of Pediatrics, Section on Breastfeeding, Committee on Nutrition. Prevention of rickets and vitamin D deficiency: new guidelines for vitamin D intake. *Pediatrics.* 2003;111:908–910

40. Caplan MS, Lickerman M, Adler L, Dietsch GN, Yu A. The role of recombinant platelet-activating factor acetylhydrolase in a neonatal rat model of necrotizing enterocolitis. *Pediatr Res.* 1997;42:779–783

41. Hamosh M. Bioactive factors in human milk. *Pediatr Clin North Am.* 2001;48:69–86

42. Kleinman RE, Walker WA. The enteromammary immune system: an important new concept in breast milk host defense. *Dig Dis Sci.* 1979;24:876–882

43. Victora CG, Smith PG, Vaughan JP, et al. Evidence for protection by breastfeeding against infant deaths from infectious diseases in Brazil. *Lancet.* 1987;2:319–322

44. Schanler RJ. The use of human milk for premature infants. *Pediatr Clin North Am.* 2001;48:207–219

45. Duncan B, Ey J, Holberg CJ, Wright AL, Martinez FD, Taussig LM. Exclusive breast-feeding for at least 4 months protects against otitis media. *Pediatrics.* 1993;91:867–872

46. Aniansson G, Alm B, Andersson B, et al. A prospective cohort study on breastfeeding and otitis media in Swedish infants. *Pediatr Infect Dis J.* 1994;13:183–188

47. Owen MJ, Baldwin CD, Swank PR, Pannu AK, Johnson DL, Howie VM. Relation of infant feeding practices, cigarette smoke exposure, and group child care to the onset and duration of otitis media with effusion in the first two years of life. *J Pediatr.* 1993;123:702–711

48. Teele DW, Klein JO, Rosner B. Epidemiology of otitis media during the first seven years of life in children in greater Boston: a prospective, cohort study. *J Infect Dis.* 1989;160:83–94

49. Paradise JL, Elster BA, Tan L. Evidence in infants with cleft palate that breast milk protects against otitis media. *Pediatrics.* 1994;94:853–860

50. Dewey KG, Heinig MJ, Nommsen-Rivers LA. Differences in morbidity between breastfed and formula-fed infants. *J Pediatr.* 1995;126:696–702

51. Wright AL, Holberg CJ, Martinez FD, Morgan WJ, Taussig LM, Group Health Medical Associates. Breast feeding and lower respiratory tract illness in the first year of life. *BMJ.* 1989;299:946–949

52. Chantry CJ, Howard CR, Auinger P. Full breastfeeding duration and associated decrease in respiratory tract infection in US children. *Pediatrics.* 2006;117:425–432

53. Friedman NJ, Zeiger RS. The role of breast-feeding in the development of allergies and asthma. *J Allergy Clin Immunol.* 2005;115:1238–1248

54. Arnold C, Makintube S, Istre GR. Day care attendance and other risk factors for invasive *Haemophilus influenzae* type B disease. *Am J Epidemiol.* 1993;138:333–340

55. Peterson GM, Silimperi DR, Chiu CY, Ward JI. Effects of age, breast feeding, and household structure on *Haemophilus influenzae* type B disease risk and antibody acquisition in Alaskan Eskimos. *Am J Epidemiol.* 1991;134:1212–1221

56. Howie PW, Forsyth JS, Ogston SA, Clark A, Florey CD. Protective effect of breastfeeding against infection. *BMJ.* 1990;300:11–16

57. Marild S, Jodal U, Hanson LÅ. Breastfeeding and urinary-tract infection [letter]. *Lancet.* 1990;336:942

58. Pisacane A, Garziano L, Mazzarella G, Scarpellino B, Zona G. Breastfeeding andurinary tract infection. *J Pediatr.* 1992;120:87–89

59. Coppa GV, Gabrielli O, Giorgi P, et al. Preliminary study of breastfeeding and bacterial adhesion to uroepithelial cells. *Lancet.* 1990;335:569–571

60. James-Ellison MY, Roberts R, Verrier-Jones K, Williams JD, Topley N. Mucosal immunity in the urinary tract: Changes in sIgA, FSC and total IgA with age and in urinary tract infection. *Clin Nephrol.* 1997;48:69–78

61. Sullivan P. Breast-feeding still faces many roadblocks, national survey finds. *CMAJ.* 1996;154:1569–1570

62. Goldblum RM, Schanler RJ, Garza C, Goldman AS. Human milk feeding enhances the urinary excretion of immunologic factors in low birth weight infants. *Pediatr Res.* 1989;25:184–188

63. Arnon SS. Infant botulism: anticipating the second decade. *J Infect Dis.* 1986;154:201–206

64. Ford RP, Taylor BJ, Mitchell EA, et al. Breastfeeding and the risk of sudden infant death syndrome. *Int J Epidemiol.* 1993;22:885–890

65. Lucas A, Cole TJ. Breast milk and neonatal necrotizing enterocolitis. *Lancet.* 1990;336:1519–1523

66. Schanler RJ, Shulman RJ, Lau C. Feeding strategies for premature infants: beneficial outcomes of feeding fortified human milk versus preterm formula. *Pediatrics.* 1999;103:1150–1157

67. Furman L, Taylor G, Minich N, Hack M. The effect of maternal milk on neonatal morbidity of very low-birth-weight infants. *Arch Pediatr Adolesc Med.* 2003;157:66–71

68. Schanler RJ, Lau C, Hurst NM, Burns PA. Randomized trial of donor human milk versus preterm formula as supplements to mothers' own milk in the feeing of extremely premature infants. *Pediatrics.* 2005;116:400–406

69. Chen A, Rogan WJ. Breastfeeding and the risk of postneonatal death in the United States. *Pediatrics.* 2004;113(5):e435–e439. Available at: http://pediatrics.aappublications.org/cgi/content/full/113/5/e435. Accessed July 3, 2007

70. Bahl R, Frost C, Kirkwood BR, et al. Infant feeding patterns and risks of death and hospitalization in the first half of infancy: multicentre cohort study. *Bull World Health Organ.* 2005;83:418–426

71. Koletzko S, Sherman P, Corey M, Griffiths A, Smith C. Role of infant feeding practices in development of Crohn's disease in childhood. *BMJ.* 1989;298:1617–1618

72. Akobeng AK, Ramanan AV, Buchan I, Heller RF. Effect of breast feeding on risk of coeliac disease: a systematic review and meta-analysis of observational studies. *Arch Dis Child.* 2006;91:39–43

73. Davis MK, Savitz DA, Graubard BI. Infant feeding and childhood cancer. *Lancet.* 1988;2:365–368

74. Martin RM, Gunnell D, Owen CG, Smith GD. Breast-feeding and childhood cancer: a systematic review with metaanalysis. *Int J Cancer.* 2005;117:1020–1031

75. UK Childhood Cancer Study Investigators. Breastfeeding and childhood cancer. *Br J Cancer.* 2001;85:1685–1694

76. Kwan ML, Buffler PA, Abrams B, Kiley VA. Breastfeeding and the risk of childhood leukemia: a meta-analysis. *Public Health Reports.* 2004;119:521–535

77. Gerstein HC. Cow's milk exposure and type I diabetes mellitus. A critical review of the clinical literature. *Diabetes Care.* 1994;17:13–19

78. Kramer MS. Does breast feeding help protect against atopic disease? Biology, methodology, and a golden jubilee of controversy. *J Pediatr.* 1988;112:181–90

79. Hanson LA, Adlerberth I, Carlsson B, et al. Host defense of the neonate and the intestinal flora. *Acta Paediatr Scand [Suppl].* 1989;351:122–125

80. Hanson LA, Ahlstedt S, Andersson B, et al. Protective factors in milk and the development of the immune system. *Pediatrics.* 1985;75:172–176

81. Saarinen UM, Backman A, Kajosaari M, Siimes MA. Prolonged breast-feeding as prophylaxis for atopic disease. *Lancet.* 1979;2:163–166

82. Kimpimäki T, Erkkola M, Korhonen S, et al. Short-term exclusive breastfeeding predisposes young children with increased genetic risk of Type I diabetes to progressive beta-cell autoimmunity. *Diabetologia.* 2001;44:63–69

83. Caicedo RA, Li N, Atkinson MA, Schatz DA, Neu J. Neonatal nutritional interventions in the prevention of type 1 diabetes. *NeoReviews.* 2005;6:e220–e226

84. Karjalainen J, Martin JM, Knip M, Ilonen J, Robinson BH, Savilahti E et al. A bovine albumin peptide as a possible trigger of insulin-dependent diabetes mellitus. *N Engl J Med.* 1992;327:302–307

85. Stuebe AM, Rich-Edwards JW, Willett WC, Manson JE, Michels KB. Duration of lactation and incidence of type 2 diabetes. *JAMA.* 2005;294:2601–2610

86. von Kries R, Koletzko B, Sauerwald T, et al. Breast feeding and obesity: cross sectional study. *BMJ.* 1999;319:147–150

87. Gillman MW, Rifas-Shiman SL, Camargo CA, et al. Risk of overweight among adolescents who were breastfed as infants. *JAMA*. 2001;285:2461–2467

88. Owen CG, Martin RM, Whincup PH, Smith GD, Cook DG. Effect of infant feeding on the risk of obesity across the life course: a quantitative review of published evidence. *Pediatrics*. 2005;115:1367–1377

89. Dewey KG, Lönnerdal B. Infant self-regulation of breast milk intake. *Acta Paediatr Scand*. 1986;75:893–898

90. Heinig MJ, Nommsen LA, Peerson JM, Lonnerdal B, Dewey KG. Intake and growth of breast-fed and formula-fed infants in relation to the timing of introduction of complementary foods: the DARLING study. Davis Area Research on Lactation, Infant Nutrition, and Growth. *Acta Paediatr*. 1993;82:999–1006

91. Stettler N, Zemel BS, Kumanyika S, Stallings VA. Infant weight gain and childhood overweight status in a multicenter, cohort study. *Pediatrics*. 2002;109:194–199

92. Singhal A, Farooqi IS, O'Rahilly S, Cole TJ, Fewtrell M, Lucas A. Early nutrition and leptin concentrations in later life. *Am J Clin Nutr*. 2002;75:993–999

93. Singhal A, Fewtrell M, Cole TJ, Lucas A. Low nutrient intake and early growth for later insulin resistance in adolescents born preterm. *Lancet*. 2003;361:1089–1097

94. Rogan WJ, Gladen BC. Breast-feeding and cognitive development. *Early Hum Dev*. 1993;31:181–193

95. Horwood LJ, Fergusson DM. Breastfeeding and later cognitive and academic outcomes. *Pediatrics*. 1998;101(1):e9. Available at: http://pediatrics.aappublications.org/cgi/content/full/101/1/e9. Accessed July 3, 2007

96. Lucas A, Morley R, Cole TJ, Lister G, Leeson-Payne C. Breast milk and subsequent intelligence quotient in children born preterm. *Lancet*. 1992;339:261–264

97. Horwood LJ, Mogridge N, Darlow BA. Cognitive, educational, and behavioral outcomes at 7 to 8 years in a national very low birthweight cohort. *Arch Dis Child Fetal Neonatal Ed*. 1998;79:F12–F20

98. Anderson JW, Johnstone BM, Remley DT. Breastfeeding and cognitive development: a meta-analysis. *Am J Clin Nutr*. 1999;70:525–535

99. Heinig MJ, Dewey KG. Health effects of breastfeeding for mothers: a critical review. *Nutr Res Rev*. 1997;10:35–56

100. McNeilly AS. Lactational amenorrhea. *Endocrinol Metab Clin North Am*. 1993;22:59–73

101. Labbok MH. Effects of breastfeeding on the mother. *Pediatr Clin North Am*. 2001;48:143–158

102. Newcomb PA, Storer BE, Longnecker MP, et al. Lactation and a reduced risk of premenopausal breast cancer. *N Engl J Med*. 1994;330:81–87

103. Rosenblatt KA, Thomas DB. Lactation and the risk of epithelial ovarian cancer. WHO Collaborative Study of Neoplasia and Steroid Contraceptives. *Int J Epidemiol*. 1993;22:192–197

104. Sowers M. Pregnancy and lactation as risk factors for subsequent bone loss and osteoporosis. *J Bone Miner Res*. 1996;11:1052–1060

105. Kalkwarf HJ, Specker BL, Bianchi DC, Ranz J, Ho M. The effect of calcium supplementation on bone density during lactation and after weaning. *N Engl J Med*. 1997;337:523–528

106. Specker BL, Tsang RC, Ho ML. Changes in calcium homeostasis over the first year postpartum: effect of lactation and weaning. *Obstet Gynecol.* 1991;78:56–62

107. Montgomery DL, Splett PL. Economic benefit of breast-feeding infants enrolled in WIC. *J Am Diet Assoc.* 1997;97:379–385

108. Cattaneo A, Ronfani L, Burmaz T, Quintero-Romero S, Macaluso A, Di Mario S. Infant feeding and cost of health care: a cohort study. *Acta Paediatr.* 2006;95:540–546

109. American Academy of Pediatrics, Committee on Drugs. The transfer of drugs and other chemicals into human milk. *Pediatrics.* 2001;108:776–789

110. Lawrence RA. *Breastfeeding: A Guide For The Medical Profession.* St Louis, MO: Mosby-Year Book Inc; 1994

111. Freed GL, Landers S, Schanler RJ. A practical guide to successful breast-feeding management. *Am J Dis Child.* 1991;145:917–921

112. Bhutani VK, Johnson L. Kernicterus in late preterm infants cared for as term healthy infants. *Semin Perinatol.* 2006;30:89–97

113. Newman TB, Liljestrand P, Escobar GJ. Infants with bilirubin levels of 30 mg/dL or more in a large managed care organization. *Pediatrics.* 2003;111:1303–1311

114. Moritz ML, Manole MD, Bogen DL, Ayus JC. Breastfeeding-associated hypernatremia: are we missing the diagnosis? *Pediatrics.* 2005;116(3):e343–e347. Available at: http://pediatrics.aappublications.org/cgi/content/full/116/3/e343. Accessed July 3, 2007

115. Neifert MR. Prevention of breastfeeding tragedies. *Pediatr Clin North Am.* 2001;48:273–297

116. American Academy of Pediatrics, Subcommittee on Hyperbilirubinemia. Management of hyperbilirubinemia in the newborn infant 35 or more weeks of gestation. *Pediatrics.* 2004;114:297–316

117. Butte NF, Garza C, Smith EO, Nichols BL. Human milk intake and growth of exclusively breast-fed infants. *J Pediatr.* 1984;104:187–195

118. Dewey KG, Heinig MJ, Nommsen LA, Peerson JM, Lonnerdal B. Growth of breast-fed and formula-fed infants from 0 to 18 months: The DARLING study. *Pediatrics.* 1992;89:1035–1041

119. Dewey KG. Nutrition, growth, and complementary feeding of the breastfed infant. *Pediatr Clin North Am.* 2001;48:87–104

120. Dewey KG, Heinig MJ, Nommsen LA, Lonnerdal B. Adequacy of energy intake among breast-fed infants in the DARLING study: relationships to growth velocity, morbidity, and activity levels. Davis Area Research on Lactation, Infant Nutrition, and Growth. *J Pediatr.* 1991;119:538–547

121. Butte NF, Smith EO, Garza C. Energy utilization of breast-fed and formula-fed infants. *Am J Clin Nutr.* 1990;51:350–358

122. de Onis M, Garza C, Onyango AW, Martorell R. WHO child growth standards. *Acta Paediatr.* 2006;95:1–104

123. Powers NG. How to assess slow growth in the breastfed infant: birth to 3 months. *Pediatr Clin North Am.* 2001;48:345–364

124. Human Milk Banking Association of North America. *Guidelines for the Establishment and Operation of a Donor Human Milk Bank.* West Hartford, CT: Human Milk Banking Association of North America; 1994

Formula Feeding of Term Infants

General Considerations

In the absence of human milk, iron-fortified infant formulas are the most appropriate substitutes for feeding healthy, full-term infants during the first year of life. Although infant formulas do not duplicate the composition of human milk, formulas are continuously improved as new nutritional information, ingredients, and technology become available. When used as the sole source of nourishment during the first 6 months of life, infant formulas meet all the energy and nutrient requirements of healthy, term infants. After 6 months of age, formulas complement the increasing variety of solid foods in the diet and continue to supply a significant part of the infant's nutritional requirements.[1,2]

Rates of Breastfeeding and Formula Feeding

A survey in 2004 found that approximately 65% of all infants born in the United States are initially breastfed in hospital.[3] This represents a decrease from a peak of 70% in 2002. Breastfeeding initiation rates are highest among women who are 25 years or older, are white, have had at least some college education, are relatively affluent, and live in the western United States. The lowest rates of breastfeeding are among black mothers who are younger than 20 years and mothers who have lower incomes or live in the southeastern United States.[3,4] Breastfeeding initiation rates do not differ between women who are employed (full- or part-time) and those who are unemployed, although employment status does affect length of breastfeeding, as might be expected. The percentage of infants who are still breastfed at 6 months of age is approximately 32%. Approximately 80% of infants are fed an infant formula or some form of whole cow milk by 1 year of age.[3] Thus, commercial infant formulas are widely available and play a substantial role in meeting the nutritional needs of infants in the United States. Because of concern that mothers may choose not to initiate breastfeeding or may stop prematurely, the American Academy of Pediatrics and other organizations have expressed disapproval of direct advertising of infant formula to the general public. Such advertising runs counter to the World Health Organization "International Code of Marketing of Breastmilk Substitutes," to which the United States is not a signatory.

Indications for the Use of Infant Formula

There are 3 indications for the use of infant formulas: (1) as a substitute (or supplement) for human milk in infants whose mothers choose not to breastfeed (or not to do so exclusively); (2) as a substitute for human milk in infants for whom breastfeeding is medically contraindicated (eg, some inborn errors of metabolism); and (3) as a supplement for breastfed infants whose intake of human milk is inadequate to support adequate weight gain. In these cases, supplementation should be instituted only after attempts to increase milk supply have proven ineffective, because the introduction of formula will lead to a decrease in milk supply. Because of the beneficial properties of human milk, mothers should be encouraged to continue breastfeeding even if formula is used as a supplement. All of the currently available infant formulas have been tested in 3- to 4-month growth and tolerance studies and are proven to provide adequate nutrition to the healthy infant when used exclusively for the first 4 to 6 months of life.

History of Infant Formula Development

Feeding the weaned infant has been a problem for centuries, and often, "wet nurses" or the unaltered milks of cows and other animals were used. The first scientific comparison of the composition of human milk and cow milk was published in 1838. After that study was published, several, often complicated, systems of altering cow milk to make it more suitable for infant feeding were developed. In 1919, Gerstenberger published a report on his 3-year experience with a cow milk formula, "synthetic milk adapted," which had levels of protein, fat, and carbohydrate similar to human milk. Commercially produced formulas soon followed.[5,6] Nevertheless, for many years, infant formulas were predominantly prepared in the home using whole or evaporated cow milk, corn syrup, and water. The protein content of these formulas was much higher than that found in human milk. The fat largely comprised saturated fatty acids, which are poorly absorbed by young infants, and small amounts of the essential fatty acids. The carbohydrate content was a mixture of lactose and the added corn syrup (dextrins, glucose polymers). Vitamins needed to be supplemented separately. The composition of infant formulas has evolved considerably over the ensuing years. Each of the macronutrients (protein, fat, and carbohydrate) has been modified in currently available preparations to approximate more closely the composition of human milk. Ongoing research continues to improve the nutritional quality of formulas.

Rationale for Development of Current Infant Formulas

Although the composition of human milk provides a basis for the composition of infant formulas, formulas do not duplicate the composition of human milk for several reasons. First, human milk contains a number of components, such as hormones, growth factors, antibodies, enzymes, and live cells, that are difficult, if not impossible, to add to infant formula. Second, infant formulas are made from cow milk and other ingredients, which often provide nutrients that are dissimilar in chemical form and composition to the corresponding nutrients in human milk. For example, although the whey-to-casein ratio of cow milk-based infant formulas can be adjusted to approximate that of human milk, the types of whey and casein proteins in cow milk and their amino acid compositions are not the same as those found in human milk. Third, whereas human milk is usually consumed within hours of being produced, infant formulas are heat-treated and must have long shelf lives, generally at least 1 year. All of these considerations make it impossible to duplicate the composition of human milk. Additionally, the bioavailability of some nutrients in infant formula may be lower than that of the nutrients in human milk. Increasingly in recent years, because of the inability to match the composition of human milk per se, the development of infant formulas has focused on trying to duplicate the growth, physiological, and developmental outcomes of the breastfed infant through formula feeding. This requires a different approach to infant formula research and development and increases the reliance on the results of randomized clinical trials rather than on compositional similarity.[7]

Regulatory agencies have implicitly recognized that infant formulas should not be identical in composition to human milk. In the United States, for example, the standards for nutrient concentrations in infant formulas (see Appendix E) are specified by the Infant Formula Act of 1980 (Pub L No. 96–359), which was amended in 1986 (Pub L No. 99–570). This act established the minimum levels of 29 nutrients and the maximum levels of 9. In the case of 19 nutrients, the minimum amount required in infant formula is above the average level found in human milk. Both branded and generic formulas are available. Although all formulas must meet the requirements set forth in the Infant Formula Act, the composition of branded and generic formulas may differ qualitatively and quantitatively within the ranges allowed by the law.

Available Forms of Infant Formula

Infant formulas are available in 3 forms: ready-to-feed, concentrated liquid, and powder. The different forms of a given product are nearly identical in nutrient composition, but small differences may exist for technical reasons. Ready-to-feed formulas for healthy, full-term infants provide 20 kcal/fluid ounce (fl oz) and approximately 670 kcal/L and are available principally in 32-fl oz containers and also in smaller-volume packages, depending on the product and manufacturer. Concentrated liquid products are available in 13-fl oz cans and, when diluted with equal amounts of water, yield 26 fl oz of standard 20-kcal/fl oz formula. Powder products are most often found in 12.9-oz and 25.7-oz cans. Depending on the manufacturer, when prepared according to instructions, the 12.9-oz can yields approximately 94 to 96 fl oz and the larger can yields approximately 188 to 190 fl oz of standard formula. Some powder products also are available in packages of single-serving packets.

Infant Formula Labels

The Infant Formula Act requires the manufacturer to ensure by analysis the amount of all 29 essential nutrients in each batch of formula and to make a quantitative declaration for each nutrient on the label. In the United States, this "label claim" for the amount of each nutrient is the minimum amount of the nutrient that will be present in the formula at the end of shelf life.* It is not the average amount of the nutrient in the formula, as is commonly thought and is the case in many other countries. Thus, the actual content of a given nutrient in a formula will always be higher than the level declared on the label. Consequently, health care professionals who need to prescribe carefully defined diets based on infant formulas are advised to contact manufacturers to obtain the average or typical amounts of the nutrient(s) of interest in the formula being used. Among other requirements of the Infant Formula Act, all labels must have detailed mixing instructions, which may differ among manufacturers' products and should be followed for the specific formula being used.

---

* This is especially important for some vitamins. Although some vitamins degrade very little over shelf life (eg, vitamin K), others, such as riboflavin, vitamin B_{12}, and vitamin C, are subject to considerable loss.

Safe Preparation of Infant Formula

All infant formulas must be manufactured in adherence to good manufacturing practices, and all production facilities are inspected at least annually by the US Food and Drug Administration (FDA). Ready-to-feed and concentrated liquid products are commercially sterile—that is, they contain no pathogenic organisms. (Liquid products may contain small numbers of nonpathogenic organisms that are capable of growing only at very high temperatures—so-called thermophiles—that may spoil the formula). Although powder products are heat-treated during manufacture and must meet strict standards regarding amounts of pathogenic organisms, they are not completely sterile and, in rare cases, may contain pathogenic organisms. Of recent concern has been the occasional presence of *Enterobacter sakazakii* in some powder infant formulas. This opportunistic organism has been the sporadic cause of severe infections in preterm infants in the early months of life and in other immunocompromised infants. For this reason, powder infant formulas generally are not recommended for these infants.

Careful preparation and handling of infant formulas are important to ensure their safety. Ready-to-feed formula should be shaken before being poured into the bottle to resuspend any mineral sediment that may have settled during storage. The normal preparation of formula from concentrated liquid products requires dilution with an equal volume of water; concentrated liquids also should be shaken before being mixed. In preparing formula from powder products, it is important to adhere closely to the manufacturers' instructions on the label; most powders of standard formulas are mixed using 1 level, unpacked scoop of powder per 2 fl oz of water. It is important to use the scoop provided by the manufacturer with the specific product and not rely on standard measuring spoons or scoops from other products, because powders from different manufacturers provide slightly different amounts of nutrients per unit of volume, and scoop sizes will vary accordingly.

For special feeding situations, both powders and concentrated liquids can be reconstituted to provide formulas with more than the standard 20 kcal/fl oz. Concentrated liquid products from all manufacturers contain 40 kcal/fl oz; consequently, the same instructions for preparation of more-concentrated formula from concentrated liquid can be used for all. These mixing instructions are shown in Appendix F, Table F-1. As mentioned previously, because powders differ among manufacturers, a single approach cannot safely be used for all powder products. Instructions for preparation of more-concentrated formulas from powder should be obtained from the manufacturer. In some instances, instructions may be available on the manufacturers' Web sites.

All formulas need to be prepared in clean containers and fed from clean bottles with clean nipples. In most cases, it is not necessary to sterilize bottles (or nipples) before mixing formula in them, especially if they have been washed in a dishwasher. Ready-to-feed formula can be poured into the bottle and fed immediately. Formula from concentrated liquid or powder can be prepared in individual bottles just before each feeding or in larger quantities in a clean container before transferring the desired amounts to individual bottles. In the latter case, use of a blender is specifically advised against. In all cases, safe, potable water needs to be used (see next paragraph). Although there are few recent data, terminal sterilization of formulas in the home seems to be performed far less frequently than in the past, possibly because of the improved level of hygiene in most homes and the practice of preparing single bottles just before feeding. The apparent abandonment of terminal sterilization increases the importance of cleanliness during preparation.

"Safe, potable water" implies that the water is both free of microorganisms capable of causing disease and low in minerals that may be detrimental. Municipal water supplies are generally free of pathogenic microorganisms. Well water needs to be tested regularly. In some cases, the use of bottled water may be the best alternative. In all cases, water to be used for preparation should be brought to a rolling boil for 1 minute; longer boiling may concentrate minerals to an undesirable degree. Instructions from most manufacturers suggest allowing the water to cool to at least 38°C (approximately 100°F) and using cool water to prepare formula. Recently, after a meeting of an expert group in 2004, the Food and Agriculture Organization of the United Nations and the World Health Organization recommended that powder formula be prepared with water that is at least 70°C (approx 158°F) to decrease the risk of infection with *E sakazakii*. Their data suggested that this approach could result in as much as a 4-log decrease in the concentrations of *E sakazakii*.[8] This recommendation has since been adopted and promulgated by other groups. A temperature of 70°C implies cooling water after boiling for no more than 30 minutes before it is used. It should be noted, however, that use of water at this temperature can cause major decreases in the concentrations of certain heat-labile nutrients, notably vitamin C; the concentrations of heat-labile nutrients in current powder formulas were formulated on the assumption of using cooler water for preparation, before these recommendations were made. Parents may also complain that the use of excessively hot water causes clumping of the formula. There is no reason not to allow water to cool fully after boiling when reconstituting concentrated liquid.

Municipal water supplies may contain variable concentrations of minerals, including fluoride, depending on the source; well water may contain high concentrations of fluoride as well as other minerals, such as copper. (Formulas prepared with well water with very high concentrations of copper have been reported to cause hepatotoxicity.) Infant formulas are produced with defluoridated water, but some of the other ingredients naturally contain fluoride. Fluoride is not specifically added during manufacturing. It has been recommended that the concentration of fluoride in formula be less than 60 to 100 µg/100 kcal (400–670 µg/L). There is no need to supplement the diet of the formula-fed infant with fluoride during the first 6 months of life. Health care professionals should ascertain the fluoride concentrations in the local water supplies of the communities in which their patients live. If the fluoride content of the municipal or well water used to prepare infant formula is high, bottled water that has been defluoridated should be used. After 6 months of age, the need for additional fluoride will depend principally on the fluoride content of the water (for recommendations, see Chapter 48: Nutrition and Oral Health).

Safe Handling and Storage of Infant Formula

Parents should be instructed to use proper hand-washing techniques whenever preparing or feeding infant formula. They also should be given guidance on proper storage of formula product remaining in the original container that will be used or mixed later and on proper storage of formula that has been prepared if it is not to be fed immediately. Once opened, cans of ready-to-feed and concentrated liquid product can generally be stored covered (with a plastic overcap or aluminum foil) in the refrigerator for no longer than 48 hours. Powder formula should be stored in a cool, dry place, not in the refrigerator (both unopened and opened cans). Once opened, cans of powder should be covered with the overcap; product can be used for up to 4 weeks if proper precautions are taken to avoid microbiologic contamination.

Prepared formula should not be left out of the refrigerator. If more than one bottle is prepared at a time, those bottles for later use should be refrigerated immediately. This is especially important for powder products prepared with hot water, because they require longer to cool to reach a safe storage temperature. Regardless, all bottles should be used within 24 hours. "Unopened" bottles of prepared formula should not be unrefrigerated for more than 2 hours before being fed. Once the feeding has begun, the contents should be fed within an hour or discarded. In the early months of life especially, infants prefer warm infant formula. This warming can be accomplished by putting the unopened bottle in a bowl of warm water for 5 to 10 minutes prior to feeding. Bottles of infant formula should not be warmed in a microwave oven. Microwave ovens can create "hot spots" in the bottle, and burns to the infant's mouth can occur despite the formula seeming to be at the right temperature when tested by the mother before feeding.

Guidelines for Length of Exclusive Formula Feeding and Supplementation With Solid Foods

Formula should be offered ad libitum, the goal being to allow the infant to regulate intake to meet his or her energy needs. The usual intake will be 140 to 200 mL/kg per day for the first 3 months of life. This intake provides 90 to 135 kcal/kg of body weight per day and should result in an initial weight gain of 25 to 30 g/day. Between 3 and 6 months of age, weight gain decreases to 15 to 20 g/day, and between 6 and 12 months of age, weight gain decreases to 10 to 15 g/day. If human milk or formula intake is adequate, healthy infants do not need additional water, except when the environmental temperature is extremely high. Although most infants thrive on formulas derived from cow milk, some infants may exhibit intolerance to these formulas. Vomiting or spitting up is common for the first few months of life and requires no change in the feeding regimen if weight gain is adequate. Constipation with slow weight gain may indicate inadequate intake of formula. When a transition from one formula to another is undertaken because of tolerance, cost, availability, or a specific desire to alter the nutrient composition of the diet, the change from one formula to another can almost always be made abruptly.

Complementary foods can be introduced between 4 and 6 months of age on the basis of developmental readiness (eg, oromotor coordination, head control) and nutritional needs of the growing infant. In addition to solid foods, continued breastfeeding or the use of infant formula for the entire first year of life, rather than feeding any form of cow milk, reduces the risk of inadequate intakes of nutrients such as zinc, the essential fatty acids, and other important long-chain, polyunsaturated fatty acids. These practices also help prevent excessive intakes of certain nutrients, such as protein and sodium, during this time.

Intact Cow Milk Protein-Based Formulas

Composition

Commercial, intact cow milk protein-based formulas have many similarities but also differ substantially from one another in sources and quantity of nutrients. Although the different manufacturers provide a rationale for formula composition, physiologically significant differences have not always been clearly demonstrated among the various products. The composition of formulas may change over time and is reflected on the formula label. In attempting to differentiate among different formulas, health care professionals should rely on the results of clinical studies rather than on composition alone whenever possible. The composition of currently available standard cow milk-derived formulas for healthy, full-term infants is presented in Appendix F, Table F-2.

Protein

Cow milk-based formulas in the United States contain protein at concentrations varying from approximately 1.45 to 1.6 g/dL. These concentrations represent almost 50% more protein than the average amount found in human milk (0.9–1.0 g/dL). The ratio between the predominant types of cow milk proteins (ie, whey proteins and casein proteins) varies considerably among these formulas. Some formulas contain cow milk protein with its unaltered whey-to-casein ratio of 18:82. Other formulas contain added cow milk whey protein in an effort to approach the whey-to-casein ratio of human milk; these have whey-to-casein ratios of between 48:52 and 60:40.[9] One cow milk-based infant formula containing 100% partially hydrolyzed whey protein also is available. As stated previously, there are compositional and functional differences between the principal whey proteins in cow milk and in human milk.[10] The predominant whey protein in cow milk is β-lactoglobulin, whereas the predominant whey protein in human milk is α-lactalbumin. Because of these and other differences in amino acid composition, compared with breastfed infants, formula-fed infants have increased serum concentrations of several amino acids, and each type of formula results in a characteristic amino acid pattern. The clinical importance of these patterns has not been demonstrated.

Fat

Fat provides approximately 40% to 50% of the energy in cow milk-based formulas and is provided by vegetable oils or a mixture of vegetable and animal fats. These blends are better absorbed than the butterfat of cow milk and provide more appropriate amounts of the essential fatty acids. Fat blends are selected to provide a balance of saturated, monounsaturated, and polyunsaturated fatty acids. Commonly used oils include coconut oil (a good source of short-, medium- and long-chain saturated fatty acids), palm and palm olein oils (a source of long-chain, saturated fatty acids), and soy, corn, and safflower or sunflower oils (rich sources of polyunsaturated fatty acids). Some manufacturers use high-oleic variants of safflower or sunflower oils to increase monounsaturated fatty acids in the fat blend. The concentrations and ratio of the 2 essential fatty acids (linoleic acid, 18:2 ω-6; and alpha-linolenic acid, 18:3 ω-3) meet current guidelines. In contrast to human milk, which is high in cholesterol, commercially available infant formulas contain little or no cholesterol; the value of adding cholesterol to infant formulas has not been demonstrated.

Determination of the ideal fatty acid composition for infant formulas has been an area of intense research, particularly with regard to the ω-6 and ω-3 essential fatty acids and their very long-chain, polyunsaturated derivatives arachidonic acid (ARA) and docosahexaenoic acid (DHA). ARA and DHA are found in a wide range of concentrations in human milk, depending on maternal diet. They also can be synthesized from their precursor essential fatty acids by both preterm and term infants. Some, but not all, clinical studies have found improved short-term performance in tests of visual and cognitive functions both in preterm and in term infants fed formulas supplemented with ARA and DHA (see Chapter 17: Fats and Fatty Acids). ARA and DHA derived from single-cell microfungi and microalgae, respectively, have been classified by the FDA as generally recognized as safe for use in infant formula when added at approved concentrations and ratios. Many infant formulas now contained added ARA and DHA, and formulas containing these fatty acids represent at least 75% of infant formula sales in the United States.

Carbohydrate

Lactose is the major carbohydrate in human milk and in most standard cow milk-based infant formulas. Lactose is hydrolyzed in the small intestine by the action of lactase, which is located on the brush border of the intestinal villus epithelial cell. Lactose appears later than other brush-border disaccharidases in the developing fetal intestine but is present in maximal amounts in full-term infants. Nevertheless, even in full-term infants, some lactose enters the large intestine, where it is fermented. The end products of fermentation are short-chain fatty acids and several gases, among them carbon dioxide and hydrogen. This fermentation helps to maintain an acidic environment in the colon, which in turn fosters an acidophilic bacterial flora that includes lactobacilli and other organisms that suppress the growth of more pathogenic organisms. In addition to lactose, some formulas for term infants also contain modified starch or other complex carbohydrates, such as maltodextrins.

Iron

Cow milk-based formulas are available in both "low-iron" and "iron-fortified" versions. By law in the United States, a formula with an iron concentration of <6.7 mg/L (<1.0mg/100 kcal) is designated as "low iron." A formula with an iron concentration ≥6.7 mg/L (≥1 mg/100 kcal) is considered iron-fortified and must be labeled as such. Commercially available infant formulas originally were low in iron. During the 1950s, in response to a high prevalence of iron deficiency among infants in the United States and to link iron with a major source of dietary energy, iron was added to infant formulas at a concentration of 12 mg/L. However, low-iron versions of milk-based formulas also continued to be available. Currently, most low-iron formulas contain approximately 4 to 6 mg/L, and the iron-fortified formulas contain between 10 mg/L and 12 mg/L. Low-iron formulas continue to be available primarily because they are recommended by some health care professionals; iron is perceived by some parents and physicians to cause constipation and other feeding problems. Well-controlled studies have consistently failed to show any increase in prevalence of fussiness, cramping, colic, gastroesophageal reflux, constipation, or flatulence with the use of iron-fortified formulas. The federally funded Special Supplemental Food Program for Women, Infants, and Children (WIC), which provides food for more than half the infants in the United States, requires the use of iron-fortified formula. One of the manufacturers of infant formulas in the United States stopped manufacturing low-iron formulas in 2007.

AAP

The American Academy of Pediatrics

sees no role for the use of low-iron formulas in infant feeding and recommends that all formulas fed to infants be iron-fortified.[11]
Pediatrics. 1999;104:119-123 (Reaffirmed November 2002)

Other Nutrients

In addition to the macronutrients (protein, fat, and carbohydrate), the other required nutrients in infant formula (ie, the major and trace minerals and vitamins) are inherent in the ingredients used to supply the macronutrients and/or are specifically added during manufacture. A number of nutrients may come from more than one ingredient. All the ingredients used to produce formulas are regulated by the FDA and must be generally recognized as safe for use in infant formula.

Since the early 1980s, infant formulas have seen the addition of other nutrients not required by the Infant Formula Act. Examples of these are taurine, an amino acid found in high concentrations in the brain and retina; nucleotides, semi-essential nutrients that have been added to many formulas and that may enhance development of immune function and promote the development of a less pathogenic intestinal flora; and the long-chain polyunsaturated fatty acids ARA and DHA. These nutrients were added only after extensive studies were performed on safety and possible efficacy and new or modified infant formula notifications were filed with the FDA. One can expect that in the coming years, additional ingredients will be added to infant formulas.

Soy Formulas

Although soy formulas date back to the 1920s, during the 1960s and 1970s, improved, better-tolerated formulas were developed that were based on more refined soy protein isolates. Soy formulas are lactose free and are useful for feeding infants who cannot tolerate milk protein or lactose. Soy formulas (see Appendix F, Table F-3) constitute approximately 20% of all formulas sold. Soy formulas support growth equivalent to that of breastfed and cow milk-based formula-fed infants.[12] Bone mineralization is similar in full-term infants fed soy and cow milk-based formulas.[13-15] Earlier formulations of currently available soy formulas were associated with an increased incidence of osteopenia in preterm infants. Data on the effects of newer formulations of soy formulas on bone mineralization in preterm infants are scarce, and consequently, the use of soy formulas in these infants should be avoided if possible. Special formulas with higher nutrient concentrations than standard milk-based or soy formulas for term infants have been developed for feeding preterm infants after discharge, and their use is preferred whenever possible.

Uses

There are several indications for the use of soy formulas. Infants for whom soy formula is indicated include those with intolerance to lactose and to milk protein (in most instances), those with galactosemia, and those whose parents are vegetarian and wish for their infant's diet to be vegetarian.

All soy formulas in the United States are lactose free and are recommended for infants with clinically significant lactose intolerance or galactosemia.[16] Lactose intolerance occurs in some infants as a result of acute gastroenteritis; soy formulas are recommended for postdiarrheal refeeding only in patients who have signs and symptoms of clinically significant lactose intolerance.[17] Those who require a lactose-free formula generally can be rechallenged with a lactose-containing formula after 1 month. Other symptoms of intolerance to cow milk-based formulas, such as colic, loose stools, spitting up, or vomiting, sometimes prompt a switch to soy formula. Most of these problems are unrelated to the formula being fed; occasionally, however, some infants respond positively to soy formulas for reasons not totally understood.

Most infants who have an immunoglobulin E-associated reaction to cow milk proteins do well when fed soy formulas (up to 85% in one prospective study).[18,19] These formulas taste better and cost less than formulas based on extensively hydrolyzed protein. Nevertheless, although soy protein does not cross-react with cow milk protein, some infants who are allergic to cow milk protein will develop allergy to soy protein as well.[18,19] Soy formulas should specifically be avoided in infants with intestinal blood loss attributable to protein sensitivity.

Composition

Protein concentrations in soy infant formulas are slightly higher than in cow milk-based formulas. In addition, methionine is added to compensate for the low concentration of this amino acid in soy protein. The fat blends in soy formulas are similar to those found in cow milk-based formulas. Lactose, the major carbohydrate of human milk and most cow milk-based formulas, is not used in soy formulas to avoid contamination with milk proteins. Carbohydrate in various soy formulas is supplied by sucrose and/or corn syrups and maltodextrins. The required concentrations of minerals and vitamins in soy formulas do not differ from those required in milk-based formulas. There are differences in the actual concentrations of a number of nutrients in the 2 types of formulas, as much because of the concentrations inherent in the ingredients used in their manufacture as because of any specific addition. For some minerals, phytates present in soy protein isolates may affect absorption, and there are increased concentrations of minerals in some soy formulas to compensate for this lower bioavailability. Soy formulas are available only in iron-fortified versions. This fact is of particular interest because of the belief by many health care professionals and parents that soy formulas are useful in the management of infants with feeding intolerance, and it belies the belief that iron is a cause of such intolerance. Carnitine, which is inherently low in soy formulas and plays a role in lipid metabolism, is added to these formulas.

Soy formulas contain phytoestrogens, which have been demonstrated to have physiological activity in rodent models. To address the possible long-term effects relating to the presence of phytoestrogens in soy formulas, a comprehensive follow-up study in 2001 compared early and later growth, pubertal development, and reproductive outcomes in 20- to 34-year-olds who had been fed cow milk-based or soy formulas as infants in a study at the University of Iowa. There were no significant differences in the outcomes of these 2 groups related to the type of formula that had been fed in infancy.[20]

AAP

The American Academy of Pediatrics states:

1. In term infants, indications for use of soy formula in place of cow milk formula include (*a*) infants with galactosemia and hereditary lactase deficiency (rare); and (*b*) situations in which a vegetarian diet is preferred.
2. Extensively hydrolyzed protein formula should be considered for infants with cow milk protein allergy, because 10% to 14% will also have soy allergy.
3. Most previously well infants with acute gastroenteritis can be managed after re-hydration with continued human milk or standard dilutions of cow milk formulas. Soy formulas may be indicated when secondary lactose intolerance occurs.
4. Soy formula has no advantage over cow milk formula as a supplement for the breastfed infant unless 1 of the indications noted previously occurs.
5. Soy formulas are not recommended for preterm infants.
6. Soy formula has no proven value in preventing or managing colic or fussiness.
7. Infants with cow milk protein-induced enteropathy or enterocolitis can be as sensitive to soy protein and should not be given soy formula they should be given formula derived from hydrolyzed protein or synthetic amino acids.
8. Soy formula is not proven to prevent atopic disease in healthy or high-risk infants.
Pediatrics. 2008;121:1062–1068

Protein Hydrolysate Formulas

Protein hydrolysate formulas may contain either partially hydrolyzed protein or extensively hydrolyzed protein. The indications for use of these 2 types of formula are distinctly different.

Infant Formula With Partially Hydrolyzed Protein

There are several infant formulas available in the US market with partially hydrolyzed protein (see Appendix F, Table F-2). They have fat blends similar to those found in other standard infant formulas. Carbohydrate is supplied by corn maltodextrins or corn syrup solids and, in some cases, lactose. These formulas are used in the United States for routine feeding of normal term infants. Because the protein is not extensively hydrolyzed, these formulas are contraindicated in the management of infants with cow milk protein allergy. Partially hydrolyzed formulas (whey protein) may be useful in the prevention of atopic dermatitis (see Chapter 34).

Infant Formulas With Extensively Hydrolyzed Protein

Uses

Formulas based on hydrolyzed casein were originally developed for infants who could not digest or were severely intolerant to intact cow milk protein. The protein in these hydrolysate formulas is extensively hydrolyzed to produce a mixture of free amino acids and dipeptides, tripeptides, and short-chain peptides that are incapable of eliciting an immunologic response in most infants. Formulas containing protein hydrolysates of this type are the preferred formulas for infants intolerant of cow milk proteins and soy proteins.[21] Because these formulas are lactose free and, in some cases, include substantial amounts of medium-chain triglycerides, they are also often useful in infants with significant malabsorption caused by gastrointestinal or hepatobiliary disease (eg, cystic fibrosis, short gut syndrome, biliary atresia, cholestasis, and protracted diarrhea). In such cases, protein hydrolysate formulas can be lifesaving and are preferable to the alternative of total parenteral nutrition. Disadvantages of protein hydrolysate formulas include their poor taste (because of the presence of specific amino acids and some peptides), greater cost, and in some cases, higher osmolalities. It should be noted that despite their taste, these formulas are generally well accepted when introduced in the early months of life, before the infant's sense of taste is well developed.

Composition

The unique compositions of the different protein hydrolysate formulas are summarized in Appendix G. In contrast to the partially hydrolyzed protein formulas discussed previously, all infant formulas with extensively hydrolyzed protein are based on casein that has been heat-treated and enzymatically hydrolyzed. The resulting hydrolysate, consisting of free amino acids and short-chain peptides of varying length, is then fortified with selected amino acids to compensate for the amino acids lost in the manufacturing process. Although in vitro tests and animal immunization studies have proven useful in the preclinical evaluation of extensively hydrolyzed proteins, the assurance of the hypoallergenicity of infant formulas containing these protein sources relies on carefully conducted clinical trials that document their efficacy in highly allergic infants and children. All infant formulas based on extensively hydrolyzed protein are lactose free. Manufacturers use sucrose, tapioca starch, corn syrup solids, and modified starches in various mixtures. Fat in some of these formulas contains varying amounts of medium-chain triglycerides to facilitate absorption of fat. Other polyunsaturated vegetable oils are used to supply essential fatty acids. Products differ significantly from each other; brochures from the manufacturers should be consulted for explanations of the differences.

Other Formulas

Other special formulas are available for infants with low birth weight (see Chapter 4: Nutritional Needs of the Preterm Infant) and for infants with inborn errors of metabolism (see Chapter 29: Inborn Errors of Metabolism).

Amino Acid-Based Formulas

Amino acid-based formulas specifically designed for infants are indicated for extreme protein hypersensitivity—when symptoms persist even when extensively hydrolyzed protein formulas are used (see Appendix G).[22,23] These formulas are more costly than cow milk protein- and soy protein-based formulas.

Follow-up Formulas

Follow-up and "toddler" formulas are available in the United States. The composition of these formulas differs from that of standard formulas (increased protein and minerals, among other differences). They are nutritionally adequate but offer no clear advantage over standard infant formula during the first year of life. The iron fortification and balance of nutrients they contain may be an advantage for toddlers receiving inadequate amounts in their solid feedings (see Appendix H, Tables H-1 and H-2).

Cow Milk

Full-fat cow milk, 1% to 2% fat cow milk, "skim" or fat-free cow milk, goat milk, evaporated milk, and other "milks" have levels of nutrients, both excesses and deficiencies, that are not well suited for meeting the infant's

nutritional requirements (see Appendix F, Table F-4), and they are not recommended for use during the first 12 months of life.[24] Of particular note, the
Centers for Disease Control and Prevention has reported that the use of cow
milk during the first year of life, or an intake of more than 750 mL (approx
25 fl oz) per day in the second year of life, is associated with iron deficiency.
Infants fed cow milk in the first 12 months of life are at risk of depleting
their iron stores and ultimately developing iron-deficiency anemia[25] because
of the low concentration and bioavailability of iron in cow milk and possible intestinal blood loss. The higher intakes of protein, sodium, potassium,
and chloride associated with the use of cow milk inappropriately increase
the renal solute load.[26] The limited amounts of essential fatty acids as well
as vitamin E, zinc, and perhaps other micronutrients may not be adequate to
prevent deficiencies. Skim milks may cause the infant to consume excessive
amounts of protein, because large volumes of these hypocaloric milks will
be ingested as the infant tries to satisfy his or her caloric needs.[27]

References

1. Montalto MB, Benson JD, Martinez GA. Nutrient intakes of formula-fed infants and infants fed cow milk. *Pediatrics.* 1985;75:343–351

2. Martinez GA, Ryan AS, Malec DJ. Nutrient intakes of American infants and children fed cow's milk or infant formula. *Am J Dis Child.* 1985;139:1010–1018

3. Abbott Laboratories. *Breastfeeding Data from the Mothers Survey.* Columbus, OH: Ross Products Division, Abbott Laboratories; 2004

4. Ryan AS, Zhou W. Lower breastfeeding rates persist among the Special Supplemental Nutrition Program for Women, Infants, and Children participants, 1978–2003. *Pediatrics.* 2006;117:1136–1146

5. Cone TE Jr. Infant feeding of paramount concern. In: *History of American Pediatrics.* Boston, MA: Little, Brown & Co; 1979:131–148

6. Schuman AJ. A concise history of infant formula (twists and turns included). *Contemp Pediatr.* 2003;20(2):91–103

7. European Society of Paediatric Gastroenterology, Hepatology and Nutrition, Committee on Nutrition. The nutritional and safety assessment of breast milk substitutes and other dietary products for infants: a commentary by the ESPGHAN Committee on Nutrition. *J Pediatr Gastroenterol Nutr.* 2001;32:256–258

8. Food and Agriculture Organization of the United Nations, World Health Organization. *Enterobacter sakazakii* and other microorganisms in powdered infant formula: meeting report. Microbiological Risk Assessment Series 10. Geneva, Switzerland: World Health Organization and Food and Agriculture Organization of the United Nations; 2004. Available at: ftp://ftp.fao.org/docrep/fao/007/y5502e/y5502e00.pdf. Accessed July 5, 2007

9. Kunz C, Lonnerdal B. Re-evaluation of the whey protein/casein ratio of human milk. *Acta Paediatr.* 1992; 81:107–112

10. Heine WE, Klein PD, Reeds PJ. The importance of alpha-lactalbumin in infant nutrition. *J Nutr.* 1991;121:277–283

11. American Academy of Pediatrics, Committee on Nutrition. Iron fortification of infant formulas. *Pediatrics.* 1999;104:119–123 (Reaffirmed November 2002)

12. Lasekan JB, Ostrom KM, Jacobs JR, et al. Growth of newborn, term infants fed soy formulas for 1 year. *Clin Pediatr (Phila).* 1999;38:563–571

13. Mimouni F, Campaigne B, Neylan M, Tsang RC. Bone mineralization in the first year of life in infants fed human milk, cow-milk formula, or soy-based formula. *J Pediatr.* 1993;122:348–354

14. Hillman LS, Chow W, Salmons SS, Weaver E, Erickson M, Hansen J. Vitamin D metabolism, mineral homeostasis, and bone mineralization in term infants fed human milk, cow milk-based formula, or soy-based formula. *J Pediatr.* 1988;112:864–874

15. Venkataraman PS, Luhar H, Neylan MJ. Bone mineral metabolism in full-term infants fed human milk, cow milk-based, and soy-based formulas. *Am J Dis Child.* 1992;146:1302–1305

16. Bhatia J, Greer FR, American Academy of Pediatrics, Committee on Nutrition. The use of soy protein-based formulas in infant feeding. *Pediatrics.* In press

17. Brown KH, Peerson JM, Fontaine O. Use of nonhuman milks in the dietary management of young children with acute diarrhea: a meta-analysis of clinical trials. *Pediatrics.* 1994;93:17–27

18. Zeiger RS, Sampson HA, Bock SA, et al. Soy allergy in infants and children with IgE-associated cow's milk allergy. *J Pediatr.* 1999;134:614–622

19. Cordle CT. Soy protein allergy: incidence and relative severity. *J Nutr.* 2004;134:1213S–1219S

20. Strom BL, Schinnar R, Ziegler EE, et al. Exposure to soy-based formula in infancy and endocrinological and reproductive outcomes in young adulthood. *JAMA.* 2001;286:807–814

21. Greer FR, Sicherer SH, Burks AW, American Academy of Pediatrics, Committee on Nutrition and Section on Allergy and Immunology. Effects of early nutritional interventions on the development of atopic disease in infants and children: the role of maternal dietary restriction, breastfeeding, timing of introduction of complementary foods, and hydrolyzed formulas. *Pediatrics.* 2008;121:183–191

22. Sampson HA, James JM, Bernhisel-Broadbent J. Safety of an amino acid-derived infant formula in children allergic to cow milk. *Pediatrics.* 1992;90:463–465

23. Kelso JM, Sampson HA. Food protein-induced enterocolitis to casein hydrolysate formulas. *J Allergy Clin Immunol.* 1993;92:909–910

24. Penrod JC, Anderson K, Acosta PB. Impact on iron status of introducing cow milk in the second six months of life. *J Pediatr Gastroenterol Nutr.* 1990;10:462–467

25. Centers for Disease Control and Prevention. Recommendations to prevent and control iron deficiency in the United States. *MMWR Recomm Rep.* 1998;47:1–29

26. Ziegler EE, Fomon SJ. Potential renal solute load of infant formulas. *J Nutr.* 1989;119:1785–1788

27. Ryan AS, Martinez GA, Krieger FW. Feeding low-fat milk during infancy. *Am J Phys Anthropol.* 1987;73:539–548

Nutritional Needs of the Preterm Infant

Although optimal nutrition is critical in the management of small preterm infants, no standard has been set for the precise nutritional needs of infants born preterm. Current recommendations for enteral (Table 4.1) and parenteral (Table 4.2) nutrition are designed to provide nutrients to approximate the rate of growth and composition of weight gain for a normal fetus of the same postconceptional age and to maintain normal concentrations of nutrients in blood and tissue.[1-2] Nearly all infants with extremely low birth weight (<1000 g birth weight) experience significant growth restriction during their stay in the neonatal intensive care unit, and although the intrauterine growth rate can be achieved, it is not typically obtained until near the time of discharge.[3,4] This is largely a result of the management of acute neonatal illnesses and gradual advancement of feeding to minimize the risk of feeding-related complications, such as necrotizing enterocolitis. If catchup growth occurs, it does not happen until well after the time of discharge.[5]

Table 4.1

Comparison of Enteral Intake Recommendations for Growing Preterm Infants in Stable Clinical Condition

Element	Consensus Recommendations*		Consensus Recommendations*	
	<1000 g/kg per day	<1000 g/100 kcal	1000–1500 g/kg per day	1000–1500 g/100 kcal
Water/fluids, mL	160–220	107–169	135–190	104–173
Energy, kcal	130–150	100	110–130	100
Protein, g	3.8–4.4	2.5–3.4	3.4–4.2	2.6–3.8
Carbohydrate, g	9–20	6.0–15.4	7–17	5.4–15.5
Fat, g	6.2–8.4	4.1–6.5	5.3–7.2	4.1–6.5
Linoleic acid, mg	700–1680	467–1292	600–1440	462–1309
Linoleate:linolenate (C18:2–C18:3)	5–15	5–15	5–15	5–15
Docosahexaenoic acid, mg	≥21	≥16	≥18	≥16
Arachidonic acid, mg	≥28	≥22	≥24	≥22
Vitamin A, IU	700–1500	467–1154	700–1500	538–1364
Vitamin D, IU	150–400	100–308	150–400	115–364
Vitamin E, IU	6–12	4.0–9.2	6–12	4.6–10.9
Vitamin K_1, μg	8–10	5.3–7.7	8–10	6.2–9.1
Ascorbate, mg	18–24	12.0–18.5	18–24	13.8–21.8

Table 4.1 *(continued)*
Comparison of Enteral Intake Recommendations for Growing Preterm Infants in Stable Clinical Condition

Element	Consensus Recommendations*		Consensus Recommendations*	
	<1000 g/kg per day	<1000 g/100 kcal	1000–1500 g/kg per day	1000–1500 g/100 kcal
Thiamine, µg	180–240	120–185	180–240	138–218
Riboflavin, µg	250–360	167–277	25–3600	192–327
Pyridoxine, µg	150–210	100–162	150–210	115–191
Niacin, mg	3.6–4.8	2.4–3.7	3.6–4.8	2.8–4.4
Pantothenate, mg	1.2–1.7	0.8–1.3	1.2–1.7	0.9–1.5
Biotin, µg	3.6–6	2.4–4.6	3.6–6	2.8–5.5
Folate, µg	25–50	17–38	25–50	19–45
Vitamin B$_{12}$, µg	0.3	0.2–0.23	0.3	0.23–0.27
Sodium, mg	69–115	46–88	69–115	53–105
Potassium, mg	78–117	52–90	78–117	60–106
Chloride, mg	107–249	71–192	107–249	82–226
Calcium, mg	100–220	67–169	100–220	77–200
Phosphorus, mg	60–140	40–108	60–140	46–127
Magnesium, mg	7.9–15	5.3–11.5	7.9–15	6.1–13.6
Iron, mg	2–4	1.33–3.08	2–4	1.54–3.64
Zinc, µg	1000–3000	337–2308	1000–3000	769–2727
Copper, µg	120–150	80–115	120–150	92–136
Selenium, µg	1.3–4.5	0.9–3.5	1.3–4.5	1.0–4.1
Chromium, µg	0.1–2.25	0.07–1.73	0.1–2.25	0.08–2.05
Manganese, µg	0.7–7.75	0.5–5.8	0.7–7.75	0.5–6.8
Molybdenum, µg	0.3	0.20–0.23	0.3	0.23–0.27
Iodine, µg	10–60	6.7–46.2	10–60	7.7–54.5
Taurine, mg	4.5–9.0	3.0–6.9	4.5–9.0	3.5–8.2
Carnitine, mg	~2.9	~1.9–2.2	~2.9	~2.2–2.6
Inositol, mg	32–81	21–62	32–81	25–74
Choline, mg	14.4–28	9.6–21.5	14.4–28	11.1–25.2

* From Tsang RC, Uauy R, Koletzko B, Zlotkin SH, eds. *Nutrition of the Preterm Infant: Scientific Basis and Practical Guidelines.* Cincinnati, OH: Digital Educational Publishing Inc; 2005:417–418.

Table 4.2
Comparison of Parenteral Intake Recommendations for Growing Preterm Infants in Stable Clinical Condition

Element	Consensus Recommendations*		Consensus Recommendations*	
	<1000 g/kg per day	<1000 g/100 kcal	1000–1500 g/kg per day	1000–1500 g/100 kcal
Water/fluids, mL	140–180	122–171	120–160	120–178
Energy, kcal	105–115	100	90–100	100
Protein, g	3.5–4.0	3.0–3.8	3.2–3.8	3.2–4.2
Carbohydrate, g	13–17	11.3–16.2	9.7–15	9.7–16.7
Fat, g	3–4	2.6–3.8	3–4	3.0–4.4
Linoleic acid, mg	340–800	296–762	340–800	
Linoleate:linolenate (C18:2–C18:3)	5–15	5–15	5–15	5–15
Vitamin A, IU	700–1500	609–1429	700–1500	700–1667
Vitamin D, IU	40–160		40–160	
Vitamin E, IU	2.8–3.5	2.4–3.3	2.8–3.5	2.8–3.9
Vitamin K_1, µg	10	8.7–9.5	10	10.0–11.1
Ascorbate, mg	15–25	13.0–23.8	15–25	15.0–27.8
Thiamine, µg	200–350	174–333	200–350	200–389
Riboflavin, µg	150–200	130–190	150–200	150–222
Pyridoxine, µg	150–200	130–190	150–200	150–222
Niacin, mg	4–6.8	3.5–6.5	4–6.8	4.0–7.6
Pantothenate, mg	1–2	0.9–1.9	1.2	1.0–2.2
Biotin, µg	5–8	1.3–7.6	5–8	5.0–8.9
Folate, µg	56	49–53	56	56–62
Vitamin B_{12}, µg	0.3	0.26–0.29	0.3	0.30–0.33
Sodium, mg	69–115	60–110	69–115	69–128
Potassium, mg	78–117	68–111	78–117	78–130
Chloride, mg	107–249	93–237	107–249	107–277
Calcium, mg	60–80	52–76	60–80	60–89
Phosphorus, mg	45–60	39–57	45–60	45–67
Magnesium, mg	4.3–7.2	3.7–6.9	4.3–7.2	4.3–8.0
Iron, µg	100–200	87–190	100–200	100–222

Table 4.2 *(continued)*
Comparison of Parenteral Intake Recommendations for Growing Preterm Infants in Stable Clinical Condition

Element	Consensus Recommendations* <1000 g/kg per day	Consensus Recommendations* <1000 g/100 kcal	Consensus Recommendations* 1000–1500 g/kg per day	Consensus Recommendations* 1000–1500 g/100 kcal
Zinc, µg	400	348–381	400	400–444
Copper, µg	20	17–19	20	20–22
Selenium, µg	1.5–4.5	1.3–4.3	1.5–4.5	1.5–5.0
Chromium, µg	0.05–0.3	0.04–0.29	0.05–0.3	0.05–0.33
Manganese, µg	1	0.87–0.95	1	1.00–1.11
Molybdenum, µg	0.25	0.22–0.24	0.25	0.25–0.28
Iodine, µg	1	0.87–0.95	1	1.00–1.11
Taurine, mg	1.88–3.75	1.6–3.6	1.88–3.75	1.9–4.2
Carnitine, mg	~2.9	~2.5–2.8	~2.9	~2.9–3.2
Inositol, mg	54	47–51	54	54–60
Choline, mg	14.4–28	12.5–26.7	14.4–28	14.4–31.1

* From Tsang RC, Uauy R, Koletzko B, Zlotkin SH, eds. *Nutrition of the Preterm Infant: Scientific Basis and Practical Guidelines.* Cincinnati, OH: Digital Educational Publishing Inc; 2005:417–418.

The quality of postnatal growth depends on the type, quantity, and quality of feedings. Preterm infants fed standard infant formulas gain a higher proportion of their weight as fat when compared with a fetus of the same maturity.[6] The use of specially formulated preterm infant formulas and preterm human milk fortifiers results in a composition of weight gain and bone mineralization closer to that of the reference fetus, as compared with infants fed standard formulas for term infants or unfortified human milk.

Randomized prospective trials of specially formulated preterm formulas have shown significant improvements in growth and cognitive development compared with standard formulas for full-term infants.[7] These findings underscore the need for the clinician to carefully plan and monitor the nutritional care of preterm infants during hospitalization and after discharge. Monitoring nutrition status is even more important in the preterm infant maintained on unfortified human milk after discharge. A consensus recommendation of nutrition experts on specific nutrient requirements in preterm infants summarizes available data and recommendations and should be referred to for more detailed information.[1]

Energy Requirements

Energy is required for body maintenance and growth. The estimated resting metabolic rate of preterm infants with minimal physical activity is lower during the first week after birth than later. In a thermoneutral environment, it is approximately 40 kcal/kg per day when the infant is parenterally fed and 50 kcal/kg per day by 2 to 3 weeks of age when the infant is fed orally. Each g of weight gain, including the stored energy and the energy cost of synthesis, requires between 3 and 4.5 kcal.[8] Thus, a daily weight gain of 15 g/kg requires a caloric expenditure of 45 to 67 kcal/kg above the 50 kcal/kg per day for the resting metabolic rate.

Estimated average energy requirements of preterm infants during the neonatal period are shown in Table 4.3.[9] It must be noted, however, that these energy requirements have largely been determined in healthy growing preterm infants at 3 to 4 weeks of age. There is relatively little information on energy requirements of sick infants and those with extremely low birth weight (<1000 g birth weight), especially in early postnatal life.

Table 4.3
Estimation of the Energy Requirement of the Infant With Low Birth Weight*

Energy	Average Estimation, kcal/kg per day
Energy expended	40–60
Resting metabolic rate	40–50†
Activity	0–5†
Thermoregulation	0–5†
Synthesis	15‡
Energy stored	20–30‡
Energy excreted	15
Energy intake	90–120

* Adapted from the Committee on Nutrition of the Preterm Infant, European Society of Paediatric Gastroenterology and Nutrition.[9]
† Energy for maintenance.
‡ Energy cost of growth.

Activity, basal energy expenditure at thermoneutrality, the efficiency of nutrient absorption, and the utilization of energy for new tissue synthesis vary among infants. These variations may be pronounced in growth-retarded infants. Energy intake by the enteral route of 105 to 130 kcal/kg per day enables most preterm infants to achieve satisfactory rates of growth. More calories may be given if growth is unsatisfactory at these intakes. Lower energy intakes can support growth if the infant is receiving total parenteral nutrition, with estimates of 60 kcal/kg per day, including protein intake, in nonventilated infants of 30 to 34 weeks' gestation in the first week of life and up to 105 to 115 kcal/kg per day, including 3 g/kg per day of protein, in infants with extremely low birth weight.[10]

Protein Amount and Type

Enteral protein intakes between 3.0 and 4.0 g/kg per day are adequate and not toxic. The estimated requirements based on the fetal accretion rate of protein are 3.5 to 4 g/kg per day, with higher protein intakes correlating with younger gestational ages. A recent study suggests that in infants with very low birth weight, a higher protein content of 3.6 g/100 kcal versus 3.0 g/100 kcal in standard formula results in increased protein accretion and weight gain without evidence of metabolic stress.[11] This finding was supported by a recent Cochrane review.[12] The type and quantity of protein in infant formulas most suitable for preterm infants has been examined in multiple studies.[13–16] In general, infants fed whey-predominant formulas had metabolic indices and plasma amino acid concentrations closer to those of infants fed pooled, mature human milk.

Soy-based formulas, as currently constituted, are not recommended for preterm infants, because optimal carbohydrate, protein, and mineral absorption and utilization are even less well documented for soy-based formulas than for those based on cow milk.[17]

Fats

Fat provides a major source of energy for growing preterm infants. In human milk, approximately 50% of the energy is from fat; in commercial formulas, fat provides 40% to 50% of the energy. These feedings provide 5 to 7 g of fat per kg per day. The saturated fat of human milk is well absorbed by the preterm infant, in part because of the distribution pattern of fatty acids on the triglyceride molecule. Palmitic acid is present in the beta position in human milk fat and is more easily absorbed than palmitic acid in the alpha position, which occurs in cow milk, most other animal fats, and vegetable oils. Lingual lipase, acting in conjunction with gastric lipase, facilitates triglyceride digestion in the stomach, and bile salt-activated lipase in breastfed preterm infants continues digestion in the duodenum. These lipase activities substitute for the low pancreatic lipase of preterm infants and seem to partly compensate for the low intraluminal bile salt concentration of preterm infants. In formula-fed preterm infants, fat absorption is increased when human milk is mixed with the formula, presumably because of the lipases in human milk.[18]

The special formulas for preterm infants contain a mixture of medium-chain triglycerides and vegetable oils rich in polyunsaturated, long-chain triglycerides, both of which are well absorbed by preterm infants.[1,2] This fat blend meets the estimated essential fatty acid requirement of at least 3% of energy in the form of linoleic acid with additional small amounts of alpha-linolenic acid. Formulas containing 10%, 30%, and 50% medium-chain triglycerides are well tolerated by preterm infants,[19] with no observed differences in weight gain or fat deposition.

Human milk contains small amounts of the fatty acids docosahexaenoic acid (DHA) and arachidonic acid (ARA). Although the capacity for endogenous synthesis of these fatty acids has been thought to be limited in neonates, stable isotope studies have demonstrated that both term and preterm infants have the capacity to synthesize DHA and ARA.[20,21] It remains unclear whether DHA and ARA can be biosynthesized in quantities sufficient to meet the needs of these infants. A variety of clinical observations suggest exogenous DHA (and ARA) may be needed for optimal development. However, studies performed over the past 15 years regarding the effects of formulas containing DHA or DHA plus ARA on visual function and neurodevelopmental outcome have produced conflicting results. These results leave largely unanswered the question of whether these fatty acids are beneficial for the preterm infant.[22,23] Despite the limited evidence of efficacy, formulas supplemented with DHA and ARA are now available and appear to be safe.[24]

Carbohydrates

Carbohydrates contribute a readily usable energy source and protect against tissue catabolism. Once the infant's condition is stabilized, the requirement for carbohydrate is estimated at 40% to 50% of calories, or approximately 10 to 14 g/kg per day.

By 34 weeks' gestation, preterm infants have intestinal lactase activities that are only 30% of term infants.[25] However, in clinical settings, lactose intolerance is rarely a problem. Human milk is usually well tolerated, possibly because preterm infants acquire a relatively efficient capacity to hydrolyze lactose in the small intestine at an earlier developmental stage that do infants in utero.[26] Glycosidase enzymes for glucose polymers are active in small preterm infants, and these polymers are well tolerated by preterm infants. Because glucose polymers add fewer osmotic particles to the formula per unit weight than does lactose, they permit the use of a high-carbohydrate formula with an osmolality <300 mOsm/kg of water. Special formulas for preterm infants contain approximately 40% to 50% lactose and 50% to 60% glucose polymers, a ratio that does not impair mineral absorption.[27]

Minerals

Sodium and Potassium

Preterm infants, particularly those with a birth weight <1500 g, have high fractional excretion rates of sodium for the first 10 to 14 days after birth, although urinary loss of sodium is also related to total fluid intake. The low sodium concentrations of human milk, formulas for term infants, or human milk fortifiers designed for the feeding of preterm infants may lead to hyponatremia if these are used initially as the sole source of sodium. Special formulas for preterm infants provide 1.7 to 2.2 mEq/kg per day of sodium at full feeding levels (Appendix I).[28] During periods of stable growth, sodium requirements are usually met with a daily intake of 2 to 3 mEq/kg per day. The potassium requirement of preterm infants seems to be similar to that of term infants, 2 to 3 mEq/kg per day.

Calcium, Phosphorus, and Magnesium

During the last trimester of pregnancy, the human fetus accrues approximately 80% of the calcium, phosphorus, and magnesium present at term. To achieve similar rates of accretion for normal growth and bone mineralization, small preterm infants require higher intakes of these minerals per kg of body weight than do term infants.[29] Current recommendations (Tables 4.1, 4.2) reflect the high daily intake requirements for these minerals. However, providing adequate amounts of these nutrients, particularly calcium and phosphorus, to infants with very low birth weight during the first few weeks of life is not always possible, particularly for those maintained on total parenteral nutrition. As a result, osteopenia is common in these infants, and fractures occur in some.[30]

Milk-based formulas used for term infants contain 53 to 76 mg of calcium/100 kcal and 42 to 57 mg of phosphorus/100 kcal. The bone mineral content in preterm infants consuming these formulas, as determined by photon absorptiometry, is less than normal fetal values.[30] However, the use of formulas specially designed for preterm infants (Appendix I) that contain

165 to 180 mg of calcium/100 kcal and 82 to 100 mg of phosphorus/100 kcal may improve the mineral balance and bone mineral content to levels similar to normal fetal values.[31,32] Preterm human milk contains approximately 40 mg of calcium/100 kcal and 20 mg of phosphorus/100 kcal. It has been associated with impaired bone mineralization and rickets. The addition of powdered or liquid human milk fortifiers has improved mineral balance and bone mineralization.[32–34]

Iron

The iron content of preterm infants at birth (75 mg/kg per day) is lower than the iron content of term infants.[35] Much of the iron is in the circulating hemoglobin; therefore, the frequent blood sampling that occurs with some preterm infants further depletes the amount of iron available for erythropoiesis. The early physiologic anemia of prematurity is not ameliorated by iron therapy. However, blood transfusions with packed red blood cells supply 1 mg/mL of elemental iron, and these transfusions may be given frequently to infants with very low birth weight.

During the first 2 weeks of life, no clear indication exists for iron supplementation. However, after 2 weeks of age, 2 to 4 mg/kg day of iron should be provided to growing preterm infants.[35] Preterm infants on iron-fortified special formulas for preterm infants do not need additional iron. However, all preterm infants (even those who are breastfed) should receive at least 2 mg/kg of iron until 12 months of age. There is no role for the use of low-iron formulas. Iron-fortified formulas can be used from the first feeding in formula-fed preterm infants.

Many controversial questions remain regarding the practice of neonatal red blood cell transfusions versus the use of recombinant human erythropoietin in the treatment of the anemia of prematurity. On the basis of a large number of clinical trials and a meta-analysis of these trials, it is impossible to clearly recommend one treatment strategy over the other. Clearly, recombinant human erythropoietin has efficacy in stimulating erythropoiesis in preterm infants, but success in the elimination or marked reduction in the need for red blood cell transfusions has not been definitively demonstrated.[36] Thus, the use of recombinant erythropoietin to prevent or treat anemia of prematurity is probably not indicated in most preterm infants, including the smallest preterm infants (birth weight <1000 g), although there is limited evidence to support its use.[37,38] If erythropoietin is used, iron supplementation up to 6 mg/kg per day is needed, because active erythropoiesis requires additional iron as a substrate.[39]

Trace Minerals

During the last trimester of pregnancy, the estimated fetal accretion of zinc is 850 µg/day.[40] Although the zinc concentration of colostrum is high, its concentration in human milk rapidly decreases to 2.5 mg/L by 1 month postpartum and 1.1 mg/L by 3 months postpartum. These concentrations of zinc are inadequate to meet the requirements of the growing preterm infant whose condition is stable, as demonstrated by reports of clinical zinc deficiency among breastfed preterm infants.[41] Current enteral recommendations for zinc are 1 to 3 mg/kg per day (Table 4.1). Currently marketed preterm and full-term infant formulas as well as human milk fortifiers provide sufficient zinc to meet these recommendations.

Copper retention by the fetus has been estimated to be 56 µg/kg per day. Human milk from mothers of preterm infants contains 58 to 72 µg/dL during the first month after birth. Preterm infants absorb copper at rates of 57% from fortified human milk to 27% from standard cow milk-based formula.[42] Copper absorption is affected by the concentration of dietary zinc. Copper deficiency has been identified among infants primarily fed cow milk or given prolonged copper-free parenteral nutrition. The recommended daily intake (Table 4.1) can be met by using human milk or preterm infant formula.[35]

The iodine content of human milk varies depending on the mother's intake, which is related to the geographic location of her food sources. Transient hypothyroidism has been reported among preterm infants receiving 10 to 30 µg/kg per day of iodine,[43] although the recommended iodine intake is 10 to 60 µg/kg per day.[35] All formulas for preterm infants will supply this amount. Currently available powdered human milk fortifiers do not contain added iodine. Human milk may not supply enough iodine by itself if the preterm infant is maintained for extended periods on human milk, although the needs for supplementation in this population have not been definitively established.

Deficiency of selenium, chromium, molybdenum, or manganese has not been reported for healthy preterm infants fed human milk.[35] Current minimum recommendations for these microminerals are based on the concentrations in human milk (see Table 4.1 and Appendix C).

Water-Soluble Vitamins

The recommended intake of water-soluble vitamins is based on the estimated amount provided by human milk and current feeding regimens, an understanding of their physiologic functions and excretion, stability during storage, and a limited amount of research data on the water-soluble vitamin needs of preterm infants (Table 4.1).

The ascorbic acid content of human milk is approximately 8 mg/100 kcal, and that of preterm infant formulas ranges from 20 to 40 mg/100 kcal. Although no reports of deficiency among preterm infants receiving these feedings have been made, no published studies have assessed the ascorbic acid status of enterally fed preterm infants. Because ascorbic acid is essential for the metabolism of several amino acids, its requirement may be increased because of the high rate of protein metabolism in the growing preterm infant. Ascorbic acid supplementation of human milk with a human milk fortifier or multivitamins will offset any losses that occur during handling and storage of human milk. Current guidelines for ascorbic acid intake are 18 to 24 mg/kg per day (Table 4.1).[44]

Thiamine (vitamin B_1) is a cofactor for 3 enzyme complexes required for carbohydrate metabolism as well as for the decarboxylation of branched-chain amino acids. The thiamine content of human milk is 29 µg/100 kcal, and that of preterm infant formulas is 200 to 250 µg/100 kcal (Appendix I). Commercially available human milk fortifiers provide an equivalent amount of thiamine when used to fortify human milk to 24 kcal/oz. Recommendations for thiamine intake range from 180 to 240 µg/kg per day.[44]

Riboflavin (vitamin B_2) is a primary component of flavoproteins that serve as hydrogen carriers in numerous oxidation-reduction reactions. Infants with a negative nitrogen balance may have increased urinary losses of riboflavin, and those requiring phototherapy may use their reserves of riboflavin in the photocatabolism of bilirubin. The riboflavin content is 49 µg/100 kcal in human milk and 150 to 620 µg/100 kcal in preterm formulas (Appendix I).

Commercially available human milk fortifiers provide 250 to 500 µg/100 kcal when used to fortify human milk to 24 kcal/oz. Because of the photosensitivity of riboflavin, its content in human milk decreases during storage and handling. Guidelines for riboflavin intake range from 250 to 360 µg/kg per day.[44] The higher intake allows for increased losses of riboflavin associated with medical problems commonly found among preterm infants.

Pyridoxine (vitamin B_6) is a cofactor for numerous reactions involved in amino acid synthesis and catabolism. The requirement for pyridoxine is directly related to protein intake. The pyridoxine content of human milk is 28 µg/100 kcal, and that of preterm formulas is 150 to 250 µg/100 kcal (Appendix I). Human milk fortifiers contain the equivalent amount when used as directed. The current guideline ranges from 150 to 210 µg/kg per day.[44]

Niacin (vitamin B_3) is a primary component of cofactors that function in numerous oxidation-reduction reactions, including glycolysis, electron transport, and fatty acid synthesis. Human milk contains 210 µg of niacin/100 kcal, and preterm formulas contain 3900 to 5000 µg of niacin/100 kcal (Appendix I). Human milk fortifiers contain the equivalent amount when used as directed. No cases of niacin deficiency have been reported among healthy preterm infants using current feeding regimens; however, no studies of niacin status among enterally fed infants are available. Recommended intake ranges from 3.6 to 4.8 mg/kg per day.[44]

Biotin is a cofactor for 4 carboxylation reactions and is active in folate metabolism. The only reports of biotin deficiency have occurred among infants supported on biotin-free parenteral nutrition for several weeks.[45] The biotin content of human milk is 0.56 µg/100 kcal, and that of preterm formulas is 3.9 to 37 µg/100 kcal (Appendix I). Powdered human milk fortifiers contain the equivalent amount when used as directed. The recommended daily intake ranges from 3.6 to 6 µg/kg per day.[44]

Pantothenic acid is a component of the acyl transfer group coenzyme A that is essential for fat, carbohydrate, and protein metabolism. Human milk provides 250 µg of pantothenic acid/100 kcal and preterm formulas contain from 1200 to 1900 µg of pantothenic acid/100 kcal (Appendix I, Table I-1), which easily provides the recommended daily intake of 1.2 to 1.7 mg/kg per day.[44] Powdered human milk fortifiers contain the equivalent amount when used as directed (Appendix I, Table I-2).

Folic acid is a cofactor that serves as an acceptor and donor of one-carbon units in amino acid and nucleotide metabolism. Folate deficiency alters cell division, particularly in tissues with rapid cell turnover, such as the intestine and bone marrow. Preterm infants are at increased risk of folate deficiency because of limited hepatic stores and rapid postnatal growth. Studies of preterm infants have shown improved folate status, assessed by red blood cell folate concentrations, among those provided supplemental folic acid.[46–48] On the basis of these studies, recommendations for folic acid intake range from 25 to 50 µg/100 kcal.[44] Human milk provides approximately 7 µg of folic acid/100 kcal. Preterm formulas contain 20 to 37 µg of folic acid/100 kcal (Appendix I). Powdered human milk fortifiers supply up to 30 µg of folic acid/100 kcal when used as directed.

Vitamin B_{12} (cobalamine) is a cofactor involved in the synthesis of DNA and the transfer of methyl groups. Clinical symptoms of deficiency have been reported among infants who were exclusively breastfed by vegetarian mothers.[49] Deficiency has not been reported among term or preterm infants born to well-nourished mothers. Vitamin B_{12} is well absorbed from human milk and infant formula. Human milk provides 0.07 µg of vitamin B_{12}/100 kcal and preterm infant formulas provide 0.25 to 0.55 µg of vitamin B_{12}/100 kcal (Appendix I). Powdered human milk fortifiers provide 0.22 to 0.79 µg of B_{12}/100 kcal when used as directed. The recommended intake is 0.3 µg/kg per day.[44]

As a group, the body's reserves of water-soluble vitamins are limited, and a continuing supply of these nutrients is essential for normal metabolism. The higher recommended intakes for preterm infants compared with those for term infants are based on higher protein requirements and reduced vitamin reserves of preterm infants associated with shortened gestation. The recommended enteral intake of water-soluble vitamins for breastfed preterm infants may be achieved by using a vitamin-containing human milk fortifier. Relatively few of these vitamins are provided by standard, oral multivitamin supplements. In formula-fed preterm infants, recommendations may be met by feeding preterm formulas that contain higher amounts of water-soluble vitamins than term formulas.

There are no guidelines for providing preterm infants with supplemental water-soluble vitamins after hospital discharge, and no published studies are available.

Fat-Soluble Vitamins

Vitamin A is a fat-soluble vitamin that promotes normal growth and differentiation of epithelial tissues. The liver is the primary storage site for vitamin A. At birth, the hepatic vitamin A content of preterm infants is low.[50] Measured values have indicated limited reserves and, in some cases, depletion. In addition, the plasma retinol concentration, retinol-binding protein (RBP) concentration, and retinol-to-RBP molar ratios of preterm infants are less than those of term infants.[51] Low vitamin A reserves in conjunction with impaired absorption, attributable to reduced hydrolysis of fats and low concentrations of intestinal carrier proteins for retinol, place the preterm infant at risk of vitamin A deficiency. The preterm infant's vitamin A status may affect the maintenance and development of pulmonary epithelial tissue. Recommendations for vitamin A intake range from 700 to 1500 IU/kg per day.[52] Supplementation of preterm infants with 1500 IU/kg per day results in normalization of serum retinol and RBP concentrations.[53] Given their high vitamin A content (10 150 IU/L, 1250 IU/100 kcal [Appendix I]), special formulas for preterm infants supply this amount. Human milk, with a vitamin A concentration of 2230 IU/L (338 IU/100 kcal), does not supply the recommended intake. Human milk fortifiers, when used as directed, provide an additional 6200 to 9500 IU/L. Several studies have indicated that normal vitamin A status reduces the incidence and severity of lung disease in the preterm infant,[53–55] although the largest study to date found that the only benefit was a reduction in oxygen requirement among the survivors at 36 weeks' postmenstrual age.[56] Although additional supplementation may be beneficial for preterm infants at risk of lung disease, clinicians must weigh the modest benefits against necessity for repeated intramuscular injections.[57]

Vitamin E is an antioxidant that actively inhibits fatty acid peroxidation in cell membranes. The vitamin E requirement increases with the amount of polyunsaturated fatty acids in the diet. Vitamin E deficiency-induced hemolytic anemia has been reported among preterm infants.[58,59] This syndrome has been associated with the use of formulas that contain high amounts of polyunsaturated fatty acids with inadequate vitamin E while providing supplemental iron, which functions as an oxidant.[60,61] Current formulas have been designed to provide a ratio of vitamin E to polyunsaturated fatty acids that prevents this problem. The enteral intake of vitamin E should be a minimum of 0.7 IU/100 kcal and at least 1 IU/g of linoleic acid. Pharmacologic doses of vitamin E for the prevention or treatment of retinopathy of prematurity, bronchopulmonary dysplasia, and intraventricular hemorrhage are not recommended. There is general consensus in the United States that the preterm infant with birth weight <1500g should receive 6 to 12 IU/kg of vitamin E per day enterally (Table 4.1).[52] The formulas for preterm infants supply 4 to 6 IU/100 kcal per day. Because the vitamin E content of mature human milk is quite variable and generally low, powdered human milk fortifiers supply the equivalent amount per 100/kcal per day.

Overt vitamin D deficiency is rare in the preterm infant in the United States, given the maternal vitamin D status and the use of supplemental vitamin D in total parenteral nutrition solutions and infant formulas. Vitamin D deficiency has been implicated in the etiology of osteopenia of prematurity, but it is apparent that the main cause of this condition is a deficiency of calcium and phosphorus.[62] The recommended enteral intake of vitamin D is between 150 and 400 IU/kg per day (Table 4.1).[29] Preterm infants with birth weight <1250 g and gestational age <32 weeks who receive a high mineral-containing cow milk-based formula and a daily vitamin D intake of approximately 400 IU maintain normal serum 25-hydroxyvitamin D concentrations and appropriately elevated 1,25-dihydroxyvitamin D concentrations for many months.[63] There is no compelling evidence to give the preterm infant any more than 400 IU/kg per day of vitamin D. Powdered human milk fortifiers and special formulas for preterm infants supply between 200 and 400 IU per day when fed in the usual amounts.

Hemorrhagic disease of the newborn infant, most commonly seen in exclusively breastfed infants, results from vitamin K deficiency.[64] As a preventive measure, an intramuscular injection of vitamin K is routinely provided after birth. In preterm infants who weigh more than 1 kg at birth, the standard prophylactic dose of 1 mg of phylloquinone is appropriate. Among infants who weigh less than 1 kg, a dose of 0.3 mg/kg of phylloquinone is recommended. Preterm formulas provide sufficient vitamin K to meet daily needs thereafter. Human milk has a low vitamin K content. The use of human milk fortifiers that contain supplemental vitamins provide the additional vitamin K needed to meet the recommended intake of 8 to 10 µg/kg per day (Table 4.1).[52]

There is little information regarding supplementation of fat-soluble vitamins after hospital discharge. For breastfed infants, supplements of vitamins A, D, and E are readily available as oral solutions. None of these supplements contain vitamin K. Supplementing formula-fed infants is more problematic, but in general, if preterm infants are discharged on standard term infant formulas, they may not receive the recommended amounts of these vitamins as discussed previously until they reach a weight of 3 kg. Thus, in the "healthy" preterm infant, it is probably not necessary to supplement with fat-soluble vitamins after attaining a weight of 3 kg. On the other hand, special formulas designed for preterm infants after discharge should supply adequate amounts of the fat-soluble vitamins (Appendix I).

Energy Density and Water Requirements

The energy density of human milk from mothers of preterm and term infants is approximately 67 kcal/dL (20 kcal/oz) at 21 days of lactation. Formulas of this energy density may be used for feeding preterm infants, but more concentrated formulas (ie, 81 kcal/dL [24 kcal/oz]) are often preferred. The increased caloric density allows smaller feeding volumes, an advantage when the gastric capacity is limited or fluid restriction is necessary. Formulas of this concentration provide most preterm infants with sufficient water for the excretion of protein metabolic products and electrolytes derived from the formula. If a higher caloric concentration is needed for special circumstances, a 100-kcal/dL (30-kcal/oz) formula is now available to mix half and half with 24-kcal/oz formula to make a 27-kcal/oz (90-kcal/dL) formula (see Appendix-I, Table I-1).

Human Milk

Human milk from the preterm infant's mother is the enteral feeding of choice. Human milk is generally well tolerated by preterm infants and has been reported to promote the earlier achievement of full enteral feeding compared with infant formula. In addition to its nutritional value, human milk provides immunologic and antimicrobial components, hormones, and enzymes that may contribute positively to the infant's health and development.[65] Nevertheless, once growth is established, the nutritional needs of the preterm infant exceed those in human milk for protein, calcium, phosphorus, magnesium, sodium, copper, zinc, folic acid, and vitamins B_2 (riboflavin), B_6 (pyridoxine), C, D, E, and K.[65,66]

Unlike infant formula, the composition of human milk varies within a single feeding (or expression), diurnally, and throughout the course of lactation. Milk from mothers of preterm infants, especially during the first 2 weeks after delivery, contains higher amounts of energy and higher concentrations of fat, protein, and sodium but slightly lower concentrations of lactose, calcium, and phosphorus compared with milk from mothers of term infants.[67] The higher fat content accounts for the higher energy density of preterm milk. The higher protein content of preterm milk expressed during the first 2 to 3 weeks of lactation may be sufficient to match the fetal growth requirement for nitrogen when consumed at very high volumes (180 to 200 mL/kg per day). However, by the end of the first month of lactation, the protein content of preterm milk is inadequate to meet the needs of most preterm infants.[68] Metabolic complications associated with the long-term use of unsupplemented human milk in preterm infants include hyponatremia at 4 to 5 weeks of age,[69] hypoproteinemia at 8 to 12 weeks of age,[65,70] osteopenia at 4 to 5 months of age,[71] and zinc deficiency at 2 to 6 months of age.[35]

To correct the nutritional inadequacies of human milk for preterm infants, human milk fortifiers are available that provide additional protein, minerals, and vitamins (Appendix I). When these supplements are added to human milk in the first postpartum month, the resultant nutrient, mineral, and vitamin concentrations are similar to those of the formulas developed for feeding preterm infants. Clinical studies of human milk fortified with commercially available powdered mixtures show metabolic and growth effects approaching those of formulas designed for infants with low birth weight.[32,34]

It has been suggested that immunologic and antimicrobial components of human milk reduce the incidence of necrotizing enterocolitis[72-74]; however, data to support this claim with donor milk or mother's own milk are limited.

Given the relative infrequency of confirmed cases of necrotizing entero-colitis in preterm infants, a very large randomized controlled trial would be necessary to demonstrate the protectiveness of human milk.

The presence of milk enzymes, such as bile salt-stimulated lipase and lipoprotein lipase, may facilitate nutrient bioavailability. In addition, feeding of human milk from the mother of a preterm infant may promote neuro-logic development. A nonrandomized study reported higher developmental scores at 18 months of age and 7.5 to 8 years of age among preterm infants fed their mother's milk than among infants fed term formula[7]; however, there were many confounding variables in this study.

Facilitating Lactation and Human Milk Handling

Mothers of preterm infants should be encouraged to provide their milk for feeding their infants. Even mothers who plan to feed infant formula at discharge are often willing to express their milk for a few days or weeks after delivery. This milk can then be used to establish enteral feeding during the early critical weeks of life when the infant's medical condition is less stable.

Mothers should begin expressing their milk within the first 24 hours after delivery. They should be given verbal and written instructions about appropriate methods for collection, storage, and handling of their milk[75] and assisted in locating a supplier for breast pumping equipment needed to establish and maintain a milk supply. Individual counseling about lactation management issues, such as pumping frequency, methods to facilitate milk let-down, and breast and nipple care, should be readily available.

Fresh milk from an infant's mother may be fed immediately or refrigerated at approximately 4°C. Refrigerated milk should be fed within 48 hours of expression. Any milk that will not be fed within 48 hours should be frozen at –20°C, immediately after it has been expressed. Freezing and heat treatment of human milk alter such labile factors as cellular elements, immunoglobulin (Ig)A, IgM, lactoferrin, lysozyme, and C3 complement. However, freezing generally preserves these factors better than heat treatment. Human milk that has been frozen retains most of its immunologic properties (except for cellular elements) and vitamin content when fed within 3 months of expression. Routine bacteriologic testing and pasteurization of human milk is not necessary when it is fed to the mother's own infant.[75]

Frozen human milk should be thawed in cool or lukewarm running tap water or in a basin of warm water. Thawing in a microwave oven is not recommended, because it reduces the concentration of IgA and decreases lysozyme activity and can produce hot spots in the milk.[76,77] Thawed human milk should be stored in a refrigerator and used within 24 hours.

A number of human milk banks in the United States and Canada provide pooled donor human milk to hospitals on prescription.* More recently, some for-profit milk banks have been established, but their operation is controversial. Donor human milk banks follow specific procedures recommended by the Human Milk Banking Association of North America for screening potential donors for infectious diseases, medical history, and lifestyle behaviors that could affect the quality of donated milk. There are no federal regulations or guidelines for banking human milk. Donor milk is pooled, pasteurized, tested for bacteria and human immunodeficiency virus (HIV), and frozen for storage. Limited supplies of frozen, raw donor milk that meet specific bacteriologic testing criteria are also available for the rare instances in which infants do not tolerate pasteurized milk. Donor milk consists primarily of term human milk and requires fortification when used as a feeding source for preterm infants. However, to date, pooled donor milk used when own mother's milk is not available, compared with specialized formulas for preterm infants, has not been demonstrated to be advantageous.[74]

As described previously, powdered milk fortifiers are available for supplementing human milk for the preterm infant (Appendix I). These are very similar in content and can be used to supplement human milk for the preterm infant up to 24 kcal/oz with a well-balanced fortifier containing protein, minerals, and vitamins. These are designed for mixing with human milk at the bedside.

Commercial Formulas for Preterm Infants

Commercial preterm infant formulas (Appendix I) have been developed to meet the unique nutritional needs of the growing preterm infant. Characteristics of this group of formulas include increased amounts of protein and minerals compared with term formulas, carbohydrate blends of lactose and glucose polymers, and fat blends containing a portion of the fat as medium-chain triglycerides. The vitamin contents of these formulas are such that, in

---

* Information about donor human milk banks in the United States and Canada is available from the Human Milk Banking Association of North America, 1500 Sunday Drive, Suite 102, Raleigh, NC 27607, (919) 787–5181. Web site: www.hmbana.org/

general, no additional multivitamin supplementation is necessary. Preterm formulas are whey-predominant, cow milk-based formulas. Preterm formulas provide 3.0 g of protein/100 kcal, which promotes a rate of weight gain and body composition similar to that of the reference fetus.[78–80]

The higher intake of calcium and phosphorus provided by preterm formulas increases net mineral retention and improves bone mineral content compared with standard term formulas.[31,32] No additional supplements of vitamin D are needed.[62]

The fat blends of preterm formulas have been designed to optimize absorption. Of the fat, 40% to 50% is provided as medium-chain triglycerides. These fats help reduce losses attributable to low intestinal lipase or bile salt concentrations. Fat blends providing 40% to 50% of the fat as medium-chain triglycerides may lead to increased plasma ketones and urinary dicarboxylic acid excretion in preterm infants, but this has not been shown to be detrimental to date.[81–82]

In 2002, the US Food and Drug Administration (FDA) alerted the pediatric medical community about reports of serious infections in infants caused by *Enterobacter sakazakii* that were traced to milk-based powdered infant formulas that were contaminated with this organism. Powdered infant formulas are not commercially sterile products. Case reports in the literature suggest that preterm infants and those with underlying medical conditions may be at the highest risk of developing infection; therefore, the FDA recommended that powdered infant formulas not be used for preterm or immunocompromised infants and that only commercially sterile liquid formulas designed specifically for preterm infants be used.[83] This prohibition did not extend to use of powdered human milk fortifiers in preterm infants, because there is no sterile alternative to their use. Caregivers were also encouraged to follow the infant formula preparation guidelines established by the American Dietetic Association (http://www.eatright.org) to minimize contamination risks during the preparation and delivery of enteral nutrition in preterm infants.

Methods of Enteral Feeding

The method of enteral feeding for each infant should be chosen on the basis of gestational age, birth weight, clinical condition, and experience of the hospital nursing personnel. Specific feeding decisions that must be made by the clinician include age to initiate feeding, type of feeding (formula, human milk), method of delivery, feeding frequency, and rate of advancement.

Even minimal enteral feedings have often been delayed when infants require high ventilatory settings or continuous positive airway pressure, have umbilical catheters, or are perceived to be at risk of necrotizing enterocolitis. However, a number of well-designed studies have identified advantages for the early introduction of low-volume, "priming" feedings (1 mL every 2–4 hours), even when some of these factors are present.[84–87] Among the benefits reported for early enteral nutrition are a decreased incidence of indirect hyperbilirubinemia, cholestatic jaundice, and metabolic bone disease; increased concentrations of gastrin and other enteric hormones; fewer days to achieve full enteral feeding; and increased weight gain. These studies have not found an increased incidence of necrotizing enterocolitis among preterm infants receiving early, minimal enteral feedings. On the basis of the available evidence, the institution of early enteral feedings should be considered for all infants with very low birth weight. Although there is no uniform definition of these so called "trophic" or "priming" feedings and these terms have been used in the literature to describe nonnutritive intakes ranging from 1 to 25 mL/kg per day, it is recommended that trophic feedings of human milk be started as soon as possible after birth.

The route of enteral feeding is determined by the infant's ability to coordinate sucking, swallowing, and breathing, which appear at approximately 32 to 34 weeks of gestation. Preterm infants of this gestational age who are alert and vigorous may be fed by nipple or offered the breast. Infants who are more preterm or critically ill require feeding by tube. Nasogastric and orogastric feedings are the most commonly used tube feedings. Use of the stomach maximizes the digestive capability of the gastrointestinal tract. A large randomized study demonstrated increased feeding intolerance and decreased growth in preterm infants fed continuously compared with those fed by bolus.[87] On the other hand, transpyloric feedings provide no improvement in energy intake or growth and may be associated with significant risks.[88] This method of feeding should be undertaken only in rare instances (ie, prolonged gastroparesis or dysmotility), and gastric feedings should be resumed as soon as possible. Gastrostomy tube feeding should be considered for infants who will be unable to nipple feed for long periods of time, to decrease negative oral stimulation associated with feeding tubes.

Infants who receive nasogastric, orogastric, or gastrostomy tube feedings may be fed on an intermittent bolus or continuous schedule. Because of the significant differences in the criteria used to define feeding intolerance in existing studies, it is difficult to compare the effect of these 2 feeding methods on feeding tolerance. Bolus feedings have been associated with cyclical hormone release that is commonly thought to be more physiological.[89] On the other hand, in a study of the duodenal motor response to feeding in preterm infants, full-strength formula given continuously over 2 hours produced a normal duodenal motility pattern, whereas the same volume administered as a 15-minute bolus feeding actually inhibited motor activity[90]; therefore, a "slow bolus" technique (ie, intermittent feedings lasting from 30 minutes to 2 hours) may be the best-tolerated feeding method. Continuous drip feedings may be better tolerated in some infants, particularly those with delayed gastric emptying and/or decreased distal motility. Decreased nutrient absorption is also a problem associated with continuous drip feeding.[91] Fat from human milk and medium-chain triglyceride additives tends to adhere to the feeding tube surfaces and reduces energy density.[92,93] Likewise, the loss of nutrients from fortifiers used to supplement human milk is increased when given in a continuous feeding.[94]

The ideal initial feeding is full-strength human milk, with full-strength formula used only when human milk is not available. There is no evidence to support use of diluted human milk or formula as the initial feeding, a strategy that only serves to decrease nutrient intake.

Parenteral Nutrition (see Table 4.2)

Parenteral administration of glucose, fat, and amino acids is an important aspect of the nutritional care of preterm infants, particularly those who weigh <1500 g. The high incidence of respiratory problems, limited gastric capacity, and intestinal hypomotility in small preterm infants dictates the need for slow advancement of the volume of enteral feedings.

Parenteral nutrition can supplement the slowly increasing enteral feedings so the total daily intake by both routes meets the infant's nutritional needs. When necessary, most nutritional requirements can be met for considerable periods by the parenteral route alone.

Fluid therapy is designed to avoid dehydration or overhydration, to provide stable electrolyte and glucose concentrations, and to avoid abnormal acid-base balance. For preterm infants with a birth weight >1500 g, fluid regimens should provide 60 to 80 mL/kg on the first day and should increase to 110 to 120 mL/kg by the fourth day of a solution containing up to 3 to 4 mEq/kg of sodium as a mixture of chloride and acetate to correct sodium losses and acidosis.[95] For infants with a birth weight of 1000 to 1500 g, a similar fluid should be given, with sodium added after serum sodium concentration decreases below 140 mg/dL. For infants with a birth weight

<1000 g, generally higher fluid intakes are necessary in the first 5 days of life, dependent on urine output and insensible water losses, which may be 5 to 7 mL/kg per hour in extreme cases.[28,95] Once full total parenteral nutrition has been achieved with a weight gain of 15 to 20 g/kg per day, fluid rates will be in the range of 140 to 160 mL/kg per day in most infants. For this active period of growth, 2 to 4 mEq/kg per day of sodium and chloride and 1.5 to 2 mEq/kg per day of potassium will be needed.[28,95] Higher intakes of sodium and chloride may be required in very preterm infants with high urinary excretion of electrolytes.

Body protein stores are lost at high rates in preterm infants who are receiving glucose alone.[96-99] At a minimum, intravenous amino acids should be provided to infants with very low birth weight at 1.5 to 2 g/kg per day as early as possible (within the first 24 hours of life) to preserve body protein stores.[100,101] Furthermore, studies have documented no clinically significant increase in metabolic acidosis, blood urea nitrogen concentration, or ammonia concentration with early amino acid administration.[102,103]

Positive nitrogen balance, which indicates an anabolic state, can occur with parenteral lipid or glucose energy intakes of 60 kcal/kg per day and amino acid intakes of 2.5 to 3.0 g/kg per day.[104] With nonprotein energy intakes of 80 to 85 kcal/kg per day and amino acid intakes of 2.7 to 3.5 g/kg per day, nitrogen retention may occur at the fetal rate.[105,106] Growth generally requires a minimum parenteral nonprotein energy intake of 70 kcal/kg per day.

Use of glucose as the sole nonprotein energy source presents several problems. Concentrations of glucose higher than 12.5 g/dL cause local irritation of peripheral veins. In addition, preterm infants with very low birth weight have poor glucose tolerance during the first days of life, with hyperglycemia (serum glucose concentration >150 mg/dL) occurring frequently when glucose infusion rates exceed 6 mg/kg per minute.[107] To avoid the potentially adverse effects of widely varying serum osmolality and osmotic diuresis from substantial glycosuria, glucose infusion rates should start at a rate less than 6 mg/kg per minute (8.6 g/kg per day). Usually, a steady increase of the glucose infusion rate stimulates endogenous insulin secretion, and an infusion rate of 11 to 12 mg/kg per minute (130 to 140 mL/kg per day of a 13-g/dL solution) is tolerated after 5 to 7 days of parenteral nutrition. Insulin has been administered to achieve an energy intake sufficient for growth.[108-110] However, the use of insulin in this situation is still considered investigational, and it may produce wide variations in blood glucose concentrations, with resulting periods of hypoglycemia, as well as some lactic acidosis.[111]

The availability of intravenous lipid preparations has allowed the provision of energy adequate for growth via peripheral veins. The lipids have a high concentration of calories (2.0 kcal/mL in the 20% preparation) but have the same osmolality as plasma and, thus, do not irritate the veins. Lipid tolerance is clearly superior with 20% compared with 10% solutions because of the lower phospholipid emulsifier content of the 20% solution; therefore, 10% intravenous lipid solutions should not be used.[112] The tolerance for parenteral lipid is lower in newborn infants than in older children and is even further decreased in the small preterm infant.[113–114] In addition, infants with restricted intrauterine growth have even lower parenteral fat tolerance than would be predicted from their gestational ages. Thus, the lipid should be administered continuously over 18 to 24 hours per day at an initial dose of 1.0 to 2.0 g/kg per day and should be increased to a maximum of 3.0 g/kg per day during the first few days of life. Fat tolerance can be assessed by measuring serum triglyceride concentrations, which should be kept less than 200 mg/dL. The role of carnitine deficiency in causing the poor tolerance of lipids in the parenterally fed preterm infant is uncertain. Blood and tissue carnitine concentrations are low in preterm infants.[115] Intravenous carnitine may enhance the preterm infant's ability to use exogenous fat for energy, although clinical studies are contradictory in demonstrating metabolic or physiologic benefit in preterm infants after addition of carnitine to parenteral nutrition solutions.[116–117] Intravenous lipids increase serum concentrations of free fatty acids, which can displace bilirubin from albumin-binding sites. However, studies have demonstrated that if parenteral lipids are provided continuously over a 24-hour period, free bilirubin is unaffected, and intravenous lipids do not need to be discontinued in jaundiced infants.[112,118]

The provision of calcium and phosphorus intravenously can be accomplished more easily with currently used amino acid mixtures with added cysteine, because cysteine lowers the pH enough to allow the addition of calcium and phosphorus in increased amounts. Fetal calcium concentration and phosphorus accretion requirements cannot generally be met with parenteral nutrition, but severe metabolic bone disease in preterm infants can be minimized by adding calcium and phosphorous to parenteral amino acid solutions containing at least 2.5 g/dL amino acids and by administering the solution at 120 to 150 mL/kg per day.[29] Each institution should establish calcium and phosphorous solubility curves for their parenteral nutrition solutions. Goals for calcium intake are 60 to 80 mg/kg per day and goals for phosphorous intake are 39 to 67 mg/kg per day. [29]

When parenteral nutrition supplements enteral feedings or is limited to 1 to 2 weeks, zinc is the only trace mineral that needs to be added. If total parenteral nutrition is required for a longer period, other trace minerals may be added; however, copper and manganese should be omitted in the presence of obstructive jaundice, and selenium and chromium should be omitted in patients with renal dysfunction.[35]

Two parenteral vitamin solutions are available for use in preterm infants in the United States. With MVI Pediatric (AstraZeneca Pharmaceuticals, Wilmington, DE), the recommended daily dose of parenteral vitamins for preterm infants is 40% of the currently available single-dose vial of the lyophilized multivitamin mixture (Table 4.4).[44,52] With INFUVITE Pediatric (Boucherville, Quebec, Canada), the 4-mL and 1-mL vials are combined at the time of total parenteral nutrition solution preparation, and 40% of the 5-mL solution (2 mL) is added. These vitamin mixtures given at this dosage provide the recommended amounts of vitamins E and K, low amounts of vitamins A and D, and excess amounts of most B vitamins. However, a more appropriate mixture is not available, and individual vitamins are not available for parenteral use. A practical problem in providing fat-soluble vitamins parenterally is adherence to the plastic tubing in intravenous administration sets, especially for vitamin A. This can be overcome in part by administering the multivitamin mixture in the lipid emulsion used for parenteral nutrition.[119]

Feeding the Preterm Infant After Discharge

With infants now leaving neonatal intensive care units with weight as low as 1500 g and/or receiving human milk as well, the nutrition of the post-discharge preterm infant has assumed new importance and is of growing concern. Even though the rate of intrauterine weight gain is often achieved before discharge with intensive dietary management, catch-up growth itself does not occur until well after discharge.[3,4] To bridge the change from preterm to standard infant formulas in formula-fed infants, "transitional" formulas with intermediate nutrient density have been developed for feeding the preterm infant as weight approaches 2000 g and the time of hospital discharge nears.[120–130] These formulas may be mixed to 22 or 24 kcal/oz. Because the vitamin content of these formulas is higher than standard infant formulas, supplemental vitamins should be discontinued. However, a recent meta-analysis of randomized controlled trials concluded that these formulas with higher energy and protein content had limited benefits at best for growth and development up to 18 months after term compared with standard infant formulas.[131] In some of the randomized trials, infants on standard formulas simply increased their volume of intake compared with the infants on the special discharge formulas, thus, largely compensating for any additional nutrients from the special transitional formulas.[126,128,130]

Table 4.4

Vitamins Provided With Total Parenteral Nutrition Solutions*

Vitamin	Amount Provided Per 2 mL
Ascorbic acid (vitamin C)	80 mg
Vitamin A (retinol)[†]	2300 USP units
Vitamin D[†]	400 USP units
Thiamine (vitamin B_1) (as the hydrochloride)	1.20 mg
Riboflavin (vitamin B_2) (as riboflavin-5-phosphate sodium)	1.4 mg
Pyridoxine (vitamin B_6) (as the hydrochloride)	1.0 mg
Niacinamide	17.0 mg
Dexpanthenol (pantothenyl alcohol)	5 mg
Vitamin E (D-α-tocopheryl acetate)	7.0 USP units
Biotin	20 µg
Folic acid	140 µg
Vitamin B_{12} (cyanocobolamin)	1.0 µg
Vitamin K_1 (phylloquinone)[†]	200 µg

* MVI Pediatric is a lyophilized, sterile powder intended for reconstitution and dilution in intravenous infusions. INFUVITE Pediatric is provided in 4-mL and 1-mL vials that can be combined for administration. For each vitamin mixture, 5 mL of reconstituted product provides the indicated amounts of the vitamins.
† Fat-soluble vitamins solubilized with polysorbate 80.

In general, there is a paucity of data on what to feed the preterm infant after hospital discharge, especially if the goal is to achieve "catch-up" growth. How fast these preterm infants (and especially those born small for gestational age) should demonstrate catch-up growth after hospital discharge is an area in critical need of research given the increased risk of these infants developing the metabolic syndrome later in life.[132–134]

More information is also needed for the preterm infant who is maintained on human milk after discharge. These infants require supplemental vitamins and iron as well as more careful monitoring of growth parameters after discharge. In infants who are maintained on standard formulas after discharge, supplemental vitamins should also be given, and any formula used should be iron fortified. However, there is no information that indicates how long after discharge these supplements should be continued.

Conclusion

Nutrition plays a major role in the ultimate well-being of the increasing number of preterm infants with very low birth weight who survive, and it is becoming clear that early nutritional intervention can have long-term consequences.[6,135] Because of the potential damage caused by inadequate nutrition during the early neonatal period, the dilemma of feeding the preterm infant is that of providing sufficient nutrition by enteral and parenteral routes to ensure optimal growth and development without inducing additional morbidity and mortality secondary to the feedings. A randomized controlled trial has demonstrated that early aggressive enteral and parenteral nutrition in sick infants with very low birth weight can improve growth outcomes without increasing the risk of all measured clinical and metabolic sequelae.[136] Although most infants with very low birth weight have achieved the intrauterine growth rate by the time of discharge, most are still less than the 10th percentile for their postconceptional age at this time. Altering these nutritional outcomes will require a more sustained effort to provide adequate nutritional support in early postnatal life, both before and after hospital discharge.

References

1. Tsang RC, Uauy R, Koletzko B, Zlotkin SH, eds. *Nutrition of the Preterm Infant: Scientific Basis and Practical Guidelines*. 2nd ed. Cincinnati, OH: Digital Educational Publishing Inc; 2005

2. American Academy of Pediatrics, Committee on Nutrition. Nutritional needs of low-birth-weight infants. *Pediatrics*. 1985;75:976–986

3. Lemons JA, Bauer CR, Oh W, et al. Very low birth weight outcomes of the National Institute of Child Health and Human Development Neonatal Research Network, January 1995 through December 1996. *Pediatrics*. 2001;107(1):e1. Available at: http://pediatrics.aappublications. org/cgi/content/full/107/1/e1. Accessed July 6, 2007

4. Ehrenkranz RA, Younes N, Lemons JA, et al. Longitudinal growth of hospitalized very low birth weight infants. *Pediatrics*. 1999;104:280–289

5. Dusick AM, Poindexter BB, Ehrenkranz RA, Lemons JA. Growth failure in the preterm infant: can we catch up? *Semin Perinatol*. 2003;27:302–310

6. Reichman B, Chessex P, Putet G, et al. Diet fat, accretion, and growth in premature infants. *N Engl J Med*. 1981;305:1495–1500

7. Morley R, Lucas A. Influence of early diet on outcome in preterm infants. *Acta Paediatr Suppl.* 1994;405:123–126

8. Roberts SB, Young VR. Energy costs of fat and protein deposition in the human infant. *Am J Clin Nutr.* 1988;48:951–955

9. Bremer HJ, Wharton BA. *Nutrition and Feeding of Preterm Infants.* Oxford, England: Blackwell Scientific Publications; 1987

10. Leitch CA, Denne SC. Energy. In: Tsang RC, Uauy R, Koletzko B, Zlotkin SH, eds. *Nutrition of the Preterm Infant: Scientific Basis and Practical Guidelines.* 2nd ed. Cincinnati, OH: Digital Educational Publishing Inc; 2005:23–44

11. Cooke R, Embleton N, Rigo J, Carrie A, Haschke, F, Ziegler E. High protein pre-term infant formula: effect on nutrient balance, metabolic status and growth. *Pediatr Res.* 2006;59:1–6

12. Premji SS, Fenton TR, Suave RS. Higher versus lower protein intake in formula-fed low birth weight infants. *Cochrane Database Syst Rev.* 2006(1):CD003959

13. Gaull GE, Rassin DK, Raiha NC, Heinonen K. Milk protein quantity and quality in low-birth-weight infants. III. Effects on sulfur amino acids in plasma and urine. *J Pediatr.* 1977;90:348–355

14. Raiha NC, Heinonen K, Rassin DK, Gaull GE. Milk protein quantity and quality in low-birthweight infants. I. Metabolic responses and effects on growth. *Pediatrics.* 1976;57:659–684

15. Kashyap S, Schulze KF, Forsyth M, et al. Growth, nutrient retention, and metabolic response in low birth weight infants fed varying intakes of protein and energy. *J Pediatr.* 1988;113:713–721

16. Rigo J, Senterre J. Significance of plasma amino acid pattern in preterm infants. *Biol Neonate.* 1987;52(Suppl 1):41–49

17. Shenai JP, Jhaveri BM, Reynolds JW, Huston RK, Babson SG. Nutritional balance studies in very low-birth-weight infants: role of soy formula. *Pediatrics.* 1981;67:631–637

18. Alemi B, Hamosh M, Scanlon JW, Salzman-Mann C, Hamosh P. Fat digestion in very low-birth-weight infants: effect of addition of human milk to low-birth-weight formula. *Pediatrics.* 1981;68:484–489

19. Bustamante SA, Fiello A, Pollack PF. Growth of premature infants fed formulas with 10%, 30%, or 50% medium-chain triglycerides. *Am J Dis Child.* 1987;141:516–519

20. Carnielli VP, Wattimena DJ, Luijendijk IH, Boerlage A, Degenhart HJ, Sauer PJ. The very low birth weight premature infant is capable of synthesizing arachidonic and docosahexaenoic acids from linoleic and linolenic acids. *Pediatr Res.* 1996;40:169–174

21. Sauerwald TU, Hachey DL, Jensen CL, Chen H, Anderson RE, Heird WC. Intermediates in endogenous synthesis of C22:6 omega 3 and C20:4 omega 6 by term and preterm infants. *Pediatr Res.* 1997;41:183–187

22. Simmer K, Patole S. Long chain polyunsaturated fatty acid supplementation in preterm infants. *Cochrane Database Syst Rev.* 2004;(1):CD000375

23. Heird WC, Lapillonne A. The role of essential fatty acids in development. *Annu Rev Nutr.* 2005;25:549–571

24. Fleith M, Candinin MT. Dietary PUFA for preterm and term infants: review of clinical studies. *Crit Rev Food Sci Nutr.* 2005;45:205–229

25. Kien CI, Heitlinger LA, Li BU, Murray RD. Digestion, absorption, and fermentation of carbohydrate. *Semin Perinatol*. 1989;13:78–87

26. Parimi P, Kalhan SC. Carbohydrates including oligosaccharides and inositol. In: Tsang RC, Uauy R, Koletzko B, Zlotkin SH, eds. *Nutrition of the Preterm Infant: Scientific Basis and Practical Guidelines*. Cincinnati, OH: Digital Educational Publishing; 2005:81–95

27. Wirth FH Jr, Numerof B, Pleban P, Neylan MJ. Effect of lactose on mineral absorption in preterm infants. *J Pediatr*. 1990;117:283–287

28. Fusch Ch, Jochum F. Water, sodium, potassium and chloride. In: Tsang RC, Uauy R, Koletzko B, Zlotkin SH, eds. *Nutrition of the Preterm Infant: Scientific Basis and Practical Guidelines*. Cincinnati, OH: Digital Educational Publishing; 2005:201–244

29. Atkinson SA, Tsang RC. Calcium, magnesium, phosphorus, and vitamin D. In: Tsang RC, Uauy R, Koletzko B, Zlotkin S, eds. *Nutrition of the Preterm Infant: Scientific Basis and Practical Guidelines*. Cincinnati, OH: Digital Educational Publishing; 2005:245–275

30. Koo WW, Sherman R, Succop P, et al. Fractures and rickets in very low birth weight infants: conservative management and outcome. *J Pediatr Orthop*. 1989;9:326–330

31. Chan GM, Mileur L, Hansen JW. Effects of increased calcium and phosphorus formulas and human milk on bone mineralization in preterm infants. *J Pediatr Gastroenterol Nutr*. 1986;5:444–449

32. Ehrenkranz RA, Gettner PA, Nelli CM. Nutrient balance studies in premature infants fed premature formula or fortified preterm human milk. *J Pediatr Gastroenterol Nutr*. 1989;8:58–67

33. Schanler RJ, Garza C. Improved mineral balance in very low birth weight infants fed fortified human milk. *J Pediatr*. 1988;112:452–456

34. Greer FR, McCormick A. Improved bone mineralization and growth in premature infants fed fortified own mother's milk. *J Pediatr*. 1988;112:961–969

35. Rao R, Georgieff M. Microminerals. In: Tsang RC, Uauy R, Koletzko B, Zlotkin SH, eds. *Nutrition of the Preterm Infant: Scientific Basis and Practical Guidelines*. Cincinnati, OH: Digital Educational Publishing; 2005:277–310

36. Strauss, RG. Controversies in the management of the anemia of prematurity using single-donor red blood cell transfusions and/or recombinant human erythropoietin. *Transf Med Rev*. 2006;20:34–44

37. Ohls RK. Erythropoietin treatment in extremely low birth weight infants: blood in versus blood out. *J Pediatr*. 2002;141:3–6

38. Zipursky A. Erythropoietin therapy for premature infants: cost without benefit? *Pediatr Res*. 2000;48:136

39. Franz AR, Mihatsch WA, Sander S, Kron M, Pohlandt F. Prospective randomized trial of early versus late enteral iron supplementation in infants with a birth weight of less than 1301 grams. *Pediatrics*. 2000;106:700–706

40. Widdowson EM, Southgate DAT, Hey E. Fetal growth and body composition. In: Lindblade B, ed. *Perinatal Nutrition*. San Diego, CA: Academic Press; 1988:3–14

41. Zlotkin SH. Assessment of trace element requirements (zinc) in newborns and young infants, including the infant born prematurely. In: Chandra RK, ed. *Trace Elements in Nutrition of Children II*. New York, NY: Raven Press; 1991:49–64

42. Ehrenkranz RA, Gettener PA, Nelli CM, et al. Zinc and copper nutritional studies in very low birth weight infants: comparison of stable isotopic extrinsic tag and chemical balance methods. *Pediatr Res.* 1989;26:298–307

43. Delange F, Dalhem A, Bourdoux P, et al. Increased risk of primary hypothyroidism in preterm infants. *J Pediatr.* 1984;105:462–469

44. Schanler R. Water-soluble vitamins for preterm infants. In: Tsang RC, Uauy R, Koletzko B, Zlotkin SH, eds. *Nutrition of the Preterm Infant: Scientific Basis and Practical Guidelines.* Cincinnati, OH: Digital Educational Publishing; 2005:173–199

45. Mock DM, deLorimer AA, Liebman WM, Sweetman L, Baker H. Biotin deficiency: an unusual complication of parenteral alimentation. *N Engl J Med.* 1981;304:820–823

46. Burland WL, Simpson K, Lord J. Response of low birthweight infants to treatment with folic acid. *Arch Dis Child.* 1971;46:189–194

47. Kendall AC, Jones EE, Wilson CI, Shinton NK, Elwood PC. Folic acid in low-birthweight infants. *Arch Dis Child.* 1974;49:736–738

48. Stevens D, Burman D, Strelling MK, Morris A. Folic acid supplementation in low birth weight infants. *Pediatrics.* 1979;64:333–335

49. Higginbottom MC, Sweetman L, Nyhan WL. A syndrome of methylmalonic aciduria, homocystinuria, megaloblastic anemia and neurologic abnormalities in a vitamin B12 deficient breast-fed infant of a strict vegetarian. *N Engl J Med.* 1978;299:317–323

50. Shenai JP, Chytil F, Stahlman MT. Liver vitamin A reserves of very low birth weight neonates. *Pediatr Res.* 1985;19:892–893

51. Shenai JP, Chytil F, Jhaveri A, Stahlman MT. Plasma vitamin A and retinol-binding protein in premature and term neonates. *J Pediatr.* 1981;99:302–305

52. Greer FR. Vitamins A, E, and K. In: Tsang RC, Uauy R, Koletzko B, Zlotkin SH, eds. *Nutrition of the Preterm Infant: Scientific Basis and Practical Guidelines.* Cincinnati, OH: Digital Educational Publishing; 2005:141–172

53. Shenai JP, Rush MG, Stahlman MT, Chytil F. Plasma retinol-binding protein response to vitamin A administration in infants susceptible to bronchopulmonary dysplasia. *J Pediatr.* 1990; 116:607–614

54. Shenai JP, Kennedy KA, Chytil F, Stahlman MT. Clinical trial of vitamin A supplementation in infants susceptible to bronchopulmonary dysplasia. *J Pediatr.* 1987;111:269–277

55. Robbins ST, Fletcher AB. Early vs delayed vitamin A supplementation in very-low-birth-weight infants. *JPEN J Parenter Enteral Nutr.* 1993;17:220–225

56. Tyson JE, Wright LL, Oh W, Kennedy KA, Mele L, Ehrenkranz RA, Stoll BJ, Lemons JA, Stevenson DK, Bauer CR, Korones SB, Fanaroff AA, Vitamin A supplementation for extremely-low-birth-weight infants *N Engl J Med.* 1999;340:1962–1968

57. Darlow BA, Graham PJ. Vitamin A supplementation for preventing morbidity and mortality in very low birthweight infants. *Cochrane Database Syst Rev.* 2002;(2):CD000501

58. Oski FA, Barness LA. Vitamin E deficiency: a previously unrecognized cause of hemolytic anemia in the premature infant. *J Pediatr.* 1967;70:211–220

59. Ritchie JH, Fish MB, McMasters V, Grossman M. Edema and hemolytic anemia in premature infants: a vitamin E deficiency syndrome. *N Engl J Med.* 1968;279:1185–1190

60. Williams ML, Shott RJ, O'Neal PL, Oski FA. Role of dietary iron and fat on vitamin E deficiency anemia of infancy. *N Engl J Med.* 1975;292:887–890

61. Gross S, Melhorn DK. Vitamin E-dependent anemia in the premature infant. *J Pediatr.* 1974;85:753–759

62. Greer FR. Osteopenia of prematurity. *Annu Rev Nutr.* 1994;14:169–185

63. Cooke R, Hollis B, Conner C, Watson D, Werkman S, Chesney R. Vitamin D and mineral metabolism in the very low birth weight infant receiving 400 IU of vitamin D. *J Pediatr.* 1990;116:423–428

64. Greer FR, Zachman RD. Neonatal vitamin metabolism: fat soluble. In: Cowett RM, ed. *Principles of Perinatal-Neonatal Metabolism.* 2nd ed. New York, NY: Springer Verlag; 1998:943–975

65. Schanler RJ, Atkinson SA. Human milk. In: Tsang RC, Uauy R, Koletzko B, Zlotkin SH, eds. *Nutrition of the Preterm Infant: Scientific Basis and Practical Guidelines.* Cincinnati, OH: Digital Educational Publishing; 2005:333–356

66. Yu VYH, Simmer K. Enteral nutrition: practical aspects, strategy, and management. In: Tsang RC, Uauy R, Koletzko B, Zlotkin SH, eds. *Nutrition of the Preterm Infant: Scientific Basis and Practical Guidelines.* Cincinnati, OH: Digital Educational Publishing; 2005:311–332

67. Atkinson SA. Effects of gestational age at delivery on human milk components. In: Jensen RG, ed. *Handbook of Milk Composition.* San Diego, CA: Academic Press; 1995:222–237

68. Lucas A, Hudson G. Preterm milk as a source of protein for low birthweight infants. *Arch Dis Child.* 1984;59:831–836

69. Engelke SC, Shah BL, Vasan U, Raye JR. Sodium balance in very low-birth-weight infants. *J Pediatr.* 1978;93:837–841

70. Ronnholm KA, Sipila I, Siimes MA. Human milk protein supplementation for the prevention of hypoproteinemia without metabolic imbalance in breast milk-fed, very-low-birth-weight infants. *J Pediatr.* 1982;101:243–247

71. Greer FR, Steichen JJ, Tsang RC. Calcium and phosphate supplements in breast milk-related rickets: results in a very-low-birth-weight infant. *Am J Dis Child.* 1982;136:581–583

72. Lucas A, Cole TJ. Breast milk and neonatal necrotising enterocolitis. *Lancet.* 1990;336:1519–1523

73. Schanler RJ, Shulman RJ, Lau C. Feeding strategies for premature infants: beneficial outcomes of feeding fortified human milk versus preterm formulas. *Pediatrics.* 1999;103:1150–1157

74. Schanler RJ, Lau C, Hurst NE, Smith EO. Randomized trial of donor human milk versus preterm formula as substitutes for mothers' own milk in the feeding of extremely premature infants. *Pediatrics.* 2005;116:400–406

75. Human Milk Banking Association of North America. *2006 Best Practice for Expressing, Storing and Handling of Mother's Own Milk in Hospital and at Home.* Raleigh, NC: Human Milk Banking Association of North America; 2006

76. Quan R, Yang C, Rubenstein S, et al. Effects of microwave radiation on anti-infective factors in human milk. *Pediatrics.* 1992;89:667–669

77. Sigman M, Burke KI, Swarner OW, Shavlik GW. Effects of microwaving human milk: changes in IgA content and bacterial count. *J Am Diet Assoc.* 1989;89:690–692

78. Putet G, Senterre J, Rigo J, Salle B. Nutrient balance, energy utilization, and composition of gain in very-low-birth-weight infants fed pooled human milk or a preterm formula. *J Pediatr.* 1984;105:79–85

79. Gross SJ. Growth and biochemical response of preterm infants fed human milk or modified infant formula. *N Engl J Med.* 1983;308:237–241

80. Schulze KF, Stefanski M, Masterson J, et al. Energy expenditure, energy balance, and composition of weight gain in low birth weight infants fed diets of different protein and energy content. *J Pediatr.* 1989;110:753–759

81. Sulkers EJ, Lafeber HN, Sauer PJ. Quantitation of oxidation of medium-chain triglycerides in preterm infants. *Pediatr Res.* 1989;26: 294–297

82. Ponder DL. Medium chain trigylceride and urinary di-carboxylic acids in newborns. *JPEN J Parenter Enteral Nutr.* 1991;93–94

83. Taylor, CJ. Health Professionals Letter on *Enterobacter sakazakii* Infections Associated with the Use of Powdered (Dry) Infant Formulas in Neonatal Intensive Care Units. April 11, 2002. US Food and Drug Administration, Center for Food Safety and Applied Nutrition, Office of Nutritional Products, Labeling and Dietary Supplements. Available at: www.cfsan.fda. gov/~dms/inf-ltr3.html. Accessed July 6, 2007

84. Berseth CL. Effect of early feeding on maturation of the preterm infant's small intestine. *J Pediatr.* 1992;120:947–953

85. Davey AM, Wagner CL, Cox C, Kendig JW. Feeding premature infants while low umbilical artery catheters are in place: a prospective, randomized trial. *J Pediatr.* 1994;124:795–799

86. McClure RJ, Newell SJ. Randomised controlled trial of trophic feeding and gut motility. *Arch Dis Child.* 1999;80:F54–F58

87. Schanler RJ, Shulman RJ, Lau C, Smith EO, Heitkemper MM. Feeding strategies for premature infants: randomized trial of gastrointestinal priming and tube-feeding method. *Pediatrics.* 1999;103:434–439

88. MacDonald PD, Skeoch CH, Carse H, et al. Randomized trial of continuous nasogastric, bolus nasogastric, and transpyloric feeding in infants of birth weight under 1400g. *Arch Dis Child.* 1992;67:429–431

89. Ansley-Green A, Adrian TE, Bloom SR. Feeding and the development of enteroinsular hormone secretion in the preterm infant. Effects of continuous gastric infusions or human milk compared with intermittent boluses. *Acta Paediatr Scand.* 1982;71:379–383

90. Baker JH, Berseth CL. Duodenal motor responses in preterm infants fed formula with varying concentrations and rates of infusion. *Pediatr Res.* 1997;42:618–622

91. Roy RN, Pollnitz RB, Hamilton JR, Chance GW. Impaired assimilation of nasojejunal feeds in healthy low-birth-weight newborn infants. *J Pediatr.* 1977;90:431–434

92. Greer FR, McCormick A, Loker J. Changes in fat concentration of human milk during delivery by intermittent bolus and continuous mechanical pump infusion. *J Pediatr.* 1984;105:745–749

93. Mehta NR, Hamosh M, Bitman J, Wood DL. Adherence of medium-chain fatty acids to feeding tubes during gavage feeding of human milk fortified with medium-chain triglycerides. *J Pediatr.* 1988;112:474–476

94. Bhatia J, Rassin DK. Human milk supplementation: delivery of energy, calcium, phosphorus, magnesium, copper, and zinc. *Am J Dis Child.* 1988;142:445–447

95. Ekblad H, Kero P, Takala J, Korvenranta H, Valimaki I. Water, sodium and acid-base balance in premature infants: therapeutical aspects. *Acta Paediatr Scand.* 1987;76:47–53

96. Denne SC, Karn CA, Ahlrichs JA, Dorotheo AR, Wang J, Liechty EA. Proteolysis and phenylalanine hydroxlyation in response to parenteral nutrition in extremely premature and normal newborns. *J Clin Invest.* 1996;97:746–754

97. Mitton SG, Calder AG, Garlick PJ. Protein turnover rates in sick, premature neonates during the first few days of life. *Pediatric Res.* 1992;30:418–422

98. Rivera A Jr, Bell EF, Bier DM. Effect of intravenous amino acids on protein metabolism of preterm infants during the first three days of life. *Pediatr Res.* 1993;33:106–111

99. Kashyap S, Heird WC. Protein requirements of low birthweight, very low birthweight, and small for gestational age infants. In: Raiha NCR, ed. *Protein Metabolism During Infancy. Nestle Nutrition Workshop Series.* Vol 33. New York, NY: Vevey/Raven Press Ltd; 1994:133–151

100. Van Lingen RA. Van Goudoever JB, Luijendijk IH, Wattimena JL, Saur PJ. Effects of early amino acid administration during total parenteral nutrition on protein metabolism in pre-term infants. *Clin Sci (Lond).* 1992;82:199–203

101. Van Goudoever JB, Colen T, Wattimena JL, Huijmans JG,Carnielli VP, Sauer PJ. Immediate commencement of amino acid supplementation in preterm infants: effect on serum amino acid concentrations and protein kinetics on the first day of life. *J Pediatr.* 1995;127:458–465

102. Thureen PJ, Melara D, Fennessey PV, Hay WW. Effect of low versus high intravenous amino acid intake on very low birth weight infants in the early neonatal period. *Pediatr Res.* 2003;53:24–32

103. Ridout E, Melara D, Rottinghaus S, Thureen PJ. Blood urea nitrogen concentration as a marker of amino-acid intolerance in neonates with birthweight less than 1250 g. *J Perinatol.* 2005;25:130–133

104. Anderson TL, Muttart CR, Bieber MA, Nicholson JF, Heird WC. A controlled trial of glucose versus glucose and amino acids in premature infants. *J Pediatr.* 1979;94:947–951

105. Duffy B, Gunn T, Collinge J, Pencharz P. The effect of varying protein quality and energy intake on the nitrogen metabolism of parenterally fed very low birthweight (less than 1600 g) infants. *Pediatr Res.* 1981;15:1040–1044

106. Zlotkin SH, Bryan MH, Anderson GH. Intravenous nitrogen and energy intakes required to duplicate in utero nitrogen accretion in prematurely born human infants. *J Pediatr.* 1981;99:115–120

107. Dweck HS, Cassady G. Glucose intolerance in infants of very low birth weight. I. Incidence of hyperglycemia in infants of birth weights 1,100 grams or less. *Pediatrics.* 1974;53:189–195

108. Binder ND, Raschko PK, Benda GI, Reynolds JW. Insulin infusion with parenteral nutrition in extremely low birth weight infants with hyperglycemia. *J Pediatr.* 1989;114: 273–280

109. Collins JW, Hoppe M, Brown K, Edidin DV, Padbury J, Ogata ES. A controlled trial of Insulin infusion and parenteral nutrition in extremely low birth weight infants with glucose intolerance. *J Pediatr.* 1991;118:921–927

110. Kanarek KS, Santeiro ML, Malone JI. Continuous infusion of insulin in hyperglycemic low-birth weight infants receiving parenteral nutrition with and without lipid emulsion. *JPEN J Parenter Enteral Nutr.* 1991;15:417–420

111. Poindexter BB, Karn CA, Denne SC. Exogenous insulin reduces proteolysis and protein synthesis in extremely low birth weight infants. *J Pediatr.* 1998;132:948–953

112. Putet G. Lipid metabolism of the micropremie. *Clin Perinatol.* 2000;27:57–69, v–vi

113. Andrew G, Chan G, Schiff D. Lipid metabolism in the neonate. I. The effects of Intralipid infusion on plasma triglyceride and free fatty acid concentrations in the neonate. *J Pediatr.* 1976;88:273–278

114. Shennan AT, Bryan MH, Angel A. The effect of gestational age on intralipid tolerance in newborn infants. *J Pediatr.* 1977;91:134–137

115. Penn D, Schmidt-Sommerfeld E, Pascu F. Decreased tissue carnitine concentrations in newborn infants receiving total parenteral nutrition. *J Pediatr.* 1981;98:976–978

116. Schmidt-Sommerfield E, Penn D. Carnitine and total parenteral nutrition of the neonate. *Biol Neonate.* 1990;58:81–88

117. Larrson LE, Olegard R, Ljung BM, Niklasson A, Rubensson A, Cederblad G. Parenteral nutrition in preterm neonates with and without carnitine supplementation. *Acta Anaesthesiol Scand.* 1990;34:501–505

118. Brans YW. Ritter DA, Kenny JD, Andrews DS, Dutton EB, Carrillo DW. Influence of intravenous fat emulsion on serum bilirubin in very low birthweight neonates. *Arch Dis Child.* 1987;62:156–160

119. Baekert PA, Greene HL, Fritz I, Oelberg DG, Adcock EW. Vitamin concentration in very low birth weight infants given vitamins intravenously in a lipid emulsion: measurement of vitamins A, D, and E and riboflavin. *J Pediatr.* 1988;113:1057–1065

120. Lucas A, Bishop NJ, King FJ, Cole TJ. Randomised trial of nutrition for preterm infants after discharge. *Arch Dis Child.* 1992;67:324–327

121. Bishop NJ, King FJ, Lucas A. Increased bone mineral content of preterm infants fed with a nutrient enriched formula after discharge from hospital. *Arch Dis Child.* 1993;68:573–578

122. Chan GM. Growth and bone mineral status of discharged very low birth weight infants fed different formulas or human milk. *J Pediatr.* 1993;123:439–443

123. Hall RT, Wheeler RE, Rippetoe LE. Calcium and phosphorus supplementation after initial hospital discharge in breast-fed infants at less than 1800 grams birth weight. *J Perinatol.* 1993;13:272–278

124. Friel JK, Andrews WL, Matthew JD, McKim E, French S, Long DR. Improved growth of very low birthweight infants. *Nutr Res.* 1993;13:611–620

125. Wheeler RE, Hall RT. Feeding of premature infant formula after hospital discharge of infants weighing less than 1800 grams at birth. *J Perinatol.* 1996;16:111–116

126. Carver JD, Wu PY, Hall RT, et al. Growth of preterm infants fed nutrient-enriched or term formula after hospital discharge. *Pediatrics.* 2001;107:683–9

127. Cooke RJ, Griffin IJ, McCormick K, Wells JC, Smith JS, Robinson SJ, Leighton M. Feeding preterm infants after hospital discharge: effect of dietary manipulation on nutrient intake and growth. *Peds Res.* 1998;43:355–360

128. Cooke RJ, Embleton ND, Griffin IJ, Wells JC, McCormick KP. Feeding preterm infants after hospital discharge: growth and development at 18 months of age. *Pediatr Res.* 2001;49:719–722

129. Lapillonne A, Salle BL, Glorieux FH, Claris O. Bone mineralization and growth are enhanced in preterm infants fed an isocaloric, nutrient enriched preterm formula through term. *Am J Clin Nutr.* 2004;80:1595–1603

130. Koo WE, Hockman EM. Post hospital discharge feeding for preterm infants: standard versus enriched milk formula on growth, bone mass, and body composition. *Am J Clin Nutr.* 2007; in press

131. Henderson G, Fahey T, McGuire W. Calorie and protein-enriched formula versus standard term formula for improving growth and development in preterm or low birth weight infants following hospital discharge. *Cochrane Database Syst Rev.* 2005;(2):CD004696

132. Euser AM, Finken MJ, Keijzer-Veen MG, Hille ET, Wit JM, Dekker FW. Associations between prenatal and infancy weight gain and BMI, fat mass, and fat distribution in young adulthood; a prospective cohort study in males and females born very preterm. Dutch POPS–19 Collaborative study Group. *Am J Clin Nutr.* 2005;81:480–487

133. Singhal A, Fewtrell M, Cole TJ, Lucas A. Low nutrient intake and early growth for later insulin resistance in adolescents born preterm. *Lancet.* 2003;361:1089–1097

134. Singhal A, Lucas A. Early origins of cardiovascular disease: is there a unifying hypothesis? *Lancet.* 2004;363:1642–1645

135. Lucas A, Morley R, Cole RJ, et al. Early diet in preterm babies and development status at 18 months. *Lancet.* 1990;335:1477–1481

136. Wilson DC, Cairns P, Halliday HL, Reid M, McClure G, Dodge JA. Randomized controlled trial of an aggressive nutritional regimen in sick very low birthweight infants. *Arch Dis Child.* 1997;77:F4–F11

5 | Complementary Feeding

Introduction

Complementary feeding is defined as providing nutrient-containing foods or liquids along with human milk[1] and includes both solid foods and infant formula.[2] Some nutritionists have restricted the term "complementary" to solid or liquid foods that do not displace (ie, reduce intake of) human milk. However, the available evidence indicates that any energy-containing foods will displace breastfeeding and reduce the intake of human milk to some extent,[1,3–6] and all such foods are referred to herein as complementary.

Complementary foods can be introduced between 4 and 6 months of age. However, the American Academy of Pediatrics (AAP) supports exclusive breastfeeding (in which all fluid, energy, and nutrients come from human milk, with the possible exception of small amounts of medicinal/nutrient supplements[1]) for minimum of 4 but preferably 6 months (Table 5.1).[7]

This chapter presents a review of the evidence bearing on complementary feeding and the timing of its introduction in the first year of life and includes a discussion of infant growth and development issues related to infant nutritional needs and complementary feeding; a review of the scientific evidence and conclusions on the relationships between key infant outcomes and the duration of exclusive breastfeeding and timing of complementary foods introduction; and a review of the energy and micronutrient requirements of complementary foods for infants 1 year and younger, including the current complementary food intake patterns in the United States and how well they meet the requirements.

Infant Growth and Development Factors

A number of factors related to an infant's growth and development underlie complementary feeding perspectives and recommendations. This section presents scientific evidence regarding these factors, including infant energy requirements; nutrients (iron, zinc, vitamin D); and infant feeding readiness.

Infant Energy Requirements

Whereas adult energy requirements are based on energy and nutrients needed to maintain the body, infants need energy for both maintenance and growth.[14] A 1973 report from the Food and Agriculture Organization of the United Nations (FAO)/World Health Organization (WHO) estimated the

Table 5.1

American Academy of Pediatrics Recommendations Relevant to the Initiation of Complementary Foods (see text for AAP recommendations on human milk)

Nutrient/Food	Subgroups	AAP Recommendations
Human milk	Most infants	Exclusive breastfeeding for minimum of 4 but preferably 6 mo.
	Infants with unique needs or feeding patterns	Individual infants may require complementary foods as early as 4 mo of age or may be unable to accept them until about 8 mo of age.[7]
Calcium	Term infants	Recommended intakes, human milk or infant formulas: First 6 mo: 210 mg/day 7–12 mo: 270 mg/day No benefit from increasing calcium content of infant formulas above these amounts.
	Preterm infants	Have higher calcium requirements than term infants. Can meet requirements using human milk plus commercial fortifiers or preterm infant formulas enriched with calcium and vitamin D. Optimal calcium concentrations and duration of use unknown.[8]
Cholesterol	Infants younger than 2 y	No restriction of fat or cholesterol; rapid growth requires high energy intake.[9]
Fluoride	Infants 6 mo and older	Supplement with 0.25 mg/day in areas with <0.3 ppm fluoride concentration in community drinking supplies (see Chapter 48).
Iron	Breastfed infants 6–12 mo	Iron from complementary foods at 6 mo of age (see Chapters 2 and 18).
	Nonbreastfed infants younger than 12 mo	Ingest iron-fortified formula (10–12 mg/L) until weaning at 12 mo of age.
	Breastfed preterm or low birth weight infant	Oral iron supplement drops at 2 mg/kg per day, 1–12 mo of age (see Chapter 4).
	Formula-fed preterm infants	May benefit from an additional iron supplement (drops) of 1 mg/kg per day.
Lactose	Children from populations with high rates of lactose malabsorption	Unwise to discourage use of milk unless children have severe diarrhea or clear intolerance; clinical problems usually manifest at 5–7 y of age.[10]
Vitamin D	All breastfed infants and nonbreastfed infants	Should have a supplement of 400 IU/day of vitamin D beginning during first 2 mo of life through childhood and adolescence unless ingesting at least 500 mL/day of vitamin D-fortified formula or milk.[11]

Table 5.1 *(continued)*
American Academy of Pediatrics Recommendations Relevant to the Initiation of Complementary Foods (see text for AAP recommendations on human milk)

Nutrient/Food	Subgroups	AAP Recommendations
Fruit juice	Infants up to 1 y of age	Should not be introduced before 6 mo of age.
		Should not be given juice in containers that allow them to consume juice easily throughout the day.
		Should not be given at bedtime.
		Should not consume unpasteurized juices.[12]
Soy protein-based formulas	Term infants whose nutritional needs are not met by human or cow milk	Isolated soy protein-based formula is a safe, effective alternative.
	Infants with documented lactose intolerance	Use is appropriate.
	Most infants with documented immunoglobulin E-mediated allergy to cow milk	Use may be appropriate.
	Preterm infants who weigh <1800 g	Use is not recommended.[13]
Water*	All infants up to 1 y of age	No data basis for minimum or maximum usual water intake recommendations; water intoxication not a discernable public health problem.
	Formula-fed infants	*During hot weather:* No recommendations.
	Infants up to 1 y of age, exclusively breastfed or partial breastfeeding eating complementary foods	Monitor for dark or decreased urine output. When present, offer solute-free water up to maximum of 225 mL/kg per day.

* AAP Committee on Nutrition advice, based on literature search pertaining to water intoxication, current recommendations from AAP materials, and opinions of pediatric nutrition experts.

energy requirements of infants by observing intakes of breastfed infants growing typically. Although energy intake varies among infants and for the same infant over the course of a day, the report found that, from 0 to 3 months of age, 850 mL per day of human milk provides an average of 120 kcal/kg. That figure decreases slightly from 3 to 5 months of age, and by 6 months, infants were deemed unable to meet complete energy requirements on human milk alone, with more active children needing more complementary food.[15]

Additional studies by Fomon and Nelson[14] and Butte et al[16] determined the body composition of reference infants to estimate the gain in energy and specific nutrients during defined age periods and provide a target value for studies of infant energy and nutrient requirements. Although specifics differ, the reference infants in both studies demonstrated that the gain in body fat is significant during the first 4 or 6 months of life, suggesting that energy requirements for growth during this period make up a substantial proportion of the total energy requirement. In fact, the percentage of first-year energy intake devoted to growth is highest (27%) from birth to 4 months of age and decreases to 5% from 6 to 12 months of age.[17] Physical and metabolic activity also require a percentage of energy intake (Fig 5.1).

In 2005,[18] data were available that allowed Butte to estimate the energy requirements of infants by measuring total energy expenditure (TEE) and energy deposition during growth, which had not been not possible in previous studies. Butte used the "doubly labeled water" method to measure TEE, which encompasses basal metabolism, thermoregulation, physical activity, and the synthetic cost of growth. The earlier work on body composition provided the measurements to estimate energy deposition. Results showed that 1985 FAO/WHO estimates of infant energy requirements,[19] which were based on observed energy intakes of infants from about 1940 to 1980 and included a 5% increment for an assumed underestimation, were 10% to 32% higher than estimates made using TEE and energy deposition based on stable isotope measurements (Table 5.2).

The WHO also provided estimates of the energy required from complementary foods at various ages and with various intakes by subtracting the amounts of energy provided by human milk from estimates of children's average energy requirements.[1] The report cautions, however, that the estimates may be inflated, because, as noted above, complementary foods displace human milk intake to some extent. Table 5.3 provides the estimates for infants and children 0 to 24 months of age living in industrialized and developing countries (Table 5.3).

Infant Nutrient Needs

Nutrient intake is a key determinant of child survival, growth, and development. Human milk is an ideal food for young infants because of its unique nutrient profile. However, feeding human milk alone may lead to insufficiencies of some nutrients, such as iron, zinc, vitamin K, and vitamin D, after a certain age.[1]

Fig 5.1
Allocation of energy expenditure during the first year of life.

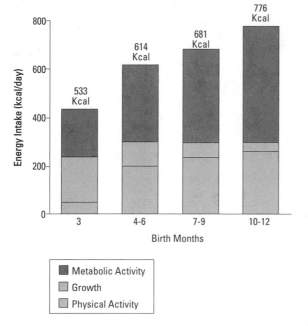

Figure drawn from data presented in Wells JC, Davies PS. Estimation of the energy cost of physical activity in infancy. *Arch Dis Child.* 1998;78:131–136 and Butte NF, Wong WW, Hopkinson JM, Heinz CJ, Mehta NR, Smith EO. Energy requirements derived from total energy expenditure and energy deposition during the first 2 y of life. *Am J Clin Nutr.* 2000;72:1558–1569.

Table 5.2
Comparing Recommended Energy Intakes in the First 2 Years of Life in Breastfed Infants*

Age Group (mo)	FAO/WHO/UNU 1985		Total Energy Expenditure Plus the Energy Cost of Growth[18]	
	kcal/kg per day	kcal/day	kcal/kg per day	kcal/day
0–2	116	520	88	404
3–5	99	662	82	550
6–8	95	784	83	682
9–11	101	949	89	830
12–23	106	1170	86	1092

FAO indicates Food and Agricultural Organization of the United Nations; WHO, World Health Organization; UNU, United Nations University.

* Table adapted from WHO.[1p49]

Table 5.3
Energy Consumed Over a Range of Human Milk Intakes and Corresponding Amount of Energy Needed From Complementary Foods in Industrialized Countries by Age*

| Age Group (mo) | Energy Consumed From Human Milk | | | Energy Needed From Complementary Foods | | |
| | Human Milk Intake (kcal/day) | | | (kcal/day) | | |
	Low	Average	High	Low	Average	High
0–2	294	490	686	110	0	0
3–5	362	548	734	188	2	0
6–8	274	486	698	408	196	0
9–11	41	375	709	789	455	121
12–23	0	313	669	1092	779	423

*Table adapted from WHO.[1p51]

Iron Needs (also see Chapter 18: Iron)
The Dietary Reference Intakes for iron in the first year are as follows[20]:

- For infants 0 to 6 months of age, the Adequate Intake is 0.27 mg/day.

- For infants 7 to 12 months of age, the Recommended Dietary Allowance is 11 mg/day.

Human milk is relatively low in iron regardless of maternal intake, containing only approximately 0.5 mg/L during the early weeks of lactation and approximately 0.35 mg/L thereafter,[21] although its bioavailability is reported to be high.[22] Many infant foods have significant inhibitors of iron absorption, but human milk has few, and more than 50% of iron from human milk is absorbed, compared with approximately 12% from cow milk-derived formula.[23] Nonetheless, a number of studies have found that exclusively breastfed infants are at risk of iron deficiency in the latter half of the first year.[24]

The prevalence of iron deficiency among infants and children has decreased in the United States, and iron-deficiency anemia is uncommon, but national data still indicate a rate of 9% to 11% among 18-month-olds.[25] Therefore, iron deficiency is a public health concern, particularly because iron is a critical nutrient for neurodevelopment. Thus, preventing iron insufficiency remains an important goal. Table 5.1 outlines AAP recommendations to prevent and treat iron deficiency for both breastfed and formula-fed infants.

Zinc Needs (also see Chapter 19: Trace Elements)
The Dietary Reference Intakes for zinc in the first years are as follows[20]:

- For infants 0 to 6 months of age, the Adequate Intake is 2 mg/day.

- For children 7 months to 3 years of age, the Recommended Dietary Allowance is 3 mg/day.

As with iron, the zinc content of human milk is relatively low, reportedly ranging from approximately 8 to 12 mg/L in the first month after birth and decreasing to approximately 1 to 3 mg/L or less at 4 to 6 months after birth.[21] Like iron, zinc bioavailability is reported to be higher from human milk than from infant formulas.[26]

In affluent populations, exclusively breastfed infants up to 6 months of age do not appear to be at higher risk of zinc deficiency than formula-fed infants[27]; however, zinc intake may be insufficient in some populations from 6 to 12 months of age. Infant risk factors for zinc deficiency include chronic diarrhea and diets low in zinc content or containing inhibitors of zinc absorption, such as dietary phytate (found in foods such as unleavened whole wheat, legumes, and corn). Zinc deficiency appears more prevalent among infants in developing countries than among those in industrialized nations.[1]

Zinc is an important nutrient for maintaining immune function, and it contributes to cell growth and repair. Zinc deficiency has been associated with impaired growth, increased susceptibility to infections, and increased risk of childhood diarrhea, the frequency of which increased in a Peruvian study by 15% per standard deviation decrease in height-to-age z score.[28] Zinc supplementation has been associated in meta-analyses with a highly significant increase in linear growth and weight gain of prepubertal children, especially among children with low initial weight or height. However, it showed no effect on the weight-for-height index. Zinc supplementation also produces a large, highly significant increase in children's serum zinc concentrations[29,30] and is associated with significantly decreased rates of diarrhea and pneumonia in developing countries.[31] Table 5.4 summarizes reported beneficial effects from zinc supplementation on mental and motor development.

Zinc supplementation has also been shown to enhance immune function in children. For example, a study of preschool children found a decrease of 45% in the incidence of acute lower respiratory infections in zinc-supplemented infants and preschool children.[37]

Table 5.4

Reported Effects of Zinc Supplementation on Mental Development and Motor Activity Patterns

Country/Study	Population	Benefits of Supplementation: Increases in
Brazil[32]	Low birth weight infants	Overall responsiveness scores
China[33]	6–9 y of age	Neuropsychological scores
Guatemala[34]	Term infants 6–9 mo of age	Time sitting up, time playing
India[35]	12–23 mo of age	Time in fast motor activities, overall activity rating, rates of energy expenditure
Canada[36]	Very low birth weight infants 6, 9, and 12 mo of age	Motor development scores

Vitamin D Needs

The recommended daily intake of vitamin D for infants and children is 400 IU of vitamin D per day.[38] The vitamin D content of human milk is low (12–60 IU/L), even with adequate maternal vitamin D intake. Observational and case studies suggest that exclusively breastfed infants in temperate climates with limited sun exposure and/or born to vitamin D-deficient mothers are at increased risk of rickets caused by vitamin D deficiency. Dark-skinned exclusively breastfed infants are at particular risk.[39,40] In addition, low maternal vitamin D intake has resulted in infants born with low total body bone mineral content and high bone resorption.[41] Currently, there is no national surveillance of nutritional rickets in the United States, but estimates based on data from the National Hospital Discharge Survey (1990–1998) suggest that 9 out of 1 million children were hospitalized with rickets.[42] Because human milk does not provide sufficient vitamin D to prevent rickets in at-risk infants, supplemental sources of vitamin D are needed. Given current concerns about risk of sunlight exposure, even for young infants, the AAP recommends that all breastfed infants receive 400 IU of vitamin D per day beginning within the first 2 months of life (Table 5.1).

Vitamin K Needs

Infant Feeding Readiness

Successful introduction of complementary foods presupposes the ability of developing infants to be nourished by, to safely ingest, and to accept such foods. Issues of digestion and absorption, neuromuscular development, and taste and texture acceptance are central. Although developmental milestones are achieved by individual infants at a range of ages, some average trends have been identified.

Full-term infants are capable of digesting complex diets of carbohydrates, starches, fats, and proteins at birth. Fat digestion is sufficient at birth to allow absorption of more than 90% of ingested fat.[24,43]

A number of feeding reflexes related to the maturation of the neuromuscular system also affect an infant's ability to handle various types of foods. For example, an infant's rooting and sucking mechanisms, usually developed at birth, facilitate breastfeeding. However, the early gag reflex may hinder ingestion of solid foods until its locus moves from the mid portion to the posterior of the tongue (usually between 3 and 7 months of age).

Truncal (vertical) stability and oral motor skills are also critical determinants of developmental readiness for complementary foods. By 4 months of age, most infants have the truncal stability to sit with support and indicate an appetite or desire for food (by opening the mouth or leaning in) or satiety (by closing the mouth or turning away), and parents can interpret their behavior correctly.[24] In addition, by 4 months of age, infants have exhibited the ability to give evidence of taste preferences and accept new tastes; rejection of new foods does not appear to occur in most infants until later in the first year.[44]

AAP

Recommendations from the American Academy of Pediatrics

Prevention of early vitamin K deficiency bleeding (VKDB) of the newborn, with onset at birth to 2 weeks of age (formerly known as classic hemorrhagic disease of the newborn), by oral or parenteral administration of vitamin K is accepted practice. In contrast, late VKDB, with onset from 2 to 12 weeks of age, is most effectively prevented by parenteral administration of vitamin K. Earlier concern regarding a possible causal association between parenteral vitamin K and childhood cancer has not been substantiated.

Pediatrics. 2003;112:191–192

Timing of Complementary Foods Introduction: Review of the Evidence on Related Health Outcomes

Recent epidemiologic evidence has shown that breastfeeding protects against gastrointestinal and, to a lesser extent, respiratory infection and that the protective effect is enhanced with greater duration and exclusivity of breastfeeding.[45-48] Prolonged and exclusive breastfeeding (at least for the first few months of life) has been associated with reduced risks of sudden infant death syndrome,[48] atopic disease,[49-51] and chronic conditions such as obesity,[52,53] type 1 diabetes mellitus,[54,55] Crohn disease,[56] and lymphoma[57,58] as well as acceleration of neurocognitive development[59-62] (see Chapter 2). It is also clear that breastfeeding protects against morbidity and mortality from infectious diseases in developing and industrialized countries, even into the second year of life.[63-65]

Although the benefits of breastfeeding are clear, data regarding how long exclusive breastfeeding should continue and when to introduce complementary foods are not definitive. For example, a WHO consultation on the optimal duration of exclusive breastfeeding supported exclusive breastfeeding for 6 months, because no adverse effects had been found on a population level and some benefits were conferred. However, the panel pointed out that the data (from 2 small controlled trials and 17 observational studies of varying quality) were insufficient to exclude some potential risks of 6-month exclusive breastfeeding. They concluded that individualized risk-benefit decisions were appropriate.[66]

Information from a recent systematic review for the WHO[67] will be described here in some detail, because it provides the most comprehensive review of the evidence that bears on the timing of the introduction of complementary foods. Yet, the authors' evaluation of the methodologic quality of included studies pointed to substantial problems. For example, the review included both controlled clinical trials and observational studies, published in any language, that compared health outcomes of full-term infants and their mothers who had exclusively breastfed for ≥6 months of age with those who had exclusively breastfed for at least 3 months and continued mixed breastfeeding until at least 6 months. Only studies with an internal comparison group were included in the review; those based on an external comparison group or reference were excluded. A total of 36 citations (articles or abstracts) were identified that met the selection criteria for the review, for a total of 20 separate studies, 9 of which were conducted in developing countries and 11 of which were conducted in industrialized countries. However, only 16 studies met selection criteria and only 2 of these were controlled trials (which did not receive high quality ratings for methodology). The other 14 were observational studies deemed of variable quality.

Another issue that has received attention in proposed timing for introduction of complementary foods has been the so-called "weanlings" dilemma, described in the 1970s and 1980s for infants in developing countries.[68,69] The dilemma centered on the risk of infection with the introduction of contaminated complementary foods versus the risk of suboptimal growth with continued exclusive breastfeeding. Growth faltering is commonly observed in developing countries after about 3 months of age,[70–72] and early calculations made by the FAO and WHO suggested that human milk alone would be inadequate to meet the energy requirements beyond 3 or 4 months of life.[15] However, more recent studies have shown that the earlier FAO/WHO energy recommendations substantially overestimate true energy requirements in infancy,[19] and exclusive breastfeeding can meet most infants' energy requirements for 6 months. Additionally, the weanlings dilemma does not apply in most industrialized countries, because uncontaminated, nutritionally adequate complementary foods are readily available, and growth faltering is relatively uncommon.

Maternal Outcomes

Two Honduran studies,[4,73] which included both term infants and infants with low birth weight, found that only 6-month exclusive breastfeeding of term infants (in contrast to 6-month exclusive breastfeeding of infants with low birth weight) resulted in greater maternal weight loss than did introduction of complementary foods at 3 to 6 months of age (–0.7±1.5 kg vs –0.1±1.5 kg). Women in the exclusive breastfeeding group who had infants with low birth weight were more likely to postpone return to menses until 6 months after birth.

Maternal risk of breast cancer decreases with the duration of breastfeeding and with each birth. The relative risk of breast cancer decreases by 4.3% (95% confidence interval [CI], 2.9–5.8; $P <.0001$) for every 12 months of breastfeeding in addition to a decrease of 7.0% (95% CI, 5.0–9.0; $P <.0001$) for each birth. The decrease in the relative risk of breast cancer associated with breastfeeding does not differ significantly among women in industrialized and developing countries and does not vary significantly by age, menopausal status, ethnic origin, the number of births a woman has had, or age when a woman's first child was born.[74]

Infant Outcomes

Weight, Length, and Head Circumference Effects

One of the potential risks posited for prolonged and exclusive breastfeeding in industrialized countries has been data that show a deceleration in weight and length gain for exclusively breastfed infants relative to the international WHO/Centers for Disease Control and Prevention (CDC) growth reference from approximately 3 to 12 months of age, with partial catch-up in the second year.[75–80] On the other hand, the first study in humans based on a randomized experiment suggests that prolonged and exclusive breastfeeding may accelerate weight and length gain in the first few months of life, with no observable deficit by 1 year of age. The authors concluded that the findings of earlier observational analyses (including their own previous observational study) may reflect either unmeasured confounding differences or a true biologic effect of formula feeding.[81]

In addition, the WHO/CDC growth reference was based on the Fels Longitudinal Study, which was conducted several decades ago on infants who were primarily formula fed, which could have led to the introduction of solid foods sooner than necessary.[82] The WHO, therefore, embarked on an ambitious international study to establish new growth standards for breastfed infants.[83] It will be important to assess the influence that these standards will have on clinical pediatric care once they are adopted widely, because they lower the reference standards for acceptable weight (ie, 5th percentile).

In a Cochrane review (2002, updated in 2006),[67] a pooled sample of breastfed infants from 6 industrialized countries,[76] a pooled analysis from 5 countries (2 industrialized, 3 developing [but in which study women were all literate and of middle- to high-socioeconomic status]),[84] and a large cohort study nested within a randomized trial in Belarus[85] reported on weight gain between 3 and 8 months of age. One of the WHO studies[84] and the Belarus study[85] controlled for size or growth in the first 3 to 4 months and other potential confounders using multilevel (mixed) regression analyses. The primary outcome of the Belarus study, based on a randomized, controlled design that provided mothers with exposure to the Baby Friendly initiatives as the intervention, was duration of exclusive breastfeeding. In addition, secondary observational outcomes were determined by comparing infants who had exclusively breastfed for 6 months with those who had exclusively breastfed for 3 months or more and those with mixed breastfeeding until at least 6 months of age. The intervention group had a rate of 8%

exclusive breastfeeding, compared with 0.6% in the control group. A high proportion (60%) of the control group was breastfeeding at 6 months.

Except for the Belarus study, no significant differences were noted in weight gain from 3 to 8 months of age, which averaged 400 to 500 g per month in both the exclusively breastfeeding and mixed breastfeeding groups. In the Belarus study, however, weight gains were much higher: 641 versus 612 g per month in the mixed breastfeeding versus exclusively breastfeeding groups.[85] Given the large weight gains in both groups in the Belarus study, the higher weight gain in the mixed breastfeeding group is not necessarily beneficial. Parallel findings were observed for length gain from 3 to 8 months of age, again with the Belarus study showing slightly but significantly more rapid length gains in the mixed breastfeeding group but with no significant differences observed in the 3 other studies. No significant differences were observed in head circumference in the Belarus study at 6 or 9 months of age, although the exclusively breastfeeding group had a significantly larger average head circumference at 12 months of age. Thus, infants exclusively breastfed for 6 months appear to grow adequately. In only the Belarus study, infants fed complementary foods before 6 months of age gained more weight and length than their exclusively breastfed counterparts.[85]

The Honduran studies discussed previously[4,73] also found equivalent growth and weight gain for 6-month exclusive breastfeeding and introduction of complementary foods at 4 months among infants with low birth weight; however, dropouts from the study had lower weights than did ongoing participants. A more recent study from India showed that stunted growth was least common among children receiving complementary foods at 3 months of age, whereas nearly two thirds of infants who exclusively breastfed until 6 months of age were stunted.[86]

Given current concerns about childhood obesity, it is also important to understand whether exclusive breastfeeding or the timing of introduction of complementary foods contribute to later adiposity. One recent US study collected information about early feeding habits from mothers of 313 children at 3 years of age and measured body composition of the children at 5 years of age. Results showed that neither breastfeeding for a longer duration nor introduction of complementary foods at 4 months of age is associated with childhood obesity at 5 years of age.[87]

Iron and Zinc Status

Few studies met the inclusion criteria for the systematic review regarding the effect of exclusive breastfeeding versus mixed breastfeeding on micronutrient status during infancy. A small Italian study[88] of hematologic outcomes included in the review reported that, at 12 months of age, infants in the exclusive breastfeeding group had a significantly higher hemoglobin concentration (117 vs 109 g/L), a nonsignificant reduction in anemia (hemoglobin concentration <110 g/L), a nonsignificantly higher ferritin concentration, and a nonsignificant reduction in the risk of a low ferritin concentration (<10 µg/L). In the Honduras trial,[89] the risk of iron deficiency at 6 months of age was low in the exclusive breastfeeding group when birth weight was >3000 g; however, the exclusive breastfeeding group exhibited a significantly lower hemoglobin concentration (104 g/L) than the group receiving iron-fortified complementary foods (109 g/L). Iron-fortified complementary feedings introduced before 6 months of age were not sufficient to prevent anemia among all the study infants. In a subsequent study of infants with low birth weight (1500–2500 g) in Honduras,[90] iron status at 6 months of age was higher in the group receiving iron-fortified complementary foods (113 g/L) than in the exclusive breastfeeding group (107 g/L). However, by 2 months of age, approximately half of the infants studied (75 of 157) had a hemoglobin concentration <100 g/L and were given iron supplements. Among infants receiving iron supplements, the exclusive breastfeeding group maintained a higher hemoglobin concentration (113 g/L) than the group receiving iron-fortified complementary foods (105 g/L). From these observations, Dewey et al[90] recommended that term infants with low birth weight be exclusively breastfed for 6 months with iron supplementation. It is evident that the duration for which the iron endowment at birth is adequate varies, and modifiers include birth weight, maternal iron status, and postnatal rate of growth.[91] Some infants will benefit from additional iron at 4 to 6 months of age. Whether the preferred source of iron should be complementary foods or medicinal preparations remains to be investigated under the characteristic environmental circumstances of the community where the infants reside.

Zinc status was reported for infants in one of the Honduran trials; no significant effect of complementary feeding was observed on the proportion of infants with a low zinc concentration (<70 µg/L) at 6 months of age.[90] As noted earlier, zinc supplementation has been found beneficial for some infants, and complementary foods (primarily meat) are required beginning between 4 and 6 months of age to prevent zinc deficiency and its consequences, including slowing of growth.[92]

Infection Risks

The Belarus study[85] found a significantly decreased risk in the exclusive breastfeeding group of 1 or more episodes of gastrointestinal infection in the first 12 months of life (adjusted risk ratio [RR] = 0.61 [95% CI, 0.41–0.93]) but not in hospitalization for gastrointestinal infection (RR = 0.79 [95% CI, 0.42–1.49]). Only 9% in the intervention group and 13% in the control group had more than 1 episode of diarrhea (95% CI, 0.41–0.91), both very low compared with original estimates that approximately 60% would have more than 1 episode. All other studies in the Cochrane review found no significant decrease in diarrhea risk with 6 months of exclusive breastfeeding,[67] and the Honduran study of infants with low birth weight found an increased prevalence of diarrhea in the group with 6 months of exclusive breastfeeding compared with the group with mixed breastfeeding (complementary feeding introduced from 4–6 months of age).[4]

Pooled results from the Belarus study,[92] an Australian study,[51] and a study from Arizona[93] showed no significant decrease in risk of upper respiratory tract infection, lower respiratory tract infection, hospitalization for respiratory infection, or otitis media with exclusive breastfeeding for 6 months.

Allergy Risks

In the Cochrane review, both the Belarus study[85] and a cohort study from Finland[94] recorded on atopic eczema at 1 year of age. The 2 studies showed statistical heterogeneity, with the Finnish study reporting a significantly reduced risk at 1 year of age (RR = 0.40 [95% CI, 0.21–0.78]) but no decrease in risk at 5 years of age. The larger Belarus study found a much lower absolute risk of atopic eczema than the Finnish study in both feeding groups and no decrease in risk with exclusive breastfeeding. Although the Finnish study also reported a decreased risk of food allergy by history at 1 year of age in the exclusive breastfeeding group, double food challenges showed no significant decrease in risk,[94] and no decrease in risk was seen at 5 years of age.[95] Neither the Australian[51] nor Belarus[85] studies found a significant decrease in recurrent (2 or more) episodes of wheezing in the exclusively breastfed group. In the Finnish study, the decrease in risk of any atopy at 5 years of age in the exclusive breastfeeding group was nonsignificant. Both the Finnish[95] and Australian[51] studies reported no decrease in risk of asthma at 5 to 6 years of age from exclusive breastfeeding. The Australian study found no decrease in risk of a positive skin-prick test result at 6 years of age in the exclusive breastfeeding group.

A group of experts conducting a systematic review of observational and interventional studies regarding dietary prevention of allergic diseases in infants and small children concluded that, for children at high risk of allergic diseases, breastfeeding combined with avoiding solid food and cow milk for at least the first 4 to 6 months of life was an effective preventive regimen.[96] However, prolonged exclusive breastfeeding for ≥9 months was reported to be associated with development of atopic dermatitis and symptoms of food hypersensitivity at 5 years of age and with symptoms of food hypersensitivity at 11 years of age in children with a family history of allergy.[97]

Developmental Effects

No studies from industrialized countries have compared neurocognitive development or behavior in exclusive breastfeeding versus mixed breastfeeding groups. However, Jain et al[98] conducted a critical review of 40 publications relating to breastfeeding and intellect. They found that 68% of the publications concluded that breastfeeding promotes intelligence but that the evidence from the higher-quality studies was less persuasive.

The 2 controlled clinical trials from Honduras reported that infants in the exclusive breastfeeding group crawled significantly sooner (an average of 0.8 months [0.3 to 1.3 months]) than those in the mixed breastfeeding group.[73] No difference was seen, however, in the mean age at which infants first sat from a lying position, and the 2 trials differed with respect to walking by 12 months of age, with a significantly lower proportion of exclusively breastfed infants not walking by 12 months of age in the first trial (RR = 0.66 [95% CI, 0.45–0.98]) but a nonsignificantly higher proportion not doing so in the second trial (RR = 1.12 [0.90–1.38]). Given the inconsistency in these results and the potential for biased maternal reporting attributable to nonblinding, no definitive conclusions can be drawn on this factor.

Conclusions: Lack of Evidence to Support or Refute Changing Current Recommendations

Study results to date suggest that there is no significant harm associated with introduction of complementary foods at 4 months of age and no significant benefit from exclusive breastfeeding for 6 months in terms of growth, development, iron/zinc nutriture (limited data), allergy, or infections. Likewise, very few studies demonstrate significant benefits of delaying complementary foods until 6 months in the industrialized world, but there is little theoretical or empirical evidence that healthy breastfed infants require complementary foods before 4 months of age. In fact, a systematic review by Lanigan et al[99] concerning the age of introduction of complementary foods to healthy, full-term infants found "a lack of clear evidence to either support or refute a change from current recommendations" for exclusive breastfeeding for 6 months for industrialized or developing nations. They did conclude, however, that the evidence suggests that subgroups, such as infants who consume low amounts of human milk and those with low birth weight, may need an earlier initiation of complementary foods.

In addition, these and other investigators who conducted reviews of multiple studies emphasized that additional randomized clinical trials and well-designed observational studies on relevant factors are needed. For example, the WHO report on complementary feeding in developing nations pointed to a particular need for controlled intervention trials in different settings assessing the effects of the timing and schedules of different complementary foods at different ages on factors such as total energy and energy consumed from human milk and complementary foods, total micronutrient intake and status, and growth/development and morbidity.[1] The Cochrane review recommended large randomized trials in industrialized and developing regions to rule out small adverse effects on growth and to confirm the reported health benefits of exclusive breastfeeding for 6 months.[67]

Complementary Foods: Desirable Nutritional Profile and Adequacy of Current Eating Patterns

Ideally, complementary foods will combine with human milk to provide the full range of nutrients needed for infant growth, development, and good health. The WHO has estimated the energy requirements from complementary foods (Table 5.3).

The WHO has also developed estimates of the amount of micronutrients needed from complimentary foods on the basis of data on the composition of human milk from women in industrialized countries and the desired nutrient density of complementary foods.[1]

Current Practices: Foods Eaten and Energy/Nutrient Adequacy

Current complementary feeding practices largely meet infants' energy and nutrient needs as discussed previously. However, some improvements in food choices would provide the foundation for sustained healthier eating habits later in life.

Currently Consumed Complementary Foods

In 2002, the Feeding Infants and Toddlers Study (FITS)[100] collected data on the food consumption patterns of 3022 US infants and toddlers by conducting telephone interviews during which parents provided 24-hour dietary recalls. The FITS data show that virtually all infants 12 months and younger consumed some form of milk—human or formula—each day; more infants consumed formula than human milk from 4 to 11 months of age. At 9 to 11 months of age, as many as 20.3% consumed cow milk (5.3% of these consumed reduced fat or nonfat) and 1.7% consumed soy milk.

The most commonly eaten solid foods were cereals (Table 5.5). Fewer than 15% of infants younger than 7 months consumed meats and other high-protein foods, but by 7 to 8 months of age, 54.9% did, increasing to 79.2% for 9- to 11-month-olds.

Table 5.5
Percentages of US Infants Consuming Cereals at Least Once a Day

Age Group	% Consuming Infant Cereals	% Consuming Noninfant Cereals
4–6 mo	64.8	0.6
7–8 mo	81.2	18.3
9–11 mo	63.8	44.3

Data from Fox MK, Devaney B, Jankowski L. Feeding infants and toddlers study: what foods are infants and toddlers eating? *J Am Diet Assoc.* 2004;104(Suppl 1):S22–S30.

In addition, the FITS found that infant eating patterns, in some ways, mirror those of older children and adults. For example, from 61.1% to 27.4% of infants 4 to 11 months of age consumed no vegetables each day, and French fries were one of the 3 most common vegetables consumed by infants 9 to 11 months of age. Approximately 24.5% of 7- to 11-month-olds ate no fruit; apples and bananas were the most commonly consumed fruits. Almost half (46%) of 7- to 8-month-olds consumed some type of dessert, sweet, or sweetened beverage daily, and the percentage increased as age increased.

Nutrient Adequacy
The FITS data show that the mean usual intake of infants 11 months and younger equals or exceeds Adequate Intake levels for all nutrients. Evidence did show that some infants 7 to 11 months of age had dietary intakes judged to be inadequate for iron (7.5% estimated prevalence) and/or zinc (4.2% estimated prevalence).[101]

Dietary Supplements
The FITS also found that, despite the overall nutrient adequacy of current eating patterns, some infants received dietary supplements—8% of those

4 to 5 months of age and 19% of those 6 to 11 months of age, with prevalence continuing to increase with age. Most received only a multivitamin and/or mineral supplement. The investigators saw no significant difference between supplement users and nonusers in mean daily intakes of nutrients or nutrient density from foods alone and few differences in consumption, although more supplement nonusers had a lower-than-estimated average requirement level of vitamin E than did supplement users. However, the FITS did find some evidence of excessive intakes of vitamin A, zinc, and folic acid in both supplement user and nonuser toddlers, and approximately 60% of older infants in both groups had excessive zinc intake.[102] These nutrients are also widely used as food fortificants.

Practical Recommendations for Initiating Complementary Foods

The following guiding principles are provided for introducing complementary foods, in part on the basis of current US practices identified in the FITS:

1. **Introduce one "single-ingredient" new food at a time,** and do not introduce other new foods for 3 to 5 days to observe for possible allergic reactions. In practice, iron-fortified infant rice cereal appears to be one of the solid foods least likely to cause an allergic reaction. The foods most commonly causing infant allergies are cow milk, hen eggs, soy, peanuts, tree nuts (and seeds), wheat, fish, and shellfish, although there is no good evidence that delaying their introduction affects the overall incidence of atopic disease in infants and children.[103] Multigrain cereals or mixed dishes, such as macaroni and cheese, are not recommended as first foods because of the difficulty in identifying the food responsible for an adverse reaction, should one occur.

2. **Choose first foods that provide key nutrients and help meet energy needs.** Although no comprehensive research has been conducted on which specific complementary foods to provide or in which order, the AAP recommends iron-fortified infant cereals and pureed meats as good first foods, because they contain ample protein, iron, and zinc. The FITS finding that iron and zinc are the nutrients most likely to be deficient in the diets of infants and toddlers in the United States emphasizes this priority. A randomized, controlled study comparing the effects of introducing meat or iron-fortified cereal as the first complementary food for exclusively breastfed infants found that meat-fed infants had substantially higher zinc intake than did cereal-fed infants. In addition, meat-fed infants had a higher rate of growth in head circumference and a possible trend toward other developmental advantages. The study also found

that the infants accepted the meat similarly to other new complementary foods.[92]

3. **Introduce a variety of foods by the end of the first year.** Although many factors affect food choices and habits, a foundation for healthy eating patterns may be established in childhood.[104] Although more guidance is needed on the timing of transitions and which foods to emphasize, feeding behaviors that minimize variety and diversity limit important sources of nutrients in the diets of young children and could compromise nutritional status. The FITS findings of low toddler consumption of fruits and vegetables, little variety in foods eaten, and high consumption of sweets, French fries, and carbonated beverages suggests the need to increase early attention to pattern of eating to maintain and promote health.[105] Introducing a wide variety of developmentally appropriate, nutrient-rich foods takes advantage of the opportunity to instill positive initial habits. Once an infant has accepted meat and cereal, strained or pureed fruits and vegetables can be added to the complementary diet. When offering a new food, parents need to provide approximately 8 to 15 exposures to enhance food acceptance.[106]

4. **Withhold cow milk (and other "milks" not specifically formulated for infants) during the first year of life.** Cow milk does not have the optimal concentration of a variety of nutrients to support the rapidly growing infant.[107] Given the FITS finding that approximately 20% of infants had received cow milk daily before 1 year of age, the 1-year message may need reinforcement. In addition, when cow milk is introduced at 1 year of age, only whole cow milk, not reduced-fat alternatives, should be offered; data from the FITS show that approximately one quarter of the cow milk served to infants and toddlers was reduced fat.[106]

5. **Ensure adequate calcium intake when transitioning to complementary foods.** Providing cow milk at the appropriate age helps boost calcium intake. However, milk consumption and calcium intake have been falling in the United States in recent years. The FITS found that by 24 months of age, some infants drank little or no milk in a day. Although mean intakes of calcium among toddlers exceeded adequate intake levels, low milk consumption may set a pattern for inadequate calcium intake in later years. For toddlers with lactose intolerance and others who do not consume cow milk products, careful planning is needed to ensure adequate calcium intake, especially because calcium-rich nondairy foods are not typically part of US toddlers' diets. Although the

AAP recommends soy "milks" as appropriate for some groups (see Table 5.1), natural soy beverages contain only small amounts of calcium. Calcium-fortified products are available, but calcium bioavailability differs among products. For example, although tricalcium phosphate-fortified soy milk was shown to have lower calcium bioavailability than cow milk in men,[108] calcium carbonate-fortified soy milk showed equivalent calcium absorption to cow milk for premenopausal women in another study.[109] Goat milk is not a recommended alternative to cow milk.[107]

6. **Do not introduce fruit juices during the first 6 months of life.** Thereafter, offer only 100% juices, limited to 4 to 6 oz daily for children 1 to 6 years of age (see Table 1). Data from the FITS and other research show that 21% of infants 4 to 6 months of age were already consuming fruit juice and that some children consume more than 6 oz per day, so these messages may need emphasis. In addition, types of fruit juices provided should be varied to maximize nutrition. For example, the highly popular apple juice is low in folate compared with orange juice.[110]

AAP

Recommendations from the American Academy of Pediatrics

The **American Academy of Pediatrics** recommends an upper limit of 4 to 6 oz of juice for children 1 to 6 years of age and 8 to 12 oz for children 7 to 18 years of age. Children should be encouraged to consume whole fruits to meet recommended levels of fruit intake. Pediatricians should routinely discuss the use of 100% fruit juice and fruit drinks and should educate parents about the differences between the two.

Pediatrics. 2001;107:1210-1213 (reaffirmed October 2006)

---

7. **Ensure safe ingestion and adequate nutrition when choosing and preparing homemade foods.**

   * Mash or puree solid foods for infants 12 months and younger so foods can be swallowed without risk of aspiration.

   * Avoid hot dogs, nuts, grapes, raisins, raw carrots, popcorn, and rounded candies in children younger than 4 years.

   * Avoid adding salt or sugar to complementary foods. Amounts of constituent nutrients are sufficient in the foods themselves to meet requirements. The addition of salt and sugar is not necessary for acceptance—that is best accomplished by repeated presentation of the food.

- Warm solid foods to body temperature, but do not heat them excessively. After microwaving food for an infant, mix the food thoroughly and check the temperature to avoid burning the infant's mouth.

- Ensure nutrient and energy sufficiency when using home-prepared foods. In a European study, investigators found that many home-prepared complementary foods were low in energy, fat, protein, iron, and zinc. In addition, nutrient content was more variable than for infants fed commercial baby foods, despite mothers' intention to provide a more nutritious diet by preparing foods at home.[111]

8. **Manage and monitor each infant individually to detect and correct for slow growth or other adverse outcomes.** For breastfed infants, this means ensuring adequate breastfeeding techniques and optimizing human milk intake and productivity by the mother before introducing complementary foods. Because of evidence that formula displaces human milk more readily than does solid food, complementary feeding of breastfed infants should focus on solid foods rather than on formula. Breastfed and formula-fed infants may have their hemoglobin concentration and mean corpuscular volume tested at 9 to 12 months of age to ensure adequate hematologic status and to initiate treatment if iron deficiency is detected.

AAP

American Academy of Pediatrics Recommendations

In the United States and Canada, processed infant foods have not been implicated in methemoglobinemia associated with food or water intake in infants. Although raw spinach and beets have a higher nitrate content than do other infant foods, one or more protective factors may prevent the extrinsic or intrinsic formation of toxic concentrations of nitrite from these foods as commercially processed for feeding of infants. Nitrate contamination of drinking water, which may occur as the result of runoff from fields fertilized with nitrates, represents a potential hazard.

AAP

The American Academy of Pediatrics Committee on Nutrition recommends the following foods as excellent sources of iron in the diet of the infant.

Fitting Iron-Rich Foods Into Different Meals Eaten by An Older Infant*

Sample meal food items[†]	Iron content (mg)[‡]
Morning meal could include:	
Baby food, rice cereal, dry, 2 tbsp	2.4
Poached egg, 1/2 large egg	0.5
Baby food or other fruit (vitamin C source)	
Morning snack could include:	
Prunes, dehydrated (low moisture), stewed, 1/8 cup	0.4
Whole wheat bread, commercially prepared, 1/4 slice	0.2
Vitamin C-fortified juice (vitamin C source)	
Mid day meal could include:	
Baby food, lamb, junior, 1/2 to 1 jar (2.5 oz)	0.6 to 1.2
Baby food, peas, strained, 1/2 jar (1.7 oz)	0.5
White bread, commercially prepared, 1/4 slice	0.2
Baby food or other fruit (vitamin C source)	
Afternoon snack could include:	
Baby food, oatmeal cereal, dry, 1 tbsp	1.6
Baby food, green beans, strained, 1/2 jar (3 oz) (vitamin C source)	0.4
Evening meal could include:	
Baby food, chicken, strained, 1/2 to 1 jar (2.5 oz)	0.5 to 1.0
Baby food, sweet potatoes, junior, 1/2 jar (3 oz)	0.3
Enriched white rice, long grain, regular, cooked (1/8 to 1/4 cup)	0.2 to 0.5
Baby food or fresh fruit (vitamin C source)	

* For example, a 6- to 12-month-old breastfed infant who is receiving no iron-fortified formula. A 6-month old infant starting solid foods would not eat the variety or quantities of foods shown here.

† Assume that an adequate quantity of human milk and other foods to meet other nutrient needs are consumed.

‡ Figures are rounded. The amount of iron obtained depends on the quantity of food that an infant actually consumes and bioavailability factors (eg, foods and beverages that may be consumed that may inhibit or enhance iron absorption of any non-heme iron).

References

1. Brown K, Dewey K, Allen L. *Complementary Feeding of Young Children in Developing Countries: A Review of Current Scientific Knowledge*. Geneva, Switzerland: World Health Organization; 1998. Document No. WHO/NUT/98.1. Available at: http://www.who.int/child-adolescent-health/publications/NUTRITION/WHO_NUT_98.1.htm. Accessed November 2, 2007

2. Foote KD, Marriott LD. Weaning of infants. *Arch Dis Child*. 2003;88:488–492

3. Cohen RJ, Brown KH, Canahuati J, Rivera LL, Dewey KG. Effects of age of introduction of complementary foods on infant breast milk intake, total energy intake, and growth: a randomized intervention study in Honduras. *Lancet*. 1994;344:288–293

4. Dewey KG, Cohen RJ, Brown KH, Rivera LL. Age of introduction of complementary foods and growth of term, low-birth weight, breast-fed infants: a randomized intervention study in Honduras. *Am J Clin Nutr*. 1999;69:679–686

5. Drewitt R, Paymon B, Whiteby S. Effect of complementary foods on sucking and milk intake in breastfed babies: an experimental study. *J Reprod Infant Psychol*. 1987;5:133–143

6. Stuff JE, Nichols BL. Nutrient intake and growth performance of older infants fed human milk. *J Pediatr*. 1989;115:959–968

7. American Academy of Pediatrics, Section on Breastfeeding. Policy statement: breastfeeding and the use of human milk. *Pediatrics*. 2005;115:496–506

8. American Academy of Pediatrics, Committee on Nutrition. Optimizing bone health and calcium intakes of infants, children, and adolescents. *Pediatrics*. 2006;117:578–585

9. American Academy of Pediatrics, Committee on Nutrition. Cholesterol in childhood. *Pediatrics*. 1998;101:141–147

10. American Academy of Pediatrics, Committee on Nutrition. Practical significance of lactose intolerance in children. *Pediatrics*. 1990;86:643–644

11. Gartner LM, Greer, FR, American Academy of Pediatrics, Section on Breastfeeding and Committee on Nutrition. Prevention of rickets and vitamin D deficiency: new guidelines for vitamin D intake. *Pediatrics*. 2003;111:908–910

12. American Academy of Pediatrics, Committee on Nutrition. The use and misuse of fruit juice in pediatrics. *Pediatrics*. 2001;107:1210–1213

13. American Academy of Pediatrics, Committee on Nutrition. The use of soy protein-based formulas in infant feeding. *Pediatrics*. In press

14. Fomon SJ, Nelson SE. Body composition of the male and female reference infants. *Annu Rev Nutr*. 2002;22:1–17

15. Food and Agriculture Organization of the United Nations and World Health Organization, Ad Hoc Expert Committee. *Energy and Protein Requirements*. Rome, Italy: Food and Agriculture Organization of the United Nations; 1973

16. Butte NF, Hopkinson JM, Wong WW, Smith EO, Ellis KJ. Body composition during the first 2 years of life: an updated reference. *Pediatr Res*. 2000;47:578–585

17. Fomon SJ, Bell EF. Energy. In: Fomon SJ, ed. *Nutrition of Normal Infants*. St Louis, MO: Mosby-Year Book; 1993:103–120

18. Butte NF. Energy requirements of infants. *Public Health Nutr*. 2005;8(7A):953–967

19. Food and Agricultural Organization of the United Nations and World Health Organization. FAO/WHO/UNU Expert Consultation. *Energy and Protein Requirements.* Geneva, Switzerland: World Health Organization; 1985. WHO Technical Report No. 724. Available at: http://www.fao.org/DOCREP/003/AA040E/AA040E00.htm. Accessed November 2, 2007

20. Institute of Medicine. *Dietary Reference Intakes for Vitamin A, Vitamin K, Arsenic, Boron, Chromium, Copper, Iodine, Iron, Manganese, Molybdenum, Nickel, Silicon, Vanadium, and Zinc.* Washington, DC: National Academies Press; 2000

21. Picciano MF. Representative values for constituents of human milk. *Pediatr Clin North Am.* 2001;48:263–264

22 Fomon SJ , Nelson SE, Ziegler EE. Retention of iron by infants. *Annu Rev Nutr.* 2000;20:273–290

23. American Academy of Pediatrics, Committee on Nutrition. Iron fortification of infant formulas. *Pediatrics.* 1999;104:119–123

24. Fomon SJ. Feeding normal infants: rationale for recommendations. *J Am Diet Assoc.* 2001;101:1002–1005

25. Centers for Disease Control and Prevention. Iron deficiency—United States, 1999–2000. *MMWR Morb Mortal Wkly Rep.* 2002;51:897–879

26. Sandstrom B, Cederblad A, Lonnerdal B. Zinc absorption from human milk, cow's milk, and infant formulas. *Am J Dis Child.* 1983;137:726–729

27. Dewey KG, Heinig MJ, Nommsen LA, Lonnerdal B. Zinc status in breastfed infants [lett]. *Lancet.* 1992;340:1417

28. Checkley W, Gilman RH, Black RE, et al. Effects of nutritional status on diarrhea in Peruvian children. *J Pediatr.* 2002;140:210–218

29. Brown KH, Peerson JM, Rivera J, Allen LH. Effect of supplemental zinc on the growth and serum zinc concentrations of prepubertal children: a meta-analysis of randomized controlled trials. *Am J Clin Nutr.* 2002;7:1062–1071

30. Peerson JM, Allen LH. Effect of zinc supplementation on children's growth: a meta-analysis of intervention trials. *Bibl Nutr Dieta.* 1998;54:76–83

31. Bhutta ZA, Black RE, Brown KH, et al. Prevention of diarrhea and pneumonia by zinc supplementation in children in developing countries: pooled analysis of randomized controlled trials. *J Pediatr.* 1999;135:689–697

32. Ashworth A, Morris SS, Lira PI, Granthan-Mcgregor SM. Zinc supplementation, mental development and behaviour in low birth weight term infants in northeast Brazil. *Eur J Clin Nutr.* 1998;52:223–227

33. Sandstead HH, Penland JG, Alcock NW, et al. Effects of repletion with zinc and other micronutrients on neuropsychologic performance and growth of Chinese children. *Am J Clin Nutr.* 1998;68:470S–475S

34. Bentley ME, Caulfield LE, Ram M, Santizo MC, Hurtado E, Rivera JA, Ruel MT, Brown KH. Zinc supplementation affects the activity patterns of rural Guatemalan infants. *J Nutr.* 1997;127:1333–1338

35. Sazawal S, Bentley M, Black RE, Dhingra P, George S, Bhan MK . Effect of zinc supplementation on observed activity in low socioeconomic Indian preschool children. *Pediatrics.* 1996;98:1132–1137

36. Friel JK, Andrews WL, Matthew JD, Long DR, Cornel AM, Cox M, McKim E, Zerbe GO. Zinc supplementation in very-low-birth-weight infants. *J Pediatr Gastroenterol Nutr.* 1993;17:97–104

37. Sazawal S, Black RE, Jalla S, Mazumdar S, Sinha A, Bhan MK. Zinc supplementation reduces the incidence of acute lower respiratory infections in infants and preschool children: A double-blind, controlled trial. *Pediatrics.* 1998;102:1–5

38. Institute of Medicine. *Dietary Reference Intakes for Calcium, Phosphorus, Magnesium, Vitamin D, and Fluoride.* Washington, DC: National Academies Press; 1997

39. Tomashek KM, Nesby S, Scanlon KS, et al. Commentary: nutritional rickets in Georgia. *Pediatrics.* 2001;107(4):e45. Available at: http://pediatrics.aappublications.org/cgi/content/full/107/4/e45. Accessed July 30, 2007

40. Kreiter SR, Schwartz RP, Kirkman HN Jr, Charlton PA, Calikoglu AS, Davenport ML. Nutritional rickets in African American breast-fed infants. *J Pediatr.* 2000;137:153–157

41. Namgung R, Tsang RC, Lee C, Han DG, Ho ML, Sierra RI. Low total body bone mineral content and high bone resorption in Korean winter-born versus summer-born newborn infants. *J Pediatr.* 1998;132:421–425

42. Weisberg P, Scanlon KS, Li R, Cogswell ME. Nutritional rickets among children in the United States: review of cases reported between 1986 and 2003. *Am J Clin Nutr.* 2004;80:1697S–1705S

43. Hamosh M. Digestion in the newborn. *Clin Perinatol.* 1996;23:191–209

44. Harris G, Thomas A, Booth DA. Development of salt taste in infancy. *Dev Psychol.* 1990;26:534–538

45. Howie PW, Forsyth JS, Ogston SA, Clark A, du V Florey CD. Protective effect of breast feeding against infection. *BMJ.* 1990;300:11–16

46. Cunningham AS, Jelliffe DB, Jelliffe EF. Breast-feeding and health in the 1980s: a global epidemiologic review. *J Pediatr.* 1991;118:659–666

47. Raisler J, Alexander C, O'Campo P. Breast-feeding and infant illness: a dose-response relationship? *Am J Public Health.* 1999;89:25–30

48. Ford RP, Taylor BJ, Mitchell EA, et al. Breastfeeding and the risk of sudden infant death syndrome. *Int J Epidemiol.* 1993;22:885–890

49. Saarinen U, Backman A, Kajosaari M, Simes M. Prolonged breast-feeding as prophylaxis for atopic disease. *Lancet.* 1979;2:163–166

50. Hide DW, Guyer BM. Clinical manifestations of allergy related to breast and cows' milk feeding. *Arch Dis Child.* 1981;56:172–175

51. Oddy WH, Holt PG, Sly PD, et al. Association between breast feeding and asthma in 6 year old children: findings of a prospective birth cohort study. *BMJ.* 1999;319:815–819

52. Kramer MS, Moroz B. Do breast feeding and delayed introduction of solid foods protect against subsequent atopic eczema? *J Pediatr.*1981;98:546–550

53. von Kries R, Koletzko B, Sauerwald T, et al. Breast feeding and obesity: cross sectional study. *BMJ.* 1999;319:147–150

54. Mayer EJ, Hamman RF, Gay EC, Lezotte DC, Savitz A, Klingensmith GJ. Reduced risk of IDDM among breastfed children. *Diabetes.* 1988;37:1625–1632

55. Owen CG, Martin RM, Whincup PH, Smith GD, Cook DG. Does breastfeeding influence risk of type 2 diabetes in later life? A quantitative analysis of published evidence. *Am J Clin Nutr.* 2006;84:1043–1054

56. Koletzko S, Sherman P, Corey M, Griffiths A, Smith C. Role of infant feeding practices in development of Crohn's disease in childhood. *BMJ.* 1989;298:1617–1618

57. Davis M, Savitz DA, Graubard BI. Infant feeding and childhood cancer. *Lancet.* 1988;2:365–368

58. Davis MK. Review of the evidence for an association between infant feeding and childhood cancer. *Int J Cancer.* 1998;11(suppl):29–33

59. Lucas A, Morley R, Cole TJ, Lister G, Leeson-Payne C. Breast milk and subsequent intelligence quotient in children born preterm. *Lancet.* 1992;339:261–264

60. Lanting CI, Fidler V, Huisman M, Touwen BC, Boersma ER. Neurological differences between 9-year-old children fed breast-milk or formula-milk as babies. *Lancet.* 1994;344:1319–1322

61. Horwood L, Fergusson D. Breastfeeding and later cognitive and academic outcomes. *Pediatrics.* 1998;101(1):e9. Available at: http://pediatrics.aappublications.org/cgi/content/full/101/1/e9. Accessed July 30, 2007

62. Anderson JW, Johnstone BM, Remley DT. Breast-feeding and cognitive development: a meta-analysis. *Am J Clin Nutr.* 1999;70:525–535

63. Jason JM, Nieburg P, Marks JS. Mortality and infectious disease associated with infant-feeding practices in developing countries. *Pediatrics.* 1984;74:702–727

64. Feachem R, Koblinsky M. Interventions for the control of diarrhoeal diseases among young children: promotion of breast-feeding. *Bull WHO.* 1984;62:271–291

65. WHO Collaborative Study Team on the Role of Breastfeeding on the Prevention of Infant Mortality. Effect of breastfeeding on infant and child mortality due to infectious diseases in less developed countries: a pooled analysis. *Lancet.* 2000;355:451–455

66. WHO. *The Optimal Duration of Exclusive Breastfeeding: Report of an Expert Consultation.* Geneva, Switzerland: World Health Organization; 2001

67. Kramer M, Kakuma R. The optimal duration of exclusive breastfeeding. *Cochrane Database Syst Rev.* 2002;(1):CD003517

68. Rowland MG, Barrell RA, Whitehead RG. Bacterial contamination in traditional Gambian weaning foods. *Lancet.* 1978;1:136–138

69. Rowland MG. The weanling's dilemma: are we making progress? *Acta Paediatr Scand Suppl.* 1986;323(Suppl):33–42

70. Waterlow JC, Thomson AM. Observations on the adequacy of breast-feeding. *Lancet.* 1979;2:238–242

71. Whitehead RG, Paul AA. Growth charts and the assessment of infant feeding practices in the western world and in developing countries. *Early Hum Dev.* 1984;9:187–207

72. Shrimpton R, Victora CG, de Onis M, Lima RC, Blossner M, Clugston G. Worldwide timing of growth faltering: implications for nutritional interventions. *Pediatrics.* 2001;107(5):e75. Available at: http://pediatrics.aappublications.org/cgi/content/full/107/5/e75. Accessed July 30, 2007

73. Dewey KG, Cohen RJ, Brown KH, Rivera LL. Effects of exclusive breastfeeding for four versus six months on maternal nutritional status and infant motor development: results of two randomized trials in Honduras. *J Nutr.* 2001;131:262–267

74. Collaborative Group on Hormonal Factors in Breast Cancer. Breast cancer and breastfeeding: collaborative reanalysis of individual data from 47 epidemiological studies in 30 countries, including 50302 women with breast cancer and 96973 women without the disease. *Lancet.* 2002;360:187–195

75. MacDonald A. Is breast best? Is early solid feeding harmful? *J R Soc Health.* 2003;123:169–174

76. World Health Organization, Working Group on Infant Growth. *An Evaluation of Infant Growth.* Geneva, Switzerland: World Health Organization, Nutrition Unit; 1994. Document No. WHO/NUT/94.8. Available at: http://whqlibdoc.who.int/hq/1994/WHO_NUT_94.8.pdf. Accessed November 2, 2007

77. Dewey KG, Peerson JM, Brown KH, et al. Growth of breast-fed infants deviates from current reference data: a pooled analysis of US, Canadian, and European data sets. *Pediatrics.* 1995;96:495–503

78. Nielsen G, Thomsen B, Michaelsen K. Influence of breastfeeding and complementary food on growth between 5 and 10 months. *Acta Paediatr.* 1998;87:911–917

79. Hediger ML, Overpeck MD, Ruan WJ, Troendle JF. Early infant feeding and growth status of US-born infants and children aged 4–71 mo: analyses from the third National Health and Nutrition Examination Survey, 1988–1994. *Am J Clin Nutr.* 2000;72:159–167

80. Haschke F, van't Hof MA. Euro-Growth references for breast-fed boys and girls: influence of breast-feeding and solids on growth until 36 months of age. Euro-Growth Study Groups. *J Pediatr Gastroenterol Nutr.* 2000;31(Suppl 1):S60–S71

81. Kramer MS, Guo T, Platt RW, et al. Breastfeeding and infant growth: biology or bias? *Pediatrics.* 2002;110:343–347

82. Whitehead RG. Paul AA. Long-term adequacy of exclusive breastfeeding: how scientific research has led to revised opinions. *Proc Nutr Soc.* 2000;59:17–23

83. World Health Organization. WHO Child Growth Standards based on length/height, weight, and age. *Acta Paediatr Suppl.* 2006;450:76–85

84. WHO Working Group on the Growth Reference Protocol, WHO Task Force on Methods for the Natural Regulation of Fertility. Growth of healthy infants and the timing, type, and frequency of complementary foods. *Am J Clin Nutr.* 2002;76:620–627

85. Kramer MS, Chalmers B, Hodnett ED, et al. Promotion of breastfeeding intervention trial (PROBIT): a randomized trial in the Republic of Belarus. *JAMA.* 2001;285:413–420

86. Padmadas SS, Hutter I, Willekens F. Weaning initiation patterns and subsequent linear growth progression among children aged 2–4 years in India. *Int J Epidemiol.* 2002;31:855–863

87. Burdette HL, Whitaker RC, Hall WC, Daniels SR. Breastfeeding, introduction of complementary foods, and adiposity at 5 y of age. *Am J Clin Nutr.* 2006;83:550–558

88. Pisacane A, De Vizia B, Valiante A, et al. Iron status in breast-fed infants. *J Pediatr.* 1995;127:429–431

89. Dewey KG, Cohen RJ, Rivera LL, Brown KH. Effects of age of introduction of complementary foods on iron status of breast-fed infants in Honduras. *Am J Clin Nutr.* 1998;67:878–884

90. Dewey KG, Cohen RJ, Brown KH. Exclusive breast-feeding for 6 months, with iron supplementation, maintains adequate micronutrient status among term, low-birthweight, breast-fed infants in Honduras. *J Nutr.* 2004;134:1091–1098

91. Meinzen-Derr JK, Guerrero ML, Altaye M, Ortega-Gallegos H, Ruiz-Palacios GM, Morrow AL. Risk of infant anemia is associated with exclusive breast-feeding and maternal anemia in a Mexican cohort. *J Nutr.* 2006;136:452–458

92. Krebs NF, Wescott JE, Butler N, Robinson C, Bell M, Hambidge KM. Meat as a first complementary food for breastfed infants: feasibility and impact on zinc intake and status. *J Pediatr Gastroenterol Nutr.* 2006;42:207–214

93. Duncan B, Ey J, Holberg CJ, Wright AL, Martinez FD, Taussig LM. Exclusive breast-feeding for at least 4 months protects against otitis media. *Pediatrics.* 1993;91:867–872

94. Kajosaari M, Saarinen U. Prophylaxis of atopic disease by six months' total solid food elimination. Evaluation of 135 exclusively breast-fed infants of atopic families. *Acta Paediatr Scand.* 1983;72:411–414

95. Kajosaari M. Atopy prevention in childhood: the role of diet: a prospective 5-year follow-up of high-risk infants with six months exclusive breastfeeding and solid food elimination. *Pediatr Allergy Immunol.* 1994;5:26–28

96. Muraro A, Dreborg S, Halken S, et al. Dietary prevention of allergic diseases in infants and small children. Part III: critical review of published peer-reviewed observational and interventional studies and final recommendations. *Pediatr Allergy Immunol.* 2004;15:291–307

97. Pesonen M, Kallio MJT, Ranki A, Siimes MA. Prolonged exclusive breastfeeding is associated with increased atopic dermatitis: a prospective follow-up study of unselected healthy newborns from birth to age 20 years *Clin Exp Allergy.* 2006;36:1011–1018

98. Jain A, Concato J, Leventhal JM. How good is the evidence linking breastfeeding and intelligence? *Pediatrics.* 2002;109:1044–1053

99. Lanigan JA, Bishop J, Kimber AC, Morgan J. Systematic review concerning the age of introduction of complementary foods to the healthy full-term infant. *Eur J Clin Nutr.* 2001;55:309–320

100. Fox MK, Pac S, Devaney B, Jankowski L. Feeding infants and toddlers study: what foods are infants and toddlers eating? *J Am Diet Assoc.* 2004;104:S22–S30

101. Devaney B, Ziegler P, Pac S, Karwe V, Barr SI. Nutrient intakes of infants and toddlers. *J Am Diet Assoc.* 2004;104:S14–S21

102. Briefel R, Hanson C, Fox MK, Novak T, Ziegler P. Feeding infants and toddlers study: Do vitamin and mineral supplements contribute to nutrient adequacy or excess among U.S. infants and toddlers? *J Am Diet Assoc.* 2006;106:S52–S65

103. Greer FR, Sicherer S, Burks AW, American Academy of Pediatrics, Section on Allergy and Immunology and Committee on Nutrition. The effects of early nutritional interventions on the development of atopic disease in infants and children: the role of maternal dietary restriction, breastfeeding, timing of introduction of complementary foods, and hydrolyzed formulas. *Pediatrics.* In press

104. Stang J. Improving the eating patterns of infants and toddlers. *J Am Diet Assoc.* 2006;106:S7–S9

105. Briefel RR, Reidy K, Karwe V, Jankowski L, Hendricks K. Toddlers' transition to table foods: impact on nutrient intakes and food patterns. *J Am Diet Assoc.* 2004;104(Suppl 1):S38–44

106. Briefel RR, Reidy K, Darwe V, Devaney B. Feeding infants and toddlers study: improvements needed in meeting infant feeding recommendations. *J Am Diet Assoc.* 2004;104(Suppl 1):S31–S37

107. Goldberg JP, Folta SC, Must A. Milk: can a "good" food be so bad? *Pediatrics.* 2002;110:826–832

108. Heaney RP, Dowell MS, Rafferty K, Bierman J. Bioavailability of the calcium in fortified soy imitation milk, with some observations on method. *Am J Clin Nutr.* 2000;71:1166–1169

109. Zhao Y, Martin BR, Weaver CM. Calcium bioavailability of calcium carbonate fortified soymilk is equivalent to cow's milk in young women. *J Nutr.* 2005;135:2379–2382

110. Skinner JD, Ziegler P, Ponza M. Transitions in infants' and toddlers' beverage patterns. *J Am Diet Assoc.* 2004;104:S45–S50

111. Stordy BJ, Redfern AM, Morgan JB. Healthy eating for infants—mothers' actions. *Acta Paediatr.* 1995;84:733–741

Feeding the Child and Adolescent

II

Feeding the Child

After infancy, children experience significant developmental progress that is fundamentally tied to the evolution and establishment of eating behavior. In contrast to infancy, however, the period from 1 year of age to puberty is a slower period of physical growth. Birth weight triples during the first year of life but does not quadruple until 2 years of age; birth length increases by 50% during the first year but does not double until 4 years of age. Although growth patterns vary in individual children, from 2 years to puberty, children gain an average of 2 to 3 kg (4.5–6.5 lb) and grow in height 5 to 8 cm (2.5–3.5 in) per year. As growth rates decrease during the preschool years, appetites decrease and food intake may appear erratic and unpredictable. Parental confusion and concern are not uncommon. Frequently expressed concerns include the limited variety of foods ingested, dawdling and distractibility, limited consumption of vegetables and meats, and a desire for too many sweets. Parental concern regarding children's eating behaviors, whether warranted or unfounded, should be addressed with developmentally appropriate nutrition information. Anticipatory guidance for parents and caregivers is key to preventing many feeding problems.

An important goal of early childhood nutrition is to ensure children's current and future health by fostering the development of healthy eating behaviors. Caregivers are called on to offer foods at developmentally appropriate moments—matching the child's age and stage of development with his or her nutrition needs. Appropriate limits for children's eating are set by adhering to a division of responsibility in child feeding.[1] Caregivers are responsible for providing a variety of nutritious foods, defining the structure and timing of meals, and creating a mealtime environment that facilitates eating and social exchange. Children are responsible for participating in choices about food selection and determining how much is consumed at each eating occasion.

Toddlerhood

Toddler eating patterns are characterized by independence in terms of both the physical skills that allow them to become mobile and to self-feed and the acquisition of language skills that enable them to verbally express eating preferences and needs. Between 7 and 12 months of age, most infants become capable of grasping food with their hands, removing food from the spoon with their lips, and making the transition to eating soft foods or those with tiny lumps without gagging.[1,2] By 15 months of age, the toddler is generally capable of self-feeding firmer table foods and drinking from a "sippy" cup without help.[2] Weaning from the bottle should occur at the beginning of toddlerhood (12–15 months of age), and bedtime bottles should be particularly discouraged because of their association with dental caries, as should bottles containing juice at any time of the day.[2] Between the first and second year, infants move from gross motor skills required for holding a spoon to developing fine motor skills needed to scoop food, dip food, and bring the spoon to the mouth with limited spilling.[1,2] Supporting self-feeding is thought to encourage the maintenance of self-regulation of energy intake and the mastery of feeding skills. Given earlier opportunities for mastery of self-feeding skills, the older toddler (2 years of age) is ready to consume most of the same foods offered to the rest of the family, with some extra preparation to prevent choking and gagging.

Toddlers are continually engaged in understanding the cause-and-effect relationship. In the eating domain, this translates into using utensils to move foods and using food and eating to elicit responses from the parent. These interactions are part of children's learning about the family's and culture's standards for behavior; children as young as 2 years of age have demonstrated the ability to evaluate their actions according to its badness or goodness in relation to parental standards for behavior.[3] An example of this type of learning is the toddler's response of "uh-oh" to dropping food or drink on the floor. Toddlers seek attention and will find ways, positive or negative, to engage the notice of parents. Helping parents focus on children's positive eating behaviors rather than on food refusals or negative conduct, will keep mealtime pleasant and productive.

Preventing Choking

Gagging and choking are realistic concerns for the toddler. The chewing and swallowing functions are not fully developed until 8 years of age, so a number of precautions should be followed to avoid choking. The toddler should be given foods that gradually build self-feeding skills—starting with soft, mashed, or ground foods and building to prepared table foods by 15 to 18 months of age. Foods that may be hard to control in the mouth and may be easily lodged in the esophagus, such as nuts, raw carrots, popcorn, and round candy, should be avoided. Other potentially problematic foods—like hot dogs, grapes, and string cheese—may be modified by cutting them into small pieces. The caregiver should always be present during feeding and children should be seated in a high chair during mealtimes. The mealtime environment ideally should be free of distractions like television, loud music, and activities. Eating in the car should be discouraged, because: 1) aiding the child quickly is difficult if the only adult present is driving; and 2) with obesity prevention in mind, eating should not be encouraged in environments that are not related to family meals (in cars, in front of television/computers, etc). Finally, analgesics used to numb the gums during teething may anesthetize the posterior pharynx; children who receive such medications should be carefully observed during feeding.

Food Acceptance

Preferences for the taste of sweet have been observed shortly after birth,[4] and young children show the capacity to readily form preferences for the flavors of energy-rich foods.[5] Acceptance of other foods, however, is not immediate and may occur only after 8 to 10 exposures to those foods in a noncoercive manner.[6-8] The findings of one study indicate that many parents are not aware of the lengthy but normal course of food acceptance in young children; approximately 25% of mothers with toddlers reported offering new foods only 1 or 2 times before deciding whether the child liked it, and approximately half made similar judgments after serving new foods 3 to 5 times.[9] Touching, smelling, and playing with new foods as well as putting them in the mouth and spitting them back out are normal exploratory behaviors that precede acceptance and even willingness to taste and swallow foods.[10] Beginning around 2 years of age, children become characteristically resistant to consuming new foods, and sometimes dietary variety diminishes to 4 or 5 well-accepted favorites. In a study of 3022 infants and toddlers ranging from 6 to 24 months of age, half of mothers with 19- to 24-month-old toddlers reported picky eating, whereas only 19% reported picky eating among 4- to 6-month-old infants.[9] It should be stressed to families that children's failure to immediately accept new foods is a normal stage of child development that, although potentially frustrating, can be dealt with effectively with knowledge, consistency, and patience.

Although toddlers are in a generally explorative phase, they can go on food "jags," during which certain foods are preferentially consumed to the exclusion of others.[11,12] Parents who become concerned when a "good eater" in infancy becomes a "fair to poor" eater as a toddler should be reassured that this change in acceptance is developmentally typical.

Preschoolers

Preschoolers have more fully developed motor skills, handle utensils and cups efficiently, and can sit at the table for meals. Since growth has slowed, their interest in eating may be unpredictable, with characteristic periods of disinterest in food. Their attention span may limit the amount of time that they can spend in the mealtime setting; however, they should be encouraged to attend and partake in family meals for reasonable periods of time (15–20 minutes)—whether they choose to eat or not.

As children move from toddlerhood to the preschool years, they become increasingly aware of the environment in which eating occurs, particularly the social aspects of eating. By interacting with and observing other children and adults, preschool-aged children become more aware of when and where eating takes place, what types of foods are consumed at specific eating occasions (ie, ice cream is a dessert food), and how much of those foods are consumed at each eating occasion (ie, "finish your vegetables"). As a consequence of this increased awareness, children's food selection and intake patterns are influenced by a variety of environmental cues, including the time of day[13]; portion size[14-16]; controlling child feeding practices, including restriction and pressure to eat[17,18]; and the preferences and eating behaviors of others.[19-21]

During the preschool period, most children have moved from eating on demand to a more adult-like eating pattern, consuming 3 meals each day as well as several smaller snacks. Although children's intake from meal to meal may appear to be erratic, total daily energy intake remains fairly constant.[22] Children show the ability to respond to the energy content of foods by adjusting their intake to reflect the energy density of the diet.[17,23] In contrast to their skills in regulation of food intake, young children do not appear to have the innate ability to choose a well-balanced diet.[11,12] Rather, they depend on adults to offer them a variety of nutritious and developmentally appropriate foods and to model the consumption of those foods.

School-Aged Children

During the school years, increases in memory and logic abilities are accompanied by reading, writing, and math skills and knowledge. This is the period in which basic nutrition education concepts can be successfully introduced. Emphasis should be placed on enjoying the taste of fruits and vegetables rather than to focus exclusively on their healthfulness, because young children tend to think of taste and healthfulness as mutually exclusive.[24] Socially, children are learning rules and conventions and also begin to develop friendships. During the period between 8 and 11 years of age, children begin making more peer comparisons, including those pertaining to weight and body shape. An awareness of the physical self begins to emerge, and comparisons with social norms for weight and weight status begin to occur. During this period, children vary greatly in weight, body shape, and growth rate, and teasing of those who fall outside the perceived norms for weight status frequently occurs. Friends and those outside the family can influence food attitudes and choices either beneficially or negatively, which can affect the nutritional status of a given child. Television is another source of influence on young children's eating, given that a majority of US school-aged children watch at least 2 hours of television each day.[25] The more time children spend watching television, the more likely they are to have higher energy intakes; consume greater amounts of pizza, salty snacks, and soda; and to be overweight than children who spend less time watching television.[25–29]

School-aged children have more freedom over their food choices and, during the school year, eat at least 1 meal per day away from the home. Choices, such as the decision to consume school lunch or a snack bar meal, may affect dietary quality.[30]

Eating Patterns and Nutrient Needs

Toddlers

Toddlers eat, on average, 7 times each day, with snacks representing approximately one fourth of daily energy intake. Between 15 and 24 months of age, approximately 59% of energy comes from table foods.[31] Milk constitutes the leading source (25%) of daily energy, macronutrients, and many vitamins and minerals, including vitamins A and D, calcium, and zinc.[32] Fruit and vegetable intake is notably absent in some toddlers. Between 28% and 33% of toddlers do not consume fruit and between 18% and 20% do not consume vegetables on a given day; French fries are the vegetable most commonly consumed by toddlers.[33]

Preschool and School-Aged Children

Fruit and vegetable intake among preschool and school-aged children is also well below current recommendations.[34,35] A majority of preschool and school-aged children do not consume recommended amounts of fiber; low-fiber fruits, such as applesauce and fruit cocktail, have the greatest contributions to daily fiber intake.[36] Alternatively, children's intakes of fat, discretionary fat, and added sugar are high.[34,35,37] Further, low micronutrient-dense foods constitute more than 30% of 8- to 18-year-old children's daily energy intake.[38] Among the top 10 food groupings contributing to children's daily energy intake are cakes, cookies, quick breads, or doughnuts; soft drinks; potato chips, corn chips, or popcorn; and sugars, syrup, or jams.[39] More energy-dense diets, defined as the amount of energy per daily amount of food and drink (g), are associated with higher energy intakes among pre-school and school-aged children.[40] Trends in eating patterns among children have been attributed to an increase in the frequency of snacking, a shift to foods consumed away from home, and increasing food portion sizes.[41–43]

Key Eating and Activity Concerns	
Toddlers and Preschoolers	School-Aged Children
• Weaning • Fluctuations in appetite • Low micronutrient intake (iron and zinc) • Juice consumption • Fruit and vegetable acceptance • Television and screen time • Routines for eating and activity	• Fruit and vegetable acceptance • High-energy snacks • Beverages and foods with added sugar • Low fiber intake • Decreased milk consumption • Television and screen time • Dieting and body image

The American Academy of Pediatrics Committee on Nutrition recommends the following foods as excellent sources of iron in the diet of the child.

Table A
Foods to Increase Iron

Selected Heme Iron Sources	
Table Food	Iron (mg of elemental iron)
Clams, canned, drained solids, 3 oz	23.8
Chicken liver, cooked, simmered, 3 oz	9.9
Oysters, Eastern canned, 3 oz	5.7
Beef liver, cooked, braised, 3 oz	5.6
Shrimp, cooked moist heat, 3 oz	2.6
Beef, composite of trimmed cuts, lean only, all grades, cooked, 3 oz	2.5
Sardines, Atlantic, canned in oil, drained solids with bone, 3 oz	2.5

AAP

Turkey, all classes, dark meat, roasted, 3 oz	2.0
Lamb, domestic, composite of trimmed retail cuts, separable lean only, choice, cooked, 3 oz	1.7
Fish, tuna, light, canned in water, drained solids, 3 oz	1.3
Chicken, broiler or fryer, dark meat, roasted, 3 oz	1.1
Turkey, all classes, light meat, roasted, 3 oz	1.1
Veal, composite of trimmed cuts, lean only, cooked, 3 oz	1.0
Chicken, broiler or fryer, breast, roasted, 3 oz	0.9
Pork, composite of trimmed cuts (leg, loin, shoulder), lean only, cooked, 3 oz	0.9
Fish, salmon, pink, cooked, 3 oz	0.8
Commercial Baby Food*	
Meat	
Baby food, lamb, junior, 1 jar (2.5 oz)	1.2
Baby food, chicken, strained, 1 jar (2.5 oz)	1.0
Baby food, lamb, strained, 1 jar (2.5 oz)	0.8
Baby food, beef, junior, 1 jar (2.5 oz)	0.7
Baby food, beef, strained, 1 jar (2.5 oz)	0.7
Baby food, chicken, junior, 1 jar (2.5 oz)	0.7
Baby food, pork, strained, 1 jar (2.5 oz)	0.7
Baby food, ham, strained, 1 jar (2.5 oz)	0.7
Baby food, ham, junior, 1 jar (2.5 oz)	0.7
Baby food, turkey, junior, (2.5 oz)	0.6
Baby food, turkey, strained, 1 jar (2.5 oz)	0.5
Baby food, veal, strained, 1 jar (2.5 oz)	0.5
Selected Non-Heme Iron Sources	
Oatmeal, instant, fortified, cooked, 1/2 cup	7.0
Blackstrap molasses,† 2 tbsp	7.4
Tofu, raw, regular, 1/2 cup	6.7
Wheat germ, toasted, 1/2 cup	5.1
Ready-to-eat cereal, fortified at different levels, 1 cup	about 4.5 to 18
Soybeans, mature seeds, cooked, boiled, 1/2 cup	4.4

(continued)

AAP

Apricots, dehydrated (low-moisture), uncooked, 1/2 cup	3.8
Sunflower seeds, dried, no hulls, 1/2 cup	3.7
Lentils, mature seeds, cooked, 1/2 cup	3.3
Spinach, cooked, boiled, drained, 1/2 cup	3.2
Chickpeas, mature seeds, cooked, 1/2 cup	2.4
Prunes, dehydrated (low-moisture), uncooked, 1/2 cup	2.3
Lima beans, large, mature seeds, cooked, 1/2 cup	2.2
Navy beans, mature seeds, cooked, 1/2 cup	2.2
Kidney beans, all types, mature seeds, cooked, 1/2 cup	2.0
Molasses, 2 tbsp	1.9
Pinto beans, mature seeds, cooked, 1/2 cup	1.8
Raisins, seedless, packed, 1/2 cup	1.6
Prunes, dehydrated (low-moisture), stewed, 1/2 cup	1.6
Prune juice, canned, 4 fluid oz	1.5
Green peas, cooked, boiled, drained, 1/2 cup	1.2
Enriched white rice, long-grain, regular, cooked, 1/2 cup	1.0
Whole egg, cooked (fried or poached), 1 large egg	0.9
Enriched spaghetti, cooked, 1/2 cup	0.9
White bread, commercially prepared, 1 slice	0.9
Whole wheat bread, commercially prepared, 1 slice	0.7
Spaghetti or macaroni , whole wheat, cooked, 1/2 cup	0.7
Peanut butter, smooth style, 2 tbsp	0.6
Brown rice, medium-grain, cooked, 1/2 cup	0.5
Commercial Baby Food*	
Vegetables	
Baby food, green beans, junior, 1 jar (6 oz)	1.8
Baby food, peas, strained, 1 jar (3.4 oz)	0.9
Baby food, green beans, strained, 1 jar (4 oz)	0.8
Baby food, spinach, creamed, strained, 1 jar (4 oz)	0.7
Baby food, sweet potatoes, junior, 1 jar (6 oz)	0.7
Baby food, sweet potatoes, strained, 1 jar (4 oz)	0.4

AAP

Cereals	
Baby food, brown rice cereal, dry, instant, 1 tbsp	1.8
Baby food, oatmeal cereal, dry, 1 tbsp	1.6
Baby food, rice cereal, dry, 1 tbsp	1.2
Baby food, barley cereal, dry, 1 tbsp	1.1

Selected Good Vitamin C Sources	
Fruits	**Vegetables**
Citrus fruits (eg, orange, tangerine, grapefruit)	Red, yellow, and green peppers
Pineapple	Broccoli
Fruit juices enriched with vitamin C	Tomato
Strawberries	Cabbage
Cantaloupe	Potato
Kiwifruit	Leafy green vegetables
Raspberries	Cauliflower

Source of iron values in foods: US Department of Agriculture, Agricultural Research Service. USDA National Nutrient Database for Standard Reference, Release 20. 2007. Nutrient Data Laboratory Home Page. Available at: http://www.ars.usda.gov/ba/bhnrc/ndl. Accessed April 17, 2008. Note: figures are rounded.

* Baby food values are generally based on generic jar, not branded jar; 3 oz table food meat = 85 g; a 2.5 oz. jar of baby food = 71 g (an infant would not be expected to eat 3 oz [about the size of a deck of cards] of pureed table meat at a meal).

† Source of iron value was obtained from a manufacturer of this type of molasses (October 2007).

Table B
Dietary Reference Intakes (DRIs) for Iron for Children

Birth to 6 months	0.27 mg/day*
7–12 months	11 mg/day†
1–3 years	7 mg/day†
4–8 years	10 mg/day†

* Adequate Intake (AI)
† Recommended Dietary Allowance (RDA)
Source: Institute of Medicine, Food and Nutrition Board. 2004. Available at: http://www.nap.edu

AAP

Table C

Fitting Iron-Rich Foods Into Different Meals Eaten by Toddlers (1 to 3 Years Old)

Sample Meal Food Items*	Iron Content (mg)†
Morning meal could include:	
Oatmeal, instant, fortified, cooked, 1/3 cup	4.7
Poached egg, 1	0.9
Vitamin-C rich fruit (vitamin C source)	
Morning snack could include:	
Prunes, dehydrated (low moisture), stewed, 1/4 cup	0.8
Whole-wheat bread, commercially prepared, 1/2 slice	0.3
Vitamin C-fortified juice (vitamin C source)	
Mid day meal could include:	
Tofu, regular, 1/4 cup	3.3
Spinach, cooked, boiled, 1/4 cup	1.6
White bread, commercially prepared, 1/2 slice	0.5
Vitamin-C rich fruit (vitamin C source)	
Afternoon snack could include:	
Chickpeas, cooked, 1/4 cup	1.2
Macaroni, whole wheat, elbow shaped (1/4 cup)	0.4
Vitamin-C rich fruit (vitamin C source)	
Evening meal could include:	
Turkey, dark meat, roasted, 1.5 oz	1.0
Green peas, cooked, 1/4 cup	0.6
Enriched white rice, long-grain, regular, cooked (1/3 cup)	0.6
Vitamin-C rich fruit (vitamin C source)	

Note: the amount of iron obtained depends on the quantity of food that a child actually consumes and bioavailability factors (eg, foods and beverages that may be consumed that may inhibit or enhance iron absorption of any non-heme iron).

* Assume that an adequate quantity of cow milk and other foods to meet other nutrient needs are consumed.

† Figures are rounded.

Energy Needs

Dietary Reference Intakes (DRIs) are a set of 4 nutrient-based reference values that can be used for planning and assessing diets of individuals and groups (see Appendix J).[44] The DRIs include data on safety and efficacy, reduction of chronic degenerative disease (rather than the avoidance of nutritional deficiency), and data on upper levels of intake (where available). The estimated average requirement (EAR) refers to the median usual intake value that is estimated to meet the requirements of one half of apparently healthy individuals of a given age and sex over time. The Recommended Dietary Allowance (RDA) refers to the level of intake that is adequate for nearly all healthy individuals of a given sex and age. When the EAR or RDA has not been established, an Adequate Intake (AI) is provided as a standard. The tolerable upper intake level (UL) is the highest level of continuing daily nutrient intake that is likely to pose no risk of adverse health effects in almost all individuals. The UL, however, is not intended to be a recommended level of intake. Using the age- and sex-specific EAR, is it possible to make a quantitative statistical assessment of the adequacy of an individual's usual intake of a nutrient and to assess the safety of an individual's usual intake by comparison with the UL.

Energy needs are most variable in children and depend on basal metabolism, rate of growth, physical activity, body size, sex, and onset of puberty (also see Chapter 13: Energy). Many nutrient requirements depend on energy needs and intake. Micronutrients that are most likely to be low or deficient in the diets of young children are calcium, iron, zinc, vitamin B_6, magnesium, and vitamin A.[45,46]

Supplements

Parents often ask health care professionals whether their children need vitamin supplements, and many routinely give supplements to their children, with recent estimates suggesting that 30% to 40% of children are given some kind of supplement.[31] The children who receive supplements are not necessarily the children who need them most, however, and in some cases, adequate amounts of the marginal nutrients, such as calcium and zinc, are not included in the supplement. Routine supplementation is not necessary for healthy growing children who consume a varied diet. For children and adolescents who cannot or will not consume adequate amounts of micronutrients from any dietary sources, the use of mineral supplements should be considered. Children at nutritional risk who may benefit from supplementation include those:

1. With anorexia or an inadequate appetite or who follow fad diets.
2. With chronic disease (eg, cystic fibrosis, inflammatory bowel disease, hepatic disease).
3. From deprived families or who suffer parental neglect or abuse.
4. Who participate in a dietary program for managing obesity.
5. Who consume a vegetarian diet without adequate intake of dairy products.
6. With failure to thrive.

Evaluation of dietary intake should be included in any assessment of the need for supplementation. If parents wish to give their children supplements, a standard pediatric vitamin-mineral product containing nutrients in amounts no larger than the DRI (EAR or RDA) poses no risk. Amounts higher than the DRI should be discouraged and counseling should be provided about the toxic effects, especially of fat-soluble vitamins. Because the taste, shape, and color of most pediatric preparations are as attractive as candy, parents should be cautioned to keep them out of reach of children. (See Chapters 17–20 for more information on vitamins and minerals.)

Dietary Fat

In recent decades, emphasis and educational efforts supporting low-fat, low-cholesterol diets for the general population have increased. A variety of health organizations, including the American Academy of Pediatrics, recommend against fat or cholesterol restriction in the first 2 years of life, when rapid growth and development require high intakes of energy. For this reason, nonfat milks are not recommended for use in children younger than 2 years. For children between 12 months and 2 years of age, low-fat dairy products should be considered for children with a body mass index (BMI) at the 85th percentile or greater or a family history of obesity. Fat intake should be gradually decreased during the toddler years so that fat intake, averaged across several days, provides approximately 30% of total energy.[47,48] Parents should be reassured that this level of intake is sufficient for adequate growth[49,50] and does not place children at increased risk of nutritional inadequacy.[37] Transitioning children's diets to provide 30% energy from fat can be achieved by substituting grain products, fruits, vegetables, low-fat milk products or other calcium-rich foods, beans, lean meat, poultry, fish, or other protein-rich foods for higher-fat foods. Because concerns have been expressed that some parents and their children may overinterpret the need to restrict their fat intakes, a lower limit of 20% of energy from fat has been established.

Dietary Guidelines for Americans

In 2005, the US Department of Agriculture (USDA) and Department of Health and Human Services updated the Dietary Guidelines for Americans (DGAs), the federal government's science-based advice to promote health and reduce risk of major chronic diseases through diet and physical activity.[51] The DGAs can be used in developing educational programs and materials for people 2 years and older. The DGAs promote 3 main concepts: (1) make smart choices from every food group; (2) find your balance between food and physical activity; and (3) get the most nutrition out of your calories.[52] Overall, the DGAs encourage Americans to eat fewer calories, be more active, and make wiser food choices. To follow the advice provided by the DGAs, parents should be encouraged to: (1) help children consume adequate amounts of fiber-rich fruits and vegetables; (2) help children consume whole-grain products often, with at least half of total grains being whole grains; (3) help children 2 to 8 years of age consume 2 cups per day of fat-free or low-fat milk or equivalent milk products and help children 9 years of age and older consume 3 cups per day; (4) enable children to engage in at least 60 minutes of physical activity on most, preferably all, days of the week; (5) offer foods that help keep total fat intake between 30% and 35% of calories for children 2 to 3 years of age and between 25% and 35% of calories for children 4 to 18 years of age; (6) choose and prepare foods and beverages with little added sugars or caloric sweeteners; (7) choose and prepare foods for children with little salt; and (8) keep foods offered to children safe by not feeding them raw (unpasteurized) milk or any products made from unpasteurized milk; raw or partially cooked eggs or foods containing raw eggs; raw or undercooked meat, poultry, fish, or shellfish; unpasteurized juices; or raw sprouts.

MyPyramid (see Appendix K, Fig K-1) is a system of educational information and interactive tools developed by the USDA to implement the DGAs. It provides personalized food-based guidance for the public and additional resources for health care professionals.[53] MyPyramid is based on both the DGAs and the DRIs from the National Academy of Sciences, keeping in mind typical food consumption patterns of Americans. MyPyramid translates nutritional recommendations into the kinds and amounts of food to eat each day. Guidance and print materials are available on the MyPyramid Web site (www.mypyramid.gov) for children 2 years and older as well as for adults.

The USDA also developed child-friendly materials to support MyPyramid called MyPyramid for Kids (See Appendix K, Fig K-2). MyPyramid for Kids provides age-appropriate information for children 6 to 11 years of age. The MyPyramid for Kids symbol represents the general proportions of food from each food group and focuses on the importance of making smart food choices every day. In addition to helping parents identify the amounts that children need from each food group, the symbol and materials can be used to convey basic nutrition concepts for feeding young children, such as variety and moderation. Daily physical activity is a prominent message in MyPyramid for Kids. To support this message, Enjoy Moving, a physical activity pyramid (http://teamnutrition.usda.gov/Resources/enjoymovingflyer.html; see Appendix K, Fig K-3), was developed to provide a more detailed, illustrated description of the types of physical activity in which children may engage. Children are encouraged to get at least 60 minutes of physical activity on most days and to do: plenty of moving whenever they can, more making their hearts work harder, enough stretching and building muscles, and less sitting around. Through an interactive Web-based game, lesson plans, colorful posters and flyers, worksheets, and valuable tips for families, MyPyramid for Kids encourages children, teachers, and parents to work together to make healthier food choices and be active every day.

In addition, the USDA has developed dietary advice for Pregnant and Breastfeeding women as part of the MyPyramid Web site (http://www.mypyramid.gov/mypyramidmoms/index.html). The interactive "MyPyramid Plan for Moms" provides personalized advice on the kinds and amounts of food to eat, taking into account the trimester of pregnancy or stage of breastfeeding. Additional information on food choices, nutritional needs, and supplements is also available on the Web site and as downloadable fact sheets.

MyPyramid was released in April 2005, and MyPyramid for Kids was released in September 2005, and they replace the original Food Guide Pyramid (1992) and Food Guide Pyramid for Young Children (1998), widely recognized nutrition education tools.

To calculate BMI for children and adolescents 2 through 19 years of age and the corresponding BMI-for-age percentile on a Centers for Disease Control and Prevention (CDC) growth chart, a calculator is available on the CDC Web site (http://apps.nccd.cdc.gov/dnpabmi/Calculator.aspx). Alternatively, a table for calculated BMI values for selected heights and weights for ages 2 to 20 years is available (http://www.cdc.gov/nccdphp/dnpa/bmi/00binaries/bmi-tables.pdf).

Nutrition Guidelines for Children*
• Make available and offer a colorful variety of fruits and vegetables for children to consume every day.
• Limit intake of foods and beverages with added sugars or salt.
• Keep total fat intake between 30% and 35% of calories for children 2 to 3 years of age and between 25% and 35% of calories for children 4 to 18 years of age.
• Offer fruits, vegetables, fat-free or low-fat dairy, and whole-grain snacks to get the most nutrition out of snacks.
• Offer child-appropriate portions.[54–58]
• Engage in at least 60 minutes of moderate to vigorous physical activity on most, preferably all, days of the week.
• Provide food that is safe (eg, by not feeding unpasteurized juices, raw sprouts, raw [unpasteurized] dairy products, raw or partially cooked eggs, and raw or undercooked meat, poultry, fish, or shellfish), especially to young children.

*Most recommendations are from the 2005 Dietary Guidelines for Americans.

Parenting and the Feeding Relationship

Feeding can be quite challenging, particularly during the toddler and pre-school years. Satter's division of responsibility—in which parents provide structure in mealtime, a healthy variety of foods, and opportunities for learning and the child ultimately decides how much and whether to eat on a given eating occasion—represents a sound theoretical basis for implementing appropriate child-feeding practices.[59]

Structure and routine for eating occasions is particularly important for the young child. Children can be moved to a more adult-like eating pattern with opportunities for consumption being centered on meals and snacks[60] (4–6 per day) and limited grazing in between. Adults should decide when food is offered or available and the child should be left to decide how much and whether they choose to eat at a given eating occasion. The physical environment should also be structured to promote healthy eating with distractions from television or other activities avoided. Ideally, eating should occur in a designated area of the home with a developmentally appropriate chair for the child. Family meals, with adults present and eating at least some of the same foods as children, provide occasions to learn and model healthful eating habits as well as opportunities to include the social aspects of eating.

The "job" of early childhood is to learn about the self and the external environment. To facilitate learning in the eating domain, parents should provide repeated opportunities for learning about new foods and about normative eating behavior. Research suggests that it takes many exposures (up to 10) to help a child accept a novel food; therefore, patience and consistency are required to facilitate children's acceptance of foods like vegetables and meats that are not sweet.[6] However, parental responsibility falls short of "getting" children to eat or like particular foods. Pressuring children to consume foods or rewarding them for consuming specific foods is counterproductive in the long run, because it is likely to build resistance and food dislikes rather than acceptance. Instead, considering mealtime from the child's perspective—where everything is new and different—and recognizing that finicky eating is a normal stage of development that children outgrow—is a more productive outlook. Parents' concerns can be diminished if the focus becomes the adequacy of children's growth rather than children's behavior at individual eating occasions.

Feeding Guidance for Parents
Parents' responsibilities include: • Choosing food. • Setting mealtime routines. • Creating positive mealtime environments that are free of distractions (television, loud music) with appropriate physical components (chairs, tables, utensils, cups, etc). • Modeling behaviors that they desire their children learn, such as consuming a varied and healthy diet. • Regarding mealtime as a time of learning and mastery with respect to eating and social skills and with respect to family and community time. Children decide which of the foods (that are selected by parents) that they will consume. They also decide how much to eat.
Parents can be reminded that: • Foods should be offered repeatedly (10 times) and patiently to establish children's acceptance of the food. • Children need a routine of 3 meals and 2 snacks per day. • Appropriate demands for mastery (such as using a spoon and drinking from a cup) facilitate children's learning and sense of accomplishment. Pressure and coercion may have short-term benefits but will ultimately make feeding more difficult and eating less rewarding and pleasurable.

Providing ample nourishment is important and can be an emotionally rewarding part of parenting. Some parents have an inability to say "no" to their toddlers' demands and use counterproductive strategies to get their children to consume certain foods. The most common strategy used to encourage young children to eat is bribery. However, the use of bribes, threats, and food restriction is adversely related to positive eating behaviors in young children and is related to higher BMI z-scores.[17,61]

Parents' feeding styles have been associated with children's dietary intake and weight status.[62–65] Authoritative feeding, characterized by adults encouraging children to eat healthy foods and allowing the child to have limited choices but stopping short of pressuring or forcing, has been associated with increased availability and intake of fruits, vegetables, and dairy and lower intake of "less nutritious" foods.[62,66] In contrast, authoritarian feeding, characterized by attempts to control children's eating, has been associated with lower intake of fruit, juices, and vegetables. Children who were told to "clean their plates" were less sensitive to physiological cues of satiety.[63] Permissive feeding, characterized by little structure in feeding, has been associated with greater intake of fat and sweet foods, more snacks, and fewer healthy food choices.[64]

Young children respond well when appropriate maturity demands are made. Children want to learn and want to eat. They also desire to participate in decisions about their own eating. Allowing them the opportunities for mastery of eating, even when it translates into extra work and mess, ultimately promotes self-regulation and autonomy building. Experience is the only established predictor of acceptance and liking. Therefore, encouraging learning—using all senses and various modes for learning (eg, food shopping and preparation; reading to children about food, eating, and cultures)—can promote more enthusiasm for trying new foods.

Special Topics

Feeding During Illness

A common treatment for acute diarrhea has been a clear liquid diet until symptoms improve. The American Academy of Pediatrics clinical practice guideline on the management of acute gastroenteritis in young children[67] recommends that only oral electrolyte solutions be used to rehydrate infants and young children and that a normal diet be continued throughout an episode of gastroenteritis (also see Chapter 28: Oral Therapy for Acute Diarrhea). Infants and young children can experience a decrease in nutritional status and the illness can be prolonged with a clear liquid diet, especially when it is extended beyond a few days.[68] Continuous or early refeeding has been shown to shorten the duration of the diarrhea. Recommendations for toddlers and preschool children include reintroduction of solid foods shortly after rehydration. Foods that are usually well tolerated include rice cereals, bananas, potatoes, eggs, rice, plain pasta, and other similar foods. Dairy products, in recommended amounts, can also be included. During viral illnesses, colds, and other acute childhood illnesses, a variety of foods should be offered according to the child's appetite and tolerance, with extra fluids provided when fever, diarrhea, or vomiting is present.

Breakfast

Nationally representative data indicate that 8% to 12% of children skip breakfast on any given day, with the numbers growing to 20% to 30% by adolescence.[69] Among school-aged children, common barriers to eating breakfast include lack of time and not being hungry in the morning.[70] Children who frequently consume breakfast have superior nutritional profiles compared with those who do not.[71] Several studies have also demonstrated positive effects of breakfast consumption on children's cognitive performance, primarily aspects of memory,[72,73] with benefits most pronounced among children at nutritional risk.[74,75] Ready-to-eat cereal is among the top contributors to fiber, folic acid, vitamin C, iron, and zinc intakes in young children's diets.[39,76] School breakfast programs, which to a large extent serve children from low-income families,[77] are associated with improvements in children's nutrient intake and overall diet quality.[78] School breakfast participation has also been associated with increases in attendance and academic performance, with benefits again most pronounced among children at nutritional risk.[79–81] The influence of breakfast consumption on body weight is unclear. Some studies have reported a protective association of breakfast consumption on BMI in children,[69,82,83] particularly for ready-to-eat breakfast cereal.[76,84] Alternatively, breakfast skippers have generally lower daily energy intakes than do breakfast eaters,[85,86] suggesting that the behavior may represent a marker of, rather than a direct contributor to, overweight.[71]

Obesity (also see Chapter 33: Obesity)

The prevalence of overweight among children has increased drastically over the past 2 decades and is alarmingly high; currently, 25% of children 2 to 18 years of age are overweight.[87] Overweight children are at increased risk of social stigmatization, hyperlipidemia, abnormal glucose tolerance, type 2 diabetes mellitus, liver disease, and hypertension.[88] Environmental influences that promote problematic eating have been given increasing attention in light of the fact that secular increases in overweight have occurred too rapidly to be explained by genetic influences alone.[89,90] Parents have an important role in the etiology of childhood overweight, because they provide children with both genes and the environment in which eating and physical activity take place. Evidence of this point is found in the fact that the tracking of childhood overweight into adulthood is particularly strong among children who have one or more overweight parents.[91]

It is recommended that children younger than 3 years with a BMI ≥85th percentile and with complications of obesity or with a BMI ≥95th percentile with or without medical complications undergo evaluation and possible treatment.[92] When possible, guidance to promote healthful eating patterns in the overweight child should be directed toward modifying the dietary intake patterns and behaviors of the family as a whole rather than targeting only the overweight child. Referring the family for nutrition and physical activity education and counseling may be useful to help parents discuss behavioral issues involved in child feeding. These discussions should focus on the types of foods that are available in the home, identifying appropriate portion sizes, and incorporating micronutrient-rich, low–energy-density foods into the child's and family's diet. Parents should also be made aware that highly restrictive approaches to child feeding are not effective but rather appear to promote the intake of restricted foods[18,93] and contribute to low self-appraisal.[94] Furthermore, parents' should be encouraged to exhibit the eating behaviors they would like their children to adopt, because children learn to model their parents' eating and behaviors.[21,30]

Increased physical activity is a critical component of childhood obesity prevention and treatment, because low-energy diets may compromise the nutrient status of growing children.[95] Sedentary behavior has been associated with overweight among children[26,28]; health care professionals should inquire about the amount of time a child spends in front of television, computers, and video monitors and encourage parents to set daily limits for their children. Caregivers have a central responsibility in this area, because they serve as role models for active lifestyles and are children's gatekeepers to opportunities to be physically active. Health care professionals should convey the importance of encouraging activity of the family as a whole as well as among individuals within the family. Children should be encouraged to participate in discussions about diet and activity modifications, both to take into account their preferences and allow them a sense of responsibility for decisions about their behavior.

Beverage Consumption

Fruit juices and soft drinks, including fruit-flavored and carbonated drinks, are increasingly common beverages consumed by young children at home and in group settings.[96] Between 1977 and 2001, soft drink intake among children 2 to 18 years of age more than doubled, largely because of increases in the average portion size consumed.[97] On any given day, 60% of toddlers consumed 100% fruit juice, with 1 in 10 children consuming more than 14 oz of 100% fruit juice daily.[98] Further, sweetened beverages are one of the top 3 contributors (4.7%) to daily energy intake in this age group, with 40% of toddlers consuming fruit drinks and 11% consuming carbonated beverages on any given day.[32] Among older children, these types of beverages provide roughly 10% of energy in 2- to 19-year-old children's diets, with soft drinks providing as much as 8% of total daily energy for adolescents.[99] Children's soft drink consumption exceeds that of 100% fruit juice by 5 years of age and that of milk by 13 years of age.[100] Soft drinks, a main source of added sugar in young children's diets,[101] have been shown to replace milk in the diet and are associated with lower intakes of key nutrients, particularly calcium (see Appendices L and M).[102–107]

Failure to thrive has been anecdotally associated with excessive intake of fruit juice,[108] and at least 1 study found carbohydrate malabsorption after consumption of fruit juices in healthy children and in children with chronic nonspecific diarrhea.[109] In addition, weight gain and adiposity have been linked to excess energy-containing beverage consumption.[110,111] For all young children, consumption of sweetened beverages should be monitored.[112] For those with either chronic diarrhea or excessive weight gain, obtaining a diet history, including the volume of fruit juice and soft drinks consumed, is useful in approaching anticipatory guidance. Intake of fruit juice should be limited to 4 to 6 oz/day for children 1 to 6 years of age.[113] For children 7 to 18 years of age, juice intake should be limited to 8 to 12 oz or 2 servings per day. Parents should be encouraged to routinely offer plain, unflavored water to children, particularly for fluids consumed outside of meals and snacks.[114]

AAP

Recommendations from the American Academy of Pediatrics

The **American Academy of Pediatrics** recommends an upper limit of 4 to 6 oz of juice for children 1 to 6 years of age and 8 to 12 oz for children 7 to 18 years of age. Children should be encouraged to consume whole fruits to meet recommended levels of fruit intake. Pediatricians should routinely discuss the use of 100% fruit juice and fruit drinks and should educate parents about the differences between the two.

Pediatrics. 2001;107:1210-1213 (Reaffirmed October 2006)

The Role of Anticipatory Guidance in Promoting Healthy Eating Behaviors

The feeding relationship is vital for its role in promoting healthy growth and development but also for its function in engendering healthy behaviors and habits that can prevent the advent of chronic disease. Beyond physiological outcomes associated with poor eating habits and environments, the feeding relationship is critical for establishing a healthy parent-child relationship. Feeding, at its best, provides opportunities for pleasure, learning, and attaining security as well as occasions for self-discovery and for learning self-control.

A healthy feeding environment requires structure, knowledge, supportive limit setting and parenting, an appreciation of children's developing capabilities, and perhaps most of all, patience. The pediatrician's role includes the timely delivery of information that links children's individual development to their nutrition needs. Each well-child visit can be structured to include nutrition guidance that is relevant to the individual child's development and growth. Information regarding a child's growth and weight status (by use of BMI curves adjusted for sex and age) and interpretation of the child's growth tracking over time is both important and enlightening for parents. Furthermore, anticipating and addressing problematic childhood behaviors (eg, neophobia and preferences for sweet-tasting foods) and framing them in a developmental light often alleviates parental overconcern. Guiding parents to establish and adopt routines for eating and physical activity from infancy through adolescence will greatly assist parents to prioritize healthy eating and activity patterns. Pediatricians can support families by offering continued encouragement and direction regarding the benefits of a varied diet, appropriate expectations for children's intake, and the importance of physical activity for children and families.

Table 6.1
Feeding Guide for Children

Food Group	Age, y						Comments
	2–3		4–8		9–12		
	Portion Size	Daily Amounts*	Portion Size	Daily Amounts*	Portion Size	Daily Amounts*	
Milk, yogurt, and cheese	1/2 cup (4 oz)	2 cups	1/2–3/4 cup (4–6 oz)	2 cups	1/2–1 cup (4–8 oz)	3 cups	Make most choices fat free or low fat. The following may be substituted for 1/2 cup fluid milk: 1/2–3/4 oz cheese, 1/2 cup low-fat yogurt, or 21/2 tbsp nonfat dry milk.
Meat, fish, poultry, dry beans, eggs, and nuts	1–2 oz	2 oz	1–2 oz	3 oz	2 oz	5 oz	Make most choices lean or low fat. The following may be substituted for 1 oz meat, fish, or poultry: 1 egg, 2 tbsp peanut butter, or 4 tbsp cooked dry beans or peas.
Vegetables Cooked Raw*	2–3 tbsp Few pieces	1 cup	3–4 tbsp Few Pieces	11/2 cups	1/4–1/2 cup Several pieces	2 cups	Include dark green and orange vegetables, such as carrots, spinach, broccoli, winter squash, or greens. Limit starchy vegetables (potatoes) to 21/2 cups weekly (11/2 cups for 2- to 3-year-olds).
Fruit Raw Canned Juice	1/2–1 small 2–4 tbsp 3–4 oz	1 cup	1/2–1 small 4–6 tbsp 4 oz	1 cup	1 medium 1/4–1/2 cup 4 oz	11/2 cups	Make less than half of total fruit choices juice.

Table 6.1 *(continued)*
Feeding Guide for Children

Food Group	2–3		4–8		9–12		Comments
	Portion Size	Daily Amounts*	Portion Size	Daily Amounts*	Portion Size	Daily Amounts*	
Grains (bread, cereal, rice, and pasta)		3 oz eq.		4 oz eq		5 oz eq	One oz eq equals a 1-oz slice of bread. The following may be substituted for 1 slice of bread: 1/2 cup spaghetti, macaroni, noodles, or rice; 5 saltine crackers; 1/2 English muffin or bagel; 1 tortilla; corn grits; or posole. Make at least 1/2 of grain intake whole grain.
Whole-grain or enriched bread	1/2–1 slice		1 slice		1 slice		
Cooked cereal	1/4–1/2 cup		1/2 cup		1/2–1 cup		
Dry cereal	1/2–1 cup		1 cup		1 cup		

* Daily amounts are from MyPyramid Plans to meet needs for sedentary children of average size at the younger end of each age range. Amounts shown are from 1000-kcal (2- to 3-year-olds), 1200-kcal (4- to 8-year-olds), and 1600-kcal MyPyramid Plans. Active, older, and larger children would need more energy and foods from each group. A specific MyPyramid Plan for a child of a specified age, gender, and activity level can be found at http://www.mypyramid.gov/. For children 9 years and older, height and weight can also be specified in selecting a MyPyramid Plan.
† Do not give to young children until they can chew well.

References

1. Carruth BR, Skinner JD. Feeding behaviors and other motor development in healthy children (2–24 months). *Am Coll Nutr.* 2002;21:88–96

2. Carruth BR, Ziegler PJ, Gordon A, Hendricks K. Developmental milestones and self-feeding behaviors in infants and toddlers. *J Am Diet Assoc.* 2004;104:S51–S56

3. Burhans KK, Dweck CS. Helplessness in early childhood: the role of contingent worth. *Child Dev.* 1995;66:1719–1738

4. Desor JA, Maller O, Turner R. Taste acceptance of sugars by human infants. *J Comp Physiol Psychol.* 1973;84:496–501

5. Kern DL, McPhee L, Fisher J, Johnson S, Birch LL. The post-ingestive consequences of fat condition preferences for flavors associated with high dietary fat. *Physiol Behav.* 1993;54:71–76

6. Sullivan S, Birch L. Pass the sugar; pass the salt: experience dictates preference. *Dev Psychol.* 1990;26:546–551

7. Wardle J, Herrera ML, Cooke L, Gibson EL. Modifying children's food preferences: the effects of exposure and reward on acceptance of an unfamiliar vegetable. *Eur J Clin Nutr.* 2003;57:341–348

8. Wardle J, Cooke LJ, Gibson EL, Sapochnik M, Sheiham A, Lawson M. Increasing children's acceptance of vegetables; a randomized trial of parent-led exposure. *Appetite.* 2003;40:155–162

9. Carruth BR, Ziegler P, Gordon A, Barr SI. Prevalence of picky eaters among infants and toddlers and their caregiver's decisions about offering a food. *J Am Diet Assoc.* 2004;104:S57–S64

10. Johnson SL, Bellows L, Beckstrom L, Anderson J. Evaluation of a social marketing campaign targeting preschool children. *Am J Health Behav.* 2007;31:44–55

11. Davis CM. Self-selection of diet by newly weaned infants. *Am J Dis Child.* 1928;36:651–679

12. Davis CM. Results of the self-selection of diets by young children. *CMAJ.* 1939;41:257–261

13. Birch LL, Billman J, Richards S. Time of day influences food acceptability. *Appetite.* 1984;5:109–116

14. Rolls BJ, Engell D, Birch LL. Serving portion size influences 5-year-old but not 3-year-old children's food intakes. *J Am Diet Assoc.* 2000;100:232–234

15. Fisher JO, Rolls BJ, Birch LL. Children's bite size and intake of an entree are greater with large portions than with age-appropriate or self-selected portions. *Am J Clin Nutr.* 2003;77:1164–1170

16. Fisher JO. Effects of age on children's intake of large and self-selected portions. *Obesity (Silver Spring).* 2007;15:403–412

17. Johnson SL, Birch LL. Parents' and children's adiposity and eating style. *Pediatrics.* 1984;94:653–661

18. Birch LL, Fisher JO. Mothers' child-feeding practices influence daughters' eating and weight. *Am J Clin Nutr.* 2000;71:1054–1061

19. Birch LL. Effects of peer models' food choices and eating behaviors on preschoolers' food preferences. *Child Dev.* 1980;51:489–496

20. Hendy HM, Raudenbush B. Effectiveness of teacher modeling to encourage food acceptance in preschool children. *Appetite.* 2000;34:61–76

21. Cutting TM, Fisher JO, Grimm-Thomas K, Birch LL. Like mother, like daughter: familial patterns of overweight are mediated by mothers' dietary disinhibition. *Am J Clin Nutr.* 1999;69:608–613

22. Birch LL, Johnson SL, Andresen G, Peters JC, Schulte MC. The variability of young children's energy intake. *N Engl J Med.* 1991;324:232–235

23. Birch LL, Deysher M. Conditioned and unconditioned caloric compensation: evidence for self-regulation of food intake by young children. *Learn Motiv.* 1985;16:341–355

24. Wardle J, Huon G. An experimental investigation of the influence of health information on children's taste preferences. *Health Educ Res.* 2000;15:39–44

25. Andersen RE, Crespo CJ, Bartlett SJ, Cheskin LJ, Pratt M. Relationship of physical activity and television watching with body weight and level of fatness among children: results from the Third National Health and Nutrition Examination Survey. *JAMA.* 1998;279:938–942

26. American Academy of Pediatrics, Committee on Public Education. Children, adolescents, and television. *Pediatrics.* 2001;107:423–426

27. Coon KA, Goldberg J, Rogers BL, Tucker KL. Relationships between use of television during meals and children's food consumption patterns. *Pediatrics.* 2001;107(1):e7. Available at: http://pediatrics.aappublications.org/cgi/content/full/107/1/e7. Accessed October 31, 2007

28. Crespo CJ, Smit E, Troiano RP, Bartlett SJ, Macera CA, Andersen RE. Television watching, energy intake, and obesity in US children: results from the Third National Health and Nutrition Examination Survey, 1988–1994. *Arch Pediatr Adolesc Med.* 2001;155:360–365

29. Wiecha JL, Peterson KE, Ludwig DS, Kim J, Sobol A, Gortmaker SL. When children eat what they watch: impact of television viewing on dietary intake in youth. *Arch Pediatr Adolesc Med.* 2006;160:436–442

30. Cullen KW, Eagan J, Baranowski T, Owens E, de Moor C. Effect of a la carte and snack bar foods at school on children's lunchtime intake of fruits and vegetables. *J Am Diet Assoc.* 2000;100:1482–1486

31. Briefel RR, Reidy K, Karwe V, Jankowski L, Hendricks K. Toddler's transition to table foods: impact on nutrient intakes and food patterns. *J Am Diet Assoc.* 2004;104:S38–S44

32. Fox MK, Reidy K, Novak T, Ziegler P. Sources of energy and nutrients in the diets of infants and toddlers. *J Am Diet Assoc.* 2006;106:S28–S42

33. Fox MK, Pac S, Devaney B, Jankowski L. Feeding infants and toddlers study: what foods are infants and toddlers eating? *J Am Diet Assoc.* 2004;104:S22–S30

34. Krebs-Smith SM, Cook A, Subar AF, Cleveland L, Friday J, Kahle LL. Fruit and vegetable intakes of children and adolescents in the United States. *Arch Pediatr Adolesc Med.* 1996;150:81–86

35. Munoz KA, Krebs-Smith SM, Ballard-Barbash R, Cleveland LE. Food intakes of US children and adolescents compared with recommendations. *Pediatrics.* 1997;100:323–329

36. Kranz S, Mitchell DC, Siega-Riz AM, Smiciklas-Wright H. Dietary fiber intake by American preschoolers is associated with more nutrient-dense diets. *J Am Diet Assoc.* 2005;105:221–225

37. Ballew C, Kuester S, Serdula M, Bowman B, Dietz W. Nutrient intakes and dietary patterns of young children by dietary fat intakes. *J Pediatr.* 2000;136:181–187

38. Kant AK. Reported consumption of low-nutrient-density foods by American children and adolescents: nutritional and health correlates, NHANES III, 1988 to 1994. *Arch Pediatr Adolesc Med.* 2003;157:789–796

39. Subar AF, Krebs-Smith SM, Cook A, Kahle LL. Dietary sources of nutrients among US children, 1989–1991. *Pediatrics.* 1998;102:913–923

40. Mendoza JA, Drewnowski A, Cheadle A, Christakis DA. Dietary energy density is associated with selected predictors of obesity in U.S. children. *J Nutr.* 2006;136:1318–1322

41. Jahns L, Siega-Riz AM, Popkin BM. The increasing prevalence of snacking among US children from 1977 to 1996. *J Pediatr.* 2001;138:493–498

42. Nielsen SJ, Siega-Riz AM, Popkin BM. Trends in energy intake in U.S. between 1977 and 1996: similar shifts seen across age groups. *Obes Res.* 2002;5:370–378

43. Bowman SA, Gortmaker SL, Ebbeling CB, Pereira MA, Ludwig DS. Effects of fast-food consumption on energy intake and diet quality among children in a national household survey. *Pediatrics.* 2004;113:112–118

44. Institute of Medicine. *Dietary Reference Intakes: Applications in Dietary Assessment.* Washington, DC: National Academies Press; 2000

45. Alaimo K, McDowell MA, Briefel RR, et al. Dietary intake of vitamins, minerals, and fiber of persons ages 2 months and over in the United States: Third National Health and Nutrition Examination Survey, Phase 1, 1988–91. *Adv Data.* 1994;258:1–28

46. Federation of American Societies for Experimental Biology, Life Sciences Research Office. *Third Report on Nutrition Monitoring in the United States: Volume 1.* Washington, DC: US Government Printing Office; 1995

47. American Academy of Pediatrics, Committee on Nutrition. Statement on cholesterol. *Pediatrics.* 1998;101:141–147

48. Krauss RM, Eckel RH, Howard B, et al. Dietary guidelines revision 2000: a statement for healthcare professionals from the nutrition committee of the American Heart Association. *J Nutr.* 2001;131:132–146

49. Obarzanek E, Hunsberger SA, Van Horn L, et al. Safety of a fat-reduced diet: the Dietary Intervention Study in Children (DISC). *Pediatrics.* 1997;100:51–59

50. Butte NF. Fat intake of children in relation to energy requirements. *Am J Clin Nutr.* 2000;72:1246S–1252S

51. US Department of Health and Human Services and US Department of Agriculture. *Dietary Guidelines for Americans 2005.* 6th ed. Washington, DC: US Government Printing Office; 2005

52. US Department of Health and Human Services and US Department of Agriculture. *Finding Your Way to a Healthier You 2005.* Washington, DC: US Government Printing Office; 2005

53. US Department of Agriculture, Center for Nutrition Policy and Promotion. MyPyramid. Available at: http://www.mypyramid.gov. Accessed October 31, 2007

54. Young LR, Nestle M. Portion sizes in dietary assessment: issues and policy implications. *Nutr Rev.* 1995;53:149–158

55. Nielsen SJ, Popkin BM. Patterns and trends in food portion sizes, 1977–1998. *JAMA.* 2003;289:450–453

56. Fox MK, Devaney B, Reidy K, Razafindrakoto C, Ziegler P. Relationship between portion size and energy intake among infants and toddlers: evidence of self-regulation. *J Am Diet Assoc.* 2006;106:77–83

57. McConahy KL, Smicikclas-Wright H, Birch LL, Mitchell DC, Picciano MF. Food portions are positively related to energy intake and body weight in early childhood. *J Pediatr.* 2002;140:340–347

58. McConahy KL, Smiciklas-Wright H, Mitchell DC, Picciano MF. Portion size of common foods predicts energy intake among preschool-aged children. *J Am Diet Assoc.* 2004;104:975–976

59. Satter E. *How to Get Your Kid to Eat...But Not Too Much.* Palo Alto, CA: Bull Publishing Co; 1987

60. Skinner JD, Ziegler P, Pac S, DeVaney B. Meal and snack patterns of infants and toddlers. *J Am Diet Assoc.* 2004;104:S65–S70

61. Faith MS, Berkowitz RI, Stallings VA, Kerns J, Storey M, Stunkard AJ. Parental feeding attitudes and styles and child body mass index: prospective analysis of a gene-environment interaction. *Pediatrics.* 2004;114(4):e429. Available at: http://pediatrics.aappublications.org/cgi/content/full/114/4/e429. Accessed October 31, 2007

62. Gable S, Lutz S. Household, parent, and child contributions to childhood obesity. *Fam Relat.* 2000;49:293–300

63. Fisher JO, Birch LL. Restricting access to palatable foods affects children's behavioral response, food selection, and intake. *Am J Clin Nutr.* 1999;69:1264–1272

64. De Bourdeaudhuij I. Family food rules and healthy eating in adolescents. *J Health Psychol.* 1997;2:45–56

65. Rhee KE, Lumeng JC, Appugliese DP, Kaciroti N, Bradley RH. Parenting styles and overweight status in first grade. *Pediatrics.* 2006;117:2047–2054

66. Patrick H, Nicklas TA, Hughes SO, Morales M. The benefits of authoritative feeding style: caregiver feeding styles and children's food consumption patterns. *Appetite.* 2005;44:243–249

67. American Academy of Pediatrics, Provisional Committee on Quality Improvement, Subcommittee on Acute Gastroenteritis. Practice parameter: the management of acute gastroenteritis in young children. *Pediatrics.* 1996;97:424–435

68. Brown KH. Dietary management of acute childhood diarrhea: optimal timing of feeding and appropriate use of milks and mixed diets. *J Pediatr.* 1991;118:S92–S98

69. Siega-Riz AM, Popkin BM, Carson T. Trends in breakfast consumption for children in the United States from 1965–1991. *Am J Clin Nutr.* 1998;67:748S–756S

70. Reddan J, Wahlstrom K, Reicks M. Children's perceived benefits and barriers in relation to eating breakfast in schools with or without Universal School Breakfast. *J Nutr Educ Behav.* 2002;34:47–52

71. Rampersaud GC, Pereira MA, Girard BL, Adams J, Metzl JD. Breakfast habits, nutritional status, body weight, and academic performance in children and adolescents. *J Am Diet Assoc.* 2005;105:743–760

72. Wesnes KA, Pincock C, Richardson D, Helm G, Hails S. Breakfast reduces declines in attention and memory over the morning in schoolchildren. *Appetite*. 2003;41:329–331

73. Mahoney CR, Taylor HA, Kanarek RB, Samuel P. Effect of breakfast composition on cognitive processes in elementary school children. *Physiol Behav*. 2005;85:635–645

74. Cueto S, Jacoby E, Pollitt E. Breakfast prevents delays of attention and memory functions among nutritionally at-risk boys. *J Appl Dev Psychol*. 1998;19:219–233

75. Simeon DT, Grantham-McGregor S. Effects of missing breakfast on the cognitive functions of school children of differing nutritional status. *Am J Clin Nutr*. 1998;49:646–653

76. Barton BA, Eldridge AL, Thompson D, et al. The relationship of breakfast and cereal consumption to nutrient intake and body mass index: the National Heart, Lung, and Blood Institute Growth and Health Study. *J Am Diet Assoc*. 2005;105:1383–1389

77. US Department of Agriculture, Food and Nutrition Service. *School Breakfast Program Participation and Meals Served*. Alexandria, VA: US Department of Agriculture; 2006

78. Bhattacharya J, Currie J, Haider SJ. *Evaluating the Impact of School Nutrition Programs: Final Report*. Washington, DC: US Department of Agriculture, Economic Research Service; 2004

79. Powell CA, Walker SP, Chang SM, Grantham-McGregor SM. Nutrition and education: a randomized trial of the effects of breakfast in rural primary school children. *Am J Clin Nutr*. 1998;68:873–879

80. Kleinman RE, Hall S, Green H, et al. Diet, breakfast, and academic performance in children. *Ann Nutr Metab*. 2002;46(Suppl 1):24–30

81. Murphy JM, Pagano ME, Nachmani J, Sperling P, Kane S, Kleinman RE. The relationship of school breakfast to psychosocial and academic functioning: cross-sectional and longitudinal observations in an inner-city school sample. *Arch Pediatr Adolesc Med*. 1998;152:899–907

82. Miech RA, Kumanyika SK, Stettler N, Link BG, Phelan JC, Chang VW. Trends in the association of poverty with overweight among US adolescents, 1971–2004. *JAMA*. 2006;295:2385–2393

83. Affenito SG, Thompson DR, Barton BA, et al. Breakfast consumption by African-American and white adolescent girls correlates positively with calcium and fiber intake and negatively with body mass index. *J Am Diet Assoc*. 2005;105:938–945

84. Albertson AM, Anderson GH, Crockett SJ, Goebel MT. Ready-to-eat cereal consumption: its relationship with BMI and nutrient intake of children aged 4 to 12 years. *J Am Diet Assoc*. 2003;103:1613–1619

85. Berkey CS, Rockett HR, Gillman MW, Field AE, Colditz GA. Longitudinal study of skipping breakfast and weight change in adolescents. *Int J Obes Relat Metab Disord*. 2003;27:1258–1266

86. Cho S, Dietrich M, Brown CJ, Clark CA, Block G. The effect of breakfast type on total daily energy intake and body mass index: results from the Third National Health and Nutrition Examination Survey (NHANES III). *J Am Coll Nutr*. 2003;22:296–302

87. Ogden CL, Flegal KM, Carroll MD, Johnson CL. Prevalence and trends in overweight among US children and adolescents. *JAMA*. 2002;288:1728–1732

88. Dietz WH. Health consequences of obesity in youth: childhood predictors of adult disease. *Pediatrics*. 1998;101:518–525

89. Hill JO, Peters JC. Environmental contributions to the obesity epidemic. *Science.* 1998;280:1371–1374

90. Poston WS, Foreyt JP. Obesity is an environmental issue. *Atherosclerosis.* 1999;146:201–209

91. Whitaker RC, Wright JA, Pepe MS, Seidel KD, Dietz WH. Predicting obesity in young adulthood from childhood and parental obesity. *N Engl J Med.* 1997;337:869–873

92. Barlow SE, Dietz WH. Obesity evaluation and treatment: expert committee recommendations. The Maternal and Child Health Bureau, Health Resources and Services Administration and the Department of Health and Human Services. *Pediatrics.* 1998;102(3):e29. Available at: http://pediatrics.aappublications.org/cgi/content/full/102/3/e29. Accessed October 31, 2007

93. Fisher JO, Birch LL. Restricting access to foods and children's eating. *Appetite.* 1999;32:405–419

94. Davison KK, Birch LL. Weight status, parent reaction, and self-concept in five-year-old girls. *Pediatrics.* 2001;107:46–53

95. Goran MI, Reynolds KD, Lindquist CH. Role of physical activity in the prevention of obesity in children. *Int J Obes Relat Metab Disord.* 1999;23:S18–S33

96. Briefel RR, Johnson CL. Secular trends in dietary intake in the United States. *Ann Rev Nutr.* 2004;24:401–31

97. Nielsen SJ, Popkin B. Changes in beverage intake between 1977 and 2001. *Am J Prev Med.* 2004;27:205–210

98. Skinner JD, Ziegler P, Ponza M. Transitions in infants' and toddlers' beverage patterns. *J Am Diet Assoc.* 2004;104:S45–S50

99. Troiano RP, Briefel RR, Carroll MD, Bialostosky K. Energy and fat intakes of children and adolescents in the United States: data from the national health and nutrition examination surveys. *Am J Clin Nutr.* 2000;72:1343S–1353S

100. Rampersaud GC, Bailey LB, Kauwell GP. National survey beverage consumption data for children and adolescents indicate the need to encourage a shift toward more nutritive beverages. *J Am Diet Assoc.* 2003;103:97–100

101. Kranz S, Smiciklas-Wright H, Siega-Riz AM, Mitchell D. Adverse effect of high added sugar consumption on dietary intake in American preschoolers. *J Pediatr.* 2005;146:105–111

102. Harnack L, Stang J, Story M. Soft drink consumption among US children and adolescents: nutritional consequences. *J Am Diet Assoc.* 1999;99:436–441

103. American Academy of Pediatrics, Committee on Nutrition. Calcium requirements of infants, children, and adolescents. *Pediatrics.* 1999;104:1152–1157

104. Fisher JO, Mitchell DC, Smiciklas-Wright H, Birch LL. Maternal milk consumption predicts the trade-off between milk and soft drinks in young girls' diets. *J Nutr.* 2001;131:246–250

105. Striegel-Moore RH, Thompson D, Affenito SG, et al. Correlates of beverage intake in adolescent girls: the National Heart, Lung, and Blood Institute Growth and Health Study. *J Pediatr.* 2006;148:183–187

106. Frary CD, Johnson RK, Wang MQ. Children and adolescents' choices of foods and beverages high in added sugars are associated with intakes of key nutrients and food groups. *J Adolesc Health.* 2004;34:56–63

107. Marshall TA, Eichenberger Gilmore JM, Broffitt B, Stumbo PJ, Levy SM. Diet quality in young children is influenced by beverage consumption. *J Am Coll Nutr.* 2005;24:65–75

108. Smith MM, Lifshitz F. Excess fruit juice consumption as a contributing factor in nonorganic failure to thrive. *Pediatrics.* 1994;93:438–443

109. Lifshitz F, Ament ME, Kleinman RE, et al. Role of juice carbohydrate malabsorption in chronic non-specific diarrhea in children. *J Pediatr.* 1992;120:825–829

110. Ludwig DS, Peterson KE, Gortmaker SL. Relation between consumption of sugar-sweetened drinks and childhood obesity: a prospective, observational analysis. *Lancet.* 2001;357:505–508

111. Welsh JA, Cogswell ME, Rogers S, Rockett H, Mei Z, Grummer-Strawn LM. Overweight among low-income preschool children associated with the consumption of sweet drinks: Missouri, 1999–2002. *Pediatrics.* 2005;115:223–229

112. Dietz WH. Sugar-sweetened beverages, milk intake, and obesity in children and adolescents. *J Pediatr.* 2006;148:152–154

113. American Academy of Pediatrics, Committee on Nutrition. The use and misuse of fruit juice in pediatrics. *Pediatrics.* 2001;107:1210–1213

114. American Academy of Pediatrics, Committee on Sports Medicine and Fitness. Climatic heat stress and the exercising child and adolescent. *Pediatrics.* 2000;106:158–159

Adolescent Nutrition

Approximately 36.5 million people in the United States (14% of the population) are 10 to 19 years of age. Because adolescents grow and develop at a different rate than children, they have unique nutritional needs. Some adolescents have insufficient intakes of calcium, iron, and vitamins A and C. Special situations, such as pregnancy, chronic disease, and physical conditioning, increase nutritional requirements of the adolescent. Some disorders seen during adolescence, such as anorexia, bulimia, and obesity, are associated with insufficient or excessive nutrient intakes.

Factors Influencing Nutritional Needs of Adolescents

The onset of puberty, with its associated increased growth rate, changes in body composition and physical activity, and onset of menstruation in girls, affects normal nutritional needs during adolescence. Increased growth rates occur in girls between 10 and 12 years of age and in boys about 2 years later, although substantial individual variability occurs. Growth in girls is accompanied by a greater increase in the proportion of body fat than in boys, and in boys, growth is accompanied by a greater increase in the proportion of lean body mass and blood volume than in girls. There are a number of tools geared specifically toward assessing adolescent nutrition.[1]

Dietary Reference Intakes

The Dietary Reference Intakes (DRIs) provide guidelines for normal nutrition of adolescent boys and girls in 2 age categories: 11 to 14 years and 15 to 18 years (Appendix J, Table J–1). The Recommended Dietary Allowances (RDAs) for energy are based on the median energy intakes of adolescents followed in longitudinal growth studies. Among adolescents, individual variability occurs in the rates of physical growth, timing of the growth spurt, and physiologic maturation. In addition, individual physical activity patterns vary widely. For these reasons, assessment of energy needs of adolescents should include consideration of appetite, growth, activity, and weight gain in relation to deposition of subcutaneous fat. Restricted food intake in the physically active adolescent results in diminished growth and a drop in the basal metabolic rate and, in girls, amenorrhea. For protein, vitamins, and minerals, the DRIs are estimates designed to meet the needs of almost all healthy adolescents; therefore, they exceed the requirements for the average person. Because of the rapid growth rate at these ages, it is recommended that fat should constitute approximately 30% of dietary calories during the first 2 decades of life.[2]

During adolescence, increases in the requirement for energy and such nutrients as calcium, nitrogen, and iron are determined by increases in lean body mass rather than an increase in body weight, with its variable fat content. On the basis of data from 570 males between 8 and 25 years of age and 450 females between 10 and 20 years of age, the male lean body mass increases from 27 to 62 kg (an average of 35 kg), and the female lean body mass increases from 24 to 43 kg (an average of 19 kg).[3,4] Assuming that the lean body contents of calcium, iron, nitrogen, zinc, and magnesium of adolescents are the same as those of adults, the daily increments of body nutrients for the growing adolescent can be estimated (Table 7.1).[5] The increments in body contents of these nutrients and the increased nutrient needs are not constant throughout adolescence but are associated with growth rate rather than chronologic age.

Table 7.1
Daily Increments in Body Content of Minerals and Nitrogen During Adolescent Growth*

Mineral	Sex	Average for 10–20 y, mg	Average at Peak of Growth Spurt, mg
Calcium	M	210	400
	F	110	240
Iron	M	0.57	1.1
	F	0.23	0.9
Nitrogen[†]	M	320	610
	F	160	360
Zinc	M	0.27	0.50
	F	0.18	0.31
Magnesium	M	4.4	8.4
	F	2.3	5.0

* Adapted from Forbes[5]
† Multiply by 0.00625 to obtain grams of protein.

Nutrition Concerns During Adolescence

The National Health and Nutrition Examination Surveys (NHANES [1971–1974, 1976–1980, and 1988–1991]) found that of all age groups, adolescents had the highest prevalence of unsatisfactory nutritional status.[6]

On the basis of dietary recall, adolescents' intakes of calcium, vitamin A, vitamin C, and iron were below the RDAs. The nutrient intakes of male adolescents were closer to the RDAs simply because they ate relatively more food, whereas female adolescents frequently dieted. Soft drinks, coffee, tea, and alcoholic beverages often replaced milk and juice. Milk intake was diminished in nonwhite adolescents, possibly because of lactose intolerance.

Food habits of adolescents are characterized by: (1) an increased tendency to skip meals, especially breakfast and lunch; (2) eating more meals outside the home; (3) snacking, especially candies; (4) consumption of fast foods; and (5) dieting. Some adhere to vegetarian diets or to extremely restrictive dietary regimens, such as Zen macrobiotic diets. Some adolescents follow fad diets and may change their eating habits frequently. These behavioral patterns are explained by the adolescents' independence and busy schedule, difficulty in accepting existing values, dissatisfaction with body image, search for self-identification, desire for peer acceptance, and need to conform to the adolescent lifestyle. As a result of typical adolescent food behaviors, the following aspects of poor nutrition are related to the adolescent's diet.

1. **Energy:** The low energy intake by many adolescents creates difficulties in planning diets that contain adequate amounts of nutrients, especially iron. The RDAs for energy do not include a safety factor for increased energy needs attributable to illness, trauma, or stress and should be considered to be only average needs. Actual needs for adolescents vary with physical activity levels and the stage of maturation.
2. **Protein:** During adolescence, protein needs, like those for energy, correlate more closely with growth pattern than with chronologic age.
3. **Calcium:** Because of accelerated muscular and skeletal growth, calcium needs are greater during puberty and adolescence than during childhood.
4. **Iron:** The need for iron is increased during adolescence to sustain the rapidly increasing lean body mass and hemoglobin mass; in female adolescents, it is needed to offset menstrual losses as well.
5. **Zinc:** Zinc is essential for growth and sexual maturation. Growth retardation and hypogonadism have been reported in adolescent boys with zinc deficiency.
6. **Vegetarianism:** Adolescents who consume no animal products are vulnerable to deficiencies of several nutrients, particularly vitamins D and B_{12}, riboflavin, protein, calcium, iron, zinc, and perhaps other trace elements (see Chapter 9).

7. **Dental caries:** Although dental caries begin in early childhood, they are a highly prevalent nutrition-related problem of adolescence. Caries are associated with low fluoride intake in childhood and frequent consumption of foods containing carbohydrates (see Chapter 48).

8. **Obesity:** Results from the 1999 NHANES report that 14% of individuals between 12 and 19 years of age were overweight. This was an increase of 3% when compared with the previous NHANES report. The major nutrition-related health problem of obesity in adolescents is discussed in Chapter 33.

9. **Conditioned deficiencies:** A number of drug-nutrient interactions have been described (Appendix N).[7] Anticonvulsant drugs, especially phenytoin and phenobarbital, interfere with the metabolism of vitamin D and can lead to rickets and/or osteomalacia; therefore, supplementation with vitamin D may be desirable. Isoniazid interferes with pyridoxine metabolism. Oral contraceptives may have effects on serum lipid concentrations—in some cases, positive; in other cases, negative—that may have some clinical significance.[8]

10. **Chronic disease:** Adolescents may have inflammatory bowel disease, diabetes mellitus type 1 or type 2, juvenile rheumatoid arthritis, and sickle cell disease, among other chronic diseases. These chronic diseases can profoundly affect nutritional status.

Nutritional Considerations During Pregnancy (also see Chapter 11)
Approximately 500 000 live births to adolescent females per year are reported; more than one tenth of the adolescents are 15 years or younger. Pregnancy is believed to cause additional stress on the nutritional status of the growing and maturing adolescent. Because the adolescent growth spurt is not complete until a few years after menarche, fetal demand for nutrients could place maternal growth in jeopardy. This is especially true in girls who mature early and in girls whose prepregnancy nutritional status is unsatisfactory. However, the nutrient requirements for the adolescent growth spurt, which wanes by the time pregnancy is possible, represent only a small amount above that considered the requirement for a nongrowing pregnant adult. Growing pregnant adolescents gain more weight than do their nongrowing adolescent counterparts. Still, growing adolescents have smaller babies than those who are not growing.[9]

Although the fetus may be protected from the vagaries of maternal diet, except in extreme malnutrition, supplementation of inadequate maternal diets with calories and nutrients results in improved maternal weight gain during pregnancy and a decrease in the prevalence of infants with low birth weight.[10] However, an extensive study of healthy pregnant women showed that protein and energy supplements did not affect birth weight, and the birth weight of infants born to adolescent mothers is similar to those born to older women, when race and maternal stature are considered.[11]

Pregnant adolescents are just as likely as other teenage girls to skip meals, ingest poor-quality snacks, eat away from home, be overly concerned about weight, and have limited food choices.[12] Deficiencies of calcium, vitamins A and C, folate, iron, and zinc—most frequently reported in the diets of adolescents—may have deleterious effects on the outcome of the pregnancy. Pregnant adolescents should be cautioned against skipping meals, especially breakfast, because skipping meals may increase the risk of ketosis. The pregnant adolescent who is a strict vegetarian may ingest insufficient protein, riboflavin, vitamin B_{12}, vitamin D, and trace minerals. Appropriate vitamin and mineral supplementation is necessary for those who habitually consume inadequate diets. Folate and iron supplementation should be recommended routinely.

A comprehensive health care program for the pregnant adolescent should include proper prenatal care, monitoring of weight gain, nutritional assessment, counseling and support, family planning, and continued schooling. Whenever possible, parents or other caregivers should be included in counseling sessions. Many adolescents respond to suggestions that incorporate ethnic foods into their eating patterns. Pregnancy may provide the educator with a unique opportunity to help the adolescent understand and improve her eating habits. Nonnutritional factors can also influence the pregnancy outcome. Pregnant women should be informed of the adverse effects of smoking and of the use of alcohol and nonessential drugs.

Nutritional Concerns for Adolescent Bone Health (also see Chapter 17)
By the time of the adolescent growth spurt, the bones of the extremities have largely completed their growth. The main bone growth associated with adolescence occurs in the axial bones and is accompanied by a large increase in bone mineral density.[13] Peak bone mineral accretion rates occur at 12.5 years for girls and 14.0 years for boys. Bone mineral density reaches its peak between the ages of 20 and 30 years and decreases thereafter.[14] Adolescence is of utmost importance with regard to long-term bone health, because fully half of the adult bone calcium is accreted during these years.[15] Factors that

influence bone growth and mineral accretion during adolescence include genetics, hormonal status, exercise, adequacy of dietary calcium and vitamin D, and general nutrition and health. Although genetic factors account for more than half of the variance in final bone mineral density, the remaining factors are amenable to manipulation.

There are a number of impediments to the teenager attaining optimal bone health. Most teenagers in the United States do not ingest the recommended daily amount of calcium (1300 g/day). The biggest factor in failure of teenagers to achieve adequate calcium intake is the general decline in dietary dairy intake during these years. The American Academy of Pediatrics recommends that adolescents consume 4 servings of dairy or the equivalent per day.[16] Many teenagers no longer drink milk for various reasons. Some are truly lactose intolerant, some do not like the taste, and others consider milk to be a "child's drink." Whatever the reason, if a teenager is not consuming dairy, alternative sources of calcium and vitamin D need to be identified. Juices and fruit drinks fortified with both these nutrients are commercially available. Green, leafy vegetables that are not high in oxalates, such as broccoli, have bioavailable calcium; spinach, because of it high oxalate concentration, is not a good source of calcium. America's youth has also become progressively less active, and the amount of "screen time" they have daily has increased. These trends are detrimental to good bone health. Weight-bearing, moderate physical activity should be encouraged.[16]

References

1. Rockett RH, Berkey CS, Colditz GA. Evaluation of dietary assessment instruments in adolescents. *Curr Opin Clin Metab Care.* 2003;6:557–562

2. Gidding SS, Dennison BA, Birch LL, et al. American Heart Association. Dietary recommendations for children and adolescents: a guide for practitioners. *Pediatrics.* 2006;117:544–559

3. Forbes GB. Growth of the lean body mass in man. *Growth.* 1972;36:325–338

4. Forbes GB. Relationship of lean body mass to height in children and adolescents. *Pediatr Res.* 1972;6:32–37

5. Forbes GB. Nutritional requirements in adolescence. In: Suskind RM, ed. *Textbook of Pediatric Nutrition.* New York, NY: Raven Press; 1981:381–391

6. Caloric and selected nutrient intakes of persons 1–74 years of age: first Health and Nutrition Examination Survey. United States, 1971–1974. *Vital Health Stat 11.* 1979;(209):1–88

7. Roe DA. Diet-drug interactions and incompatibilities. In: Hathcock JN, Coon J, eds. *Nutrition and Drug Interrelations.* New York, NY: Academic Press; 1978:319–345

8. Unintended serum lipid level changes induced by some commonly used drugs. *Drug Ther Perspect.* 2001;17:11–15

9. Scholl TO, Hediger ML, Schall JI, Khoo CS, Fischer RL. Maternal growth during pregnancy and the competition for nutrients. *Am J Clin Nutr.* 1994;60:183–188

10. Chez RA. Nutritional factors in pregnancy affecting fetal growth and subsequent infant development. In: Suskind RM, Lewinter-Suskind L, eds. *Textbook of Pediatric Nutrition.* 2nd ed. New York, NY: Raven Press; 1993:1–7

11. Rush D, Stein Z, Susser M. A randomized controlled trial of prenatal nutritional supplementation in New York City. *Pediatrics.* 1980;65:683–697

12. Garn SM, Petzold AS. Characteristics of the mother and child in teenage pregnancy. *Am J Dis Child.* 1983;137:365–368

13. Southard RN, Morris JD, Mahan JD, et al. Bone mass in healthy children: measurement with quantitative DXA. *Radiology.* 1991;179:735–738

14. Steelman J, Zeitler P. Osteoporosis in pediatrics. *Pediatr Rev.* 2001;22:56–65

15. Theintz G, Buchs B, Rizzoli R, et al. Longitudinal monitoring of bone mass accumulation in healthy adolescents: evidence for a marked reduction after 16 years of age at the levels of lumbar spine and femoral neck in female subjects. *J Clin Endocrinol Metab.* 1992;75:1060–1065

16. Greer FR, Krebs NF, American Academy of Pediatrics, Committee on Nutrition. Optimizing bone health and calcium intakes of infants, children, and adolescents. *Pediatrics.* 2006;117:578–585

8 Cultural Considerations in Feeding Children

Introduction

One of the 2 overriding goals of *Healthy People 2010,* the set of health objectives for the nation, is to eliminate health disparities by addressing the needs of a population with expanding cultural diversity.[1] This goal recognizes the growing number and population of ethnic and racial groups in the United States, including individuals from the Caribbean, Central and South America, Asia, Southeast Asia, South Pacific islands, Africa, Russia, and other former Soviet Republic block countries. It is projected that by the year 2050, minorities will represent one-half of the population of the United States.[2] Newly arriving groups bring and retain their cultural identities that encompass long-held traditions and customs, including health beliefs and behaviors that often present challenges to health care professionals. Food choices and eating habits, an elemental part of one's culture, are among the most potent and emotional elements of these traditions, values, and behaviors.

Culture is a dynamic process that is both learned and shared and reflects values, practices, and habits passed down from one generation to the next.[3-6] Food and eating are among the most deep-seated cultural behaviors in life and are reflected in the way we feel and think about, value, choose, and share our food as well as when, how, and with whom we eat. Especially during early and middle childhood, family environments are key for the development of food preferences, patterns of food intake, eating styles, and activity preferences and patterns that shape children's growth, development, and health. However, from a cultural-ecological perspective, caregivers make conscious choices about behavior regarding infant and child feeding practices and act within a system of environmental constraints and opportunities.[7] Thus, caregivers also show adaptive behavior as manifested in the changing of feeding practices within new environments, as occurs with migration or contacts with different cultures and situations.

Feeding the infant as well as the young child is often approached from the narrow viewpoint that the young child is the passive receiver of food and depends on the mother's ability to adequately fulfill this role or not, and the mother's feeding of her child is rarely seen in the total context of her life. A cultural-ecological perspective for child feeding requires that attention be focused not only on the individual decision makers, the mother, and household but also on the characteristics of the environment in which the decisions are made. Mothers may be influenced in their choices of feeding practices by economic considerations and food availability, allocation of time, health characteristics and concerns, the presence of alternative care-givers, beliefs and values related to social acceptability of the choices, and advice from other people and media sources.[7] Understanding the cultural context of the mother and child will help health care professionals give appropriate and effective nutrition advice.

Importance of Addressing Cultural Food Practices

Cultural patterns are significant, because feeding patterns, the food and beverages consumed, and how these are given or served determine health and nutritional status and, especially in the case of children, provide opportunities for social, emotional, and educational development.[8,9] Optimal health, which incorporates balanced nutrition, is a highly significant factor in enabling an infant to grow as an individual into a healthy, well-adjusted, and productive adult.

A major concern about feeding practices of infants and young children in the United States is the growing problem of childhood overweight and obesity, with a high prevalence of these conditions in immigrant groups as well as other sectors of the population. Counseling to address feeding practices and lifestyles that lead to overweight and obesity is required and will only be effective if the cultural aspects of infant and child feeding and nutrition are understood and addressed by health care professionals.

Understanding Cultural Food Practices: Challenges for Health Care Professionals

The beliefs and perceptions of mothers, families, and children may be similar to or completely different from those of the health care professional. To bridge this gap, health care professionals who are sensitive to the cultural issues of their patients and willing to learn from them are better able to address their health and nutritional problems. Health care professionals who are knowledgeable in understanding the depth of these practices or who are culturally sensitive will more likely succeed in counseling patients to improve the health of children and their families.

As families migrate, there are necessary changes in their cultural food patterns, health beliefs, and behaviors and lifestyles. This process of acculturation may occur relatively rapidly, slowly, or not at all, frequently leading to a mixture of traditional and "modern" cultures. As a result, counseling and advising parents about nutrition and feeding requires listening to what the parent is saying and observing responses and reactions to questions asked. Interventions, if any, require an integrated cultural approach.

Within every culture, there are individuals who do not necessarily embrace the same set of values, beliefs, and behaviors, and the degree of changes and adaptations to the local context vary. Thus, some cultural groups are more homogenous than others. Examples of more homogenous groups include some Muslim and Hasidic Jewish groups comprising children and families who adhere to a defined set of religious and dietary laws or customs, like fasting on certain days or completely avoiding certain foods like pork and pork products. In comparison, other cultural groups, such as Hispanic immigrants and black people in the United States, have a wider range of cultural practices in relation to the feeding of their children.

Infant Feeding: Foundation of Eating Behavior

Eating is a learned process that begins at birth, starting with the first food and the very first feeding. These practices are reinforced with each and every subsequent feeding. For example, for the breastfed infant, there is the physical, emotional, and social bonding and attachment that begins to evolve between mother and infant. What foods an infant or young child is fed, the climate or environment in which feeding occurs, and the feelings and attitudes of the person who does the feeding all reflect the cultural practices of both mother and child. Because feeding an infant is defined within the cultural framework of the mother and family, it is important to understand the meaning of food and eating within this context, especially its strong role as a determinant of later food patterns and practices of a child.

Breastfeeding Practices

Cultural perceptions toward breastfeeding an infant vary considerably. Optimal breastfeeding practices as promoted by the World Health Organization include exclusive breastfeeding during the first 6 months and continued breastfeeding during the second year of life.[10] These practices are uncommon in North America, and the reasons for breastfeeding or not vary across different cultures. Breastfeeding is frequently the cultural norm in many countries of origin of immigrants in the United States. Mothers in countries such as Colombia[11] or Peru[12] consider human milk the best and other milks or formula second best. When these substitutes are given, it is primarily because the mother perceives she has insufficient milk or caregivers believe that the infant requires other liquids to satisfy thirst or prevent or treat colic.[12] Perceived negative effects on the mother's health or a new pregnancy are also common reasons for weaning. Black mothers[13] and white higher-income mothers in the United States have also given insufficient milk production as a reason for not breastfeeding.[14]

Negative changes have generally occurred with breastfeeding practices in the process of acculturation with migration. Although Hispanic infants in the United States are more likely to have been breastfed than non-Hispanic infants, the prevalence of breastfeeding is much lower than populations in their countries of origin, and studies show that the vast majority of children of Hispanic mothers in the United States also receive infant formula.[15] Children of Spanish-speaking Mexican American mothers are more likely to breastfeed than English-speaking Mexican mothers,[16] and mothers emigrating from Mexico to the United States are more likely to breastfeed than those born in the United States.[17] Similarly, Pakistani mothers in the United Kingdom breastfed much less than did those in Pakistan. Reasons given for this difference included cultural factors, such as peer pressure and social acceptance, as well as the promotion of formula feeding in the United Kingdom.[18] Another example of changes in breastfeeding habits has been seen in Hmong refugee families in the United States who formula feed instead of breastfeeding their infants.[19] The Hmong traditionally have the child-raising custom of "hlu" that caters to the child's desires; thus, formula feeding may cause infants to be given too much milk.

In a study of black mothers and their infants in North Carolina, only 14% were breastfed for more than 3 months.[13] These mothers did not believe that breastfeeding is better for an infant's health than formula feeding. White mothers have reported not initiating breastfeeding because it restricts their lifestyle,[14,20,21] whereas reasons given by black mothers were the inconvenience, pain, and physical discomfort associated with breastfeeding.[20,21] White mothers of higher socioeconomic status also said that fathers could not participate in the feeding of a breastfed child.[14]

Breastfeeding during the second year of life continues to be advantageous to a child's health and nutrition.[10] Breastfeeding during the second year is low among Hispanic (12%) and non-Hispanic (6%) populations in the United States.[15] Again, this contrasts with practices in countries of origin, where it is common for mothers to continue to breastfeed during the second year of life as internationally recommended.[10] The median duration of breastfeeding in Peru, for example, is 21 months[22]; mothers in urban Peru breastfeed their children during the second year of life to ensure a source of good nutrition and to protect the child when ill or with a poor appetite. Mothers wean their children when they feel that the children are eating enough food.[23]

These different breastfeeding practices reflect some of the many different cultural perspectives that need to be addressed in the promotion of breastfeeding.

Introduction of First Foods

For optimal nutrition, health, and development, first complementary foods should be introduced at 4 to 6 months of age (preferably 6 months of age) with the continuation of breastfeeding through or beyond the first birthday. However, the age at which first foods are introduced to an infant and the type of food offered varies considerable and is largely determined by cultural practices and perceptions. These relate to perceptions of the infant's physical and neurological maturity and developmental milestones, the child's size, the process of maturation of the eating and digestive system, interpretation of the child's signs of interest in food, and the expectations of the caregiver and other family members toward the infant's process of independence, among other factors.[24] Cultural perceptions regarding this process vary considerably. For instance, in urban Peru, infants are perceived to be reaching out and showing interest in food from around 3 to 4 months of age, and caregivers respond by giving first foods, whereas the same signs are interpreted as readiness at 7 or 8 months of age in rural populations of the country.[12,22]

Developmental factors that influence the choice of food in Hispanic cultures as well as in other cultures include the child's ability to swallow and the process of "forming the stomach,"[25] reflected in the choice of a soft consistency of foods, such as soups, a practice also observed in Hispanic populations in the United States,[15] which may result in nutritionally inadequate foods and a late introduction of lumpy foods leading to later feeding difficulties.[26] Mashed and strained foods are considered appropriate for infants who do not have teeth, a belief common to many populations, including white mothers in the United States[14] and populations in Peru.[25] Meats are considered by Peruvian mothers to be too hard for infants to eat until 10 or 11 months of age, although chicken liver is considered appropriate because of its soft texture.

Mothers do select nutritious foods for their young children, yet there are different cultural perceptions as to what is nutritious. Examples include soups, considered nutritious by Peruvian mothers, because the "goodness" is thought to be extracted from the food ingredients into the broth during boiling; soups are a typical first food. Hispanic populations in the United States often prefer fruit as a preferred first food, and white populations consider vegetables as appropriate first foods.[13] Hispanic mothers of children 2 to 4 years of age in the United States[27] and mothers of infants in urban Peru[25] both expressed a concern about "processed" foods and considered "natural" foods best, which affects their food choices.

The introduction of first foods requires trial and error and perseverance on the part of the caregiver. Non-Hispanic mothers have been seen to be more perseverant than Hispanic mothers, offering new foods more frequently before deciding that their infant did not like the food.[28] These cultural attitudes toward the introduction of first foods are important considerations to be taken into account in nutrition counseling.

Infant and Toddler Foods

Early flavor and food experiences of Hispanic infants in the United States have been shown to differ from those of non-Hispanic infants in several ways.[15] Hispanic infants younger than 1 year were more likely to be eating pureed baby foods daily, and at 6 to 11 months, Hispanic infants were less likely to be eating noninfant cereals than non-Hispanic infants. Cultural family foods, such as soups, rice, beans, and tortillas, were introduced during the second year, and infants were more likely to eat fresh fruits and fruit-flavored beverages and fewer canned foods than non-Hispanic children, consistent with practices in Mexico. Hispanic mothers commented that preparing traditional and culturally specific foods is important to them.[27] Hispanic children tended to have heightened sweet and sodium preferences.[13]

Studies have shown that Hispanic toddlers in the United States consume a higher proportion of daily energy intake from carbohydrates and a lower proportion of energy from fats than do non-Hispanic toddlers,[29] with differences between English-speaking and Spanish-speaking families, indicating a process of acculturation. Hispanic toddlers have a lower intake of calcium and a higher intake of sodium than do non-Hispanic toddlers.

Hispanic mothers have expressed different attitudes toward foods on coming to the United States.[30] Mothers mentioned a liking for "junk" food and commented that in their country of origin, vegetables were considered animal food and it is difficult for them to get used to eating them in the United States. Also, because they never had enough meat in their countries, they now think it is the best and most delicious type of food to prepare.

Many immigrant populations value their traditional foods and consider them part of their cultural identity, especially staple foods. Rice is a predominant food for 9- to 12-month old toddlers in Pakistan but not so for Pakistani toddlers in the United Kingdom.[18] Other weaning foods were cereals and eggs followed by vegetables and fruit for Pakistani children in Pakistan, compared with vegetables, fruit, and convenience foods for Pakistani children in the United Kingdom. However, mothers expressed confusion and uncertainly with respect to hidden ingredients in convenience foods, preferring vegetarian options or sweet foods to avoid the possibility of eating foods prohibited by their religion. Because of this, many mothers postponed their child's introduction to traditional family foods at a critical age, which resulted in subsequent rejection when the child was older, a phenomenon that has occurred commonly with American Indian/Alaska Native families and has led to less nutritious diets. This uncertainty about appropriate foods during the toddler years is a concern of many different ethnic groups and, like appropriate first foods, needs to be addressed with parents.

Meals and Snacks

Infants starting complementary feeding at 4 to 6 months of age need to eat semisolid or solid foods 2 to 3 times a day, and this increases to 3 meals and 1 to 2 snacks during the second year of life.[10] In general, young children in the United States consume food several times a day. Infants and toddlers of both Hispanic and non-Hispanic families have been observed to eat a mean of 7 times a day, with a range of 4 to 12 snacks,[31] and this is consistent with eating patterns found in Mexico.[32] The total daily energy intake was similar between these ethnic groups, but there were differences in the source of energy at the different feeding times by ethnic group and age of the children. Notably, snacks provided a high proportion (25%) of the daily energy intake, and Hispanic toddlers had a higher intake of carbohydrate and lower intake of fat at lunch. Snacks provided more fiber in the Hispanic toddler diet because of a higher rate of eating fresh fruit, especially in the afternoon. A typical lunch was hot dogs and French fries for non-Hispanic toddlers and cooked potatoes and raw vegetables followed by sweets for Hispanic toddlers. Low-income Hispanic mothers in one study expressed an ambivalence about adhering to a regular schedule for meals,[28] in contrast to mothers in a study in urban Peru, where a structured meal was considered best for toddlers, children, and adolescents.[33]

Snacking in other countries shows a variety of cultural practices. In urban Peru, similar to Mexico, toddlers, especially those who are breastfed, are given snacks several times a day, and snacks contribute significantly to energy intake, whereas toddlers in Ghana, as in many other developing countries, eat less often, consume more energy at meals, and consume little food later in the day.[34] Different practices regarding the relative importance and types of foods served at snacks and meals require different emphases when providing advice to parents about how to improve their children's dietary patterns.

Young Child Feeding

Ensuring that a young child consumes a balanced diet is a challenge for all caregivers. Giving infants and children nutritious foods and getting their children to eat are goals for most mothers of different ethnic groups. In a study of 2- to 5-year-old children, Hispanic mothers placed significant value on "eating enough," thus pressuring their children to eat. They were also concerned about having nutritious foods for their children and providing foods their children liked and that are easy and quick to prepare.[27] Middle-income white and black mothers were concerned about providing enough vegetables and portion sizes, and middle-income white mothers were concerned about high-fat foods. All groups were concerned about too many sweets. Middle-income white mothers were challenged to get their children to eat a "balanced" diet and enough food but "not too much." Black mothers mentioned drinks before a meal as a challenge. Variety of food in the infant diet is valued by all ethnic groups, and establishing good feeding habits early in life was mentioned specifically by higher-income white mothers.[14] Strategies used to introduce new foods and a mother's response to children's specific alternative food requests are frequently influenced by culture.[27]

Feeding Style

Perhaps one of the most important cultural aspects of child feeding is the difference in feeding styles that caregivers use with their infants and young children. Feeding style is critical in determining the food that a child eats and the feeding patterns he or she develops for the future. Feeding style includes family eating patterns, whether mealtimes are shared or the child eats separately. Parental interactions during feeding include the degree of control over the child's eating and emotional aspects of feeding a child.[13]

On the basis of the work of Birch et al,[35] Bentley[13] observed the following feeding styles among black mothers of infants and toddlers in North Carolina: (1) laissez faire, in which the mother has little interaction with the child during feeding and enforces no limits regarding food; (2) pressuring or controlling, in which the caregiver worries that the child is eating too little or tries to soothe the child; (3) restrictive/controlling, in which the caregiver limits a child to healthy food and the amount of food given; and (4) responsive feeding, in which caregivers are attentive to the child's cues and set appropriate limits. Responsive feeding is considered to be the most appropriate feeding style and is based on the concepts of psychosocial care.[10,21,36] A range of feeding styles is seen between and within different cultures. Typically, a laissez faire style has been observed in rural India, Central America,[37] and the rural highlands of Peru,[38] where infants receive little physical help or verbal encouragement, in part because they are encouraged to be independent from an early age and fend for themselves when the next baby is born. This feeding style often leads to inadequate food intake and undernutrition.[38] With migration to the cities, there is a change from the laissez fair style to a more controlling style and efforts to pressure the child to eat.

Among the black mothers in the North Carolina study,[13] there was a high prevalence of pressuring behaviors—for example, mothers said they frequently tried to get their infants to finish their food and they praised them after each bite. When the child was perceived to be thin, more pressure to eat was applied, similar to that described in Hispanic populations in the United States.[27,39] The laissez faire feeding style was also observed. Mothers propped up the infant's feeding bottle, and half of the mothers reported watching television while feeding their children, and they were less likely to limit their children's intake of sweet or junk food. This feeding style was associated with perceived fatter children in contrast to that observed in rural populations of developing countries, where it is associated with undernutrition.[13] Mothers exhibiting restrictive behaviors frequently controlled how much their children ate and some were concerned that they would eat too much if another person fed them, and they seldom let their children eat sweets or junk food. Mothers who exhibited a responsive feeding style monitored their child's feeding and kept track of how much junk foods, high-fat foods, and sweet foods their children ate and reported being attentive to their children while they were eating.

Strategies to get children to eat vary among different ethnic or cultural groups. Special snacks or treats are used as rewards, bribes, or pacifiers across cultures, and foods such as ice cream, gelatin, popcorn, or cookies are common devices. Common strategies used by low-income Hispanic mothers were bribes regarding television, playing, or dessert[28] and are perceived by the mothers as effective forms of discipline rather than force. The mother's own upbringing influences many attitudes toward feeding. In one study, Hispanic mothers recalled that they had to eat everything when they were children. Mexican American mothers have also been observed to encourage their sons to eat more than their daughters.[40]

The type of verbal interaction during a meal is an integral component of feeding style and varies considerably between cultures. There may be little verbal interaction during feeding, as in rural communities of Peru or India[38]; orders or commands given to the child during feeding, such as in urban Peru; or a responsive verbal interaction, with praising and giving positive comments about the food and the child, as reported by black mothers in North Carolina.[13]

Across different cultures, there is balance between pleasing children and giving foods considered healthy, and where this balance lies depends on the different cultures. In France, parental feeding styles tend to exclude between-meal snacks, because it is believed that children should learn to eat what adults eat. In contrast, in the United States, the predominant attitude is that food choices are determined by what the child likes.[13]

Body Image and Expectations

How a mother perceives her child, especially in terms of body size—such as normal weight, overweight, or underweight—is important, because it can influence her feeding of the child. In the North Carolina study,[13] black mothers often thought their children were thin when they were not or that their children were not fat when in fact they were at the higher end of the weight distribution. The latter perception is also seen in higher-income white mothers.[27] These perceptions are important, because they are related to the parental feeding styles: the perceived thin children were pressed to eat more, and fatter children were fed with a laissez faire style.[13]

Thinness has been mentioned as being especially worrisome to immigrant Hispanic mothers of 2- to 5-year-olds, who considered that undernutrition and intestinal infections were greater threats to a child's health than overweight, reflecting the concern for undernutrition seen commonly in their country of origin.[27,30] Thin children are considered to be more disease prone, whereas a little extra weight is thought to help the child recover from illness. Moderate overweight is what parents perceive as looking best or healthiest. But even more than weight, healthy children are considered to be those who have a happy expression, sit upright, and have healthy skin and hair.[30] In several reports, Hispanic parents believed that good health and what foods their children ate were more important than their weight, but they didn't want their children to be underweight.[27] Black mothers generally believed children would outgrow their overweight or that having a high weight in childhood is healthy. They tended to believe that genetics is an important determinant of overweight (as well as environment).[27] Hispanic mothers considered that environment was a major determinant of over-weight,[27] and for mothers in Pennsylvania, fatness in babies was not valued, because they believed that fat babies would become fat adults.[14] These are examples of cultural perceptions that need to be addressed to reduce the risk of overweight and obesity. This is especially the case for Hispanic families, for whom developing an acceptance of thin as well as a "chubby" appearance may be essential to help mothers more readily accept healthy changes, putting emphasis on improved diet and physical activity and happy children rather than weight outcomes.[30]

Feeding and Child Characteristics

Fussy or difficult children demand special attention from caregivers to ensure that they eat sufficient food. How a mother perceives her child's emotional and behavioral characteristics and how she reacts and responds to the child's temperament or fussiness varies across cultures. In a study of black adolescents conducted in Baltimore, the child characteristics that most influenced feeding decisions were body size, crying, sleeping patterns, and appetite.[41] Studies have found that fussy or irritable infants of black mothers are more likely to be fed to quiet them, thus leading to rapid weight gain.[41,42] A mother's perception of an easy temperament in her child and her own flexibility in caregiving have been related to longer duration of breastfeeding.[43] Black and white mothers cite children's changing likes and dislikes of foods as well as normal development and the introduction of new foods as reasons for difficult feeding for 2- to 5-year-olds.[27] Only Hispanic mothers mentioned that breaking routines and illness could be a cause of difficult feeding.

Black mothers in North Carolina described an infant who had a huge appetite and was always reaching for food as a "greedy" child. Grandmothers tended to use "greedy" as a positive quality, whereas young mothers did not want their infants to be greedy.[13] Yet, most respondents preferred a greedy child to a picky one.[41] Thus, the connotations of words used to describe a child can vary between and within cultures and need to be understood by the health care professional.

Specific Cultural Food Beliefs

In many cultures, there are specific beliefs around certain foods or groups of foods. Health care professionals typically classify foods by food groups on the basis of the food pyramid in the United States. Different cultural groups may classify foods differently, such as foods that are prepared or eaten together or foods that are considered good or unsuitable for infants or according to their taste rather than their nutritional value or function.[44]

Among some groups, a rather complex system of food categories has existed for centuries and is woven into the lives of families on the basis of body image and functions.[45] An example of this concept is the "hot" and "cold" humoral system common in Central and South America, in which foods are perceived as part of the balance for the health of an individual. Disease occurs when there is an imbalance between the hot and cold. When these are in balance, it is thought the result is a positive state of health for an individual.[46] The label of hot and cold has nothing to do with the temperature of the food but with the properties of food and illness states on body function. An illness such as diarrhea may be considered a hot or cold condition according to its perceived etiology, and foods with the opposite property would be given to counteract the illness. Examples of hot foods in the highlands of Peru are herbs or toasted wheat, and many tubers and fruits are considered cold foods unless they have been left in the sun or processed in a way that changes them into hot/warm foods.[44,47]

Some foods are thought to have some magical or healing properties or contain special ingredients to improve one's health. One example of this belief is the practice of mixing raw eggs with malta (a beverage containing less than 0.5% alcohol/12 oz) by Puerto Rican individuals, who believe this drink will enhance a child's appetite and, hence, promote growth.[48] Frog's blood is considered a good medicine for anemia in Peru[33]; eggs are believed to cause stubbornness in young children in the Lao People's Democratic Republic.[49]

Sources of Advice on Child Feeding

Different cultures give different weight to the sources of advice of the child's primary caregiver regarding infant and child feeding. In some cultures, advice from the health care professional may be the most influential; in others, family members may be considered the most important and credible sources. It is helpful to understand who influences a mother and to take this into account in counseling. In Hispanic cultures, the opinions of the mother's own mother are frequently a major influence,[13] and this is often observed in black adolescent mothers.[21,41]

The role of the father and his influence on child feeding practices varies between cultures. Male partners of white mothers have been reported to be more likely to influence white mothers than black partners of black mothers and to encourage the early introduction of solids.[20]

Pakistani mothers in both the United Kingdom and Pakistan received advice on weaning food practices from family and friends, and especially in Pakistan, from the extended family, principally from grandmothers and other mothers in the family, and this advice often contradicted that given by health care professionals. Pakistani mothers in the United Kingdom expressed a lack of confidence because of the conflicting advice given by relatives, confusion among health care professionals, and the wide variety of baby foods available in the stores.[18]

Table 8.1
Some Cultural Differences to be Considered in Counseling

Breastfeeding/ formula feeding	Perceptions of breastfeeding, reasons for not breastfeeding
	Breastfeeding versus formula feeding
	Who initiates and ends a feed (mother, child)
	Opinions of other family members
	Previous experiences, peer and social influences
	Attentiveness and interactions during feeding, attention on the child, other activities of the mother while breastfeeding or bottle feeding
Introduction of first foods	Perception of child's readiness for food: age, signs, maturity
	Perceptions of appropriate first foods: consistency, types of foods and reasons
	Perceptions toward trying different foods
Complementary (weaning) foods	Introduction and use of traditional foods
	Food selection, home prepared, commercial foods
	Preferences for sweet or savory, etc
	Preference for high carbohydrate, fat, or nutrient-rich foods
	Perceptions of processed and commercially available foods affecting food choices
	Introduction of new foods
	What is considered a balanced and varied diet
	How much should be eaten

Table 8.1 *(continued)*
Some Cultural Differences to be Considered in Counseling

Meals and snacks	Frequency of feeding
	Relative importance of meals and snacks
	Perceptions to meal structure
	Types of snacks, variations in the morning or afternoon
	Drinks and meals
Feeding style	Type of feeding style: laissez faire, pressuring or controlling, restrictive controlling, responsive feeding
	How children are encouraged to eat: bribes, treats
	Personal history of how mother was fed as a child
	Verbal interaction during feeding
	Pleasing children versus health foods
Body image	Perceptions of normal, underweight, overweight
	Concerns of underweight or overweight
	Perceptions and ideals of a healthy child
	Perceptions of determinants of overweight
Child characteristics	Perceptions of temperament and fussy children
	Reasons for and responses to difficult feeding
	Perceptions of child appetite
Specific food beliefs	Religious or ethnic beliefs about prohibited or special foods
	Use of certain foods in health or illness
Source of advice	Who influences the mother
	Importance of grandmother, extended family, and peers and what happens in situations when influential family members are not available for advice
	Influence of father, health care professional

Understanding as much as possible of the cultural context of the mothers, children, and families and positioning advice within the context relevant for each family will help health care professionals to be as effective as possible in assisting families to make appropriate food, diet, and feeding choices for optimal health and development of their children.

References

1. US Department of Health and Human Services. *Healthy People 2010.* Conf ed. Washington, DC: US Department of Health and Human Services; 2000

2. United States Census Bureau. Census projections, April 1996. Available at: http://www.census.gov. Accessed August 7, 2007

3. Kittle PM, Sucher K. *Food and Culture in America.* Florence, KY: Van Nostrand Reinhold; 1990

4. Pelto G. Cultural issues in maternal and child health and nutrition. *Soc Sci Med.* 1987;25:553–559

5. Terry RD. Needed: a new appreciation of culture and food behavior. *J Am Diet Assoc.* 1994;94:501–503

6. Monses ER. Respecting diversity helps America eat right. *J Am Diet Assoc.* 1993;92:282

7. Pelto GH. Perspectives on infant feeding: decision-making and ecology. *Food Nutr Bull.* 1981;3(3):16–29

8. Novello AC, Degraw C, Kleinman DV. Healthy children ready to learn: an essential collaboration between health and education. *Public Health Rep.* 1992;10:3–15

9. US Department of Education. *Preparing Young Children for Success: Guideposts for Achieving Our First National Goal.* Washington, DC: Dept Education; 1991

10. Pan American Health Organization/World Health Organization. *Guiding Principles for Complementary Feeding of the Breastfed Child.* Geneva, Switzerland: Pan American Health Organization/World Health Organization; 2003. Available at: http://www.paho.org/English/AD/FCH/NU/Guiding_Principles_CF.pdf. Accessed November 2, 2007

11. Alvarado BE, Tabares RE, Delisle H, Zunzunegui MV. [Maternal beliefs, feeding practices and nutritional status in Afro-Colombian infants.] [Article in Spanish.] *Arch Latinoam Nutr.* 2005;55:55–63

12. Carrasco Saenz N, Vega Sanchez SM, eds. *Evaluación de la Situación de la Lactancia Materna y Alimentación Complementaria en el Perú – 2001.* Lima, Peru: CEPREN/Red Peruana de Lactancia Materna; 2001

13. Lederman SA, Akabas SR, Moore BJ, et al. Summary of the presentations at the Conference on Preventing Childhood Obesity, December 8, 2003. *Pediatrics.* 2004;114(Suppl 1):1146–1173

14. Adair L. Feeding babies: mothers' decisions in urban US setting. *Med Anthropol.* 1983;4:1–19

15. Mennella JA, Ziegler P, Briefel R, Novak T. Feeding Infants and Toddlers Study: the types of foods fed to Hispanic infants and toddlers. *J Am Diet Assoc.* 2006;106(Suppl 1):S96–S106

16. John AM, Martorell R. Incidence and duration of breast-feeding in Mexican-American infants, 1970–1982. *Am J Clin Nutr.* 1989;50:868–874

17. Romero-Gwynn E, Carias L. Breast-feeding intentions and practice among Hispanic mothers in southern California. *Pediatrics.* 1989;84:626–632

18. Sarwar T. Infant feeding practices of Pakistani others in England and Pakistan. *J Hum Nutr Diet.* 2002;15:419–428

19. Culhane-Pera KA, Naftali ED, Jacobson C, Xiong ZB. Cultural feeding practices and child-raising philosophy contribute to iron-deficiency anemia in refugee Hmong children. *Ethn Dis.* 2002;12:199–205

20. McLorg PA, Bryant CA. Influence of social network members and health care professionals on infant feeding practices of economically disadvantaged mothers. *Med. Anthropol.* 1989;10:265–278

21. Pelto GH, Levitt E, Thairu L. Improving feeding practices: current patterns, common constraints, and the design of interventions. *Food Nutr Bull.* 2003;24:45–82

22. National Institute of Statistics and Information. *Demographic and Health Family Survey, 2000.* Lima, Peru: Instituto Nacional de Estadistica e Informatica; 2001:163–186

23. Marquis GS, Diaz J, Bartolini R, Creed de Kanashiro H, Rasmussen KM. Recognizing the reversible nature of child-feeding decisions: breastfeeding, weaning and relactation patterns in a shanty town community of Lima, Peru. *Soc Sci Med.* 1998;47:645–656

24. Alder EM, Williams FL, Anderson AS, Forsyth S, Florey Cdu V, van der Velde P. What influences the timing of the introduction of solid foods to infants? *Brit J Nutr.* 2004;92:527–531

25. Liria R, Bartolini R, Abad M, Creed-Kanashiro H. Mothers' perceptions towards the feeding of animal sources foods to infants, Lima, Peru [abstr 285.6]. Paper presented at FASEB Experimental Biology; April 2–6, 2005; San Diego, CA

26. Northstone K, Emmett P, Nethersole F, ALSPAC Study Team. Avon Longitudinal Study of Pregnancy and Childhood. The effect of age of introduction to lumpy solids on foods eaten and reported feeding difficulties at 6 and 15 months. *J Hum Nutr Diet.* 2001;14:43–54

27. Sherry B, McDivitt J, Birch LL, et al. Attitudes, practices, and concerns about child feeding and child weight status among socioecomically diverse white, Hispanic, and African-American mothers. *J Am Diet Assoc.* 2004;104:215–221

28. Kaiser LL, Martinez NA, Harwood JO, Garcia LC. Child feeding strategies in low-income Latino households: focus group observations. *J Am Diet Assoc.* 1999;99:601–603

29. Briefel R, Zeigler P, Novak T, Ponzo M. Feeding Infants and Toddlers Study: characteristics and usual nutrient intake of Hispanic and non-Hispanic infants and toddlers. *J Am Diet Assoc.* 2006;106:S84–S95

30. Crawford PB, Gosliner W, Anderson C, et al. Counseling Latina mothers of preschool children about weight issues: suggestions for a new framework. *J Am Diet Assoc.* 2004;104:387–394

31. Ziegler P, Hanson C, Ponza M, Novak T, Hendricks K. Feeding infants and toddlers study: meal and snack intakes of Hispanic and Non-Hispanic infants and toddlers. *J Am Diet Assoc.* 2006;106:S107–S123

32. Garcia ES, Kaiser LL, Dewey KG. Self-regulation of food intake among rural Mexican preschool children. *Eur J Clin Nutr.* 1990;44:371–380

33. Creed-Kanashiro HM, Bartolini RM, Fukumoto MN, Uribe TG, Robert RC, Bentley ME. Formative research to develop a nutrition education intervention to improve dietary iron

intake among women and adolescent girls through community kitchens in Lima, Peru. *J Nutr Suppl.* 2003;133(11 Suppl 2):3987S–3991S

34. Marquis GS, Penny ME, Colecraft EK, Lozada MF. A comparison of patterns of breastfeeding and complementary feeding in Peru and Ghana. *Adv Exp Med Biol.* 2004;554:293–298

35. Birch LL, Davison KK. Family environmental factors influencing the developing behavioral controls of food intake and childhood overweight. *Pediatr Clin North Am.* 2001;48:893–907

36. Engle PL, Bentley M, Pelto G. The role of care in nutrition programmes: current research and a research agenda. *Proc Nutr Soc.* 2000;59:25–35

37. Engle PL, Zeitlin M. Active feeding behavior compensates for low interest in food among young Nicaraguan children. *J Nutr.* 1996;126:1808–1016

38. Bentley ME, Engle P, Penny ME, et al. Care and nutrition: differences in feeding style and infant nutrition status among low-income urban and rural Peru caregivers. *FASEB J.* 2000;Abstr. 356.2

39. Anderson CB, Hughes SO, Fisher JO, Nicklas TA. Cross-cultural equivalent of feeding beliefs and practices: the psychometric properties of child feeding questionnaire among Blacks and Hispanics. *Prev Med.* 2005;41:521–531

40. Olvera-Ezzell N, Power TG, Cousins JH. Maternal socialization of children's eating habits: strategies used by obese Mexican-American mothers. *Child Dev.* 1990;61:395–400

41. Bentley M, Gavin L, Black MM, Teti L. Infant feeding practices of low income, African-American, adolescent mothers: an ecological, multigenerational perspective. *Soc Sci Med.* 1999;49:1085–1100

42. Carey WB. Temperament and increased weight gain in infants. *J Dev Behav Pediatr.* 1985;6:128–131

43. Vandiver TA. Relationship of mothers' perceptions and behavior to the duration of breastfeeding. *Psychol Rep.* 1997;80(3 Pt 2):1375–1384

44. Creed-Kanashiro H. Peru: the rural community of Chamis and the urban suburb of San Vicente in Cajamarca. In: Kuhnlein H, Pelto GH, eds. *Culture, Environment and Food to prevent Vitamin A Deficiency.* Ottawa, Ontario: International Development Research Centre; Boston, MA: International Nutrition Foundation for Developing Countries; 1997. Available at: http://www.unu.edu/unupress/food2/UIN07E/uin07e00.htm. Accessed November 2, 2007

45. Risser AL, Mazur LJ. Use of folk remedies in a Hispanic population. *Arch Pediatr Adolesc Med.* 1995;149:978–981

46. Ikeda J, Wright J. Pediatrics in a culturally diverse society. *Pediatric BASICS.* 1996;76:10–17

47. Creed-Kanashiro H, Fukumoto M, Jacoby E, Verzosa C, Bentley M, Brown KH. Use of recipe trials and anthropological techniques for the development of a home prepared weaning food in the central highlands of Perú. *J Nutr Educ.* 1991;23:30–35

48. Jelliffe DB. *Child Nutrition in Developing Countries: A Handbook for Fieldworkers.* Washington, DC: Department of Health, Education, and Welfare; 1968

49. Gillespie A, Creed-Kanashiro HM, Srivongsa D, Sayakoummane D, Galloway R. Consulting with caregivers: using formative research to improve maternal and newborn care and infant and young child feeding in the Lao People's Democratic Republic. In: *Health, Nutrition and Population, Discussion Paper.* Washington, DC: The World Bank; 2004

9   Nutritional Aspects of Vegetarian Diets

Vegetarianism, according to the *Merriam–Webster Dictionary,* is defined as "the theory or practice of living on a diet made up of vegetables, fruits, grains, nuts, and sometimes eggs or dairy products." Vegetarianism is a way of life for many individuals for various reasons. Because there can be potentially serious implications for the growing pediatric and adolescent population secondary to self-imposed or misguided limitations, it behooves the pediatrician to assess the nutritional status of vegetarian patients to ensure their optimal health and growth and provide anticipatory guidance to prevent any potential deficits.

A true vegetarian is a person who does not eat meat, fish, or fowl or products containing these foods. The eating patterns of vegetarians may vary considerably. Vegetarians are a heterogenous group of individuals falling in different categories, as shown in Table 9.1. In fact, many so-called vegetarians eat some meat, fish, or seafood products. A lacto-ovo vegetarian eats grains, vegetables, fruits, legumes, seeds, nuts, dairy products, and eggs but excludes meat, fish, or fowl. The lacto vegetarian excludes eggs as well as meat, fish, and fowl. The eating pattern of a vegan, or total vegetarian, is similar to the lacto vegetarian diet, with the exclusion of dairy and all products of animal origin, including gelatin and honey. A macrobiotic diet is based largely on grains, legumes, and vegetables. Fruits, nuts, and seeds are consumed to a lesser extent.[1] However, some individuals on a macrobiotic diet also consume limited amounts of fish. A sproutarian eats primarily

Table 9.1
Types of Vegetarians[26]

Classic Vegetarians	New Vegetarians
Lacto-ovo vegetarians	Low meat vegetarians
Lacto vegetarians	Almost vegetarians
Ovo vegetarians	Semivegetarians
Vegans	Pesco vegetarians
Raw food eaters	Pollo vegetarians
Sproutarians	Pudding vegetarians
Fruitarians	
Macrobiotic vegetarians	
Anthroposophic vegetarians	

sprouted seeds (eg, bean sprouts, wheat, or broccoli sprouts) supplemented with other raw foods. Fruitarianism involves fruits, berries, juices, grains, nuts, seeds, legumes, and a few vegetables. A raw food diet excludes anything cooked above 118°F; this is the temperature at which enzymes begin to be destroyed.[2] People leading an anthroposophic lifestyle have a diet comprising vegetables spontaneously fermented by lactobacilli and a restriction on antibiotics, antipyretics, and immunizations.[3] Each of these eating styles has different implications on the nutrition and health of children and adolescents. Therefore, it is important for the health care professional or nutritionist to determine which groups of foods are actually consumed and which are avoided and the degree of conviction and adherence to the dietary pattern so as to provide appropriate recommendations.

Various reasons for choosing a vegetarian diet are listed in Table 9.2. Some may practice vegetarianism for more than one reason. Health considerations, concern for the environment, animal welfare activism, economic considerations, and religious beliefs are some of the reasons for choosing vegetarianism. Economic reasons alone are usually not involved, because in the United States, a wide variety of both plant and animal foods are widely available and inexpensive. However, some immigrants from developing countries (eg, mainland China, India, Pakistan, and Southeast Asia) may

Table 9.2
Reasons for Vegetarian Lifestyle[26]

Health	Religion
Performance	Ethics
Economical reasons	Animal rights
Environmental concerns	Cosmetics
Hygiene	Social influence
Moral	New age

maintain vegetarian eating patterns based on tradition, habit, and religious beliefs. Other reasons for eating vegetarian diets include concerns about the risks of omnivorous diets and the negative publicity about bacterial foodborne disease from animal foods. There is a group of moral vegetarians who avoid meat because they believe it involves animal cruelty or environmental degradation or because of political reasons.[4] Ecological reasons involving views that the environmental effect of meat and poultry production is an inefficient use of the planet's resources motivate others.[5] Some have religious (eg, Seventh-Day Adventists, some Hindus, Jains, and Buddhists) or philosophical beliefs (macrobiotics, transcendental meditators, anthroposophists, some yogic groups) that encourage various types of vegetarian diets and/or other food avoidances.

Trends

A survey from 2003 found that approximately 2.8% of the US adult population (260 million people) consistently follow a vegetarian diet,[6] of which 0.9% were vegans. Approximately 2% of 6- to 17-year-old children and adolescents in the United States are vegetarians, and approximately 0.5% of these are vegans.[7] As the popularity of vegetarian diets increase, many parents encourage their children to join them in these eating patterns.[8]

As with any dietary pattern, the degree of adherence to vegetarian patterns varies, and thus, overall nutrient intake differs from one vegetarian to the next. Most dietary patterns can be accommodated while fulfilling nutrient needs with appropriate dietary planning on the basis of scientific principles of sound nutrition. Most vegetarian parents welcome such advice. However, when goals are zealously pursued and nutrition principles are ignored, the health consequences can be unfortunate, especially for infants and young children.[9] Overall, it is possible to provide a balanced diet to vegetarians and vegans.[10]

The extent and degree of animal food restriction does not always predict either the extent of other food avoidances or the divergences in lifestyle and philosophical beliefs from nonvegetarians, although there is some correspondence. Generally, vegetarians with the most restrictive diets have the largest number of reasons for their eating styles, and their dietary patterns are most closely interwoven into their philosophical and belief systems.

A position paper of the American Dietetic Association and Dietitians of Canada states that appropriately planned vegetarian diets are healthful and nutritionally adequate and provide health benefits in the prevention and treatment of certain diseases.[11] A vegetarian, including vegan, diet can also meet current Recommended Dietary Allowances (RDAs) for protein, iron, zinc, calcium, vitamin D, riboflavin, vitamin B_{12}, vitamin A, omega-3 fatty acids, and iodine. In some cases, use of fortified foods or supplements can be helpful in meeting recommendations for individual nutrients. Well-planned vegan and other types of vegetarian diets are appropriate for all stages of the life cycle, including during pregnancy, lactation, infancy, childhood, and adolescence. Vegetarian diets have been shown to offer numerous advantages, including lower amounts of saturated fat, cholesterol, and animal protein and higher amounts of carbohydrates, fiber, magnesium, vitamins C and E,[12] carotenoids, and phytochemicals.[13] Vegetarians have been reported to have lower body mass indices than nonvegetarians.

Although vegetarians can also suffer from coronary artery disease, hypertension, type 2 diabetes mellitus, and prostate and colon cancer, the incidence of these diseases are lower than in omnivores. There may be other advantages in addition to an improved lipid profile[14] from vegetarian diets. A study evaluating circulating E-selectin concentrations, which include circulating intercellular adhesion molecule and circulating vascular adhesion molecule, in vegetarian and control adults showed that low circulating E-selectin concentrations in vegetarians may reflect the favorable cardiovascular risk profile of this group.[15] There is overwhelming epidemiologic evidence that consumption of a high amount of fruits and vegetables is associated with reduced mortality from cardiovascular disease,[16,17] stroke,[18] cancer,[19] and other causes.[20] In part, this may simply indicate that consumption of a high amount of fruits and vegetables is a marker of a healthy lifestyle, but there is also strong evidence from in vitro studies and clinical trials that micronutrients and other components of fruits and vegetables have beneficial biologic effects. Most attention has focused on antioxidants,[21] B group vitamins, minerals, and fiber, but several strands of evidence now indicate that increased intake of salicylates may be another benefit of fruit and vegetable consumption.[22] Lawrence and colleagues have reported that urinary excretion of salicyluric acid and salicylic acid is significantly increased in vegetarians compared with nonvegetarians.[23] They previously reported that serum salicylic acid was also significantly increased in vegetarians compared with nonvegetarians.[24] Interestingly, urinary excretion of salicylic acid of vegetarians was similar to that of nonvegetarians consuming 75 or 150 mg of aspirin/day, although salicyluric acid excretion was substantially greater in the nonvegetarian aspirin group. The concentrations of salicylic acid seen in vegetarians have been shown to inhibit COX-2 in vitro,[25] and it is plausible that dietary salicylates may contribute to the beneficial effects of a vegetarian diet, whereas it seems unlikely that most people who consume a mixed diet will achieve sufficient dietary intake of salicylates to have a therapeutic effect.

Additional Implications of Vegetarianism

The lifestyle of vegetarians is different from omnivores in 3 major ways. First, they are more likely to practice abstinence or moderation in alcohol consumption as well as other stimulating products, including nicotine. Second, they tend to be engaged in increased physical activities. Third, overall, plant foods are less calorie dense and, thus, predispose to less obesity and many be compatible with healthier outcome in sedentary individuals. So the overall benefit may be from vegetarian lifestyle rather than diet alone.[26] It is generally believed that all these factors account for its advantages, although the issues of the vegetarian lifestyle involving ecological, social (ethical, moral, philosophical), and economical concerns are beyond the scope of this discussion.

Another example of such perceived benefit has been reported in children with anthroposophic lifestyle. An anthroposophic lifestyle involves a high intake of organically produced food items, including spontaneously fermented vegetables, and foods containing live lactobacilli. In addition, a restrictive use of antibiotics, antipyretics, and immunizations is common in these families.[27] A study evaluating gut flora in children younger than 2 years with this lifestyle in comparison to those with a traditional lifestyle reported that microflora-associated characteristics were different between the 2 groups. Such diversity in the innate population of bacteria may contribute to lower prevalence of atopic disease. This could be secondary to a combination of probiotics[28] and restriction of antibiotics, leading to inhibition of immunoglobulin E, as shown in animal studies.[29] In an open-label study in adults with refractory atopic dermatitis, alternative therapy with a low-energy vegetarian diet caused striking improvement in the severity of dermatitis and laboratory parameters, such as lactate dehydrogenase-5 activity and number of peripheral eosinophils. Although the exact beneficial ingredient from the diet was difficult to determine on the basis of this study, the vegetarian diet was believed to contribute partially to the improvement by inhibiting eosinophil differentiation and of prostaglandin E_2 by monocytes.[30]

There may be a concern regarding lower intake of vitamin B_{12}, vitamin D, calcium, zinc, and riboflavin in vegetarians—especially vegans. A Polish study suggested that prepubertal vegetarian children had lower concentrations of leptin, a polypeptide that plays a role in bone growth, maturation, and weight regulation in comparison with their omnivore counterparts,[31] which may contribute to reduced bone growth and development in childhood. These preliminary observations need further corroboration in the future. A vegan diet may put children at risk of vitamin A deficiency and subsequent keratomalacia, anemia, and protein and zinc deficiency if proper evaluation and education of the family is not performed.[32] The overall belief that patients following vegan or vegetarian diets suffer from nutritional deficiencies is false, as reports of specific malnutrition in these populations are rare.[33]

Dietary practices among vegetarians are varied; hence, individual assessment of dietary intakes is important. Such assessments can be best made by using a 24- to 72-hour food recall and food frequency questionnaire.[34] Tips for balanced meal planning are shown in Table 9.3. Health care professionals and nutritionists can educate vegetarians about food sources of specific nutrients, food purchase and preparation, and any dietary modifications that may be necessary to meet individual needs. Menu planning for vegetarians can be simplified by use of a food guide that specifies food groups and serving sizes as shown in Fig 9.1 to 9.3. Such guidance is of particular importance in planning adequate meals for pediatric patients of all ages to ensure proper growth and development.

Table 9.3
Tips for Meal Planning[10]

1. Encourage a variety of foods from Fig 9.1–9.3
2. The number of servings in each group is for minimum daily intakes as shown in Fig 9.1 and 9.2. Choose more foods from any of the groups to meet energy needs.
3. A serving from the calcium-rich food group provides approximately 10% of adult daily requirements. Choose 8 or more servings a day. These also count toward servings from other food groups in the guide. For example, 1/2 cup (125 mL) of fortified fruit juice counts as a calcium-rich food and also counts toward servings from the fruit group.
4. Include 2 servings every day of foods that supply omega-3 fatty acids. Foods rich in omega-3 fat are found in the legumes/nuts group and in the fats group. A serving is 1 tsp (5 mL) of ground Flaxseed oil, 3 tsp (15 mL) of canola or soybean oil, 1 tbsp (15 mL) of ground Flaxseed, or 1/4 cup (60 mL) of walnuts. Olive and canola oil are the best choices for cooking.
5. Equivalent servings of nuts and seeds can replace servings from the fats group.
6. Vitamin D from daily sun exposure or through fortified foods or supplements. Cow milk and some brands of soy milk and breakfast cereals are fortified with vitamin D.
7. Include at least 3 good food sources of vitamin B_{12} daily (eg, 1 tbsp [15 mL] of Red Star Nutritional Yeast–Vegetarian Support, 1 cup [250 mL] of fortified soy milk, 1/2 cup [125 mL] of cow milk, 3/4 cup [185 mL] of yogurt, 1 large egg, 1 oz of fortified breakfast cereal, or 1–1-1/2 oz of fortified meat analog). If these foods are not consumed regularly (at least 3 servings/day), a daily vitamin B_{12} supplement of 5–10 µg or a weekly dose of 2000 µg is recommended.
8. Consume sweets or alcohol in moderation. Use foods in the vegetarian food guide to get most of calories.

Fig 9.1
Vegan pyramid.

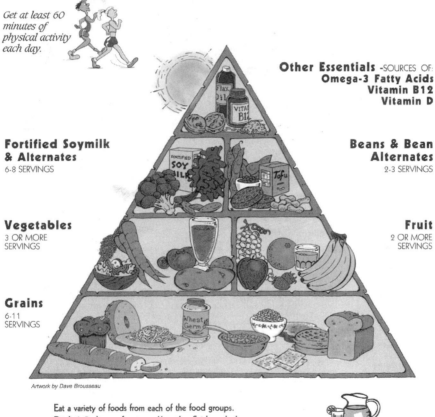

VEGAN FOOD GUIDE
DAILY PLAN FOR HEALTHY EATING

Get at least 60 minutes of physical activity each day.

Other Essentials -SOURCES OF:
Omega-3 Fatty Acids
Vitamin B12
Vitamin D

Fortified Soymilk
& Alternates
6-8 SERVINGS

Beans & Bean
Alternates
2-3 SERVINGS

Vegetables
3 OR MORE
SERVINGS

Fruit
2 OR MORE
SERVINGS

Grains
6-11
SERVINGS

Artwork by Dave Brousseau

Eat a variety of foods from each of the food groups.
Drink 6-8 glasses of water and/or other fluids each day.
Limit intake of concentrated fats, oils, and added sugars, if used.

Reproduced with permission from Messina et al.[10]

Fig 9.2
Vegetarian food guide pyramid.

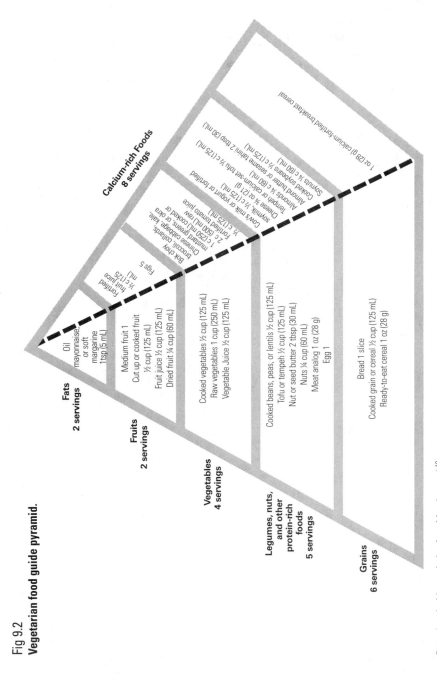

Fats
2 servings

Oil
mayonnaise
or soft
margarine
1 tsp (5 mL)

Fruits
2 servings

Medium fruit 1
Cut up or cooked fruit
½ cup (125 mL)
Fruit juice ½ cup (125 mL)
Dried fruit ¼ cup (60 mL)

Vegetables
4 servings

Cooked vegetables ½ cup (125 mL)
Raw vegetables 1 cup (250 mL)
Vegetable Juice ½ cup (125 mL)

**Legumes, nuts,
and other
protein-rich
foods
5 servings**

Cooked beans, peas, or lentils ½ cup (125 mL)
Tofu or tempeh ½ cup (125 mL)
Nut or seed butter 2 tbsp (30 mL)
Nuts ¼ cup (60 mL)
Meat analog 1 oz (28 g)
Egg 1

**Grains
6 servings**

Bread 1 slice
Cooked grain or cereal ½ cup (125 mL)
Ready-to-eat cereal 1 oz (28 g)

Calcium-rich Foods
8 servings

1 oz (28 g) calcium-fortified breakfast cereal

Almonds ¼ c (60 mL)
Cooked soybeans ½ c (125 mL)
Soynuts ¼ c (60 mL)

Tempeh or calcium-set tofu ½ c (125 mL)
Almond butter or sesame tahini 2 tbsp (30 mL)

Cheese ¾ oz (21 g)
Cow's milk or yogurt or fortified
soymilk ½ c (125 mL)

Bok choy
broccoli, collards, kale,
Chinese cabbage, kale,
mustard greens, or okra
1 c (250 mL) cooked or
2 c (500 mL) raw

Fortified tomato juice
½ c (125 mL)

Fortified
fruit juice
½ c (125
mL)

Figs 5

Reproduced with permission from Messina et al.[10]

Fig 9.3
Vegetarian food guide rainbow.

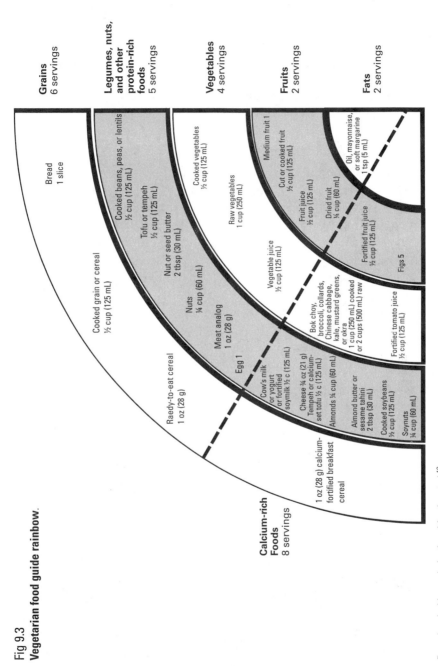

Grains
6 servings

Bread
1 slice

Cooked grain or cereal
½ cup (125 mL)

Ready-to-eat cereal
1 oz (28 g)

Legumes, nuts, and other protein-rich foods
5 servings

Cooked beans, peas, or lentils
½ cup (125 mL)

Tofu or tempeh
½ cup (125 mL)

Nut or seed butter
2 tbsp (30 mL)

Nuts
¼ cup (60 mL)

Meat analog
1 oz (28 g)

Egg 1

Vegetables
4 servings

Cooked vegetables
½ cup (125 mL)

Raw vegetables
1 cup (250 mL)

Vegetable juice
½ cup (125 mL)

Bok choy, broccoli, collards, Chinese cabbage, kale, mustard greens, or okra
1 cup (250 mL) cooked or 2 cups (500 mL) raw

Fortified tomato juice
½ cup (125 mL)

Fruits
2 servings

Medium fruit 1

Cut or cooked fruit
½ cup (125 mL)

Fruit juice
½ cup (125 mL)

Dried fruit
¼ cup (60 mL)

Fortified fruit juice
½ cup (125 mL)

Figs 5

Fats
2 servings

Oil, mayonnaise, or soft margarine
1 tsp (5 mL)

Calcium-rich Foods
8 servings

1 oz (28 g) calcium-fortified breakfast cereal

Cow's milk or yogurt (or fortified soymilk ½ c (125 mL)

Cheese ¾ oz (21 g)
Tempeh or calcium-set tofu ½ c (125 mL)

Almonds ¼ cup (60 mL)

Almond butter or sesame tahini
2 tbsp (30 mL)

Cooked soybeans
½ cup (125 mL)

Soynuts
¼ cup (60 mL)

Reproduced with permission from Messina et al.[10]

Nutrient Intake Guidelines

Some basic guidelines are used to determine the requirements of nutrients for healthy vegetarians. The recommendations for calories are the same as for the general population. The recommendations for nutrient intakes are increased by 2 standard deviations above the RDA average to overcompensate for potential deficiencies in intake and ensure the adequacy of nutrients.[32] Furthermore, recommendations for the same nutrient can vary in different countries. In addition, the variations in bioavailability of foods determine actual assimilation of the nutrient.

Whole Foods Concept

The concept of eating whole foods is an integral part of vegetarian diets. The principle behind this concept is that almost any kind of food processing can lead to loss of nutrients, with the exception of preparation of fermented foods. For example, processing whole grains to white flour leads to a loss of minerals, vitamins, phytochemicals, and dietary fibers by 75% to 95%.[26] Whole-grain products contain almost an ideal combination of nutrients to meet human needs, although they are deficient in calcium and vitamin C. Such losses occur with processing most other foods as well. Similarly, in frozen food preparation, there is a 20% to 30% loss of nutrients. Moreover, as long as the products are kept frozen, the nutrients are preserved rather well, but with heating frozen food, certain additional nutrients losses occur.[26]

Nutritional Considerations

Energy

Children with adequate energy intakes will grow at a predictable rate. Studies of vegan children have indicated that their energy intake is close to the recommended amount[35] or that of nonvegetarian controls.[36] During infancy and weaning, the amount of food needed to meet energy needs on vegan diets may be beyond gastric capacity, unless the child is fed frequently.[37] Concentrated sources of calories that are acceptable for older infants and children include soy products, legumes, oils, nuts, nut butters, and fruit juices.[38]

Protein

Despite the low caloric density of strict vegetarian diets, especially if weaning from the breast occurs relatively early, food intakes are usually sufficient to support protein needs.[39] Plant protein can meet energy requirements when a variety of plant foods are consumed. Complementary proteins need not be consumed at the same meal, as long as an assortment of foods is eaten during the day.[40] A recent meta-analysis of nitrogen balance studies in adults found no significant difference in protein needs on the basis of the source of dietary proteins.[41] Other studies have shown that considering the low digestibility of plant proteins, the protein requirements would be 30% to 35% more for vegan infants, 20% to 30% more for vegan 2- to 6-year-olds, and 15% to 20% more for vegan children 6 years and older.[42]

The 5 major food sources of plant protein are legumes, cereals, nuts and seeds, fruits, and vegetables. Each of these has nutritional advantages and disadvantages. For example, legumes and cereals provide relatively large amounts of quality protein but must be cooked or processed to enhance their palatability and to remove substances that decrease digestibility,[43] such as tough skins, amylase inhibitors, lectins, and tannins. Protein quantity, quality, and digestibility are all of potential concern, especially when vegan-vegetarian diets are used during infancy. The quality of plant proteins varies. A standard method for determining protein quality is the protein digestibility corrected amino acid score. Using this method, isolated soy protein is shown to meet protein needs as effectively as animal protein, unlike wheat protein, which is almost 50% less usable than animal protein.[44] The amount of lysine is lower in all plant foods than in animal foods. The amounts of sulfur-containing amino acids methionine and cysteine are lower in legumes and fruits. The amount of the essential amino acid threonine is lower in cereals, and tryptophan content tends to be lower in fruits than in most animal foods.[45] Therefore, if parents feed diets that are adequate in food energy and select a variety of plant foods with proteins that complement one another, vegetarian children should be able to receive an adequate amount of protein to grow and thrive.

Fat

Although dietary fat intakes of vegetarian children older than 2 years (between 25% and 35% of calories) are a little lower than those of omnivores, effects on growth appear to be small.[46] However, when dietary fat is below approximately 15% of calories, special care must be taken to ensure that recommended intakes of essential fatty acids are met. At least 3% of energy should be from linoleic acid (omega-3 fatty acid), and 1% of energy should be from linolenic acid (omega-6 fatty acid).[47] The recommended ratio of omega-6 fatty acids to omega-3 fatty acids is in the range of 2:1 to 4:1.[48] Linoleic acid is found in seeds, nuts, and grains. Alpha-linolenic acid is found in the green leaves of plants and in phytoplankton and algae, in certain seeds, and in nuts and legumes, such as flax, canola, walnuts, hazelnuts, and soy. These can be converted into more highly unsaturated fatty acids, including arachidonic acid (ARA), eicosapentaenoic acid (EPA), and docosahexaenoic acid (DHA).[49] ARA and EPA serve as precursors for the eicosanoids. Tentative recommended intakes for these polyunsaturated fatty acids range from 3% to 10% of total energy intakes. ARA is found in animal foods, such as meat, poultry, and eggs. EPA and DHA are largely found in fish and seafood. Vegan-vegetarians have no direct sources of these long-chain omega-3 fatty acids in their diets and, thus, must convert alpha-linolenic acid to them.[50] There is concern that pregnant women who follow vegan, vegetarian, or macrobiotic diets and consume little or no fish or other animal foods may not obtain enough of these fatty acids, especially during pregnancy and in early infancy when breastfeeding.[51] Risks are thought to be especially high if infants are preterm, because their capacity to desaturate alpha-linolenic acid to DHA may be limited.[52] Such individuals may need DHA supplements, either from fish oils or from cultured microalgae. Algae sources of DHA have been shown to positively affect blood concentrations of DHA and of EPA through retroconversion.[53] However, such supplements should only be dispensed under a physician's direction, because they are also potent anticoagulants.

Fiber

Recent recommendations for dietary fiber have been made on the basis of its function as a source of energy. Depending on age and gender, recommended daily fiber intake for 1- to 3-year-olds is 19 g/day, for 4- to 8-year-olds is 25 g/day, and for adolescents is up to 38 g/day.[45] In very small children, the sheer bulk and low energy density of such a high-fiber diet may make consumption of sufficient energy difficult for the child and may inhibit absorption of some minerals.[35] The sieving or mashing of cereals, pulses, and vegetables that are fed to infants can increase their digestibility, and partial replacement of whole-grain cereals with more highly refined cereals that are lower in fiber can further increase energy intakes and decrease bulk if this is a problem in small children. Lacto-ovo vegetarian children usually consume adequate, but not excessive, amounts of dietary fiber.

Vitamins

Vitamin A/Beta-Carotene

Because plant foods contain only dietary carotenoids, vitamin A requirements can be met by 3 servings a day of plant foods rich in beta-carotene, such as leafy or deep yellow or orange vegetables and fruits. Absorption of beta-carotene is less efficient when plant foods are in the raw, unprepared state[54] than when the foods are cooked, chopped, or pureed or when small amounts of fat are added in preparation or consumed with the food.[55]

Riboflavin

Intakes of riboflavin appear to be similar in vegetarians and omnivores.[11] Riboflavin has occasionally been deficient in people on severely restricted macrobiotic diets, but it is not a problem in other forms of vegetarianism. Good sources include nutritional yeast, wheat germ, soy, fortified cereals, and enriched grains.

Folic Acid

Usually, vegetarians who consume high amounts of vegetables and fruits as well as other plant foods have adequate intakes of folic acid. However, those who consume vegetables that are usually braised or fried at high temperature and who rarely drink fruit juices or eat grain products fortified with folic acid may be at risk. Additionally, postmenarchal adolescent girls who are capable of becoming pregnant should consume 400 µg of folic acid as a supplement or in fortified foods in addition to usual food sources of the nutrient.[56]

Vitamin B_{12}

No plant foods, unless fortified, or certain sea vegetables contain vitamin B_{12}. Lacto-ovo vegetarians get sufficient amounts of vitamin B_{12} if dairy products are consumed on a regular basis. Studies indicate that some strict vegans are deficient in Vitamin B_{12},[57,58] and vegetarian diets typically are high in folic acid, which masks hematologic symptoms of deficiency earlier on, leading to late diagnosis. In such situations, presentation involves neurologic symptoms.[59,60] Absorption is effective when small amounts of vitamin B_{12} are consumed at regular intervals.[61] Regular intake of vitamin B_{12}-fortified foods or permitting dairy products should be encouraged in vegetarians and especially in mothers of breastfed infants.

Vitamin D

Vitamin D concentrations are dependent on sunlight exposure and intake of vitamin D-rich foods or supplements. Infants and children synthesize vitamin D less efficiently.[62] Foods such as cow milk, some types of soy milk, rice milk, and breakfast cereals that are enriched with vitamin D_2 (ergocalciferol) and/or vitamin D_3 (cholecalciferol [animal based]) should be consumed. Intake of such fortified foods along with sun exposure, whenever possible and in a safe manner, should be encouraged. Vitamin D_2 is less bioavailable than vitamin D_3; thus, the requirements are increased for certain types of vegetarians.[63] If sunlight exposure and intake of fortified foods are insufficient, then supplements are recommended.

Minerals

Iron

Iron is vital at all ages, and there is a risk of iron deficiency during infant growth, the adolescent growth spurt, and pregnancy. The iron nutritional status of vegetarian infants and children varies. Iron deficiency is by far the most common of the micronutrient deficiencies exhibited by vegetarian children.[62] It is particularly common in children consuming vegan diets, because plant foods contain nonheme iron as opposed to heme iron in animal sources. Nonheme iron is more sensitive to inhibitors of iron absorption, such as phytates, calcium, herbal teas, cocoa, some spices, and fiber. Vitamin C and other organic acids in fruits and vegetables enhance the absorption of iron. Recommended iron intakes for vegetarians are 1.8 times those of nonvegetarians because of the lower bioavailability of iron in a vegetarian diet,[64] and although vegetarians have lower iron stores, their serum ferritin concentrations are usually within the normal range.[65,66] Incidence of iron-deficiency anemia among vegetarians is similar to nonvegetarians.[55] Although many studies have been short-term, there is evidence that adaptation to low intakes takes place over a longer term and involves increased absorption and decreased losses.[67,68]

Zinc

Approximately half of the zinc in American diets comes from meat, poultry, and fish.[69] Foods such as red meat contain large amounts of zinc and protein, which enhances zinc bioavailability. Human milk contains zinc in a bioavailable form, but it does not contain enough zinc for infants older than 6 months, so breastfed infants of this age should consume foods containing zinc. The bioavailability of relatively rich plant sources of zinc, such as whole-grain cereals, soy, beans, lentils, peas, and nuts, tends to be low, because most of them also contain large amounts of phytate and fiber, which inhibit zinc absorption.[70] In lacto-ovo vegetarians, zinc absorption is approximately a third less than in omnivores.[71]

The requirement for zinc may be as much as 50% greater among strict vegetarians.[31] Vegetarian diets also tend to be lower in zinc than are omnivorous diets. When daily requirements for zinc are increased, as they are in infants and children, the risk of suboptimal zinc nutritional status is increased, because the ability to increase zinc absorption is limited.[72] Because the presence of inhibitors is highest in vegan diets, vegans are at special risk. Despite this, zinc supplementation is not recommended, because clinical signs of deficiency are rare among vegetarians, even in children younger than 24 months.[73] Good plant sources of zinc are yeast-fermented whole-grain breads (the phytic acid content is reduced) and zinc-fortified infant and adult cereals.

Calcium

Calcium intakes of vegans tend to be lower than lacto vegetarians and nonvegetarians.[74] Although oxalates, phytates, and fiber in plant foods decrease calcium availability, research shows that the bioavailability of calcium from plant foods and soy products at times is higher than that from milk.[75] Calcium is present in a large number of plant and fortified foods, such as broccoli, Chinese cabbage, collards, kale, okra, and turnip greens.

Consumption of soy products appeared to favor bone health in mature animals.[76] For children who consume soy products, calcium-fortified products are recommended. If children's diets do not contain adequate sources of dietary calcium, supplements may be advisable.

Iodine

Iodine deficiency is not commonly noted in vegetarian children since the introduction of easily available and widely used iodized salt. Vegans whose diets are restricted to kosher or sea salts, which are generally not iodized, and who also have a substantial intake of goitrogens, such as broccoli, mustard, kale, turnips, etc are at risk of iodine deficiency. For these children, especially for those living in iodine-poor areas,[77] iodine-fortified foods can be recommended.

Carnitine and Taurine

Carnitine and taurine concentrations in the serum are decreased in lacto-ovo vegetarian and vegan diets; however, the functional significance of the serum concentrations of these substances is not apparent; therefore, supplementation does not appear to be warranted.[78,79]

Vegetarian Diets for Special Populations

Infants

Infants receiving human milk or commercial formula have diets that contain adequate sources of energy and nutrients, such as iron, vitamin B_{12}, and vitamin D and have normal growth. The milk of vegetarian women is similar in nutrient composition to that of nonvegetarians. Vegetarian women should be encouraged to breastfeed like all other women. Soy formula is the only option for vegan infants who are not being breastfed. Soy milk, rice milk, homemade formulas, cow milk and goat milk should not be used to replace human milk or commercial formulas during infancy, because they do not contain the proper amounts of macronutrients or micronutrients.[11]

Guidelines for the introduction of semisolid/solid foods are similar for vegetarian and nonvegetarians.[80] Infants older than 6 months are potentially at the greatest risk of overt deficiency states related to inappropriate restrictions of the diet, although deficiencies of vitamins B_{12} and essential fatty acids may appear earlier.[81,82] They are particularly vulnerable during the weaning period if fed a macrobiotic diet and may experience psychomotor delay in some instances.[83,84] Attempting to anticipate these problems for vegetarian families by explaining the principles of providing calorie-dense foods at the time of weaning is important so the increased bulk of vegetarian diets does not interfere with adequate consumption of energy, protein, and other nutrients.

Children

Except those on severely restricted diets such as vegan nonmacrobiotic diets,[85] vegetarian children exhibit growth comparable with their omnivore peers.[86] Average calorie and protein intake generally meets or exceeds recommendations. Vegan children may have slightly more protein needs than nonvegan children because of differences in protein digestibility and amino acid profile in certain plant proteins,[51] but this is usually met with a variety of plant foods.[51] Importance of proper intake of calcium, zinc, and iron should be emphasized.[42]

Adolescents

Whether adolescents have only recently begun practicing a vegetarian diet or whether they have been vegetarian from the beginning of their lives, nutritional imbalance can have major health effects in later life. Vegetarianism is a behavior reported with disordered eating attitudes and behaviors according to some studies[87,88] but not others.[89,90] A vegetarian diet is adopted by some young women as a means of weight control.[91] Adolescent vegetarians were significantly more likely to exhibit bulimic behaviors in a Minnesota study.[92] A study of 131 college undergraduates revealed that vegetarians displayed a higher dietary restraint than nonvegetarians, complicating the normalization of eating. Therefore, vegetarian practices may be a marker to help identify those with tendencies toward eating disorders or obsession with weight.[93]

Early detection of disordered eating is vital so that preventive action or intervention can be implemented before such behaviors become persistent. It is, therefore, important to determine identifiable factors associated with eating disorders. Klopp et al[94] reported that, although no differences in eating attitudes and behaviors between self-reported vegetarian and nonvegetarian college women were demonstrated, adolescent vegetarians were at greater risk of unhealthy and extreme weight control behaviors than were control adolescents.[94] Male vegetarians appear more vulnerable in this regard. Vegetarianism among adolescents may, therefore, be a signal for preventive intervention. Adolescents who choose to become vegetarians may also need to know the right method to do so (see Table 9.4), because they have poor calcium intake across all groups, with only 30% of children and adolescents meeting the recommended 1300 mg of calcium intake per day.

Table 9.4

Modifications to the Vegetarian Food Guide (Fig 9.2 and 9.3) for Children, Adolescents, and Pregnant and Lactating Women[10]

Stage	Food Group*: B12-Rich Foods (Servings)	Beans/Nuts/ Seeds/ Egg (Servings)	Calcium-Rich Foods (Servings)
Child[†]	2	5	6
Adolescent[‡]	2	6	10
Adolescent[§]	3	6	10

* The number of servings in each group is the minimum amount needed. The minimum number of servings from other groups is not different from the vegetarian food guide (Fig 9.2 and 9.3). Additional foods can be chosen from any of the groups in the vegetarian food guide to meet energy needs.

[†] 4 to 8 y.

[‡] 9 to 13 y.

[§] 14 to 18 y.

In a Turkish study to evaluate the prevalence of eating disorders in vegetarians, abnormal eating habits, low self-esteem, high social physique anxiety, and high trait anxiety were detected in Turkish adolescent vegetarians between 7 and 21 years of age.[95] Data from a study conducted between fish-eating vegetarians and omnivores demonstrate that long-term adherence to a vegetarian diet is associated with maintained leanness and a lower body mass index.[96]

Athletes

With increasing interest in the potential health benefits of vegetarian diets in athletes, it is relevant to consider dietary practices that influence athletic performance. Athletes can meet their protein needs with a vegetarian diet.[97,98] Although long-term controlled studies are needed, a well-planned and appropriately supplemented vegetarian diet appears to support requirements of athletes effectively.[99] Female vegetarian athletes should be informed about an increased risk of nonanemic iron deficiency, which may limit endurance performance.[100] Vegetarian athletes have a lower mean muscle creatine concentration and, hence, are likely to experience greater performance increments after creatine loading in activities that rely on adenosine triphosphate/phosphocreatine systems.[101] Trainers and coaches need to be aware of the use of a vegetarian diet as a form of weight control, and appropriate steps should be taken to investigate that a balanced vegetarian diet be followed to ensure the good health of these athletes.

Developmentally and Neurologically Delayed Children

It is possible to provide oral and/or enteral feeding to tube-fed pediatric patients with swallowing problems. A list of appropriate formulas for use in vegetarian and vegan diets at different ages is provided in Table 9.5.

Table 9.5
Formulas for Gastrostomy Tube Feeds

Vegetarian		Vegan	
<1 y	≥1 y	<1 y	≥1 y
Alimentum*	Kindercal[†]	Isomil*	Elecare*
Enfamil[†]	Next Step[†]	Neocate[‖]	Isomil 2*
Nutramigen[†]	Nutren Jr 1.0/2.0[‡]	ProSobee[†]	Neocate Jr/One[‖]
Pregestimil[†]	PediaSure*	Nestlé Good Start Soy[‡]	L-Emental[¶]
Similac*	Peptamen Jr[‡]	RCF*	Tolerex[‡]
EnfaCare[†]	Similac 2*		Vivonex Plus/Ten[‡]
Nestlé Good Start[‡]	Ensure/Plus[§]		Nestlé FAA[‡]
	Jevity[§]		Next Step Soy[†]
	Isocal[†]		

* Abbott Nutrition, Columbus, OH
[†] Mead Johnson, Evansville, IN
[‡] Nestlé, Glendale, CA
[§] Abbott Laboratories, Abbott Park, IL
[‖] Nutricia North America, Rockville, MD
[¶] Hormel Health Labs, Savannah, GA

Conclusion

Vegetarian diets can meet the nutritional needs of children and adolescents if appropriately planned and monitored by a health care professional or nutritionist. Table 9.6 lists a few useful Web sites for use by vegetarian families and pediatricians. The current database of vegetarian studies convincingly indicate that plant-based diets have numerous health benefits. In addition to maintaining awareness of various relevant nutritional issues, health care professionals may need to be familiar with availability of various foods and social, cultural, and ideological systems present in their communities.

Table 9.6
List of Useful Vegetarian Web Sites

http://www.kidshealth.org/parent/nutrition_fit/nutrition/vegetarianism.html http://www.americanheart.org/presenter.jhtml?identifier=4777 http://www.nal.usda.gov/fnic/pubs/bibs/gen/vegetarian.htm

References

1. Kushi M. *The Book of Macrobiotics: The Universal Way of Health, Happiness, and Peace.* Rev ed. Tokyo, Japan: Japan Publications; 1986

2. Corliss R. Should we all be vegetarians? *Time.* 2002;160(3):48–56

3. Edmunds F. The way of Rudolf Steiner. In: *An Introduction to Anthroposophy.* Rev ed. East Sussex, England: Sophia Books; 2005:3–27

4. Fessler DM, Arguello AP, Mekdara JM, Macias R. Disgust sensitivity and meat consumption: a test of an emotivist account of moral vegetarianism. *Appetite.* 2003;41:31–41

5. Amato PR, Partridge SA. *The New Vegetarians: Promoting Health and Protecting Life.* New York, NY: Plenum Press; 1989

6. The Vegetarian Resource Group. How many vegetarians are there? Available at: http://www.vrg.org/journal/vj2003issue3/vj2003issue3poll.htm. Accessed August 8, 2007

7. The Vegetarian Resource Group. How many teens are vegetarian? How many kids don't eat meat? Available at: http://www.vrg.org/journal/vj2001jan/2001janteen.htm. Accessed August 8, 2007

8. Smith J, Dwyer JT. Vegetarian diets for children. In: Dershewitz RA, ed. *Ambulatory Pediatric Care.* 3rd ed. Philadelphia, PA: Lippincott Raven Publishers; 1999:106–112

9. Jacobs C, Dwyer JT. Vegetarian children: appropriate and inappropriate diets. *Am J Clin Nutr.* 1988;48:811–818

10. Messina V, Melina V, Mangels AR. A new food guide for North American vegetarians. *J Am Diet Assoc.* 2003;103:771–775

11. American Dietetic Association, Dietitians of Canada. Position of the American Dietetic Association and Dietitians of Canada: vegetarian diets. *J Am Diet Assoc.* 2003;103:748–765

12. Jacob RA, Burri BJ. Oxidative damage and defense. *Am J Clin Nutr.* 1996;63:985S–990S

13. Janelle KC, Barr SI. Nutrient intakes and eating behavior scores of vegetarian and nonvegetarian women. *J Am Diet Assoc.* 1995;95:180–186, 189

14. Richter V, Rassoul F, Hentschel B, et al. Age-dependence of lipid parameters in the general population and vegetarians. *Z Gerontol Geriatr.* 2004;37:207–213

15. Purschwitz K, Rassoul F, Reuter W, et al. [Soluble leukocyte adhesion molecules in vegetarians of various ages.] [Article in German.] *Z Gerontol Geriatr.* 2001;34:476–479

16. Joshipura KJ, Hu FB, Manson JE, et al. The effect of fruit and vegetable intake on risk for coronary heart disease. *Ann Intern Med.* 2001;134:1106–1114

17. Liu S, Manson JE, Lee IM, et al. Fruit and vegetable intake and risk of cardiovascular disease: the Women's Health Study. *Am J Clin Nutr.* 2000;72:922–928

18. Joshipura KJ, Ascherio A, Manson JE, et al. Fruit and vegetable intake in relation to risk of ischemic stroke. *JAMA.* 1999;282:1233–1239

19. Key TJ, Allen NE, Spencer EA, Travis RC. The effect of diet on risk of cancer. *Lancet.* 2002;360:861–868

20. Key TJ, Fraser GE, Thorogood M, et al. Mortality in vegetarians and nonvegetarians: detailed findings from a collaborative analysis of 5 prospective studies. *Am J Clin Nutr.* 1999;70:516S–524S

21. John JH, Ziebland S, Yudkin P, Roe LS, Neil HA. Effects of fruit and vegetable consumption on plasma antioxidant concentrations and blood pressure: a randomised controlled trial. Oxford Fruit and Vegetable Study Group. *Lancet.* 2002;359:1969–1674

22. Hare LG, Woodside JV, Young IS. Dietary salicylates. *J Clin Pathol.* 2003;56:649–650

23. Lawrence JR, Peter R, Baxter G, Robson G, Graham B, Paterson B. Urinary excretion of salicyluric and salicylic acids by non-vegetarians, vegetarians and patients taking low dose aspirin. *J Clin Pathol.* 2003;56:651–653

24. Blacklock CJ, Lawrence JR, Malcolm EA, Wiles D. Salicylic acid in the serum of subjects not taking aspirin. Comparison of salicylic acid concentrations in the serum of vegetarians, non-vegetarians, and patients taking low dose aspirin. *J Clin Pathol.* 2001;54:553–555

25. Xu XM, Sansores-Garcia L, Chen XM, Matijevic-Aleksic N, Du M, Wu KK. Suppression of inducible cyclo-oxygenase 2 gene transcription by aspirin and sodium salicylate. *Proc Natl Acad Sci U S A.* 1999;96:5292–5297

26. Leitzmann C. Vegetarian diets: what are the advantages? *Forum Nutr.* 2005;57:147–156

27. Alm JS, Swartz J, Bjorksten B, et al. An anthroposophic lifestyle and intestinal microflora in infancy. *Pediatr Allerg Immunol.* 2002;13:402–411

28. Kalliomaki M, Salminen S, Arvilommi H, Kero P, Koskinen P, Isolauri E. Probiotics in primary prevention of atopic disease: a randomised placebo-controlled trial. *Lancet.* 2001;357:1076–1079

29. Matsuzaki T, Yamazaki R, Hashimoto S, Yokokura T. The effect of oral feeding of *Lactobacillus casei* strain Shirota on immunoglobulin E production in mice. *J Dairy Sci.* 1998;81:48–53

30. Tanaka T, Kouda K, Kotani M, et al. Vegetarian diet ameliorates symptoms of atopic dermatitis through reduction of the number of peripheral eosinophils and of PGE2 synthesis by monocytes. *J Physiol Anthropol Appl Hum Sci.* 2001;20:353–361

31. Ambroszkiewicz J, Laskowska-Klita T, Klemarczyk W. Low levels of osteocalcin and leptin in serum of vegetarian prepubertal children. *Med Wieku Rozwoj.* 2003;7:587–591

32. Colev M, Engel H, Mayers M, Markowitz M, Cahill L. Vegan diet and vitamin A deficiency. *Clin Pediatr (Phila).* 2004;43:107–109

33. Moilanen BC. Vegan diets in infants, children, and adolescents. *Pediatr Rev.* 2004;25:174–176

34. Dunham L, Kollar LM. Vegetarian eating for children and adolescents. *J Pediatr Health Care.* 2006;20:27–34

35. Fulton JR, Hutton CW, Stitt KR. Preschool vegetarian children. Dietary and anthropometric data. *J Am Diet Assoc.* 1980;76:360–365

36. Sanders TA, Purves R. An anthropometric and dietary assessment of the nutritional status of vegan preschool children. *J Hum Nutr.* 1981;35:349–357

37. Truesdell DD, Acosta PB. Feeding the vegan infant and child. *J Am Diet Assoc.* 1985;85:837–840

38. Dietz WH, Dwyer JT. Nutritional implications of vegetarianism for children. In: Suskind RM, ed. *Textbook of Pediatric Nutrition.* New York, NY: Raven Press; 1981:179–188

39. Millward DJ. The nutritional value of plant-based diets in relation to human amino acid and protein requirements. *Proc Nutr Soc.* 1999;58:249–260

40. Young VR, Pellet PL. Plant proteins in relation to human protein and amino acid nutrition. *Am J Clin Nutr.* 1994;59:1203S–1212S

41. Rand VM, Pellet PL, Young VR. Meta-analysis of nitrogen balance studies for estimating protein requirements in healthy in adults. *Am J Clin Nutr.* 2003;77:109–127

42. Messina V, Mangels AR. Considerations in planning vegan diets: children. *J Am Diet Assoc.* 2001;101:661–669

43. Bishnoi S, Khetarpaul N. Protein digestibility of vegetables and field peas (*Pisum sativum*). Varietal differences and effect of domestic processing and cooking methods. *Plant Foods Hum Nutr.* 1994;46:71–76

44. Young VR, Fajardo L, Murray E, Rand WM, Scrimshaw NS. Protein requirements of man: comparative nitrogen balance response within the submaintenance-to-maintenance range of intakes of wheat and beef proteins. *J Nutr.* 1975;105:534–542

45. Institute of Medicine. *Dietary Reference Intakes for Energy, Carbohydrate, Fiber, Fat, Fatty Acids, Cholesterol, Protein, and Amino Acids (Macronutrients).* Washington, DC: National Academies Press; 2005

46. Attwood CR. Low-fat diets for children: practicality and safety. *Am J Cardiol.* 1998;82:77T–79T

47. World Health Organization and Food and Agricultural Organization of the United Nations. *Expert Consultation on Diet, Nutrition and the Prevention of Chronic Diseases.* Geneva, Switzerland: World Health Organization; 2003. Available at: http://www.who.int/hpr/nutrition/26Aprildraftrev1.pdf. Accessed November 2, 2007

48. Kris-Etherton PM, Taylor DS, Yu-Poth S, et al. Polyunsaturated fatty acids in the food chain in the United States. *Am J Clin Nutr.* 2000;71:179S–188S

49. Bremer RR, Peluffo RO. Regulation of unsaturated fatty acid biosynthesis. I. Effect of unsaturated fatty acid of 18 carbons on the microsomal desaturation of linoleic acid into gamma-linolenic acid. *Biochem Biophys Acta.* 1969;176:471–479

50. Sanders TA, Manning J. The growth and development of vegan children. *J Hum Nutr Diet.* 1992;5:11–21

51. Sanders TA, Ellis FR, Dickerson JW. Study of vegans: the fatty acid composition of plasma choline phosphoglycerides, erythrocytes, adipose tissue, and breast milk, and some indicators of susceptibility to ischemic heart disease in vegans and omnivore controls. *Am J Clin Nutr.* 1978;31:805–813

52. Boulton TJ, Magarey AM. Effects of differences in dietary fat on growth, energy and nutrient intake from infancy to eight years of age. *Acta Pediatr.* 1995;84:146–150

53. Conquer JA, Holub BJ. Supplementation with an algae source of docosahexanoic acid increases (ω-3) fatty acid status and alters selected risk factors for heart disease in vegetarian subjects. *J Nutr.* 1996;126:3032–3039

54. Sabate J, Ratzin-Turner RA, Brown JE. Vegetarian diets: description and trends. In: Sabate J, ed. *Vegetarian Nutrition.* Boca Raton, FL: CRC Press; 2001:3–17

55. Ribaya-Mercado JD. Influence of dietary fat on beta-carotene absorption and bioconversion into vitamin A. *Nutr Rev.* 2002;60:104–110

56. Institute of Medicine. *Dietary Reference Intakes for Thiamin, Riboflavin, Niacin, Vitamin B_6, Folate, Vitamin B_{12}, Pantothenic Acid, Biotin, and Choline.* Washington, DC: National Academies Press; 1998

57. Donaldson MS. Metabolic vitamin B12 status on a mostly raw vegan diet with follow up using tablets, nutritional yeast, or probiotic supplements. *Ann Nutr Metab.* 2000;44:229–234

58. Hermann W, Schorr H, Purschwitz K, Rassoul F, Richter V. Total homocysteine, vitamin B(12), and total antioxidant status in vegetarians. *Clin Chem.* 2001;47:1094–1101

59. Gilois C, Wierzbicki AS, Hirani N, et al. The hematological and electrophysiological effects of cobalamin. Deficiency secondary to vegetarian diets. *Ann N Y Acad Sci.* 1992;669:345–348

60. Weiss R, Fogelman Y, Bennett M. Severe vitamin B12 deficiency in an infant associated with a maternal deficiency and a strict vegetarian diet. *J Pediatr Hematol Oncol.* 2004;26:270–271

61. Nathan I, Hackett AF, Kirby S. The dietary intake of a group of vegetarian children aged 7–11 years compared with matched omnivores. *Br J Nutr.* 1996;75:533–544

62. Institute of Medicine. *Dietary Reference Intakes for Calcium, Phosphorous, Magnesium, Vitamin D, and Fluoride.* Washington, DC: National Academies Press; 1997

63. Trang HM, Cole DE, Rubin LA, Pierratos A, Siu S, Vieth R. Evidence that vitamin D3 increases serum 25-hydroxyvitamin D more efficiently than does vitamin D2. *Am J Clin Nutr.* 1998;68:854–858

64. Institute of Medicine. *Dietary Reference Intakes for Vitamin A, Vitamin K, Arsenic, Boron, Chromium, Copper, Iodine, Iron, Manganese, Molybdenum, Nickel, Silicon, Vanadium, and Zinc.* Washington, DC: National Academies Press; 2000

65. Donovan UM, Gibson RS. Iron and zinc status of young women aged 14 to 19 years consuming vegetarian and omnivorous diets. *J Am Coll Nutr.* 1995;14:463–472

66. Haddad EH, Berk LS, Kettering JD, Hubbard RW, Peters WR. Dietary intake and biochemical, hematologic, and immune status of vegans compared with nonvegetarians. *Am J Clin Nutr.* 1999;70:586S–593S

67. Hunt JR, Roughead ZK. Nonheme-iron absorption, fecal ferritin excretion, and blood indexes of iron status in women consuming controlled lactoovovegetarian diets for 8 weeks. *Am J Clin Nutr.* 1999;69:944–952

68. Hunt JR, Roughead ZK. Adaptation of iron absorption in men consuming diets with high or low iron bioavailability. *Am J Clin Nutr.* 2000;71:94–102

69. Subar AF, Krebs-Smith SM, Cook A, Kahle LL. Dietary sources of nutrients among US adults, 1989 to 1991. *J Am Diet Assoc.* 1998;98:537–547

70. Harland BF, Oberleas D. Phytate in foods. *World Rev Nutr Diet.* 1987;52:235–259

71. Hunt JR, Matthys LA, Johnson LK. Zinc absorption, mineral balance and blood lipids in women consuming controlled lactoovovegetarian and omnivorous diets for 8 weeks. *Am J Clin Nutr.* 1998;67:421–430

72. Gibson RS. Content and bioavailability of trace elements in vegetarian diets. *Am J Clin Nutr.* 1994;59(Suppl):1223S–1232S

73. Taylor A, Redworth EW, Morgan JB. Influence of diet on iron, copper, and zinc status in children under 24 months of age. *Biol Trace Element Res.* 2004;97:197–214

74. Weaver C, Proulx WR, Heaney R. Choices for achieving adequate dietary calcium with a vegetarian diet. *Am J Clin Nutr.* 1999;70:543S–548S

75. Heaney RP, Dowell MS, Rafferty K, Bierman J. Bioavailability of calcium in fortified soy imitation milk, with some observations on method. *Am J Clin Nutr.* 2000;71:1166–1169

76. Ishida H, Uesugi T, Hirai K, et al. Preventive effects of the plant isoflavones, diadzin and genistin, on bone loss in ovariectomized rats fed a calcium-deficient diet. *Biol Pharm Bull.* 1998;21:62–66

77. Remer T, Neubert A, Manz F. Increased risk of iodine deficiency with vegetarian nutrition. *Br J Nutr.* 1999;81:45–49

78. Lombard KA, Olson AL, Nelson SE, Rebouche CJ. Carnitine status of lactoovovegetarians and strict vegetarian adults and children. *Am J Clin Nutr.* 1989;50:301–306

79. Laidlaw SA, Shultz TD, Cecchino JT, Kopple JD. Plasma and urine taurine levels in vegans. *Am J Clin Nutr.* 1988;47:660–663

80. Mangels AR, Messina V. Considerations in planning vegan diets: infants. *J Am Diet Assoc.* 2001;101:670–677

81. Sanders TA, Reddy S. Vegetarian diets and children. *Am J Clin Nutr.* 1994;59(Suppl): 1176S–1181S

82. Sanders TA. Essential fatty acid requirements of vegetarians in pregnancy, lactation, and infancy. *Am J Clin Nutr.* 1999;70:555S–559S

83. Sanders TA. Vegetarian diets and children. *Pediatr Clin North Am.* 1995;42:955–965

84. Dagnelie PC, Vergote FJ, van Staveren WA, van den Berg H, Dingjan PG, Hautvast JG. High prevalence of rickets in infants on macrobiotic diets. *Am J Clin Nutr.* 1990;51:202–208

85. Dusseldorf MV, Arts ICW, Bergsma JS, De Jong N, Dagnelie PC, Van Staveren. Catch up growth in children fed a macrobiotic diet in early childhood. *J Nutr.* 1996;26:2977–2983

86. Hebbelinck M, Clarys P. Physical growth and development of vegetarian children and adolescents. In: Sabate J, ed. *Vegetarian Nutrition.* Boca Raton, FL: CRC Press; 2001:173–193

87. Freeland-Graves JH, Greninger SA, Graves GR, Young RK. Health practices, attitudes, and beliefs of vegetarians and non vegetarians. *J Am Diet Assoc.* 1986;86:913–918

88. Worsley A, Skrzypiec G. Teenage vegetarianism: prevalence, social and cognitive contexts. *Appetite.* 1998;30:151–170

89. Barr SI, Broughton TM. Relative weight, weight loss efforts and nutrient intakes among health-conscious vegetarian, past vegetarian and non vegetarian women ages 18 to 50. *J Am Coll Nutr.* 2000;19:781–788

90. Larrson CL, Klock KS, Nordrehaug Astrom A, Haugejorden O, Johansson G. Lifestyle-related characteristics of young low-meat consumers and omnivores in Sweden and Norway. *J Adolesc Health.* 2002;31:190–198

91. Gillbody SM, Kirk SF, Hill AJ. Vegetarianism in young women: another means of weight . control? *Int J Eat Disord.* 1999;26:87–90

92. Neumark-Sztainer D, Story M, Resnick MD, Blum RW. Adolescent vegetarians. A behavioral profile of a school-based population in Minnesota. *Arch Pediatr Adolesc Med.* 1997;151:833–838

93. Klopp SA, Heiss CJ, Smith HS. Self-reported vegetarianism may be a marker for college women at risk for disordered eating. *J Am Diet Assoc.* 2003;103:745–747

94. Perry CL, Mcguire MT, Neumark-Sztainer D, Story M. Characteristics of vegetarian adolescents in a multi-ethnic urban population. *J Adolesc Health.* 2001;29:406–416

95. Bas M, Karabudak E, Kiziltan G. Vegetarianism and eating disorders: association between eating attitudes and other psychological factors among Turkish adolescents. *Appetite.* 2005;44:309–315

96. Phillips F, Hackett AF, Stratton G, Billington D. Effect of changing to a self selected vegetarian diet on anthropometric measurements in UK adults. *J Hum Nutr Diet.* 2004;17:249–255

97. Nieman DC. Physical fitness and vegetarian diets: is there a relation? *Am J Clin Nutr.* 1999;70:570S–575S

98. American Dietetic Association, Dietitians of Canada, and American College of Sports Medicine. Position of the American Dietetic Association, Dietitians of Canada, and American College of Sports Medicine: nutrition and athletic performance. *J Am Diet Assoc.* 2000;1543–1556

99. Barr SI, Rideout CA. Nutritional considerations for vegetarian athletes. *Nutrition.* 2004;20:696–703

100. Snyder AC, Dvorak LL, Roepke JB. Influence of dietary iron source on measures of iron status among female runners. *Med Sci Sports Exerc.* 1989;21:7–10

101. Burke DG, Chilibeck PD, Parise G, Candow DG, Mahoney D, Tarnopolsky M. Effect of creatine and weight training on muscle creatine and performance in vegetarians. *Med Sci Sports Exerc.* 2003;35:1946–1955

Sports Nutrition

Introduction

Participation in sports and athletics is very important in the lives of many American youth and their families. In the 2003 Youth Risk Behavior Survey, 64% of male high school students and 51% of female high school students reported participation on an organized sports team during the previous 12 months.[1] However, this statistic does not capture the concomitant increase in intensity of athletic involvement for many of these young athletes. This intensity may lead some young athletes to an increased interest in nutrition as a possible contributor to improved performance, but it also may make them more susceptible to dietary fads and use of supplements or ergogenic aids to achieve their sports-related goals.

The goal of this chapter is to provide evidence-based information regarding the role of nutrition in young athletes. As much as possible, the information is based on results from studies performed in the pediatric population. The key points covered in this chapter include: the use of fluids and macronutrients to provide fuel for and enhance recovery from exercise and physical exertion, the role of select vitamins and minerals in the young athlete's diet, issues related to weight loss and weight gain in the athlete, and information regarding nutritional supplements commonly used by young athletes.

Fueling the Workout

One of the basic tenets of sports nutrition is to ensure adequate fuel and fluid to optimize athletic efforts. The preferred fuel for physical activity depends on the intensity and duration of the physical effort. Fat is the primary fuel source during very low levels of activity, such as walking, but does not provide enough adenosine triphosphate (ATP) to fuel the level of physical activity required by most sports.

For activities lasting less than 10 to 30 seconds, the ATP/phosphocreatine system is the primary fuel substrate. As activity continues, muscle glycogen stores become an important fuel source, especially for the intermittent activity that is so prevalent in most youth sports. However, some authors state that preadolescents have not yet fully developed their glycolytic capacity and, therefore, may remain more dependent on fat as a fuel source for a given level of exertion compared with adolescents and adults.[2]

After 10 to 20 minutes of aerobic-level activity, blood glucose becomes an increasingly important energy source and is particularly important for athletes involved in endurance activity. An overview of fuel requirements during exercise can be found at http://cellinteractive.com/ucla/nutrition_101/phys_lect6.html.

Carbohydrates

For most youth sports activities, carbohydrates fulfill the bulk of fuel requirements. Therefore, adequate carbohydrate intake and stores are keys to successful athletic pursuits. Carbohydrate recommendations for adult athletes are 6 to 10 g/kg per day.[3] This is likely an appropriate range for many adolescents as well and has significant overlap with the general recommendation in young athletes that at least 50% of caloric intake should be from carbohydrates.[2] However, multiple studies have shown that child and adolescent athletes often consume significantly less.[2,4,5] Convincing athletes to increase carbohydrate intake to cover the caloric demand of activity can be a "hard sell" for some athletes, who are often used to functioning on far less. However, when carbohydrate intake is inadequate, the metabolic response is to catabolize muscle to provide needed fuel. In these cases, it is often helpful to educate the athlete that the muscle and strength they are working so hard to gain is being broken down and used as an expendable fuel source.

Carbohydrates should be ingested throughout the course of the day, but they are particularly important during the times surrounding athletic activity (Table 10.1). Before working out, carbohydrates are important to bolster blood glucose and muscle glycogen stores. It is generally recommended that athletes have a high-carbohydrate meal (approx 4 g of carbohydrate/kg for adults and adolescents) approximately 3 to 4 hours before training.[6] Because most school-aged athletes have sports practice after school, lunch often becomes an important pretraining meal. In addition, a high-carbohydrate snack (approx 0.5–1 g of carbohydrate/kg) is recommended approximately 1 to 2 hours before training.

In some individuals, carbohydrate ingestion and subsequent insulin release in the hour before activity may lead to decreased availability of lipids and of liver glucose and possible subsequent hypoglycemia.[6] This effect raises the question of the possible role of the glycemic index (GI) of different carbohydrates in the pre-exercise meal. Most studies in adults have demonstrated that pre-exercise meals with a higher GI result in increased carbohydrate oxidation and decreased fat oxidation relative to meals with a lower GI.[7–9] However, most of these studies have not demonstrated any significant changes in performance, and none of these studies have been performed in children. At this point, individual preference and tolerance should dictate pre-exercise carbohydrate choice.

Table 10.1
Dietary Recommendations Before, During, and After Physical Exercise

3–4 h before exercise	Carbohydrate: 4 g/kg
1–2 h before exercise	Carbohydrate: 0.5–1 g/kg
	Fluid: 90–180 mL if weight <40 kg 180–360 mL if ≥40 kg
During exercise (especially if >1 h duration)	Carbohydrate: 0.7 g/kg per h, divided every 15–20 min
	Fluid: 150 mL every 20 min if weight approx 40 kg 250 mL every 20 min if weight approx 60 kg
After exercise	Carbohydrate: 1–1.5 g/kg
	Fluid: replace losses: 450–680 mL/0.5 kg of body weight lost
	Protein: approx 0.2–0.4 g/kg

Intake of carbohydrates during activity appears to be beneficial. This has been well established for activities lasting longer than 60 minutes, but there is accumulating evidence that this may also be true during shorter periods of activity as well.[3] It is currently recommended that endurance athletes consume 0.7 g of carbohydrate/kg per hour divided into 15- to 20-minute intervals. The type and form of carbohydrate can be dictated by the athlete's preference and gastric tolerance. Hydration with recommended volumes of a 6% to 8% carbohydrate-containing sports drink during exercise can also provide the recommended amount of carbohydrates.

Many scholastic athletes train 1 to 2 hours/day at least 5 days/week. For athletes training at this frequency, the postexercise meal becomes very important in replenishing diminished muscle glycogen, which becomes the primary fuel source for the next day's workout. In addition, the postexercise meal appears to have an important role in sparing muscle from postexercise catabolism. The postexercise meal is best ingested as soon as possible after exercise, when muscles are most sensitive to the effects of insulin and glycogen synthesis is maximized.[3] It is currently recommended that athletes ingest 1 to 1.5 g of carbohydrate/kg immediately after exercise, which can be repeated 2 and 4 hours later.

Some authors suggest that a postexercise meal with a high GI further enhances glycogen synthesis and leads to a more anabolic hormonal profile.[10–12] However, data are conflicting on performance effects.[13] On the basis of current data, the quantity and timing of postexercise carbohydrates appear to be far more important determinants of glycogen replenishment than the GI of postexercise meal.

"Carbohydrate loading" describes a regimen used by endurance and ultraendurance athletes to increase muscle glycogen content before competition. There are several regimens in common use, which usually involve decreasing physical activity and increasing carbohydrate amounts in the diet for several days before event participation. One 2002 study found that 10 g of carbohydrate/kg (using foods with a high GI) combined with physical inactivity resulted in maximal muscle glycogen stores after only 1 day.[14] However, despite documented increases in muscle glycogen with carbohydrate loading, studies do not show benefit in terms of athletic performance when compared with controls who follow the dietary recommendations outlined in Table 10.1.[15,16]

Fluids

Maintenance of fluid volume is very important in optimizing physical performance, especially for endurance activities. Fluid requirements are highly variable depending on intensity of training, climatic conditions, and the intrinsic sweat rate and acclimatization of the athlete. In the adolescent population, older and male athletes tend to have higher sweat rates than younger and female athletes. Studies document sweat rates ranging from 510 to 1260 mL/hour; however, in a case report, a 17-year-old male had a sweat rate of 2.5 L/hour.[2] Although thirst is often recognized when dehydration approaches 3% to 5%, aerobic performance begins to drop off at approximately 1% dehydration.[17] Anaerobic performance is also affected by dehydration, but it appears to be less sensitive to fluid status than aerobic efforts.[18–20]

Given the variation in sweat losses, fluid recommendations should encourage athletes to monitor their own fluid status. Young athletes should maintain euhydration throughout the day, which can be readily accomplished by having the athlete drink enough to keep urine light yellow or clear in color. In preparation for physical training, athletes should prehydrate 1 to 2 hours before training (90–180 mL for children <40 kg, 180–390 mL for children ≥40 kg).[21] This allows for gastric emptying and absorption into the vascular system before exertion begins. Once exercise begins, athletes should then maintain hydration by ingesting fluid at 15- to 20-minute intervals, even if they do not feel thirsty (approximately 150 mL every 20 min for a 40-kg athlete, 250 mL every 20 min for a 60-kg athlete).[22] See Table 10.1 for a summary of fluid recommendations.

Athletes can be educated to weigh themselves before and after working out (making sure to remove sweat-soaked clothing). In adults, recommendations include fluid consumption of up to 150% of weight lost during exercise.[3] This is moderated slightly for the pediatric population; athletes weighing <40 kg are advised to replenish approximately 100% of weight lost (ie, 480 mL of fluid per pound lost).[21] Future intake can then be adjusted to avoid these losses in subsequent practice sessions.

Multiple studies have demonstrated that young athletes will often not maintain euhydration without interventions designed to encourage fluid intake.[21,22] This may include structuring the practice setting so that ad lib fluid intake and designated fluid breaks are encouraged. Children are also more likely to drink appropriate fluid volumes if they are provided fluid that is flavored, colored, and contains 6% to 8% carbohydrate.[2,22,23] Addition of 10 to 20 mmol of sodium/L also appears to enhance palatability and increase volume ingested.

Over the past several years, there has been increasing recognition of exertional hyponatremia in endurance athletes. Although this has generated much press and much concern among some athletic governing bodies, it is mainly a phenomenon found in endurance and ultraendurance efforts of more than 4 hours in duration. There is some speculation that there may be athletes with undiagnosed variants of cystic fibrosis who lose unusually high amounts sodium in their sweat.[24] It has been proposed that these athletes may be at increased risk of exertional hyponatremia and muscle cramping and may benefit from sodium-containing beverages during exercise. This is an area of ongoing study.

Gastric Tolerance

When advising athletes on fuel and fluid ingestion before and during exercise, some will complain about stomach upset when trying to implement these changes. During exercise, gastric emptying often slows, which may increase the risk of stomach upset. This is often particularly true in running athletes and those exercising at a high intensity.

For many athletes, "gastric tolerance" is something that can be trained by starting with small volumes of food and/or fluid ingested several hours ahead of time. The athletes then slowly advance the time and volume ingested until goal intake is met.

In addition, it may be helpful to review some of the following strategies to enhance stomach emptying[3]:

- Solutions of 4% to 8% carbohydrate empty from the stomach faster than either water or higher-carbohydrate content drinks/juices. Table 10.2 has further information on commonly used fluid replacements.

- Tepid solutions empty faster than ice-cold solutions.

- Stomachs containing at least 600 mL empty faster than empty stomachs.

- Sucrose/glucose sources empty faster than fructose sources. In addition, some athletes experience gastric upset with fructose-containing foods or beverages. Athletes may want to experiment with a variety of carbohydrates to find what works best for them.

Table 10.2
Carbohydrate and Sodium Content of Selected Fluids

Product	kcal/240 mL	% Carbohydrate	g Carbohydrate /240 mL	Primary Carbohydrate type	Sodium mEq/L
AllSport*	70	8	20	Fructose	10
Gatorade[†]	50	6	14	Sucrose	20
Powerade[‡]	70	8	19	Fructose	10
Apple juice	125	16	38	Fructose	4
Grape juice	170	18	42	Fructose	4

*Monarch Beverage Company, Atlanta, GA.
[†]Gatorade, Chicago, IL.
[‡]The Coca-Cola Co, Atlanta, GA.

Building Blocks for Recovery

During the 24 to 48 hours after working out, the body repairs the microtrauma induced during a rigorous exercise session. This repair process results in hypertrophy and increased strength of skeletal muscle and other tissues and requires the following:

- Adequate protein intake to provide the "building blocks" for muscle growth and tissue repair;

- Adequate carbohydrate intake to avoid further muscle catabolism; and

- Adequate sleep and rest from additional physical stress.

Young athletes often do not appreciate the role of rest in physical training. Athletes who persist in not giving their body appropriate rest and repair time between training sessions will not experience optimal gains in performance. They also are at increased risk of injury and development of overtraining syndrome.

Protein

Many adolescent athletes are highly interested in the role protein plays in building strength and muscle. The current Recommended Dietary Allowances (RDAs) for protein are 0.8 g/kg per day in adults, 0.85 g/kg per day in 14- to 18-year-olds, and 0.95 g/kg per day in 4- to 13-year-olds.[25] This higher value in children and adolescents accommodates the protein requirements for growth and development. Research in adults has demonstrated that athletes have increased protein requirements relative to the sedentary population, and this is probably true in younger athletes as well. Increased protein requirements are likely attributable in part to increased protein turnover as well as utilization of some amino acids (especially the branched-chain amino acids) for fuel. Current evidence supports the following protein recommendations in adults[3] (for reference, the average US daily intake is 1.4 g/kg per day):

- Resistance-trained athletes: 1.2 to 1.7 g/kg per day
- Endurance-trained athletes: 1.2 to 1.4 g/kg per day

Although there is a paucity of data on the pediatric athlete, the increased protein requirements for growth and athletic activity are probably cumulative but not necessarily additive. Protein contents for several common foods and supplements can be found in Table 10.3.

Protein ingested before a workout is likely to be metabolized as fuel and may increase stomach upset in some athletes. There is some evidence in young adult athletes that adding protein to carbohydrates ingested shortly before exercise may decrease exercise-induced muscle catabolism.[26] However, any role for protein in the pre-exercise meal is secondary to the importance of adequate carbohydrates. Protein is best ingested after workouts and during meals throughout the day to provide a steady stream of amino acids for tissue repair. Several studies have demonstrated that adding some protein to post-exercise meals increases release of insulin and growth hormone and decreases muscle catabolism.[26] Carbohydrate-to-protein ratios in these studies are generally approximately 3:1 to 5:1.

Table 10.3

Protein Content of Some Common Foods/Supplements Used by Athletes

Food	Protein (g)
Meats/eggs	
Hamburger (3 oz, extra lean)	24
Chicken, roasted (3 oz)	21
Tuna (3 oz, water packed)	20
Egg (1 large)	6
Dairy	
Cottage cheese (1/2 cup, low-fat)	14
Yogurt (8 oz)	12
Milk (8 oz, whole or skim)	8
Nonfat dry milk (2 tbsp)	3
Beans/legumes	
Tofu (1/2 cup)	10
Peanut butter (2 tbsp)	10
Lentils (1/2 cup, cooked)	9
Black beans (1/2 cup)	8
Grains	
Pasta (1 cup, cooked)	7
Bread (whole wheat, 2 slices)	5
Other	
Protein supplements (per serving)	20–35
Promax* bar	20
Clif[†] bar (peanut butter flavor)	12
Carnation Instant Breakfast[‡] (with 8 oz skim milk)	12
PowerBar[§]	10
Ensure[||] (8 oz)	9
Snickers[¶] bar	4
Nutrigrain[#] bar	2

*Promax Nutrition Corp, Concord, CA.
[†] Clif Bar Inc, Berkeley, CA.
[‡] Nestlé, Glendale, CA.
[§] PowerBar, Glendale, CA.
[||] Abbott Laboratories, Abbott Park, IL.
[¶] Masterfoods USA, Hackettstown, NJ.
[#] Kellogg Co, Melbourne, Australia.

Micronutrients

Minerals

Iron

The body is very good at conserving iron, except in menstruating females. In endurance and ultraendurance events, some athletes will lose small amounts of iron via sweat or through the gastrointestinal or genitourinary tracts. However, these losses are compensated with enhanced dietary absorption and are likely not clinically significant in most young athletes.[27] Dietary iron recommendations are the same in both the athletic and nonathletic populations, and the prevalence of inadequate intake is high in both groups.[2,28] This is particularly true in females; approximately half of all females older than 12 years in the United States consume less than 55% of the RDA of iron.

The primary concern with inadequate iron intake is the development of iron-deficiency anemia. Once again, there is a similar prevalence in both athletes and nonathletes. However, one of the first signs of iron-deficiency anemia is decreased exercise tolerance; therefore, athletes may present for screening more frequently than nonathletes.

Multiple hematologic changes occur with physical training. This includes initial expansion of plasma volume and subsequent increase in red cell mass. Appropriate increase in red cell mass certainly depends on adequate iron stores, but studies looking at additional effects of low iron stores on athletic performance have had inconsistent results.[27,29,30] Multiple methodologic limitations likely confound many of the studies looking at nonanemic iron depletion and athletic performance. A rigorous 2001 study in elite adolescent athletes found an aerobic performance benefit with adequate iron supplementation (100 mg elemental iron twice/day) in athletes with low iron stores.[30] A key finding was that this performance improvement occurred in the absence of significant changes in red cell mass or other hematologic measures. However, further studies are certainly needed, and expert opinions remain divided on the relationship between nonanemic iron deficiency and performance.[2,27–29]

There should be a low threshold for checking hemoglobin and hematocrit and performing iron studies in athletes presenting with fatigue or decreases in performance. Possible changes in laboratory values in young athletes include an "athletic pseudoanemia" attributable to increased plasma volume and hemodilution, especially at the initiation of training, and "runner's macrocytosis," a reactive reticulocytosis attributable to increased mechanical hemolysis. Both of these conditions are diagnoses of exclusion. Ferritin is often used as a marker for iron stores in the body, but it is subject to a variety of influences in athletes and is an unreliable measure of iron status.[27] Serum transferrin receptor appears to be more consistently associated with iron stores and is not subject to changes resulting from growth and physical activity.[31]

Although iron supplementation is common in young athletes, it is not without risk and should be reserved for those cases of documented iron deficiency in which symptoms, performance, and laboratory values are followed during treatment.[27]

Calcium

As with iron, inadequate intake of calcium is common in both athletes and nonathletes. In childhood and adolescence, calcium intake and weight-bearing exercise are both important components in achieving peak bone mass, but the interactions between the 2 are still not clear.[32] Although calcium requirements do not appear to change with athletic participation, athletes do place increased stress across their skeletal system compared with nonathletes. This results in increased bone mass accretion as long as there is adequate calcium, vitamin D, protein, and caloric intake. In athletes who do not meet these dietary requirements, this adaptation may not occur, and the athlete may be at increased risk of development of stress injuries to bones.

Female athletes whose energy intake is too low to support their caloric requirements will often suppress estrogen production, possibly resulting in pubertal delay or oligomenorrhea or amenorrhea. This combination of low caloric intake and decreased estrogen production results in diminished bone formation. This condition has come to be known as "the female athlete triad."[33,34] Although adequate dietary or supplemental calcium remains important in these athletes, increased caloric intake appears to be the key in reversing the loss of bone mineral density.

Zinc/Magnesium

Athletes who are restricting calories, particularly females, may be at increased risk of inadequate intake of zinc and magnesium. Magnesium deficiency has been shown to contribute to suboptimal athletic performance in a variety of settings, but no benefits with supplementation has been found in athletes with adequate magnesium status.[28]

Vitamins

Vitamins A, C, and E

There is significant interest in the role these antioxidants may play in reducing oxidative damage to muscle and other tissues during exercise. However, athletes already have enhanced antioxidant mechanisms, and it is unclear how exogenous antioxidants may affect this population. This is an area of very active research in adults, but there are currently few data in the pediatric population.

Several studies in child and adolescent athletes have examined increased oxidant stress during exercise, and 1 study examined possible attenuation of that stress with vitamin supplementation.[35,36] However, these results were strictly in laboratory markers of cellular oxidation and injury, and there was no demonstrated effect on health or performance in vivo. Although minimization of tissue injury appears to be universally desirable, there is some theoretic concern that reducing the amount of microinjury during exertion may shortchange post-training protein synthesis and training adaptations.[28]

B Vitamins

B vitamins are involved in a broad range of energy-generating and other functions in the body. There is some evidence in adults to suggest that athletes have increased turnover and utilization of B vitamins. The American College of Sports Medicine and the American Dietetic Association currently support intake of up to twice the RDA for B vitamins in athletic adults.[3] It is unclear whether this is applicable to young athletes as well.

For most of the B vitamins, intake generally parallels calorie ingestion.[3,28] Therefore, athletes who are eating a variety of foodstuffs and are not restricting calories are likely ingesting adequate amounts. The exception to this may be vegetarians, who may need some nutritional guidance to meet their vitamin B_{12} needs. Despite the role B vitamins play in energy metabolism, supplementation in nondeficient individuals does not appear to produce any benefit to athletic performance.[28]

Determination of Optimal Body Weight in Young Athletes

For a given athlete in a given sport, there is a range of body weights that can support optimal performance. The specific weight range may change depending on sport, developmental stage, body composition, and a variety of factors intrinsic to the individual. But the basic relationship holds that body weights at either extreme are associated with a drop in athletic performance.[37] Although this relationship may appear somewhat self-evident, it conflicts with some commonly held beliefs in the sports community. In some sports, many athletes and coaches perceive that competing at the lowest possible weight is advantageous, possibly because of appearance concerns, increased strength-mass ratio, or the desire to compete in a lower weight class. Other sports often encourage athletes to gain weight to enhance performance, especially in contact/collision sports, such as football.

Weight and body mass index are 2 common measures in pediatric offices, but neither is a good measure of athletic performance or of body fat in athletes.[37] Other measures of body composition, such as skin-fold measures and hydrostatic weighing, may give more accurate ranges of body fat in young athletes. However, their use is limited in that optimal body composition measures for athletic performance have not been determined. Sports performance measures (ie, speed, agility, jump height, etc) are far better gauges than body composition measures in determining optimal body weight for a given athlete. If body composition measures are clinically indicated, they should be obtained no more than twice per year.[38]

Principles of Weight Gain in Young Athletes

Despite the growing epidemic of obesity in American youth, many adolescent males are actively seeking to gain weight. In some contact/collision sports, increased body mass does confer some advantage, especially if lean body mass is increased relative to fat mass. In adolescents, significant gains in lean body mass require:

1. Endogenous anabolic hormones to support hypertrophy of muscle and lean tissue;
2. Physical training (especially resistance training) sufficient to stimulate protein synthesis, with appropriate recovery between sessions;
3. Sufficient carbohydrate intake to support training and minimize muscle catabolism; and
4. Sufficient protein intake to support tissue repair and hypertrophy.

In examining these factors, it is evident that most females and preadolescent males should not expect to make the same gains as postadolescent males. Genetic factors and training history also play large roles in determining the rate and amount of lean mass accretion. A reasonable goal for most adolescents who are attempting to gain weight is approximately 1 lb of lean body mass/week.[37] For athletes who are currently maintaining their weight, this requires an additional 300 to 400 kcal/day and maintenance of 1.5 to 1.8 g of protein/kg per day. Intakes higher than this or weight gain in excess of 1.5% of body weight/week will likely produce increased gains of fat mass.[37] See Table 10.4 for practical recommendations on weight gain in young athletes.

Table 10.4
Strategies for Weight Gain

Training
Resistance training is a key aspect of making gains in lean mass: • For muscle hypertrophy: multiple sets of 8–15 repetitions/set • For strength/power gain: multiple sets of 4–6 repetitions/set Appropriate rest: • Strength training for a given body part should be done on nonconsecutive days

Nutrition

Calories:
• Increase intake by 300–400 kcal/day over any increased expenditures
Protein:
• Maintain 1.5–1.8 g/kg per day
Practical recommendations to attain above:
• Increase frequency of meals/snacks
   Do not skip breakfast
   Aim to eat 5–9 times/day
• Increase size of meals/portions
• Change dietary composition to include foods with higher caloric density. Examples of ways to enhance calorie/protein content of foods in diet:
   Enrich milk with nonfat dry milk, instant breakfast, other flavorings
   Reconstitute canned soup with evaporated milk instead of water
   Choose cranberry, grape, or pineapple juice instead of orange or grapefruit juice
   Add dried fruits and/or nuts to hot cereal, sandwich fillings, etc
   Create sandwiches with thick-sliced, dense bread instead of white bread
Fat: Consider increasing fat content of diet if:
• Difficulty gaining weight or ingesting adequate calories after implementing above recommendations
• No contraindications/other risk factors for a higher-fat diet
Weight gain supplements (ie, "weight gainers"):
• May provide between 500–2000 kcal/serving
   If used as directed, will often result in excessive fat gains
   Often with 20–35 g of protein/serving
   Fat content variable
• For young athletes, liquid food products (eg, Ensure [Abbott Laboratories, Abbott Park, IL], Carnation Instant Breakfast [Nestlé, Glendale, CA]) are reasonable options
   Regulated by US Food and Drug Administration and widely available
   2 servings/day often provide appropriate calories and protein to support lean tissue growth

Principles of Weight Loss in Young Athletes

In contrast to the desire for increased body weight as described previously, many athletes instead strive to lose weight. Weight loss practices of athletes can be loosely divided into those techniques that produce rapid loss of fluid weight (also known as "cutting weight") and those that result in reductions in lean tissue or fat mass.

Rapid loss of fluid weight, especially prevalent in wrestling, has come under close scrutiny in the past decade. These practices are potentially life threatening, and many techniques previously used to produce rapid dehydration have now been regulated by the National Federation of State High School Associations (www.nfhs.org). Most states have developed programs to determine appropriate weight classifications for individual athletes. These programs are usually based on measures of body composition and hydration obtained at the beginning of the season, but specifics vary from state to state. Details can be accessed via links from the National Federation of State High School Associations Web site (www.nfhs.org).

A variety of additional weight loss practices are used to produce longer-term changes in body mass. Athletes who desire to lose weight should be instructed in the importance of maintaining lean mass as much as possible during this process. Loss of lean mass results in possible reductions in strength and performance as well as a reduction in caloric expenditure attributable to resulting decreases in resting metabolic rate. In athletes who are currently maintaining their weight, weight loss should not exceed 1.5% of total body weight/week (usually 1–2 lb/week). Weight loss of 1 lb/week requires a caloric deficit of 3500 kcal/week, which is best achieved by a combination of a reduction in caloric intake and an increase in caloric expenditure.

Once weight goals are met, weight maintenance should be emphasized. Cyclic fluctuations in weight should be strongly discouraged, as they tend to produce significant decreases in metabolic rate and lean body mass over time.[37] Some young athletes who seek to lose weight may benefit from consultation with a knowledgeable sports nutritionist (lists of American Dietetic Association-certified nutritionists with a particular interest in sports can be found through the Sports, Cardiovascular, and Wellness Nutritionists Web site [www.scandpg.org]).

Although athletic participation is often associated with improvements in nutritional status and body image, an increased prevalence of disordered and restrictive eating behavior in a variety of subpopulations of athletes has been well documented.[37]

Vegetarian Athletes

Approximately 2% of children 6 to 17 years of age identify themselves as vegetarian, and up to 6% report that they have eliminated beef or pork from their diet.[39] Although questions are often raised about athletic performance in vegetarians, most studies show that vegetarian athletes who consume a well-planned diet demonstrate no change in athletic performance compared with their meat-eating peers.[39] The challenge in a diet devoid of meat or animal products is the greater effort required to ensure daily intake of a full complement of essential amino acids and adequate amounts of vitamin B_{12}, iron, and calcium. This amount of planning is difficult for many children and adolescents. However, as long as nutritional requirements are met, the dietary source does not seem to matter with regard to supporting athletic performance. Many vegetarian athletes, particularly at higher performance levels, may benefit from consultation with a sports nutritionist (www.scandpg.org).

Dietary Supplements/Ergogenic Aids

Comparison and competition among peers is an inevitable part of youth and adolescence. This is especially true in the realm of sport and athletic participation, in which the desire for competitive advantage or for rapid performance gains may lead to experimentation with a variety of ergogenic aids. This often includes a number of dietary supplements. In a 2004 Texas study, 74% of surveyed high school students reported use of a dietary supplement.[40] Other recent North American studies found that approximately half of surveyed high school students reported use of dietary supplements, and in general, athletes reported higher rates than nonathletes.[40–43] The most commonly used supplements were vitamins and minerals. Use of other supplements, including protein, amino acids, creatine, and stimulants, ranged from approximately 5% to 20%.[40–42]

Despite the prevalence of supplement use, there is a paucity of data on the safety and efficacy of dietary supplements in young athletes. Knowledge of the effects of performance-enhancing aids is based almost solely on studies in adults, which may or may not be applicable to a pediatric population. The American Academy of Pediatrics (AAP) has taken a firm stand against the use of performance-enhancing substances in young athletes, citing both safety and ethical concerns.[44] The AAP states that pediatricians should directly ask their athletic patients about supplement use and should be prepared to provide unbiased information about risks and benefits.

Protein Supplements

Protein supplementation is very common in young athletes, and most protein supplements contain 20 to 35 g of protein/serving (see Table 10.2 for dietary comparisons). Although manufacturers of these supplements sometimes make claims about the superiority of one protein type over another (eg, whey vs soy), the evidence is less clear-cut. Some studies appear to demonstrate that as long as the full complement of essential amino acids is provided, protein type does not appear to confer an advantage in building muscle or strength.[39,45,46] However, a 2005 report stated that young men fed milk protein during a 12-week resistance training program appeared to demonstrate increased amino acid uptake compared with a soy-fed group.[47] No significant differences in strength were found, but the authors ascribed importance to a trend toward greater lean mass in the milk-fed group. Other authors agree that protein type may produce some difference in muscle growth[48]; however, the clinical and performance significance of these differences is not yet known.

Convenience is the primary advantage of protein supplements, and cost and taste are the primary drawbacks. As with all supplements, product purity and quality are variable depending on manufacturer. One low-cost way to supplement protein for athletes who have difficulty achieving optimal intake is to enrich foods or beverages in the diet with nonfat powdered milk. This provides 3 g of protein/2 tablespoons of powder, which may be added to milk, cereal, sandwiches, pasta sauce, etc.

"Weight Gainers"

These popular supplements are often higher-calorie versions of the protein supplements described previously, and their content is highly variable. Carbohydrates (usually maltodextrin) and/or fats are added to increase the calorie count, with some preparations containing up to 2000 kcal/serving. They are often supplemented with significant amounts of vitamins and minerals and may contain additional herbal or other ingredients. The instructions for these products often direct the consumer to drink 1 to 2 servings/day in addition to regular meals. However, as described in the earlier section on weight gain, this caloric increase will typically result in significant increases in fat mass, which is often not the desired effect. See Table 10.4 for additional recommendations on weight gain.

Amino Acid Supplements

Amino acid supplements may contain either individual or combinations of select amino acids (eg, branched-chain amino acids), as compared with protein supplements, which typically contain all the essential amino acids. A recent study in adolescents suggests that supplementation with certain amino acids is at least as common as protein supplementation.[40]

Interest in these supplements seems to follow a cyclical pattern driven by interest in a succession of amino acids with purported performance benefits.[49] Amino acids of recent interest among athletes have included glutamine (reported to enhance immune function), branched-chain amino acids (reported to spare muscle glycogen in endurance athletes), and carnitine (reported to enhance lipolysis).[29,49] One amino acid of particular interest has been arginine. It is found either in the form of l-arginine or of arginine alpha-ketoglutarate (which is reported to enhance the arginine moiety absorption). Arginine has been reported to increase growth hormone release and to stimulate production of nitric oxide, a vasodilator.[29,50] Although exogenous arginine may assist in maintenance of lean body mass in critically ill patients, it has not been shown to improve athletic performance or body composition in otherwise healthy individuals.[50]

On the basis of current evidence, supplementation of individual or selected amino acids in otherwise healthy athletes is unnecessary and potentially problematic. Ingestion of an excess of one amino acid may impair the absorption of others, and some amino acids are toxic when taken in supraphysiologic amounts.[49]

Creatine

Creatine is a metabolite of arginine that is used widely among athletes as a dietary supplement. In the pediatric population, use appears to increase with age, with up to 44% of 12th-grade athletes reporting creatine supplementation in a New York study.[51] Creatine monophosphate is the most commonly used form, for which sales in the United States exceeded $400 million (2.5 million kg) in the year 2000.[52] See Table 10.5 for common creatine use patterns.

Creatine is primarily stored in skeletal muscle as phosphocreatine, where it rephosphorylates ATP during the initial 10 to 30 seconds of physical activity. It is fairly unique among current "purported ergogenic aids" in that the body of evidence appears to favor some performance benefit from its use, but only in select situations. The primary benefit seems to occur in activities of <30 seconds' duration,[29,52,53] and the gain in performance appears to be approximately 5% to 10%.[54] One of the few studies looking at creatine use in adolescence found a 10% to 30% improvement in several sprint tests and in vertical jump height as compared with placebo.[55]

Table 10.5
Creatine Supplementation: Common Dosing Schedules and Dietary Comparisons

Several different strategies for use have emerged[53]:
• Loading and maintenance:
Load: 20 g/day (5 g, 4 times/day) for 5-7 days
Maintenance: 3-5 g/day for 4-16 wk
• Low dose: 2-3 g/day (demonstrated to increase intramuscular creatine concentration over course of a month and maintain concentrations during supplementation)
For comparison purposes:
• Meat, poultry, and fish contain 2-5 g of creatine/lb.
• Adult liver synthesizes up to 1-2 g of creatine/day.
• 70-kg adult loses 2 g of creatine/day as creatinine.
• Average mixed diet in United States provides 1 g of creatine/day.

Weight-bearing activities may be negatively affected by the 1- to 3-kg weight gain that is commonly seen with creatine use.[53,56] The weight gain associated with creatine use was previously believed to be primarily water, however, studies document significant increases in lean tissue in subjects who have used creatine in conjunction with resistance training.[26,53] It is unclear whether this is attributable to an anabolic effect of creatine or whether it merely reflects the increased training capacity secondary to its effect in ATP regeneration.

There does appear to be significant interindividual variability in the effects of creatine use, leading some to propose that there are "responders" and "nonresponders" to supplemental creatine.[53,56] Uptake of creatine by skeletal muscle is dependent on creatine concentrations within the muscle. Biopsy studies in subjects who are not using creatine supplements reveal that some individuals have creatine concentrations that approach the muscle's maximum carrying capacity, whereas others have significantly less.[57] Those with the lowest creatine concentrations experience the greatest increases in creatine content with supplementation; however, it is unclear whether these changes in muscle content correlate with changes in athletic performance.

Current theory is that the differences in intramuscular creatine concentrations are attributable to dietary choice (ie, eating meat). This is consistent with the finding that vegetarians generally appear to have lower concentrations of muscle creatine, and that these concentrations do increase with exogenous creatine supplementation.[39,58] A 2003 placebo-controlled study in vegetarians and omnivores demonstrated strength gains that correlated with changes in intramuscular creatine.[58] A smaller study found insignificant differences between vegetarians and meat eaters in anaerobic cycling performance after creatine supplementation.[59]

Gastric upset is the most common adverse effect reported with creatine use.[60] Other adverse events include case reports of exacerbation of underlying renal disease, elevation of blood pressure, lower leg compartment pressures, and concerns about possible increased risks of heat illness and dehydration. However, the short-term studies to date and accumulating anecdotal experience do not appear to reveal significant, reproducible adverse effects in healthy adults. Data on long-term use in young athletes are currently lacking.

The evidence favoring creatine as an ergogenic aid with minimal adverse effects adds to its appeal for many young athletes. Many studies have demonstrated widespread creatine use among high school athletes, particularly among males. However, it is important to note that the literature favoring performance enhancement is primarily based on evidence in adults, and no study has demonstrated any benefit in generalized "on-field" performance outside the laboratory or weight room.

Other Supplements

The evidence-based literature cannot keep up with the pace of the development and dissemination of information about dietary supplements and ergogenic aids. The Internet is a common source of nutritional information—and misinformation—for young athletes, and availability of an appropriate Internet resource can be helpful for the clinician as well as for the athlete and his or her family. Two good resources include:

- The Food and Nutrition Information Center of the US Department of Agriculture National Agricultural Library (www.nal.usda.gov/fnic). The Web site includes links to "dietary supplements" and "fitness, sports, and sports nutrition," and serves as a portal for a spectrum of information on dietary supplements and ergogenic aids.

- Choices in Sports (www.drugfreesport.com/choices). The Web site includes information on supplements and ergogenic aids and is tailored for collegiate athletes but is also applicable to many adolescent and high-school athletes as well.

In young athletes, the most powerful combination for improving athletic performance includes nutrition fundamentals, appropriate coaching and practice, and the onset of puberty. Changes in strength, speed, endurance, and athletic proficiency that come with maturation dwarfs even the most optimistic results of performance enhancement with any dietary supplement.

References

1. Grunbaum JA, Kann L, Kinchen S, Ross J, et al. Youth risk behavior surveillance—United States, 2003. *MMWR Surveill Summ.* 2004;53:1–96

2. Petrie HJ, Stover EA, Horswill CA. Nutritional concerns for the child and adolescent competitor. *Nutrition.* 2004;20:620–631

3. American Dietetic Association, Dietitians of Canada, American College of Sports Medicine. Position of the American Dietetic Association, Dietitians of Canada, and American College of Sports Medicine: nutrition and athletic performance. *J Am Diet Assoc.* 2000;100:1543–1556

4. Ziegler PJ, Nelson JA, Jonnalagadda SS. Nutritional and physiological status of U.S. national figure skaters. *Int J Sport Nutr.* 1999;9:345–360

5. Hinton PS, Sanford TC, Davidson MM, Yakushko OF, Beck NC. Nutrient intakes and dietary behaviors of male and female collegiate athletes. *Int J Sport Nutr Exerc Metab.* 2004;14:389–405

6. Hargreaves M, Hawley JA, Jeukendrup A. Pre-exercise carbohydrate and fat ingestion: effects on metabolism and performance. *J Sports Sci.* 2004;22:31–38

7. Sparks MJ, Selig SS, Febbraio MA. Pre-exercise carbohydrate ingestion: effect of the glycemic index on endurance exercise performance. *Med Sci Sports Exerc.* 1998;30:844–849

8. Stannard SR, Constantini NW, Miller JC. The effect of glycemic index on plasma glucose and lactate levels during incremental exercise. *Int J Sport Nutr Exerc Metab.* 2000;10:51–61

9. Wee SL, Williams C, Gray S, Horabin J. Influence of high and low glycemic index meals on endurance running capacity. *Med Sci Sports Exerc.* 1999;31:393–399

10. Burke LM, Kiens B, Ivy JL. Carbohydrates and fat for training and recovery. *J Sports Sci.* 2004;22:15–30

11. Siu PM, Wong SH. Use of the glycemic index: effects on feeding patterns and exercise performance. *J Physiol Anthropol Appl Human Sci.* 2004;23:1–6

12. Suzuki M. Glycemic carbohydrates consumed with amino acids or protein right after exercise enhance muscle formation. *Nutr Rev.* 2003;61:S88–S94

13. Stevenson E, Williams C, McComb G, Oram C. Improved recovery from prolonged exercise following the consumption of low glycemic index carbohydrate meals. *Int J Sport Nutr Exerc Metab.* 2005;15:333–349

14. Bussau VA, Fairchild TJ, Rao A, Steele P, Fournier PA. Carbohydrate loading in human muscle: an improved 1 day protocol. *Eur J Appl Physiol.* 2002;87:290–295

15. Burke LM, Hawley JA, Schabort EJ, St Clair Gibson A, Mujika I, Noakes TD. Carbohydrate loading failed to improve 100-km cycling performance in a placebo-controlled trial. *J Appl Physiol.* 2000;88:1284–1290

16. Ivy JL. Role of carbohydrate in physical activity. *Clin Sports Med.* 1999;18:469–484, v

17. Wilk B, Yuxiu H, Bar-Or O. Effect of body hypohydration on aerobic performance of boys who exercise in the heat. *Med Sci Sports Exerc.* 2002;34(5 Suppl):S48

18. Yoshida T, Takanishi T, Nakai S, Yorimoto A, Morimoto T. Dehydration threshold for the decrease in aerobic and anaerobic fitness during out-door exercise in the heat. *Med Sci Sports Exerc.* 1999;31(5 Suppl):S308

19. Maxwell NS, Gardner F, Nimmo MA. Intermittent running: muscle metabolism in the heat and effect of hypohydration. *Med Sci Sports Exerc*. 1999;31:675–683

20. Oppliger RA, Case HS, Horswill CA, Landry GL, Shelter AC. American College of Sports Medicine position stand: weight loss in wrestlers. *Med Sci Sports Exerc*. 1996;28:ix–xii

21. Casa DJ, Yeargin SW. Avoiding dehydration among young athletes. *ACSM Health Fitness J*. 2005;9:20–23

22. American Academy of Pediatrics, Committee on Sports Medicine and Fitness. Climatic heat stress and the exercising child and adolescent. *Pediatrics*. 2000;106:158–159

23. Wilk B, Brien E, Bar-Or O. Carbohydrate drink content and voluntary drinking pattern in boys exercising in the heat. *Med Sci Sports Exerc*. 1999;31(5 Suppl):S299

24. Loud KJ, Field AE, Micheli LJ. Primary care of the elite or elite-emulating adolescent male athlete. *Adolesc Med*. 2003;14:647–661, vii

25. United States Department of Agriculture, Food and Nutrition Information Center. Dietary reference intakes (DRI) and recommended daily allowances (RDA): Dietary reference intakes: macronutrients. www.nalusda.gov/fnic/etext/000150.html (accessed 4/13/2006).

26. Kreider RB. Dietary supplements and the promotion of muscle growth with resistance exercise. *Sports Med*. 1999;27:97–110

27. Zoller H, Vogel W. Iron supplementation in athletes—first do no harm. *Nutrition*. 2004;20:615–619

28. Lukaski HC. Vitamin and mineral status: effects on physical performance. *Nutrition*. 2004;20:632–644

29. Ciocca M. Medication and supplement use by athletes. *Clin Sports Med*. 2005;24:719–738, x–xi

30. Friedmann B, Weller E, Mairbaurl H, Bartsch P. Effects of iron repletion on blood volume and performance capacity in young athletes. *Med Sci Sports Exerc*. 2001;33:741–746

31. Takala TI, Suominen P, Lehtonen-Veromaa M, et al. Increased serum soluble transferrin receptor concentration detects subclinical iron deficiency in healthy adolescent girls. *Clin Chem Lab Med*. 2003;41:203–208

32. Greer FR, Krebs NF, American Academy of Pediatrics, Committee on Nutrition. Optimizing bone health and calcium intakes of infants, children, and adolescents. *Pediatrics*. 2006;117:578–585

33. Ireland ML, Ott SM. Special concerns of the female athlete. *Clin Sports Med*. 2004;23:281–298, vii

34. Lerand SJ, Williams JF. The female athlete triad. *Pediatr Rev*. 2006;27(1):e12–e13. Available at: http://pedsinreview.aappublications.org/cgi/content/full/27/1/e12. Accessed August 9, 2007

35. Cavas L, Tarhan L. Effects of vitamin-mineral supplementation on cardiac marker and radical scavenging enzymes, and MDA levels in young swimmers. *Int J Sport Nutr Exerc Metab*. 2004;14:133–146

36. Anyanwu EC, Ehiri JE, Kanu I. Biochemical evaluation of antioxidant function after a controlled optimum physical exercise among adolescents. *Int J Adolesc Med Health*. 2005;17:57–66

37. American Academy of Pediatrics, Committee on Sports Medicine and Fitness. Promotion of healthy weight-control practices in young athletes. *Pediatrics* 2005;1557–1564

38. NCAA Committee on Competitive Safeguards. Assessment of Body Composition in *NCAA Sports Medicine Handbook 2005–06*. National Collegiate Athletics Association: Indianapolis. 2005:32–26

39. Barr SI, Rideout CA. Nutritional concerns for vegetarian athletes. *Nutrition*. 2004;20:696–703

40. Herbold NH, Vazquez IM, Goodman E, Emans SJ. Vitamin, mineral, herbal and other supplement use by adolescents. *Topics Clin Nutr*. 2004;19:266–272

41. Kayton S, Cullen RW, Memken JA, Rutter R. Supplement and ergogenic aid use by competitive male and female high school athletes. *Med Sci Sports Exerc*. 2002;34(5 Suppl):193

42. Bell A, Dorsch KD, McCreary DR, Hovey R. A look at nutritional supplement use in adolescents. *J Adolesc Health*. 2004;34:508–516

43. Dorsch KD, Bell A. Dietary supplement use in adolescents. *Curr Opin Pediatr*. 2005;17:653–657

44. American Academy of Pediatrics, Committee on Sports Medicine and Fitness. Use of performance-enhancing substances. *Pediatrics*. 2005;115:1103–1106

45. Haub MD, Wells AM, Tarnopolsky MA, Campbell WW. Effect of protein source on resistive-training-induced changes in body composition and muscle size in older men. *Am J Clin Nutr*. 2002;76:511–517

46. Tipton KD, Elliott TA, Cree MG, Wolf SE, Sanford AP, Wolfe RR. Ingestion of casein and whey proteins result in muscle anabolism after resistance exercise. *Med Sci Sports Exerc*. 2004;36:2073–2081

47. Phillips SM, Hartman JW, Wilkinson SB. Dietary protein to support anabolism with resistance exercise in young men. *J Am Coll Nutr*. 2005;24:134S–139S

48. Lemon PW, Berardi JM, Noreen EE. The role of protein and amino acid supplements in the athlete's diet: does type or timing of ingestion matter? *Curr Sports Med Rep*. 2002;1:214–221

49. Williams MH. Facts and fallacies of purported ergogenic amino acid supplements. *Clin Sports Med*. 1999;18:633–649

50. Paddon-Jones D, Borsheim E, Wolfe RR. Potential ergogenic effects of arginine and creatine supplementation. *J Nutr*. 2004;134 (10 suppl):2888S–2894S

51. Metzl JD, Small E, Levine SR, Gershel JL. Creatine use among young athletes. *Pediatrics*. 2001;108:421–425.

52. Ellender L, Linder MM. Sports pharmacology and ergogenic aids. *Prim Care Clin Office Pract*. 2005;32:277–292

53. Calfee R, Fadale P. Popular ergogenic drugs and supplements in young athletes. *Pediatrics*. 2006;117(3):e577–e589. Available at: http://pediatrics.aappublications.org/cgi/content/full/117/3/e577. Accessed August 9, 2007

54. Fomous CM, Costello RB, Coates PM. Symposium: conference on the science and policy of performance-enhancing supplements. *Med Sci Sports Exerc*. 2002;34:1685–1690

55. Ostojic SM. Creatine supplementation in young soccer players. *Int J Sport Nutr Exerc Metab*. 2004;14:95–103

56. Schwenk TL, Costley CD. When food becomes a drug: nonanabolic nutritional supplement use in athletes. *Am J Sports Med*. 2002;30:907–916

57. Harris RC, Soderlund K, Hultman E. Elevation of creatine in resting and exercised muscle of normal subjects by creatine supplementation. *Clin Sci (Lond)*. 1992;83:367–374

58. Burke DG, Chilibeck PD, Parise G, Candow DG, Mahoney D, Tarnopolsky M. Effect of creatine and weight training on muscle creatine and performance in vegetarians. *Med Sci Sports Exerc*. 2003;35:1946–1955

59. Shomrat A, Weinstein Y, Katz A. Effect of creatine feeding on maximal exercise performance in vegetarians. *Eur J Appl Physiol*. 2000;82:321–325

60. Bemben MG, Lamont HS. Creatine supplementation and exercise performance: recent findings. *Sports Med*. 2005;35:107–125

The optimal nutritional support of a mother and her developing fetus begins before conception. This poses a challenge for pediatricians caring for pregnant adolescents. Approximately 1 million teenagers become pregnant in the United States each year. Of these pregnancies, 51% end in live births, 35% end in induced abortion, and 14% result in a miscarriage or stillbirth.[1] Although birth rates to adolescents decreased in the 1990s, the teenage birth rate in 1996 (54.7 live births/1000) was still higher than the rate in 1980.[2] The pregnant adolescent is more likely to be a member of a poor or low-income family (83%), to be unmarried (72%), and to have an unplanned pregnancy (>90%). One third of adolescents who become parents—mothers as well as fathers—were themselves the product of an adolescent pregnancy.

Adolescent pregnancy is associated with an increased risk of medical complications, such as low birth weight, neonatal death, maternal mortality, pregnancy-induced hypertension, and sexually transmitted infections; the youngest adolescents appear to be at greatest risk.[1] A low prepregnancy body mass index (BMI), low gestational weight gain, anemia, and a poor-quality diet are related to poor pregnancy outcomes among adolescents. Early prenatal care, including assessment of nutritional status, is of paramount importance for pregnant adolescents. Assessment of nutritional status should identify individuals who are significantly underweight or overweight as well as those with conditions such as bulimia, anorexia, pica, hypovitaminosis, or hypervitaminosis and special dietary habits, such as vegetarianism.

Assessment of Nutritional Status

Underweight women are at increased risk of reproductive problems.[3] Not only is fertility compromised, but also, the likelihood of preterm delivery and intrauterine growth restriction (IUGR) is increased. In addition, Apgar scores of offspring of underweight women are more frequently low. The condition of being underweight is potentially modifiable, because it is often related to abusive dieting practices or exercise programs. A woman motivated toward increasing her body weight-for-height status may achieve her goal within a relatively short period (3 to 6 months).

Overweight women are at greater risk than normal-weight women for an unsatisfactory course or outcome of pregnancy.[4,5] Numerous studies have shown that obese women are at higher risk of prenatal complications, such as gestational diabetes, infertility, hypertension, and pyelonephritis. They are also more likely to experience prolonged labor followed by difficult vaginal delivery and, thus, more frequently deliver by cesarean section. The incidence of adverse perinatal outcomes is likewise higher.

The weight status of a woman planning to become pregnant may be evaluated by her prepregnancy BMI, defined as weight (in kg) divided by height^2 (in m^2) (Table 11.1).[6]

Table 11.1
Classification of Adult Maternal Prepregnancy Body Mass Index (BMI)[6]

Classification	BMI
Underweight	<19.8
Normal weight	19.8–26.0
Overweight	>26.0–29.0
Obese	>29.0

During adolescence, the categories of weight in Table 11.1 are referenced by percentiles because of continued linear growth during those years. Reference BMI values for females by age for underweight (<25th percentile), normal weight (25th–85th percentile), at risk of overweight (85th–95th percentile), and overweight (>95th percentile) are found in Appendix D.

Guidelines for Gestational Weight Gain

Substantial evidence indicates that optimal birth weight is influenced by gestational weight gain. Methodologically acceptable studies have been virtually unanimous in reporting a positive relationship between birth weight and gestational weight gain. However, maternal prepregnancy BMI is a strong effect modifier of this relationship. A number of studies have demonstrated an increased risk of IUGR with low total gestational weight gain.[7-9] Others have observed a specific risk associated with low weight gain during the second trimester[10,11] and/or the third trimester of pregnancy[12,13] (Table 11.2). On the other hand, the increased risk of having large-for-gestational-age infants is associated with excessive gestational weight gain in very obese (BMI >35) women (Table 11.3).[14] Obese women are more likely to have pregnancy complications of diabetes, hypertension, preeclampsia, arrest of labor, fetal distress, and cesarean delivery. The recognized relationship between gestational weight gain and birth weight underlies the 1990 Institute of Medicine (IOM)[6] recommendations for weight gain on the basis of prepregnancy BMI.

Weight gains associated with optimal birth weights and least neonatal morbidity were determined. Recommended ranges for gestational weight gain by prepregnancy BMI are shown in Table 11.4.

Table 11.2
Relative Risk (and 95% Confidence Intervals) of Intrauterine Growth Retardation Based on Low Trimester Weight Gain in Women with Low, Normal, or High BMI*

Trimester Weight Gain	Maternal BMI		
	Low (<19.8)	Normal (<19.8–26.0)	High (>26.0)
1st trimester: <0.1 kg/wk	0.88 (0.50–1.57)	1.31 (0.88–1.95)	1.02 (0.50–2.08)
2nd trimester: <0.3 kg/wk	2.68 (1.46–4.94)	1.92 (1.29–2.87)	1.88 (1.03–3.43)
3rd trimester: <0.3 kg/wk	2.07 (1.22–3.51)	2.12 (1.48–3.04)	1.53 (0.86–2.74)

*Low weight gain was defined as <0.1 kg/wk, and <0.3 kg/wk, <0.3 kg/wk in the first, second, and third trimesters, respectively.[13]

Table 11.3
High Birth Weight Associated With Excessive Maternal Gestational Weight Gain in Obese Women[14]

Maternal Variables	Gestational Weight Gain Range				
	Loss (n = 51)	1–7 kg (n = 153)	7–12 kg (n = 146)	12–16 kg (n = 97)	>16 kg (n = 80)
Mean birth weight (g)	3302	3192	3337	3506	3453
Number of infants small for gestational age*	2 (4.0%)	6 (3.9%)	8 (5.6%)	3 (3.1%)	3 (3.8%)
Number of infants large for gestational age*	6 (12.0%)	18 (11.8%)	27 (18.8%)	25 (25.8%)	19 (23.8%)

*Data as N (%).

Table 11.4
Recommended Total Gestational Weight Gain Ranges for Pregnant Women by Prepregnancy BMI[6]

Prepregnancy BMI	Recommended Gestational Weight Gain
Underweight (BMI <19.8)	12.5–18 kg (28–40 lb)
Normal weight (BMI 19.8–26.0)	11.5–16 kg (25–35 lb)
Overweight (BMI 26.0–29.0)	7–11.5 kg (15–25 lb)
Obese (BMI >29.0)	At least 6 kg (at least 15 lb)

There is concern that excessive gestational weight gain contributes to the increasing incidence of obesity among women in the United States. According to the 1999–2000 National Health and Nutrition Examination Surveys, 54.3% of women of reproductive age (20–39 years) are classified as overweight (BMI ≥25), and 28.4% are classified as obese (BMI ≥30). In recent decades, the average gestational weight gain has increased among American women. Average gestational weight gain increased from approximately 9 kg in the 1940s–1960s to 12–14 kg in the 1970s–1990s.[6] For most women, weight retention at 6 to 18 months after birth is 1 to 2 kg over preconceptional weight.[15,16] However, pregnancy substantially increases weight in a subset of women. Childbearing results in long-term weight gain, but it is unknown whether weight gain is caused by pregnancy itself or changes in behaviors and activities related to child rearing.

Studies demonstrate that approximately 50% of women receive no advice or inappropriate advice regarding gestational weight gain. A large survey of American women revealed that 27% received no medical advice regarding gestational weight gain.[17] Among those who received advice, 14% were advised to gain less than the recommended amount of weight, and 22% were advised to gain more than the recommended amount of weight. The odds of being advised to gain more than recommended were higher in the high-BMI group, which is concerning, because overweight women are already at risk of obesity and of delivering infants with high birth weight. In addition, black women in the survey were more likely than white women to have been advised to gain less than the recommended amount of weight, which also is concerning, because black women are at greater risk of delivering infants with low birth weight, and gaining an insufficient amount of weight can increase this risk. Survey findings showed that the advice given and the target weight were strongly associated with actual gain, and no advice was associated with gaining weight outside IOM recommendations. These findings indicate that greater efforts are needed to improve medical advice about gestational weight gain.

During the period from 1990 to 1996, gestational weight gain was studied in populations participating in the Special Supplemental Nutrition Program for Women, Infants, and Children (WIC) in Indiana, Kansas, Massachusetts, Minnesota, and Nebraska.[18] The findings indicated that 34% of WIC participants gained weight within the IOM-recommended range, 22% to 23% gained less than the recommended amount, and 42% to 43% gained more than the recommended amount.[18] Excessively high gestational weight gain was observed in young, primiparous, and overweight women. IOM recommendations apparently have had an effect on reducing inadequate gestational weight gain among WIC participants, but closer attention should be paid to preventing excessive gain.

Nutrient Needs During Pregnancy

Energy

Energy requirements during pregnancy increase as a result of increases in basal and activity energy expenditure and energy deposition in the newly acquired fetal and maternal tissues. Obligatory energy needs of the fetus, uterus, placenta, and mammary glands have been estimated to represent only 15% of the total requirement; the remainder supports energy needs for maintenance, work, and maternal fat deposition.

Basal energy expenditure increases during pregnancy as a result of the metabolic contribution of the uterus and fetus and increased work of the heart, lungs, and kidney. The increased basal metabolic rate (BMR) is one of the major components of the increased energy requirement during pregnancy.[19] Variation in energy expenditure between individuals is largely attributable to differences in fat-free mass, which in pregnancy comprises the expanded plasma, high-energy-requiring fetal and uterine tissues, and moderate- energy-requiring skeletal muscle mass.[19] In late pregnancy, approximately half of the increment in basal energy expenditure can be attributed to the fetus.[19] BMR of pregnant women has been measured longitudinally in a number of studies using a Douglas bag, ventilated hood, or whole-body respiration calorimeter.[20–24] Cumulative changes in BMR throughout pregnancy ranged from 29 636 to 50 300 kcal. This amounts to approximately 106 to 180 kcal/day.

Until late gestation, the gross energy cost of standardized nonweight-bearing activity does not significantly change. In the last month of pregnancy, the gross energy cost of cycling was increased on the order of 10%.[25] The energy cost of standardized weight-bearing activities, such as treadmill walking, was unchanged until 25 weeks of gestation, after which it increased by 19%.[25] Standardized protocols, however, do not allow for behavioral changes in pace and intensity of physical activity, which may occur and conserve energy during pregnancy. The doubly labeled water method has been used in 5 studies of well-nourished, pregnant women to measure free-living total energy expenditure (TEE).[21,26–29] TEE increased from approximately 2200 to 2400 kcal/day before pregnancy to 2700 kcal/day in the third trimester. Activity energy expenditure or physical activity level decreased by the 36th week of gestation, compared with levels before pregnancy.

Gestational weight gain includes the products of conception (fetus, placenta, and amniotic fluid), and accretion of maternal tissues (uterus, breasts, blood, extracellular fluid, and adipose tissue). The energy cost of deposition can be calculated from the amount of protein and fat deposited. Hytten[19] made theoretical calculations on the basis of a weight gain of 12.5 kg, of which 3.8 kg is fat and 925 g is protein, and a birth weight of 3.4 kg (Table 11.5). The energy cost of pregnancy was calculated from the energy deposition plus the energy cost of maintaining maternal and fetal tissues. The cumulative total gain of 85 000 kcal was divided by gestational duration to yield an increment of approximately 300 kcal/day.

Table 11.5
Theoretical Energy Costs of Pregnancy by Gestational Weeks[19]

Nutrient	Energy Equivalence (kcal/day)				Cumulative total (kcal)
	Wk 0–10	Wk 10–20	Wk 20–30	Wk 30–40	
Protein	3.6	10.3	26.7	34.2	5186
Fat	55.6	235.6	207.6	31.3	36 329
Oxygen consumption	44.8	99.0	148.2	227.2	35 717
Total net energy	104.0	344.9	382.5	292.7	77 234
Allowance for digestibility (+10%)	114	379	421	322	84 957

Fat gains associated with weight gains within the IOM-recommended ranges were measured in 200 women using a 4-component body composition model (Table 11.6).[30] The total energy deposition between 14 and 37+ weeks of gestation was calculated on the basis of an assumed protein deposition of 925 g and energy equivalences of 5.65 kcal/g of protein and 9.25 kcal/g of fat. Mean fat gain in normal-weight women concurred with Hytten's theoretical model.

The estimated energy requirement during pregnancy was derived from the sum of the TEE of the woman in the nonpregnant state, the median change in TEE, and the energy deposition in maternal and fetal tissues.[31]

Using empirical data on the longitudinal changes in the body composition of well-nourished pregnant women, total energy deposition was calculated from a mean fat gain of 3.7 kg plus an assumed deposition of 925 g of protein, applying energy equivalencies of 5.65 kcal/g of protein and 9.25 kcal/g of fat. Mean energy deposition was equal to 39 862 kcal or 180 kcal/day. The median change in TEE was 8 kcal/gestational week. Because TEE changes little and weight gain is minor, no additional energy intake is recommended during the first trimester. An estimated 340 and 452 kcal/day higher than the nonpregnant estimated energy requirement are required during the second and third trimesters, respectively.

Table 11.6
Energy Deposition During Pregnancy Measured by a Four-Component Body Composition Model in 200 Women[30]

Prepregnancy BMI Category	Recommended Gestational Weight Gain (kg)	Actual Gestational Weight Gain (kg)	Fat Gain (kg)	Energy Deposition (kcal) (as Fat and Protein)
Underweight (BMI <19.8)	12.5–18	12.6	6.0	60 726
Normal (BMI 19.8–26.0)	11.5–16	12.1	3.8	40 376
High (BMI >26.0–29.0)	7–11.5	9.1	2.8	31 126
Obese (BMI >29.0)	6	6.9	−0.6	−324

Protein

Protein requirements increase during pregnancy as a result of the increase in protein turnover and protein deposition in the fetus, uterus, expanded maternal blood volume, mammary glands, and skeletal muscle.[6] The amount of protein accretion is estimated to be 925 g.[19] Whole-body protein turnover, measured by leucine and glycine kinetics, is augmented in the second and third trimesters compared with first-trimester and prepregnancy rates.[32–34]

Estimation of the additional protein required during pregnancy was based on increased maintenance needs estimated by nitrogen balance and total body protein deposition estimated from potassium retention.[31] The total additional protein required was 0, 14.7, and 27.3 g/day during the first, second, and third trimesters of pregnancy, respectively. Given the minimal amount of changes during the first trimester, no increase in requirement was stipulated. The estimated average requirement was set at 21 g/day higher than prepregnancy protein requirements for the last 2 trimesters of pregnancy. For pregnant adolescents, the additional needs for protein were assumed to be the same as for adult women. To cover the needs of all pregnant adolescents and adults, the recommended dietary allowance (RDA) was set at twice the coefficient of variation (12%) in protein requirements or at 25 g/day of additional protein.

Table 11.7
Estimated Energy Requirement (EER)* During Pregnancy[31]

Age Category	Increase in Energy Expenditure	Energy Deposition (as Fat and Protein)
Adolescents, 14–18 y		
1st trimester	0	0
2nd trimester	160	180
3rd trimester	272	180
Adults, 19–50 y		
1st trimester	0	0
2nd trimester	160	180
3rd trimester	272	180

*EER of pregnancy is the EER of nonpregnant state plus increase of energy expenditure and energy required for fat and protein deposition during pregnancy.

Dietary Fats

Arachidonic acid (ARA) concentrations in red blood cell phospholipids decrease during pregnancy, but whether this is a normal physiologic response to pregnancy or a reflection of dietary inadequacy of omega-6 fatty acids is uncertain.[35] Because of the lack of evidence for determining the requirement during pregnancy, the IOM recommended an adequate intake at the median linoleic intake of pregnant women in the United States: 13 g/day for pregnant adolescents and adults.

Similarly, lower docosahexaenoic acid (DHA) concentrations in plasma and red blood cells have been reported for pregnant women; however, it is uncertain whether this reflects declining DHA status.[35] Supplementation with fish oil during pregnancy can increase blood concentrations of DHA in the mother and newborn infant, but no apparent physiological benefit to the infant has been found.[36] Population studies have suggested that a higher intake of eicosapentaenoic acid from fish oil and other marine foods is associated with higher birth weights and longer gestational duration.[37] Because data on omega-3 fatty acids are insufficient, the adequate intake for pregnancy was based on the median intake of alpha-linolenic acid of pregnant women in the United States: 1.4 g/day for pregnant adolescents and adults.[31]

Dietary Carbohydrates

To ensure the supply of glucose for the fetal brain and maternal brain, the estimated average requirement for available carbohydrate was estimated from that for nonpregnant women (100 g/day) plus the additional amount required during the third trimester (35 g/day). To allow for individual variation, the RDA for available carbohydrate was set at 175 g/day for pregnant adolescents and adults.[31]

Iron

Iron functions in the body as an integral part of many proteins, including hemoglobin. Approximately two thirds of the iron in the body is in hemoglobin, and the remainder is in other heme proteins (myoglobin, cytochromes), iron-sulfur enzymes (flavoproteins), and storage and transport vehicles (ferritin, transferrin). Insufficient dietary iron during pregnancy can result in iron-deficiency anemia. Epidemiologic evidence demonstrates that maternal anemia is associated with higher mortality, preterm delivery, low birth weight, and increased perinatal infant mortality.[38] High hemoglobin concentrations at delivery also are associated with adverse outcomes of preterm birth, low birth weight, and fetal death. High hemoglobin concentrations are a result of decreased plasma volume attributable to maternal hypertension and eclampsia. Although fetal needs take precedence over mother's iron needs, infants born to mothers with severe anemia have lower iron stores. Maternal anemia may further limit iron stores of the infant born preterm or with low birth weight.

Iron needs increase during pregnancy, even though menstruation does not occur and intestinal absorption of this mineral is enhanced. Dietary iron requirement during pregnancy covers basal losses, deposition in fetal and maternal tissues, and expansion of hemoglobin concentration.[38] Basal losses are estimated to be 250 mg over the 280 days of pregnancy. Approximately 315 mg of iron is deposited in fetal and placental tissues, and the expansion of hemoglobin concentration accounts for 500 mg. Accounting for individual variability and an efficiency of absorption of 25%, the RDA was set at 27 mg/day.[38] This can be supplied by the diet if substantial effort is made to consume iron-rich foods. Unfortunately, this challenge can be substantial for women who wish to moderate their intake of red meat or otherwise choose a diet with limited iron sources. The median iron intake of pregnant women in the United States is 15 mg/day, which indicates a need for supplementation. The IOM recommended that pregnant women receive an oral iron supplement of 30 mg/day during the second and third trimesters of pregnancy.[6] Most prenatal vitamin and mineral supplements supply this recommended amount of iron in the form of ferrous salts.

When therapeutic amounts of iron (>30 mg/day) are given to treat anemia, supplementation with approximately 15 mg of zinc and 2 mg of copper is recommended, because the iron may interfere with the absorption and utilization of these trace elements.[6]

Calcium

Calcium is required not only for bone mineralization but also for vascular contraction and vasodilation, muscle contraction, nerve transmission, and glandular secretion. During pregnancy, the fetus accretes approximately 25 to 30 g of calcium, with maximum accretion rates in the third trimester. Changes in maternal calcium homeostasis provide for fetal accretion of calcium.[39] Calcium absorption and urinary calcium excretion increase by approximately twofold in pregnant women. Bone resorption as well as bone formation are increased during pregnancy, as reflected in the 50% to 200% increase in bone turnover markers. Total serum calcium concentration decreases, with a slight increase at term. These changes in calcium homeostasis are mediated in part by the increase in calcitropic hormone 1,25-dihydroxyvitamin D. The major physiological adaptation to meet the increased calcium requirement of pregnancy is the increased efficiency of calcium absorption.

The effect of pregnancy on maternal bone mineral status has been studied in only a few prospective studies, and the results are conflicting.[39] Some have reported increases in bone mineral in the total body and cortical bone, others have reported decreases in bone mineral in sites rich in trabecular bone, and still others have observed no changes at all.

Dietary calcium intake does not appear to affect bone mineral changes during pregnancy.[40] Although studies are limited, maternal calcium supplementation appears to have little effect on pregnancy-induced changes in calcium and bone metabolism in well-nourished women.

The effect of calcium supplementation in reducing the incidence of pregnancy-induced hypertension remains controversial. A meta-analysis of 14 randomized trials involving 2459 women showed significant reductions in systolic and diastolic blood pressure, and the odds ratio for preeclampsia in women receiving calcium supplement (1500–2000 mg) compared with placebo was 0.38.[41] The US Trial of Calcium for Preeclampsia Prevention involving 4589 nulliparous pregnant women on a calcium supplement of 2000 mg/day did not reveal a decrease in incidence of preeclampsia or high blood pressure.[42] In contrast, a randomized trial in Australia demonstrated a beneficial effect of calcium supplementation (1800 mg/day) on the incidence of preeclampsia.[43] Although no definite recommendation can be made based on these conflicting results, it does appear that some women at risk of preeclampsia may benefit from calcium supplementation. Further studies are needed to identify these susceptible individuals. A beneficial effect of calcium supplementation (2000 mg/day) on the incidence of preterm delivery and low birth weight was observed in a randomized trial involving 189 adolescents[44] and should be confirmed with further studies.

Because of the adaptive maternal responses to fetal calcium needs, it was concluded that there is no need for increased calcium intake, provided dietary calcium intake is adequate for maximizing bone accretion in the nonpregnant state. The recommended intake or adequate intake of calcium during pregnancy is 1300 mg/day for adolescents 14 to 18 years of age and 1000 mg/day for women 19 to 50 years of age.[40]

Zinc

Zinc is essential for structural integrity of proteins and regulation of gene expression. The additional zinc requirement during pregnancy reflects zinc accretion in newly synthesized maternal and fetal tissues. Changes in intestinal zinc absorption appear to be the primary homeostatic adjustment in zinc metabolism to meet the increased demand for zinc, but this has been technically difficult to prove in women.[45] In experimental animal models, zinc deficiency limits fetal growth and, if severe, causes teratogenic abnormalities. In humans, teratogenic effects have been observed in pregnancies of women with untreated acrodermatitis enteropathica. Maternal zinc deficiency in animals and humans has been associated with infertility, hypertension, prolonged labor, intrapartum hemorrhage, preterm delivery, IUGR, and embryonic or fetal death, although reports have been inconsistent.[38,45]

Randomized, controlled intervention trials of supplemental zinc yield equivocal results, partly because of issues of subject compliance, sample size, indicators of zinc status, and control for confounding variables.[45] Of 12 trials, 6 showed no effect of the supplement; 2 demonstrated an improvement in fetal growth; and 4 showed a reduction in delivery complications, pregnancy-induced hypertension, preterm delivery, or IUGR. Zinc supplementation increased birth weight, head circumference, and gestational age in black women whose plasma zinc concentration was below the median for their population at 20 weeks of gestation.[46]

On the basis of maternal and fetal zinc accumulation of 2.7 mg/day[47] and a fractional absorption of 27%,[48] the RDA for zinc during pregnancy was set at 13 mg/day for adolescents 14 to 18 years of age and 11 mg/day for women. Factors that interfere with zinc absorption (ie, high dietary phytate, fiber, and calcium; high doses of supplemental iron; gastrointestinal diseases) or placental transport of zinc (ie, smoking, alcohol abuse, and an acute stress response to stress or infection) can cause a secondary zinc deficiency. Pregnant women with these conditions may benefit from a zinc supplement providing approximately 25 mg/day.[45]

Iodine

Iodine is an essential constituent of the thyroid hormones thyroxine and triiodothyronine, which regulate essential enzymatic and metabolic processes. Iodine deficiency results in delayed growth and development, mental retardation, hypothyroidism, goiter, and cretinism. Goiter is the earliest clinical manifestation of iodine deficiency during pregnancy. Serum thyroglobin and thyroid-stimulating hormone concentrations also increase.

The daily accumulation of iodine by the newborn infant is estimated to be 75 μg/day, with close to 100% daily turnover.[38] From studies conducted in iodine-deficient areas, it is estimated that 160 μg/day prevented goiter in pregnant women. Accounting for individual variability, the RDA for pregnancy was set at 220 μg/day to prevent goiter in most pregnant women.[38]

In the United States, the median urinary iodine concentration of pregnant women was 173 μg/L (95% confidence interval [CI], 75–229 μg/L) in 2001–2002, well within the normal range established by the World Health Organization (150–248 μg/L). However, the lower 95% CI was less than the lower boundary of the World Health Organization range. Therefore, the American Thyroid Association recommends that women receive 150 μg iodine supplements daily during pregnancy and lactation and that all prenatal vitamin/mineral preparations contain 150 μg of iodine until additional data are available.

Vitamins

Vitamin A

Vitamin A is essential for normal vision, gene expression, reproduction, embryonic development, growth, and immune function. Vitamin A deficiency in pregnancy is associated with preterm birth, IUGR, and low birth weight.[6]

The RDAs for vitamin A during pregnancy of 750 µg/day for adolescents 14 to 18 years of age and 770 µg/day for women 19 to 50 years of age are based on the accumulation of vitamin A in the fetal liver and on the assumption that the liver contains half the body's vitamin A when liver stores are low and a 70% efficiency of absorption.[38] Although most fetal vitamin A is accumulated during the last trimester, it can be stored in the mother's liver and later mobilized for fetal and maternal needs. Therefore, the recommended vitamin A intake is for the entire pregnancy.

Excessive consumption of vitamin A appears to be teratogenic.[49] Adverse drug reaction reports filed with the US Food and Drug Administration confirm that circumstances of excessive exposure to vitamin A during pregnancy may interfere with normal embryonic development. The critical period appears to be the first trimester of pregnancy. Birth defects are related to the cranial neural crest cells and include craniofacial malformations and abnormalities of the central nervous system except neural tube defects. The hazardous level of vitamin A intake likely varies from one woman to another; concern should begin when the daily intake of vitamin A (through foods or supplements) exceeds the tolerable upper limit for adults set at 3000 µg/day.[38]

Folate

Folate functions as a coenzyme in single-carbon transfer reactions involved in nucleic and amino acid metabolism. The term folate includes synthetic folic acid in fortified foods and dietary supplements and naturally occurring forms in food. Since January 1998, all enriched cereal-grain products in the United States have been fortified to contain 140 µg/100 g to achieve a projected mean increase of 100 µg of folic acid/day in the US population.[50] Because of differences in bioavailability of food folate and synthetic folic acid, the dietary folate equivalent is used to convert synthetic folic acid to a quantity equivalent to the amount in food; 1 µg of dietary folate equivalent is equal to 1 µg of food folate, which is equal to 0.5 µg of folic acid on an empty stomach or 0.6 µg of folic acid with a meal.

Because of the marked increase in single-carbon transfer reactions, including those associated with nucleotide synthesis and, thus, cell division in maternal and fetal tissues, folate requirements increase during pregnancy. The increase in cell division is seen in the fetus, placenta, red blood cell expansion, uterus, and mammary glands. Folate is actively transferred to the fetus; cord blood concentrations of folate are higher than maternal blood concentrations. Inadequate dietary folate and low serum folate concentrations are associated with poor pregnancy outcomes.[51] Inadequate folate intake can eventually result in megaloblastic anemia.

The current RDA for folate during pregnancy was based on population-based studies and a controlled metabolic study.[52] It was apparent that low dietary folate plus 100 µg/day of supplemental folate was inadequate to maintain normal folate status in a significant number of pregnant women. Therefore, the RDA was set at 300 µg/day or 600 µg/day of dietary folate equivalents. On the basis of population and clinical studies, this amount is sufficient to maintain normal folate status in 97% to 98% of pregnant women.

The IOM recommendation for women capable of becoming pregnant is to consume 400 µg/day of folate from fortified foods and/or a supplement as well as food folate from a varied diet.[52] (The RDA for all other women is 400 µg/day of dietary folate equivalents.) This preventive measure is based on evidence that a >50% decrease in risk of neural tube defects was observed for women who took a folate supplement of 360 to 800 µg/day in addition to consuming 200–300 µg/day of dietary folate. A larger dose of folate (4000 µg/day) beginning at least 1 month before conception and continuing through the first trimester has been recommended by the Centers for Disease Control (CDC)[53] and endorsed by the American Academy of Pediatrics (AAP)[54] to prevent neural tube defects in women who have previously delivered an infant with a neural tube defect. Women should be advised not to attempt to achieve the 4000-µg dose from over-the-counter or prescription multivitamin preparations because of the risk of ingesting harmful amounts of other vitamins. Also, the patient should understand that folate supplementation did not prevent all neural tube defects in clinical trials; therefore, prenatal neural tube defect testing should still be considered.

Vitamin C

Vitamin C functions as an antioxidant and cofactor for enzymes involved in the biosynthesis of collagen, carnitine, and neurotransmitters. Plasma concentrations of vitamin C decrease with the progression of pregnancy, probably as a result of hemodilution.[55] The placenta takes up the oxidized form of ascorbic acid and delivers the reduced form to the fetus.[56] Vitamin C deficiency is associated with increased risk of infections, preterm rupture of membranes, preterm birth, and eclampsia.[57] The fetus is subject to maternal status, as evidenced by lower amniotic fluid concentrations of vitamin C in pregnant smokers than in nonsmokers.[58]

The RDA for vitamin C is increased by 10 mg/day to allow for adequate fetal transfer. Higher amounts are recommended for women who use illicit drugs, cigarettes, alcohol, and aspirin regularly. Although there is no firm evidence of vitamin C toxicity during pregnancy, megadoses can result in high concentrations in the fetus, with possible induction of fetal hemolysis and oxidative damage in preterm infants.[57]

Vitamin E

Vitamin E functions as an antioxidant that prevents propagation of lipid peroxidation. Plasma concentrations of vitamin E increase during pregnancy along with total lipids. Placental transfer of vitamin E appears to be relatively constant throughout pregnancy.[59] Neither vitamin E deficiency nor toxicity has been reported in pregnant women. There is no evidence that maternal supplementation prevents hemolytic anemia in preterm infants. The RDA for pregnancy is assumed to be same as that for nonpregnant women.[57]

Vitamin Supplementation

A varied diet in accordance with the US dietary guidelines can meet all vitamin and nutrient needs associated with pregnancy; however, women whose dietary practices seem to be less than satisfactory may benefit from a prenatal vitamin supplement.[6] Special circumstances in which specific supplements are recommended include:

- Vitamin D: 10 µg (400 IU) daily is recommended for complete vegetarians (those who consume no animal products) and others with a low intake of vitamin D-fortified milk; vitamin D status is a special concern for women at northern latitudes in winter and for others with minimal exposure to sunlight and, thus, at risk of reduced synthesis of vitamin D in the skin.

- Vitamin B_{12}: 20 µg daily is recommended for complete vegetarians.

- Vitamin B_6: Supplements of vitamin B_6 may prevent nausea and vomiting in early pregnancy, because vitamin B_6 catalyzes a number of reactions involving neurotransmitter production.[60,61] In 1991, results of a randomized, double-blind, placebo-controlled study were reported in which vitamin B_6 supplementation was evaluated for its effect on nausea and vomiting in early pregnancy.[62] Results indicated that women with mild to moderate nausea did not benefit from B_6 supplementation. However, women with severe nausea and vomiting showed a substantial reduction in their symptoms. Therefore, some benefit may be derived from B_6 supplementation for women with problematic nausea and vomiting during early pregnancy.

Alcohol

Consumption of alcohol adversely affects fetal development. Fetal alcohol syndrome is estimated to occur in approximately 1 to 2 infants per 1000 live births in the United States.[63] More moderate drinkers may produce offspring with fetal alcohol effects[64]; such women also demonstrate a higher rate of spontaneous abortion, abruptio placentae, and having infants with low birth weight. All women planning for conception should be advised to avoid consumption of alcoholic beverages. Women with a known addiction to alcohol should be strongly encouraged to enroll in a treatment program and practice contraception if treatment is unsuccessful. Rehabilitation of women who are addicted to alcohol after conception may not prevent adverse embryonic development, but it may positively affect the growth of the fetus.

Caffeine

The effect of caffeine on the course and outcome of pregnancy is still controversial. Research using animals indicates that excessive amounts of caffeine intake increase the incidence of congenital malformations; the effects of consuming smaller quantities (eg, 3 to 5 cups of coffee per day) have not been satisfactorily studied. Human observational data suggest that excessive caffeine intake is associated with an increased risk of miscarriage, even accounting for concurrent smoking. Thus, common sense should prevail, and women considering pregnancy could legitimately be advised to use caffeine in moderation if they choose to use it at all.[65]

Metabolic Disorders

Discussing existing metabolic disorders may be critical to the health of both mother and infant. Examples of disorders for which early intervention is effective are maternal phenylketonuria and type 1 diabetes mellitus. Metabolic control of both diseases involves conscientious dietary manipulation well before the critical period of embryonic development. In the case of the woman with phenylketonuria, restriction of dietary phenylalanine is mandatory while satisfying the protein and other nutrient requirements of mother and fetus; evidence indicates that the IQ of the offspring is inversely related to the maternal serum phenylalanine concentration during pregnancy.[66] The woman with type 1 diabetes mellitus must control blood glucose concentrations through careful food selection and scheduled meal timing in concert with the administration of insulin. By so doing, the risk of spontaneous abortion and congenital defects in the offspring can be markedly reduced.[67,68]

Gestational diabetes mellitus (GDM) is defined as "carbohydrate intolerance of variable severity with onset or first recognition during the present pregnancy."[69] GDM is a heterogeneous disorder in which age, obesity, and genetic background contribute to the severity of the disease. Women with GDM are at risk of later developing type 2 diabetes mellitus. Only a 1.6% incidence of islet-cell antibodies is found using a specific monoclonal antibody in women with GDM.[70] In the management of women with GDM, treatment modalities aimed at improving insulin sensitivity may be useful. Changes in diet, exercise, and achievement of desirable gestational weight gain should be encouraged to improve insulin sensitivity. Self-monitoring of glucose, daily checking of urinary ketones, and exercise to enhance insulin sensitivity are integral components of many programs for women with GDM. Insulin therapy is initiated if the fasting blood glucose concentration exceeds target values.

Guidelines for daily energy intake to support a desirable gestational weight gain have been provided for women with GDM. The American College of Obstetricians and Gynecologists recommends energy intakes of 35 to 40, 30, 24, and 12 to 15 kcal/kg for women with a current pregnancy weight <80%, 80% to 120%, 120% to 150%, and >150% of ideal body weight, respectively.[69] The American Diabetes Association (ADA) has published similar guidelines.[71] On the basis of 24-hour measurements of total energy expenditure in women with GDM,[72] recommendations of energy intakes ≤25 kcal/kg per day would be unlikely to cover the free-living daily energy expenditure of these overweight women.

Caloric restriction has resulted in improved glycemic control in obese women with GDM.[73,74] With calorie-restricted diets, the incidence of macrosomia was 6%, versus 23% in untreated controls. Knopp[73] studied obese women with GDM prescribed diets of 2400 kcal/day, 1600 to 1800 kcal/day (33% reduction), or 1200 kcal/day (50% reduction). Glycemic control improved on both calorie-restricted diets, but ketonuria increased twofold to threefold in the 50% calorie reduction group. Potentially deleterious effects of ketonemia on fetal development and subsequent infant intellectual performance warrant avoidance of ketonemia.[75] IQ was inversely correlated with plasma concentrations of beta-hydroxybutyrate and fatty acids but not with concentrations of acetonuria in the third trimester.[75] Although maternal weight gain and fetal macrosomia may be decreased, the safety of calorie restriction in the management of GDM has not been established, and thus, it is not recommended by the American College of Obstetricians and Gynecologists.[69]

Specific recommendations for diet composition have not been made for women with GDM. The American Dietetic Association states that the percentage of carbohydrate is dependent on individual eating habits and the effect on blood glucose, and the percentage of fat depends on assessment and treatment goals.[71] This position acknowledges the need for individualization of dietary treatment. Several programs have successfully used diets consisting of 40% to 50% carbohydrate, 20% protein, and 30% to 40% fat.[76] The lower carbohydrate blunts the postprandial hyperglycemia. In 1 study, diet-controlled patients with GDM were randomly assigned to a low-carbohydrate diet (<42%) or a high-carbohydrate diet (45%–50%).[77] Carbohydrate restriction improved glycemic control, decreased the insulin requirement, decreased the incidence of large-for-gestational-age infants, and decreased cesarean deliveries for cephalopelvic disproportion and macrosomia. Exercise has also been shown to improve glycemic control.[78,79] Preventive measures should be aimed at improving insulin sensitivity in women predisposed to GDM.

Additional Dietary and Lifestyle Concerns

Food Cravings and Aversions

Most women change their diets during the course of pregnancy. Some changes are based on medical advice, others on folk medical beliefs, and others on changes in preference and appetite that may be idiosyncratic or culturally patterned. The health care professional should be aware that culturally sanctioned changes in diet may affect a woman's willingness to follow prescribed dietary regimens.

The most commonly avoided foods during pregnancy are also excellent sources of animal protein: milk, meats, pork, and liver. Cravings and aversions are powerful urges toward or away from foods, including foods about which women experience no unusual attitudes outside of pregnancy. The most commonly reported craved foods are sweets and dairy products. The most commonly reported aversions are alcohol, caffeinated drinks, and meats. However, cravings and aversions are not limited to any particular foods or food groups.[80] Pica may result in lead toxicity to mother and fetus if lead-containing paint is ingested.

The nutritional significance of these food-related behaviors is difficult to evaluate. Available information has often been collected in an anecdotal or uncontrolled manner. Thus, limited detailed information exists about dietary alterations that appear to be detrimental. As a result, quantifying the nutritional effect of restrictive beliefs, avoidances, cravings, and aversions is difficult. The nutritional importance of such practices cannot be assessed without reference to the rest of the woman's diet. Overall, however, most cravings result in decreased intake of alcohol, caffeine, and animal protein. Cravings and aversions are not necessarily deleterious.[80]

Herbal Teas

Pregnant women should be discouraged from unlimited consumption of herbal teas, because the composition and safety of most herbal teas are un-known. Rather than seek approval from the US Food and Drug Administration, most manufacturers of herbal tea preparations stopped marketing the mixtures as medicine and simply list the ingredients on the label.[81] Because of the lack of safety testing, pregnant women should be cautious of herbal tea mixtures. They should be advised to choose only products in filtered tea bags and, to avoid displacing more nutritious beverages, to limit herbal tea consumption to 2 servings of 8 oz per day.

Food Additives and Contaminants

The teratogenicity of specific common food additives would be a major concern if the US Food and Drug Administration did not require animal testing of new additives for their potential to cause birth defects. Some food contaminants are recognized as harmful to a developing fetus. Examples include heavy metals, chlorinated dioxin derivatives, and the fungal toxin aflatoxin. By law, no chemical that is found to be a carcinogen in humans or animals can be used as a food additive. There are no reports of birth defects from food additives used in commercial food products in the United States. Noncommercial foods, however, such as fish caught in polluted waters, can contain high amounts of mercury and other chemicals toxic to the fetus (see Chapter 53). States in which this is a problem have advisories about sport fish consumption, and these should be read with care by the pregnant woman. Although government and industry undertake significant efforts to control contamination of food and water, they cannot eliminate all risks of exposure during pregnancy.

Exercise During Pregnancy

In the absence of medical or obstetric complications, pregnant women who engage in a moderate level of physical activity can maintain cardiovascular and muscular fitness throughout pregnancy. In the absence of either medical or obstetric complications, 30 minutes or more of moderate exercise a day on most, if not all, days of the week is recommended for pregnant women.[82] Recreational and competitive athletes with uncomplicated pregnancies can remain active during pregnancy. Information on strenuous exercise is scarce, and women who engage in such activities should be closely supervised by a health care professional. Inactive women and those with complications should be evaluated before recommendations are made. Women with GDM may benefit from exercise.

Because of the physiological changes in the pregnant woman, some physical activities are not recommendable, such as contact sports; scuba diving; and recreational sports with a high risk of falling, such as gymnastics, downhill skiing, and vigorous racket sports. Medical and obstetric contraindications to exercise include hemodynamically significant heart disease, restrictive lung disease, incompetent cervix/cerclage, multiple gestation at risk of preterm labor, persistent second- or third-trimester bleeding, placenta previa after 26 weeks of gestation, preterm labor, pre-eclampsia/pregnancy-induced hypertension, or ruptured membranes. Relative contradictions to aerobic exercise during pregnancy include severe anemia, unevaluated cardiac arrhythmia, chronic bronchitis, extreme morbid obesity, BMI <12, extremely sedentary lifestyle, IUGR, heavy smoking, and poorly controlled type 1 diabetes mellitus, hypertension, seizure disorder, or hyperthyroidism.

The effects of vigorous exercise on the pregnant woman and the fetus have been the source of considerable debate. Physical fitness enthusiasts have championed maintenance of vigorous activity during pregnancy, but others have urged caution. A series of well-conducted studies of the effects of vigorous exercise on pregnancy outcome[83–86] concluded that very active women were no more likely to have a spontaneous abortion than were more sedentary women, and they seemed to have fewer difficulties during labor and delivery; however, their infants were smaller. The longer-term consequences of smaller size on later health and well-being of the neonate are unknown. Until more data are available, pregnant women should be advised to exercise moderately during the third trimester.

References

1. American Academy of Pediatrics, Committee on Adolescence. Adolescent pregnancy—current trends and issues. *Pediatrics.* 1999;103:516–520

2. Ventura SJ, Mathews TJ, Curtin SC. Declines in teenage birth rates, 1991–98: update of national and state trends. *Natl Vital Stat Rep.* 1998;48:1–7

3. Garbaciak JA Jr, Richter M, Miller S, Barton JJ. Maternal weight and pregnancy complications. *Obstet Gynecol.* 1985;152:238–245

4. Kleigman RM, Gross T. Perinatal problems of the obese mother and her infant. *Obstet Gynecol.* 1985;66:299–306

5. Kleigman RM, Gross T, Morton S, Dunnington R. Intrauterine growth and postnatal fasting metabolism in infants of obese mothers. *J Pediatr.* 1984;104:601–607

6. Institute of Medicine. *Nutrition During Pregnancy.* Washington, DC: National Academies Press; 1990

7. Lechtig A, Habicht JP, Delgado H, Klein RE, Yarbrough C, Martorell R. Effect of food supplementation during pregnancy on birthweight. *Pediatrics.* 1975;56:508–520

8. Kramer MS. Determinants of low-birth weight: methodological assessment and meta-analysis. *Bull World Health Organ.* 1987;65:663–737

9. Naeye RL. Teenaged and pre-teenaged pregnancies: consequences of the fetal-maternal competition for nutrients. *Pediatrics.* 1981;67:146–150

10. Abrams B, Selvin S. Maternal weight gain pattern and birth weight. *Obstet Gynecol.* 1995;86:163–169

11. Hickey CA, Cliver SP, McNeal SF, Hoffman HJ, Godenberg RL. Prenatal weight gain patterns and birth weight among nonobese black and white women. *Obstet Gynecol.* 1996;88:490–496

12. Scholl TO, Hediger ML, Ances IG, Belsky DH, Salmon RW. Weight gain during pregnancy in adolescence: Predictive ability of early weight gain. *Obstet Gynecol.* 1990;75:948–953

13. Strauss RS, Dietz WH. Low maternal weight gain in the second or third trimester increases the risk for intrauterine growth retardation. *J Nutr.* 1999;129:988–993

14. Bianco AT, Smilen SW, Davis Y, Lopez S, Lapinski R, Lockwood CJ. Pregnancy outcome and weight gain recommendations for the morbidly obese woman. *Obstet Gynecol.* 1998;91:97–102

15. Greene GW, Smiciklas-Wright H, Scholl TO, Karp RJ. Postpartum weight change: how much of the weight gained in pregnancy will be lost after delivery? *Obstet Gynecol.* 1988;71:701–707

16. Gunderson EP, Abrams B. Epidemiology of gestational weight gain and body weight changes after pregnancy. *Epidemiol Rev.* 1999;21:261–275

17. Cogswell ME, Scanlon KS, Fein SB, Schieve LA. Medically advised, mother's personal target, and actual weight gain during pregnancy. *Obstet Gynecol.* 1999;94:616–622

18. Schieve LA, Cogswell ME, Scanlon KS. Trends in pregnancy weight gain within and outside ranges recommended by the Institute of Medicine in a WIC population. *Maternal Child Health J.* 1998;2:111–116

19. Hytten FE. Weight gain in pregnancy. In: Hytten FE, Chamberlain G, eds. *Clinical Physiology in Obstetrics.* 2nd ed. Oxford, England: Blackwell Scientific Publications; 1991:173–203

20. National Research Council. *Recommended Dietary Allowances.* 10th ed. Washington, DC: National Academies Press; 1989

21. Goldberg GR, Prentice AM, Coward WA, et al. Longitudinal assessment of energy expenditure in pregnancy by the doubly labeled water method. *Am J Clin Nutr.* 1993;57:494–505

22. Forsum E, Sadurskis A, Wager J. Resting metabolic rate and body composition of healthy Swedish women during pregnancy. *Am J Clin Nutr.* 1988;47:942–947

23. Spaaij CJK. The Efficiency of Energy Metabolism During Pregnancy and Lactation in Well-Nourished Dutch Women [dissertation]. Wageningen, The Netherlands: Wageningen University; 1993

24. van Raaij JM, Vermaat-Miedema SH, Schonk CM, Peek ME, Hautvast JG. Energy requirements of pregnancy in The Netherlands. *Lancet.* 1987;2:953–955

25. Prentice AM, Spaaij CJ, Goldberg GR, et al. Energy requirements of pregnant and lactating women. *Eur J Clin Nutr.* 1996;50:S82–S111

26. Forsum E, Kabir N, Sadurskis A, Westerterp K. Total energy expenditure of healthy Swedish women during pregnancy and lactation. *Am J Clin Nutr.* 1992;56:334–342

27. Goldberg GR, Prentice AM, Coward WA, et al. Longitudinal assessment of the components of energy balance in well-nourished lactating women. *Am J Clin Nutr.* 1991;54:788–798

28. Kopp-Hoolihan LE, van Loan MD, Wong WW, King JC. Longitudinal assessment of energy balance in well-nourished, pregnant women. *Am J Clin Nutr.* 1999;69:697–704

29. Butte NF, Wong WW, Treuth MS, Ellis K, O'Brian Smith E. Energy requirements during pregnancy based on total energy expenditure and energy deposition. *Am J Clin Nutr.* 2004;79:1078–1087

30. Lederman SA, Paxton A, Heymsfield SB, Wang J, Thornton J, Pierson RN Jr. Body fat and water changes during pregnancy in women with different body weight and weight gain. *Obstet Gynecol.* 1997;90:483–488

31. Institute of Medicine. *Dietary Reference Intakes for Energy, Carbohydrate, Fiber, Fat, Fatty Acids, Cholesterol, Protein, and Amino Acids (Macronutrients).* Washington, DC: National Academies Press; 2005

32. Thompson GN, Halliday D. Protein turnover in pregnancy. *Eur J Clin Nutr.* 1992;46:411–417

33. Jackson AA. Measurement of protein turnover during pregnancy. *Hum Nutr Clin Nutr.* 1987;41:497–498

34. Fitch WL, King JC. Protein turnover and 3-methylhistidine excretion in non-pregnant, pregnant and gestational diabetic women. *Hum Nutr Clin Nutr.* 1987;41:327–339

35. Ghebremeskel K, Min Y, Crawford MA, et al. Blood fatty acid composition of pregnant and nonpregnant Korean women: red cells may act as a reservoir of arachidonic acid and docosahexaenoic acid for utilization by the developing fetus. *Lipids.* 2000;35:567–574

36. Connor WE, Lowensohn R, Hatcher L. Increased docosahexaenoic acid levels in human newborn infants by administration of sardines and fish oil during pregnancy. *Lipids.* 1996;31:S183–S187

37. Olsen SF, Hansen HS, Jensen B, Sorensen TL. Pregnancy duration and the ratio of long-chain n-3 fatty acids to arachidonic acid in erythrocytes from Faroese women. *J Intern Med Suppl.* 1989;731:185–189

38. Institute of Medicine. Vitamin A. In: *Dietary Intakes for Vitamin A, Vitamin K, Arsenic, Boron, Chromium, Copper, Iodine, Iron, Manganese, Molybdenum, Nickel, Silicon, Vanadium, and Zinc.* Washington, DC: National Academies Press; 2001:82–161

39. Prentice A. Calcium in pregnancy and lactation. *Annu Rev Nutr.* 2000;20:249–272

40. Institute of Medicine. *Dietary Reference Intakes for Calcium, Phosphorus, Magnesium, Vitamin D, and Fluoride.* Washington, DC: National Academies Press; 1997

41. Bucher HC, Guyatt GH, Cook RJ, et al. Effect of calcium supplementation on pregnancy-induced hypertension and preeclampsia. *JAMA.* 1996;275:1113–1117

42. Levine RJ, Hauth JC, Curet LB, et al. Trial of calcium to prevent preeclampsia. *N Engl J Med.* 1997;337:69–76

43. Crowther CA, Hiller JE, Pridmore B, et al. Calcium supplementation in nulliparous women for the prevention of pregnancy-induced hypertension, preeclampsia and preterm birth: an Australian randomized trial. FRACOG and the ACT Study Group. *Aust N Z J Obstet Gynaecol.* 1999;39:12–18

44. Villar J, Repke JT, Belizan JM, Pareja G. Calcium supplementation reduces blood pressure during pregnancy: results of a randomized controlled clinical trial. *Obstet Gynecol.* 1987;70:317–322

45. King JC. Determinants of maternal zinc status during pregnancy. *Am J Clin Nutr.* 2000;71:1334S–1343S

46. Goldenberg RL, Tamura T, Neggers Y. The effect of zinc supplementation on pregnancy outcome. *JAMA.* 1995;274:463–468

47. Swanson CA, King JC. Zinc and pregnancy outcome. *Am J Clin Nutr.* 1987;46:763–771

48. Fung EB, Ritchie LD, Woodhouse LR, Roehl R, King JC. Zinc absorption in women during pregnancy and lactation: a longitudinal study. *Am J Clin Nutr.* 1997;66:80–88

49. Rosa F, Wilk AL, Kelsey FO. Teratogen update: vitamin A congeners. *Teratology.* 1986;33:355–364

50. US Food and Drug Administration. Food standards: amendment of standards of identity for enriched grain products to require addition of folic acid; final rule. *Fed Regist.* 1996;61(44):8781–8797. Codified at 21 CFR §136, 137, 139 (1996)

51. Scholl TO, Hediger ML, Shall JI, Khoo CS, Fischer RL. Dietary and serum folate: their influence on the outcome of pregnancy. *Am J Clin Nutr.* 1996;63:520–525

52. Institute of Medicine. Thiamin. In: *Dietary Reference Intakes for Thiamin, Riboflavin, Niacin, Vitamin B6, Folate, Vitamin B12, Pantothenic Acid, Biotin, and Choline.* Washington, DC: National Academies Press; 1998:58–86

53. Centers for Disease Control and Prevention. Use of folic acid for prevention of spina bifida and other neural tube defects—1983–1991. *MMWR Morb Mortal Wkly Rep.* 1991;40:513–516

54. American Academy of Pediatrics, Committee on Genetics. Folic acid for the prevention of neural tube defects. *Pediatrics.* 1999;104:325–327

55. Morse EH, Clarke RP, Keyser DE, Merrow SB, Bee DE. Comparison of the nutritional status of pregnant adolescents with adult pregnant women. I. Biochemical findings. *Am J Clin Nutr.* 1975;28:1000–1013

56. Choi JL, Rose RC. Transport and metabolism of ascorbic acid in human placenta. *Am J Physiol.* 1989;257:C110–C113

57. Institute of Medicine. Vitamin C. In: *Dietary Reference Intakes for Vitamin C, Vitamin E, Selenium, and Carotenoids.* Washington, DC: National Academies Press; 2000:95–185

58. Barrett B, Gunter E, Jenkins J, Wang M. Ascorbic acid concentration in amniotic fluid in late pregnancy. *Biol Neonate*. 1991;60:333–335

59. Abbasi S, Ludomirski A, Bhutani VK, Weiner S, Johnson L. Maternal and fetal plasma vitamin E to total lipid ratio and fetal RBC antioxidant function during gestational development. *J Am Coll Nutr*. 1990;9:314–319

60. Schuster K, Bailey LB, Mahan CS. Morning sickness and vitamin B_6 status of pregnant women. *Hum Nutr Clin Nutr*. 1985;39:75–79

61. Schuster K, Bailey LB, Mahan CS. Effect of maternal pyridoxine X HCl supplementation on the vitamin B-6 status of mother and infant and on pregnancy outcome. *J Nutr*. 1984;114:977–988

62. Sahakian V, Rouse D, Sipes S, Rose N, Niebyl J. Vitamin B_6 is effective therapy for nausea and vomiting of pregnancy: a randomized double-blind placebo-controlled study. *Obstet Gynecol*. 1991;78:33–36

63. Abel EL, Sokol RJ. Incidence of fetal alcohol syndrome and economic impact of FAS-related anomalies. *Drug Alcohol Depend*. 1987;19:51–70

64. Little RE, Wendt JK. The effects of maternal drinking in the reproductive period: an epidemiologic review. *J Subst Abuse*. 1991;3:187–204

65. Worthington-Roberts BS, Williams SR. *Nutrition in Pregnancy and Lactation*. 5th ed. St Louis, MO: Mosby; 1993

66. Levy HL, Waisbren SE. Effects of untreated maternal phenylketonuria and hyperphenylalaninemia on the fetus. *N Engl J Med*. 1983;309:1269–1274

67. Fuhrmann K, Reiher H, Semmler K, Fischer F, Fischer M, Glockner E. Prevention of congenital malformations in infants of insulin-dependent diabetic mothers. *Diabetes Care*. 1983;6:219–223

68. Mills JL, Simpson JL, Driscoll SG, et al. Incidence of spontaneous abortion among normal women and insulin-dependent diabetic women whose pregnancies are identified within 21 days of conception. *N Engl J Med*. 1988;392:1617–1623

69. American College of Obstetricians and Gynecologists, Committee on Technical Bulletins. ACOG technical bulletin. Diabetes and pregnancy. *Int J Gynecol Obstet*. 1995;48:331–339

70. Catalano PM, Tyzbir ED, Sims EA. Incidence and significance of islet cell antibodies in women with previous gestational diabetes. *Diabetes Care*. 1990;13:478–482

71. Fagen C, King JD, Erick M. Nutrition management in women with gestational diabetes mellitus: A review by ADA's Diabetes Care and Education Dietetic Practice Group. *J Am Diet Assoc*. 1995;95:460–467

72. Butte NF. Carbohydrate and lipid metabolism in pregnancy: normal compared with gestational diabetes mellitus. *Am J Clin Nutr*. 2000;71:1256S–1261S

73. Knopp RH, Magee MS, Raisys V, Benedetti T. Metabolic effects of hypocaloric diets in management of gestational diabetes. *Diabetes*. 1991;40(Suppl 2):165–171

74. Magee MS, Knopp RH, Benedetti TJ. Metabolic effects of a 1200-kcal diet in obese pregnant women with gestational diabetes. *Diabetes*. 1990;39:234–240

75. Rizzo T, Metzger BE, Burns WJ, Burns K. Correlations between antepartum maternal metabolism and intelligence of offspring. *N Engl J Med*. 1991;325:911–916

76. Miller EH. Metabolic management of diabetes in pregnancy. *Semin Perinatol.* 1994;18:414–431

77. Major CA, Henry MJ, De Veciana M, Morgan MA. The effects of carbohydrate restriction in patients with diet-controlled gestational diabetes. *Obstet Gynecol.* 1998;91:600–604

78. Jovanovic-Peterson L, Peterson CM. Exercise and the nutritional management of diabetes during pregnancy. *Obstet Gynecol Clin North Am.* 1996;23:75–86

79. Bung P, Artal R, Khodiguian N, Kjos S. Exercise in gestational diabetes. *Diabetes.* 1991;40:182–185

80. US Assembly of Life Sciences. *Alternative Dietary Practices and Nutritional Abuses in Pregnancy: Proceedings of a Workshop.* Washington, DC: National Academies Press; 1982

81. Larkin T. Herbs are often more toxic than magical. *FDA Consum.* October 1983;17(8):4–10

82. American College of Obstetricians and Gynecologists. ACOG committee opinion. Exercise during pregnancy and the postpartum period. *Obstet Gynecol.* 2002;99:171–173

83. Clapp JF III, Dickstein S. Endurance exercise and pregnancy outcome. *Med Sci Sports Exerc.* 1984;16:556–562

84. Clapp JF III. The effects of maternal exercise on early pregnancy outcome. *Am J Obstet Gynecol.* 1989;161:1453–1457

85. Clapp JF III. The course of labor after endurance exercise during pregnancy. *Am J Obstet Gynecol.* 1990;163:1799–1805

86. American College of Obstetricians and Gynecologists. Exercise during pregnancy and the postnatal period. *ACOG Bull.* 1985;87

12 Fast Foods, Organic Foods, Fad Diets

Fast Food

Fast Food and the Fast Food Industry

There is no standard definition of fast food. If you ask children in Vietnam, they are likely to point to a street vendor selling pho; if you ask children in Peru, they are likely to tell you anticuchos, a spicy bit of grilled beef heart sold on a skewer on the street. In the United States, however, fast food restaurants are associated with hamburgers and French fries, hot dogs, pizza, fried chicken, or ice cream; orders can be placed and picked up within a few minutes and be taken away or consumed on the premises. Generally, fast food is eaten without cutlery, and fast-food restaurants have no wait staff. Failure to have a standardized definition makes it difficult to compare studies.

The growth of the fast-food industry in this country has been phenomenal. The origin of the fast food restaurant is unclear. In the early 1930s, hamburger restaurants destined to become fast-food restaurant chains were established. By 1970, there were approximately 30 000 fast food restaurants; in 2001, there were approximately 222 000, with annual sales of $130 billion. By 2010, it is estimated that 53% of food dollars will be spent away from home.[1] Fast-food outlets are ubiquitous and can be found in local communities, public schools, and even hospitals.

In 2002, Americans spent nearly half of their food dollars outside the home, totaling $415 billion dollars. Expenditures at fast-food restaurants accounted for 37.9% of total sales.[2] It is projected that by 2010, 53% of food dollars will be spent away from home.[1] Because there is no agreed on definition of fast food, it is difficult to determine the prevalence of people eating fast food; however, up to 37% of adults and 42% of children consume fast food on a given day.[3] Eating at fast-food restaurants is especially prevalent among adolescents.[4]

Characteristics of Fast Food

Foods available outside the home tend to be high in energy and fat compared with foods eaten at home, and fast-food restaurant meals have different quantities of fat and calories than do meals from full-service restaurants.[5] Fast-food restaurants tend to provide large portions of foods that are high in energy, fat, sugar, and salt. The latter may appeal to primordial tastes.

Fast-food restaurants tend to promote meals low in fruit, vegetables, and dairy products.[4] Foods available at fast-food restaurants tend to be poor in nutrients and may compromise diet quality.[3,6-8] Table 12.1 shows food consumption in children 2 to 18 years of age at different locations. It is clear from the table that fast foods contribute few servings of fruit, vegetables, whole grains, and dairy foods to the diets of children.

Table 12.1
Food Consumption at Different Locations: All Children 2 to 18 Years of Age

Item	All Food	Home	Per Day Restaurant	Fast Food	School	Others
Food energy (kcal)	1932	1305	74	210	171	172
Added sugar (tsp)	23.08	15.60	0.85	2.37	1.42	2.84
Discretionary fat (g)	54.88	34.98	2.46	6.99	5.58	4.87
Soft drinks, tea, etc (oz)	17.46	11.44	0.81	2.45	0.54	2.22
Total grains (servings)	6.89	4.72	0.24	0.82	0.55	0.56
Whole grains (servings)	0.96	0.81	0.01	0.02	0.05	0.07
Nonwhole grains (servings)	5.93	3.91	0.23	0.80	0.50	0.49
Vegetables (servings)	2.60	1.47	0.14	0.51	0.28	0.20
Dark green/deep yellow (servings)	0.18	0.15	0.01	0.00	0.01	0.01
Tomatoes (servings)	0.39	0.24	0.02	0.06	0.04	0.03
Potatoes: fried (servings)	0.82	0.26	0.05	0.34	0.12	0.04
Potatoes: other (servings)	0.33	0.25	0.01	0.01	0.03	0.04
Others (servings)	0.87	0.58	0.05	0.09	0.08	0.07
Fruit group (servings)	1.63	1.30	0.03	0.02	0.17	0.12
Dairy group (servings)	1.96	1.38	0.05	0.14	0.29	0.11
Milk (servings)	1.47	1.11	0.02	0.03	0.24	0.07
Meat group (oz lean cooked)	3.88	2.59	0.19	0.49	0.28	0.32

Source: 1994–1996 Continuing Survey of Food Intakes by Individuals, Daily Intake, 2-day Averages. Available at: http://www.ers.usda.gov/Briefing/DietAndHealth/data/foods/table7.htm.

Portion sizes are a critical issue for controlling energy intake. Restaurant portions may offer close to the Recommended Dietary Allowance for food-group servings in a single entrée. In infants, toddlers, and children up to 3 years of age, food intake is self-regulated.[9] By 4 years of age, increased portion size increases consumption.[10] Fisher et al demonstrated that children consumed 25% more of an entrée when the large portion was presented on their plates.[11] In general, the amount of food on a plate influences consumption and lessens self-monitoring of intake; in a restaurant setting, increased portion size contributes to increased energy intake. It has also been shown that portion size and energy density of food act independently to increase intake.[12]

Relationship of Weight to Fast Food

The parallel growth of the fast-food industry with the obesity epidemic has led to the preconceived idea that fast food is a causative agent. Cross-sectional studies have shown that the frequency of fast-food consumption was associated with weight status in children and adults.[13] In the CARDIA Study on 3031 young adults, changes in frequency of fast-food consumption were associated with changes in body weight in white individuals but not in black individuals.[7] A study of 7745 girls and 6610 boys (9 to 14 years of age) suggested that children who consumed greater quantities of fried foods away from home were heavier, had higher total energy intakes, and overall poorer diet quality than those who did not.[14]

There are few longitudinal studies looking at the relationship between fast food intake and weight.[15,16] French et al[15] showed in young adult women that the consumption of 1 fast-food meal a week was associated with an extra 56 kcal/day and a weight gain of 0.72 kg over a 3-year period. In a longitudinal study of 101 girls 8 to 12 years of age, the frequency of eating quick-service food at baseline was positively associated with change in body mass index (BMI) z-score on follow-up at 11 to 19 years of age.[16]

Children who ate fast food were shown to consume an average of 187 kcal/day more than children who did not, and on days when fast food was eaten, the children ate an average of 126 kcal more than on days that they did not.[6] The question, therefore, is that if consuming fast-food meals is causally related to the obesity epidemic, why is it that not all children who eat fast food are overweight? In part, this may relate to how often they eat fast food and how many calories they consume when they do. Recently, it was suggested that overweight adolescents consume more energy at fast-food restaurants than their leaner counterparts (1860 vs 1458 kcal) and that they ate more energy overall on days when fast food was eaten. Overweight adolescents were less likely to compensate for their higher energy intake.

Although data suggest that fast-food consumption may be related to BMI, more longitudinal studies and randomized control trials are needed, particularly with a larger sample of children from various ethnic groups and geographic locations, before any definitive conclusions can be made. However, reducing the frequency of fast-food consumption may be a strategy for individuals to decrease total energy intake, providing that there is no compensation for consuming more energy at other times of the day. One study found that 75% of adolescents reported eating at a fast-food restaurant during the previous week.[4]

Societal Influences on Fast-Food Consumption

Children and adolescents live in a media-saturated environment. Two thirds of children and adolescents 8 to 18 years of age have a television in their bedroom; black youth are more likely to have a television in their room than either Hispanic or white youth. Television is often a constant presence; in households with youth 8 to 18 years of age, almost half (47%) report that the television is on "most of the time," regardless of whether anyone is watching. Two thirds (65%) of adolescents report that the television is on during meals.[17] Increased television viewing has been associated with increased energy intake,[15,18] and adolescents who watch more television eat more high-fat foods and fast food.[15] An association between exposure to food advertisements and increased weight in children has been demonstrated, although study findings are inconsistent. The potential role of the media in childhood obesity has been reviewed recently.[19]

Over the past decade, there has been aggressive food marketing to children and adolescents. US adolescents spend $140 billion a year; children younger than 12 years spend another $25 billion, but they influence another $200 billion of spending per year. It is projected that adolescents spend nearly $13 billion at fast-food outlets.[20] The food industry spends more than $11 billion on advertising, with approximately $3 billion spent on fast foods. Fast food and snack foods dominate television advertising targeted at children. In 1 study, children viewed an average of 21.3 commercials per hour, amounting to a viewing time of more than 10 minutes every hour. Food advertisements accounted for 47.8% of these commercials, and 91% of advertised foods are high in fat, sugar, or salt.[21]

Before the age of 10 years, many children do not understand that the purpose of advertising is to sell them a product.[22] Studies on children's choices have shown consistently that children exposed to advertising choose advertised food products at significantly higher rates than do those not exposed.[23] Some advertising campaigns targeted to children are remarkably successful; Ronald McDonald was introduced as the spokesman for McDonald's in 1963 and today is recognized by nearly 96% of American children.

Environmental Influences on Choice of Fast Foods

An obesogenic environment has been implicated in the dramatic increases in the prevalence of overweight in children of all racial and ethnic groups. Children and adolescents have access to fast-food restaurants in their neighborhoods, at school, and in the workplace.

Locations of fast-food restaurants have been implicated in the childhood obesity epidemic. In Chicago, it was shown that the median distance from any school to the nearest fast-food restaurant was 0.52 km and that 78% of schools had at least 1 fast-food restaurant within 800 m. It was estimated that there were 3 to 4 times as many fast-food restaurants within 1.5 km from schools than would be expected if the restaurants were randomly distributed throughout the city.[24] The effect that proximity of fast-food restaurants has on schools is not clear, although it is assumed that intake of these foods would be increased. There is evidence to suggest that there are more fast-food restaurants in areas where obesity is common[25] or where there are higher rates of cardiac disease.[26] Other studies have failed to show a link.[27–29] Burdette and Whitaker,[28] for example, showed that there was no relationship to the prevalence of overweight and the location of fast-food restaurants; however, their study was limited to preschool children. Further studies are needed to assess more fully the link between obesity in children and adolescents and the location of fast-food outlets.

Virtually all schools, public and otherwise, participate in the National School Lunch Program (NSLP), and approximately 50% of schools participate in the National School Breakfast Program. Schools participating in these programs are required to provide meals that meet the US Dietary Guidelines for Americans. Students participating in the NSLP have a higher nutrient intake than students who do not. Participation in the NSLP decreases with age, with 66% of elementary school students but only 40% of high-school students participating; overall, over the past decade, participation has decreased. Middle and high schools often sell alternative options, including soft drinks and candy, to increase their profits; 17% of these schools have fast-food outlets as a lunch alternative.[30] Less than 15% of parents and teachers think that fast-food options should be available for school lunch.[31] It is important to provide children with healthy food options at school.

Most high-school students hold part-time jobs. At any given time, approximately one third of all high school students are employed. Restaurant work, particularly at fast-food outlets, and retail sales work account for approximately 60% of all student jobs.[20] These worksites may provide employee food discounts or free beverages during the work day, and many adolescents may eat meals on site during their shifts.

Other Factors Contributing to Fast-Food Intake

The family is a major influence on what children and adolescents eat. The traditional pattern of the family eating at the kitchen table has changed, with fewer families eating meals together. Approximately 46% of family food expenditures were on food and beverages outside the home, with 34% of the total food dollars spent on fast foods.[32] There has been an increase in the number of single-parent households and a substantial growth in maternal employment in the past few decades. Currently, 74% of mothers with children 6 to 17 years of age are employed outside the house. Of these mothers, 77% work full-time and 23% work part-time. Working parents and single parents have less time to prepare meals. Reliance on fast foods is a convenient and relatively cheap alternative for these parents to feed their families.

Accessibility of Nutrient Information on Food Consumed Away From Home

Americans are less likely to be aware of ingredients and nutrient content of foods prepared away from home compared with foods prepared in their own homes.[33] Although the majority of people (62%) support a mandatory labeling law for fast foods, only 57.9% rated nutrition as important when buying fast food.[34] Consumers also believe that, when eating out, it is less important to consider nutritional quality of food than when eating at home, and they are less willing to sacrifice taste.[35]

The current nutrition labeling laws exempt much of the food consumed away from home from mandatory labeling requirements. However, under current nutrition-labeling regulations, restaurants may make specific nutrient content claims, provided that they substantiate the claims with relevant nutrition information if sought by consumers. Limited studies suggest that fast-food restaurant claims of healthy food are accurate.[36]

It is important to provide all consumers with nutrient information on foods purchased away from home. Pressured by lawsuits and public interest groups, the Menu Education and Labeling Act was introduced into the US House of Representatives on November 5, 2003. An amendment to the Federal Food, Drug, and Cosmetic Act, this bill would mandate that at a minimum, energy, fat, saturated fat, trans-fat, and sodium contents of menu items would be available to the consumer. This bill never became law. Similar proposals have been made previously. A National Academy of Sciences study that coincided with the National Labeling and Education Act of 1990 recommended mandatory labeling for food consumed away from home.[37] Padberg[38] proposed developing a "meal nutrition quality index" to rate entrées on restaurant menus.

The benefits of nutrition labeling are unclear. When 106 adolescents (11 to 18 years of age) were asked to order from 3 different restaurant menus with and without energy and fat content posted beside each menu item, most of them did not modify their ordering behavior. Of the 27 who rated themselves as too fat or slightly overweight, only 9 (33%) changed their orders.[39] Some studies have suggested that providing consumers information on the energy and fat content did not affect food choice.[40] Other studies have suggested a paradoxical relationship in which, when informed of the energy content of foods eaten away from home, people selected higher-energy options.[41] For any nutrition-labeling initiative to be successful, the public will need appropriate nutrition education.

Corporate Responsibility

McDonald's has been called "the most dominant fast food chain on the planet," and it has taken major steps to improve the food it offers and to inform the public of the nutrient content of the food. In March 2004, McDonald's announced that "supersized" beverages (42 oz, 410 kcal) and fries (7 oz, 610 kcal) would no longer be available by the end of 2004, except in promotions. In October 2005, McDonald's announced it would begin printing nutrition facts on food packages, and at the 2006 Winter Olympics, McDonald's unveiled the new packages. The new packaging was implemented in North America, Europe, Asia, and Latin America in the first half of 2006. Public interest groups are pressuring the company to post nutrition information in its restaurants. Fast-food restaurants, including McDonald's, Burger King, Wendy's, Subway, KFC, and Domino's Pizza, have nutrition information available on their Web sites and in their restaurants, but it is hoped that other fast-food restaurants will follow McDonald's lead in product labeling.

Most fast-food restaurant chains employ a dietitian or a fitness specialist at the corporate level. Providing healthful options in fast-food restaurants is not new. Table 12.2 provides a list of good selections at fast-food restaurants. But when healthy food options are available at fast-food restaurants, do people purchase them? Wendy's introduced its salad bar in 1979, Burger King test-marketed vegetarian burgers in the 1980s, and McDonald's introduced McLean Burgers in 1992; McDonald's discontinued its McLean Burgers and Wendy's discontinued its salad bar because of lack of consumer demand. At Burger King, Whoppers outsell Veggie Burgers at a rate of 100 to 1, and for every salad sold, consumers purchase 10 Whoppers.

Table 12.2
Selected Good Choices at Fast-Food Restaurants*

Food	Energy (kcal)	Total Fat (g)	Saturated Fat (g)	Cholesterol (mg)	Sodium (mg)
Jack in the Box					
Asian Chicken Salad	140	1.0	0	25	470
Chicken Caesar Salad	220	8.0	4.0	55	1030
KFC					
Oven Roasted Twister	380	8.0	1.5	60	1390
Caesar Side Salad	50	3.0	2.0	10	135
Seasoned Rice	150	1.0	0	0	640
McDonald's					
Hamburger	260	9.0	3.5	30	530
Premium Grilled Chicken Classic	420	9.0	2.0	80	1240
Chicken McNuggets (6 piece)	250	15	3.0	35	670
Small French Fries	250	13	2.5	0	140
Fruit and Walnut Salad	310	13	2.0	5	85
Apple Dippers With Low Fat Caramel	100	0.5	0	5	40
Kiddie Cone	45	1	0.5	5	20
Hotcakes (2)	600	17	4	20	620
Pizza Hut (1-slice servings)					
12" Thin Crust Veggie Lovers	180	7	3	15	480
12" Thin Crust Chicken Supreme	200	7	3.5	25	740
12" Thin Crust Cheese only	200	8	4.5	25	490
12" Medium Hand Tossed Veggie	220	6	3	15	490
14" Fit and Delicious Diced Chicken	160	4	2	15	420
Subway					
6-in Ham	290	5.0	1.5	20	1280
6-in Roast Beef	290	5.0	2.0	15	920
6-in Veggie Delight	230	3.0	1.0	0	520
6-in Sweet Onion Chicken Teriyaki	370	5.0	1.5	50	1220
Grilled Chicken/Spinach Salad	140	3.0	1.0	50	450
Subway Club	160	4.0	1.0	35	880
Chicken and Dumpling Soup	130	4.5	2.5	30	1030
Minestrone Soup	90	4.0	1.0	20	1180
Berry Lishus (small)	110	0	0	0	30
Taco Bell					
Chicken Ranchero Taco Fresco Style	170	4	1	25	560
Grilled Steak Soft Taco	170	5	1.5	15	560
Bean Burrito Fresco Style	350	8	2	0	1220
Chicken Supreme Chicken Burrito Fresco Style	350	8	2	25	1270
Fresco Style Spicy Chicken Soft Taco	190	7	2	20	640
Wendy's					
Small Chili	220	6.0	2.5	35	780
Junior Frosty	160	4.0	2.5	15	75
Mandarin Oranges	80	0	0	0	15
Sour Cream and Chives Potato	320	4.0	2.5	10	50

* Nutrient information is per serving and from company Web sites (accessed April 14, 2006). Salads are without dressing (low fat is available), and sandwiches are without mayonnaise. Fast food restaurants also have 1% milk and juice for other good choices. Note: Almost all entrees and sides have high sodium content.

Other ventures into healthful options by fast-food chains have been more successful. Most chains have changed some of their preparation methods and added some new, healthier choices. In 2004, McDonald's improved their child-targeted "Happy Meals" by allowing options of 1% milk or 100% apple juice instead of soft drinks and apple dippers instead of French fries. All major hamburger chains have switched from beef fat to vegetable shortening for all frying; although this does not reduce energy intake, it does reduce the saturated fat in the product. Restaurant chains are also working to reduce the sodium content of some foods. As can be seen in Table 12.2, even good choices at fast-food restaurants are high in sodium. Virtually all chains now offer grilled and broiled foods alongside their fried dishes; for example, Burger King removed half the fat from its BK Broiler Chicken Sandwich, and Wendy's added a Grilled Chicken Sandwich. Subway advertises that 8 of its sandwiches have 6 g of fat or less (kcal range 167 for the Veggie Delight to 279 for the Teriyaki Chicken); they also use a celebrity spokesperson to promote their products and weight loss. Salads are available at most fast-food restaurants; although, as with all salad options, dressing can add significant amounts of energy and fat. Despite the finding that salads appear to be meeting with greater consumer acceptance than earlier attempts at health foods,[42] hamburgers and French fries continue to be the leader in sales volume.[3]

Other chains have instituted other public health efforts. For example, Subway has teamed with *My Weekly Reader*, the largest and oldest educational magazine for students, to produce "One Body! One Life! Eat Fresh! Get Fit!"—an in-school curriculum designed to stress the importance of healthy eating and exercise. McDonald's has several major initiatives to increase physical activity in children.

Responsible advertising to children must also be part of the corporate plan to improve the nation's health. This can be accomplished by advertising healthier menu options to children, emphasizing the importance of milk and other nutrient-dense foods in the diet, and clearly identifying what is being advertised on corporate Web sites. Sweden and Norway have an explicit ban on advertising targeted to children younger than 12 years. Although accessibility to global media through cable and the Internet dilute the effect of this somewhat, it is still an important step.

Recommendations Regarding Fast Food

Fast-food restaurants are an integral and pervasive part of our society. Three of 10 consumers state that meals away from home, including fast food meals, are essential to the way they live. As stated previously, eating at fast-food restaurants is especially prevalent among adolescents.[4] Restrictive feeding practices in children are associated with an increased preference for forbidden foods[43] and an increased intake when these foods are available.[44] Thus, it is important not to restrict fast food totally from the diets of children and adolescents if the children wish to eat it occasionally. Parents, with the help of nutrition professionals, must teach children and adolescents to make the best choices at fast-food restaurants. It is also important that we promulgate healthy foods in schools and limit the number of fast food options to be sure that more healthful choices are available. It is also critical that nutrition information be available for all fast foods.

Organic Foods

What Are Organic Foods?

The Organic Foods Production Act of 1990 (Title XXI of the 1990 Farm Bill) mandated that the United States Department of Agriculture (USDA) (1) establish national standards governing the marketing of certain agricultural products as organically produced products; (2) assure consumers that organically produced products meet a consistent standard; and (3) facilitate interstate commerce in fresh and processed food that is organically produced. Foods covered by this act are fruits, vegetables, mushrooms, grains, dairy products, eggs, livestock feed, meats, poultry, fish and other seafood, and honey.

Regulations for organic foods were proposed in 1997 and modified in 1998, and the first national standards were adopted in 2001. By October 21, 2002, 12 years after the Organic Foods Production Act was enacted, consumers buying foods bearing the USDA Organic Seal (Fig 12.1) were assured that the food was produced and handled according to set standards. The Organic Seal can appear only on foods that are at least 95% organic; this means that a raw or processed agricultural product must contain (by weight or fluid volume, excluding water and salt) at least 95% of organically produced or processed agricultural products. Products with less than 70% of organic ingredients may list specific organically produced ingredients on the side panel of the product packaging but may not make any organic claims on the front panel. The name and address of the government-approved certifier must be on all products that contain at least 70% organic ingredients. Use of the USDA Organic Seal is voluntary, and there is a fine of up to $10 000 per violation for misuse.

Fig 12.1
The US Department of Agriculture Organic Seal.

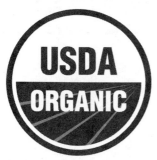

Available at: http://www.ams.usda.gov/nop/Consumers/Seal.html.

"Organic" is a production term and does not refer to characteristics of the foods themselves. Organic crop standards include that land has had no prohibited substances applied to it for at least 3 years before the harvest of an organic crop. Use of genetic engineering, ionizing radiation, and sewage sludge is prohibited. Soil fertility and crop nutrients are managed through tillage and cultivation practices, crop rotations, and cover crops; soils can be supplemented with animal and crop waste materials and allowed synthetic materials. Crop pests, weeds, and diseases are controlled primarily through management practices including physical, mechanical, and biologic controls. When these practices are not sufficient, a biological, botanical, or synthetic substance approved for use on the national list (http://www.ams.usda.gov/nop/NationalList/FinalRule.html) may be used.

Purchasing Trends for Organic Foods

Once sold only in premium markets, organic foods are now widely available in conventional supermarkets year-round. Consumer preference for organic foods is associated with perceived benefits for environmental protection, animal welfare, food safety, and especially, personal health.[45,46] Organic farmers have expressed greater concern for environmental problems associated with agriculture than have conventional farmers.

Consumer demand for variety, convenience, and quality in fresh produce has boosted sales of organic foods and pressured farmers to expand acreage devoted to organic foods. In the past decade, the US organic food industry has grown substantially. In 2003, organic foods accounted for nearly $10.4

billion or approximately 1.8% of total food sales in the United States; this figure was up from $3.5 billion in 1996. By 2010, sales of organic foods are estimated to increase to $23.8 billion or 3.5% of total food sales.[47] Organic fruits and vegetables have a higher market-penetration rate, accounting for 4.5% of total sales.

Organic produce is purchased at a premium price, with the cost of many vegetables consistently exceeding 100% of conventional produce.[48] For example, in a 17-month period during 2000–2001, the prices of organic broccoli, carrots, and mesclun were 130%, 125%, and 110%, respectively, of their conventional counterparts.[49] The top-selling organic fruits and vegetables are tomatoes, carrots, peaches, squash, leafy vegetables, apples, potatoes, and bananas.[48] Strawberries, beans, broccoli, and oranges are also high-selling organic produce items. Infants, children, and adolescents all commonly consume these foods. Households with children younger than 18 years are more likely to purchase organic produce than others.[50] Buyers and consumers are clearly willing to pay more for perceived benefits of organic foods. It is noteworthy that for organic baby food, the organic label is more important to consumers than the nutrient content.[51]

Nutrients and Phytochemicals in Organic Versus Conventional Foods

There is a widespread belief that organic foods are healthier and safer than conventional foods.[45,46] Because considerations of the effects of organic growing systems on nutrient bioavailability and nonnutrient components have received little attention, this belief does not have a science base. Many published studies comparing the nutrient content of organic to conventional produce have methodologic flaws. Moreover, it is difficult to compare studies performed over time, because regulations, recommendations, and analytical techniques have varied.

Several recent literature reviews[52–54] have considered the differences between nutrient content of organic and conventional foods. The most consistent finding was higher amounts of vitamin C, especially in leafy green vegetables, peaches, tomatoes, and potatoes[55]; however, only 21 (58%) of 36 studies examined showed higher concentrations of vitamin C in organic produce. No differences were found in mineral, trace element, or vitamin B concentrations in organic versus conventional produce.[52]

Evaluation of phytochemical content of organic foods compared with conventionally grown ones has received almost no attention. One could argue that organic farming places plants under more stress than conventional farming practices and that plants would be expected to respond by producing higher amounts of defensive chemicals. A recent report in the United Kingdom concluded that organic crops have higher amounts of phytochemicals, including lycopene in tomatoes, polyphenols in potatoes, flavonols in apples, and resveratrol in red wine.[56] Sporadic reports of increased phytochemicals in organic fruits and vegetables suggest that defense-related secondary metabolites of plants, such as polyphenols, could be 10% to 50% higher than in conventional plants.[57] The potential health benefit of these differences is not clear.

Overall, there is no convincing evidence that organic foods differ significantly in nutrient content when compared with conventional foods.[58] The Institute of Food Technologists Expert Panel on Food Safety and Nutrition and the USDA do not promulgate organically grown food as more nutritious than conventional foods. Health benefits of consuming recommended amounts of produce cannot be underestimated, but there is no indication that organic foods offer an advantage over conventional ones.

Nitrate Content of Organic Versus Conventional Foods

An article in *US News and World Reports*[59] suggested that consumers believed that organic foods were free of the hazardous materials found in conventional foods. Nitrate is the main form of nitrogen fertilizer applied to crops. Nitrogenous fertilizers can, in turn, leech into the groundwater and contaminate well water and increase the nitrate content of food. Nitrate has low toxicity; however, conversion of nitrates to nitrites or nitrosamines can cause adverse health effects. Nitrate-contaminated well water and vegetables high in nitrates have been shown to cause methemoglobinemia in infants.[60] The maximum contaminant concentration for nitrates is based on concentrations that reduce the risk of methemoglobinemia. The effects of the exposure to nitrates in drinking water on the incidence of birth defects, especially neural tube defects and cardiac anomalies, have also been reported[61]; however, the effect nitrate had in these studies was equivocal.

Nitrosamines can initiate and promote cancer, and more than 250 nitrosamines have been shown to cause cancer in laboratory animals. Evidence on whether nitrates cause cancer in humans is controversial and contradictory. For example, exposure to nitrates has been associated with childhood leukemia but not with brain tumors or testicular cancer.

Lower nitrate concentrations have been found in some organically grown crops when compared with conventional ones, especially in leafy green vegetables.[53,58] Lower levels of nitrates have been shown for organically grown lettuce and rocket but not for arugula. Cereals, fruits, and bulb vegetables did not show any consistent difference in nitrate concentration.[55] In general, concentrations of nitrates in plant foods are inconsistent and depend on the producer, crop, season in which the plants are grown, storage conditions, geographic location, and postharvest processing. Thus, it seems that the use of organic farming to reduce dietary nitrate intake and with the goal of reducing carcinogenesis is premature.

Pesticides (also see Chapter 53)
A detailed look at the affects of pesticides and health is beyond the scope of this chapter; however, some discussion is warranted. The 1993 National Research Council report on pesticides in the diets of infants and children recognized that children have higher exposures and increased susceptibility to environmental toxicants, including pesticides (Table 12.3).[62] Children also tend to have diets high in foods that are potentially high in pesticide residues, including juices, fruits, and vegetables.[62]

Table 12.3
Increased Risk to Children of Environmental Agents

Children have disproportionally higher exposures to many environmental agents.	Per unit weight, children drink more water, eat more food, and breathe more air than adults. Putting objects in their mouths and crawling or playing on the floor or ground also potentially contribute to higher exposures to pesticides.
A child's ability to metabolize, detoxify, or excrete environmental agents differs from adults.	Ironically, in some instances, children are protected against some agents, because they cannot make active metabolites required for toxicity.
Developmental processes are easily disrupted during rapid growth and development before and after birth.	
Children have more years of future life and, thus, more time to develop diseases initiated by early exposures.	

Adapted with permission from Landrigan PJ, Kimmel CA, Correa A, Eskenazi B. Children's health and the environment: public health issues and challenges for risk assessment. *Environ Health Perspect.* 2004;112:257–265.

The Food Quality Protection Act of 1996 (Pub L No. 104-170) amended the Federal Insecticide, Fungicide, and Rodenticide Act and the Federal Food, Drug, and Cosmetic Act and set high standards to protect infants and children from pesticide risks. Under the Federal Insecticide, Fungicide, and Rodenticide Act, the Environmental Protection Agency (EPA) registers pesticides for use in the United States and prescribes labeling and other regulatory requirements to prevent unreasonable adverse effects on health or the environment. Under the Federal Food, Drug, and Cosmetic Act, the EPA establishes tolerances (maximum legally permissible amounts) for pesticide residues in food. The US Food and Drug Administration (FDA) enforces tolerances for most foods; the USDA Food Safety and Inspection Service enforces tolerances for meat, poultry, and some egg products.

The Food Quality Protection Act explicitly requires the EPA to address risks to infants and children and to publish a specific safety finding before a tolerance can be established. It also provides for an additional safety factor (tenfold, unless reliable data show that a different factor will be safe) to ensure that tolerances are safe for infants and children and requires collection of better data on food consumption patterns, pesticide residue levels, and pesticide use.

The Organic Seal does not guarantee that the food products are free of pesticides. In the United States, to be certified organic, no pesticides can have been applied to the land for at least 3 years; in addition, a "sufficient buffer zone" must also be in place to reduce the risk of contamination from conventional farming operations. Products can still become contaminated with pesticides. The persistence of pesticides in the environment was recently shown when organochlorine insecticides were shown to contaminate root crops[63] and tomatoes,[64] despite having been off the market for 20 years. Pesticide contamination of organic foods can occur from cultivation of previously contaminated soil, percolation of chemicals through soils, wind-drift, or groundwater or irrigation water or during transport, processing, or storage.

Organic foods have been shown to be contaminated by pesticide residues; however, they are much less likely to be contaminated by pesticide residues than foods grown using conventional methods.[58,65] One report that compared results from 3 studies showed that organic crops are 10 times less likely to be contaminated with multiple pesticide residues.[65] It should be stated clearly that detection of permitted pesticides is low—often undetectable—in both organic and conventional foods.[55]

Consumption of organic foods is often assumed to reduce health risks by reducing exposure to pesticide residues.[66] It is clear that children can be exposed to pesticides via the diet.[67] Intuitively, it would seem that eating organic produce will affect concentrations of pesticide residues in children; however, there are almost no data supporting this. Several recent studies have used biological monitoring to examine dietary exposures to pesticides in children.[67–69] In a study of 39 children 2 to 5 years of age, it was shown that children eating primarily organic produce had significantly lower concentrations of total dimethyl metabolites in their urine than did children eating conventional diets.[68] In a crossover study of 23 children 3 to 11 years of age, Lu et al[69] showed that children consuming a conventional diet during phases 1 (days 1–3) and 3 (days 9–15) of the study had significantly higher organophosphorus pesticide concentrations than when they ate an organic diet (phase 2, days 4–8). Although small, these studies provide tantalizing information about the potential effect that consuming organic foods has on pesticide concentrations of children. What they do not show is a long-term health benefit.

Are There Other Health Concerns With Organic Foods?

The relationship between the consumption of organic foods and improved long-term health is unknown. Ironically, the use of composted manure and the reduced use of fungicides and antibiotics in organic food production could lead to a higher rate of contamination by microorganisms or microbial products. Like other evaluations of organic produce, whether it is more susceptible to microbial contamination or whether it takes up microbial contamination from organic manure is controversial. It is clear, however, that organic foods are not free from microbial contamination. Organically grown chickens have not been demonstrated to have less *Salmonella*[70,71] or *Camplyobacter*[71] organisms than either conventional or free-range chickens. *Listeria monocytogenes* and *Escherichia coli* have been demonstrated on organically grown lettuce.[72] These studies suggest that foods bearing the Organic Seal must be treated, handled, and prepared in a manner aimed at reducing the risk of foodborne illness.

Fad Diets

What Is a Fad Diet?

"Fad" refers to something that enjoys temporary popularity. Fad diets have been described variously as diets that make unrealistic claims, promise a "quick fix" and rapid weight loss, or eliminate foods or food groups, often stating that these foods are toxic. One problem with these diets is that they are usually undertaken without medical advice or under medical supervision. This is of special concern for children and adolescents. The percentage of overweight in children and adolescents 6 to 19 years of age in 2002 was 16%, a figure that has nearly tripled from 1980. It is not surprising, therefore, that children and their parents may be driven to weight-loss regimens, including those that are untested or unsuitable for children or adolescents.

The Institute of Medicine defines successful long-term weight loss as "a 5% reduction in initial body weight (IBW) that is maintained for at least 1 year."[73] This is inconsistent with goals and expectations of most dieters,[74] who are looking for the aforementioned "quick fix," which leads many dieters to turn to self-prescribed weight-loss regimens. In 2001, a search on www.amazon.com with the key words "weight loss" yielded 1214 books[74]; today, a similar search yields 2252 books and a search on "diet books" yields 2871. The overwhelming majority of these books describe what can be termed a "fad diet." Table 12.4 describes how to determine whether a popular diet is actually a fad diet.

Fad diets can be generally categorized as very low carbohydrate and, hence, high in fat; moderate carbohydrate, which may (or may not) incorporate principles of the glycemic index in carbohydrate selection; and high carbohydrate and, hence, low fat (Table 12.5; Appendix O). Low-carbohydrate diets have emerged as perhaps the most popular of the fad diets. It is inconceivable that children and adolescents have not heard of low-carbohydrate diets, although they may not associate them with fad diets or even with weight loss. A Google search using the terms "low-carbohydrate diets" returned 3 950 000 Web pages.

Low-Carbohydrate Diets

Although none of the fad diets have been studied adequately or long-term, low-carbohydrate diets are among the best studied of the fad diets. *Atkins' New Diet Revolution*, a very low-carbohydrate diet, is perhaps the most recognizable of these diets. Atkins diet books have sold more than 45 million copies over a 40-year period. The theory of this diet is that reduced carbohydrate intake will lower insulin concentrations, allow unrestrained lipolysis, increase lipid oxidation, and initiate ketone production, which will in turn suppress appetite. The *Atkins' Diet* is divided into 4 main phases: induction, leading to rapid initial weight loss; ongoing weight loss when initial weight loss slows; premaintenance, with slow weight loss; and lifetime maintenance. The amount of carbohydrates and the percent of energy from carbohydrates ranges from 15 g (3%) in the induction phase to 116 g (22%) of energy in the maintenance phase. Energy levels are lowest during the induction phase (1152 kcal) and highest during maintenance.[74]

Do people lose weight on Atkins and other low carbohydrate diets? Yes, they do. Studies have shown repeatedly that, in the short-term, low-carbohydrate diets cause weight loss. In a 2003 review of the literature, Bravata et al[75]

Table 12.4
How to Determine Whether a Diet is a Fad Diet

	Comment	Example: *Sugar Busters*
Step 1	Keep an open but informed mind. Many of the diets available on the market today are fad diets, but many are not. Do not automatically dismiss a popular diet as a fad diet.	*Sugar Busters* by H. Leighton Steward, Morrison C. Bethea, MD, Sam S. Andrews, MD, and Luis A Balart, MD
Step 2	Look at the authors and their qualifications—are they trained in medicine or nutritional sciences or are they celebrity spokespeople?	3 medical doctors lend credence to this diet.
Step 3	Evaluate the overall tone of the writing—is it professional or is it biased?	The writing is casual, even for a popular press book—"How do I avoid getting arteriosclerosis? The answer is easy. Don't live long enough." And, "When the liver goes, 'Adios, amigo'" are examples of this casual tone.
Step 4	Understand the premise of the diet—is the diet low carbohydrate, low energy, low fat, or something else?	Is the effect of the diet biologically plausible? Yes and no. The diet is based on the glycemic index but makes comments like "insulin is toxic."
Step 5	Does the peer-reviewed literature support the effectiveness of the diet? Or do the authors rely on testimonials?	The authors of this book rely principally on testimonials; however, it should be noted that articles linking weight loss to eating low-glycemic-index foods are beginning to appear in the peer-reviewed literature. Long-term studies on the safety and effectiveness of these diets are lacking. There are other comments in the book that are of concern. For example, "Yet the standard diet recommended for patients with or at risk for coronary disease is to consume 80 to 85% of calories from carbohydrates with very low amounts of fat and protein!" This is not consistent with recommendations from the National Cholesterol Education Program.
Step 6	Look at the claims the authors make. If it seems too good to be true...it probably is not true.	There are no fantastic claims for this diet.

Table 12.4 *(Continued)*
How to Determine Whether a Diet is a Fad Diet

	Comment	Example: *Sugar Busters*
Step 7	Are any foods or supplements required for the diet? Are the authors of the diet selling their own foods or supplements? Are any health risks associated with the supplements?	There is a line of *Sugar Buster* products.
Step 8	Are foods or food groups omitted?	Foods with high glycemic indices are omitted from this diet. Eliminating foods with simple sugars is an effective weight loss strategy; however, many wholesome foods like bananas, beets, and carrots are also eliminated.
Step 9	Is this diet potentially dangerous?	The diet is low in dairy and potentially low in fruits, vegetables, and fiber. The cumbersome schedule outlined for eating what fruits are allowed may limit intake.
Step 10	Are there any health warnings associated with the diet?	Yes, the authors do suggest that more carbohydrate foods may be needed for individuals with strenuous exercise schedules. There is no mention that people with type 1 diabetes may need to adjust their insulin schedule. This diet should not be used by people with renal failure.
Step 11	Does the diet imply that weight loss can be maintained without physical activity and permanent lifestyle changes?	The diet encourages permanent lifestyle changes.
Step 12	Are there any good points associated with the diet?	Yes, there are many elements of this diet that can lead to weight loss. By omitting high-energy simple carbohydrates like cake, candy, and alcohol, followers can eliminate many calories and lead to weight loss. *Sugar Busters* works principally because it is low energy.

Is this a fad diet? Yes, although elimination of foods high in simple sugars is likely to result in weight loss.

identified 43 studies using randomized research designs, including 24 controlled trials and 19 randomized crossover trials, and another 17 studies that used a nonrandomized design. This was a difficult task, because there is no standard definition for the carbohydrate content of a low-carbohydrate diet.

Table 12.5
Type, Energy Breakdown, and Examples of Popular Weight Loss Diets

Type	Energy Breakdown			Examples
	Fat (% kcal)	Carbohydrate (% kcal)	Protein (% kcal)	
Very low carbohydrate	55–65	<20	25–30	*Dr. Atkins' New Diet Revolution,*[*] *Protein Power,*[†] *The Carbohydrate Addict's Diet*[‡]
Low carbohydrate combined with glycemic index	Approx 30	Approx 40	Approx 30	*Ann Louise Gittleman's Guide to the 40/30/30 Phenomenon,*[§] *Sugar Busters,*[ǁ] *A Week in the Zone*[¶]
Moderate carbohydrate	20–35	55–60	15–20	*US Dietary Guidelines,*[#] *MyPyramid,*[**] DASH[††]
High carbohydrate	<10–19	>65	10–20	*Dr. Dean Ornish's Program for Reversing Heart Disease,*[‡‡] *The New Pritikin Program*[§§]

[*] Atkins RC. *Dr. Atkins' New Diet Revolution.* New York, NY: Avon Books Inc; 1992
[†] Eades MR, Eades MD. *Protein Power.* New York, NY: Bantam Books; 1996
[‡] Heller RF, Heller RF. *The Carbohydrate Addict's Diet.* New York, NY: Penguin Books; 1991
[§] Gittleman AL. *Ann Louise Gittleman's Guide to the 40/30/30 Phenomenon.* Chicago, IL: Contemporary Books; 2002
[ǁ] Steward HL, Bethea MC, Andrews SS, Balart LA. *The New Sugar Busters.* Ballantine Books; 2003
[¶] Sears B. *A Week in the Zone.* New York, NY: Harper Collins Publishers; 2000
[#] http://www.health.gov/dietaryguidelines/dga2005/document. Accessed April 12, 2006
[**] http://www.usda.gov/cnpp/pyramid.html. Accessed April 12, 2006
[††] http://www.nhlbi.nih.gov/health/public/heart/hbp/dash/new_dash.pdf. Accessed April 12, 2006
[‡‡] Ornish D. *Eat More, Weigh Less.* New York, NY: Harper Paperback Books; 1993
[§§] Pritikin R. *The Pritikin Weight Loss Breakthrough.* New York, NY: Signet; 1999

Randomized controlled trials have compared weight loss from low-carbohydrate and low-fat diets. Most studies have been short-term, but some have begun to look at longer-term outcomes. All diets resulted in weight loss[76–78]; in the short-term (6 months), low-carbohydrate diets resulted in more weight loss than low-fat diets, although the difference was modest. Longer-term, the picture is not as clear. Most studies show by 1 year, there was no longer a significant difference between low-fat or low-carbohydrate diets,[76–78] whereas other studies suggest low-carbohydrate diets still show more of a weight loss.[79] In general, there is a high dropout rate in all these studies, although there is a suggestion that participants on low-carbohydrate diets have higher retention rates,[80] possibly leading to higher levels of compliance.

The rapid weight loss seen at the outset with most low-carbohydrate diets results from diuresis as a result of mobilization of glycogen stores. It is unclear what actually causes the longer-term weight loss seen in subjects on a low-carbohydrate diet. Authors of the diet books suggest it is because ketosis suppresses appetite or because the high protein amounts suppress hunger and increase satiety. None of these factors has been confirmed, although most studies suggest that protein preloads significantly increased subjective ratings of satiety.[81] In massively obese adolescents, protein content of diets did not confer any benefit.[82] It is generally assumed in the scientific community, however, that these diets are effective because they are low in energy, diet duration, and starting weight. Freedman[74] reported energy levels of the Atkins' induction diet (1152 kcal), the *Carbohydrate Addict's Diet* (1476 kcal), and *Sugar Busters* (1462 kcal). Clearly, the overwhelming majority of people will lose weight at these lower energy levels. It has also been suggested that low-carbohydrate diets have less variety and are, therefore, less palatable, leading people to eat less.

Are There Health Advantages of Low-Carbohydrate Diets?

If the end justifies the means, these diets can be said to have health advantages, the principal one being that they result in weight loss. Weight loss is usually rapid at the outset, which may "jump start" some dieters and make them more likely to comply with a weight loss regimen. Lean body mass appears to be spared during weight loss.[83] Because low-carbohydrate diets are generally associated with higher intakes of total fat, saturated fat, and cholesterol, as a result of the protein being provided mainly by animal sources, there were initial concerns that they would adversely affect lipid profiles, but at least in the short-term, these have proven to be unfounded. Some short-term studies have suggested that low-carbohydrate and low-glycemic load diets have improved lipid profiles in children,[84] adolescents,[84,85] and adults.[86] The most notable improvements are in high-density lipoprotein cholesterol and triglyceride concentrations; the diets do not appear as effective in lowering low-density lipoprotein cholesterol concentrations. Other studies have failed to show significant improvement in lipid concentrations.

Health Concerns of Low-Carbohydrate Diets

Short-term effects have been summarized by Freedman et al[74] and include bad taste, constipation, diarrhea, dizziness, headache, nausea, thirst, tiredness, weakness, and fatigue. It is unclear whether these are related to the low energy content of the diets or the composition of the diet. Ketoacidosis has also been reported.[87] There is also some evidence that in children, dietary restraint may be associated with decreased cognitive function.[88]

Over a longer term, low-carbohydrate diets or other fad diets do not provide adequate energy for growth. This is a concern in ketogenic diets used to treat some children with epilepsy (discussed later) or, under medical supervision, some severely overweight children and adolescents.

Low-carbohydrate diets or other fad diets do not meet the dietary recommendations for children and adolescents[89,90] and, therefore, are not recommended for unsupervised use. Fruit and vegetable consumption in children is already low, with some studies showing that when French fries are excluded, fewer than 20% of children ate the recommended number of fruits and vegetables a day.[91] If children were to follow a low-carbohydrate diet, this problem would be exacerbated. Consumption of fruits and vegetables has been inversely related to the risk of some cancers, coronary heart disease, hypertension, stroke, type 2 diabetes mellitus, obesity, and all-cause mortality. Dairy foods are also omitted from low-carbohydrate diets. In the US Dietary Guidelines report, calcium has been identified as a nutrient of concern, because intake is low in many groups. Because low-carbohydrate diets are low in these wholesome foods, they also provide lower-than-recommended amounts of vitamins A, E, and B_6; folate; thiamin; calcium; magnesium; iron; potassium; and dietary fiber.[74] For children older than 2 years, a diet containing fruits and vegetables, whole grains, low-fat and nonfat dairy products, beans, fish, and lean meats is needed to maintain health and support growth.[90]

The high-protein aspects of these diets, coupled with the lack of fruits and vegetables, pose concerns about bone health. Observational studies suggest that the alkaline-forming properties of fruits and vegetables mediate the body's acid-base balance to improve bone health.[92] This may be especially important with the high renal acid loads that may occur with low-carbohydrate diets. There is also controversy regarding whether high-protein diets in patients without renal disease damages the kidneys, although there is no substance to these claims. Studies have not been performed in children or adolescents. It is clear that children with existing renal disease or diabetes with microalbuminuria or clinical albuminuria should not attempt a high-protein diet.

Do Calories From Carbohydrates Facilitate Weight Gain?

Bray said succinctly, "A calorie is a calorie."[93] But is there something different about calories from carbohydrates? Traditionally, diets balanced in macronutrients have been recommended for weight loss, and these have been shown to be efficacious. Studies conducted in the 1970s and early 1980s suggested that people given isoenergetic diets in which the macronutrient amounts had been altered lost more weight when the diets were very low in carbohydrates.[94]

Other Types of Fad Diets

Very low-fat diets, such as the Pritikin diet or the Ornish diet, may not constitute a "fad diet," but nevertheless are worthy of mention. These diets contain <10% of energy from fat and are both contraindicated in children. These diets are primarily fruits, vegetables, and grains with nonfat dairy or soy, egg whites, and small amounts of sugar and white flour. The Pritikin Diet allows no more than 3.5 oz of lean beef, poultry, or fish a day. Like their low-carbohydrate counterparts, these diets are low in energy. The Ornish diet has been estimated at less than 1300 kcal/day[74] and the new Pritikin program recommends 1000 to 1200 kcal/day. Weight loss is the result of a reduction in fat and lean body mass. As with other low-energy diets, there are concerns that children may not have adequate energy to grow. Very low-fat diets are also deficient in vitamins E, D, and B_{12} and zinc.[74]

Dieting Behavior in Children and Adolescents

Dieting for weight loss is common in adolescents, especially girls. In the National Adolescent and School Health Survey of 8th- and 10th-grade students, 61% of girls and 28% of boys reported dieting in the previous year.[95] These figures are similar to the Minnesota Adolescent Health survey, in which 62% of girls and 20% of boys in grades 7 to 12 reported dieting behavior.[96] In a study of 105 overweight children 6 to 13 years of age, 60% reported attempting at least 1 weight-loss diet.[97] It is important to note that many adolescents who diet have BMI within the normal range for height.[98] Very few studies have asked adolescents who diet whether they have ever followed a "fad diet." One report of 146 high-school students revealed that 36.5% of boys and 73.6% of girls had tried to lose weight; however, of these, none of the boys and only 4.5% of the girls reported following a fad diet.[99] In Calderon's study, the term "fad diet" was described for the participants; however, it is possible that adolescents may not understand what constitutes a diet or fad diet or even that low-carbohydrate diets are usually classified as fad diets.

Very concerning is that girls as young as 5 years have reported body dissatisfaction, which is associated with the likelihood of dieting at 9 years of age.[100] Between 34% and 65% of 5-year-old girls have ideas about dieting[101] and have expressed concerns about gaining weight.[102]

Many factors, including parent's attitudes and practices about diet and weight,[101] peer pressure, and teasing or bullying by other children, influence a child's perception of body image or decision to diet. Mothers, in particular, have an influence on girl's perceptions of dieting; thus, it is especially important that parents model healthy eating; however, all caregivers responsible for feeding children should also serve as good role models. Girls' perceptions of weight and shape are significantly affected by the mass media.[103] In 1 study of 5th- to 12th-grade students (n = 548), 69% of students reported that magazines influenced their idea of a perfect body shape and 47% reported wanting to lose weight because of pictures in magazines.[103] Use of unhealthful weight-loss practices in high-school students was associated with reading women's beauty and fashion magazines.[104] Adolescents who diet are more likely to become overweight as adults,[98] suggesting a need to teach healthy eating at home and in schools rather than having students resort to use of short-term weight-loss diets, fad or otherwise.

An unresolved question is whether dieting behavior, especially in adolescent girls, leads to disordered eating.[105,106] Studies tend to be small; longitudinal studies are uncommon, and findings are inconsistent.[105–107] Patton et al[107] found that adolescent girls who dieted at a severe level were 18 times more likely to develop an eating disorder than those who did not diet, and girls who dieted at a more moderate level were 5 times more likely to develop an eating disorder than those who did not diet. Killen et al[108] also showed that girls with the highest level of dieting were more likely to develop disordered eating. A 5-year longitudinal study that followed adolescents (n = 2516; 45% boys) for a 5-year period[106] showed that both adolescent boys and girls who used unhealthy weight-control behaviors were at increased risk of binge eating with loss of control. Clearly, a large proportion of adolescents have tried to lose weight either through diet or by more extreme weight-loss measures, including self-induced vomiting or use of laxatives, whereas estimates for eating disorders in girls (at higher risk than boys) is between 1% and 4%.

Nutrient Intake in Restricted Eating

It is a challenge to attain a nutrient-dense, low-energy diet. It is also difficult to attain nutrient adequacy on diets that provide a limited variety of foods, as may occur on carbohydrate-restricted diets. Low-carbohydrate diets limit the variety of foods that can be eaten and, therefore, may be difficult to follow long-term. In general, low-carbohydrate diets require supplementation because these diets are low in vitamins E, A, and B_6; thiamin; folate; calcium; magnesium; iron; potassium; and dietary fiber.[74] Few studies have looked at the effect that low-carbohydrate diets have on the intake of children or adolescents. Dietary intake data from 568 children 10 years of age in the Bogalusa Heart Study were stratified into 4 levels of carbohydrate intake: <45%, 45% to 50%, 50% to 55%, and >55% of energy. Investigators found that children in the low-carbohydrate group ate more meat, whereas children in the high-carbohydrate group ate more desserts and candy but also more fruit, grains, and milk.[109] The 1990 Ontario Health Survey collected dietary information via a food frequency questionnaire on 5194 adolescents 12 to 18 years of age. Low-carbohydrate diets were consumed by 27.6% of males and 24.1% of females. Fruit and vegetable intake was low, and cholesterol and total fat intake was high in adolescents consuming these diets. Overweight status, smoking, and alcohol use were also associated with consuming a low-carbohydrate diet.[110]

Medically Supervised Low-Carbohydrate Diets in Children: Lessons for Fad Diets?
High-fat (90% of energy), low-carbohydrate (3% of energy) ketogenic diets are used to control seizures in children with epilepsy that is refractory to more traditional treatment (see Chapter 47: The Ketogenic Diet). Energy restriction up to 75% of recommendations is also a feature of these diets.[111] Children with higher concentrations of urinary ketones seem to have better seizure control than do subjects reporting variable ketosis.[112] Children on these diets may be deficient in calcium, magnesium, and iron. A major concern about these diets is that they adversely affect growth.[112] Recently, it was shown that the higher the concentration of urinary ketones, the more severely growth was affected.[112] Although low-carbohydrate diets, such as the Atkins diet, are not as severe as the standard ketogenic diet, they do induce ketosis and, in small studies, have been used successfully to reduce seizures in infants, children, adolescents, and adults.[113]

Early-onset adverse effects of ketogenic diets include hypertriglyceridemia, transient hyperuricemia, hypercholesterolemia, various infectious diseases, symptomatic hypoglycemia, hypoproteinemia, hypomagnesemia, repetitive hyponatremia, low concentrations of high-density lipoprotein cholesterol, aspiration pneumonia, hepatitis, acute pancreatitis, and persistent metabolic acidosis. Late-onset adverse effects include growth abnormalities, osteopenia, renal stones, cardiomyopathy, secondary hypocarnitinemia, and iron-deficiency anemia.[114] This suggests that diets, including low-carbohydrate fad diets that induce ketosis, have the potential to cause potentially severe adverse reactions in children and should not be undertaken lightly or without medical supervision.

Very low-energy ketogenic diets, introduced in the 1980s, for weight loss in moderately to severely overweight children and adolescents make no pretense of being nutritionally adequate. These diets usually provide approximately 650 to 750 kcal/day along with 80 to 100 g of protein and 25 g of carbohydrate and fat and must be supplemented with potassium, calcium, and a multivitamin.[115] These diets are effective in inducing weight loss and, with short-term use (1–5 months), are not associated with growth abnormalities; however, with longer-term use, there may be some growth slowing. These low-energy diets are also associated with decreased bone mineral density.[115] These diets should not be undertaken unless under the guidance of a medical team. Children and adolescents who self-select a similar diet should be counseled against this choice.

Recommendations Regarding Fad Diets

No unsupervised weight loss program should be undertaken by children or adolescents. Fad diets have been shown to be neither safe nor efficacious in children. Most children would be better served with medically supervised programs that rely on behavior modification techniques to improve diet and lifestyle. Because of the potential link to dieting, notably severe dieting and eating disorders, education programs should be established to alert children and adolescents to potential dangers of fad diets.

Botanical and Herbal Products

Background

Complementary and alternative medicine (CAM) and health care practices are defined simply as those that are not currently part of conventional medicine. Included among these practices is phytotherapy, or using plant-derived substances to treat or prevent disease. Technically, plant parts, including leaves, stems, flowers, berries, rhizomes, or roots, are called botanicals. They are valued for their therapeutic qualities, flavor, or scent. The terms "herb" and "herbals" are often used interchangeably with botanicals; however, by definition, herbs are nonwoody seed-producing plants that die to the ground at the end of the growing season.

The Dietary Supplement Health and Education Act of 1994 (Pub L No. 103–417) created a new framework for dietary supplements by defining them as "a vitamin, mineral, herb or other botanical, amino acid, a dietary substance for use by man to supplement the diet by increasing the total dietary intake; or a concentrate, metabolite, constituent, extract, or combination of any ingredient described in clause."* These products are considered safe until proven otherwise. Before marketing a new dietary supplement, the manufacturer must only provide "reasonable assurance" that no ingredient "presents a significant or unreasonable risk of illness or injury." This assurance must be presented to the FDA 75 days before marketing a new product. Although the FDA does not regulate dietary supplements, they can withdraw them from the market. Dietary supplements must bear on the label "This statement has not been evaluated by the Food and Drug Administration. This product is not intended to diagnose, treat, cure, or prevent disease." Structure function claims are also allowed on labels. Safety information and health risk of herbals is presented in Table 12.6.

Table 12.6
Health Risks and Safety Ratings of Herbals

Health Risks of Herbal Remedies	
Indirect Risks	People on herbal medicines should have been treated with conventional medications
Direct Health Risks	
Type A reactions	Predictable problems—didn't follow information provided on the package—usually took too high a dose
Type B reactions	Unpredictable—herb taken at the recommended dosage, but a person could have adverse effects anyway
Type C reactions	Developed an adverse reaction secondary to long-term therapy (eg, senna—with long-term therapy, it no longer works)
Type D reactions	Delayed effects—carcinogenic or teratogenic
Herbal Classifications: http://www.ibismedical.com/interact/Inter7.html	
Class 1:	Herbs that can be consumed safely when appropriately used
Class 2:	Herbs for which the following use restrictions apply, unless directed otherwise by and expert in herbal therapy
(2a)	For external use only
(2b)	Not for pregnant women
(2c)	Not for lactating women
(2d)	Other specific restrictions noted
Class 3:	Herbs for which enough data exist to recommend this labeling: "To be used only under the supervision of an expert qualified in the appropriate use of this substance." Labeling must include use information: dose, contraindications, potential adverse effects and drug interactions, and other relevant information related to the safe use of this herb.

* http://www.fda.gov/opacom/laws/dshea.html#sec3

Herbal medicines are widely available from drug stores, supermarkets, and the Internet. By 1996, Americans spent more than $3 billion on herbal products. But there is evidence that the market is decreasing. Herbal sales in the 52-week period ending January 2, 2005, were $257 514 900*; this is a decrease of 7.4% from 2004. Despite the general downward market trend, multiherbal preparation sales increased 29.1% in the same time period. Sales from Wal-Mart or from other market channels, health and natural food stores, mail order companies, multilevel marketing companies, health care professionals, warehouse buying clubs, and convenience stores are not included.

Herbal Medicines

Herbal medicines are available in several forms. Children often receive teas or tisanes, which are made by pouring boiling water over herbal parts, like leaves or flowers, and allowing them to steep. Decoctions are similar, made by boiling parts of the herb, usually woody parts like roots or bark, in water and then straining and drinking the extract. Tinctures are hydroalcoholic or glycerol solutions that usually contain 1 or 2 g of active ingredients per 10 mL of solution. Fluid extracts contain a ratio of 1 part solvent to 1 part herb; these are more concentrated than tinctures. Powdered herbs can be pressed into tablets or made into capsules. Salves, ointments, shampoos, and poultices can also be used for external use. Aromatherapy uses inhalation of volatile oils from herbs to treat illnesses or reduce stress.

Aside from their classification as dietary supplements, herbal medicines differ from conventional medicines in other ways. In common with other plant extracts, herbals are not limited to a single agent, and the actual therapeutic component(s) and mechanism(s) of action may not be known. Herbals can be grown, harvested, processed, and sold by anyone. The concentration of active ingredients can be influenced by growing conditions, time of harvest, and storage and processing. The species used may be in question if herbs are harvested locally using common names. Finally, herbal medicines have not been subjected to the rigorous clinical trials that traditional medicines have.

Caveat emptor (let the buyer beware) clearly applies when purchasing an herbal supplement. Of 59 commercially available Echinacea preparations that were evaluated, the assayed species content was consistent with labeled content in 31 (52%) of the samples, and 6 (10%) had no Echinacea at all. Of the 21 standardized preparations assessed, 9 (43%) met the quality standard

* http://www.herbalgram.org/herbalgram/articleview.asp?a=2828

described on the label.[116] A larger study of 880 products, including Echinacea, St John wort, *Ginkgo biloba*, garlic, saw palmetto, ginseng, goldenseal, aloe, Siberian ginseng, and valerian, 43% were consistent with a benchmark in ingredients and recommended daily dose, 20% were consistent in ingredients only, and 37% were either not consistent or label information was insufficient.[117] A recent review of 81 randomized controlled trials showed that 12 manufacturers (15%) reported performing tests to quantify actual contents, and only 3 (4%) provided adequate data to compare actual with expected content values of at least 1 chemical constituent.[118] Herbal medicines can also be contaminated with other drugs, including scopolamine or barbiturates, or heavy metals, including lead.

Use of Botanicals by Children and Adolescents

Seventy percent of the world's sick or injured children are treated, often by a physician, using CAM, including traditional herbal medicines. In the United States, use of botanicals is self-selected. Most studies have shown that the use of CAM, including botanicals, by children and adolescents is common, with more than 70% of some populations using CAM.[119] Children who take herbals often take more than one product. The youngest child reported to be given herbal therapy was 5 months of age and received catnip tea for a cold. CAM use among pediatric populations appears to be increasing, especially among children with chronic or recurrent conditions.[119] Use of botanicals reported in pediatric surgical patients varies greatly, ranging from as few as 3.5% or 4%[120] to as many as 12.8% of children using herbs before surgery.[121] Echinacea was the most commonly reported herbal used. Up to 42% of these children were also taking conventional medications. The recommended preoperative discontinuation times of botanical vary, but in general, it is recommended that herbals be discontinued 2 weeks in advance of elective surgery.

Aloe vera, chamomile, garlic, peppermint, lavender, cranberry, ginger, Echinacea, lemon balm/grass, licorice root, goldenseal, St John wort, gingko, sweet oil, and milk thistle are common botanicals taken by children (and their caregivers).[122–124] Echinacea is the most prevalent herbal taken by children presenting for elective surgery. Nontraditional and potentially toxic products, such as turpentine, pine needles, and cow chip tea, have also been reported.[122] Table 12.7 reviews herbals commonly used in pediatric populations.

Table 12.7
Herbs and Herbal Products That Are Commonly Used by Pediatric Populations

Herb	Use	Comments
Aloe (*Aloe ferox*)	Internal: purgative External: burns and other skin conditions	Internal use is contraindicated in children younger than 12 years because of potential for diarrhea, dehydration, and electrolyte loss.
Chamomile (*Chamaemelum nobilis*)	Internal uses: gastrointestinal distress—indigestion, colic, heartburn, anorexia, diarrhea External: swelling, inflammation	Allergic reactions. Inhibits cytochromes, potentially leading to drug interactions or toxicities. May be effective in treatment of infantile colic.
Cranberry (*Vaccinium macrocarpon*)	Primarily used for urinary tract infections, also used for *Helicobacter* infections	Appears safe, but excess amounts can lead to stomach upset and diarrhea.
Echinacea (*Echinacea angustifolio*; *Echinacea purpurea*)	Colds, flu, coughs, bronchitis, fever, immune stimulant	Not recommended for individuals with autoimmune disorders. Allergic reactions may occur in some individuals. No benefit for upper respiratory infection has been shown for children 2 to 11 years of age.
Garlic (*Allium sativum*)	Internal: colds, bronchitis, fever, hypertension, dyslipidemia External: antibacterial, antifungal	Not well studied in children. Possible adverse effects include allergic reaction, stomach disorders, odor of skin or breath, diarrhea, and rash. Dysrhythmias have also been reported.
Ginger (*Zingiber officinale*)	Antinausea, motion sickness, indigestion, anti-inflammatory, headache	Has been used in children undergoing cancer chemotherapy. Allergic reactions are seen, as is heartburn, if taken in excess. Ginger may interfere with blood clotting, although there are no reports of interactions with blood-thinning medications; there is a report of a ginger and drug bezoar small bowel obstruction.
Ginkgo (*Ginkgo biloba*)	Asthma, bronchitis, tinnitus, multiple sclerosis, memory improvement	Adverse effects include headache, nausea, gastrointestinal upset, diarrhea, dizziness, and allergic skin reactions. There is an increased risk of bleeding, and ginkgo is contraindicated in patients taking anticoagulants.
Goldenseal (*Hydrastis canadensis*)	Internal use: colds, flu, inflammation of mucous membranes External use: antiseptic, antimicrobial	Often used in conjunction with Echinacea to treat colds. The safety of goldenseal in children is unknown; however, many preparations contain berberine, an alkaloid that disrupts normal flora in the gastrointestinal tract.
Lavender (*Lavandula species*)	Internal use: sleep aid External use: insect bites, headaches (rub), acne, burns, inflammation	Allergic reactions have been reported.

Table 12.7 *(Continued)*
Herbs and Herbal Products That Are Commonly Used by Pediatric Populations

Herb	Use	Comments
Lemon balm (*Melissa officinalis*)	Nervous disorders, sleep aid, colic	Although there are no known contradictions, children with "nervous disorders" and in need of sleep aid should be seen by a physician.
Licorice root (*Glycyrrhiza glabra*)	Cough, sore throat, hoarseness, bronchitis, canker sores, stomach or duodenal ulcers	May promote hypertension, edema, and hypokalemia; has mild estrogenic effects. Contraindicated with diabetes, liver disease, hypertension, heart disease, or depression. Note: licorice root is not licorice candy.
Milk thistle (*Silybum marianum*)	Antihepatotoxicity, anti-inflammatory	Interactions with many drugs, including erythromycin, statins, sedatives, and phenothiazines. Adverse effects include gastrointestinal distress, headache, pruritus, rash, hives, eczema, and insomnia.
Peppermint (*Mentha piperita*)	Carminative, indigestion, nausea, colds, cough, bronchitis	Should not be applied to the face or nose of infants or young children.
St. John wort (*Hypericum perforatum*)	Depression, anti-inflammatory.	Has not been studied adequately in children; however, other antidepressants have been shown to induce suicidal ideation, and in children, all antidepressants should be used under a doctor's supervision only. Can increase the effect of prescription antidepressants, and can interact with drugs used for HIV or cancer treatment, birth control, or organ rejection. May cause sun sensitivity.

Botanicals are used by children and adolescents because of dissatisfaction with conventional medicine, fear of adverse effects of conventional medicine, perceived benefits, and the belief that herbals are "more natural" and, therefore, safer than conventional medications. A profile of pediatric populations most likely to use botanicals has not been well established; however, in general, children of parents who used botanicals and children with chronic diseases are more likely to use botanicals.[120,125] CAM use was greater with increasing parental or child age[125] and in Hispanic or Asian children or adolescents than in white children or adolescents.

Fewer than 50% of children or adolescents or their parents inform health care professionals about herbal use, because they do not believe botanicals would have adverse effects or that they could interact with conventional medications. Many of those who did try to discuss use of botanicals with health care professionals were not given information to help them make an informed decision about use and got information from friends or relatives instead.[122] Although most pediatricians surveyed believe their patients use CAM, few ask about use.[126] Physicians with a higher comfort level discussing CAM therapies with patients were more likely to discuss them with patients; however, fewer than 5% of physicians surveyed felt very knowledgeable about CAM, and most believe that they need more education.[126] Because use of botanicals can pose health risks, especially in children, it is crucial that physicians are knowledgeable about them and ask parents and children about use.

Botanical Use and Potential Risks and Benefits in Children With Chronic Health Problems

CAM use, including the use of botanicals, is up to 3 times more common in children with chronic disease, including asthma, inflammatory bowel disease, and cancer[120,125] or recurrent disease. It is especially important to assess potential benefits and risks in these children.

Up to 29% of children with asthma use botanicals; those who do are significantly more likely than nonusers to have persistent asthma, to be on high-dose inhaled or oral steroids, to have poor or very poor control of symptoms, and to have more frequent doctor visits. They also had more adverse reactions to bronchodilators.[127] Although some treatments, like quail eggs, are benign, others, like lobelia, possibly pennyroyal mint, and tree tea oil, are potentially toxic.[128] The most dangerous herbal treatment reported was Ephedra* and albuterol.[122]

Approximately 14% of children and young adults with inflammatory bowel diseases used botanicals; parental CAM use and the number of adverse reactions to conventional medications were predictors of use in children. Only a minority of parents believed that CAM treatments were very efficacious. Botanicals had the potential to adversely interact with other conventional therapy.[129]

A wide variety of CAM therapies are used by children with cancer, with up to 35% using herbals.[130] In most surveys, these therapies are used as adjunct therapies rather than primary ones. Parents identified a need for additional information on CAM for their children, but most did not discuss them with physicians. The most common botanicals used in cancer patients along with potential adverse reactions for surgical patients were recently reviewed.[131] Ginger, as an anti-emetic, may be of benefit in pediatric populations undergoing chemotherapy treatments.

* Ephedra was withdrawn from the US market April 12, 2004.

Safety of Botanicals in Children

A wide variety of drug-herbal and food-herbal adverse effects and toxicities have been reported from herbal medicines; however, very little is known about the safety and efficacy of botanicals in children. Of major concern is that in the United States, herbals are self-prescribed, usually without an understanding of their potential toxicity or adverse effects. Moreover, dosages for children are unclear.

Infants and children differ from adults in the absorption, distribution, metabolism, and excretion of drugs, including herbals. Their developing central nervous system and immune system may make them more susceptible to adverse effects of herbals. Paradoxically, children have larger livers than adults and may be more efficient in detoxifying substances,[132] but the growing number of reports of hepatotoxicity of herbals is also of concern.[133] Laxatives, such as aloe and senna, and diuretics, including fennel and licorice root, have the potential to cause dehydration and electrolyte imbalances in infants and young children.[132] Children are also at high risk of developing allergic reactions to commonly used herbs, such as Echinacea and chamomile, both members of the Compositae family.

The effect of long-term exposures of herbals on the fetus and breast-feeding infant is unknown. Woolf[132] reviewed a case of a newborn whose mother drank senecionine-containing herbal tea daily during her pregnancy. The infant was born with hepatic vaso-occlusive disease; senecionine is one of the pyrrolizidine alkaloids associated with hepatic venous injury. Comfrey is an example of an herb containing pyrrolizidine; although comfrey has a long history of herbal use, in 2001, the FDA recommended that it be removed from the market.

The German Commission E listed aloe, buckthorn, camphor, cajeput oil, cascara sagrada bark, eucalyptus leaf and oil, fennel oil, horseradish, mint oils (external), nasturtium, rhubarb root, senna, and watercress as contraindicated in children. However, more research is clearly needed to establish the safety and efficacy of botanicals in children.

Recommendations Regarding Botanical and Herbal Products

Herbal medicines have been used for centuries and are still used by the majority of the world's children. As use in the United States continues to grow, it is critical that reliable information be available to parents, adolescents, and physicians. Rigorous scientific studies should be conducted to determine the safety and efficacy of phytotherapy in children and adolescents. Courses on CAM, including phytotherapy, should be offered as part of the education of pediatricians and pharmacists, and doctors should be prepared to discuss CAM therapies with their patients.

Table 12.8
Reliable Sources of Information About Herbs

Books
Foster S, Tyler VE. *Tyler's Honest Herbals: A Sensible Guide to the Use of Herbs and Related Remedies.* 4th ed. New York, NY: MJF Books/Fine Communications; 2007
PDR for Herbal Medicines. 3rd ed. Montvale, NJ: Medical Economics Co; 2004
Robbers JE, Tyler VE. *Tyler's Herbs of Choice: The Therapeutic Use of Phytomedicinals.* 2nd ed. New York, NY: Haworth Herbal Press; 1999
Herr SM. *Herb-Drug Interaction Handbook.* 3rd ed. Nassau, NY: Church Street Books; 2002
Online Databases
Agricola: http://agricola.nal.usda.gov
Amazon Plants Tropical Plant Database: http://www.rain-tree.com/plants.htm
Botanical Dermatology Database: http://bodd.cf.ac.uk
Community of Science: http://www.cos.com
Cyberbotanica: Plant Compounds and Ethnobotanical Databases: http://biotech.icmb.utexas.edu/botany
Dr. Duke's Phytochemical and Ethnobotanical Databases: http://www.ars-grin.gov/duke
Garden Gate: Roots of Botanical Names: http://garden-gate.prairienet.org/botrts.htm
Medical Herbalism: Poisonous Plant Database: http://medherb.com/POISON.HTM
Medicinal Plant Databases: http://www.floridaplants.com/mdata.htm
Medicinal and Poisonous Plant Databases: http://www.biologie.uni-hamburg.de/b-online/ibc99/poison
NAPRALERT: http://www.cas.org/ONLINE/DBSS/napralertss.html
Native American Ethnobotany Database: http://herb.umd.umich.edu
Natural Standard: http://www.naturalstandard.com
Plants Database: http://plants.usda.gov
Plants for a Future Database Search: http://www.ibiblio.org/pfaf/D_search.html
Poisonous Plant Database (PLANTOX): http://www.cfsan.fda.gov/~djw/plantox.html
PubMed: http://www.ncbi.nlm.nih.gov
Reliable Information About Botanicals on the Internet
American Herbalist Guild: http://www.americanherbalistsguild.com
American Herbal Products Association: http://www.ahpa.org
American Botanical Council: http://www.herbalgram.org
Herb Research Foundation: http://www.herbs.org
Food and Drug Administration: http://www.fda.gov
MedLine Plus Health Information Drugs and Supplements: http://www.nlm.nih.gov/medlineplus/druginformation.html
National Center for Complementary and Alternative Medicine: http://nccam.nih.gov
Office of Dietary Supplements, National Institutes of Health: http://dietary-supplements.info.nih.gov
World Health Organization: http://www.who.int/en

References

1. National Restaurant Association. Quickservice Restaurant Trends, 2002. Available at: http://www.restaurant.org/research. Accessed April 14, 2006

2. Steward H, Blisard N, Bhuyan S, Nayga RM Jr. *The Demand for Food Away from Home. Full-Service or Fast Food.* Washington, DC: Economic Research Service, US Department of Agriculture; 2004. Agricultural Economic Report No. 829

3. Paeratakul S, Ferdinand DP, Champagne CM, Ryan DH, Bray GA. Fast-food consumption among US adults and children: dietary and nutrient intake profile. *J Am Diet Assoc.* 2003;103:1332–1338

4. French SA, Story M, Neumark-Sztainer D, Fulkerson JA, Hannan P. Fast food restaurant use among adolescents: associations with nutrient intake, food choices and behavioral and psychosocial variables. *Int J Obes Relat Metab Disord.* 2001;25:1823–1833

5. Lin B, Frazao E. Nutritional quality of foods at and away from home. *Food Rev.* 1997;May/Aug:33–40

6. Bowman SA, Gortmaker SL, Ebbeling CB, Pereira MA, Ludwig DS. Effects of fast-food consumption on energy intake and diet quality among children in a national household survey. *Pediatrics.* 2004;113:112–118

7. Pereira MA, Kartashov AI, Ebbeling CB, et al. Fast-food habits, weight gain, and insulin resistance (the CARDIA study): 15-year prospective analysis. *Lancet.* 2005;365:36–42

8. Schmidt M, Affenito SG, Striegel-Moore R, et al. Fast-food intake and diet quality in black and white girls: the National Heart, Lung, and Blood Institute Growth and Health Study. *Arch Pediatr Adolesc Med.* 2005;159:626–631

9. Fox MK, Devaney B, Reidy K, Razafindrakoto C, Ziegler P. Relationship between portion size and energy intake among infants and toddlers: evidence of self-regulation. *J Am Diet Assoc.* 2006;106(1 Suppl 1):S77–S83

10. Rolls BJ, Engell D, Birch LL. Serving portion size influences 5-year-old but not 3-year-old child's food intakes. *J Am Diet Assoc.* 2000;100:232–234

11. Orlet Fisher J, Rolls BJ, Birch LL. Children's bite size and intake of an entrée are greater with large portions than with age-appropriate or self-selected portions. *Am J Clin Nutr.* 2003;77:1164–1170

12. Diliberti N, Bordi PL, Conklin MT, Roe LS, Rolls BJ. Increased portion size leads to increased energy intake in a restaurant meal. *Obes Res.* 2004;12:562–568

13. Bowman SA, Vinyard BT. Fast food consumption of U.S. adults: impact on energy and nutrient intakes and overweight status. *J Am Coll Nutr.* 2004;23:163–168

14. Taveras EM, Berkey CS, Rifas-Shiman SL, et al. Association of consumption of fried food away from home with body mass index and diet quality in older children and adolescents. *Pediatrics.* 2005;116(4):e518–e524. Available at: http://pediatrics.aappublications.org/cgi/content/full/116/4/e518. Accessed August 13, 2007

15. French SA, Harnack L, Jeffrey RW. Fast food restaurant use among women in the Pound of Prevention study: dietary, behavioral and demographic correlates. *Int J Obes Relat Metab Disord.* 2000;24:1353–1359

16. Thompson OM, Ballew C, Resnicow K, et al. Food purchased away from home as a predictor of change in BMI z-score among girls. *Int J Obes Relat Metab Disord.* 2004;28:282–289

17. Ozer EM, Brindis CD, Millstein SG, Knopf DK, Irwin CE Jr. *America's Adolescents: Are They Healthy?* 2nd ed. San Francisco, CA: University of California, San Francisco, National Adolescent Health Information Center; 1998

18. Crespo CJ, Smit E, Troiano RP, Bartlett SJ, Macera CA, Anderson RE. Television watching, energy intake, and obesity in US children: results from the third National Health and Nutrition Examination Survey, 1988–1994. *Arch Pediatr Adolesc Med.* 2001;155:360–365

19. The Henry J. Kaiser Family Foundation. *The Role of Media in Childhood Obesity.* Kaiser Family Issue Brief February 2004. Available at: http://epsl.asu.edu/ceru/Articles/CERU-0402-202-OWI.pdf. Accessed August 13, 2007

20. Story M, Neumark-Sztainer D, French S. Individual and environmental influences on adolescent eating behaviors. *J Am Diet Assoc.* 2002;102(3 Suppl):S40–S51

21. Taras HL, Gage M. Advertised foods on children's television. *Arch Pediatr Adolesc Med.* 1995;149:649–652

22. Oates C, Blades M, Gunter B, Don J. Children's understanding of television advertising: a qualitative approach. *J Mark Commun.* 2003;9(2):59–71

23. Coon KA, Tucker KL. Television and children's consumption patterns. A review of the literature. *Minerva Pediatr.* 2002;54:423–436

24. Austin SB, Melly SJ, Sanchez BN, Patel A, Buka S, Gortmaker SL. Clustering of fast-food restaurants around schools: a novel application of spatial statistics to the study of food environments. *Am J Public Health.* 2005;95:1575–1581

25. Block JP, Scribner RA, DeSalvo KB. Fast food, race/ethnicity, and income: a geographic analysis. *Am J Prev Med.* 2004;27:211–217

26. Alter DA, Eny K. The relationship between the supply of fast-food chains and cardiovascular outcomes. *Can J Public Health.* 2005;96:173–177

27. Sturm R, Datar A. Body mass index in elementary school children, metropolitan area food prices and food outlet density. *Public Health.* 2005;119:1059–1068

28. Burdette HL, Whitaker RC. Neighborhood playgrounds, fast food restaurants, and crime: relationships to overweight in low-income preschool children. *Prev Med.* 2004;38:57–63

29. Jeffery RW, Baxter J, McGuire M, Linde J. Are fast food restaurants an environmental risk factor for obesity? *Int J Behav Nutr Phys Act.* 2006;3:2

30. Pateman BC, McKinney P, Kann L, Small ML, Warren CW, Collins JL. School food service. *J Sch Health.* 1995;65:327–332

31. Kubik MY, Lytle LA, Story M. Soft drinks, candy, and fast food: What parents and teachers think about the middle school food environment. *J Am Diet Assoc.* 2005;105:233–239

32. Putnam JJ, Allshouse JE. *Food Consumption, Prices and Expenditures, 1970–1997.* Washington, DC: Economic Research Service, US Department of Agriculture; 1999. Statistical Bulletin No. 965. Available at: http://www.ers.usda.gov/Publications/SB965/sb965.pdf. Accessed November 2, 2007

33. Variyam JN. *Nutrition Labeling in the Food-Away-From-Home Sector: An Economic Assessment.* Washington, DC: Economic Research Service, US Department of Agriculture; 2005. ERS Report No. 4. Available at: http://www.ers.usda.gov/publications/err4/err4.pdf. Accessed November 2, 2007

34. O'Dougherty M, Harnack LJ, French SA, Story M, Oakes JM, Jeffery RW. Nutrition labeling and value size pricing at fast-food restaurants: a consumer perspective. *Am J Health Promot.* 2006;20:247–250

35. Guthrie JF, Lin BH, Frazao E. Role of food prepared away from home in the American diet, 1977–78 versus 1994–96: changes and consequences. *J Nutr Educ Behav.* 2002;34:140–150

36. Root AD, Toma RB, Frank GC, Reiboldt W. Meals identified as healthy choices on restaurant menus: an evaluation of accuracy. *Int J Food Sci Nutr.* 2004;55:449–454

37. Porter DV, Earl RO, eds. *Nutrition Labeling: Issues and Directions for the 1990s.* Washington, DC: National Academies Press; 1990

38. Padberg D. Nutritional Labeling for Food-Away-From-Home. Paper presented at the New Economic Approaches to Consumer Welfare and Nutrition Conference; January 14–15, 1999; Alexandria VA. Available at: http://www.ag.uiuc.edu/famc/Jan99conf/PDFdocs/padberg1.pdf. Accessed April 14, 2006

39. Yamamoto JA, Yamamoto JB, Yamamoto BE, Yamamoto LG. Adolescent fast food and restaurant ordering behavior with and without calorie and fat content menu information. *J Adolesc Health.* 2005;37:397–402

40. Stubenitsky K, Aaron J, Catt S, Mela D. The influence of recipe modification and nutritional information on restaurant food acceptance and macronutrient intakes. *Public Health Nutr.* 2000;3:201–9

41. Aaron JI, Evans RE, Mela DJ. Paradoxical effect of a nutrition labelling scheme in a student cafeteria. *Nutr Res.* 1995;15:1251–1261

42. Horovitz B. What's next: fast-food giants hunt for new products to tempt consumers. *USA Today.* July 3, 2002:A-01

43. Birch LL, Zimmerman S, Hind H. The influence of social-affective context on preschool children's food preferences. *Child Dev.* 1980;51:856–861

44. Fisher JO, Birch LL. Restricting access to palatable foods affects children's behavioral response, food selection, and intake. *Am J Clin Nutr.* 1999;69:1264–1272

45. Magnusson MK, Arvola A, Hursti UK, Aberg L, Sjoden PO. Choice of organic foods is related to perceived consequences for human health and to environmentally friendly behaviour. *Appetite.* 2003;40:109–117

46. Shepherd R, Magnusson M, Sjoden PO. Determinants of consumer behavior related to organic foods. *Ambio.* 2005;34:352–359

47. National Business Journal, SPINS. *The NBJ/SPINS Organic Foods Report.* San Diego, CA: Penton Media Inc; 2004

48. Oberholtzer L, Dimitri C, Greene C. *Price Premiums Hold on as U.S. Organic Produce Market Expands.* Washington, DC: Economic Research Service, US Department of Agriculture; 2005. Outlook Report No. VGS-308-1. Available at: http://www.ers.usda.gov/publications/vgs/may05/VGS30801/VGS30801.pdf. Accessed November 2, 2007

49. Sok E, Glaser L. Tracking wholesale prices for organic produce. *Agricultural Outlook.* 2001;(285)7–8. Available at: http://www.ers.usda.gov/publications/agoutlook/oct2001/ao285d.pdf. Accessed November 2, 2007

50. Thompson G, Kidwell J. Explaining the choice of organic produce: cosmetic defects, prices, and consumer preferences. *Am J Agric Econ.* 1998;80:277–278

51. Harris JM. Consumers pay a premium for organic baby foods. *Food Rev.* 1997;20:13–16

52. Woese K, Lange D, Boess C, Werner Bogl K. A comparison of organically and conventionally grown foods—results of a review of the relative literature. *J Sci Food Agric.* 1997;74: 281–293

53. Williams CM. Nutritional quality of organic food: shades of grey or shades of green? *Proc Nutr Soc.* 2002;61:19–24

54. Worthington V. Effect of agricultural methods on nutritional quality: a comparison of organic with conventional crops. *Altern Ther Health Med.* 1998;4:58–69

55. Magkos F, Arvaniti F, Zampelas A. Organic food: Buying more safety or just piece of mind? A critical review of the literature. *Crit Rev Food Sci Nutr.* 2006;46:23–56

56. Heaton S. *Organic Farming, Food Quality and Human Health: A Review of the Evidence.* Bristol, England: Soil Association; 2001

57. Brandt K, Molgaard JP. Organic agriculture: does it enhance or reduce the nutritional value of plant foods? *J Sci Food Agric.* 2001;81:924–931

58. Bourn D, Prescott J. A comparison of the nutritional value, sensory qualities, and food safety of organically and conventionally produced foods. *Crit Rev Food Sci Nutr.* 2002;42:1–34

59. Marcus MB. Organic foods offer peace of mind—at a price. *US News & World Rep.* 2001;130(2):48–50

60. Sanchez-Echaniz J, Benito-Fernandez J, Mintegui-Raso S. Methemoglobinemia and consumption of vegetables in infants. *Pediatrics.* 2001;107:1024–1028

61. Croen LA, Todoroff K, Shaw GM. Maternal exposure to nitrate from drinking water and diet and risk for neural tube defects. *Am J Epidemiol.* 2001;153:325–331

62. National Research Council. *Pesticides in the Diets of Infants and Children.* Washington DC: National Academies Press; 1993

63. Benbrook CM. Organochlorine residues pose surprisingly high dietary risks. *J Epidemiol Community Health.* 2002;56:822–823

64. Gonzales M, Miglioranza KS, Aizpun de Moreno JE, Moreno VJ. Occurrence and distribution of organochlorine pesticides (OCPs) in tomato (*Lycopersicon esculentum*) crops from organic production. *J Agric Food Chem.* 2003;51:1353–1359

65. Baker BP, Benbrook CM, Groth E III, Lutz Benbrook K. Pesticide residues in conventional, integrated pest management (IPM)-grown and organic foods: insights from three US data sets. *Food Addit Contam.* 2002;19:427–446

66. Williams PR, Hammitt JK. A comparison of organic and conventional fresh produce buyers in the Boston area. *Risk Anal.* 2000;20:735–746

67. MacIntosh DL, Kabiru C, Echols SL, Ryan PB. Dietary exposure to chlorpyrifos and levels of 3,5,6 trichloro-2-pyridinol in urine. *J Expo Anal Environ Epidemiol.* 2001;11:279–285

68. Curl CL, Fenske RA, Elgethun K. Organophosphorus pesticide exposure of urban and suburban preschool children with organic and conventional diets. *Environ Health Perspect.* 2003;111:377–382

69. Lu C, Toepel K, Irish R, Fenske RA, Barr DB, Bravo R. Organic diets significantly lower children's dietary exposure to organophosphorus pesticides. *Environ Health Perspect.* 2006;114:260–263

70. Bailey JS, Cosby DE. Salmonella prevalence in free-range and certified organic chickens. *J Food Prot.* 2005;68:2451–2453

71. Cui S, Ge B, Zheng J, Meng J. Prevalence and antimicrobial resistance of Campylobacter spp. and Salmonella serovars in organic chickens from Maryland retail stores. *Appl Environ Microbiol.* 2005;71:4108–111

72. Loncarevic S, Johannessen GS, Rorvik LM. Bacteriological quality of organically grown leaf lettuce in Norway. *Lett Appl Microbiol.* 2005;41:186–189

73. Institute of Medicine. *Weighing the Options: Criteria for Evaluating Weight Management Programs.* Thomas PR, ed. Washington, DC: National Academies Press; 1995

74. Freedman MR, King J, Kennedy E. Popular diets: a scientific review. *Obes Res.* 2001;9(Suppl 1):1S–40S

75. Bravata DM, Sanders L, Huang J, et al. Efficacy and safety of low-carbohydrate diets. A systematic review. *JAMA.* 2003;289:1837–1850

76. Brehm BJ, Seeley RJ, Daniels SR, D'Alessio DA. A randomized trial comparing a very low carbohydrate diet and a calorie-restricted low fat diet on body weight and cardiovascular risk factors in healthy women. *J Clin Endocrin Metab.* 2003;88:1617–1623

77. Fleming, RM. The effect of high-, moderate-, and low-fat diets on weight loss and cardiovascular disease risk factors. *Prev Cardiol.* 2002;5:110–118

78. Foster GD, Wyatt HR, Hill JO, et al. A randomized trial of a low-carbohydrate diet for obesity. *N Engl J Med.* 2003;348:2082–2090

79. Stern L, Iqbal N, Seshadri P, et al. The effects of low-carbohydrate versus conventional weight loss diets in severely obese adults: one-year follow-up of a randomized trial. *Ann Intern Med.* 2004;140:778–785

80. Yancy WS Jr, Olsen MK, Guyton JR, Bakst RP, Westman EC. A low-carbohydrate, ketogenic diet versus a low-fat diet to treat obesity and hyperlipidemia. A randomized, controlled trial. *Ann Intern Med.* 2004;140:769–777

81. Halton TL, Hu FB. The effects of high protein diets on thermogenesis, satiety and weight loss: a critical review. *J Am College Nutr.* 2004;23:373–385

82. Rolland-Cachera MF, Thibault H, Souberbielle JC, et al. Massive obesity in adolescents: dietary interventions and behaviours associated with weight regain at 2 y follow-up. *Int J Obes Relat Metab Disord.* 2004;28:514–519

83. Brehm BJ, Spang SE, Lattin BL, Seeley RJ, Daniels SR, D'Alessio DA. The role of energy expenditure in the differential weight loss in obese women on low-fat and low-carbohydrate diets. *J Clin Endocrinol Metab.* 2005;90:1475–1482

84. Slyper A, Jurva J, Pleuss J, Hoffmann R, Gutterman D. Influence of glycemic load on HDL cholesterol in youth. *Am J Clin Nutr.* 2005;81:376–379

85. Starc TJ, Shea S, Cohn LC, Mosca L, Gersony WM, Deckelbaum RJ. Greater dietary intake of simple carbohydrate is associated with lower concentrations of high-density-lipoprotein cholesterol in hypercholesterolemic children. *Am J Clin Nutr.* 1998;67:1147–1154

86. Volek JS, Sharman MJ, Forsythe CE. Modification of lipoproteins by very low-carbohydrate diets. *J Nutr.* 2005;135:1339–1342

87. Shah P, Isley WL. Ketoacidosis during a low-carbohydrate diet. *N Engl J Med.* 2006;354:97–98

88. Brunstrom JM, Davison CJ, Mitchell GL. Dietary restraint and cognitive performance in children. *Appetite.* 2005;45:235–241

89. Gidding SS, Dennison BA, Birch LL, et al. Position of the American Heart Association. Dietary recommendations for children and adolescents: a guide for practitioners. *Pediatrics.* 2006;117:544–559

90. Nicklas TA, Johnson R. Dietary guidance for healthy children aged 2 to 11 years. *Am Diet Assoc.* 2004;104:660–677

91. Dennison BA, Rockwell HL, Baker SL. Fruit and vegetable intake in young children. *J Am Coll Nutr.* 1998;17:371–378

92. McGartland CP, Robson PJ, Murray LJ, et al. Fruit and vegetable consumption and bone mineral density: the Northern Ireland Young Hearts Project. *Am J Clin Nutr.* 2004;80: 1019–1023

93. Bray GA. Low-carbohydrate diets and realities of weight loss. *JAMA.* 2003;289:1853–1855

94. Rabast U, Kasper H, Schonborn J. Comparative studies in obese subjects fed carbohydrate-restricted and high carbohydrate 1,000-calorie formula diets. *Nutr Metab.* 1978;22:269–277

95. Story M, Rosenwinkel K, Himes JH, et al. Demographic and risk factors associated with chronic dieting in adolescents. *Am J Dis Child.* 1991;145:994–998

96. Serdula MK, Collins E, Williamson DF, Anda RF, Pamuk E, Byers TE. Weight control practices of U.S. adolescents and adults. *Ann Intern Med.* 1993;119:667–671

97. Tanofsky-Kraff M, Faden D, Yanovski SZ, Wilfley DE, Yanovski JA. The perceived onset of dieting and loss of control eating behaviors in overweight children. *Int J Eat Disord.* 2005;38:112–122

98. Field AE, Austin SB, Taylor CB, et al. Relation between dieting and weight change among preadolescents and adolescents. *Pediatrics.* 2003;112:900–906

99. Calderon LL, Yu CK, Jambazian P. Dieting practices in high school students. *J Am Diet Assoc.* 2004;104:1369–1374

100. Davison KK, Markey CN, Birch LL. A longitudinal examination of patterns in girls' weight concerns and body satisfaction from ages 5 to 9 years. *Int J Eat Disord.* 2003;33:320–332

101. Abramovitz BA, Birch LL. Five-year-old girl's ideas about dieting are predicted by their mothers' dieting. *J Am Diet Assoc.* 2000;100:1157–1163

102. Feldman W, Feldman E, Goodman JT. Culture versus biology: children's attitudes toward thinness and fatness. *Pediatrics.* 1988;81:190–194

103. Field AE, Cheung L, Wolf AM, Herzog DB, Gortmaker SL, Colditz GA. Exposure to the mass media and weight concerns among girls. *Pediatrics.* 1999;103(3):e36. Available at: http://pediatrics.aappublications.org/cgi/content/full/103/3/e36. Accessed August 13, 2007

104. Thomsen SR, Weber MM, Brown LB. The relationship between reading beauty and fashion magazines and the use of pathogenic dieting methods among adolescent females. *Adolescence.* 2002;37:1–18

105. Irving LM, Neumark-Sztainer D. Integrating primary prevention of eating disorders and obesity: feasible or futile? *Prev Med.* 2002;34:299–309

106. Neumark-Sztainer D, Wall M, Guo J, Story M, Haines J, Eisenberg M. Obesity, disordered eating, and eating disorders in a longitudinal study of adolescents: How do dieters fare 5 years later? *J Am Diet Assoc.* 2006;106:559–568

107. Patton GC, Selzer R, Coffee C, Carlin JB, Wolfe R. Onset of adolescent eating disorders: population based cohort study over 3 years. *BMJ.* 1999:318:765–768

108. Killen JD, Taylor CB, Hayward C, et al. Weight concerns influence the development of eating disorders: a four year prospective study. *J Consult Clin Psychol.* 1996;64:936–940

109. Nicklas TA, Myers L, Farris RP, Srinivasan SR, Berenson GS. Nutritional quality of a high carbohydrate diet as consumed by children: The Bogalusa Heart Study. *J Nutr.* 1996;126:1382–1388

110. Greene-Finestone LS, Campbell MK, Evers SE, Gutmanis IA. Adolescents' low-carbohydrate-density diets are related to poorer dietary intakes. *J Am Diet Assoc.* 2005;105:1783–1788

111. Freeman JM, Kelly MT, Freeman JB. *The Epilepsy Diet Treatment: An Introduction to The Ketogenic Diet.* 2nd ed. New York, NY: Demos Vermande; 1996

112. Peterson SJ, Tangney CC, Pimentel-Zablah EM, Hjelmgren B, Booth G, Berry-Kravis E. Changes in growth and seizure reduction in children on the ketogenic diet as a treatment for intractable epilepsy. *J Am Diet Assoc.* 2005;105:718–725

113. Kossoff EH, McGrogan JR, Bluml RM, Pillas DJ, Rubenstein JE, Vining EP. A modified Atkins diet is effective for the treatment of intractable pediatric epilepsy. *Epilepsia.* 2006;47: 421–424

114. Kang HC, Chung DE, Kim DW, Kim HD. Early- and late-onset complications of the ketogenic diet for intractable epilepsy. *Epilepsia.* 2004;45:1116–1123

115. Willi SM, Oexmann MJ, Wright NM, Collop NA, Key LL Jr. The effects of a high-protein, low-fat, ketogenic diet on adolescents with morbid obesity: Body composition, blood chemistries, and sleep abnormalities. *Pediatrics.* 1998;101:61–67

116. Gilroy CM, Steiner JF, Byers T, Shapiro H, Georgian W. Echinacea and truth in labeling. *Arch Intern Med.* 2003;163:699–704

117. Garrard J, Harms S, Eberly LE, Matiak A. Variations in product choices of frequently purchased herbs: caveat emptor. *Arch Intern Med.* 2003;163:2290–2295

118. Wolsko PM, Solondz DK, Phillips RS, Schachter SC, Eisenberg DM. Lack of herbal supplement characterization in published randomized controlled trials. *Am J Med.* 2005;118:1087–1093

119. Sanders H, Davis MF, Duncan B, Meaney FJ, Haynes J, Barton LL. Use of complementary and alternative medical therapies among children with special health care needs in southern Arizona. *Pediatrics.* 2004;111:584–587

120. Noonan K, Arensman RM, Hoover JD. Herbal medication use in the pediatric surgical patient. *J Pediatr Surg.* 2004;39:500–503

121. Lin YC, Bioteau AB, Ferrair LR, Berde CB. The use of herbs and complementary and alternative medicine in pediatric preoperative patients. *J Clin Anesth.* 2004;16:4–6

122. Lanski SL, Greenwald M, Perkins A, Simon HK. Herbal therapy use in a pediatric emergency department population: expect the unexpected. *Pediatrics*. 2003;111:981–985

123. Lohse B, Stotts JL, Priebe JR. Survey of herbal use by Kansas and Wisconsin WIC participants reveals moderate, appropriate use and identifies herbal education needs. *J Am Diet Assoc*. 2006;106:227–237

124. Wilson KM, Klein JD, Sesselberg TS, et al. Use of complementary medicine and dietary supplements among U.S. adolescents. *J Adolesc Health*. 2006;38:385–394

125. Ottolini MC, Hamburger EK, Loprieato JO, et al. Complementary and alternative medicine use among children in the Washington, DC area. *Ambul Pediatr*. 2001;1:122–125

126. Kemper KJ, O'Connor KG. Pediatricians' recommendations for complementary and alternative medical (CAM) therapies. *Ambul Pediatr*. 2004;4:482–487

127. Shenfield G, Lim E, Allen H. Survey of the use of complementary medicines and therapies in children with asthma. *J Paediatr Child Health*. 2002;38:252–257

128. Mazur LJ, De Ybarrondo L, Miller J, Colasurdo G. Use of alternative and complementary therapies for pediatric asthma. *Tex Med*. 2001;97:64–68

129. Heuschkel R, Afzal N, Wuerth A, et al. Complementary medicine use in children and young adults with inflammatory bowel disease. *Am J Gastroenterol*. 2002;97:382–388

130. Neuhouser ML, Patterson RE, Schwartz SM, Hedderson MM, Bowen DJ, Standish LJ. Use of alternative medicine by children with cancer in Washington state. *Prev Med*. 2001;33:347–354

131. Kumar NB, Allen K, Bell H. Perioperative herbal supplement use in cancer patients: potential implications and recommendations for presurgical screening. *Cancer Control*. 2005;12:149–157

132. Woolf AD. Herbal remedies and children: Do they work? Are they harmful? *Pediatrics*. 2003;112:240–246

133. Pak E, Esrason KT, Wu VH. Hepatotoxicity of herbal remedies: an emerging dilemma. *Prog Transplant*. 2004;14:91–96

Micronutrients and Macronutrients

III

13 Energy

Energy is defined as the capacity to do work or to produce a change in matter. Applied to nutrition, energy refers mainly to the chemical energy derived from foods, principally from oxidative metabolism of the macronutrients fat, carbohydrate, and protein. Energy is required for all the biochemical and physiologic functions that sustain life—for instance, respiration, circulation, maintenance of electrochemical gradients across cell membranes, and maintenance of body temperature—as well as for growth and physical activity.[1-3] Inadequate intake of energy inevitably has adverse consequences, even if other nutrient requirements are met.

Although in a strict sense, energy is not a nutrient (ie, fat, carbohydrate, and protein are the substances ingested), it is useful to think in terms of the energy requirement of an individual, which an international working group defined as "that level of energy intake from food which will balance energy expenditure when the individual has a body size and composition, and level of physical activity, consistent with long-term good health; and which will allow for the maintenance of economically necessary and socially desirable physical activity. In children and pregnant or lactating women the energy requirement includes the energy needs associated with the deposition of tissues or secretion of milk at rates consistent with good health."[3] In the United States, the kilocalorie (kcal) has been the most widely used unit of energy in nutrition; however, as use of Systeme International Units becomes more widespread, energy expressed in terms of kilojoules (kJ) will become more common (1 kcal = 4.184 kJ).

In any individual, energy partitioning can be described by the following relationship[1-5]:

$$\text{energy intake} = \text{energy excretion} + \text{energy expenditure} + \text{energy storage.}$$

Most clinical problems involving energy balance can be approached by systematic evaluation of the terms in this equation, although specific macronutrient effects on metabolism may need to be considered in certain clinical settings.[6,7] "Digestible energy" refers to gross energy intake minus energy lost in the feces. "Metabolizable energy" is gross energy intake minus energy excreted in feces and urine and is the value used for food labeling. Inadequate energy intake may be a consequence of insufficient provision of appropriate food by the child's caregivers or may be attributable to problems inherent to the child (eg, neurological, behavioral, or certain gastrointestinal disorders). Fecal excretion of fat usually accounts for most of the energy excretion, although in some instances, carbohydrate and nitrogenous losses also may be clinically important. Clinically significant increased energy excretion most commonly is secondary to intestinal, pancreatic, or hepatobiliary disorders that result in macronutrient maldigestion and/or malabsorption. In some situations (eg, diabetes mellitus, ketosis), energy losses in urine may be significant.

Energy expenditure includes energy expended for basal metabolic requirements, the thermic effect of food ingestion, energy expended for activity, and energy expended for thermoregulation.[1-5] Resting energy expenditure (REE) is the energy expended by a person at rest in a thermoneutral environment (ie, an environmental temperature at which the metabolic rate and, therefore, oxygen consumption are at a minimum). Basal metabolic rate is energy expenditure under standard conditions—after a 12- to 18-hour fast, awake but quietly lying down (in early morning on awakening), in a thermoneutral environment, and bodily and mentally at rest. The basal metabolic rate reflects energy required for vital body processes during physical, emotional, and digestive rest and tends to be somewhat lower (10% to 20%) than REE.[1] Important factors that affect energy expenditure at rest include age, body size and composition, and the presence of morbidity (eg, infection, fever, trauma).

"Nonactivity thermogenesis" refers to increases in energy expenditure above the REE that are not due to physical activity, including the effects of food intake, cold exposure, thermogenic agents, and psychological influences. The thermic effect of feeding (TEF), or specific dynamic action, is the increase in energy expenditure resulting from ingestion of food; it typically constitutes 5% to 10% of energy ingested. The TEF is attributable mainly to the obligatory metabolic costs of processing a meal, which include nutrient digestion, absorption, transport, and storage. The remaining facultative TEF is the component of the TEF not accounted for by known energy costs that may be related to stimulation of the sympathetic nervous system, increased futile cycle activity (net hydrolysis of adenosine triphosphate and the generation of heat via a cycle of phosphorylation and dephosphorylation catalyzed by enzymes that normally function in separate pathways), cell membrane pump activity, or changes in hormonal status. Energy required to maintain body temperature depends on environmental temperature. Beyond infancy, little additional energy is needed between environmental temperatures of 20°C and 30°C. Outside these limits, an additional 5% to 10% of total energy may be necessary to maintain body temperature. The thermoneutral temperature range is higher for neonates, particularly for those born preterm.

Any estimate of total energy requirements must consider energy expenditure attributable to physical activity. Activity thermogenesis includes exercise-related activity thermogenesis and "nonexercise activity thermogenesis" (NEAT), which includes energy expenditure attributable to spontaneous daily physical activities, such as sitting, standing, walking, and fidgeting.[8] In almost all individuals, NEAT constitutes the major portion of activity thermogenesis and is the most variable component of total energy expenditure. Interindividual differences in NEAT resulting from seemingly subtle differences in amount of fidgeting or posture allocation may have a significant effect on overall energy balance.[9,10] The physical activity level, which is defined as total energy expenditure divided by basal energy expenditure, is frequently used to quantify physical activity.[1,8] Estimates of energy expenditure for physical activities vary. Examples of energy expenditure while performing various activities are given in Chapter 10: Sports Nutrition.

Energy expenditure is determined in several ways, most commonly by indirect calorimetry, in which oxygen consumption and carbon dioxide production are measured. The doubly labeled water method, which provides an indirect measure of carbon dioxide production, has been used to estimate total energy expenditure in a number of research settings.[1] The respiratory quotient is the ratio of carbon dioxide production to oxygen consumption and varies depending on substrate utilization (ie, the relative contributions of carbohydrate, fat, and protein catabolism to total expenditure). The respiratory quotient for fat is approximately 0.7; for protein, approximately 0.85; for carbohydrate, 1.0; and for lipogenesis (conversion of carbohydrate to stored fat), >1. The ingestion or administration of a high proportion of calories as carbohydrates may cause difficulties for children with respiratory insufficiency, because excess carbon dioxide is produced. This is especially true if the energy intake from carbohydrates exceeds the energy expenditure.

The energy cost of growth also is a component of total energy requirements. This is important in energy balance, primarily during infancy. During infancy, the energy cost of growth is approximately 5 kcal/g of new tissue. The energy needed for growth represents approximately 35% of total energy intake at 1 month of age, decreases to approximately 3% at 12 months of age because of slower growth, and remains almost negligible until the onset of puberty, when it increases to approximately 4% (approximately 8.7–12 kcal/g gained depending on the composition of the tissue accreted).[1]

A number of formulas, tables, and nomograms have been developed to estimate the energy expenditure or energy requirements of infants, children, and adults on the basis of such factors as weight, height, age, sex, and body surface area. Previous recommendations for energy intake during the first 2 years of life likely overestimated actual requirements, because significantly lower mean energy intakes of healthy breastfed infants in this age group were reported.[5,11–13] Recently developed equations for estimation of energy requirements are given in Table 13.1. The potential fallibility of such estimates in individual instances, particularly in disease states, should not be forgotten. For instance, equations used for predicting energy expenditure in healthy infants may underestimate energy expenditure in infants with cystic fibrosis.[11]

Table 13.1
Estimated Energy Requirements[1]

Age	Estimated Energy Requirements*
0–3 mo	$(89 \times \text{weight [kg]} - 100) + 175$ kcal
4–6 mo	$(89 \times \text{weight [kg]} - 100) + 56$ kcal
7–12 mo	$(89 \times \text{weight [kg]} - 100) + 22$ kcal
13–36 mo	$(89 \times \text{weight [kg]} - 100) + 20$ kcal
Boys 3 through 8 y	$88.5 - (61.9 \times \text{age [y]}) + \text{PA} \times (26.7 \times \text{weight [kg]} + 903 \times \text{height [m]}) + 20$ kcal
Girls 3 through 8 y	$135.3 - (30.8 \times \text{age [y]}) + \text{PA} \times (10.0 \times \text{weight [kg]} + 934 \times \text{height [m]}) + 20$ kcal
Boys 9 through 18 y	$88.5 - (61.9 \times \text{age [y]}) + \text{PA} \times (26.7 \times \text{weight [kg]} + 903 \times \text{height [m]}) + 25$ kcal
Girls 9 through 18 y	$135.3 - (30.8 \times \text{age [y]}) + \text{PA} \times (10.0 \times \text{weight [kg]} + 934 \times \text{height [m]}) + 25$ kcal

*Total energy expenditure + energy deposition.

PA indicates the physical activity coefficient:

For boys 3 through 18 years of age:

PA = 1.00 (sedentary, estimated physical activity level 1.0–1.4)

PA = 1.13 (low active, estimated physical activity level 1.4–1.6)

PA = 1.26 (active, estimated physical activity level 1.6–1.9)

PA = 1.42 (very active, estimated physical activity level 1.9–2.5)

For girls 3 through 18 years of age:

PA = 1.00 (sedentary, estimated physical activity level 1.0–1.4)

PA = 1.16 (low active, estimated physical activity level 1.4–1.6)

PA = 1.31 (active, estimated physical activity level 1.6–1.9)

PA = 1.56 (very active, estimated physical activity level 1.9–2.5)

Although food intake is the result of complex interactions among central nervous system regulating regions (mainly hypothalamic) and peripheral neural (ie, vagal) and humoral (eg, gut peptides and insulin) signals and environmental factors, energy balance at all ages is regulated with a fair degree of precision. This is reflected in the observation that most infants and children grow in regular fashion, and many adults maintain stable body weight for long periods. Infants appear to eat to satisfy energy needs and will compensate for low food-energy density and poor digestibility by increasing food intake.[4] Observations of young children fed ad libitum while recovering from malnutrition showed that their voracious appetites abated as they approached normal weight for height.[14] Despite the usual balancing of energy intake against energy expenditure and energy needs for growth,[15] obesity (see Chapter 33), a consequence of long-term energy intake in excess of energy requirements, has become alarmingly prevalent among children in the United States.

Recent recommendations of acceptable macronutrient distribution ranges suggest that adults should get 45% to 65% of their energy intake from carbohydrates (with added sugars representing no more than 25% of total energy intake), 20% to 35% from fat, and 10% to 35% from protein. Acceptable ranges for children are similar to those for adults except that infants and younger children need a slightly higher proportion of fat (25% to 40%).[1] The average diet of individuals in the United States supplies 12% to 15% of calories from protein. Carbohydrate, fat, and alcohol provide the remainder of calories; alcohol may account for as much as 10% of the total calories in adults. Although an appropriate balance of total calories and protein is required for adequate growth, especially in response to malnutrition, the importance of energy intake is underscored by the observations that the speed of recovery from severe infantile malnutrition is more closely related to energy than to protein intake[16] and that pregnancy outcomes can be improved as much by additional calories as by protein supplements.[17] Many common pathologic entities may alter energy requirements, interfere with nutrient availability, or affect substrate utilization. Provision of adequate energy may be especially important in certain clinical settings, particularly if a patient's ability to regulate intake is impaired. During infancy, childhood, and adolescence, if energy intake is adequate relative to energy expenditure and energy excretion, adequate energy should be available for sufficient energy storage. The growth rate, in fact, serves as a good "bioassay" for the adequacy of energy intake. Careful consideration of the factors affecting energy balance (ie, energy intake, energy excretion, energy expenditure, and energy storage) can often clarify seemingly complex clinical problems.

References

1. Institute of Medicine. *Dietary Reference Intakes for Energy, Carbohydrate, Fiber, Fat, Fatty Acids, Cholesterol, Protein, and Amino Acids (Macronutrients)*. Washington, DC: National Academies Press; 2005

2. Pellett PL. Food energy requirements in humans. *Am J Clin Nutr.* 1990;51:711–722

3. Food and Agriculture Organization of the United Nations, World Health Organization. FAO/WHO/UNU Expert Consultation. *Energy and Protein Requirements.* Geneva, Switzerland: World Health Organization; 1985. WHO Technical Report No. 724

4. Fomon SJ. *Nutrition of Normal Infants.* St Louis, MO: Mosby-Year Book, Inc; 1993

5. Butte, NF. Meeting energy needs. In: Tsang RC, Zlotkin SH, Nichols BL, Hansen JW, eds. *Nutrition During Infancy: Principles and Practice.* 2nd ed. Cincinnati, OH, Digital Educational Publishing; 1997:57–82

6. Krieger JW, Sitren HS, Daniels MJ, Langkamp-Henken B. Effects of variation in protein and carbohydrate intake on body mass and composition during energy restriction: a meta-regression 1. *Am J Clin Nutr.* 2006;83:260–274

7. Feinman RD, Fine EJ. "A calorie is a calorie" violates the second law of thermodynamics. *Nutr J.* 2004;3:9

8. Levine JA. Nonexercise activity thermogenesis (NEAT): environment and biology. *Am J Physiol Endocrinol Metab.* 2004;286(5):e675–e685

9. Levine JA, Schleusner SJ, Jensen MD. Energy expenditure of nonexercise activity. *Am J Clin Nutr.* 2000;72:1451–1454

10. Levine JA, Lanningham-Foster LM, McCrady SK, et al. Interindividual variation in posture allocation: possible role in human obesity. *Science.* 2005;307:584–586

11. Thomson MA, Bucolo S, Quirk P, Shepherd RW. Measured versus predicted resting energy expenditure in infants: a need for reappraisal. *J Pediatr.* 1995;126:21–27

12. Butte NF, Wong WW, Garza C, et al. Energy requirements of breast-fed infants. *J Am Coll Nutr.* 1991;10:190–195

13. Butte NF, Wong WW, Hopkinson JM, Heinz CJ, Mehta NR, Smith EO. Energy requirements derived from total energy expenditure and energy deposition during the first 2 y of life. *Am J Clin Nutr.* 2000;72:1558–1569

14. Ashworth A. Growth rates in children recovering from protein-calorie malnutrition. *Br J Nutr.* 1969;23:834–845

15. Forbes GB, Brown MR. Energy need for weight maintenance in human beings: effect of body size and composition. *J Am Diet Assoc.* 1989;89:499–502

16. Waterlow JC. The rate of recovery of malnourished infants in relation to the protein and calorie levels of the diet. *J Trop Pediatr.* 1961;7:16–22

17. Lechtig A, Delgado H, Lasky R, et al. Maternal nutrition and fetal growth in developing countries. *Am J Dis Child.* 1975;129:553–556

14 Protein

Proteins are the major structural and functional components of all cells in the body. They are macromolecules that comprise 1 or more chains of amino acids that vary in their sequence and length and are folded into specific 3-dimensional structures. The sizes and conformations of proteins, therefore, are infinitely diverse and complex, and this enables them to serve an extensive variety of functions in the cell. Dietary protein provides the amino acids required for both the synthesis of body proteins and the production of other nitrogenous compounds with important functional roles, such as glutathione, creatine, hemes, nucleotides, hormones, nitric oxide, bile acids, and some neurotransmitters. Amino acids can exist as various stereoisomers in nature. Only the L-amino acids are biologically active and can be incorporated into proteins. Body proteins also can be catabolized and serve as an energy source when energy intake, in particular carbohydrate intake, is inadequate.

From the dietary perspective, it is the amino acid composition of a protein that is its most relevant property, although for some, the structure can dictate digestibility—for example, keratin, an insoluble protein that makes up hair, skin, and nails. Protein digestion begins in the stomach through the activity of pepsin in the presence of hydrochloric acid. In the young infant, pepsin and acid production are low, but this does not appear to limit the digestibility of protein. Protein digestion continues in the presence of pancreatic enzymes in the duodenum and enzymes in the brush border of the jejunum and proximal ileum. Some of these enzymes, such as enterokinase, also have low activity during the newborn period, but the low activity does not appear to limit protein digestion. Digestion results in the hydrolysis of proteins to oligopeptides and amino acids that are absorbed. Oligopeptides are hydrolyzed to amino acids by enzymes in the cells of the intestinal epithelium. Protein that escapes digestion in the small intestine, including secreted proteins and sloughed-off intestinal cells, can be broken down by bacteria in the colon, and the resulting ammonia can be absorbed and incorporated into amino acids.

Absorbed amino acids are first transported from the intestine to the liver and then enter the general amino acid pool of the body in the plasma and exchange with tissue pools. Some amino acids are used directly by the intestine itself, as an energy source, to synthesize gut proteins or in the production of other nitrogen-containing biological molecules. In the growing organism, an influx of amino acids to the tissues from the diet rapidly stimulates protein synthesis.[1,2] This response is dampened as the organism matures, and in adults, protein consumption primarily reduces protein breakdown with only a moderate response in protein synthesis.[3,4] Dietary amino acids consumed in excess of the body's needs cannot be stored. The nitrogen component of amino acids is converted to urea, and the remaining keto acids are used directly for energy production or converted to glucose and fat when energy intake is adequate. Therefore, blood urea nitrogen concentration is a good indicator of recent protein intake when hydration and renal function are normal. The stimulation of protein synthesis by the influx of amino acids from the diet, together with the body's inability to store excess dietary amino acids, are primary reasons for the recommendation that in infants and children, the daily protein requirement should be consumed over several meals at regular intervals throughout the day.

Body proteins and the other nitrogenous compounds are continuously degraded and resynthesized. Several times more endogenous protein is turned over every day than is usually consumed. The rate of turnover can be rapid, as in bone marrow and in gastrointestinal mucosa, or it can be slow, as in muscle and collagen. Protein turnover also changes with age; it is highest during early life, when tissues are maturing and their growth rates are at their highest.[4] Amino acids released from the breakdown of endogenous proteins are recycled, but this process is not completely efficient. Amino acids that are not reused are catabolized or lost in urine, feces, sweat, desquamated skin, hair, and nails. These losses create an obligatory requirement for dietary amino acids in addition to any requirement for the net accretion of body protein. This obligatory fraction constitutes the maintenance or basal needs of the organism, and once growth has ceased, this fraction represents an individual's entire protein requirement. The magnitude of these basal losses is dictated by the individual's total lean mass and their basal metabolic rate.

Amino acids are usually categorized into 3 groups: indispensable, dispensable, and conditionally indispensable. Amino acids for which carbon skeletons cannot be synthesized de novo in adults are regarded as indispensable (essential) amino acids and must be provided by the diet; they include leucine, isoleucine, valine, threonine, methionine, phenylalanine, tryptophan, lysine, and histidine. To sustain normal growth and the maintenance of the body's protein mass after the requirements for indispensable amino acids have been met, the additional dietary nitrogen required must be provided as dispensable (nonessential) amino acids. Dispensable amino acids are those that can be synthesized in the body from other amino acids or nitrogen-containing molecules. These are usually divided into 2 categories:

the truly dispensable amino acids and the conditionally indispensable ones. Conditionally indispensable amino acids and other nutrients are those that ordinarily can be synthesized, but an exogenous source is required under certain circumstances. The designation varies according to the age of the individual and the presence of genetic or acquired disease conditions. For all humans, alanine, aspartic acid, asparagine, serine, and glutamic acid can be classified as dispensable. Arginine, glutamine, proline, glycine, cysteine, and tyrosine are in the conditionally indispensable category. Cysteine, tyrosine, and arginine must be provided in the diets of the preterm and newborn infant because of the immaturity of the enzyme activities necessary for their synthesis from precursors. Glycine is required for the synthesis of creatine, porphyrins, glutathione, nucleotides, and bile salts; therefore, the requirement for this amino acid during times of rapid growth is relatively high.[5] Glycine is present in relatively small amounts in milk and may be a conditionally essentially amino acid for the preterm and newborn infant. Various disease conditions can also interfere with the synthesis of amino acids that can normally be synthesized from other amino acids. Arginine is essential in patients with defects of the urea cycle. Cysteine may be essential in patients with hepatic disease or homocystinuria. Tyrosine is essential for people with phenylketonuria and may be required for patients with hepatic disease. Glutamine is the preferred fuel for rapidly dividing cells, such as enterocytes and lymphocytes. Thus, during times of critical stress, such as after surgical procedures, nonsurgical trauma, or sepsis, or in patients with gastrointestinal mucosal injury, large amounts of glutamine are synthesized by the skeletal muscle from the amino acids of skeletal muscle proteins. Opinions are divided on the benefits of supplementary glutamine in these instances.[6] Taurine and carnitine are amino acids that serve important and specific functions in the cell but are not incorporated into proteins. They can be synthesized by the body from cysteine and lysine, respectively, and are present in a mixed diet containing proteins of animal origin. The rates of synthesis in infants fed by total parenteral nutrition or receiving synthetic formulas devoid of taurine and carnitine may be insufficient to meet all of their needs and necessitate dietary supplementation.[7,8] Nearly all infant formulas today contain added taurine.

Recommended Dietary Intake for Protein and Amino Acids

The amount of protein that should be eaten is expressed in a number of different ways according to the information it is meant to convey, how the values are derived, and the purpose for which the information will be used. The Recommended Dietary Allowance (RDA) for protein is the average daily intake of protein that meets the nutrient needs of most healthy individuals in a particular life stage and gender group (Appendix J, Table J-1).[9-11] The RDA is derived from:

1. The estimated average requirement (EAR) for protein. The EAR is the daily protein intake that meets the protein needs of 50% of all healthy individuals of a specific age and gender. The physiologic requirement is defined as the lowest level of protein intake needed to replace losses from the body when energy intake is in balance (maintenance requirement). In growing individuals and pregnant and lactating women, the protein requirement also includes the protein required for tissue accretion and milk production at a level associated with good health. The need for growth decreases from approximately 55% of total intake over the first 3 months of life to 10% or less by 8 years of age and accounts largely for the reduction with age in protein requirements (Table 14.1). These intakes assume that the protein source is of high quality on the basis of its amino acid composition.

2. The variability in protein needs for specific population groups. The RDA defines the protein needs of 97.5% of a particular age group. Thus, the EAR must be increased to account for variability in the requirements among groups of similar individuals. This includes the variation in maintenance needs, the variation in protein accretion rate (if relevant), and the variation in the efficiency with which dietary protein is accumulated. It is important to note that because of this adjustment, the RDA exceeds the protein needs of most individuals within a specified group.

Table 14.1
Contribution of Maintenance and Growth to Protein Needs of Infants and Children[10,13,14]

Age	Protein Gain* (g/[kg·day^{-1}])	Intake (% of Total)	
		Growth	Maintenance
0.5–3 mo	0.49	55	45
3–6 mo	0.30	43	57
6–12 mo	0.18	31	69
1–3 y	0.10	20	80
4–8 y	0.046	10	90

* Average for boys and girls.

For some nutrients and/or certain populations, the scientific data (either average intakes or their variability) for estimating an EAR are not sufficiently robust to make a definitive recommendation. In these cases, a level defined as an adequate intake (AI) is used. This value is based on the average protein intake of a group of individuals who appear to be healthy and in a good nutritional state. The recommendation for daily protein and amino acid intake of infants from birth to 6 months falls in this category and is based on the average daily protein intake of infants fed principally with human milk.

The new Dietary Reference Intake guidelines[10] define 2 additional parameters that should be taken into consideration in the evaluation of diets and in making dietary recommendations: the tolerable upper intake level and the acceptable macronutrient distribution ranges (AMDR). No tolerable upper intake levels have been set for protein or amino acid intakes because of the absence of sufficient data on which to base recommendations; this does not imply that high levels are not harmful. The AMDRs were developed because of the increasing evidence that the dietary source from which individuals obtain their energy may play a role in the development of chronic diseases. Protein, fats, and carbohydrates can substitute for one other as sources of dietary energy; thus, for a given energy intake, if the proportion of one varies, so must the others. The AMDR for protein is the proportion of the total energy intake that is protein and that is associated with a reduced risk of chronic disease. The AMDR for protein is 5% to 20% of total energy intake in 1- to 3-year-old children and 10% to 30% of total energy intake for 4- to 18-year-old children. Intakes below these ranges increase the risk of protein energy malnutrition and its consequences, including impaired growth and immune function. Intakes above the AMDR may increase the risk of chronic diseases, such as osteoporosis, renal stones, coronary artery disease, and obesity.

For the 9 indispensable amino acids, EARs and RDAs have been developed for individuals from 7 months to 18 years of age, and AIs have been determined for infants 6 months or younger. The requirement for methionine is frequently given as a composite value for total sulfur amino acids (ie, methionine and cysteine, the latter being a metabolic product of methionine catabolism). Thus, the requirement for cysteine is dependent on sufficient methionine being present in the diet to meet the needs of both amino acids, although it is clear that in some circumstances, such as infancy, the metabolism of methionine to cysteine may not be sufficient to meet the entire cysteine requirement. Similarly, the requirements for phenylalanine and tyrosine, the aromatic amino acids, are pooled because tyrosine can be formed from the metabolism of phenylalanine.

Methods of Determining Protein and Amino Acid Requirements

Protein

Protein requirements and balance data are frequently measured and expressed on the basis of nitrogen content. On average, nitrogen constitutes 16% of the weight of a protein, although the exact value varies from protein to protein. The recommendations for protein intakes have used a factor of 6.25 to convert g of nitrogen to g of protein.

Protein needs have been estimated using various approaches.[9–12] During the first 6 months of life, human milk is the optimal source of protein for infants and, when freely fed, is sufficient to sustain good health and optimal growth. Thus, the average intake of breastfed infants has been used to define the AI for this age group. The intake of infants was determined by test weighing and the average protein content of human milk.

Recommendations for dietary protein intakes of infants older than 6 months have been estimated using the factorial method. The factorial method evaluates separately for individuals of different ages, sizes, and genders, considers the body's protein needs for maintenance and growth, and adjusts for the efficiency with which dietary protein is used.

Maintenance protein requirements are derived from nitrogen balance studies. This method involves determination of the difference between the intake and excretion of nitrogen (in urine, feces, sweat, and minor losses via other routes) for 1 to 3 weeks or longer. Several different amounts of a quality protein source, such as milk or egg, legume and cereal mixes, or mixed vegetable and animal sources, are tested at a constant and adequate energy intake. From the relationship between intake and balance (intake minus excretion), the amount of nitrogen required for maintenance (zero balance) is extrapolated.

To the maintenance requirements, additional amounts of protein that would be sufficient to support appropriate body protein gains have been added. The mean rate of protein gain during growth has been estimated from the body composition data of children from 9 months to 3 years of age[13] and from 4 to 18 years of age.[14] In both studies, body composition was measured using a combination of water dilution, determination of whole-body potassium concentration, and dual-energy absorptiometry. The conversion of dietary protein to body proteins, however, is not 100% efficient. In growing individuals, the slope of the relationship between balance and intake provides a measure of the efficiency with which dietary protein is used for growth (58% from 0.5 to 13 years of age; 43% from 14 to 18 years of age[10]). Thus, the amount of dietary protein needed for growth must be adjusted to account for this inefficiency.

Amino Acids

Estimation of amino acid requirements can be determined by a number of approaches, including measurement of nitrogen balance and plasma amino acid concentrations as well as direct kinetic measurements of amino acid oxidation using stable-isotope-labeled amino acids as tracers and balance and indicator amino acid oxidation with balance. The values obtained, however, vary depending on the method used. Because of this uncertainty, together with the paucity of direct measurements of amino acid metabolism in the pediatric population, a factorial approach was used to estimate individual amino acid EAR from 0.5 to 18 years of age. For infants through 6 months of age, AIs have been defined on the basis of data from breastfed infants.[9-12] These were calculated from the average volume of milk consumed and the amino acid composition of human milk proteins of normally growing, healthy infants.

To define the growth component of the requirement for individual amino acids, the factorial approach uses data for tissue protein accretion and the amino acid composition of body tissues corrected for the inefficiency of dietary utilization. Because the maintenance protein requirement does not vary with age in children and the values are very similar to adult values (expressed per unit of body weight), the values for the maintenance component of the amino acid requirements are based on adult maintenance values. The adult values are derived from direct measurements of amino acid kinetics and yield a different amino acid pattern from that of body proteins. Hence, because the total amount of amino acid deposited decreases with age, the composition of amino acids required changes (reflected in Table 14.2); the indispensable amino acids represent approximately 42% of the tissue amino acid pattern but only 23% of the maintenance pattern.[12]

The RDA for amino acids adjusts the EAR to include an allowance for variability in the population in growth and maintenance requirements.

Table 14.2
Amino Acid Scoring Patterns Based on the Estimated Average Requirements (EAR) for Protein and Indispensable Amino Acids*[10]

	mg/g Protein		
Amino Acid	Infants	Children (1–3 y)	Adults (≥18 y)
Histidine	23	18	17
Isoleucine	57	25	23
Leucine	101	55	52
Lysine	69	51	47
Methionine + cysteine	38	25	23
Phenylalanine + tyrosine	87	47	41
Threonine	47	27	24
Tryptophan	18	7	6
Valine	56	32	29
Total indispensable amino acids	495	287	262

* Indispensable amino acid EAR/EAR for protein for an individual age group.

Protein Quality

In many respects, the ultimate test of the protein quality from a particular food is its ability to support appropriate growth of the individual consuming that food protein. When human milk is no longer the only source of protein, the quality and digestibility of food protein becomes important. Because of wide variation in amino acid composition and digestibility, proteins differ in their ability to provide nitrogen and amino acids required for growth and maintenance. The amino acid composition of the food consumed is important, because if the content of a single indispensable amino acid is insufficient to meet an individual's need for that amino acid, it will limit the ability of the body to utilize the remaining amino acids in the diet, even if the total amount of protein consumed would appear to be adequate. The recommendations for protein intake assume that the sources of protein are highly digestible (>95%) and that the indispensable amino acid composition closely meets human needs. These properties apply to animal proteins, such as egg protein, milk protein, meat, and fish, whereas vegetable proteins often have a lower digestibility (70%–80%) and often provide inadequate amounts of lysine (cereals) or sulfur amino acids (legumes) (for examples, see Table 14.3).[9,10] Although plant proteins are generally of a lower quality than proteins of animal origin, equivalent amino acid patterns can be achieved by mixing plant proteins from different sources, such as legumes and cereals. Processing of foods can also increase or decrease the digestibility of dietary proteins. An important example is the chemical modification to lysine with cooking, which renders it unavailable. Thus, to apply the recommendations for protein intake to mixed diets containing protein sources other than animal-based foods, it is necessary to adjust for the protein digestibility and correct for the adequacy of the amino-acid composition of the food.

Table 14.3
Mean Values for Digestibility and Amino Acid Scores of Various Protein Sources[10,15]

Protein Source	True Digestibility* (%)	Amino Acid Score by Age†	
		6 mo–1 y	School Age
Whole egg (hen)	97	0.74 (trp)	1.36 (his)
Cow milk	95	0.52 (thr)	0.90 (thr)
Beef (cooked)	94	0.54 (trp)	1.39 (trp)
Corn, whole	85	0.41 (lys)	0.55 (lys)
Rice, white, cooked	88	0.59 (lys)	0.80 (lys)
Wheat, flour, whole	86	0.40 (lys)	0.54 (lys)
Wheat, flour, refined	96	0.37 (lys)	0.50 (lys)
Peanut butter	95	0.40 (lys)	0.55 (lys)
Beans, navy cooked	78	0.60 (S)	0.91 (S)
Soy protein isolate	95	0.75 (S)	1.14 (S)
Rice + beans	78	0.70 (trp)	1.02 (lys)

* True digestibility in man (%) = $\dfrac{\text{Nitrogen intake} - (\text{Fecal N on test protein} - \text{Fecal N on nonprotein diet}) \times 100}{\text{Nitrogen intake}}$

A factor of 6.25 is used to convert nitrogen to protein.

† The amino acid score for various protein sources was derived using the amino acid requirement pattern shown in Table 14.2. The amino acid of the protein sources was obtained from the US Department of Agriculture Nutrient Database for Standard Reference, Release 19, 2006. The abbreviation shown in parenthesis is for the most limiting amino acid: trp indicates tryptophan; his, histidine; thr, threonine; lys, lysine; S, cysteine + methionine. Values >1 indicate that the protein source contains relatively more of that amino acid than the ideal reference protein.

For the purpose of evaluating the adequacy of the amino acid content of food proteins, an amino-acid scoring pattern that ideally must be provided by dietary protein can be derived by dividing the indispensable amino acid

EAR by the EAR for protein for an individual age group (Table 14.2).[10] Thus, an ideal protein is one containing all the indispensable amino acids in amounts sufficient to meet requirements without any excess. For infants to 1 year of age, the amino-acid pattern of human milk proteins is considered the ideal and, provided the protein requirement is met with milk, the amino acid intake will be appropriate. The scoring pattern for children older than 1 year is significantly different from that for infants because of the smaller and different requirement pattern for growth. Thus, as maintenance requirements come to dominate, the requirement for indispensable amino acids diminishes. Because the scoring pattern is similar for young children and adults, the most recent recommendations propose that the scoring pattern for children from 1 to 3 years of age also be used in the assessment of the diets of adolescents and adults.[10]

The effectiveness with which an absorbed dietary protein can meet the indispensable amino acid requirement is determined by the protein's amino acid score (Table 14.3). This is determined by the amino acid that least meets the individual's amino acid requirements. To determine the amino acid score, the amount of an amino acid in 1 g of the protein of interest is divided by the amount in 1 g of the reference protein for the relevant population (Table 14.2). The amino acid that has the lowest score is the limiting amino acid, and its value represents the amino acid score of that specific protein.

$$\text{amino acid score} = \frac{\text{mg of limiting amino acid in 1 g of food protein}}{\text{mg of amino acid in 1 g of reference pattern}}$$

The amino acid score corrected for the digestibility of the protein is termed the protein digestibility corrected amino acid score (PDCAAS)[9,10,15]:

$$\text{PDCAAS (\%)} = \text{true digestibility} \times \text{amino acid score} \times 100$$

Of the indispensable amino acids, only 4 are likely to affect the quality of a food protein: lysine, the sulfur amino acids (methionine + cysteine), threonine, and tryptophan. Examples of the amino acid score for various protein sources if they were the only protein source in the diet of a young child are shown in Table 14.3. In the formulation of special-purpose diets in clinical practice, the scoring patterns for all essential amino acids should be considered.

Protein Requirements

Because of the differences in the quality of proteins available in the diet and other factors, such as age, gender, activity levels, and methodologic limitations, confidence in the recommendations for protein and amino acid intakes for individuals or populations is somewhat tenuous. Nonetheless, recommendations are needed to guide the design of diets and the content of educational programs in nutrition and for planning specific intervention programs. The recommendations for protein are categorized by life stage and gender, because among healthy individuals, these are the 2 primary parameters that are responsible for variations in the body's need for protein. The pediatric stage of life has been subdivided into 6 groupings (ages are approximate): infancy (0–6 months and 7–12 months), toddlerhood (1 to 3 years), early childhood (4 to 8 years), puberty (9 to 13 years), and adolescence (14 to 18 years). Differences between boys and girls are only defined for the adolescent group.[10]

Infants

The optimal food for full-term infants is human milk, and the AAP recommends exclusive breastfeeding for a minimum of 4 months but preferably for 6 months. Current recommendations are based on the average value determined from a number of different studies of exclusively breastfed infants. These results indicate that, on average, infants to 6 months of age consume 0.78 L of milk per day.[10] The protein content of human milk is the lowest of any species, with reported values varying from 9 to 14 g/L of true protein after the first few weeks postpartum, and an average value of 11.7 g/L was used to calculate the AI for protein. Milk also contains a significant amount of nonprotein nitrogen compounds, such as free amino acids, urea, and creatine, which constitute 20% to 27% of the nitrogen in human milk, or 2 to 3 g/L. The proportion of the nonprotein nitrogen that is bioavailable and spares the utilization of milk protein amino acids is uncertain; estimates from 46% to 61% have been proposed.[11] The protein composition of human milk, in which the whey proteins, rather than the casein proteins, are the dominant protein constituents, is exceptional because of its high cysteine content and high cysteine-methionine ratio (Appendix C). The nonprotein nitrogen component of human milk also contains substantial quantities of taurine, which is virtually absent from cow milk but is added to commercially prepared infant formulas.

Although the protein content of human milk is less than that of commercial infant formulas, human milk proteins have a high nutritional quality and are digested and absorbed more efficiently than cow milk proteins. Thus, a 6-kg infant ingesting 780 mL/day of human milk receives approximately 9.1 g of protein. This is approximately 1.52 g/kg per day of high-quality protein, which is the AI for infants up to 6 months of age. Because of the uncertainty of its availability, the contribution of nonprotein nitrogen is not included. On the other hand, data from infants freely fed commercial formulas indicate that they consume more on the order of 2 g/kg per day.[11,12] The consensus from a number of studies seems to be that although the total weight and lean mass gain of infants fed formula is higher than for exclusively breastfed infants, especially after 3 months of age, this difference is not attributable specifically to the higher protein content of formulas but instead results from their higher food intake in general. Thus, after adjusting for differences in energy intake, differences in growth rate attributable to milk source are no longer evident.[10,11] There is no indication that the lower protein intake of breastfed infants has adverse effects. Protein intake of breastfed infants appears to satisfy the requirements for maintenance and growth without an amino acid or solute excess.

Commercial infant formulas for term infants in the United States contain a protein equivalent of 14 to 16 g/L or 2.1–2.5 g/100 kcal (Appendix F, Table F-2). This concentration is higher than for human milk and provides a margin of safety for the lower digestibility of cow milk proteins. Additionally, most cow milk-based commercial infant formulas are supplemented with bovine whey to create a whey protein-to-casein ratio similar to that of human milk. Although the specific proteins of bovine whey differ considerably from those of human whey, the amino acid composition (especially for cysteine and methionine) of these "humanized" formulas is closer to that of human milk proteins than are formulas with the whey protein-to-casein ratio of cow milk. Soy-based formulas contain even higher amounts of protein (17–22 g/L) to compensate for their even lower digestibility of proteins.[16]

For 7- to 12-month-old infants, nitrogen balance and body composition data are available, from which average requirements can be derived. Maintenance requirements for children from 9 months to 14 years of age were determined to be similar; thus, a constant value equivalent to 0.688 g/kg per day is suggested for all ages. The growth requirement over this 6-month age range (corrected for the efficiency of utilization of dietary protein for growth [ie, 58%]) yielded a value of 0.312 g/kg per day, so the EAR for the older infant was estimated at 1 g/kg per day, and the RDA is 1.2 g(kg per day. This is slightly lower than the measured AI of healthy older infants (1.6 g/kg per day) fed human milk supplemented with weaning foods.

Children

For preschool and school-aged children, there is a continuing decrease in protein needs relative to body weight. This reflects the decreasing contribution of the growth requirement relative to the constant maintenance requirement. Current protein allowances have been derived from estimates of the average requirements by the factorial method and by assuming that the variability of protein needs among individual children is the same as that of other age groups.

There are few data on the amino acid requirements of children and adolescents, and again, these have been derived using the factorial approach. The requirement for growth (calculated from body composition measurements) contributes only a small proportion of total needs after the first few years of life (Table 14.1). Because maintenance protein requirements have been demonstrated to change little with age, the amino acid requirement for maintenance has been based on the EAR for adults determined by direct amino acid oxidation measurements, which are generally believed to be more accurate than those derived from measuring obligatory losses or based on maintenance protein requirements at nitrogen equilibrium.

The amino acid requirement values for the 1- to 3-year-old are only slightly higher than for adults. Thus, the scoring pattern for dietary proteins will also be very similar. Thus, the recommendation has been made that the reference amino acid pattern for preschool children should be used for assessing the protein components of foods for all individuals older than 1 year.[10] Food consumption surveys in the United States have established that the amino acid patterns and digestibility of proteins in foods commonly consumed is uniform from 1 year of age on and that no adjustment to the RDA is required for individuals consuming a typical US diet.[10] However, appropriate corrections must be made if a diet of lower quality than any acceptable reference protein is customarily consumed.[9]

Adolescents

Few data are available on the protein requirements of adolescents specifically. Values have been estimated using the factorial approach, using the adult value for maintenance needs (0.656 g/kg per day) estimated from nitrogen balance studies. The growth component is derived from body composition studies corrected for the efficiency of utilization derived from the nitrogen balance studies (47%). Although the growth spurt is small relative to body size, the values are slightly higher for boys than girls; thus, the calculated EAR for 14- to 18-year-old boys is 0.73 g/kg per day, compared with

0.71 g/kg per day for girls of the same age. However, the RDA is the same for adolescent boys and girls: 0.85 g/kg per day. There have been no further developments in identifying any specific amino acid needs for adolescents, and the same recommendations as for children have been adopted.

Factors Affecting Dietary Protein Requirements

Dietary requirements for protein are affected by a variety of factors, including gender, age, growth, pregnancy, lactation, illness, the adequacy of other nutrients in the diet, and possibly, genetic variation. These factors influence in various ways the maintenance needs of the organism and the efficiency with which amino acids can be used for growth. The primary factor that influences protein requirements is energy intake. All balance measurements and recommendations are based on the assumption that energy needs are adequately met. When energy intake is inadequate, proteins are catabolized for the provision of energy, effectively increasing protein requirements.

Protein requirements for pregnancy are increased to meet the need for maternal and fetal tissue deposition.[9,10] During the first trimester, the amount of tissue growth is insignificant, and requirements are the same as for nonpregnant females. During the second and third trimesters of pregnancy, higher protein intakes are required for both tissue deposition and the maintenance needs of the deposited, metabolically active tissue and the fetus. The EAR to meet these needs is 0.88 g/kg per day, or 33% higher than for adult women, and the RDA for pregnancy is 1.1 g/kg per day. Whether adolescent mothers have different needs from adult mothers has not been definitively established, and no separate recommendation has been made. Protein supplementation studies demonstrating improved birth outcomes support the benefit of higher, but not excessive, protein intakes during pregnancy.[17]

Additional dietary protein also is required for lactation to supply amino acids for the production of milk proteins and nonprotein nitrogen. These values are adjusted for the efficiency of dietary protein utilization. The published recommendations specify the increase in the protein intake over the nonlactating value for adolescent girls and women that are necessary at different stages of lactation. Again, similar values (EAR, 1.05 kg/day; RDA, 1.3 kg/day) have been proposed for adolescent and adult females, even though the requirements for the nonpregnant adolescent are slightly higher than the adult.

There are no data on the amino acid requirements of pregnancy and lactation specifically, so it is generally assumed that the indispensable amino acid needs are increased in the same proportions as the increased protein needs.

Infections and stressful stimuli, such as severe thermal or physical injury, are among factors that increase individual protein and amino acid needs.[9] In these conditions, maintenance needs are increased because of increased rates of protein and amino acid catabolism and increased losses, such as those that occur with burns. These responses are frequently compounded by a loss of appetite and reduced food intake. Despite the clear-cut evidence for a greater protein need during periods of infection and stress, exact recommendations are not available. On the basis of some studies, a reasonable estimate is a 20% to 30% increase in total protein after an infection (30% to 50% in the case of diarrhea) and during the recovery period, which is 2 to 3 times longer than the duration of the illness.[18]

Although athletic activity and heavy physical work increase energy needs, whether the need for protein is also increased once the energy needs are met is not clear. In theory, both endurance and resistance exercise increase protein and amino acid needs. With endurance exercise training, an acute increase in branched-chain amino acid oxidation has been measured, but in the resting state, a decrease has been observed and overall nitrogen balance is maintained when the RDA for protein is consumed, provided that energy intake is sufficient.[19] This is commensurate with the observation that endurance/aerobic exercise does not build muscle and improves protein utilization. Resistance exercise, in contrast, promotes muscle hypertrophy. Athletes undertaking intense endurance or resistance exercise appear to require 1.2 to 1.7 g/kg per day to remain in nitrogen balance.[20] Nonetheless, chronic studies in which higher amounts of protein have been provided have not been able to demonstrate significantly greater increases in muscle mass.[21] Recent studies have demonstrated that the timing of the feed in relation to the exercise bout, the amino acid composition of the protein, and the digestibility of the protein may interact to determine the degree of muscle anabolism.[22,23] Well-controlled studies in which the effects of these dietary variables on muscle accretion have been followed chronically have not been performed. It is fair to say, however, that provided individuals consume a well-balanced diet (in which approximately 15%–20% of the total energy content is made up of proteins), the increased food consumption that usually accompanies the increased energy needs of physical activity ensures that protein intake also is increased. Thus, any increased needs will be met without the need for specific supplements or a change in the composition of the diet. Increased protein intake, in itself, will not increase skeletal muscle protein deposition.

Protein requirements are increased in infants and children undergoing catch-up growth.[9,11] The additional amount of protein that must be supplied depends on the desired rate and composition of weight gain. With intensive supplementation, rates of weight gain up to 20 g/kg per day can be achieved in severely wasted infants. The protein needs for depositing 1 g of tissue/kg per day depend on the composition of the tissue gain. Assuming a composition of 14% protein and that the efficiency of conversion of dietary protein to body protein is 70% during catch-up growth, 0.2 g/kg per day of protein above the maintenance protein requirement will be needed. Along with the additional protein, energy must also be supplemented to support catch-up growth. The level of energy supplementation that is needed varies depending on whether the child is wasted or not. Weight gain in a wasted child will have a larger proportion of fat, which carries a greater energy cost than an equivalent weight of lean body mass. However, when refeeding malnourished children by supplementing with both protein and energy, careful consideration must also be given to the overall protein-to-energy ratio of the diet, because it will influence the composition of the tissues deposited. Because children who are very wasted are often stunted, feedings with high protein-to-energy ratios to minimize the likelihood of excessive fat deposition are preferable. Catch-up growth also increases the requirements for micronutrients, such as zinc, magnesium, iron, and copper. Thus, the intake of these nutrients must be increased to maximize the efficiency of dietary protein utilization.

Effects of Insufficient and Excessive Protein Intake

Protein-energy malnutrition encompasses a wide spectrum of conditions, with kwashiorkor, the result of a greater deficiency of protein than energy intake, at one end of the spectrum, and marasmus, resulting primarily from an inadequate energy intake, at the other. Especially in kwashiorkor, the condition is often precipitated by the development of conditions that increase the child's protein needs, such as an infection or diarrhea. A marginally adequate diet, as weaning diets often can be in developing countries, does not meet these increased needs. Although protein-energy malnutrition is observed even in industrialized countries, such as the United States, the cause is usually associated with the presence of clinical conditions that decrease food intake or impair the digestion or absorption of food.

The effects of excessive dietary protein have not been studied extensively, and the findings are equivocal.[24] Extremely high protein intakes increase obligatory fluid loss, and if the fluid is not adequately replaced, dehydration can occur; this can be a concern in warmer climates, especially when activity levels are high. High intakes of protein, especially casein, by small infants can result in acidosis, aminoacidemia, and cylindruria. Although in adults, some studies have shown a correlation between protein intake and the prevalence of atherosclerosis or the risk of cancer, these findings have not been consistent. The positive associations seem to be more prevalent when meat is the source of dietary protein, and thus, a causative role for protein itself is uncertain. High protein intakes increase urinary calcium excretion, and consequently, it was believed that high protein intakes would promote bone demineralization or increase the risk of kidney stone formation. Recent prospective studies, however, have not been able to establish a causal relationship. The extent to which these findings and recommendations are pertinent to children is unknown. Given the paucity of data and the inconsistent nature of the conclusions derived from them, the only safe recommendation that can be made regarding high protein intakes is that the maximal amounts of protein intake should be dictated by the overall macronutrient composition of the diet and should fall within the AMDR.[24]

References

1. Denne SC, Kalhan S. Leucine metabolism in human newborns. *Am J Physiol.* 1987;253: e608–e615

2. Denne SC, Rossi EM, Kalhan SC. Leucine kinetics during feeding in normal newborns. *Pediatr Res.* 1991;30:23–27

3. Matthews DE. Observations of branched-chain amino acid administration in humans. *J Nutr.* 2005;135:1580S–1584S

4. Waterlow JC, Jackson AA. Nutrition and protein turnover in man. *Br Med Bull.* 1981;37:5–10

5. Jackson AA. The glycine story. *Eur J Clin Nutr.* 1991;45:59–65

6. Alpers DH. Glutamine: do the data support the cause for glutamine supplementation in humans? *Gastroenterology.* 2006;130:S106–S116

7. Lourenco R, Camilo ME. Taurine: a conditionally essential amino acid in humans? An overview in health and disease. *Nutr Hosp.* 2002;17:262–270

8. Borum PR. Carnitine in neonatal nutrition. *J Child Neurol.* 1995;10(Suppl 2):S25–S31

9. FAO/WHO/UNU Expert Consultation. Protein and Amino Acid requirements in Human Nutrition. WHO Technical Bulletin #724. Geneva, Switzerland: World Health Organization; 2007

10. Institute of Medicine. Protein and amino acids. In: *Dietary Reference Intakes for Energy, Carbohydrates, Fiber, Fat, Fatty Acids, Cholesterol, Protein, and Amino Acids (Macronutrients).* Washington, DC: National Academies Press; 2005:589–768

11. Dewey KG, Beaton G, Fjeld C, Lonnerdal B, Reeds P. Protein requirements of infants and children. *Eur J Clin Nutr.* 1996;50(Suppl 1):S119–S147

12. Rigo J, Ziegler EE. *Protein and Energy Requirements in Infancy and Childhood*. Basel, Switzerland: Karger; and Vevey, Switzerland: Nestlé Nutrition Institute; 2006

13. Butte NF, Hopkinson JM, Wong WW, Smith EO, Ellis KJ. Body composition during the first 2 years of life: an updated reference. *Pediatr Res*. 2000;47:578–585

14. Ellis KJ, Shypailo RJ, Abrams SA, Wong WW. The reference child and adolescent models of body composition. A contemporary comparison. *Ann N Y Acad Sci*. 2000;904:374–382

15. Food and Agriculture Organization of the United Nations, World Health Organization. *Protein Quality Evaluation*. Rome, Italy: Food and Agriculture Organization of the United Nations; 1991

16. Lonnerdal B. Nutritional aspects of soy formula. *Acta Paediatr Suppl*. 1994;402:105–108

17. Dubois S, Coulombe C, Pencharz P, Pinsonneault O, Duquette MP. Ability of the Higgins Nutrition Intervention Program to improve adolescent pregnancy outcome. *J Am Diet Assoc*. 1997;97:871–878

18. Scrimshaw NS. Effect of infection on nutritional status. *Proc Natl Sci Counc Repub China B*. 1992;16:46–64

19. Gaine PC, Viesselman CT, Pikosky MA, et al. Aerobic exercise training decreases leucine oxidation at rest in healthy adults. *J Nutr*. 2005;135:1088–1092

20. Lemon PW. Effects of exercise on dietary protein requirements. *Int J Sport Nutr*. 1998; 8:426–447

21. Lemon PW, Proctor DN. Protein intake and athletic performance. *Sports Med*. 1991;12: 313–325

22. Lemon PW, Berardi JM, Noreen EE. The role of protein and amino acid supplements in the athlete's diet: does type or timing of ingestion matter? *Curr Sports Med Rep*. 2002;1:214–221

23. Tipton KD, Wolfe RR. Protein and amino acids for athletes. *J Sports Sci*. 2004;22:65–79

24. Institute of Medicine. Macronutrients and healthful diets. In: *Dietary Reference Intakes for Energy, Carbohydrates, Fiber, Fat, Fatty Acids, Cholesterol, Protein, and Amino Acids (Macronutrients)*. Washington, DC: National Academies Press; 2005;769–879

15 Carbohydrate and Dietary Fiber

Carbohydrate provides 50% to 60% of the calories consumed by the average American. Although relatively little carbohydrate is needed in the diet, carbohydrate spares protein and fat being metabolized for calories. The principal dietary carbohydrates are sugars and starches. Sugars (simple carbohydrates) include monosaccharides (glucose, galactose, and fructose) and disaccharides (lactose, sucrose, maltose, and trehalose). Starches (complex carbohydrates—polysaccharides) are the storage carbohydrates of plants and consist of sugars (eg, glucose) linked together.

Digestion of Disaccharides and Starches

Lactose and sucrose are hydrolyzed to monosaccharides via lactase and sucrase, respectively (Fig 15.1). Lactase activity increases substantially during the third trimester, whereas sucrase activity is already at levels found at birth by the onset of the last trimester.[1,2] Starch digestion is more complex. The production of amylase by the pancreas increases to mature levels during the first year of life.[3] Salivary, and more likely, mucosal enzymes (glucoamylase, sucrase, isomaltase) are responsible for starch digestion in young infants.[3,4] Pancreatic and salivary amylase hydrolyze the interior alpha-1,4 bonds (Fig 15.1). Glucoamylase sequentially cleaves alpha-1,4 bonds from the nonreducing end of the molecule (Fig 15.1).[5] Glucoamylase is most active against starches between 5 and 9 glucose residues in length.[5] Isomaltase (alpha-dextrinase) and sucrase also have some activity in this regard. Isomaltase is primarily responsible for cleaving the alpha-1,6 bonds.

Absorption of Monosaccharides

The end products of disaccharide and starch digestion are monosaccharides. These are absorbed in the small intestine. The transport of monosaccharides into and out of the intestinal epithelial cell is accomplished via transporters.[6] Glutamate transporter (GLUT) 1 actively transports glucose and galactose across the brush border, whereas GLUT 5 is responsible for passive absorption of fructose. GLUT 2 releases the sugars across the basolateral membrane of the enterocyte. Carbohydrates that are not absorbed in the small intestine are fermented by colonic bacteria and converted to short-chain fatty acids, which are in turn absorbed by the colon.[7]

Fig 15.1

Pancreatic and salivary amylase hydrolyze interior alpha-1,4 bonds (⚭).Glucoamylase sequentially cleaves alpha-1,4 bonds from the non-reducing end of the molecule. The reducing end is designated: ⬤ Isomaltase and sucrase also have some activity in this regard. Isomaltase is primarily responsible for cleaving the alpha-1,6 bonds ( ). Lactose and sucrose are hydrolyzed by their respective hydrolases. The monosaccharides are transported across the epithelial surface by various active or passive means and then extruded across the basolateral membrane.

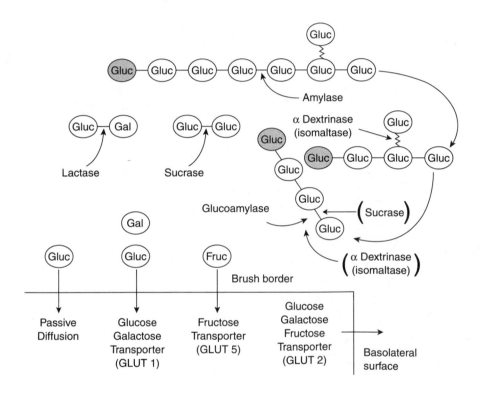

Metabolism of Glucose

Dietary carbohydrates are converted to glucose in the liver. It is the most abundant carbohydrate. Most glucose is metabolized for energy.[8] Quantitatively, the brain is the largest utilizer of glucose as an energy source. There are few data that allow the limits of carbohydrate intake to be defined.[8] Amino acids and glycerol from lipids can be converted to glucose. However, in the case of amino acids, this potentially shunts substrate away from protein synthesis. Glucose synthesis from both amino acids and glycerol is not very metabolically efficient. Estimates of minimum glucose requirements based on cerebral glucose utilization are shown in Table 15.1.

The upper limits of glucose requirements should be defined by the amount that defines a minimal need for fat and protein and maximum glucose oxidation rates (Table 15.2).[8] These are theoretical limits, because they presume the minimal intake of protein and fat with glucose providing essentially all energy needs. However, doing so can be associated with adverse effects, such as hyperglycemia.

Table 15.1
Estimates of Glucose Consumption by the Brain*

	Body Weight (kg)	Brain Weight (g)	Glucose Consumption		
			$(mg \cdot kg^{-1}) \cdot min^{-1}$	$(g \cdot kg^{-1}) \cdot day^{-1}$	g/day
Newborn	3.2	399	6.0	11.5	37
1 year	10.0	997	7.0	10.1	101
5 years	19.0	1266	4.7	6.8	129
Adolescent	50.0	1360	1.9	2.7	135
Adult	70.0	1400	1.0	1.4	98

* Adapted from Kalhan and Kilic.[8]

Table 15.2
Upper Limit* of Carbohydrate Intake for Infants and Children[†]

Age	Total Energy Expenditure[‡] $(kcal \cdot kg^{-1}) \cdot day^{-1}$	Carbohydrate Equivalent[§] $(g \cdot kg^{-1}) \cdot day^{-1}$
Newborn	73	19
1–3 y	85	22
4–6 y	68	18
12–13 y	55	14
18–19 y	44	12
Adult	35	9

* Upper limit should be determined by the minimal need for protein and fat obtained. Therefore, the upper limits described here are theoretically maximal to meet all the energy needs.

† Adapted from Kalhan and Kilic.[8]

‡ Average of data for boys and girls. Estimate based on double-labeled water method.

§ Carbohydrate equivalent = total energy expenditure/3.8, assuming each g of carbohydrate yields 3.8 kcal.

Glucose that is not immediately oxidized can be polymerized to form glycogen. Current data suggest that in the human newborn infant, gluconeogenesis appears soon after birth and contributes 30% to 70% to glucose produced.[9] As noted above, most glucose is used by the central nervous system. Storage and mobilization of glycogen are under the hormonal control of insulin and glucagon (see Chapter 31: Hypoglycemia, and Chapter 30: Diabetes Mellitus). During periods of fasting, the liver and kidney can mobilize glucose from glycogen. If fasting is prolonged, hepatic glycogen stores will be drained in a few hours, and gluconeogenesis from lactate, alanine, glycerol, and glutamine must be stimulated to maintain euglycemia.[10] The newborn infant has approximately 34 g of glycogen, only 6 g of which is in the liver and is accumulated during the last weeks of fetal life. Hepatic glycogen is totally depleted during the first few days postnatally and then reaccumulates. Carbohydrate-free diets lead to ketosis, as does fasting. Ketosis occurs when carbohydrate intake drops below approximately 10% of total calories. It occurs more readily in children than in adults during fasting or when extremely low-carbohydrate diets are consumed. Low-carbohydrate diets and low-carbohydrate, high-fat diets (the ketogenic diet [see Chapter 47]) have been used in the treatment of epilepsy and as a diagnostic test for ketotic hypoglycemia.

In addition to glycogen stores in the liver and skeletal muscle, the body contains carbohydrate in many different forms. These include mucopolysaccharides (structural carbohydrates that are important constituents of connective and collagenous tissues) and components of nucleic acids, glycoproteins, glycolipids, and various hormones and enzymes.

Recently, abnormalities in these structural carbohydrates have been associated with specific symptoms or disorders. Genetic defects in glycoprotein metabolism usually result in neurologic symptoms. However, defects in glycoprotein biosynthesis (the carbohydrate-deficient glycoprotein syndromes) also manifest as hypoglycemia, protein-losing enteropathy, and hepatic pathology.[11] In these conditions, the N-glycosylation pathway is affected, resulting in alterations in the number or structure of sugar chains on the proteins. The diagnosis often can be made via isoelectric focusing of transferrin.[11]

Lactose

Lactose is present in almost all mammalian milks and is the major carbohydrate consumed by young infants.[12] However, at an early age, infants in the United States are fed a variety of other carbohydrates, including sucrose, natural and modified starches, starch hydrolysates, and small amounts of monosaccharides and indigestible carbohydrate (ie, fiber). Lactase, an enzyme on the brush border of the enterocyte in the small intestine, hydrolyzes the disaccharide lactose into the monosaccharides glucose and galactose.

Although a congenital form of lactase deficiency exists (also termed primary lactase deficiency), it is extremely rare. It manifests at birth in the presence of a lactose-containing diet. Much more commonly, lactase activity begins to decrease in a genetically programmed fashion so that by adulthood in many ethnic groups, it is low.[13] The highest prevalence of low lactase activity is found in the Far East. The prevalence in the United States varies according to ethnicity; it is approximately 15% to 25% in white people, approximately 80% in black people, approximately 53% in Hispanic people, and approximately 90% in Asian people.[13] The age at which lactase activity begins to decrease also is related to ethnicity. In the United States, the decrease usually begins to occur around 3 to 7 years of age; ethnic groups with a higher prevalence of lactase deficiency typically have an earlier decrease. People with low lactase activity often do not have symptoms of lactose intolerance, such as flatulence, bloating, abdominal pain, and nausea and diarrhea (also see Chapter 1).[14] In fact, most people with low lactase activity can tolerate some lactose intake, particularly when it is part of a meal.

Symptoms of lactase intolerance are caused by lactose that escapes digestion in the small intestine and passes into the colon, where it is fermented by enteric bacteria forming organic acids, hydrogen, carbon monoxide, and methane.[15] The gases may cause bloating and pain, and the unabsorbed sugar and acids may cause an increase in osmotic pressure, which may result in osmotic diarrhea. Lactose malabsorption may be detected by an increase in expired breath hydrogen after lactose ingestion.[16] As noted previously, however, the likelihood of developing symptoms depends on the amount of residual lactase activity, the amount of lactose ingested, and the composition of the meal.

Lactase activity also can be diminished secondary to mucosal injury in the small intestine (also termed secondary lactase deficiency). This occurs most commonly in infants with viral gastroenteritis. It is a consequence of damage to the intestinal villi and resolves with resolution of the illness. In the otherwise healthy infant, lactase deficiency may not be clinically significant. For example, most infants with rotavirus are not lactose intolerant.[17]

However, infants who have had inadequate weight gain or prolonged diarrhea may have clinical lactose intolerance until the illness resolves. Using a lactose-free formula until the infant recovers from diarrhea may be beneficial.[18] The intolerance usually lasts 1 to 2 weeks, except in severe cases. Carbohydrate malabsorption (including that from lactose) is detected by testing the pH of the stool by using phenaphthazine paper (pH <5.5 indicates carbohydrate fermentation attributable to malabsorption) and testing for glucose (on the basis of copper reduction) using the same products used to test for glucose in the urine. The glucose derives from the breakdown of lactose by the colonic flora. It is important to test the watery part of the stool, because the formed part of the stool is likely to give a false-negative result. This test can be used to detect the presence of other sugars, such as sucrose and starches, because bacteria will degrade some proportion of these sugars to glucose. Detectable carbohydrate malabsorption should be treated to reduce fluid losses resulting from osmotic diarrhea with the consequent risks of dehydration and acidosis.

Very preterm (<32 weeks' gestation) infants may be a special case in which lactose intolerance may be clinically significant. Preterm infants do not digest lactose as well as other sugars, such as glucose polymers.[19] Recent studies suggest that the feeding of formula containing lactose as the sole carbohydrate to very preterm infants may be associated with an increased risk of feeding intolerance and that the risk of feeding intolerance is inversely related to lactase activity.[20,21] However, one study in preterm infants reported increased lactase activity in breastfed infants compared with formula-fed infants.[21] Thus, lactose feeding from human milk may be less problematic than from formula.[21]

Starches

As noted above, starches are the storage carbohydrate of plants consisting of amylose (a linear [1-4] glucan) and amylopectin (a [1-4] glucan with [1-6] branch points). Starches that contain 10 or more sugars linked glycosidically in branched or unbranched chains are arbitrarily termed polysaccharides. The larger the starch, the less osmotically active.

Corn syrup is a generic term for products derived from cornstarch by hydrolysis with acid or enzymes. These products are classified according to their chemical-reducing power relative to glucose, which has a dextrose equivalent (DE) of 100%. The DE of corn syrups ranges from less than 20% to more than 95%. A low-DE corn syrup is somewhat hydrolyzed and is, therefore, more like starch than a high-DE corn syrup. Glucose polymer (or maltodextrin) is another term for corn syrup that has been hydrolyzed to (usually) a high-DE carbohydrate. They often are added to formulas to provide additional calories without greatly increasing the osmolality of the feeding. Approximately 20% to 25% of infants in the United States are fed lactose-free soy isolate formulas containing sucrose or corn-syrup solids or a combination of both as the carbohydrate source(s).

Modified food starches possess certain technical properties, such as altered viscosity and "mouth feel," freeze-thaw stability, gel clarity, and stability in acid products. In animal models, caloric availability of modified food starches is similar to unmodified starches. Modified food starches appear to be safe and reasonably well digested by human infants, although concern has been raised about the long-term implications of their feeding.[22,23] Many powdered special formulas and strained foods contain modified corn or tapioca starches. Special formulas may provide approximately 15% of total calories in the form of modified starch, which is used to facilitate suspension of insoluble nutrients during feeding. The amount of modified starch in a few commercial infant desserts may amount to as much as 45% of the total content of the solids.

Fiber

Fiber, also called bulk or roughage, is defined as the endogenous components of plant materials in the diet that are resistant to digestion by enzymes produced by humans.[24,25] Fiber is composed predominantly of nonstarch polysaccharides and nonpolysaccharides (mainly lignins). Nonstarch polysaccharides include cellulose and noncellulosic polysaccharides (eg, hemicelluloses, pectins, gums, mucilages). This definition excludes other substances in the plant materials, such as phytates, cutins, saponins, lectins, proteins, waxes, silicon, and other organic constituents. Fibers are present in the cell walls of all plants.

Fiber also is classified as soluble (some hemicelluloses, pectins, gums, and mucilages) or insoluble (most hemicelluloses, celluloses, and lignins). Soluble fiber, found in beans, fruits, psyllium, and oat products, dissolves in water. Soluble fiber is metabolized in the colon and, to a lesser extent, in the small intestine by the enzymatic action of anaerobic bacteria. Soluble fibers have been shown to increase stool size moderately; decrease intestinal transit time, gastric emptying, and glucose absorption; and decrease serum cholesterol (see "Potential Benefits of Fiber Intake," p 350).[26,27] Insoluble fiber, found in whole-grain products and vegetables, does not dissolve. It consists of nondigestible polysaccharide and lignins. The intestinal flora does not significantly metabolize insoluble fibers. Insoluble fibers significantly increase fecal bulk, decrease intestinal transit time, delay glucose absorption, and slow the process of starch hydrolysis.[26,27]

Crude fiber refers to the residue left after strong acid and base hydrolysis of plant material. This process dissolves pectin, gums, mucilages, and most of the hemicellulose. Thus, crude fiber is mainly a measure of cellulose and lignin and tends to underestimate the total amount of fiber in the food. Most food composition tables give only crude fiber values. Appendix P lists the fiber content of common foods. It has been estimated in adults that 5% to 10% of dietary starch is "resistant starch," which is not digested in the small intestine and, therefore, reaches the colon in its intact form.[28] Young infants have a limited ability to digest starches, such as those in cereal.[29–31] Dietary fiber and related compounds are summarized in Table 15.3.

Table 15.3
Dietary Fiber and Related Compounds*

Components

Major Components
   Nonstarch polysaccharides
      Celluloses
      Noncelluloses: hemicelluloses, pectins, gums, mucilages
   Nonpolysaccharides: lignins

Minor components   Phytates, cutins, saponins, lectins, protein, waxes, silicon

Related components
   Resistant starch and protein
   Lignans

Classification of Solubility
Soluble (highly fermented): pectins, gums, mucilages, and some hemicelluloses
Insoluble (poorly fermented): celluloses, lignins, and most hemicelluloses

* Adapted from Kim.[25]

Potential Benefits of Fiber Intake

The current interest in fiber was stimulated in part by the suggestion that fiber could help prevent certain diseases common in the United States, such as cancer of the colon, irritable bowel syndrome, constipation, obesity, and coronary heart disease. Epidemiologic studies noted that Africans in rural areas where fiber intake was high rarely had these diseases. However, as urban migration has increased, the adoption of Western habits and dietary patterns has coincided with the increased incidence of Western diseases. A high-fiber diet increases fecal bulk, produces softer and more frequent stools, and speeds transit through the intestine.

A number of hypotheses have been promulgated regarding how increased dietary fiber could reduce the risk of colorectal carcinoma. These include dilution of potential carcinogens, reduced contact time with carcinogens because of faster transit, and inhibition of tumor cell lines.[25] Initial review of the data suggested a protective effect in some populations but not in others.[25] Recent studies call into question the efficacy of fiber in preventing recurrence of colorectal cancer.[32]

Increasing fiber intake has been used as a treatment in children with recurrent abdominal pain.[33] In a double-blind study, supplementation with corn fiber was associated with a 50% decrease in the frequency of abdominal pain.[33] Because of its ability to hold water, increasing fiber intake reduces the risk of constipation. It has been estimated that 5 to 7 g/day is needed to facilitate normal stooling in children.[34]

Obesity is less prevalent in populations that consume most carbohydrate as complex carbohydrate and have a high fiber intake. The lower energy density of this type of diet may increase satiety. However, in many cultures in which this type of diet is common, the total energy intake is low by Western standards. Given the increasing prevalence of childhood obesity in the United States, there is interest on the role of fiber in reducing the risk of obesity.[35] There are several explanations for the role of fiber in preventing obesity, but none have been proven unequivocally. These include effects on: 1) reducing food intake because of earlier satiety achieved with a larger volume in the stomach and intestine but reduced caloric density compared with a high-fat diet as well as slower gastric emptying; 2) reducing absorption of carbohydrate and protein (but not fat) related to faster transit through the small intestinal; and 3) flattening the insulin response curve to carbohydrate, thereby reducing the appetite stimulating effects of insulin.[35]

Interpretation of the potential relationship between fiber intake and the development of obesity in children is problematic because of a lack of data and limitations on the interpretation of available data. For example, fiber and carbohydrate intake in 1 study were not separated from one another.[35] There is some preliminary evidence that fiber supplementation may aid in weight reduction for children with obesity.[35,36] Clearly, more work is needed in this area.

Atherosclerosis has its origins in childhood. Fatty streaks begin in the coronary arteries at about the age of 10 years and in the abdominal aorta at

2 years of age.[37,38] Given that studies suggest a direct correlation between the percent of calories from saturated fat and cholesterol in children's diets and their blood cholesterol concentration, the potential effects of fiber on reducing blood lipids and, thereby, the risk of heart disease are of great interest.[37]

The lipid-lowering effect is seen with soluble fiber but not with the insoluble form (see Table 15.3). A review of the current data strongly suggests that the addition of soluble fiber to a step 1 lipid-lowering diet can reduce further certain fractions of blood lipids and/or increase serum high-density lipoprotein (HDL) concentration.[37] The degree of reduction, the fraction of lipid that is reduced, and the effect on serum HDL concentration may be dependent on the type of soluble fiber used. Supplementation with psyllium appeared to decrease the low-density lipoprotein concentration and increase the HDL concentration in serum in 48 children 2 to 11 years of age with moderate hypercholesterolemia.[37,39]

Potential Adverse Effects of Fiber Intake

Objections have been made to an increased fiber intake for children. One of the concerns has been that fiber may compromise intake of other nutrients. It has been shown in young infants that addition of cereal in the amounts used to treat gastroesophageal reflux decreases total daily formula intake.[30] On the other hand, the addition of a soy polysaccharide to infant formula does not appear to affect the intake of infants with diarrhea.[40]

Another concern is that fiber supplementation will affect the absorption of nutrients, particularly micronutrients. Some plant foods contain phytate (inositol hexaphosphate), which serves as the storage form of phosphorus for plants and may form insoluble compounds with minerals such as calcium, iron, copper, magnesium, and zinc, rendering them unavailable for normal absorption and metabolism.[41] Although phytate is destroyed in the process of leavening bread, it remains intact in many foods, such as legumes and grains. Consumption of primarily plant-based diets is considered to be a major etiologic factor for mineral deficiencies on a global basis.

Although it is possible that children on high-fiber diets may have a deficiency of these minerals, especially in situations in which mineral intake is low, children in the United States on a varied, complete dietary regimen are unlikely to have mineral deficiencies regardless of fiber intake.[41] Some foods also contain oxalic acid (spinach, rhubarb, chards, etc), which interferes with absorption of iron and calcium, especially in individuals on high-fiber diets.[41] A review of the data suggests that addition of fiber to an otherwise normal omnivorous diet for a child in the United States does not adversely affect micronutrient status, including that of iron.[41] This has recently been confirmed by a study in adolescents using dietary recall to evaluate fiber intake.[42]

Current Dietary Recommendations

It has been recommended that between 6 and 12 months of age, whole cereals, green vegetables, and legumes be introduced gradually, increasing the fiber in the diet to 5 g/day by the first birthday.[43] With the introduction of solid foods into the diet of the older child, whole-grain cereals, breads, fruits, and vegetables should be included. Recommendations for providing increased fiber to children are given in Appendix P.

The American Health Foundation has set forth a recommendation for the amount of fiber in a child's diet.[44] The recommendation for children older than 2 years is an intake of fiber approximately equivalent to the child's age plus 5 g/day. A safe range was believed to be age plus 10 g/day.[44] This "age plus 5" guideline results in a gradual increase of fiber intake over time, with 17-year-olds eating 22 g/day. The amount recommended for an older adolescent is also within the range recommended by the National Cancer Institute.[41] These recommendations were endorsed at a conference on dietary fiber in childhood.[45] More recently, the US Department of Health and Human Services and US Department of Agriculture published the *Dietary Guidelines for Americans, 2005,* which recommended a total fiber intake of ≥14 g/1000 kcal consumed.[46] The Institute of Medicine report on Dietary Reference Intakes in 2002 established the Recommended Dietary Allowance for fiber for children. Table 15.4 provides the daily recommended fiber intake by age and gender.[47] Currently, a diet that emphasizes high-fiber, low-calorie foods to the exclusion of the other common food groups is not recommended for children.

Table 15.4
Daily Recommended Intake of Fiber[47]

Gender/Age	Fiber (g)
1–3 y	19
4–8 y	25

9–13 y
  Female
  Male
	
	26
	31

14–18 y
  Female
  Male
	
	26
	38

References

1. Weaver LT, Laker MF, Nelson R. Neonatal intestinal lactase activity. *Arch Dis Child.* 1986;61:896–869

2. Antonowicz I, Chang SK, Grand RJ. Development and distribution of lysosomal enzymes and disaccharidases in human fetal intestine. *Gastroenterology.* 1974;67:51–58

3. Raul F, Lacroix B, Aprahamian M. Longitudinal distribution of brush border hydrolases and morphological maturation in the intestine of the preterm infant. *Early Hum Dev.* 1986;13: 225–234

4. Shulman RJ, Kerzner B, Sloan HR, et al. Absorption and oxidation of glucose polymers of different lengths in young infants. *Pediatr Res.* 1986;20:740–743

5. Eggermont E. The hydrolysis of naturally occurring alpha-glucosides by the human intestinal mucosa. *Eur J Biochem.* 1969;9:483–487

6. Ferraris RP, Diamond J. Regulation of intestinal sugar transport. *Physiol Rev.* 1997;77: 257–302

7. Cummings JH, Macfarlane GT. Colonic microflora: nutrition and health. *Nutrition.* 1997;13:476–478

8. Kalhan SC, Kilic I. Carbohydrate as nutrient in the infant and child: range of acceptable intake. *Eur J Clin Nutr.* 1999;53:S94–S100

9. Kalhan S, Parimi P. Gluconeogenesis in the fetus and neonate. *Semin Perinatol.* 2000;24: 94–106

10. Halliday D, Bodamer OA. Measurement of glucose turnover—implications for the study of inborn errors of metabolism. *Eur J Pediatr.* 1997;156:S35–S38

11. Freese HH. Disorders in protein glycosylation and potential therapy: tip of an iceberg? *J Pediatr.* 1998;133:593–600

12. American Academy of Pediatrics, Committee on Nutrition. Practical significance of lactose intolerance in children: supplement. *Pediatrics.* 1990;86(Suppl):643–644

13. Sahi T. Genetics and epidemiology of adult-type hypolactasia. *Scand J Gastroenterol Suppl.* 1994;202:7–20

14. Carroccio A, Montalto G, Cavera G, Notarbatolo A. Lactose intolerance and self-reported milk intolerance: relationship with lactose maldigestion and nutrient intake. Lactase Deficiency Study Group. *J Am Coll Nutr.* 1998;17:631–636

15. American Academy of Pediatrics, Committee on Nutrition. The practical significance of lactose intolerance in children. *Pediatrics.* 1978;62:240–245

16. Strocchi A, Corazza GR, Ellis CJ, Gasbarrini G, Levitt MD. Detection of malabsorption of low doses of carbohydrate: accuracy of various breath H2 criteria. *Gastroenterology.* 1993;105:1404–1410

17. Rings EH, Grand RJ, Buller HA. Lactose intolerance and lactase deficiency in children. *Curr Opin Pediatr.* 1994;6:562–567

18. Caballero B, Solomons NW. Lactose-reduced formulas for the treatment of persistent diarrhea. *Pediatrics.* 1990;86:645–646

19. Shulman RJ, Feste A, Ou C. Absorption of lactose, glucose polymers, or combination in premature infants. *J Pediatr.* 1995;127:626–631

20. Griffin MP, Hansen JW. Can the elimination of lactose from formula improve feeding tolerance in premature infants? *J Pediatr.* 1999;135:587–592

21. Shulman RJ, Schanler RJ, Lau C, Heitkemper M, Ou C-N, Smith EO. Early feeding, feeding tolerance, and lactase activity in preterm infants. *J Pediatr.* 1998;133:645–649

22. Filer LJ Jr. Modified food starch—an update. *J Am Diet Assoc.* 1988;88:342–344

23. Lanciers S, Mehta DI, Blecker U, Lebenthal E. Modified food starches in baby foods. *J Pediatr.* 1998;65:541–546

24. Asp NG. Definition and analysis of dietary fiber. *Scand J Gastroenterol Suppl.* 1987;129: 16–20

25. Kim YI. AGA technical review: impact of dietary fiber on colon cancer occurrence. *Gastroenterology.* 2000;118:1235–1257

26. Muir JG, Yeow EG, Keogh J, et al. Combining wheat bran with resistant starch has more beneficial effects on fecal indexes than does wheat bran alone. *Am J Clin Nutr.* 2004;79:1020–1028

27. Hillemeier C. An overview of the effects of dietary fiber on gastrointestinal transit. *Pediatrics.* 1995;96:997–999

28. Stephen AM, Haddad AC, Phillips SF. Passage of carbohydrate into the colon. Direct measurements in humans. *Gastroenterology.* 1983;85:589–595

29. Bianchi Porro G, Parente F, Sangaletti O. Lactose intolerance in adults with chronic unspecific abdominal complaints. *Hepatogastroenterology.* 1983;30:254–257

30. Shulman RJ, Boutton TW, Klein PD. Impact of dietary cereal on nutrient absorption and fecal nitrogen loss in formula-fed infants. *J Pediatr.* 1991;118:39–43

31. Shulman RJ, Gannon N, Reeds PJ. Cereal feeding and its impact on the nitrogen economy of the infant. *Am J Clin Nutr.* 1995;62:969–972

32. Alberts DS, Martinez ME, Roe DJ, et al. Lack of effect of a high-fiber cereal supplement on the recurrence of colorectal adenomas. Phoenix Colon Cancer Prevention Physicians' Network. *N Engl J Med.* 2000;342:1156–1162

33. Feldman W, McGrath P, Hodgson C, Ritter H, Shipman RT. The use of dietary fiber in the management of simple, childhood, idiopathic, recurrent abdominal pain. Results in a prospective, double-blind, randomized, controlled trial. *Am J Dis Child.* 1985;139:1216–1218

34. Anderson JW, Smith BM, Gustafson NJ. Health benefits and practical aspects of high fiber diets. *Am J Clin Nutr.* 1994;59(5 Suppl):1242S–1247S

35. Kimm SY. The role or dietary fiber in the development and treatment of childhood obesity. *Pediatrics.* 1995;5:1010–1014

36. Gropper SS, Acosta PB. The therapeutic effect of fiber in treating obesity. *J Am Coll Nutr.* 1987;6:533–535

37. Kwiterovich PO. The role of fiber in the treatment of hypercholesterolemia in children and adolescents. *Pediatrics.* 1995;96:1005–1009

38. Strong JP, McGill HC Jr. The natural history of coronary atherosclerosis. *Am J Pathol.* 1962;40:37–49

39. Williams CL, Spark A, Haley N, Axelrad C, Strobino B. Effectiveness of a psyllium-enriched step I diet in hypercholesterolemic children. *Circulation.* 1991;84:2–6

40. Vanderhoof JA, Murray ND, Paule CL, Ostrom KM. Use of soy fiber in acute diarrhea in infants and toddlers. *Clin Pediatr (Phila)*. 1997;36:135–139

41. Williams CL, Bollella M. Is a high-fiber diet safe for children? *Pediatrics*. 1995;96:1014–1019

42. Nicklas TA, Myers L, O'Neil C, Gustafson N. Impact of dietary fat and fiber intake on nutrient intake of adolescents. *Pediatrics*. 2000;105(2):e21. Available at: http://pediatrics.aappublications.org/cgi/content/full/105/2/e21. Accessed August 15, 2007

43. Agostoni C, Riva E, Giovannini M. Dietary fiber in weaning foods of young children. *Pediatrics*. 1995;96:1002–1005

44. Williams CL, Bollella M, Wynder EL. A new recommendation for dietary fiber in childhood. *Pediatrics*. 1995;96:985–958

45. American Academy of Pediatrics. A summary of conference recommendations on dietary fiber in childhood. Conference on Dietary Fiber in Childhood, New York, May 24, 1994. *Pediatrics*. 1995;96(5 Pt 2):S1023–S1028

46. US Department of Health and Human Services, US Department of Agriculture. *Dietary Guidelines for Americans, 2005*. 6th ed. Washington, DC: US Government Printing Office; 2005

47. Institute of Medicine. *Dietary Reference Intakes for Energy, Carbohydrate, Fiber, Fat, Fatty Acids, Cholesterol, Protein, and Amino Acids (Macronutrients)*. Washington, DC: National Academies Press; 2005

16 Fats and Fatty Acids

General Considerations

The absolute fat requirement of the human species is the amount of essential fatty acids needed to maintain optimal fatty acid composition of all tissues and normal eicosanoid synthesis. At most, this requirement is no more than approximately 5% of an adequate energy intake. However, fat accounts for approximately 50% of the nonprotein energy content of both human milk and currently available infant formulas. This is thought to be necessary to ensure that total energy intake is adequate to support growth and optimal utilization of dietary protein. In theory, the energy supplied by fat could be supplied by carbohydrate, from which all fatty acids except the essential ones can be synthesized, but in practice, it is difficult to ensure an adequate energy intake without a fat intake considerably in excess of the requirement for essential fatty acids. In part, this is because the osmolality of such a diet containing simple carbohydrates (eg, mono- and disaccharides) will be sufficiently high to result in diarrhea, and such a diet containing more complex carbohydrates may not be fully digestible, particularly during early infancy. Moreover, because approximately 25% of the energy content of carbohydrate that is converted to fatty acids is consumed in the process of lipogenesis, metabolic efficiency is greater if nonprotein energy is provided as a mixture of fat and carbohydrate rather than predominately carbohydrate. Fat also facilitates the absorption, transport and delivery of fat-soluble vitamins and, in addition, is an important satiety factor. Considering these issues, participants in a recent workshop concluded that the lower limit of fat intake that can be recommended for infants and young children is 15% of total energy intake but that a more practical recommendation is approximately 30% of energy intake.[1] These issues are important in consideration of the age at which a prudent (ie, lower-fat) diet to reduce the risks of cardiovascular disease is recommended (see Chapter 45).

Dietary Fats

Triglycerides account for the largest proportion of dietary fat. Structurally, these have 3 fatty acid molecules esterified to a molecule of glycerol. They usually contain at least 2, often 3, different fatty acids. Other dietary fats include phospholipids, free fatty acids, monoglycerides and diglycerides, and sterols and other nonsaponifiable compounds. Together, these account for less than 2% of most dietary fats, including the fat of human milk.

Naturally occurring fatty acids generally contain from 4 to 26 carbon atoms. Some of these are saturated (ie, no double bonds in the carbon chain), some are monounsaturated (ie, 1 double bond) and some are polyunsaturated (ie, 2 or more double bonds). All have common names but, by general convention, are identified by their number of carbon atoms, their number of double bonds and the site of the first double bond from the terminal methyl group of the molecule. For example, palmitic acid, a saturated, 16-carbon fatty acid, is designated 16:0, and oleic acid, an 18-carbon, monounsaturated fatty acid with the single double bond located between the ninth and tenth carbon from the methyl terminal, is designated 18:1 ω-9. Linoleic acid, 18:2 ω-6, is an 18-carbon fatty acid with 2 double bonds, the first between the sixth and seventh carbon from the methyl terminal. The common names as well as the shorthand numerical designations of a number of common fatty acids are shown in Table 16.1.

Table 16.1
Common Names and Numerical Nomenclature of Selected Fatty Acids

Common Name	Numerical Nomenclature
Caprylic acid	8:0
Capric acid	10:0
Lauric acid	12:0
Myristic acid	14:0
Palmitic acid	16:0
Stearic acid	18:0
Oleic acid	18:1 ω-9*
Linoleic acid	18:2 ω-6*
Arachidonic acid	20:4 ω-6*
Linolenic acid[†]	18:3 ω-3*
Eicosapentaenoic acid	20:5 ω-3*
Docosahexaenoic acid	22:6 ω-3*

* ω-9, ω-6, and ω-3 are used interchangeably with n-9, n-6, and n-3.

† Usually designated α-linolenic acid to distinguish it from 18:3 ω-6 or γ-linolenic acid.

Unsaturated fatty acids are folded at the site of each double bond; in this configuration, they are said to be in the "cis" form. During processing, the molecules may become unfolded, transforming them to "trans fatty acids," which have been implicated in development of atherosclerosis. In general, the amount of trans fatty acids in infant formulas and foods is low; however, some processed fats (eg, margarines) may have a higher content. The trans fatty acid content of human milk also is reasonably low unless the mother's diet is high in trans fatty acids.

Fat Digestion, Absorption, Transport, and Metabolism

At birth, the infant must adjust from using carbohydrate as the major energy source to using a mixture of carbohydrate and fat. Hence, some aspects of fat digestion and metabolism are not fully developed, even at term. However, most term infants have sufficient fat digestive capacity to adjust satisfactorily. The limitations of fat digestion are somewhat more serious in the preterm infant, but there is little evidence that these infants have significant limitations beyond the first few weeks of life.

Fat digestion begins in the stomach, where lingual lipase hydrolyzes short- and medium-chain fatty acids from triglycerides and gastric lipase hydrolyzes long- as well as medium- and short-chain fatty acids.[2] The intragastric release of fatty acids with formation of monoglycerides delays gastric emptying and also facilitates emulsification of fat in the intestine. Further, some of the released short- and medium-chain fatty acids can be absorbed directly from the stomach.[3] On entry into the duodenum, the monoglycerides and free fatty acids stimulate release of a number of enteric hormones; among these is cholecystokinin, which stimulates contraction of the gall bladder and secretion of pancreatic enzymes.[4] Lingual and gastric lipases are largely inactivated in the duodenum and fat digestion continues through the action of pancreatic lipase and colipase, which may be somewhat limited during the first several weeks of life. Like lingual and gastric lipase, pancreatic lipase hydrolyzes triglycerides into free fatty acids and a monoglyceride.

Human milk contains 2 additional lipases, lipoprotein lipase and bile salt-stimulated lipase. The former is essential for formation of milk lipid in the mammary gland but plays little role in intestinal fat digestion.[5] The latter is present in much larger amounts. It is stable at a pH as low as 3.5 if bile salts are present, and it is not affected by intestinal proteolytic enzymes.[6] However, it is heat labile and, hence, is inactivated by pasteurization. This is thought to be a major factor in the poor fat absorption of infants fed pasteurized human milk.

Bile salt-stimulated lipase hydrolyzes triglyceride molecules into free fatty acids and glycerol rather than into free fatty acids and a monoglyceride. In theory, the bile salt-stimulated lipase of human milk can substitute for limited pancreatic lipase[7]; however, this does not appear to be of great importance for fat digestion of most infants. On the other hand, because bile salt-stimulated lipase is much more effective than pancreatic lipase in hydrolyzing esters of vitamin A, the primary form of this vitamin in human milk and most other foods, it may be important for optimal vitamin A absorption.[6]

The bile acids released by contraction of the gall bladder help emulsify the intestinal contents, thereby facilitating triglyceride hydrolysis and fat absorption. They are released primarily as salts of taurine or glycine and, hence, have both a water-soluble and a lipid-soluble portion. Alone, bile salts are poor emulsifiers, but in combination with monoglycerides, fatty acids, and phospholipids, they are quite effective. Thus, the fat hydrolysis that occurs in the stomach is an important adjunct to intestinal fat digestion.

The rate of synthesis of bile salts by newborn infants is less than that of adults and the bile salt pool of newborn infants is only approximately one fourth that of adults.[8] However, an intraduodenal concentration of bile salts below 2-to-5 mmol, the critical concentration required for the formation of micelles, is unusual.[9] Bile salts are actively reabsorbed in the distal ilium and transported back to the liver and eventually reappear in bile.[10] This enterohepatic circulation occurs approximately 6 times daily, with loss of only approximately 5% of the bile salts with each circulation.[11]

The mono- and diglycerides and long-chain fatty acids resulting from lipolysis as well as phospholipids, cholesterol, and fat-soluble vitamins are insoluble in water but are solubilized by physicochemical combination with bile salts to form micelles.[11] Because of their amphophilic nature, bile salts aggregate with their hydrophobic region to the interior, or core, of the micelle and their hydrophilic region to the exterior. The components of the micelle are transferred into the enteric mucosal cell, where long-chain fatty acids and monoglycerides are re-esterified into triglycerides and subsequently combined with protein, phospholipid, and cholesterol to form chylomicrons or very low-density lipoproteins. In this form, they enter the intestinal lymphatics, then the thoracic duct, and finally, the peripheral circulation.

Medium-chain triglycerides can be absorbed into the enteric cells without being hydrolyzed.[11] However, they also are rapidly hydrolyzed in the duodenum, and because the released medium-chain fatty acids are relatively soluble in the aqueous phase of the intestinal lumen, they can be absorbed without being incorporated into micelles. This makes them particularly useful in treatment of infants and children with a variety of pancreatic, hepatic, biliary, and intestinal disorders.

In general, long-chain unsaturated fatty acids are absorbed more readily than long-chain saturated fatty acids. The ease of absorption of palmitic acid (16:0), the most common dietary saturated fatty acid, is further related to its position in the triglyceride molecule.[12] The 2-monoglyceride of palmitic acid is well absorbed, but free palmitic acid released from the terminal positions of the triglyceride molecule is not. The palmitic acid content of human milk is esterified primarily to the 2-position of glycerol, and this probably accounts for its better absorption from human milk than from formulas containing butterfat. Synthetic fats, which contain palmitic acid primarily in the 2-position, are available[13-15] but, as yet, have not been used extensively in infant formula.[16]

In the circulation, chylomicrons acquire a specialized apoprotein from high-density lipoproteins.[11] This enables the triglycerides of the chylomicron to be hydrolyzed by lipoprotein lipase, the major enzyme responsible for intravascular hydrolysis of chylomicrons and very low-density lipoproteins.[17] Lipoprotein lipase is synthesized in most tissues, and the flow of fatty acids to tissues reflects its activity on the tissue's capillary bed. Concentrations of lipoprotein lipase are somewhat low in preterm and small-for-gestational-age infants,[18] but this does not appear to impose major difficulties except, perhaps, in tolerance of intravenously administered lipid emulsions.

The phospholipids and most of the apoproteins remaining after hydrolysis of chylomicron triglyceride are transferred to high-density lipoprotein, and the remainder of the apoproteins are transferred to other lipoprotein particles. This reduces the chylomicron to a fraction of its original mass, resulting in a chylomicron remnant that is removed from the circulation by specialized hepatic receptors.

Essential Fatty Acids

Fatty acids with double bonds in the ω-6 and ω-3 positions cannot be synthesized endogenously by the human species.[19] Therefore, specific ω-6 and ω-3 fatty acids or their precursors with double bonds at these positions (ie, linoleic acid [LA], 18:2 ω-6 and alpha-linolenic acid [ALA], 18:3 ω-3) must be provided in the diet. The precursor fatty acids are metabolized by the same series of desaturases and elongases to longer-chain, more unsaturated fatty acids,[20] referred to collectively as long-chain polyunsaturated fatty acids (LCPUFAs). This pathway is outlined in Fig 16.1. Important metabolites of 18:2 ω-6 and 18:3 ω-3 include 18:3 ω-6 (gamma-linolenic acid [GLA]), 20:3 ω-6 (dihomogamma-linolenic acid [DHLA]), 20:4 ω-6 (arachidonic acid [ARA]), 20:5 ω-3 (eicosapentaenoic acid [EPA]), and 22:6 ω-3 (docosahexaenoic acid [DHA]).

Fig 16.1
Metabolism of ω-6 and ω-3 fatty acids.

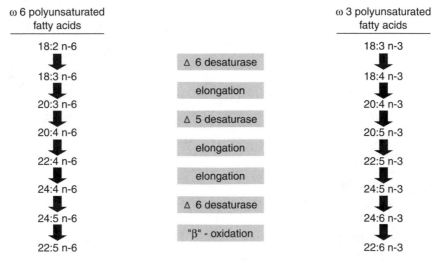

LA and ALA are present in many vegetable oils (see Table 16.2). In vivo, they are found in storage lipids, cell membrane phospholipids, intracellular cholesterol esters, and plasma lipids. The longer-chain, more unsaturated fatty acids synthesized from these precursors, in contrast, are found primarily in specific cell membrane phospholipids. DHLA, ARA, and EPA are immediate precursors of eicosanoids,[19,21] each being converted to a different series with different biologic activities and/or functions.

The same series of desaturases and elongases that catalyze desaturation and elongation of ω-6 and ω-3 fatty acids also catalyze desaturation and elongation of ω-9 fatty acids. The substrate preference of these enzymes is ω-3, ω-6, and finally, ω-9.[20] Thus, competition between the ω-9 fatty acids and either the ω-6 or ω-3 fatty acids is not an issue unless LA and/or ALA concentrations are low, as occurs in deficiency states. In this case, oleic acid (18:1 ω-9) is readily desaturated and elongated to eicosatrienoic acid (20:3 ω-9). The ratio of this fatty acid to 20:4 ω-6 (ie, the triene-tetraene ratio) is a useful diagnostic index of ω-6 fatty acid deficiency. This ratio usually is <0.1; a ratio of >0.4 is usually cited as indicative of deficiency,[22] but most believe that an even lower value (eg, >0.2) might be more reasonable. In the few documented cases of isolated 18:3 ω-3 deficiency in which it was measured, the triene-tetraene ratio was not elevated.

Table 16.2
Fatty Acid Composition of Common Vegetable Oils*

Fatty Acid	Canola	Corn	Coconut	Palm Olein	Safflower†	Soy	High-Oleic Sunflower
6:0–12:0	—	0.1	62.1	0.2	—	—	—
14.0	—	0.1	18.1	1.0	0.1	0.1	—
16:0	4.0	12.1	8.9	39.8	6.8	11.2	3.7
18:0	2.0	2.4	2.7	4.4	2.4	0.4	5.4
18:1 ω-9	55.0	32.1	6.4	42.5	12.5	22.0	81.3
18:2 ω-6	26.0	50.9	1.6	11.2	76.8	53.8	9.0
18:3 ω-3	10.0	0.9	—	0.2	0.1	7.5	—
Other	2.0	1.0	—	<1.6	<1.0	<1.0	<1.0

* Percent of total fatty acids (g/100 g).

† High-oleic safflower oil: approx 77% 18:1 and 12.5% 18:2.

LA (18:2 ω-6) has been recognized as an essential nutrient for the human species for more than 75 years.[23,24] The most common symptoms of deficiency are poor growth and scaly skin lesions. These symptoms are usually preceded by an increase in the triene-tetraene ratio of plasma lipids. It is now clear that ALA (18:3 ω-3) also is an essential nutrient. In animals, deficiency of this fatty acid results in visual and neurological abnormalities.[25-28] Neurological abnormalities also were observed in a human infant who had been maintained for several weeks on a parenteral nutrition regimen lacking ALA[29] and in elderly nursing home residents who were receiving intragastric feedings of an elemental formula with no ALA.[30]

Although symptoms related to deficiency of the 2 series of fatty acids seem to differ, many studies on which the description of ω-6 fatty acid deficiency are based used a fat-free or very low-fat diet rather than a diet deficient in only 18:2 ω-6. Thus, there may be some overlap in the symptoms of LA and ALA deficiency. The clinical symptoms of ω-6 fatty acid deficiency can be corrected by LA or ARA; those related to ALA deficiency can be corrected by ALA, EPA, or DHA. Thus, it is not clear whether LA and ALA serve specific functions other than as precursors of LCPUFAs.

LA usually constitutes between 8% and 20% of the total fatty acid content of human milk, and ALA usually constitutes between 0.5% and 1%.[31] Human milk also contains small amounts of a number of longer-chain, more unsaturated metabolites of both fatty acids, primarily ARA (20:4 ω-6) and DHA (22:6 ω-3). Maternal diet has a marked effect on the concentration of all fatty acids in human milk. The concentration of DHA in the milk of women consuming a typical North American diet is generally in the range of 0.1% to 0.3% of total fatty acids and the concentration of ARA ranges from 0.4% to 0.6%.[31] The milk of vegetarian women contains less DHA,[32] and that of women whose dietary fish consumption is high or who take DHA supplements is higher.[33-35] The ARA content of human milk is less variable and appears to be less dependent on maternal ARA intake, perhaps reflecting the relatively high LA intake of most populations.

Corn, coconut, safflower, and soy oils, as well as high-oleic safflower and sunflower oils and palm olein oil, are commonly used in the manufacture of infant formulas (see Table 16.2). All except coconut oil contain adequate amounts of LA, but only soybean oil contains an appreciable amount of ALA (6%–9% of total fatty acids). Canola oil, a component of many formulas available outside the United States, contains somewhat less LA and more ALA. Until recently, little emphasis was placed on the ALA content of infant formulas, and many with virtually no ALA were available. Current recommendations specify minimal intakes of LA ranging from 2.7% to 8% of total fat and maximum intakes ranging from 21% to 35% of total fatty acids.[36,37] The most recent recommendations for the minimum and maximum contents of ALA in term infant formulas are 1.75% and 4% of total fatty acids, respectively.[37] To maintain a reasonable balance between the 2 fatty acids, it is recommended that the LA-ALA ratio be between approximately 5 to 6 and 15 to 16.[36,37] The term and preterm infant formulas currently available in the United States contain approximately 20% of total fatty acids as LA and approximately 2% as ALA; hence, their LA-ALA ratios are approximately 10.

Long-Chain Polyunsaturated Fatty Acids
LCPUFAs are fatty acids with a chain length of more than 18 carbons and 2 or more double bonds. Those of primary interest for infant nutrition are

ARA and DHA, the plasma and erythrocyte lipid contents of which are higher in breastfed than formula-fed infants.[38-41] Because human milk contains these fatty acids but, until recently, formulas did not, the lower content of these fatty acids in plasma lipids of formula-fed infants were interpreted to indicate that the infant cannot synthesize enough of these fatty acids to meet ongoing needs. Past and concurrent observations of better cognitive function of breastfed versus formula-fed infants[42-45] focused attention on the possibility that the lower cognitive function of formula-fed infants might be related, in part, to inadequate intake of LCPUFAs.

This possibility is supported by the facts that ARA and DHA are the major ω-6 and ω-3 fatty acids of neural tissues[46-48] and that DHA is a major component of retinal photoreceptor membranes.[48] Further, the major supply of these fatty acids to the fetus during development is from maternal plasma.[49,50] Thus, the need for these fatty acids of the preterm infant who is born before or during the third trimester of pregnancy and, therefore, receives a limited supply of LCPUFA before birth is thought to be greater than that of the term infant. However, the daily rates of accumulation of these fatty acids in the developing central nervous system change minimally between mid-gestation and 1 year of age.[48]

On the basis of postmortem studies,[51-53] the cerebral content of DHA, but not ARA, is minimally but significantly lower in formula-fed term infants. However, the DHA content of the retina does not differ between breastfed and formula-fed infants,[53] perhaps because the concentration of this fatty acid in the retina reaches adult levels at approximately term, whereas adult concentrations in the cerebrum are not reached until much later.[48] In one of the postmortem studies, the cerebral DHA content of formula-fed infants reflected the ALA content of the formula the infant received before death.[52] This is consistent with data from studies in piglets showing that ALA intakes less than 0.7% of total energy result in low brain concentrations of DHA[54] as well as studies in infants showing a positive relationship between ALA intake and rates of DHA synthesis.[55]

Both term and preterm infants can convert LA to ARA and ALA to DHA.[55-60] This has been established by studies in which the precursor fatty acids labeled with stable isotopes of either carbon (^{13}C) or hydrogen (^{2}H) were administered to the infant and blood concentrations of the labeled fatty acids as well as labeled metabolites of each were measured by gas chromatography/mass spectroscopy (see Fig 16.1). The studies of Sauerwald et al[55,59] and Uauy et al[60] suggest that the overall ability of preterm infants to convert LA and ALA to LCPUFAs is at least as good as that of term infants.

On the other hand, there is considerable variability in conversion among both preterm and term infants fed the same formula. Moreover, because measurements of enrichment have been limited to plasma, which represents only a small fraction of the body pool of precursor as well as product fatty acids and may not be representative of fatty acid pools of other tissues, including the central nervous system, the amount of LCPUFAs that either preterm or term infants can synthesize is not known.

The higher DHA concentrations of plasma and erythrocyte lipids of breastfed infants and infants fed formulas supplemented with LCPUFAs versus infants fed unsupplemented formulas, including those with a relatively high ALA content,[38–41,61–63] suggest that the amounts of LCPUFAs formed endogenously are less than the amounts provided by human milk or supplemented formulas. However, the extent to which the concentration of individual LCPUFAs in plasma reflects the content of these fatty acids in tissues, particularly the brain, is not known.

In this regard, animal studies show that the concentration of LCPUFAs in plasma is much less highly correlated with the concentration of these fatty acids in brain than with the concentration in erythrocytes and liver.[64] In contrast, postmortem studies in human infants show a weak, but statistically significant, correlation between erythrocyte and brain concentrations of DHA.[53] Correlation between the concentration of this fatty acid in erythrocyte membranes and the concentrations in other tissues was not reported. Studies in isolated cell systems suggest that precursors of DHA are transferred from plasma to astrocytes, where they are converted to DHA, which is subsequently transferred to neurons.[65,66] This pathway for direct synthesis of DHA within the central nervous system appears to occur in vivo in some animal species,[67] but the extent to which it occurs in humans is not known.

Importance of LCPUFAs in Development

The findings discussed previously, although far from definitive, are compatible with the possibility that failure to provide preformed LCPUFAs during early infancy and perhaps longer may compromise development of tissues/organs with a high concentration of these fatty acids, particularly 22:6 ω-3. However, the specific roles of LCPUFAs in normal development are not clear.[68–71] These fatty acids affect gene transcription and may produce posttranslational modifications. Moreover, many are precursors of eicosanoids, which, in turn, modify a number of processes. These fatty acids also have other effects on signal transduction, and the amount of these fatty acids in cell membranes can modify membrane fluidity, membrane thickness, and the microenvironment of the membrane as well as interactions between the fatty acid and membrane proteins. Such changes, in turn, can affect receptor function, and the fatty acids also may exert direct effects on receptor function. Although the degree of unsaturation of membrane fatty acids affects fluidity, this effect is most marked by substituting a monounsaturated or polyunsaturated fatty acid for a saturated fatty acid. In 22:6 ω-3 deficiency, 22:5 ω-6 replaces 22:6 ω-3 with little effect on fluidity. Possible mechanisms for the effects of LCPUFAs have been reviewed recently by Uauy et al,[68] Lauritzen et al,[69] Heird and Lapillonne,[70] and McCann and Ames.[71]

Despite the lack of a clear mechanism of the role of LCPUFAs in development, a number of studies over the past several years have focused on differences in visual acuity and neurodevelopmental indices between breastfed and formula-fed infants as well as between infants fed LCPUFA-supplemented and unsupplemented formulas. Because human milk contains a number of factors other than LCPUFAs that might affect visual acuity and/or neurodevelopmental indices, studies comparing breastfed versus formula-fed infants cannot help resolve the specific role of LCPUFAs in infant development. On the other hand, studies taking advantage of the natural variability in milk contents of LCPUFAs or enhanced variability secondary to maternal supplementation and, hence, differences in LCPUFA intake of the recipient infants[72–75] provide important insights. The following discussions of the effect of LCPUFA intake on visual function and on cognitive/behavioral development are limited to findings from these types of studies and findings from studies in which LCPUFA-supplemented versus unsupplemented formulas were compared.

LCPUFA Intake and Visual Function

Early studies in rodents established the importance of ω-3 fatty acids for normal retinal function,[25,28] and subsequent studies established this in primates.[26,27] More recently, studies have focused on the effect of ω-3 fatty acids on retinal function and/or overall visual function of human infants. However, whereas the abnormal retinal/visual function of ω-3 fatty acid-deficient animals clearly resulted from an inadequate intake of 18:3 ω-3 and were partially reversed by adding this fatty acid or DHA, more recent studies in human infants have focused primarily on the effects of 22:6 ω-3 intake on retinal and/or visual function. Studies have been conducted in both term and preterm infants and have used both behaviorally based and electrophysiologically based methods for assessing visual function.

The most commonly used behaviorally based method for assessing visual acuity, the Teller Acuity Card procedure, is based on the innate tendency to look toward a discernible pattern rather than a blank field.[76-78] This rapid measure of resolution acuity combines forced-choice and operant preferential looking procedures. The subject is shown a series of cards with stripes (gratings) of different widths on one side and a blank field on the other and his or her looking behavior is observed through a peephole in the center of the card. Cards with wider stripes are shown initially followed by cards with progressively decreasing stripe widths. The subject's visual acuity is the finest grating toward which he or she clearly looks preferentially (ie, the finest grating that he or she is able to resolve).

The electrophysiologically based tests use visual evoked potentials (VEPs), which measure the activation of the visual cortex in response to visual information that is processed by the retina and transmitted to the visual cortex.[79,80] The presence of a reliable evoked response indicates that the stimulus information was resolved up to the visual cortex, where the response is processed. Use of VEPs to assess visual acuity requires measuring the electrical potentials of the visual cortex in response to patterns of contrast reversal with vertical square wave gratings or checkerboards. The frequency of the gratings or checkerboards is decreased from low (large) to high (small), and the visual acuity threshold is estimated by linear regression of the VEP amplitudes versus the frequency, or size, of the grating or checkerboard stimulus.[79,80] Data are recorded as the $\log_{10}$ of the minimum angle of resolution (logMAR), which is the smallest grating that results in a measurable amplitude. Thus, smaller logMAR values indicate better visual acuity. A rapid VEP method (sweep VEP) has been developed for use in infant populations.[81]

The standard VEP also allows assessment of latency, or the time between presentation of a stimulus and the peak of the electrical potential. This reflects the rate of transmission of the stimulus and, hence, should be useful for assessing the effects of LCPUFAs (or other intervention). However, it has been used for this purpose by only a few investigators,[75,82-85] perhaps because it does not provide a direct assessment of acuity.

Electroretinography, unlike the aforementioned procedures that measure the response of the entire visual system, measures only the activity of the retina.[86,87] This method is somewhat more invasive and time consuming than the other methods and has been used to assess effects of LCPUFAs in only a few studies.[80,88] The primary components of electroretinography generated in response to a flash of light are the a-wave, which is produced by hyperpolarization of the photoreceptor, and the b-wave, which reflects the subsequent activation of retinal neurons. Performance is quantified by parameters[87,89] such as the threshold (the minimal intensity of light necessary to elicit a small amplitude), the implicit time or peak latency (the time from the presentation of a brief flash of light to the response peak), the maximal amplitude, and the sensitivity (the intensity of light that elicits a response of half the maximal amplitude).

Meta-analyses of data from studies using both behavioral and electro-physiological methods of assessment in both term and preterm infants were reported in 2000.[90,91] Data from behaviorally based tests of visual acuity obtained in randomized studies of term infants fed 22:6 ω-3-supplemented versus unsupplemented formula show a statistically significant advantage of the supplemented formula at 2 months of age but not at other ages. Data from randomized studies using electrophysiological methods of assessment in term infants fed 22:6 ω-3-supplemented versus unsupplemented formula showed no statistically significant advantages at any age.[90]

A relatively large multicenter study[92] that was not included in the meta-analysis showed no advantage of 22:6 ω-3 plus 20:4 ω-6 supplementation (0.14% and 0.46% of total fatty acids, respectively) on visual acuity as assessed by the Teller Acuity Card procedure at 2, 4, 6, or 12 months of age. Other recent studies of different designs have shown an apparent relationship between 22:6 ω-3 intake and visual acuity measured by the Teller Acuity Card procedure. In one such study,[74] term infants were breastfed exclusively for at least 3 months after birth and then weaned to a standard formula. Visual acuity at 2 and 12 months but not at 4 or 6 months of age was significantly correlated with the 22:6 ω-3 concentration of erythrocyte phosphatidylethanolamine at 2 months of age. In addition, infants with an erythrocyte phosphatidylethanolamine concentration of 22:6 ω-3 in the upper tertile at 2 months of age had significantly better acuity at 2 and 12 but not at 4 and 6 months of age than those whose erythrocyte phosphatidyle-thanolamine concentration of 22:6 ω-3 was in the lowest tertile.

Birch et al[93] recently reported results of a randomized controlled trial of supplemented (0.36% of total fatty acids as 22:6 ω-3 and 0.72% 20:4 ω-6) versus unsupplemented formula after near-exclusive breastfeeding (1 feeding/day of formula allowed) for the first 6 weeks of life. Visual acuity of the 2 groups, measured by sweep VEP, was similar at enrollment, but that of the supplemented group was better at 17, 26, and 52 weeks of age. Random dot stereoacuity of the supplemented group also was better at 17 weeks but not at 26 or 52 weeks of age. Random dot stereopsis, which reflects processing in the visual cortex, is not present before 3 months of age but develops rapidly from 3 to 5 months of age and is thought to be particularly sensitive to differences in maturation of the visual cortex between 3 and 5 months of age. If so, and if adequate 22:6 ω-3 is necessary for optimal maturation, a dietary source of this fatty acid between 3 and 5 months (approx 12 and 20 weeks) of age should enhance development of random dot stereopsis.

In a similar study, Hoffman et al[94] assigned infants to the same formulas after 4 to 6 months (approx 16–24 weeks) rather than after 6 weeks of near-exclusive breastfeeding. Visual acuity of the supplemented group, assessed by sweep VEP, was better at 12 months of age, but there was no difference in random dot stereoacuity between the 2 groups, presumably because both groups were still breastfed during the period of rapid development of the visual cortex required for optimal stereopsis. These findings suggest that 22:6 ω-3 may be needed beyond 4 to 6 months of age, the maximum duration of supplementation in most previous studies. This possibility is further supported by another study by the same group.[95] In this study, 6-month-old primarily breastfed infants were assigned randomly to receive complementary foods with or without 22:6 ω-3-enriched egg yolk (83 mg/day vs 0 mg/day). Visual acuity of the control group, assessed by sweep VEP, improved from 0.49 logMAR at 6 months of age to 0.29 logMAR at 12 months of age, whereas that of the 22:6 ω-3-supplemented group improved from 0.48 logMAR to 0.14 logMAR, suggesting that the rate of retrieval and/or visual cortex maturation was more rapid in the supplemented group. The 22:6 ω-3 concentration of erythrocyte lipids of the control group decreased by 21% between 6 and 12 months of age, whereas that of the supplemented group increased by 34%. VEP acuity of the total population at 12 months of age was significantly correlated with the erythrocyte lipid concentration of 22:6 ω-3, further supporting the potential benefit of 22:6 ω-3 beyond 6 months of age.

Finally, a retrospective study of 435 children showed that stereoacuity was better at 3.5 years of age in children who had been breastfed for at least 4 months than in those who had been formula-fed.[96] In addition, stereoacuity at 3.5 years of age was greater in breastfed infants of mothers who ate oily fish during pregnancy (and, presumably, had a higher concentration of DHA in their milk) than in those whose mothers did not.

The aforementioned meta-analysis of data from randomized studies in preterm infants showed an advantage of 22:6 ω-3-supplemented versus unsupplemented formula on both behaviorally based and electrophysiologically based measurements of visual acuity.[91] Advantages with behaviorally based tests were apparent at 2 and 4 months post-term, and advantages with electrophysiologically based measurements were apparent at 4 months post-term only. A recent randomized, controlled trial in preterm infants,[97] when analyzed according to intent to treat, showed no advantage of 22:6 ω-3 and 20:4 ω-6 supplementation (0.26% and 0.42% of total fatty acids, respectively, from birth to term and then 0.16% and 0.42%, respectively, through the first year of life) on visual acuity at 2, 4, or 6 months of age as assessed by the Teller Acuity Card procedure or VEP. However, post-hoc analysis showed an advantage of supplementation on sweep VEP acuity of a subset of infants at 6 but not at 4 months post-term.

In another multicenter study, supplemented (0.36% of total fatty acids as 22:6 ω-3 and 0.72% as 20:4 ω-6) or unsupplemented formula was fed to preterm infants for an average of approximately 28 days during hospitalization.[98] Not surprisingly, there was no difference in visual acuity at either 48 or 57 weeks' postmenstrual age as assessed by the Teller Acuity Card procedure. Electrophysiological assessments were not performed.

In yet another study,[85] preterm infants were assigned randomly to receive an unsupplemented versus a supplemented formula (0.34% and 0.70% of total fatty acids as 22:6 ω-3 and 20:4 ω-6, respectively, both from single-cell oils) until a corrected age of 6 months. Visual acuity of the 2 groups, assessed by the Teller Acuity Card procedure, did not differ at 3, 6, 12, or 24 months of age. VEP latency and amplitude of the 2 groups, assessed at 3 and 12 months of age, also did not differ.

Recent Cochrane reviews of much, but not all, of the data cited previously conclude that there are no consistent effects of LCPUFAs on visual acuity of either term[99] or preterm infants.[100] Gibson et al,[101] reviewing most reported randomized controlled trials of supplemented versus unsupplemented formulas in both term and preterm infants in 2001, concluded that evidence for a beneficial effect of LCPUFA supplementation on visual function of preterm infants was "reasonably compelling" but that evidence of a beneficial effect on visual function of term infants was less so. Clearly, there is no consensus concerning the effect of LCPUFA supplementation on visual function of either term or preterm infants.

LCPUFAs and Cognitive/Behavioral Development
Most studies addressing the cognitive/behavioral development of infants fed LCPUFA-supplemented versus unsupplemented formulas have used the Bayley Scales of Infant Development, which are considered the "gold standard" for assessing global abilities of infants from birth to about 42 months

of age. The Bayley Scales provide the standardized mental development index (MDI) and psychomotor development index (PDI). However, they are intended to distinguish between "normal" and "abnormal," not degrees of either. Thus, unless cognitive and/or psychomotor function as assessed by the Bayley Scales early in life is definitely abnormal, the relationship between these early scores and later function is poor.[102]

The Fagan Test of Infant Intelligence also has been used, either alone or in combination with the Bayley Scales. This test, which assesses novelty preference,[103] involves showing the infant a single image (usually a face) for a standardized, age-based period and then showing this image paired with a "novel" one. If the infant has "learned" the original image before to the novelty test, the typical response is to look selectively toward the novel versus the familiar image. Scores on this test during infancy are somewhat more predictive of later cognitive function than scores on the Bayley Scales of Infant Development; however, its internal consistency (reproducibility), unlike that of the Bayley Scales, is relatively poor.[104] Look duration during the familiarization and the paired comparison phases of the test also is a modest predictor of both concurrent performance on other tests during infancy and later tests of intelligence[104]; shorter look durations during the familiarization phase predict better concurrent as well as subsequent cognitive performance.

One or both of these tests has been used to evaluate the effect of LCPUFA supplementation on cognitive/behavioral development. Some of the studies using these tests have shown advantages of LCPUFA supplementation with both tests, some studies have shown advantages with one but not the other, and still others have shown advantages with neither. Available studies in term infants were reviewed in 1998 by an expert panel appointed by the Life Sciences Research Organization to assess the nutrient requirements for term infant formulas.[37] These studies were criticized by consultants to the panel for including too few infants, failing to control adequately for confounding factors, failing to assess function at more than one age, failing to examine individual differences in development, and failing to follow the infants for a sufficiently long period (eg, none of the studies available at that time included data beyond 1 year of age). Partially on the basis of these criticisms, the panel did not recommend addition of LCPUFA to term infant formulas but suggested that the issue be re-evaluated in about 5 years.

The randomized trials in term infants published since 1998[92,105–107] have not resolved many of these criticisms. The trials have differed with respect to the source of LCPUFA supplementation, the duration of supplementation, the amounts of 22:6 ω-3 and 20:4 ω-6 supplemented, and the ratio of 22:6 ω-3 to 20:4 ω-6. There also were differences in the 18:2 ω-6 and 18:3 ω-3 contents of the control and experimental formulas. The variance in Bayley MDI and PDI scores also varied among studies, being smallest in the study that showed an advantage of 22:6 ω-3 and 20:4 ω-6 supplementation for the first 4 months of life on the Bayley MDI score at 18 months of age.[105]

Fewer studies are available in preterm infants fed LCPUFA-supplemented versus unsupplemented formulas, and these are subject to many of the same criticisms levied against the studies in term infants. The available data, including those from recently reported, large, multicenter studies,[97,98] suggest that preterm infants may be more likely to benefit from supplementation than term infants. However, it is important to note that this conclusion is based, in part, on post-hoc analyses of data from selected groups of the study populations (eg, infants who received only the assigned formula rather than the assigned formula plus human milk, infants who weighed less than 1250 g at birth, infants whose parents were English speaking). Analysis of data according to how the infants were randomized shows few differences in any outcome variable among groups. The study of van Wezel-Meijler et al[85] showed no difference in scores on the Dutch version of the Bayley Scales of Infant Development at 3, 6, 12, or 24 months of age between infants who were assigned to receive supplemented (0.34% and 0.70% of 22:6 ω-3 and 20:4 ω-6, respectively) versus unsupplemented formulas through 6 months' corrected age.

A few methods other than the Bayley Scales of Infant Development and the Fagan Test of Infant Intelligence have been used to assess the effects of LCPUFAs on cognitive/behavioral development. Willats et al[108] found that term infants assigned to receive a formula supplemented with both 22:6 ω-3 and 20:4 ω-6 versus an unsupplemented formula had better visual habituation scores at 4 months of age and performed better on a means-end, problem-solving test at 10 months of age. The supplemented group not only had more intentional solutions to items of this test but also scored higher than those assigned to the control formula, findings that have been related to higher IQ scores later in childhood.

Innis et al,[74] studying breastfed term infants with a range of 22:6 ω-3 and 20:4 ω-6 as well as 18:2 ω-6 and 18:3 ω-3 intakes and, hence, a range of plasma and erythrocyte lipid 22:6 ω-3 and 20:4 ω-6 concentrations, found no statistically significant relationships between 22:6 ω-3 and 20:4 ω-6 status at 2 months of age when all infants were exclusively breastfed and scores on an object-search test at either 6 or 12 months of age. There also was no statistically significant relationship between infant 22:6 ω-3 or 20:4 ω-6 status at 2 months of age and novelty preference or Bayley MDI or PDI scores at either 6 or 12 months of age. However, there was a positive relationship between the 22:6 ω-3 concentration of plasma phospholipid and erythrocyte phosphatidylethanolamine at 2 months of age and ability to discriminate nonnative retroflex and phonetic contrasts at 9 months of age. This finding was interpreted as indicating more rapid language development in those with higher plasma and erythrocyte lipid concentrations of 22:6 ω-3 at 2 months of age.

Two other studies of the effect of maternal 22:6 ω-3 supplementation and, hence, intake of 22:6 ω-3 by the breastfeeding infant are relevant. Gibson et al[72] supplemented breastfeeding mothers with varying amounts of 22:6 ω-3 and achieved human milk 22:6 ω-3 concentrations ranging from 0.1% to 1.7% of total fatty acids and, hence, a wide range in 22:6 ω-3 concentrations of infant plasma lipids. There was no relationship between the 22:6 ω-3 concentration of milk or infant plasma lipids and VEP acuity at either 12 or 16 weeks of age, but Bayley MDI scores correlated weakly with milk 22:6 ω-3 content at 12 but not at 24 months of age.

Jensen et al[109] assigned breastfeeding mothers to receive 22:6 ω-3 (approx 250 mg/day) as an algal-derived triglyceride or a control oil containing no 22:6 ω-3 for the first 4 months after birth. At 4 months of age, plasma phospholipid 22:6 ω-3 concentration of infants whose mothers had received 22:6 ω-3 was approximately 50% higher than that of infants whose mothers received the control oil, but there was no difference in visual acuity between the 2 groups at either 4 or 8 months of age whether assessed by sweep VEP or the Teller Acuity Card procedure. There also was no difference between groups in scores on a variety of neurodevelopmental tests at either 12 or 18 months of age. However, at 30 months of age, the mean Bayley PDI score of the group whose mothers received 22:6 ω-3 was 8 points higher than that of the group whose mothers received the control oil ($P < .01$).

Helland et al,[73] examining the effect of supplementing women with either cod liver oil (approx 1.2 g/day of 22:6 ω-3 and 0.8 mg/da of 20:5 ω-3) or corn oil from week 18 of pregnancy until 3 months after delivery, found that children whose mothers received cod liver oil scored higher at 4 years of age on the Mental Processing Composite of the Kaufman Assessment Battery for Children (106.4 ± 7.4 [n = 48]) than children whose mothers received corn oil (102.3 ± 11.3 [n = 36]). Maternal 22:6 ω-3 intake during pregnancy was the only variable in a multiple regression model that was related significantly to the mental processing scores of the children at 4 years of age.

In a somewhat similar study, Malcolm et al[75] assigned pregnant women to receive fish oil (approx 200 mg of DHA/day [n = 50]) or control oil capsules (n = 50) from week 15 of pregnancy through term. The 22:6 ω-3 concentration of maternal erythrocytes at birth was approximately 50% higher in the supplemented group, but the 22:6 ω-3 concentration of umbilical cord erythrocytes of the 2 groups did not differ and there was no difference in erythrocyte 22:6 ω-3 concentrations of the 2 groups at either 50 or 66 weeks' postconceptional age. On the other hand, infants with higher erythrocyte 22:6 ω-3 concentration at birth had shorter pattern-evoked VEP latencies at 50 and 66 weeks' postconceptional age, suggesting more rapid nerve conduction.

LCPUFAs and Other Aspects of Central Nervous System Development

The effects of LCPUFA supplementation on other aspects of brain function and/or development also have been examined. With respect to effects on brain auditory evoked potentials, studies in preterm infants[82,83,110] showed no effect of 22:6 ω-3-supplemented versus unsupplemented formulas. One of these studies[92] showed that supplemented infants had slower peripheral nerve conduction than infants fed human milk but not slower than infants fed the control formula.

Bouwstra et al[110] investigated the effect of supplemented (0.3% of total fatty acids as 22:6 ω-3 and 0.45% as 20:4 ω-6 from a mixture of egg yolk, tuna oil, and fungal oil) versus unsupplemented formula during the first 2 months of life on the quality of general movements, which is thought to be an index of the overall quality of brain function in young infants. At 3 months of age, the unsupplemented group had mildly abnormal general movements significantly more often (31%) than either the supplemented group (19%) or a breastfed group (20%) that was studied concurrently; however, the frequency of "normal optimal" movements did not differ between supplemented and unsupplemented groups (18% and 21%, respectively) and was less in both than in the breastfed group (34%).

Only one study has examined the effect of LCPUFA supplementation on structural brain development.[85] In this study, preterm infants were assigned randomly to receive either a standard formula (n = 20) or a formula supplemented with 0.34% and 0.70% of total fatty acids as 22:6 ω-3 and 20:4 ω-6, respectively (n = 22), both from single-cell oils, until a corrected age of 6 months. Brain structural development, assessed by magnetic resonance imaging at 3 and 12 months' corrected age, did not differ between groups at either age. This method assesses the degree of myelination, and in this study, neither global myelination nor myelination of the cerebral visual system differed between groups. Although the LCPUFA content of myelin is low, myelin deposition is dependent on close interaction among neurons, their axons, and their oligodendrocytes, all of which are rich in LCPUFAs. Thus, myelination is thought to reflect the functional maturity of all of these components.

Effects of LCPUFAs on Growth

The observation in the early 1990s that preterm infants assigned to a formula supplemented with fish oil (0.3% of total fatty acids as 20:5 ω-3 and 0.2% as 22:6 ω-3) versus an unsupplemented formula weighed less and had a lower weight-for-length at various times during the first year of life[111] generated considerable concern and continues to do so. In this study, weight at 12 months' corrected age was correlated with plasma phospholipid 20:4 ω-6 concentration at various times during the first year of life.[112] This led to the assumption that the lower rate of weight gain was related in some way to the 20:5 ω-3 content of the fish oil.

Interestingly, a smaller study also conducted in the early 1990s did not show differences in growth between supplemented and unsupplemented preterm infants, although the supplemented group received even more of a similar fish oil.[63] However, the duration of this study may not have been sufficient to permit detection of weight differences. Additional studies primarily in preterm infants[113,114] also have shown an adverse effect of ω-3 fatty acids on growth. However, no study in which the formula contained ARA as well as ω-3 fatty acids has shown such an effect.

In contrast to observations of an adverse effect of ω-3 fatty acids on growth, Innis et al[98] reported a more rapid rate of growth in preterm infants fed a formula supplemented with both 22:6 ω-3 (0.33% of fat as an algal oil) and 20:4 ω-6 (0.6% of fat as a fungal oil) versus a formula supplemented with only 22:6 ω-3 (0.34% of fat as an algal oil) or an unsupplemented formula for at least 28 days before hospital discharge and followed until 57 weeks' postmenstrual age. Another recent study also showed a positive growth effect of formulas supplemented with both 22:6 ω-3 and 20:4 ω-6.[115] In this study, weight of supplemented preterm infants was greater than that of control infants from 66 through 118 weeks' postmenstrual age and equal to that of breastfed term infants at 118 weeks postmenstrual age. Length of this group also was greater than that of the control group at 79 and 92 weeks' postmenstrual age and equal to that of breastfed term infants by 79 weeks' postmenstrual age.

The reason(s) for an inhibitory effect of ω-3 fatty acids or, perhaps, a stimulatory effect of ω-6 fatty acids on growth are not clear. Possibilities that have been suggested include inhibition of desaturation and elongation of 18:2 ω-6 to 20:4 ω-6 by the ω-3 fatty acids, inhibition of eicosanoid synthesis from 20:4 ω-6 by the intake of preformed 20:5 ω-3 or endogenous synthesis of 20:5 ω-3 from a moderately high intake of 18:3 ω-3, and effects of ω-3 and ω-6 fatty acids on transcription of genes controlling lipolysis and lipogenesis.[116]

A recent meta-analysis of growth data from 14 (from a total of 21 known trials) generally high-quality trials that involved LCPUFA supplementation of infant formula fed to term infants found no evidence that such supplementation influences the growth of term infants in either a negative or a positive way.[117] Subgroup analyses showed that neither supplementation with only ω-3 LCPUFA nor source of LCPUFA supplementation affected infant growth. This analysis of data from 1846 infants should put to rest the question of growth inhibition by ω-3 LCPUFA.

Other Adverse Effects of LCPUFAs

In addition to concerns about adverse effects of ω-3 fatty acids on growth, a number of theoretical concerns related to the known biologic effects of ω-6 and ω-3 LCPUFAs must be considered.[118] Among these is the possibility that supplementation with highly unsaturated oils will increase the likelihood of oxidant damage. This is because peroxidation occurs at the site of double bonds, making membranes with unsaturated fatty acids more vulnerable to oxidant damage. Thus, it is possible that LCPUFA supplementation will increase the incidence of conditions thought to be related to oxidant damage (eg, necrotizing enterocolitis, bronchopulmonary dysplasia, retrolental fibroplasia). There also is concern that unbalanced supplementation with ω-3 and/or ω-6 LCPUFA will result in altered eicosanoid metabolism with potential effects on a variety of physiological mechanisms (eg, blood clotting, infection). Further, a higher concentration of polyunsaturated fatty acids in muscle cell membranes has been related to enhanced insulin sensitivity,[119] and specific LCPUFAs have been shown to inhibit as well as to enhance transcription of a variety of genes.[120] There are few data to either support or allay these theoretical concerns with respect to the small amounts of LCPUFAs that are added to infant formulas.

Three recently reported, relatively large, randomized, controlled, double-blind studies in preterm infants[97,98,115] have shown no difference in the incidence of bronchopulmonary dysplasia, necrotizing enterocolitis, or other neonatal conditions between infants receiving supplements of either DHA or both ARA and DHA from a variety of sources (single-cell oils, low-eicosapentaenoic acid fish oil, egg yolk triglyceride) and infants receiving unsupplemented formula. Further, as discussed previously, no difference in growth was observed. Together, these studies included more than 750 infants assigned to supplemented or unsupplemented formulas. Thus, despite the relative absence of definitive data concerning the validity of a number of the specific theoretical safety concerns related to the known biologic effects of LCPUFAs,[118] the fact that supplementation of formulas with the amounts of DHA and ARA used in the studies of preterm infants cited previously did not result in a greater incidence of conditions thought to be related etiologically to the theoretical concerns suggests that the amounts and the sources of LCPUFA used in these studies are safe.

Sources for LCPUFA Supplementation

Available sources for LCPUFA supplementation include egg yolk lipid, phospholipid, and triglyceride, all of which contain ω-6 as well as ω-3 LCPUFA, fish oils, and oils produced by single-cell organisms (ie, microalgal and fungal oils). Aside from the early reports of an adverse effect of fish oil on growth of infants (see next section), few untoward effects of the available supplements have been noted. In vitro and animal studies of toxicity also have revealed little toxicity of any of these sources. In fact, the US Food and Drug Administration has recently accepted the conclusion of a manufacturer of a combination of algal and fungal oils as well as that of a manufacturer of a combination of low-eicosapentaenoic acid tuna and a fungal oil that their products are generally regarded as safe sources of DHA and ARA for addition to formulas intended for normal infants.

Supplementation of Infant Formulas With LCPUFAs

The American Academy of Pediatrics has no official position on supplementation of term or preterm infant formulas with LCPUFAs. The Life Sciences Research Organization Expert Panel on Nutrient Composition of Term Infant Formulas recommended neither a minimum nor maximum content of either ARA or DHA.[37] The Life Sciences Research Organization Expert Panel on Nutrient Composition of Preterm Formulas specified a maximum amount of ARA and DHA for preterm infant formulas but did not specify a minimum amount of either fatty acid.[121] In contrast, regulatory and advisory groups from other countries recommend that infant formulas, particularly those intended for preterm infants, be supplemented with these 2 fatty acids,[36] and such formulas are now available in most countries, including the United States. It has been estimated that approximately 75% of the term formulas and 100% of the preterm formulas sold in the United States are supplemented with DHA and ARA.

The evidence for efficacy of supplementing term infant formulas with these fatty acids is only minimally, if at all, different from that available to the Life Sciences Research Organization term formula panel in 1998, but the evidence for efficacy of supplementation of preterm formulas is more convincing. Few studies in preterm infants have failed to document at least transient advantages of supplementation on visual acuity, and many studies suggest that there are advantages with respect to level of general development. Moreover, most of the theoretical safety concerns expressed earlier have been resolved. Most notably, no recent study has documented an adverse effect of formulas supplemented with both ARA and DHA on growth, and supplementation with DHA alone or DHA plus ARA does not appear to result in a higher incidence of conditions such as necrotizing enterocolitis, retrolental fibroplasia, and bronchopulmonary dysplasia, which theoretically might be higher with addition of these bioactive compounds to formulas.

Finally, considering the marked variability among infants of apparent conversion of ALA to DHA and LA to ARA, it is conceivable that some infants will benefit from supplementation, whereas others will not. Such a scenario certainly would help explain the marked variability in outcomes documented by virtually every study. It also is likely that any beneficial effects of LCPUFA supplementation will be subtle and possibly not detectable with available methodology.

References

1. Bier DM, Brosnan JT, Flatt JP, et al. Report of the IDECG Working Group on lower and upper limits of carbohydrate and fat intake. International Dietary Energy Consultative Group. *Eur J Clin Nutr.* 1999;53(Suppl):S177–S178

2. Hamosh M. A review. Fat digestion in the newborn: role of lingual lipase and preduodenal digestion. *Pediatr Res.* 1979;13:615–622

3. Faber J, Goldstein R, Blondheim O, et al. Absorption of medium chain triglycerides in the stomach of the human infant. *J Pediatr Gastroenterol Nutr.* 1988;7:189–195

4. Linscheer WG, Vergroesen AJ. Lipids. In: Shils ME, Young VR, eds. *Modern Nutrition in Health and Disease.* 7th ed. Philadelphia, PA: Lea & Febiger; 1988:72–107

5. Hernell O, Olivecrona T. Human milk lipases. I. Serum-stimulated lipase. *J Lipid Res.* 1974;15:367–374

6. Hernell O, Blackberg L, Fredrikzon B, Olivecrona T. Bile salt stimulated lipase in human milk and lipid digestion during the neonatal period. In: Lebenthal E, ed. *Textbook of Gastroenterology and Nutrition in Infancy.* Vol 1. New York, NY: Raven Press; 1981:465–471

7. Hernell O. Human milk lipases. III. Physiological implications of the bile salt-stimulated lipase. *Eur J Clin Invest*. 1975;5:267–272

8. Watkins JB, Ingall D, Szczepanik P, Klein PD, Lester R. Bile salt metabolism in the newborn. Measurement of pool size and synthesis by stable isotope technique. *N Engl J Med*. 1972;288:431–434

9. Watkins JB. Lipid digestion and absorption. *Pediatrics*. 1985;75(1 Pt 2):151–156

10. Hofmann AF, Roda A. Physicochemical properties of bile acids and their relationship to biological properties: an overview of the problem. *J Lipid Res*. 1984;25:1477–1489

11. Gray GM. Mechanisms of digestion and absorption of food. In: Sleisenger MH, Fordtran JS, eds. *Gastrointestinal Disease. Pathophysiology, Diagnosis, Management*. 3rd ed. Philadelphia, PA: W.B. Saunders; 1983:844–858

12. Filer LJ Jr., Mattson FH, Fomon SJ. Triglyceride configuration and fat absorption by the human infant. *J Nutr*. 1969;99:293–298

13. Carnielli VP, Luijendijk IH, van Beek RH, Boerma GJ, Degenhart HJ, Sauer PJ. Effect of dietary triacylglycerol fatty acid positional distribution on plasma lipid classes and their fatty acid composition in preterm infants. *Am J Clin Nutr*. 1995;62:776–781

14. Carnielli VP, Luijendijk IHT, van Goudoever JB, et al. Feeding premature newborn infants palmitic acid in amounts and stereoisomeric position similar to that of human milk: effects on fat and mineral balance. *Am J Clin Nutr*. 1995;61:1037–1042

15. Carnielli VP, Luijendijk IH, van Goudoever JB, et al. Structural position and amount of palmitic acid in infant formulas: effects on fat, fatty acid, and mineral balance. *J Pediatr Gastroenterol Nutr*. 1996;23:553–560

16. Lucas A, Quinlan P, Abrams S, Ryan S, Meah S, Lucas PJ. Randomised controlled trial of a synthetic triglyceride milk formula for preterm infants. *Arch Dis Child Fetal Neonatal Ed*. 1997;77:F178–F184

17. Bensadoun A. Lipoprotein lipase. *Annu Rev Nutr*. 1991;11:217–237

18. Griffin EA, Bryan MH, Angel A. Variations in intralipid tolerance in newborn infants. *Pediatr Res*. 1983;17:478–481

19. Innis SM. Essential fatty acids in growth and development. *Prog Lipid Res*. 1991;30:39–103

20. Holman RT. Nutritional and biochemical evidences of acyl interaction with respect to essential polyunsaturated fatty acids. *Prog Lipid Res*. 1986;25:29–39

21. Oliw E, Granström E, Änggärd E. The prostaglandins and essential fatty acids. In: Pace-Asciak C, Granström E, eds. *Prostaglandins and Related Substances*. Amsterdam, The Netherlands: Elsevier Science;1983:1–44

22. Holman RT. The ratio of trienoic: tetraenoic acids in tissue lipids as a measure of essential fatty acid requirement. *J Nutr*. 1960;70:405–410

23. Burr GO, Burr MM. A new deficiency disease produced by the rigid exclusion of fat from the diet. *J Biol Chem*. 1929;82:345–367

24. Hansen AE, Steward RA, Hughes G, Soderhjelm L. The relation of linoleic acid to infant feeding. *Acta Paediatr*. 1962;137:1–41

25. Benolken RM, Anderson RE, Wheeler TG. Membrane fatty acids associated with the electrical response in visual excitation. *Science*. 1973;182:1253–1254

26. Neuringer M, Connor WE, Van Petten C, Barstad L. Dietary omega 3 fatty acid deficiency and visual loss in infant Rhesus monkeys. *J Clin Invest.* 1984;73:272–276

27. Neuringer M, Connor WE, Lin DS, Barstad L, Luck S. Biochemical and functional effects of prenatal and postnatal omega 3 fatty acid deficiency on retina and brain in rhesus monkeys. *Proc Natl Acad Sci U S A.* 1986;83:4021–4025

28. Wheeler TG, Benolken RM, Anderson RE. Visual membranes: specificity of fatty acid precursors for the electrical response to illumination. *Science.* 1975;188:1312–1314

29. Holman RT, Johnson SB, Hatch TF. A case of human linolenic acid deficiency involving neurological abnormalities. *Am J Clin Nutr.* 1982;35:617–623

30. Bjerve KS, Fischer S, Alme K. Alpha-linolenic acid deficiency in man: effect of ethyl linolenate on plasma and erythrocyte fatty acid composition and biosynthesis of prostanoids. *Am J Clin Nutr.* 1987;46:570–576

31. Jensen RG. Lipids in human milk. *Lipids.* 1999;34:1243–1271

32. Sanders TAB, Reddy S. The influence of a vegetarian diet on the fatty acid composition of human milk and the essential fatty acid status of the infant. *J Pediatr.* 1992;120:S71–S77

33. Henderson RA, Jensen RG, Lammi-Keefe CJ, et al. Effect of fish oil on the fatty acid composition of human milk and maternal and infant erythrocytes. *Lipids.* 1992;27:863–869

34. Makrides M, Neumann MA, Gibson RA. Effect of maternal docosahexaenoic acid (DHA) supplementation on breast milk composition. *Eur J Clin Nutr.* 1996;50:352–357

35. Jensen CL, Maude M, Anderson RE, Heird WC. Effect of docosahexaenoic acid supplementation of lactating women on the fatty acid composition of breast milk lipids and maternal and infant plasma phospholipids. *Am J Clin Nutr.* 2000;71(suppl):292S–299S

36. ESPGAN Committee on Nutrition. Comment on the content and composition of lipids in infant formulas. *Acta Paediatr Scand.* 1991;80:887–896

37. Raiten DJ, Talbot JM, Waters JH. LSRO Report: Assessment of nutrient requirements for infant formulas. *J Nutr.* 1998;128:2059S–2293S

38. Carlson SE, Rhodes PG, Ferguson MG. Docosahexaenoic acid status of preterm infants at birth and following feeding with human milk or formula. *Am J Clin Nutr.* 1986;44:798–804

39. Innis SM, Akrabawi SS, Diersen-Schade DA, Dobson MV, Guy DG. Visual acuity and blood lipids in term infants fed human milk or formulae. *Lipids.* 1997;32:63–72

40. Jørgensen MH, Hernell O, Lund P, Holmer G, Michaelsen KF. Visual acuity and erythrocyte docosahexaenoic acid status in breast-fed and formula-fed term infants during the first four months of life. *Lipids.* 1996;31:99–105

41. Ponder DL, Innis SM, Benson JD, Siegman JS. Docosahexaenoic acid status of term infants fed breast milk or infant formula containing soy oil or corn oil. *Pediatr Res.* 1992;32:683–688

42. Lucas A, Morley R, Cole TJ, et al. Early diet in preterm babies and developmental status at 18 months. *Lancet.* 1990;335:1477–1481

43. Lucas A, Morley R, Cole TJ. Randomised trial of early diet in preterm babies and later intelligence quotient. *BMJ.* 1998;317:1481–1487

44. Morrow-Tlucak M, Haude RH, Ernhart CB. Breastfeeding and cognitive development in the first 2 years of life. *Soc Sci Med.* 1988;26:635–639

45. Rogan WJ, Gladen BC. Breastfeeding and cognitive development. *Early Hum Dev*. 1993;31:181–193

46. Clandinin MT, Chappell JE, Leong S, Heim T, Swyer PR, Chance GW. Intrauterine fatty acid accretion rates in human brain: implications for fatty acid requirements. *Early Hum Dev*. 1980;4:121–129

47. Clandinin MT, Chappell JE, Leong S, Heim T, Swyer PR, Chance GW. Extrauterine fatty acid accretion in infant brain: implications for fatty acid requirements. *Early Hum Dev*. 1980;4:131–138

48. Martinez M. Tissue levels of polyunsaturated fatty acids during early human development. *J Pediatr*. 1992;120:S129–S138

49. Berghaus TM, Demmelmair H, Koletzko B. Fatty acid composition of lipid classes in maternal and cord plasma at birth. *Eur J Pediatr*. 1998;157:763–768

50. Dutta-Roy AK. Transport mechanisms for long-chain polyunsaturated fatty acids in the human placenta. *Am J Clin Nutr*. 2000;71:315S–322S

51. Farquharson J, Cockburn F, Patrick WA, Jamieson EC, Logan RW. Infant cerebral cortex phospholipid fatty acid composition and diet. *Lancet*. 1992;340:810–813

52. Jamieson EC, Abbasi KA, Cockburn F, Farquharson J, Logan RW, Patrick WA. Effect of diet on term infant cerebral cortex fatty acid composition. *World Rev Nutr Diet*. 1994;75:139–141

53. Makrides M, Neumann MA, Byard RW, Simmer RK, Gibson RA. Fatty acid composition of brain, retina, and erythrocytes in breast- and formula-fed infants. *Am J Clin Nutr*. 1994;60:189–194

54. Arbuckle LD, MacKinnon MJ, Innis SM. Formula 18:2(n-6) and 18:3(n-3) content and ratio influence long-chain polyunsaturated fatty acids in the developing piglet liver and central nervous system. *J Nutr*. 1994;124:289–298

55. Sauerwald T, Hachey DL, Jensen CL, Chen H, Anderson RE, Heird WC. Effect of dietary alpha-linolenic acid intake on incorporation of docosahexaenoic and arachidonic acids into plasma phospholipids of term infants. *Lipids*. 1996;31:S131–S135

56. Carnielli VP, Wattimena DJ, Luijendijk IH, Boerlage A, Degenhart HJ, Sauer PJ. The very low birth weight premature infant is capable of synthesizing arachidonic and docosahexaenoic acids from linoleic and linolenic acids. *Pediatr Res*. 1996;40:169–174

57. Demmelmair H, von Schenck U, Behrendt E, Sauerwald T, Koletzko B. Estimation of arachidonic acid synthesis in full term neonates using natural variation of 13C content. *J Pediatr Gastroenterol Nutr*. 1995;21:31–36

58. Salem N Jr., Wegher B, Mena P, Uauy R. Arachidonic and docosahexaenoic acids are biosynthesized from their 18-carbon precursors in human infants. *Proc Natl Acad Sci USA*. 1996;93:49–54

59. Sauerwald TU, Hachey DL, Jensen CL, Chen H, Anderson RE, Heird WC. Intermediates in endogenous synthesis of C22:6 omega 3 and C20:4 omega 6 by term and preterm infants. *Pediatr Res*. 1997;41:183–187

60. Uauy R, Mena P, Wegher B, Nieto S, Salem N Jr. Long chain polyunsaturated fatty acid formation in neonates: effect of gestational age and intrauterine growth. *Pediatr Res*. 2000;47:127–135

61. Carlson SE, Cooke RJ, Rhodes PG, Tyson JE, Hoffman DR. Long-term feeding of formulas high in linolenic acid and marine oil to very low birth weight infants: phospholipid fatty acids. *Pediatr Res.* 1991;30:404–412

62. Uauy RD, Birch DG, Birch EE, et al. Effect of dietary omega-3 fatty acids on retinal function of very-low-birth-weight neonates. *Pediatr Res.* 1990;28:485–492

63. Uauy RD, Hoffman DR, Birch EE, et al. Safety and efficacy of omega-3 fatty acids in the nutrition of very-low-birth-weight infants: soy oil and marine oil supplementation of formula. *J Pediatr.* 1994;124:612–620

64. Rioux FM, Innis SM, Dyer R, MacKinnon M. Diet-induced changes in liver and bile but not brain fatty acids can be predicted from differences in plasma phospholipid fatty acids in formula- and milk-fed piglets. *J Nutr.* 1997;127:370–377

65. Moore SA, Yoder E, Murphy S, Dutton GR, Spector AA. Astrocytes, not neurons, produce docosahexaenoic acid (22:6 omega-3) and arachidonic acid (20:4 omega-6). *J Neurochem.* 1991;56:518–524

66. Moore SA. Cerebral endothelium and astrocytes cooperate in supplying docosahexaenoic acid to neurons. *Adv Exp Med Biol.* 1993;331:229–233

67. Pawlosky RJ, Denkins Y, Ward G, Salem N Jr. Retinal and brain accretion of long-chain polyunsaturated fatty acids in developing felines: the effects of corn oil-based maternal diets. *Am J Clin Nutr.* 1997;65:465–472

68. Uauy R, Hoffman DR, Peirano P, Birch DG, Birch EE. Essential fatty acids in visual and brain development. *Lipids.* 2001;36:885–895

69. Lauritzen L, Hansen HS, Jorgensen MH, Michaelsen KF. The essentiality of long chain n-3 fatty acids in relation to development and function of the brain and retina. *Prog. Lipid Res.* 2001;40:1–94

70. Heird WC, Lapillonne A. The role of essential fatty acids in development. *Annu Rev Nutr.* 2005;25:549–571

71. McCann JC, Ames BN. Is docosahexaenoic acid, an n-3 long-chain polyunsaturated fatty acid, required for development of normal brain function? An overview of evidence from cognitive and behavioral tests in humans and animals. *Am J Clin Nutr.* 2005;82:281–295

72. Gibson RA, Neumann MA, Makrides M. Effect of increasing breast milk docosahexaenoic acid on plasma and erythrocyte phospholipid fatty acids and neural indices of exclusively breastfed infants. *Eur J Clin Nutr.* 1997;51:578–584

73. Helland IB, Smith L, Saarem K, Saugstad OD, Drevon CA. Maternal supplementation with very-long-chain n-3 fatty acids during pregnancy and lactation augments children's IQ at 4 years of age. *Pediatrics.* 2003;111(1):e39–e44. Available at: http://pediatrics.aappublications.org/cgi/content/full/111/1/e39. Accessed August 20, 2007

74. Innis SM, Gilley J, Werker J. Are human milk long-chain polyunsaturated fatty acids related to visual and neural development in breast-fed term infants? *J Pediatr.* 2001;139:532–538

75. Malcolm CA, McCulloch DL, Montgomery C, Shepherd A, Weaver LT. Maternal docosahexaenoic acid supplementation during pregnancy and visual evoked potential development in term infants: a double blind, prospective, randomised trial. *Arch Dis Child Fetal Neonatal Ed.* 2003;88:F383–F390

76. Dobson V. Clinical applications of preferential looking measures of visual acuity. *Behav Brain Res.* 1983;10:25–38

77. Dobson V, Teller DY. Visual acuity in human infants: a review and comparison of behavioral and electrophysiological studies. *Vision Res.* 1978;18:1469–1483

78. McDonald MA, Dobson V, Sebris SL, Baitch L, Varner D, Teller DY. The acuity card procedure: a rapid test of infant acuity. *Invest Ophthalmol Vis Sci.* 1985;26:1158–1162

79. Sokol S, Hansen VC, Moskowitz A, Greenfield P, Towle VL. Evoked potential and preferential looking estimates of visual acuity in pediatric patients. *Ophthalmology.* 1983;90:552–562

80. Uauy R, Birch E, Birch D, Peirano P. Visual and brain function measurements in studies of n-3 fatty acid requirements of infants. *J Pediatr* 1992;120:S168–S180

81. Norcia AM, Tyler CW. Spatial frequency sweep VEP: visual acuity during the first year of life. *Vision Res.* 1985;25:1399–1408

82. Bougle D, Denise P, Vimard F, Nouvelot A, Penneillo MJ, Guillois B. Early neurological and neuropsychological development of the preterm infant and polyunsaturated fatty acids supply. *Clin Neurophysiol.* 1999;110:1363–1370

83. Faldella G, Govoni M, Alessandroni R, et al. Visual evoked potentials and dietary long chain polyunsaturated fatty acids in preterm infants. *Arch Dis Child.* 1996;75:F108–F112

84. Jensen CL, Prager TC, Fraley JK, Chen H, Anderson RE, Heird WC. Effect of dietary linoleic/alpha-linolenic acid ratio on growth and visual function of term infants. *J Pediatr.* 1997;131:200–209

85. van Wezel-Meijler G, van der Knaap MS, Huisman J, Jonkman EJ, Valk J, Lafeber HN. Dietary supplementation of long-chain polyunsaturated fatty acids in preterm infants: effects on cerebral maturation. *Acta Paediatr.* 2002;91:942–950

86. Hood DC, Birch DG. The a-wave of the human electroretinogram and rod receptor function. *Invest Ophthalmol Vis Sci.* 1990;31:2070–2081

87. Naka KI, Rushton WA. S-potentials from colour units in the retina of fish (Cyprinidae). *J Physiol.* 1966;185:536–555

88. Birch DG, Birch EE, Hoffman DR, Uauy RD. Retinal development in very-low-birth-weight infants fed diets differing in omega-3 fatty acids. *Invest Ophthalmol Vis Sci.* 1992;33:2365–2376

89. Hood DC, Birch DG. The A-wave of the human electroretinogram and rod receptor function. *Invest Ophthalmol Vis Sci.* 1990;31:2070–2081

90. SanGiovanni JP, Berkey CS, Dwyer JT, Colditz GA. Dietary essential fatty acids, long-chain polyunsaturated fatty acids, and visual resolution acuity in healthy fullterm infants: a systematic review. *Early Hum Dev.* 2000;57:165–188

91. SanGiovanni JP, Parra-Cabrera S, Colditz GA, Berkey CS, Dwyer JT. Meta-analysis of dietary essential fatty acids and long-chain polyunsaturated fatty acids as they relate to visual resolution acuity in healthy preterm infants. *Pediatrics.* 2000;105:1292–1298

92. Auestad N, Halter R, Hall RT, et al. Growth and development in term infants fed long-chain polyunsaturated fatty acids: a double-masked, randomized, parallel, prospective, multivariate study. *Pediatrics.* 2001;108:372–381

93. Birch EE, Hoffman DR, Castañeda YS, Fawcett SL, Birch DG, Uauy RD. A randomized controlled trial of long-chain polyunsaturated fatty acid supplementation of formula in term infants after weaning at 6 wk of age. *Am J Clin Nutr.* 2002;75:570–580

94. Hoffman DR, Birch EE, Castañeda YS, et al. Visual function in breast-fed term infants weaned to formula with or without long-chain polyunsaturates at 4 to 6 months: a randomized clinical trial. *J Pediatr.* 2003;142:669–677

95. Hoffman DR, Theuer RC, Castaneda YS, et al. Maturation of visual acuity is accelerated in breast-fed term infants fed baby food containing DHA-enriched egg yolk. *J Nutr.* 2004;134:2307–2313

96. Williams C, Birch EE, Emmett PM, Northstone K. Avon Longitudinal Study of Pregnancy and Childhood Study Team. 2001. Stereoacuity at age 3.5 y in children born full-term is associated with prenatal and postnatal dietary factors: a report from a population-based cohort study. *Am J Clin Nutr.* 2001;73:316–322

97. O'Connor DL, Hall R, Adamkin D, et al. Growth and development in preterm infants fed long-chain polyunsaturated fatty acids: a prospective, randomized controlled trial. *Pediatrics.* 2001;108:359–371

98. Innis SM, Adamkin DH, Hall RT, et al. Docosahexaenoic acid and arachidonic acid enhance growth with no adverse effects in preterm infants fed formula. *J Pediatr.* 2002;140:547–554

99. Simmer K. Long chain polyunsaturated fatty acid supplementation in infants born at term. *Cochrane Database Syst Rev.* 2001;(4):CD000376

100. Simmer K, Patole S. Long chain polyunsaturated fatty acid supplementation in preterm infants. *Cochrane Database Syst Rev.* 2004;(1):CD000375

101. Gibson RA, Chen W, Makrides M. Randomized trials with polyunsaturated fatty acid interventions in preterm and term infants: functional and clinical outcomes. *Lipids.* 2001;36:873–883

102. McCall RB, Mash CW. Long-chain polyunsaturated fatty acids and the measurement and prediction of intelligence (IQ). In: Dobbing J, ed. *Developing Brain and Behaviour: The Role of Lipids in Infant Formula.* London, England: Academic Press; 1997:295–338

103. Fagan III, JF, Singer LT. Infant recognition memory as a measure of intelligence. *Adv Infancy Res.* 1983;2:31–78

104. Colombo J. Individual differences in infant cognition: methods, measures, and models. In: Dobbing J, ed. *Developing Brain and Behaviour: The Role of Lipids in Infant Formula.* London, England: Academic Press; 1997:339–385

105. Birch EE, Garfield S, Hoffman DR, Uauy RD, Birch DG. A randomized controlled trial of early dietary supply of long-chain polyunsaturated fatty acids and mental development in term infants. *Dev Med Child Neurol.* 2000;42:174–181

106. Lucas A, Stafford M, Morley R. Efficacy and safety of long-chain polyunsaturated fatty acid supplementation of infant-formula milk: a randomised trial. *Lancet.* 1999;354:1948–1954

107. Makrides M, Neumann MA, Simmer K, Gibson RA. A critical appraisal of the role of dietary long-chain polyunsaturated fatty acids on neural indices of term infants: a randomized, controlled trial. *Pediatrics.* 2000;105:32–38

108. Willats P, Forsyth JS, DiModugno MK, Varma S, Colvin M. Effect of long-chain polyunsaturated fatty acids in infant formula on problem solving at 10 months of age. *Lancet.* 1998; 352:688–691

109. Jensen CL, Voigt RG, Prager TC, et al. Effects of maternal docosahexaenoic acid intake on visual function and neurodevelopment in breastfed term infants. *Am J Clin Nutr.* 2005;82:125–132

110. Bouwstra H, Dijck-Brouwer DA, Wildeman JA, et al. Long-chain polyunsaturated fatty acids have a positive effect on the quality of general movements of healthy term infants. *Am J Clin Nutr.* 2003;78:313–318

111. Carlson SE, Cooke RJ, Werkman SH, Tolley EA. First year growth of preterm infants fed standard compared to marine oil n-3 supplemented formula. *Lipids.* 1992;27:901–907

112. Carlson SE, Werkman SH, Peeples JM, et al. Arachidonic acid status correlates with first year growth in preterm infants. *Proc Natl Acad Sci U S A.* 1993;90:1073–1077

113. Carlson SE, Werkman SH, Tolley EA. Effect of long-chain n-3 fatty acid supplementation on visual acuity and growth of preterm infants with and without bronchopulmonary dysplasia. *Am J Clin Nutr.* 1996;63:687–689

114. Ryan AS, Montalto MB, Groh-Wargo S, et al. Effect of DHA-containing formula on growth of preterm infants to 59 weeks postmenstrual age. *Am J Hum Biol.* 1999;11:457–467

115. Clandinin MT, Van Aerde JE, Merkel KL, et al. Growth and development of preterm infants fed infant formulas containing docosahexaenoic acid and arachidonic acid. *J Pediatr.* 2005;146:461–468

116. Lapillonne A, Clarke SD, Heird WC. Plausible mechanisms for effects of long-chain polyunsaturated fatty acids on growth. *J Pediatr.* 2003;143:S9–S16

117. Makrides M, Gibson RA, Udell T, Reid K. Supplementation of infant formula with long-chain polyunsaturated fatty acids does not influence the growth of term infants. International LCPUFA Investigators. *Am J Clin Nutr.* 2005;81:1094–1101

118. Heird WC. Biological effects and safety issues related to long-chain polyunsaturated fatty acids in infants. *Lipids.* 1999;34:207–214

119. Borkman M, Storlien LH, Pan DA, Jenkins AB, Chisholm PJ, Campbell LV. The relationship between insulin sensitivity and the fatty-acid composition of skeletal-muscle phospholipids. *N Engl J Med.* 1993;328:238–244

120. Clarke SD, Jump DB. Polyunsaturated fatty acid regulation of hepatic gene transcription. *J Nutr.* 1996;126 (4 Suppl):1105S–1109S

121. Klein CJ. Nutrient requirements for preterm infant formulas. *J Nutr.* 2002;132(6 Suppl 1): 1395S–1577S

17 Calcium, Phosphorus, and Magnesium

Basic Physiology/Homeostasis

The minerals calcium, magnesium, and phosphorus participate in many of the body's most important functions. These elements play prominent roles in energy processes and transport of metabolites in a host of molecular biochemical reactions. In addition, calcium and phosphorus constitute the principal components of the skeleton in the form of hydroxyapatite $Ca_{10}(PO_4)_6(OH)_2$. Magnesium, which is mainly an intracellular cation, is a cofactor in a wide variety of enzymatic reactions. Thus, these minerals are essential nutrients for life processes and for forming the mineral skeleton.[1-3]

Calcium sources include milk and other dairy products, animal bones, and in lesser amounts, a number of vegetables (Appendix Q, Table Q-1). In addition, calcium is widely found in fortified food products, such as breakfast cereals and fruit juices. Phosphorus is abundantly available from virtually all animal and vegetable sources. Magnesium, like phosphorus, is abundant in animal and plant cells. Together, these 3 elements constitute 98% of body minerals by weight. Bone accounts for 99% of the calcium, 80% of the phosphorus, and 60% of the magnesium.

Both calcium and phosphorus appear in the serum and extracellular fluid in low concentrations. The calcium concentration is closely controlled in a narrow range of 2.13 to 2.63 mmol/L (8.5–10.5 mg/dL). Approximately half of the calcium in the serum is bound to albumin at normal levels of the latter; the remainder is ionized. The ionized fraction is the physiologically active portion, and in health, the concentration is constant. If hypoalbuminemia should occur, the total calcium concentration decreases, but the ionized portion remains undisturbed. The phosphorus concentration varies and is dependent on age and diet. Normal ranges are 1.6 to 2.4 mmol/L (5.0–7.5 mg/dL) in infants, 1.3 to 1.78 mmol/L (4–5.5 mg/dL) in older children, and 0.8 to 1.6 mmol/L (2.5–4.5 mg/dL) in adults.[4]

Calcium is regulated by various hormones (parathyroid hormone, calcitonin, vitamin D) and a number of organs or tissues (skin, small intestine, kidney, and bone). The gastrointestinal tract regulates calcium absorption; a portion of the calcium is absorbed by passive diffusion and a portion of it is actively transported. Parathyroid hormone enhances serum calcium concentration primarily by releasing calcium from bone. The concentration of ionized calcium in the fluid perfusing the parathyroid gland is a major determinant of the rate of synthesis and release of this hormone. Calcitonin, a hormone elaborated by the parafollicular cells of the thyroid, inhibits bone reabsorption.[4-6] Vitamin D_3 is synthesized in the skin from 7-dehydrocholesterol on exposure to sunlight. The kidney is an important site of action of parathyroid hormone and is also the site of synthesis of the active form of vitamin D, 1,25-dihydroxyvitamin D.

Vitamin D facilitates transcellular calcium intestinal absorption. To achieve this effect, it must undergo sequential hydroxylation in the liver to calcidiol and in the kidney to the final product, calcitriol (1,25-dihydroxyvitamin D).[7,8] Calcidiol (25-hydroxyvitamin D) represents the primary circulatory and storage form of vitamin D. Anticonvulsant drugs, such as phenobarbital and phenytoin, can interfere with vitamin D hydroxylation and metabolism, increasing the daily requirement. The large reservoir of calcium in bone is important in maintaining calcium homeostasis, because a portion of bone calcium exchanges readily with the calcium of extracellular fluid.

Physical activity is an important determinant of bone health. Evidence suggests that in children, a combination of adequate mineral intake and weight-bearing physical activity are optimal for bone formation and mineralization.[9] Disuse osteoporosis, as may occur in children with chronic illnesses, also leads to marked bone loss.

Bone formation and calcium metabolism are also regulated via genetic factors that are only partially understood. Recent data implicate specific vitamin D receptor genes as affecting calcium absorption in children.[10] Other data indicate that race and gender also affect calcium absorption.[11,12]

Vitamin D facilitates transcellular calcium intestinal absorption. To achieve this effect, it must undergo sequential hydroxylation in the liver to calcidiol and in the kidney to the final product, calcitriol (1,25-dihydroxyvitamin D).[4,8] Calcidiol (25-hydroxyvitamin D) represents the primary storage form of vitamin D. Anticonvulsant drugs, such as phenobarbital and phenytoin, can interfere with vitamin D hydroxylation and metabolism, increasing the daily requirement.

Less is known about the regulation of phosphorus. Phosphorus is absorbed efficiently in the small intestine, and its absorption is inhibited by aluminum-containing antacids. Phosphorous is filtered and reabsorbed in the kidney, and parathyroid hormone inhibits its renal reabsorption. A significant aspect of phosphorus regulation is by renal excretion such that renal insufficiency leads to decreased renal phosphate excretion and hyperphosphatemia.[8]

Only a small fraction of total body magnesium is present in serum. The normal serum total magnesium concentration 1.6 to 2.5 mg/dL (0.67–1.04 mmol/L). Approximately half of this magnesium is bound to protein, principally albumin. Magnesium homeostasis is maintained partly by control of intestinal absorption but also by control of renal excretion. Magnesium appears to be absorbed principally in the ileum by 3 mechanisms: passive diffusion, "solvent drag," and probably, by active transport. Absorption of magnesium is inversely related to intake and is minimally affected by vitamin D.

Parathyroid hormone decreases renal reabsorption of filtered magnesium. Release of parathyroid hormone is modestly suppressed by increased concentrations of magnesium in extracellular fluid, an action that may be mediated by an increase in calcium in the cytosol of parathyroid cells. Conversely, acute (but not chronic) hypomagnesemia stimulates the release of parathyroid hormone.[8,13–16]

Transient neonatal hypomagnesemia has been observed in association with both hypocalcemia and hyperphosphatemia but is uncommon. Transient neonatal hypomagnesemia is more common in infants with intrauterine growth retardation and infants of mothers with diabetes, hypophosphatemia, or hyperparathyroidism. Magnesium supplements may be required for these infants. Rarely, severe hypomagnesemia associated with convulsions occurs in early infancy as a result of a genetically determined disorder of magnesium metabolism. This disorder probably results from a defective intestinal absorption of magnesium. Long-term magnesium supplementation is necessary.[14]

Calcium Requirements

The specific requirements for calcium intake by full-term infants, children, and adolescents have been extensively reviewed in recent years[8,17] and affirmed by the American Academy of Pediatrics. The most current recommendations for adequate calcium intake are shown in Table 17.1.

Multiple approaches are used to assess the requirements for these minerals in children, including the following: (1) measurement of calcium balance in children with various levels of calcium intake; (2) measurement of bone mineral content by dual-energy absorptiometry or other techniques in groups of children before and after calcium supplementation; and (3) epidemiologic studies relating bone mass or fracture risk in children and adults with childhood calcium intake.[17] The interactions of these factors make identification of a single optimal daily calcium "requirement" for all children impossible.[18]

Table 17.1
Recommendations for Adequate Dietary Calcium Intake in the United States

Age	Calcium Intake, mg/day (mmol/day)
0–6 mo*	210 (5.3)
7–12 mo†	270 (6.8)
1–3 y	500 (12.5)
4–8 y	800 (20.0)
9–18 y	1300 (32.5)
19–50 y	1000 (25)
50 to >70 y	1200 (30)

The Food and Nutrition Board of the National Academy of Sciences (NAS) released recommended dietary allowances for calcium in 1997. The term "Adequate Intake" was applied to calcium recommendations. Application of the Adequate Intake is similar to that of the recommended dietary allowance. The American Academy of Pediatrics recommends that the NAS guidelines should be the primary guidelines used.

* The 1997 NAS report used data based on younger infants (0–6 mo) who are fed human milk exclusively.

† The 1997 NAS report was based on the assumption that older infants (6 mo–1 y) would be consuming a diet of human milk and solid foods, which would be similar to that of formula-fed infants at this age.

Reprinted from Greer FR, Krebs NF, and American Academy of Pediatrics, Committee on Nutrition.[17]

The calcium balance technique involves measuring the effects of any given calcium intake on the net retention of calcium by the body. This approach is commonly used to estimate minimal requirement. Its usefulness is based on the principle that all retained calcium is used, and calcium that is not used is excreted and, thus, unnecessary. In children, optimizing calcium retention from the diet should lead to the highest degree of skeletal mineralization and, thus, decrease the relative risk of osteoporosis in adults.[18–21]

The substantial limitations involved in obtaining and interpreting data about calcium balance are well known. These include substantial technical problems with measuring calcium excretion and the difficulty obtaining dietary intake control in children. These problems have been partly overcome by the development of stable isotopic methods to assess calcium absorption and excretion.[20] Because most data are from studies in infants and adolescent girls, more data are needed to establish the "optimal" level of calcium retention at different ages. At very low calcium intakes in adolescents (ie, <600 mg/day), increased fractional absorption and decreasing urinary excretion of calcium occur. However, these adaptations are not able to prevent much lower amounts of total calcium absorption and retention than calcium intakes closer to recommended amounts.[22]

A major advance in the field during the last 25 years has been improved methods of measuring total body and regional bone mineral content by various radiologic techniques. Currently, the technique used in the majority of studies is dual-energy absorptiometry. This technique can rapidly measure the bone mineral content and bone mineral density of the entire skeleton or of regional sites with a minimal radiation exposure. Furthermore, recent enhancements in the precision of the technique have made it particularly suitable for assessing the short- and long-term effects of calcium supplementation on bone mass in children of all ages.[23,24] Nonetheless, substantial limitations in current dual-energy absorptiometry technology have led to increased interest in the use of newer techniques, including quantitative computed tomography and bone ultrasonography.[25] These require further evaluation in children but may provide additional information about bone structure and strength and, in the case of ultrasonography, may be more readily available for bedside use in intensive care settings.

Preterm Infants

The accretion of calcium and phosphorus increase exponentially in utero during the third trimester. Inadequate mineral intake places preterm infants at risk of the condition called osteopenia of prematurity. It is a common problem in infants weighing less than 1000 g at birth who have relatively low intakes of calcium and phosphorus. The frequency of osteopenia is also increased in preterm infants who require long-term parenteral nutrition or who require medications, such as diuretics, which may adversely affect mineral metabolism.[26] In small preterm infants fed by parenteral nutrition, the danger of calcium-phosphorus precipitation in the solution limits the amount of these minerals that can be administered intravenously. As a result, prenatal retention rates of calcium and phosphorus are not achieved.[27]

The presence of severe osteopenia can be assessed by direct radiologic evaluation. Increased lucency of the cortical bone with or without epiphyseal changes is characteristic of significant osteopenia. Although the presence of a fracture can be the presenting sign of osteopenia of prematurity, most infants with decreased bone mineralization, including some with severe rickets, do not have fractures.

Human milk is relatively low in calcium and phosphorus relative to the in utero accretion rates of these minerals. Although minerals are well absorbed from human milk (60%–70%), the net retention rates of calcium and phosphorus are far below those in utero and can lead to the development of undermineralized bones. Supplementary calcium and phosphorus are needed to sustain optimal calcium balance. Currently, several commercial mineral supplements (for breastfed infants) and special formulas are marketed in the United States for use by preterm infants (see Appendix I, Tables I-1 and I-2). Use of these products has led to net calcium retention comparable with that achieved in utero.[28] After preterm infants are discharged from the hospital, there may be benefits to providing a higher mineral intake than is available from human milk or from routine cow milk-based formulas,[29-31] although the ideal population and magnitude of benefits is uncertain. This is particularly true for infants who weighed less than 1500 g at birth and/or required oxygen or fluid restriction after hospital discharge. Multiple strategies are in clinical use for this situation, without clear identification of an optimal approach.

Full-Term Infants and Children

The optimal primary nutritional source during the first year of life for healthy full-term infants is human milk. No available evidence shows that exceeding the amount of calcium retained by the exclusively breastfed full-term infant during the first 6 months of life or the amount retained by the breastfed infant supplemented with solid foods during the second 6 months of life is beneficial to achieving long-term increases in bone mineralization. Cow milk-based formulas contain more calcium than does human milk. Relatively greater calcium concentrations are found in specialized formulas, such as soy formulas and casein hydrolysate formulas, to account for the potential lower bioavailability of the calcium from these formulas relative to cow milk-based formula.[14] Recent data demonstrate that the fractional absorption of calcium from some formulas is similar to that of human milk. Thus, the much higher calcium content in such formulas leads to greater net calcium retention than with human milk.[32,33]

Some variations exist in the amount of calcium absorbed by infants consuming different formulas and the bone mineral mass accumulated during infancy.[34,35] Similarly, studies comparing the bone mineral content of full-term infants during the first year of life have generally found a slightly greater value for those fed infant formulas than those fed human milk, likely because of the usual greater net calcium, retention as noted previously.[32,33,36] However, no data suggest such a difference is maintained through adolescence, and there is no evidence at present that these differences lead to clinically significant differences in bone mass.[37] Longer-term studies are needed to evaluate these issues, but at the present time, the bone mass of the breast-fed infant remains the reference standard for appropriate bone mineral mass accumulation in infancy.

Few data are available about the calcium requirements of children before puberty. Calcium retention is relatively low in toddlers and slowly increases as puberty approaches. The benefits of intakes above the Adequate Intake (AI) in this age group are uncertain. High calcium intake may negatively affect other minerals, especially iron, although adaptation to this effect may occur.[38] Because these minerals are important for growth and development and may be marginal in toddlers and preschool children, more data regarding the risks and benefits of higher calcium intake are needed before it can be recommended before puberty.

Perhaps of most importance in young children is the development of eating patterns that will be associated with adequate calcium intake later in life. As such, it is important that families learn to identify the calcium content of foods (see Appendix Q, Table Q-2) on the basis of the food label and incorporate this information into their food-buying habits. The most readily available source of calcium is dairy products (70%–80% of calcium content in US diets).

Preadolescents and Adolescents

Most research in children about calcium requirements has been directed toward 9- to 18-year-old females. The efficiency of calcium absorption is increased during puberty, and most bone formation occurs during this period. Data from balance studies suggest that for most healthy children in this age range, the maximal net calcium balance (plateau) is approached with intakes of approximately 1300 mg/day. That is, at intakes higher than 1300 mg/day, almost all of the additional calcium is excreted and not used; at lower intakes, the skeleton may not receive as much calcium as it can use, and peak bone mass may not be achieved.[8] Virtually all the data used to establish this intake amount are from white children; minimal data are available for other ethnic groups.

Numerous controlled trials have found an increase in the bone mineral content in children in this age group who have received calcium supplementation.[8,39-43] However, the available data suggest that if calcium intake is augmented only for relatively short periods (ie, 1 to 2 years), there may be minimal or no long-term benefits to establishing and maintaining a maximum peak bone mass.[44,45] Even longer-term increased intake of calcium may only lead to relatively small benefits in bone.[42] Recent results indicate that calcium supplementation may be more beneficial in some subgroups of children, such as those with early puberty or those of greater height.[42,46,47] The implications of such findings for dietary guidance are unclear. In general, the available data emphasize the importance of a well-balanced diet in achieving adequate calcium intake and in establishing dietary patterns with a calcium intake at or near recommended amounts throughout childhood and adolescence.[17]

In addition to calcium intake, exercise is an important aspect of achieving maximal peak bone mass. There is evidence that childhood and adolescence may represent an important period for achieving long-lasting skeletal benefits from regular exercise.[41] Recent data support the possibility that low bone mass may be a contributing factor to some fractures in children.[48]

Although virtually all data regarding the importance of calcium intake have focused on the bone health benefits, emerging evidence from studies in adults and some in children suggest that calcium intake may be important in the regulation of both blood pressure and weight.[49-51] This is a dynamic field of investigation, and firm conclusions cannot be reached at this time.

It is recommended that pediatricians actively discuss issues of bone health with families during routine visits. Such discussions are recommended at 2 to 3 years of age, 8 to 9 years of age, and later during adolescence. An emphasis should be placed on preventing inadequate calcium intake, encouraging weight-bearing exercise, and ensuring adequate vitamin D status.[17]

Adolescent Pregnancy and Lactation

At birth, the fetus contains approximately 30 g of calcium. This represents approximately 2.5% of typical maternal body calcium stores.[14] Evidence suggests that, in adult women, much of this 30 g comes from increases in dietary calcium absorption during pregnancy.[52] A recent study demonstrated a similar increase in calcium absorption during pregnancy in adolescents.[53]

During lactation, a period of 6 months of exclusive breastfeeding would lead to an additional 45 g of calcium secreted by the mother. Although some of this is accounted for by decreased urinary calcium excretion during lactation, there is extensive evidence demonstrating a loss of maternal bone calcium during lactation.[54-56] In adults, however, bone remineralization occurs after weaning, and neither pregnancy nor lactation is associated with persistent bone loss. Because of recent data demonstrating that calcium supplementation is not effective in preventing lactation-associated bone loss or enhancing postweaning bone mass recovery,[54] recent dietary recommendations do not suggest increases in calcium for healthy adult women who are pregnant or lactating higher than the 1000 mg/day recommended for nonlactating adult women.

The situation for pregnant and lactating adolescents is less clear. Current guidelines do not recommend an intake higher than the age-appropriate maximum for adolescents (1300 mg/day) who are either pregnant or lactating.[8] Recent data demonstrated a shorter fetal femur length in pregnant black adolescents with low dairy intake, compared with those with higher intakes.[57] This is consistent with earlier similar data demonstrating a lower bone mineral density associated with low calcium intake during pregnancy in adults.[58]

At the present time, the available evidence supports the recommendation that the benefits of breastfeeding greatly outweigh any demonstrated risks to adolescents in terms of achieving either optimal growth or peak bone mass.[53,59] No available data suggest that calcium intakes higher than the recommended amounts are beneficial to pregnant or lactating adolescents. However, it should be noted that these recommended intake amounts are far higher than those typical of the diet of most adolescents.

Phosphorous Requirements

As with calcium, the recommended intake of phosphorus for infants was based on usual dietary intakes of breastfed infants. These values are 100 mg/day from ages 0 to 6 months and 275 mg/day from ages 7 through 12 months. The higher value in older infants reflects the considerable contribution of solid foods to usual phosphorus intakes of these infants. There are few data on which to base estimates of phosphorus requirements for older children. Dietary guidelines[8] used a factorial approach based on limited estimates of phosphorus absorption, excretion, and accretion to determine average requirements. An allotment of an additional 20% was provided to calculate the Recommended Dietary Allowance. Using this method, values for the Recommended Dietary Allowance of 460 mg/day for children 1 through 3 years of age and 500 mg/day for children 4 through 8 years of age were derived. These values are well below typical intakes for children of these ages, suggesting that deficient phosphorus intake is an uncommon problem in small children.

For adolescents, both the factorial method and estimates of intake needed to maintain typical serum phosphorus concentrations were used to determine intake guidelines. A value of 1250 mg/day was calculated for boys and girls 9 through 18 years of age.[8] This value is much closer to typical intakes for adolescents and reflects the rapid bone and muscle growth during this time period.

Magnesium Requirements

Current dietary guidelines for infants are based on the intakes of breastfed infants. The recommended intakes are 30 mg/day for infants in the first 6 months of life and 75 mg/day from 7 through 12 months. Commercial cow milk-based infant formulas are generally higher in magnesium concentration (40–50 mg/L) than is human milk (34 mg/L). Soy-based formulas may have even higher amounts of magnesium (50–80 mg/L).[8,10] In a large series of studies, Fomon and Nelson reported approximately 40% absorption of magnesium in infants fed soy or milk-based formulas (based on total intake of 53–59 mg/day), with a net retention of 9 to 10 mg/day.[8,14]

Few metabolic balance studies have been performed for magnesium in children, especially those between 1 and 8 years of age. On the basis of limited available data, it appears that a magnesium intake of 5 mg/kg per day should lead to positive magnesium balances in most children. Using average weight-for-age data, this leads to an AI of 80 mg/day for ages 1 through 3 years, 130 mg/day for ages 4 through 8 years, and 240 mg/day for ages 9 through 13 years. For adolescents 14 through 18 years of age, slightly greater average intakes are needed (5.3 mg/kg per day) to account for increased pubertal magnesium needs. Differences in average weights of boys and girls were used to calculate AIs of 410 mg/day for boys and 360 mg/day for girls.[8]

Because of efficient homeostatic mechanisms, especially renal conservation of magnesium, low dietary magnesium intake alone does not usually cause clinically apparent magnesium deficiency. Magnesium deficiency is, however, quite common in young children with protein-energy malnutrition, especially when accompanied by gastroenteritis. Muscle magnesium is depressed, but serum magnesium concentration may be normal. Hypomagnesemia sometimes occurs in malabsorption syndromes, and magnesium depletion may develop in subjects with severe diarrhea. Convulsions are the most clearly documented feature of hypomagnesemia, with or without total body magnesium deficiency in infants and young children. Neuropsychiatric disorders are well documented in magnesium-depleted adults. Hypocalcemia associated with magnesium deficiency may be the result of defective synthesis or release of parathyroid hormone. Hypokalemia also occurs secondarily to magnesium deficiency.[60]

Numerous conditions may be related to subacute magnesium deficiency. For example, recent evidence has linked magnesium deficiency with insulin resistance and worsening diabetic regulation. Increased blood pressure, migraines, and inadequate bone mineralization may also be linked to habitually low magnesium intake, although data for these relationships continues to be incomplete.[8]

Dietary Sources: Calcium and Phosphorus

Knowledge of dietary calcium sources is a first step toward increasing the intake of calcium-rich foods. The largest source of dietary calcium for most people is milk and other dairy products. Most vegetables contain calcium, although at low density. Therefore, relatively large servings are needed to equal the total intake achieved with typical servings of dairy products. The bioavailability of calcium from vegetables is generally high. An exception is spinach, which is high in oxalate, making the calcium virtually nonbioavailable. Several products have been introduced that are fortified with calcium. These products, most notably orange juice, are fortified to achieve a calcium concentration similar to that of milk. Breakfast foods also are commonly fortified with minerals, including calcium. The gap between the recommended calcium intakes and the typical intakes of children and adolescents is substantial. A list of foods relatively high in calcium is given in Appendix Q, Table Q-1. Most adolescents, especially females, have calcium intakes below recommended amounts (see Table 17.1). Preoccupation with being thin is common in this age group, especially among females, as is the misconception that all dairy foods are fattening. Many children and adolescents are unaware that low-fat milk contains at least as much calcium as does whole milk.

For children with lactose intolerance, several alternatives exist. Lactose intolerance is more common in black, Hispanic, and Asian individuals than in white individuals. Many children with lactose intolerance can drink small amounts of milk without discomfort. Other alternatives include the use of other dairy products, such as solid cheeses and yogurt, which may be better tolerated than milk. Lactose-free and low-lactose milks are also available.[61]

In general, dietary sources of calcium, including fortified foods, are preferred to calcium supplementation via pill or similar nondietary supplements, because the range of nutrients and the establishment of good dietary habits are enhanced by use of dietary calcium sources. Furthermore, nutrient interactions may be decreased and tolerance may be greater for minerals provided from food sources.

Dietary Sources: Magnesium

Quantities in infant formulas range from 40 to 70 mg/L (3.3–5.8 mEq/L). Whole grains, beans, and legumes are good sources. Because magnesium is a component of chlorophyll, green, leafy vegetables are high in magnesium. Other dietary sources include milk, eggs, and meat. Depending on its "hardness," water may also contribute significantly to dietary magnesium intake.

References

1. Cohn SH, Vaswani A, Zanzi I, Aloia JF, Roginsky MS, Ellis KJ. Changes in body chemical composition with age measured by total-body neutron activation. *Metabolism*. 1976;25:85–95

2. Widdowson EM, Spray CM. Chemical development in utero. *Arch Dis Child*. 1951;26: 205–214

3. Widdowson EM, McCance RA, Spray CM. The chemical composition of the human body. *Clin Sci*. 1951;10:113–125

4. Broadus AE. Mineral balance and homeostasis. In: Favus MJ, ed. *Primer on the Metabolic Bone Diseases and Disorders of Mineral Metabolism*. 5th ed. New York, NY: Raven Press; 2003:105–111

5. Salle BL, Delvin EE, Lapillonne A, Bishop NJ, Glorieux FH. Perinatal metabolism of vitamin D. *Am J Clin Nutr*. 2000;71:1317S–1324S

6. Bronner F, Pansu D. Nutritional aspects of calcium absorption. *J Nutr*. 1999;129:9–12

7. Kim Y, Linkswiler HM. Effect of level of protein intake on calcium metabolism and on parathyroid and renal function in the adult human male. *J Nutr*. 1979;109:1399–1404

8. Institute of Medicine. *Dietary Reference Intakes for Calcium, Phosphorus, Magnesium, Vitamin D, and Fluoride*. Washington, DC: National Academies Press; 1997

9. Specker BL, Mulligan L, Ho M. Longitudinal study of calcium intake, physical activity, and bone mineral content in infants 6–18 months of age. *J Bone Miner Res*. 1999;14:569–576

10. Abrams SA, Griffin IJ, Hawthorne KM, et al. Vitamin D receptor Fok1 polymorphisms affect calcium absorption, kinetics, and bone mineralization rates during puberty. *J Bone Miner Res*. 2005;20:945–953

11. Wigertz K, Palacios C, Jackman LA, et al. Racial differences in calcium retention in response to dietary salt in adolescent girls. *Am J Clin Nutr*. 2005;81:845–850

12. Abrams SA, O'Brien KO, Liang LK, Stuff JE. Differences in calcium absorption and kinetics between black and white girls age 5–16 years. *J Bone Miner Res*. 1995;10:829–833

13. Hardwick LL, Jones MR, Brautbar N, Lee DB. Magnesium absorption: mechanisms and the influence of vitamin D, calcium, and phosphate. *J Nutr*. 1991;121:13–23

14. Fomon SJ, Nelson SE. Calcium, phosphorus, magnesium, and sulfur. In: Fomon SJ, ed. *Nutrition of Normal Infants*. St Louis, MO: Mosby-Year Book Inc; 1993:192–218

15. Shils ME. Magnesium in health and disease. *Annu Rev Nutr*. 1988;8:429–460

16. Yamamoto T, Kabata H, Yagi R, Takashima M, Itokawa Y. Primary hypomagnesemia with secondary hypocalcemia: report of a case and review of the world literature. *Magnesium*. 1985;4:153–164

17. Greer FR, Krebs NF, American Academy of Pediatrics, Committee on Nutrition. Optimizing bone health and calcium intakes of infants, children, and adolescents. *Pediatrics*. 2006;117:578–585

18. Miller GD, Weaver CM. Required versus optimal intakes: a look at calcium. *J Nutr*. 1994;124(8 Suppl):1404S–1405S

19. Jackman LA, Millane SS, Martin BR, Wood OB, McCabe GP, Peacock M, Weaver CM. Calcium retention in relation to calcium intake and postmenarcheal age in adolescent females. *Am J Clin Nutr*. 1997;66:327–333

20. Abrams SA, Stuff JE. Calcium metabolism in girls: current dietary intakes lead to low rates of calcium absorption and retention during puberty. *Am J Clin Nutr*. 1994;60:739–743

21. Abrams SA, Grusak MA, Stuff J, O'Brien KO. Calcium and magnesium balance in 9–14-y-old children. *Am J Clin Nutr*. 1997;66:1172–1177

22. Abrams SA, Griffin IJ, Hicks PD, Gunn SK. Pubertal girls only partially adapt to low dietary calcium intakes. *J Bone Min Res*. 2004 ;19:759–763

23. Ellis KJ, Abrams SA, Wong WW. Body composition in a young multiethnic female population. *Am J Clin Nutr*. 1997;65:724–731

24. Christiansen C, Rodbro P, Nielsen CT. Bone mineral content and estimated total body calcium in normal children and adolescents. *Scand J Clin Lab Invest*. 1975;35:507–510

25. Wren TA, Liu X, Pitukcheewanont P, Gilsanz V. Bone densitometry in pediatric populations: discrepancies in the diagnosis of osteoporosis by DXA and CT. *J Pediatr*. 2005;146:776–779

26. Atkinson SA. Human milk feeding of the micropremie. *Clin Perinatol*. 2000;27:235–247

27. Prestridge LL, Schanler RJ, Shulman RJ, Burns PA, Laine LL. Effect of parenteral calcium and phosphorus therapy on mineral retention and bone mineral content in very low birth weight infants. *J Pediatr*. 1993;122:761–768

28. Schanler RJ, Abrams SA. Postnatal attainment of intrauterine macromineral accretion rates in low birth weight infants fed fortified human milk. *J Pediatr*. 1995;126:441–447

29. Carver JD, Wu PY, Hall RT, et al. Growth of preterm infants fed nutrient-enriched or term formula after hospital discharge. *Pediatrics*. 2001;107:683–689

30. Hawthorne KM, Griffin IJ, Abrams SA. Current issues in nutritional management of very low birth weight infants. *Minerva Pediatr*. 2004;56:359–372

31. Lapillonne A, Salle BL, Glorieux FH, Claris O. Bone mineralization and growth are enhanced in preterm infants fed an isocaloric, nutrient-enriched preterm formula through term. *Am J Clin Nutr*. 2004;80:1595–1603

32. Abrams SA, Griffin IJ, Davila PM. Calcium and zinc absorption from lactose-containing and lactose-free infant formulas. *Am J Clin Nutr*. 2002;76:442–446

33. Abrams SA, Wen J, Stuff JE. Absorption of calcium, zinc and iron from breast milk by five- to seven-month-old infants. *Pediatr Res*. 1997;41:384–390

34. Nelson SE, Frantz JA, Ziegler EE. Absorption of fat and calcium by infants fed a milk-based formula containing palm olein. *J Am Coll Nutr*. 1998;17:327–332

35. Koo WW, Hammami M, Margeson DP, Nwaesei C, Montalto MB, Lasekan JB. Reduced bone mineralization in infants fed palm olein-containing formula: a randomized, double-blinded, prospective trial. *Pediatrics*. 2003;111:1017–1023

36. Specker BL, Beck A, Kalkwarf H, Ho M. Randomized trial of varying mineral intake on total body bone mineral accretion during the first year of life. *Pediatrics.* 1997;99(6):e12. Available at: http://pediatrics.aappublications.org/cgi/content/full/99/6/e12. Accessed August 21, 2007

37. Young RJ, Antonson DL, Ferguson PW, Murray ND, Merkel K, Moore TE. Neonatal and infant feeding: effect on bone density at 4 years. *J Pediatr Gastroenterol Nutr.* 2005;41:88–93

38. Ames SK, Gorham BM, Abrams SA. Effects of high vs low calcium intake on calcium absorption and incorporation of iron by red blood cells in small children. *Am J Clin Nutr.* 1999;70:44–48

39. Lloyd T, Andon MB, Rollings N, et al. Calcium supplementation and bone mineral density in adolescent girls. *JAMA.* 1993;270:841–844

40. Lee WT, Leung SS, Leung DM, Cheng JC. A follow-up study on the effects of calcium-supplement withdrawal and puberty on bone acquisition of children. *Am J Clin Nutr.* 1996;64:71–77

41. Lloyd T, Petit MA, Lin HM, Beck TJ. Lifestyle factors and the development of bone mass and bone strength in young women. *J Pediatr.* 2004;144:776–782

42. Matkovic V, Goel PK, Badenhop-Stevens NE, et al. Calcium supplementation and bone mineral density in females from childhood to young adulthood: a randomized controlled trial. *Am J Clin Nutr.* 2005;81:175–188

43. Matkovic V, Landoll JD, Badenhop-Stevens NE, et al. Nutrition influences skeletal development from childhood to adulthood: a study of hip, spine, and forearm in adolescent females. *J Nutr.* 2004;134:701S–705S

44. Lanou AJ, Berkow SE, Barnard ND. Calcium, dairy products, and bone health in children and young adults: a reevaluation of the evidence. *Pediatrics.* 2005;115:736–743

45. Abrams SA. Calcium supplementation during childhood: long-term effects on bone mineralization. *Nutr Rev.* 2005;63:251–255

46. Abrams SA, Griffin IJ, Hawthorne KM, Liang L. Height and height Z-score are related to calcium absorption in 5 to 15 yr-old girls. *J Clin Endocrinol Metab.* 2005;90:5077–5081

47. Chevalley T, Rizzoli R, Hans D, Ferrari S, Bonjour P. Interaction between calcium intake and menarcheal age on bone mass gain: an eight-year follow-up study from prepuberty to postmenarche. *J Clin Endocrinol Metab.* 2005;90:44–51

48. Goulding A, Cannan R, Williams SM, Gold EJ, Taylor RW, Lewis-Barned NJ. Bone mineral density in girls with forearm fractures. *J Bone Miner Res.* 1998;13:143–148

49. Dixon LB, Pellizzon MA, Jawad AF, Tershakovec AM. Calcium and dairy intake and measures of obesity in hyper- and normocholesterolemic children. *Obes Res.* 2005;13:1727–1738

50. Huang TT, McCrory MA. Dairy intake, obesity, and metabolic health in children and adolescents: knowledge and gaps. *Nutr Rev.* 2005;63:71–80

51. Lorenzen JK, Molgaard C, Michaelsen KF, Astrup A. Calcium supplementation for 1 y does not reduce body weight or fat mass in young girls. *Am J Clin Nutr.* 2006;83:18–23

52. Heaney RP, Skillman TG, Calcium metabolism in normal human pregnancy. *J Clin Endocrinol Metab.* 1971;33:661–670

53. O'Brien KO, Nathanson MS, Mancini J, Witter FR. Calcium absorption is significantly higher in adolescents during pregnancy than in the early postpartum period. *Am J Clin Nutr.* 2003;78:1188–1193

54. Kalkwarf HJ, Specker BL, Bianchi DC, Ranz J, Ho M. The effect of calcium supplements on bone density during lactation and after weaning. *N Engl J Med.* 1997;337:523–528

55. Kalkwarf HJ, Specker BL. Bone mineral loss during lactation and recovery after weaning. *Obstet Gynecol.* 1995;86:26–32

56. Hopkinson JM, Butte NF, Ellis K, Smith EO. Lactation delays postpartum bone mineral accretion and temporarily alters its regional distribution in women. *J Nutr.* 2000;130: 777–783

57. Chang SC, O'Brien KO, Nathanson MS, Caulfield LE, Mancini J, Witter FR. Fetal femur length is influenced by maternal diary intake in pregnant African American adolescents. *Am J Clin Nutr.* 2003;77:1248–1254

58. Koo WW, Walters JC, Esterlitz J, Levine RJ, Bush AJ, Sibai B. Maternal calcium supplementation and fetal bone mineralization. *Obstet Gynecol.* 1999;94:577–582

59. Bezerra FF, Mendonca LM, Lobato EC, O'Brien KO, Donangelo CM. Bone mass is recovered from lactation to postweaning in adolescent mothers with low calcium intakes. *Am J Clin Nutr.* 2004;80:1322–1326

60. Rude RK. Magnesium deficiency: a cause of heterogeneous disease in humans. *J Bone Miner Res.* 1998;13:749–758

61. Heymann MB, American Academy of Pediatrics, Committee on Nutrition. Lactose intolerance in infants, children, and adolescents. *Pediatrics.* 2006;118:1279–1286

Iron

Iron deficiency is the most common nutritional deficiency in the United States, affecting mainly older infants, young children, adolescent girls after onset of menarche, and women of childbearing age. The risk of iron deficiency in the developing child increases at ages when iron intake is low; when iron losses increase, usually as a result of blood loss; or when iron demand is increased during rapid expansion of the blood volume associated with growth spurts. Frequently, 2 or more of these processes are present, putting further stress on iron homeostasis. Preterm infants, infants with growth retardation, and infants of mothers with diabetes are born with low iron stores and are at risk of earlier postnatal iron deficiency than infants born without these risk factors. Young children are the most susceptible to iron deficiency as a result of an increased iron requirement related to rapid growth during the first 2 years of life and a relatively low iron content in most infant diets when iron is not added by supplementation or fortification. According to results of the 1999–2002 National Health and Nutrition Examination Survey (NHANES), 9.2% of children between the ages of 1 and 3 years have evidence of iron deficiency on the basis of iron biochemistry test results, and 2.34% have iron-deficiency anemia.[1] Children 3 to 11 years of age are at less risk of iron deficiency until the onset of the rapid growth period that occurs during puberty. Adolescent females are at greater risk of iron deficiency because of blood lost through menstruation. Adolescent athletes also have a higher rate of iron deficiency. The NHANES conducts biyearly analyses, but a compendium NHANES IV has not yet been published. Given the general decline in rates of iron deficiency over the past 4 decades with increased public awareness and fortification of infant formulas, another decrease in rates can be expected. Nevertheless, the national objective to achieve an iron deficiency rate of less than 3% by the year 2000 was not achieved and remains the target for 2010.

Significant improvements have been made in the iron nutritional status of infants and young children in the United States. Iron deficiency during childhood became a public health issue during the late 1960s with the recognition that the amount of iron in cow milk and infant formula was insufficient to support erythropoiesis during the first 2 years of life. At that time, breastfeeding rates were at a low point and infant formulas were not supplemented with additional iron. Breastfeeding and formula feeding were recommended for the first 6 months of life, and cow milk was consumed during the second 6 months. Fortification of infant formulas to a concentration of 12 mg of elemental iron/L was the logical response and reflected a strategy of "building iron stores" during the first 6 months of life to ensure adequate iron status through the following 6 to 12 months. This logic is now largely antiquated as the American Academy of Pediatrics (AAP) and other bodies have recommended breastfeeding or, alternatively, formula feeding for the first 12 months with no exposure to cow milk until after the first birthday. Given the longer exposure to these iron-sufficient nutrient sources and avoidance of potential gastrointestinal blood loss induced by early cow milk exposure, it is unlikely that iron-fortified formulas need to be supplemented to a level of 12 mg/L. Indeed, one study showed that infants maintain sufficient iron stores on formulas with iron contents as low as 4 mg/L, although markers of iron metabolism indicate that they must upregulate iron accretion rates to do so.[2] Another study demonstrated no substantial increase in iron incorporation into red blood cells between infants fed formulas containing 8 mg/L and those fed formulas containing 12 mg/L.[3] The current Life Sciences Research Office recommendations are that formula-fed term infants should consume formula with an iron concentration of 3 to 11 mg/L. The AAP policy statement on iron fortification of infant formulas recommends that the manufacture of low-iron formulas be discontinued and that infant formulas be fortified with 4.0–12 mg/L of iron.[4] Currently, term infant formulas marketed in the United States contain between 4.5 and 12 mg/L of iron.

Several studies have demonstrated a significant decrease in the prevalence of anemia as a result of the public health initiative, although a baseline rate continues to exist.[1,5] This encouraging trend of improved iron status related to better dietary practices during infancy underscores the importance of primary prevention for the control of childhood iron deficiency.

One consequence of the lower prevalence of iron-deficiency anemia is the limited ability to use anemia as a screening indicator for iron deficiency. Because iron deficiency is becoming a less common cause of anemia in general, the presence of anemia is increasingly a poorer predictor for iron deficiency. In addition, investigators have begun to define potential neurobehavioral deficits in preanemic iron-deficient children,[6] suggesting that the brain becomes iron deficient before anemia is detected. Recent efforts by the World Health Organization, Centers for Disease Control and Prevention (CDC), and NHANES have endeavored to generate new sensitive and specific tests to screen for preanemic iron deficiency.[7,8] These may include metrics, such as serum transferrin concentration, or the ratio of serum transferrin concentration to ferritin concentration. Therefore, approaches to maintain optimal childhood iron nutrition should continue the emphasis on primary prevention with sound iron nutrition during pregnancy, infancy, and adolescence (in females) and selective use of anemia testing for the subset of children whose background indicates a greater risk of iron deficiency. In newborn infants, these subsets include preterm infants and infants with intrauterine growth retardation, because they are born with lower total body iron stores than term infants and those with size appropriate for gestational age. Whereas term infants have adequate iron stores to sustain them for 4 months after birth, preterm infants and those with intrauterine growth retardation mobilize all of their iron stores within 2 months if unsupplemented. In infancy, these subsets include infants fed low-iron formula and breastfed infants older than 6 months not receiving iron supplementation as well as children living at or below the poverty level. In adolescents, the subset includes postmenarchal girls and those on low- or no-meat diets.

Consequences of Iron Deficiency

The most well-known consequence of iron deficiency is anemia. However, unless severe (hemoglobin concentration <8 g/dL), anemia in itself does not constitute a grave threat to health. Rather, it is an indicator of the severity of iron deficiency. Most children with iron deficiency are not anemic (characterized by low serum ferritin concentrations reflecting low iron stores and high serum transferrin concentrations indicating activation of cellular iron uptake mechanisms). A smaller proportion of children have the more advanced finding of iron-deficiency anemia. It is important to recognize that anemia represents the most severe end of the iron-deficiency spectrum, because iron is prioritized to the red blood cells at the expense of all other tissues, including the brain. The limitation of screening for iron deficiency by routine hemoglobin testing is that by the time anemia is diagnosed, the neurologic consequences have likely already occurred.

Among the major consequences of iron deficiency that have been studied, the evidence that significant iron deficiency adversely affects child development and behavior is of greatest concern. There are now 40 studies that have investigated the adverse effect of early iron deficiency on neurodevelopmental outcome.[9] Both cognitive and motor deficits have been documented.[10] Developmental deficits, to some extent, can be corrected with iron treatment.[11] However, evidence also showed that some neurologic and cognitive deficits were not reversible with iron treatment and persisted up to 10 years after iron treatment.[10,12] The threat of irreversible developmental delay resulting from a temporary nutritional deficiency emphasizes the importance of prevention. It is the tissue-level iron deficiency that likely results in neurobehavioral consequences.

Another health consequence of iron deficiency is enhanced absorption and brain accretion of other divalent cations, including those that can be detrimental to health, such as lead and manganese. Animal and human studies have demonstrated that gastrointestinal absorption of lead increases with the severity of iron deficiency.[13,14] Clinical and epidemiologic studies also demonstrate an association between an elevated blood lead concentration and iron deficiency.[13] Because childhood lead poisoning is a well-documented cause of neurologic and developmental deficits, iron deficiency appears to contribute to this problem directly and indirectly though increased absorption of lead.

Iron Metabolism and Factors Affecting Iron Balance

Iron in the body exists in 2 major forms: functional and stored. Most of the functional iron is in the form of heme iron as hemoglobin and myoglobin. A number of important enzymes, including those controlling cellular respiration, dopamine synthesis, and central nervous system myelination, require iron, even though these account for less than 1% of the total body iron. The stored iron in the form of ferritin and hemosiderin accumulates when a positive iron balance exists; stored iron can be mobilized to meet iron requirements when intake is low. Factors that affect iron stores, intake, and loss will determine iron status and the risk of iron deficiency. In all age groups, the major determining factors for iron requirements are 1) expansion of the red cell mass with growth; 2) increase in tissue iron for enzymatic processes; 3) expansion of the storage pool (particularly in the 7- to 18-month age range); and 4) compensation for iron losses in stool. Additional losses attributable to menstrual blood loss must be accounted for in adolescent girls.

Iron Stores

Infants are born with a relatively large endowment of iron stores compared with other species. The amount of iron in storage is proportional to birth weight or size. On average, the iron stores in a term infant of appropriate size for gestational age can meet the iron requirement until 4 to 6 months of age.[15] For this reason, anemia screening for iron deficiency before 4 to 6 months of age is of little value. Because preterm infants and those with low birth weight are born with much less stored iron and because they experience a greater rate of growth during infancy, their iron stores become depleted much earlier than those of term infants, often by 2 to 3 months of age. Therefore, preterm infants and those with low birth weight are more vulnerable to iron deficiency. Twenty-six to 86% of preterm infants weighing <1500 g at birth are at risk of iron deficiency if fed a diet containing less than 2 mg/kg per day of iron. After the exhaustion of iron stores and up to 24 months of age, maintaining substantial iron stores, even when iron intake is adequate, is difficult because of the increased iron required for rapid growth. During this period, a low or depleted iron store per se, as reflected by low serum ferritin concentration, does not meet the definition of iron-deficiency anemia but does classify the child as iron deficient. After the liver iron stores are depleted, as reflected by a ferritin concentration below the 5th percentile for age, iron-related physiologic functions are compromised. After 2 years of age, as growth velocity is decreased to a lower baseline, iron stores start to accumulate, and the risk of iron deficiency decreases until the teenage years, when increased blood loss during menses puts girls at increased risk.

Iron Intake and Factors Affecting Iron Absorption

An adult man absorbs approximately 1 mg/day of iron, an amount equivalent to iron losses through desquamation of intestinal and skin cells. Infants between 4 and 12 months of age, on average, absorb almost as much: 0.8 mg/day. However, in contrast to the adult, three fourths of this amount is needed for growth and one fourth is needed to replace losses in infants. The dietary source of iron strongly influences the efficiency of its absorption. The amount of iron absorption from a variety of foods ranges from less than 1% to, in the case of human milk, more than 50%. Preterm infants absorb approximately 33% of dietary iron. Foods of vegetable origin are at the lower end of the range for absorption efficiency, dairy products are in the middle, and meat is at the upper end. Approximately 4% of the iron in fortified infant formulas is absorbed, and approximately 10% of the small amount of iron in unfortified formulas or whole milk is absorbed. The content of iron in human milk is comparable with that of unmodified cow milk (ie, not iron-fortified formula), but up to 50% of the iron in human milk can be absorbed. Therefore, human milk may be a more bioavailable source of iron than nonfortified formula or cow milk. However, the potential better absorption efficiency of human milk does not entirely compensate for the relatively low iron content. By about 6 months of age, term breastfed infants require an additional source of iron in their diets to meet their iron requirement. Infants born preterm and/ or with low birth weight or those with rapid growth in the early months of life or with some medical conditions may benefit from an additional source of iron before 6 months. Because milk-based diets constitute most of the energy consumed during the first year of life, the iron content of various milk products and their absorption efficiency is a strong predictor of iron nutrition status.[16] For practical purposes, infants who consume primarily iron-fortified formula have approximately an 8% risk of iron deficiency and less than 1% risk of iron-deficiency anemia. Those consuming nonfortified formula or whole cow milk have a 30% to 40% risk of iron deficiency by 9 to 12 months of age. Infants who are exclusively breastfed have a 20% risk of iron deficiency and a 6% risk of iron-deficiency anemia by 9 to 12 months of age.

In the United States, major nonmilk sources of iron in the infant diet are iron-fortified cereal and meats. The absorption of reduced iron of small particle size, used to fortify infant cereals, is estimated to be approximately 4%. Meat is a good source of iron, because most iron is in the form of heme iron, which has an absorption efficiency of 10% to 20%—2 to 3 times of that of nonheme iron (2%–7%). Nonheme iron found in plant foods and fortified food products is less well absorbed, and the absorption is strongly influenced by other foods ingested at the same meal. Ascorbic acid and an unknown component of meat are among the most potent enhancers of nonheme iron absorption. Tea, bran, and milk tend to inhibit nonheme iron absorption from the meal with which they are consumed. Normally, the diet contains 5 to 20 times the amount of iron absorbed. Table 18.1 lists the major enhancers and inhibitors of iron absorption.

Table 18.1
Enhancers and Inhibitors of Iron Absorption

Enhancers of Iron Absorption	Inhibitors of Iron Absorption
Ascorbic acid (vitamin C)	Reduced gastric acidity
Heme source of iron (meats)	Phytic acid (legumes, rice, and grains)
Iron deficiency	Vegetable protein (independent of phytates)
Ferritin iron	Polyphenols (tea, oregano, red wine)
	Other divalent cations (calcium, zinc)

Iron Loss
The normal turnover of intestinal mucosa with some blood loss can be regarded as physiologic, and this blood loss is considered in the daily requirement. For the same reason, normal menstrual blood loss is an obligatory or physiologic loss. However, health care professionals should be sensitive to

the fact that menstrual blood losses are widely variable among and within individuals. This factor, combined with a high prevalence of consumption of diets that are low in iron, defines the increased risk of iron deficiency in adolescent girls. A careful menstrual and dietary history are an essential part of the routine pediatric visit for adolescent girls. Heavy menstrual blood loss would be considered greater than or equal to 80 mL/month.[17]

The most common reason for abnormal blood loss in infants and younger children is the sensitivity of some children to the protein in cow milk, resulting in increased gastrointestinal occult blood loss.[18] For this reason, consumption of whole cow milk carries 2 risk factors for iron deficiency during infancy: low iron content and increased fecal blood loss in some infants.

In some tropical countries, hookworm infection is a major cause of gastrointestinal blood loss, but this is not a problem in the United States. Gastrointestinal disorders, such as peptic ulcer disease and inflammatory bowel disease, can obviously cause increased blood loss and, therefore, iron loss. Furthermore, treatment of peptic ulcer disease with antacids, H_2-receptor antagonists, or proton pump inhibitors will decrease rates of iron absorption.

Assessment of Iron Status

A number of laboratory tests can be used to assess iron nutritional status, including determining serum ferritin concentration, free erythrocyte protoporphyrin concentration, zinc protoporphyrin-heme ratio, transferrin saturation, serum transferrin receptor concentration, hemoglobin or hematocrit concentration, and red cell indices, such as mean corpuscular volume. These tests reflect different aspects of iron metabolism and together can characterize the iron nutritional status as a spectrum, from overload to severe deficiency. The earliest finding when iron intake does not match iron requirements results in a decrease in serum ferritin concentration, which, under most circumstances, reflects decreased liver iron stores. Intervention at that time most likely prevents any physiologic consequences of iron deficiency, including anemia. However, serum ferritin concentration testing is not widely available, and factors other than low iron stores, such as an inflammatory process, can alter the results. For these reasons, the CDC has not advocated its use as a general screening tool for iron deficiency despite its advantage of early detection compared with determining hemoglobin concentration.[17] After the ferritin concentration has decreased, evidence of preanemic disordered erythropoiesis occurs with increases in serum transferrin and protoporphyrin concentrations. Again, these assessments are not currently designed for large-scale population screening but can be used to assess the iron status of specific at-risk patients. The CDC and AAP currently recommend periodic assessment of hemoglobin or hematocrit concentrations as screening tools for iron deficiency, although anemia represents the most severe end of the iron-deficiency spectrum. Table 18.2 details the sequence of events when iron delivery does not meet iron demand and the subsequent effects on the major tests available for clinical application.

Table 18.2
The Effect of Evolving Iron Deficiency on Clinical Markers

Early: mobilization of serum and storage iron to support erythropoiesis
• Decreased serum iron concentration
• Decreased percent total iron-binding capacity saturation
• Decreased ferritin concentration (after at least 1 week)
Middle: compensatory effects to increase cellular iron delivery
• Increased serum transferrin receptor concentration
• Increased transferrin concentration (with further decrease in percent total iron-binding capacity saturation)
Moderately late: preanemic compromised erythropoiesis
• Increased zinc protoporphyrin concentration
• Reduced mean corpuscular volume
• Reduced mean corpuscular hemoglobin concentration
• Increased red blood cell distribution width
Late: iron-deficiency anemia
• Reduced hemoglobin concentration

Screening for Iron Deficiency

Although a number of biochemical tests can be used to define iron deficiency, for practical purposes, anemia screening by determining hemoglobin or hematocrit concentration is the main approach in a general pediatric setting. This is likely to change in the near future as standards for preanemic markers, such as serum transferrin receptor concentration, serum ferritin concentration, and their ratio are generated for all age groups. Anemia is defined as a hemoglobin or hematocrit concentration below the 5th percentile of an age- and sex-specific US representative sample after excluding people with biochemical evidence of iron deficiency (Table 18.3). On the basis of this definition, even in a population free of iron deficiency, approximately 5% of the children would be expected to meet the criteria for anemia. This type of baseline or statistical anemia among healthy children becomes a substantial source of false-positive

Table 18.3
Fifth Percentile Cutoffs for Various Measures of Iron Deficiency in Childhood[17,20–25]

Age (y)	Hgb, g/dL	Hct (%)	MCV (fL)	ZnPP (µg/dL)	RDW (%)	%TIBC saturation	Ferritin (µg/L)
Newborn	<14.0	<42	NA	NA	NA	NA	<40
0.5–2.0	<11.0	<32.9	<77	>80	>14	<16	<15
2.0–4.9	<11.1	<33.0	<79	>70	>14	<16	<15
5.0–7.9	<11.5	<34.5	<80	>70	>14	<16	<15
8.0–11.9	<11.9	<35.4	<80	>70	>14	<16	<15
12.0–15.0 (male)	<12.5	<37.3	<82	>70	>14	<16	<15
12.0–15.0 (female)	<11.8	<35.7	<82	>70	>14	<16	<15
>15.0 (male)	<13.3	<39.7	<85	>70	>14	<16	<15
>15.0 (female)	<12.0	<35.7	<85	>70	>14	<16	<15

Hgb indicates hemoglobin concentration; Hct, hematocrit concentration; MCV, mean corpuscular volume; ZnPP, zinc protoporphyrin concentration; RDW, red blood cell distribution width; %TIBC, percent total iron-binding capacity; NA, not applicable (no standards available).

cases of iron deficiency when iron-deficiency anemia is uncommon. The other assessments listed previously or a trial response to iron supplementation can be used as adjunctive evidence to confirm or rule out iron deficiency. Beyond iron deficiency, a number of other common causes of mild anemia exist. Among younger children, current and recent infection can cause mild anemia. Among black and certain Asian populations in the United States, mild hereditary anemia, such as thalassemia traits, can play a role. A common reason for suspecting mild anemia is the imprecision of determining hemoglobin concentration related to capillary blood sampling or the accuracy of the instrument. For this reason, confirmation of anemia by a second test or by venous puncture can eliminate many false-positive results. Table 18.4 summarizes some of the common reasons for anemia. Evidence is increasing that black children and adults have lower hemoglobin concentrations than do their white counterparts and that this difference is not attributable to differences in iron status.[19] For this reason, if the purpose of anemia screening is to detect children with the likelihood of iron deficiency, the hemoglobin cutoff value for black children can be adjusted downward by 0.3 g/dL of hemoglobin or 1% of hematocrit to achieve a comparable screening performance for iron deficiency.

Table 18.4
Major Causes of Anemia or Reasons for Low Hemoglobin or Hematocrit Concentrations

True Anemia
Iron deficiency Anemia related to recent or current infections Hereditary defects in red blood cell production or hemoglobinopathies Thalassemia trait, sickle cell trait, glucose-6-phosphate dehydrogenase deficiency Chronic illness or inflammatory conditions
False Anemia
Technical anemia: result of inadequate testing instrument or inadequate capillary blood sampling Statistical anemia or normal variation: the criteria for anemia are set at a level at which some   healthy children can be classified as anemic

Adapted from Yip R. Changing characteristics of iron nutritional status in the United States. In: Filer LJ, ed. *Dietary Iron: Birth to Two Years.* New York, NY: Raven Press; 1989:37–61

In recent years, a simplified outpatient laboratory method to measure erythrocyte protoporphyrin concentration, the hematofloramever method, has been used for screening for childhood lead poisoning. Because most children with high erythrocyte protoporphyrin concentrations have iron deficiency, this simplified test can also be used for screening for iron deficiency, although the lack of ubiquity of the hematofloramever currently keeps it from replacing determination of hemoglobin concentration as a screening tool. An advantage of the method is that results are likely increased in iron deficiency before anemia is present.[16] Only a minority of children with increased erythrocyte protoporphyrin concentration actually have high blood lead concentrations. The screening cutoff for erythrocyte protoporphyrin concentration is 35 µg/dL of whole blood or 3.0 µg/g of hemoglobin. Blood lead testing programs use erythrocyte protoporphyrin concentration as a screening test for lead poisoning; however, this test is still useful in screening for iron deficiency.

Diagnosis of Iron Deficiency
Anemia screening enables the identification of children who are at risk of iron deficiency. However, because anemia is not specific for iron deficiency, only a presumptive diagnosis can be made. Two approaches can be used to diagnose iron deficiency when a child has anemia. One approach is to use the hemoglobin response to oral iron treatment as a diagnosis of iron deficiency. An increase of the hemoglobin concentration by 1.0 g/dL or more by the 1-month follow-up is a positive response. The other approach

is the application of one or more of the iron-related tests for biochemical evidence of iron deficiency. Among the multiple tests that can be used, determination of serum ferritin concentration appears to be the best confirmatory test. A low serum ferritin concentration (<15 µg/L) is the most specific laboratory finding for iron deficiency. It should be noted that serum ferritin concentrations are increased during inflammatory states. A normal or high ferritin concentration may occur in an iron-deficient child and would be considered a false-negative result in the diagnosis of iron deficiency. Assessments of acute phase responses, such as C-reactive protein concentration or erythrocyte sedimentation rate, may provide insight into interpreting serum ferritin concentrations that are normal or high when the degree of suspicion of iron deficiency is also high. If a child with anemia does not experience a substantial hemoglobin response after 1 month of oral iron treatment, the laboratory evaluation for iron deficiency is also indicated. Beyond biochemical tests such as serum ferritin concentration, a complete blood cell count is also helpful. The mean corpuscular volume, red blood cell count, and red blood cell distribution width can provide valuable clues for differentiating iron deficiency from other forms of microcytic anemia or other types of anemia.[18]

Specific Recommendations

Because dietary intake during infancy is a strong determinant of iron status for older infants and younger children, the specific recommendations emphasize the role of a dietary approach for the primary prevention of iron deficiency in younger children. The epidemiologic evidence indicates that secondary prevention through anemia screening and treatment is of limited value among children who had a sound infant diet and can best be used for children who are at higher risk of iron deficiency.[2,4,14]

Dietary Recommendations

The Institute of Medicine recently published dietary reference intakes (DRIs) for all nutrients and age groups.[26] The DRIs include 3 categories that are relevant to iron intakes in children. Recommended Dietary Allowances (RDAs) describe the average nutrient intakes required daily to ensure that 97% to 98% of the population in a given age category is sufficient in that nutrient. The Estimated Average Requirement (EAR) is the average nutrient intake required each day to meet the requirements of 50% of the individuals in that age group. The RDA is typically 2 standard deviations above the EAR and usually calculates to approximately 20% higher than the EAR. The EAR and RDA are, thus, population-data based whenever possible. When an RDA cannot be established—for example, in the case of iron intake in 0- to 6-month-old infants (because of the variable absorption of iron from human milk vs formula)—an Adequate Intake (AI) is estimated.

The AI for iron in 0- to 6-month-old infants is 0.27 mg/day on the basis of the content of iron in human milk, its high bioavailablility, and the assumption that the vast majority of breastfed infants remain iron sufficient for the first 4 to 6 months of life. The EARs and RDAs for iron in children older than 6 months are presented in Table 18.5.

Table 18.5
Institute of Medicine Guidelines[26] for EARs and RDAs for Iron Intake in Children From 0.5 to 18 Years of Age

Age (y)	EAR (mg/day)	RDA (mg/day)
0.5 to 1.0	6.9	11.0
1.0 to 3.0	3.0	7.0
4.0 to 8.0	4.1	10.0
9.0 to 13.0 (male)	5.9	8.0
14.0 to 18.0 (male)	7.7	11.0
9.0 to 13.0 (female)	5.7	8.0
14.0 to 18.0 (female)	7.9	15
14.0 to 18.0 (pregnant female)	23.0	27.0

Dietary Recommendations for Infants and Children Younger Than 3 Years

The DRI for infants 0 to 6 months of age assume that newborn infants have adequate iron stores to last 4 to 6 months and that there is no detriment to using iron stores during that time, nor should there be an effort to accumulate iron stores in preparation for the continued growth between 7 and 12 months of age. Thus, the DRI of 0.27 mg/day of highly absorbable iron from human milk is defensible. However, it is clear that by 4 to 6 months of age, iron stores are waning, and the following recommendations reflect this concern.

Breastfed Infants
1. Breastfed term infants with size appropriate for gestational age need a supplemental source of iron (approx 1 mg/kg per day) starting at 4 to 6 months of age, preferably from complementary foods. The AAP

supports exclusive breastfeeding (in which all fluid, energy, and nutrients come from human milk, with the possible exception of small amounts of medicinal/nutrient supplements[1]) for minimum of 4 but preferably 6 months, at which time complementary foods may be introduced. Iron-fortified infant cereal and/or meats are good sources of iron for initial introduction of iron-containing food. An average of 2 servings (½ oz or 15 g of dry cereal per serving) is needed to meet the daily iron requirement.

2. If a term breastfed infant is unable to consume sufficient iron from dietary sources after 6 months of age, elemental iron (1 mg/kg per day) can be used.

3. For breastfed preterm infants or those with low birth weight, an oral iron supplement (elemental iron) in the form of drops (2 mg/kg once per day) should be given starting at 1 month until 12 months of age. The dose of iron (1 mg/kg) in a vitamin preparation with iron is not likely to provide sufficient iron for the preterm breastfed infant.

4. For all infants younger than 12 months, only iron-fortified formula (10–12 mg/L) should be used for weaning or for supplementing human milk.

Formula-Fed Infants

1. For term and preterm infants, only iron-fortified formula should be used during the first year of life, regardless of the age when infant formula is started. All soy-based formulas are iron fortified to 12 mg/L. Current preterm infant and preterm discharge formulas also contain 12 mg/L of iron and, thus, supply approximately 1.8 mg/kg per day to the average preterm infant consuming 150 mL/kg per day of formula. This dose is less than the recommended 2 to 4 mg of iron/kg per day. Therefore, formula-fed preterm infants may benefit from an additional 1 mg/kg per day of iron, which can be administered as either iron drops or in a vitamin preparation with iron.

2. No common medical indication exists for the use of a low-iron formula. The AAP has recommended that the manufacture of low-iron formulas be discontinued and that all infant formulas contain at least 4 mg/L of iron. Currently, all formulas sold in the United States contain at least 4.5 mg/L. Although some believe that iron-fortified formulas increase gastrointestinal symptoms, no scientific evidence supports this belief, so using formula that is not fortified with iron for healthy infants is not justified.

Solid Foods

The specific recommendations related to solid foods are more crucial for breastfed infants than for formula-fed infants to ensure adequate iron nutrition.

1. Introduce iron-fortified infant cereal or meat between 4 and 6 months of age or when the child is developmentally ready (able to sit up and swallow such food). The iron content of selected foods is listed in Appendix R.

Iron Supplements

Iron can be supplemented in multiple forms (Table 18.6). The choice of preparation should be determined by the health care professional on the basis of whether the supplement is for prophylaxis or treatment.

Table 18.6

Common Over-the-Counter Preparations Used for Iron Supplementation in Pediatric Practice

Product (Distributor)	Iron Concentration (mg of Elemental Iron/mL)	Usual Daily Dose
Baby Vitamin Drops with Iron (Goldline Laboratories, Miami, FL)	10	1 mL
Ferrous sulfate drops (Fer-In-Sol, Mead Johnson, Evansville, IN and various generics)	25 (125 mg/mL ferrous sulfate)	2–6 mg/kg per day of elemental iron
Multi Vit Drops with Iron (Barre-National, Baltimore, MD)	10	1 mL
Poly-Vi-Sol with Iron Drops (Mead Johnson, Evansville, IN)	10	1 mL
Polyvitamin drops with iron (various generics)	10	1 mL
Tri-Vi-Sol with Iron Drops (Mead Johnson, Evansville, IN)	10	1 mL
Vi-Daylin ADC Vitamins + Iron Drops (Ross, Columbus, OH)	10	1 mL

Sources: Drug Facts and Comparisons Online (www.drugfacts.com) and Lexi-Comps *Pediatric Dosage Handbook*, 14th Ed.

Milk

1. Avoid the use of regular cow milk, goat milk, or soy milk for the milk-based part of the diet before 12 months of age.
2. For young children, avoid excessive milk intake, which can displace the desire for food items with greater iron content. A milk intake of

24 oz/day is sufficient to meet the daily calcium requirement of children 1 to 5 years of age.

Dietary Recommendations for Young Children

Iron deficiency and iron-deficiency anemia continue to be a problem into the second postnatal year, with an incidence of approximately 10%.[17,19,27] The cause of this high incidence is unknown but may relate to the large numbers of infants born with low iron stores (infants of diabetic mothers, infants with intrauterine growth retardation, and preterm infants) or to those with low dietary intake of iron in the first postnatal year (breastfed infants, infants fed low-iron formula, and infants switched to cow milk before 12 months of age). The rate is unacceptably high for public health purposes, and reasonable attempts should be made to reduce it. It may be prudent to supplement high-risk children with iron in the form of a daily vitamin containing iron during the second year, especially if the child does not have a source of meat-based iron in the diet.

Screening and Treatment of Iron-Deficiency Anemia

Anemia Screening

Two options for screening for anemia are available, although neither achieves a degree of precision that is desirable at the population level.[28] The universal screening option is for communities and populations in which a significant level of iron-deficiency anemia exists or for infants whose diet puts them at risk of iron deficiency. Selective screening is for communities or practices with low rates of anemia (5% or less) and generally good infant dietary practices related to iron nutrition. Selective screening is also targeted at the subset of children who have a less-than-satisfactory diet, for example, early introduction of cow milk or use of low-iron formula, or who have particular medical risks, such as preterm birth or low birth weight.

- Option 1: Universal screening. Initial measurement of hemoglobin or hematocrit concentration for all full-term infants between 9 and 12 months of age and a second screening 6 months after the initial screening at 15 to 18 months of age.

- Option 2: Selective screening. Same schedule as universal screening except that only infants and children deemed to be at risk are screened. Infants at risk include preterm infants, infants with low birth weight infants, infants not receiving iron-fortified formula, and breastfed infants older than 6 months who are not consuming a diet with adequate iron content.

Anemia screening before 6 months of age is of little value for the detection of iron deficiency, because iron stores are adequate for most infants except the preterm infant. In the preterm infant, iron stores at birth are sufficient for 2 to 3 months postnatally. Although no official recommendations exist for screening for iron status in preterm infants, it may be prudent to screen these infants at approximately 4 months of age. The highest risk group appears to be infants born before 32 weeks' gestation who were not transfused or who received recombinant erythropoietin and were subsequently not supplemented with iron. After 2 years of age, routine screening is not indicated, because few children in the United States have iron-deficiency anemia after this time. For children at risk of iron deficiency because of special health needs, a low-iron diet (eg, nonmeat diet), or environmental factors (eg, poverty or limited access to food), annual screening for anemia can be considered between 2 and 5 years of age.

Treatment and Follow-up

1. Anemia (low hemoglobin or hematocrit concentration) detected by capillary blood sampling should be confirmed by subsequent measurement of hemoglobin and hematocrit concentration. After confirmation of anemia, the presumptive iron-deficiency anemia can be treated with oral (elemental) iron, 3 to 6 mg/kg per day, for 4 weeks.

2. Repeat the hemoglobin or hematocrit concentration measurement in 4 weeks. An increase of the hemoglobin concentration of more than 1 g/dL or of the hematocrit concentration of more than 3% confirms iron-deficiency anemia. Continue iron treatment for another 2 months and recheck the measurements. Assess the hemoglobin or hematocrit concentration about 6 months after successful treatment.

3. If the hemoglobin or hematocrit concentration does not increase after 4 weeks of iron treatment, further laboratory evaluation is indicated. This recommendation assumes that the child is not ill, because illness, such as upper respiratory tract infection, otitis, and diarrhea, can cause a significant reduction in the hemoglobin and hematocrit concentrations. Two suggested tests are:

   • Red blood cell indices by electronic blood counter: A low mean corpuscular volume (<70 fL) and red blood cell count (<4.0 x 10^{12}/L) suggest iron deficiency, and a low mean corpuscular volume (<70 fL) and relatively high red blood cell count (>4.8 x 10^{12}/L) suggest hereditary anemia, such as thalassemia trait; red blood cell distribution width more than 17 suggests iron deficiency; a normal red blood cell distribution width is consistent with thalassemia trait.

- Serum ferritin concentration: A serum ferritin concentration below 15 µg/L confirms iron deficiency. A value equal to or higher than 15 µg/L suggests that a cause other than iron deficiency is more likely responsible for the anemia.

Recommendations for School-Aged Children

Preadolescent school-aged children are at less risk of iron deficiency in the United States unless their diet is very restricted. For this reason, routine anemia screening may not be necessary. Selective anemia screening is indicated for children who consume a strict vegetarian diet and are not receiving an iron supplement.

Adolescents

Adolescent males are at risk near the peak growth period when iron stores may not meet the demand of rapid growth. However, iron-deficiency anemia generally corrects itself after the growth spurt. For adolescent females, menstrual blood loss increases the risk of iron deficiency. For this reason, anemia screening of adolescent females is indicated.

1. Males: Screen for anemia during routine physical examination during the peak growth period.
2. Females: Screen for anemia during all routine physical examinations.

Treatment and Follow-up for Anemia

As with younger children, an oral iron trial for 4 weeks should be performed. If substantial increases in the hemoglobin or hematocrit concentration are not seen, laboratory evaluation is indicated.

> **AAP**
>
> ### The American Academy of Pediatrics states:
>
> 1. Full-term infants have sufficient iron for 4 to 6 months. Human milk contains very little iron. Exclusively breastfed infants are at risk of iron deficiency by 6 months. Because infants may be exclusively breastfed for extended periods of time, it is judicious to supplement with oral iron, 1 mg/kg per day, beginning at 4 months of age when some infants (but not all) will begin to exhaust their iron stores. In partially breastfed infants, the proportion of human milk and formula is uncertain; therefore, partially breastfed infants should receive supplemental iron as well. Most formula-fed infants get sufficient iron through fortification of the formula and appropriate complementary foods. Usually, full-term infants fed iron-fortified formula do not need additional iron until 12 months of age. For all infants, consideration should be given to meat early as a complementary food, to augment the iron supply as well as other minerals including zinc, magnesium, and potassium.
> 2. Preterm infants should receive supplemental iron. Preterm infants fed human milk need 2 mg/kg per day from 1 month to 12 months of age. Exceptions to this practice would include infants who have received multiple transfusions of packed red blood cells.
> 3. Toddlers 1 to 3 years of age should be encouraged to eat meats and vegetables that contain iron and fruits that augment the absorption of iron. Total intake of iron should be 7 mg/day. Toddlers with iron deficiency or iron-deficiency anemia should receive a therapeutic iron supplement. This can be given as iron drops or as a component of a multivitamin. Liquid is suitable for 12 to 24 months of age; chewable multivitamins can be used for children 2 to 3 years of age. Children should be tested at appropriate intervals to determine whether iron deficiency or iron-deficiency anemia has resolved or persists.
> 4. The current practice of screening for iron-deficiency anemia between 9 and 12 months of age is inadequate. Universal screening should be performed at approximately 12 months of age and again at approximately 18 months of age, with a screening test that will more accurately identify toddlers with iron deficiency or iron-deficiency anemia. Screening is usually accomplished with a heme profile, but determining hemoglobin, serum ferritin, and C-reactive protein is a better screening test. The ideal screening for iron-deficiency anemia is a hemoglobin and serum transferrin receptor test. The American Academy of Pediatrics Committee on Nutrition strongly encourages the development of transferrin receptor standards for use with this assay in infants and children.
>
> *Pediatrics.* 2008; in press

References

1. Centers for Disease Control and Prevention. National Health and Nutrition Examination Survey, 1999–2000. Available at: http:www.cdc.gov/nchs/nhanes.htm. Accessed August 24, 2007

2. Lonnerdal B, Hernell O. Iron, zinc, copper and selenium status of breast-fed infants and infants fed trace element fortified milk-based infant formula. *Acta Paediatr.* 1994;83: 367–373

3. Fomon SJ, Ziegler EE, Serfass RE, Nelson SE, Frantz JA. Erythrocyte incorporation of iron is similar in infants fed formulas fortified with 12 mg/L or 8 mg/L of iron. *J Nutr.* 1997;127:83–88

4. American Academy of Pediatrics, Committee on Nutrition. Iron fortification of infant formulas. *Pediatrics.* 1999;104:119–123

5. Dallman PR, Yip R. Changing characteristics of childhood anemia. *J Pediatr.* 1989;114: 161–164

6. Angulo-Kinzler RM, Peirano P, Lin E, Algarin C, Garrido M, Lozoff B. Twenty-four-hour motor activity in human infants with and without iron deficiency anemia. *Early Hum Dev.* 2002;70:85–101

7. World Health Organization, Centers for Disease Control and Prevention. *Assessing the Iron Status of Populations.* A Report of a Joint World Health Organization/Centers for Disease Control and Prevention Technical Consultation on the Assessment of Iron Status at the Population Level. Geneva, Switzerland; April 6–8, 2004. Available at: http://www.who.int/mediacentre/news/notes/2004/anaemia/en/index.html. Accessed August 24, 2007

8. Cook JD, Flowers CH, Skikne BS. The quantitative assessment of body iron. *Blood.* 2003;101:3359–3364

9. Nokes C, van den Bosch C, Bundy DAP. *The Effects of Iron Deficiency and Anemia on Mental and Motor Performance, Educational Achievement and Behavior in Children: An Annotated Bibliography.* Washington, DC: International Nutritional Anemia Consultative Group; 1998. Available at: http://www.idpas.org/pdf/119AEffectsofIronDeficiency.pdf. Accessed November 2, 2007

10. Lozoff B, Jimenez E, Hagen J, Mollen E, Wolf AW. Poorer behavioral and developmental outcome more than 10 years after treatment for iron deficiency in infancy. *Pediatrics.* 2000;105(4):e51. Available at: http://pediatrics.aappublications.org/cgi/content/full/105/4/e51. Accessed August 24, 2007

11. Idjradinata P, Pollitt E. Reversal of developmental delays in iron-deficient anemic infants treated with iron. *Lancet.* 1993;341:1–4

12. Algarin C, Peirano P, Garrido M, Pizarro F, Lozoff B. Iron deficiency anemia in infancy: long-lasting effects on auditory and visual system functioning. *Pediatr Res.* 2003;53:217–223

13. Centers for Disease Control and Prevention. *Preventing Lead Poisoning in Young Children.* Atlanta, GA: Centers for Disease Control and Prevention; 1985. Report No. 99-2230. Available at: http://www.cdc.gov/nceh/lead/publications/books/plpyc/plpyc_history/CLP_1985.pdf. Accessed November 2, 2007

14. Erikson KM, Shihabi ZK, Aschner JL, Aschner M. Manganese accumulates in iron deficient rat brain regions in a heterogenous fashion and is associated with neurochemical alterations. *Biol Trace Elem Res.* 2002;87:143–156

15. Dallman PR, Siimes MA, Stekel A. Iron deficiency in infancy and childhood. *Am J Clin Nutr.* 1980;33:86–118

16. Pizarro F, Yip R, Dallman PR, Olivares M, Hertrampf E, Walter T. Iron status with different infant feeding regimens: relevance to screening and prevention of iron deficiency. *J Pediatr.* 1991;118:687–692

17. Centers for Disease Control and Prevention. Recommendations to prevent and control iron deficiency in the United States. *MMWR Recomm Rep.* 1998;47(RR-3):1–29

18. Ziegler EE, Fomon SJ, Nelson SE, et al. Cow milk feeding in infancy: further observations on blood loss from the gastrointestinal tract. *J Pediatr.* 1990;116:11–18

19. Johnson-Spear MA, Yip R. Hemoglobin difference between black and white women with comparable iron status: justification for race-specific anemia criteria. *Am J Clin Nutr.* 1994;60:117–121

20. Looker AC, Dallman PR, Carroll MD, Gunter EW, Johnson CL. Prevalence of iron deficiency in the United States. *JAMA.* 1997;277:973–976

21. Dallman PR, Looker AC, Johnson CL, Carroll M. Influence of age on laboratory criteria for the diagnosis of iron deficiency anemia and iron deficiency in infants and children. In: Hallberg L, Asp NG, eds. *Iron Nutrition in Health and Disease.* London, United Kingdom: John Libby & Co; 1996:65–74

22. Oski FA. Iron deficiency in infancy and childhood. *N Engl J Med.* 1993;329:190–193

23. Centers for Disease Control and Prevention. CDC criteria for anemia in children and childbearing-aged women. *MMWR Morb Mortal Wkly Rep.* 1989;38:400–404

24. Piomelli S. The diagnostic utility of erythrocyte porphyrins. *Hematol Oncol Clin North Am.* 1987;1:419–430

25. Hallberg L, Bengtsson C, Lapidus L, Lindstedt G, Lundberg PA, Hulten L. Screening for iron deficiency: an analysis based on bone-marrow examinations and serum ferritin determinations in a population sample of women. *Br J Heaematol.* 1993;85:787–798

26. Institute of Medicine. Iron. In: *Dietary Reference Intakes for Vitamin A, Vitamin K, Arsenic, Boron, Chromium, Copper, Iodine, Iron, Manganese, Molybdenum, Nickel, Silicon, Vanadium and Zinc.* Washington, DC: National Academies Press; 2000:290–393

27. Bogen DL, Duggan AK, Dover GJ, Wilson MH. Screening for iron deficiency by dietary history in a high-risk population. *Pediatrics.* 2000;105:1254–1259

28. Biondich PG, Downs SM, Carroll AE, et al. Shortcomings in infant iron deficiency screening methods. *Pediatrics.* 2006;117:290–294

19 Trace Elements

An element is considered to be a trace element when it constitutes less than 0.01% of total body weight. Trace elements are essential to metabolic processes, because they are components of many enzyme systems and act as integral components of metalloenzymes or cofactors for enzymes activated by metal ions. Trace element deficiencies have been reported in humans and can be deleterious to health, growth, and development. Because effects of deficiency are frequently most severe during periods of rapid growth, trace element deficiencies are of special concern to pediatricians. Thirteen trace elements are believed to be nutritionally important for higher animals. These trace elements, in order of importance to children, are iron, zinc, copper, fluoride, iodine, selenium, manganese, chromium, cobalt, molybdenum, nickel, silicon, and vanadium. All these trace elements are discussed in this chapter, except iron and fluoride, which are discussed in Chapters 18 (Iron) and 48 (Nutrition and Oral Health), respectively.

The Food and Nutrition Board of the Institute of Medicine has recently established Dietary Reference Intakes (DRIs) for humans for zinc, copper, manganese, chromium, iodine, molybdenum, and selenium. The DRIs are a framework containing 4 sets of standards: estimated average requirements (EARs), Recommended Dietary Allowances (RDAs), adequate intakes (AIs), and tolerable upper intake levels (upper levels or ULs).[1] The RDA is the nutrient intake that is sufficient to meet the needs for nearly all individuals (approx 97%) in an age and gender group. The RDAs (or, if not yet established, the AIs) of the major trace minerals discussed in this chapter are shown in Table 19.1 (see also Appendix J). The table also summarizes biochemical actions, effects of deficiency, effects of excess, and food sources of the trace elements.

Zinc

Basic Science/Background

Zinc is an essential cofactor for many enzymes with a multitude of functions.[2] These enzymes are involved in nucleic acid and protein metabolism. In many species, including humans, zinc deficiency limits growth prenatally and in infants and children. The exact mechanism behind the decreased growth is not known, but zinc is an integral part of DNA and RNA polymerase, several transcription factors (in so-called "zinc-fingers"), and enzymes involved in energy metabolism, all possibly contributing to lower cellular activity during zinc deficiency. Cells and tissues that are turning over rapidly are first affected; the immune system, the intestinal mucosa, and the skin are impaired early during zinc deficiency. Zinc is vitally important for proper immune function,[3] including skin and its barrier function and humoral and cellular immunity, and also for mucosal integrity, which may explain the positive effects of zinc supplements that have been observed on acute and chronic diarrhea[4-6] and other diseases.[7-9] Zinc has also been shown to have a positive effect on physical activity of preschool children[10] and on cognition and development,[11,12] which is possibly attributable to the involvement of zinc in neuropsychological development.[13]

Zinc is absorbed in the small intestine by active transport, and there is homeostatic regulation of absorption both by uptake and endogenous secretion.[14] This is achieved by 2 families of zinc transporters, the ZIP family (ZIP 1–5), largely regulating zinc import into cells, and the ZnT family (ZnT1–14), regulating zinc efflux and intracellular compartmentalization.[15-17] Factors regulating these transporters are still poorly characterized, but zinc intake has an effect by up- or down-regulating their expression. Zinc is transported in serum bound to serum albumin and alpha-2-macroglobulin, and further homeostasis of zinc metabolism occurs in the liver.

Zinc Deficiency

Severe zinc deficiency in infants and children is uncommon and characterized by acro-orificial skin lesions, diarrhea, increased susceptibility to infection, and slow growth.[18] These features are found in the autosomal-recessive genetic disorder of zinc metabolism, acrodermatitis enteropathica (AE), which causes severe zinc deficiency by decreased cellular retention of zinc. A mutation in ZIP4, a key zinc transporter in the brush-border membrane that regulates zinc uptake into the enterocyte, causes AE.[19] The signs of AE are similar to those of dietary zinc deficiency, and affected patients require daily zinc supplements for alleviation of all symptoms. In children with AE, the proper daily dose may be difficult to determine, particularly during periods of rapid growth, and there is a risk of excessive doses causing copper deficiency.[20] Most likely, a daily dose of 20 to 30 mg/day will be adequate to meet zinc requirements of infants and children with AE. Recovery from zinc deficiency is rapid after introduction of oral zinc; the violent dermatitis is often in complete remission within 4 to 5 days. Severe zinc deficiency may also be observed in preterm infants, particularly those with mothers with a defect in mammary gland zinc secretion[21] (see "Zinc Requirements").

Table 19.1
Trace Elements

Name (Abbreviation)/ Normal Serum Concentrations	Biochemical Action	Effects of Deficiency	Effects of Excess	Recommended Dietary Allowance or Adequate Intake*	Food Sources
Zinc (Zn)/ 0.75–1.20 mg/L or 11.5–18.5 µmol/L	Components of many enzymes and transcription factors	Anorexia, hypogeusia, retarded growth, delayed sexual maturation, impaired wound healing, skin lesions	Few toxic effects; may aggravate marginal copper deficiency	**Infants** 0–6 mo: 2 mg/day* 7–12 mo: 3 mg/day **Children** 1–3 y: 3 mg/day 4–8 y: 5 mg/day **Adolescent males** 9–13 y: 8 mg/day 14–18 y: 11 mg/day **Adolescent females** 9–13 y: 8 mg/day 14–18 y: 9 mg/day	Oysters, liver, meat, cheese, legumes, whole grains
Copper (Cu)/ 1.10–1.45 mg/L or 11–22 µmol/L	Constituent of ceruloplasmin; component of key metalloenzymes; role in connective tissue biosynthesis	Sideroblastic anemia, retarded growth, osteoporosis, neutropenia, decreased pigmentation	Few toxic effects; Wilson disease, liver dysfunction	**Infants** 0–6 mo: 0.20 mg/day* 7–12 mo: 0.22 mg/ day* **Children** 1–3 y: 0.34 mg/day 4–8 y: 0.44 mg/day **Adolescents** 9–13 y: 0.70 mg/day 14–18 y: 0.89 mg/ day	Shellfish, meat, legumes, nuts, cheese
Manganese† (Mn)/ 4–12 µg/L or 73–210 nmol/L	Activator of metal-enzyme complexes important for synthesis of polysaccharides and glycoproteins; constituent of pyruvate carboxylase and Mn-superoxide dismutase	Human: not documented; animals: growth retardation, ataxia of newborn, bone abnormalities, reduced fertility	Few toxic effects; neurologic manifestations from industrial contamination and in long-term total parenteral nutrition	**Infants** 0–6 mo: 0.003 mg/ day* 7–12 mo: 0.6 mg/ day* **Children** 1–3 y: 1.2 mg/day 4–8 y: 1.5 mg/day **Adolescent males** 9–13 y: 1.9 mg/day 14–18 y: 2.2 mg/day **Adolescent females** 9–13 y: 1.6 mg/day 14–18 y: 1.6 mg/day	Nuts, whole grains, tea

Table 19.1 *(Continued)*
Trace Elements

Name (Abbreviation)/ Normal Serum Concentrations	Biochemical Action	Effects of Deficiency	Effects of Excess	Recommended Dietary Allowance or Adequate Intake*	Food Sources
Selenium (Se)/ 30–75 µg/L or 0.35–1.00 µmol/L	Component of enzymes: glutathione peroxidase and deiodinase	Humans: cardiomyopathy; animals: hepatic necrosis, muscular dystrophy, exudative diathesis, pancreatic fibrosis	Irritation of mucous membranes (nose, eyes, upper respiratory tract), pallor, irritability, indigestion	**Infants** 0–6 mo: 15 µg/day* 7–12 mo: 20 µg/day* **Children** 1–3 y: 20 µg/day 4–8 y: 30 µg/day **Adolescents** 9–13 y: 40 µg/day 14–18 y: 55 µg/day	Seafood, meat, whole grains
Chromium (Cr)	Required for maintenance of normal glucose metabolism; potentiates the action of insulin	Humans: impairment of glucose utilization; animals: impaired growth, disturbances of carbohydrate, protein, and lipid metabolism	Few toxic effects; humans: not well documented; animals: growth retardation, hepatic and kidney damage	**Infants** 0–6 mo: 0.2 µg/day* 7–12 mo: 5.5 µg/day* **Children** 1–3 y: 11 µg/day 4–8 y: 15 µg/day **Adolescent males** 9–13 y: 25 µg/day 14–18 y: 35 µg/day **Adolescent females** 9–13 y: 21 µg/day 14–18 y: 24 µg/day	Meat, cheese, whole grains, brewer's yeast
Cobalt (Co)	Component of vitamin B_{12}	Humans: unknown; animals: anemia, growth retardation	Few toxic effects; polycythemia, myocardial degeneration	Not established	Green leafy vegetables

Table 19.1 (Continued)
Trace Elements

Name (Abbreviation)/ Normal Serum Concentrations	Biochemical Action	Effects of Deficiency	Effects of Excess	Recommended Dietary Allowance or Adequate Intake*		Food Sources
Molybdenum (Mo)	Component of enzymes involved in production of uric acid (xanthine oxidase) and in oxidation of aldehydes and sulfides	Humans: unknown; animals: growth retardation, anorexia	Humans, gout-like syndrome, antagonist of copper	**Infants** 0–6 mo: 2 μg/day* 7–12 mo: 3 μg/day* **Children** 1–3 y: 17 μg/day 4–8 y: 22 μg/day	**Adolescents** 9–13 y: 34 μg/day 14–18 y: 43 μg/day	Meats, grains, legumes
Iodine (I)	Component of thyroid hormones (triiodothyronine and thyroxine), enzymes involved in production of	Goiter, impaired mental function, delayed development	"Toxic goiter"	**Infants** 0–6 mo: 110 μg/day* 7–12 mo: 130 μg/day* **Children** 1–3 y: 90 μg/day 4–8 y: 90 μg/day	**Adolescents** 9–13 y: 120 μg/day 14–18 y: 150 μg/day	Iodized salt, dairy products, saltwater fish, seafood

* For healthy breastfed infants, the adequate intake is the mean intake.
† Whole blood, rather than serum, concentration.

Mild zinc deficiency in infants was first described by Walravens and Hambidge and others, who found slower-than-normal growth[22] and lower plasma zinc concentrations[23] in male formula-fed infants than in breastfed infants. Fortification of formula to a zinc content of 5.8 mg/L led to normal growth. Several recent studies have shown a positive effect of zinc supplements on the growth of infants and children,[24-26] but others have failed to show an effect.[27] Zinc status at baseline, dose given, growth rate, infections, compliance, and other factors may affect the outcome.[28] Whether the growth impairment in children with suboptimal zinc status is attributable to effects on hormonal mediators of growth, reduced appetite and food intake, or more frequent infections is not yet known. Preterm infants are born with lower stores of zinc, and a recent study on such infants showed beneficial effects of zinc supplementation on their growth rate.[29]

During the last decade, the significance of zinc deficiency in childhood growth, morbidity, and mortality has been recognized by a number of large-scale randomized, controlled supplementation trials in developing countries, and zinc deficiency has been estimated to be a leading cause of preventable deaths in children worldwide.[30] Meta-analysis showed that zinc supplementation of children was associated with significantly increased height and weight and that the effects were strongest in children with stunting.[27] Pooled analysis of trials evaluating the effect of daily zinc supplementation on infectious disease reported a robust decrease (approx 40%) in treatment failure and death related to diarrhea and pneumonia,[6,9] and a recent study showed a similar effect of weekly zinc supplements (70 mg) on young children.[31] The consistent positive effects on diarrhea prompted the inclusion of zinc into oral rehydration solution,[32] which showed beneficial effects on stool output and diarrhea duration.[33] Zinc.supplements may also reduce the risk of malaria, but only a limited number of trials have been conducted to date.[34]

Mild to moderate zinc deficiency can be difficult to diagnose because of the lack of specific features. Slow growth, frequent infections, minor rashes, lack of appetite, and compromised immune function may be suggestive of zinc deficiency. Zinc status is often evaluated by measurement of the plasma or serum zinc concentration. However, neither is a sensitive indicator, and infection, stress, growth rate, and other factors can affect these values.[35] Hair zinc concentration is sometimes used but it is difficult to analyze and may be affected by factors other than zinc status.[36] When zinc deficiency is suspected, a zinc supplementation trial (usually 1 mg/kg per day) may result in a response.[37] The supplement can be administered as a solution of zinc acetate (30 mg of zinc acetate in 5 mL of water). Intravenous requirements of infants have been estimated to 100 µg/kg per day, and the recommended amount for preterm infants is 300 µg/kg per day.[38] Infants with cystic fibrosis have been shown to have low plasma zinc and abnormal zinc homeostasis[39] and may, therefore, have a higher requirement for zinc. Children with Crohn disease and sickle cell disease may also benefit from zinc supplements.[40,41]

Zinc Requirements

Zinc intake from human milk varies during lactation as the human milk zinc content decreases but is usually around 0.5 to 1.0 mg/day. Infant formulas are usually fortified with zinc to an amount higher than that of human milk (to compensate for lower bioavailability). Thus, intake is usually around 3 to 5 mg/day (or 1 mg/kg per day). Lower zinc intakes may be adequate for healthy term infants, because human milk zinc content as low as 1.1 mg/L does not cause zinc deficiency.[42] However, the safety margin may not be high; some women produce milk with a lower-than-normal amount of zinc, and this has been shown to cause overt zinc deficiency.[43] This is of particular concern in preterm infants, because their rapid growth increases their zinc requirement. In preterm infants, deficiency resulting from low milk content of zinc can be precipitated quickly. The cause of the lower-than-normal milk zinc content is not known, but maternal zinc supplementation does not increase the content of zinc in the milk. A recent study showed that some women with abnormally low milk zinc content have a genetic defect in ZnT-2, one of the transporters regulating mammary zinc metabolism.[44] It is not yet known how common this specific mutation is among afflicted mothers. It should be noted that infants becoming zinc deficient as a result of their mothers' low milk zinc content do not require zinc supplements after weaning, because weaning foods usually provide enough zinc.

The RDA of zinc for older (7–12 months of age) infants and toddlers (1–3 years of age) is 3 mg/day. Exclusively breastfed infants ingest only 0.4 to 0.6 mg of zinc/day at 6 months of age without signs of zinc deficiency.[45] We still know little about the infant's capacity to homeostatically regulate zinc metabolism, but several of the zinc transporters described previously are affected by zinc intake and zinc status. Stable isotope studies in infants suggest that zinc absorption is increased and fecal losses are decreased when zinc intake is low.[14] It is obvious that zinc intakes of infants and children often are low, which emphasizes the need for zinc-containing foods, such as meats and possibly zinc-fortified cereals.

Dietary Sources/Bioavailability

Zinc absorption from human milk has been shown to be high compared with absorption from cow milk-based formula or cow milk.[46] The higher bioavailability of zinc from human milk may be because zinc is loosely bound to citrate and serum albumin in human milk[47] but tightly bound to casein in cow milk and cow milk-based formula. Citrate-bound zinc is readily absorbed, and the limited digestive capacity of neonates may be sufficient to release zinc from serum albumin but possibly inadequate for complete digestion of casein, resulting in unabsorbed zinc.[48] Zinc absorption from soy formula and infant cereals is even lower than from cow milk-based formula, most likely because of the high phytate content of these diets.[46,49] Phytic acid contains several negative charges and can bind divalent cations like zinc, iron, and calcium. Because humans cannot digest phytate to any significant degree, fecal zinc losses will increase. Because removal of phytate increases zinc absorption considerably,[50] efforts are being made to reduce the phytate content of staple foods (corn, rice, barley) by fermentation, precipitation, phytase treatment, or genetic selection.[51] However, such products are not yet commercially available. High intake of phytate-containing foods (cereals, legumes) limiting zinc absorption, combined with low intake of zinc-rich foods such as meat, is the major reason for the high prevalence of low zinc status in developing countries. Appendix S shows the zinc content of common household foods.

The high level of iron fortification in most formulas has been implicated to have a negative effect on zinc absorption. However, this concern may be unfounded, because an iron-zinc ratio found in infant formula does not appear to affect zinc absorption.[52] However, when oral supplements are given, iron is likely to partially inhibit zinc absorption,[52] and combined supplements of iron and zinc have been shown to be less effective in preventing low zinc status in infants than has zinc supplementation alone.[53] This needs to be considered when determining the appropriate dose and ratio of iron to zinc to use in supplements.

During the second 6 months of life, zinc requirements remain relatively high, and the amount of zinc provided from human milk may be inadequate. The content of zinc in human milk is about 2 to 3 mg/L during early lactation, but by 6 months after birth, the content usually is only approximately 0.5 mg/L.[54] The quantity of zinc provided from human milk may be too low to meet the requirement; however, another likely reason for the beneficial effect of zinc supplements on growth of these infants may be that phytate-containing weaning foods reduce the bioavailability of zinc from human milk. It is apparent that zinc intake is a limiting factor during recovery from malnutrition and during rapid catch-up growth after stunting.[55] This fact was considered when new recommendations for complementary foods were issued by the World Health Organization/United Nations Children's Fund.[56]

Zinc Toxicity

Acute zinc toxicity is rare but may occur from ingestion of pharmacologic preparations of zinc. Symptoms are usually diarrhea and vomiting. Consumption of zinc supplements in quantities of 50 mg/day or higher may cause anemia resulting from zinc interfering with copper absorption and inducing copper deficiency. Copper deficiency was detected in an adolescent boy with AE given excessive amounts of zinc daily.[20]

Copper

Basic Science/Background

Copper is an essential trace element and functions as a cofactor in several physiologically important enzymes, such as lysyl oxidase, elastase, monoamine oxidases, cytochrome oxidase, ceruloplasmin, and Cu,Zn-superoxide dismutase.[57] Lysyl oxidase and elastase are involved in connective tissue synthesis and collagen cross-linking, cytochrome oxidase in the electron transport system and energy metabolism, ceruloplasmin (ferroxidase) in iron metabolism, and superoxide dismutase is an antioxidant and scavenger of free radicals. The signs of copper deficiency can all be related to impaired activities of these enzymes.[57,58] Knowledge regarding copper absorption and homeostasis has been limited, but several novel copper transporters (ATP7A, ATP7B, Ctr1) were discovered recently,[57] which provide a better understanding of normal copper metabolism as well as genetic disorders of copper metabolism.

Copper Deficiency

An x-linked recessive genetic disorder of copper metabolism, Menkes syndrome, usually manifests soon after birth and is characterized by pallor, anemia, steely hair, and a progressive degeneration of the brain.[59] Patients become copper deficient at a very young age, and aggressive treatment with copper should be used, but the long-term outcome for these patients is not good.[59,60] The gene was identified by work on mouse models of Menkes disease,[61] and the defective protein is a P-type adenosine triphosphatase, ATP7A, which is involved in cellular copper metabolism, particularly the export of copper out of the cell.[62] Thus, copper is blocked in the enterocyte and little copper is transported into the systemic circulation, resulting in severe copper deficiency.

Risks of copper deficiency include low stores in the liver of preterm infants, rapid growth rate, malabsorption syndromes, and increased copper losses, but the deficiency is usually not precipitated unless the dietary intake of copper also is low.[57,63] Preterm infants have substantially lower hepatic stores of copper (which mainly accumulate during the third trimester); these prenatal stores are normally used during neonatal life by copper being incorporated into ceruloplasmin and exported into the blood stream, causing an early increase in serum copper and ceruloplasmin.[64] Thus, many of the first cases of copper deficiency were preterm infants that had been fed low-copper diets (usually cow milk) for prolonged periods. Because preterm infants have low copper stores, suboptimal copper status has been suggested, and some studies show lower Cu,Zn-superoxide dismutase activities than in term infants.[65] Recent experiments in transgenic neonatal mice overexpressing Cu,Zn-superoxide dismutase who were exposed to oxygen showed that high superoxide dismutase activity protected against retinopathy as compared with wild-type mice,[66] supporting that oxygen radicals are a major causative factor in oxygen-induced retinopathy and that superoxide dismutase is protective. Whether lower-than-normal superoxide dismutase levels in preterm infants increase the risk of oxygen-induced retinopathy is not yet known. Copper deficiency has also been found in malnourished infants and children.[57] Signs of copper deficiency include neutropenia, hypochromic anemia (which does not respond to iron supplementation), bone abnormalities, skin disorders, and depigmentation of skin and hair.[57,58] The immune system is affected, reflected by decreased phagocytic capacity of neutrophils and impaired cell immunity.[67] The anemia is caused by low concentrations of ceruloplasmin, or as it more correctly should be called, ferroxidase. This enzyme is needed in several steps leading to the incorporation of iron into hemoglobin. Patients with the recently discovered genetic defect "aceruloplasminemia" have normal copper status but have pronounced iron-deficiency anemia[68] resulting from decreased release of iron from stores and, therefore, diminished incorporation of iron into developing erythrocytes. It is also likely that iron absorption is decreased during copper deficiency as a result of decreased activity of hephaestin, a copper-dependent ferroxidase in the intestine that is important in the uptake of iron into the portal vein.[69]

Recovery of copper-deficient infants or children when treated with copper (2 to 3 mg of copper sulfate as 1% solution daily or infusion) is usually rapid. Clinical parameters that are used to assess copper status include serum copper and ceruloplasmin concentration, hair copper concentration, and erythrocyte superoxide dismutaseconcentration.[58] In infants older than 1 or 2 months, serum copper concentrations lower than 0.5 μg/mL or ceruloplasmin concentrations lower than 15 μg/100 mL should be considered abnormally low. However, serum copper and ceruloplasmin concentrations are not very responsive to marginal copper deficiency and are affected by other conditions, such as infection, which may increase the concentrations. The concentration of hair copper also has limited value, because it may be affected by external factors.[36] The erythrocyte concentration of superoxide dismutase has been suggested as a good indicator of long-term copper status,[58] but the measurement has not reached routine clinical use.

Copper Requirement

The copper intake of infants is usually low because human milk contains only 0.2 to 0.4 mg copper/L, and infant formulas are usually fortified to a similar content (0.4 to 0.6 mg/L).[63] This amount of copper intake appears adequate in healthy term infants, because copper deficiency is rare.[18] In fact, even formula that had not been fortified with copper and only contained 0.08 mg/L resulted in adequate copper status in term infants.[70] The World Health Organization has set the minimum recommended intake for infants at 60 μg/kg per day, and the current RDA for copper is 200 μg/day.[1]

After weaning, cereals and other foods provide more copper than does milk, and copper intake increases rapidly. Studies on older infants and children[71] indicate that copper intake at this age meets the requirements for growth and maintenance. Although there has been some concern that drinking water may be excessively high in copper in some areas, either because of the environment (copper mining areas) or copper pipes, infants fed formula at the current maximum copper intake according to the World Health Organization (2 mg/L) exhibited no negative signs after 6 months of exposure.[72]

Dietary Sources/Bioavailability

Copper absorption in infants is high (approx 80%) and does not appear to be dependent on age.[73] Increasing the copper intake of infants did not affect copper absorption, suggesting no or limited homeostatic regulation at young age.[73] Stable isotope studies in preterm infants,[74] balance studies in term infants,[75] and radioisotope studies in experimental animals[76] demonstrate higher bioavailability of copper from human milk than from cow milk-based formula and cow milk. Copper in human milk seems to be bound to serum albumin, whereas casein binds most copper in cow milk, possibly explaining the lower bioavailability.[47] Copper bioavailability from soy formula and infant cereals appears to be even lower, although phytate present in these products does not seem to have the same strong inhibitory effect on the absorption of copper as found for zinc.[77] Dietary factors known to affect copper absorption negatively include high amounts of ascorbic acid, zinc, iron, and cysteine. However, amounts of these nutrients used in infant diets are moderate and usually exert no pronounced effects on copper absorption[78] Some types of heat processing of infant formula, however, may have a negative effect on copper absorption,[79] possibly by formation of unabsorbable complexes.

Copper Toxicity

Acute copper toxicity is rare and is usually caused by the consumption of contaminated foods or beverages or accidental or deliberate ingestion of large quantities of copper salts.[80] Symptoms include nausea, vomiting, and diarrhea. Chronic toxicity is also rare but appears in geographic clusters. Indian childhood cirrhosis has been reported in families that were consuming milk boiled or stored in brass or copper containers.[81] Children consuming such milk may consume copper up to 1 mg/kg per day, which is enough to explain the observed liver damage. In the Austrian Tyrol, infants and children were reported to have died from liver cirrhosis caused by high chronic copper intake.[82,83] In these cases, inheritance followed the typical pattern of a Mendelian recessive trait, suggesting that these individuals were particularly sensitive to copper exposure. This was supported by the observation that many children were found who had no liver damage but had received similar amounts of copper. Sporadic cases have been reported in other areas, and some of these cases have occurred in consanguineous marriages.[84] Cases were much more frequent in boys, and a genetic origin is possible. Whether a genetic disorder of copper metabolism is present in patients with liver cirrhosis is not known but should be explored in the light of the new findings of copper transporters in humans.

Wilson disease is another autosomal-recessive genetic disorder of copper metabolism that results in toxic effects of copper. In patients with Wilson disease, excessive amounts of copper accumulate in the body, particularly in the liver and brain, and clinical symptoms include liver cirrhosis, eye lesions (Kayser-Fleisher ring), kidney malfunction, and neurological problems.[85] Despite very high concentrations of copper in the liver, serum copper and ceruloplasmin concentrations are low. Treatment includes a variety of chelating agents (eg, penicillamine and triethylenetetramine), oral treatment with large doses of zinc to reduce copper absorption,[86] and hepatic transplantation for advanced cases. This disorder of copper metabolism has also been shown to be caused by a defective transporter, in this case ATP7B,[87] which is responsible for copper trafficking to excrete excess copper into the biliary canicular system. Several different mutations of ATP7B have been described, and the severity of the disease varies with the type of mutation.[88] Genotyping of presymptomatic infants and children is, therefore, important for early and appropriate medical intervention. Copper absorption does not appear to be dysregulated in these patients; rather, tissue copper metabolism, particularly in the liver, is affected, causing excessive cellular accumulation of copper.[85] The outcome for these patients under treatment is usually good, but continuous monitoring of copper, zinc, and iron status is needed.

Manganese

Basic Science/Background

The essentiality of manganese in humans has not been fully established, although it has been determined for most other species. Manganese is a necessary cofactor for some enzymes, including arginase, glutamate-ammonia ligase, manganese superoxide dismutase, and pyruvate carboxylase. Several other enzymes contain manganese, but research has shown that magnesium ions can replace manganese with maintained enzyme activity.[89] Only one potential case of human manganese deficiency has been described,[90] and it is possible that manganese deficiency does not occur in infants and children and that, instead, concern should be directed toward toxic effects of manganese (or overload).

Manganese Requirements

Requirements for manganese of infants and children are likely very small, and the current AI for infants 0 to 6 months of age is 3 µg/day.[1] However, for 9- to 13-year-old children, the AI is 1.6 to 1.9 mg/day; this considerably higher amount reflects the fact that manganese at this age is retained by the body to a very limited extent (see next paragraph).

Assessment of Status

Manganese status is difficult to assess because of the very low concentrations of manganese in biological tissues and fluids; blood concentrations are only 10 µg/L, and serum concentrations are approximately 1 µg/L,[91] making analysis impossible for most laboratories. Because few of the manganese-dependent enzymes are found in blood, they have no value in the evaluation of manganese status.

Dietary Sources/Bioavailability

The concentration of manganese in human milk is very low, only 4 to 8 μg/L.[92] Most of this manganese is bound to the major iron-binding protein in human milk, lactoferrin.[93] Cow milk and cow milk-based formula are about 10 times higher in manganese concentration (30–60 μg/L), and soy formula is approximately 50 to 75 times higher in manganese than human milk.[94] Although in the past, some formulas were fortified with manganese and, in some cases, were quite high in manganese,[91] the current amounts of manganese in cow milk-based formula and soy formula reflect the natural amounts of manganese in the protein sources used. Of potential concern is the increasing use of soy and rice beverages labeled "milks" for feeding infants. These beverages contain 2 to 17 times the amount of manganese of soy formula and exceed the UL for children 1 to 3 years of age (there is no established UL for infants).[95]

Drinking water can contain significant concentrations of manganese,[96] and 6% of US wells have been shown to contain >300 μg/L of manganese.[97] This source needs to be taken into account when estimating the manganese intake of children and also of infants fed powdered formula diluted in such water.

Manganese Toxicity

Although the bioavailability of manganese from human milk appears high relative to that from cow milk-based formula and soy formula,[98] there is little regulation of manganese uptake at young ages, and absorption is strongly correlated with dietary intake.[99] Thus, the body burden of absorbed and retained manganese will be much larger in infants fed cow milk-based formula or, in particular, soy formula than in breastfed infants.[94] This is reflected in higher whole-blood manganese concentrations in formula-fed infants.[100]

Toxic effects of manganese in human adults are manifested by central nervous system dysfunction, such as lack of coordination and balance, mental confusion, and muscle cramps.[101] The major site for the toxic effects of manganese is the extrapyramidal part of the brain, and several symptoms resemble those of Parkinson disease. Although most reports on manganese toxicity in humans are on workers exposed to manganese by inhalation, there are cases of manganese toxicity in children who have ingested high doses of manganese.[102,103] In such cases, lack of attention, poor memory test results, and an epileptic syndrome were described. It has been shown in young animals that the brain may be particularly sensitive to manganese. Ingestion of modest amounts of manganese (per body weight similar to amounts consumed by infants fed soy formula) during early life caused a dose-dependent depletion of striatum dopamine and adverse effects on motor development and behavior in rats.[104] The dopaminergic system is sensitive to manganese exposure, possibly explaining the effects on motor and memory functions. Recently, a negative correlation between blood manganese concentration and cord blood monoamine metabolites was reported in healthy women.[105] It was also shown that cord blood manganese concentration was negatively correlated to nonverbal psychomotor scores in 3-year-old children of these women. A study of 10-year-old children in Bangladesh showed that household water manganese concentration associated with lower intellectual function (Wechsler Intelligence Scale) in a dose-dependent manner.[96] In the United States, some household wells have water manganese concentrations exceeding 300 µg/L, the current lifetime health advisory level set by the US Environmental Protection Agency. It should be noted that soy formulas usually contain amounts of manganese exceeding this level. Behavioral studies in infant rhesus monkeys exposed to high amounts of manganese in soy formula show that these infant monkeys engaged in less play behavior and more affiliative clinging and had shorter wake cycles and shorter daytime inactivity than controls,[106] suggesting signs of attention-deficit/hyperactivity disorder.

Children receiving long-term parenteral nutrition may be at risk of excessive manganese exposure, because these solutions are commonly high in manganese.[107] In such patients, cholestatic disease and nervous system disorders have been associated with high blood concentrations of manganese. The normal homeostatic mechanisms of the liver and gut are bypassed in these patients, leading to hypermanganesemia, and a reduction in the manganese concentration of parenteral nutrition solutions has been advocated.[108] Manganese is excreted via bile, which explains the finding of elevated plasma manganese concentrations in children with biliary obstruction.[109]

Balance studies in infants show that breastfed infants accumulate little manganese, whereas formula-fed infants are in positive balance.[75] Little is known about the threshold for development of toxic effects of manganese, but because manganese absorption is high at young ages,[99] the possibility should be considered. This high absorption of manganese may be accentuated because manganese absorption increases substantially during iron deficiency,[94] which is not uncommon in children. Another concern is the recent interest in adding manganese compounds to gasoline (as an antiknock agent), which would further increase environmental exposure to this element. Weaning foods are usually good sources of manganese, and manganese intake increases dramatically after weaning. However, mechanisms for manganese excretion appear to become more efficient at this age, and only a small fraction of absorbed manganese may be retained by the body.

Selenium

Basic Science/Background

Selenium is an integral and necessary part of a limited number of proteins, such as selenium-dependent glutathione peroxidase, selenoprotein P in serum, and iodothyronine-5'-deiodinase. In these proteins, selenium is specifically incorporated into the proteins as selenocysteine because of a unique transfer RNA using a specific serine codon.[110] Thus, the number of selenocysteine residues in each protein is tightly regulated. Selenium can also be incorporated nonspecifically into methionine. The human diet consists of organic selenium (largely selenomethionine) and inorganic selenium in the form of selenite and selenate. Knowledge is limited about the metabolism of these different forms of selenium in humans, but they appear to be metabolized quite differently.[111,112] Glutathione peroxidase participates in the antioxidant defense and helps to scavenge free radicals that may cause tissue damage. Selenium is an integral part of cellular glutathione peroxidase, serum glutathione peroxidase, and a membrane-bound form of glutathione peroxidase, but there are also selenium-independent glutathione peroxidases.[110] Type I iodothyronine-5'-deiodinase catalyzes the conversion of thyroxine to triiodothyronine in liver and other tissues[113] and is, therefore, involved in thyroid function. In children with goiter, selenium deficiency limited their response to iodine supplementation and, therefore, the improvement in thyroid size and function.[114]

Selenium Deficiency

The essentiality of selenium in human nutrition was discovered recently, although there has been knowledge regarding selenium deficiency in animals for quite some time. In a province of China, Keshan, a cardiomyopathy of unknown etiology led to high mortality in children.[115] Because the pathologic changes of Keshan disease had similarities to the signs of selenium deficiency in cattle and the soil was found to be low in selenium, a large study evaluated the effects of selenium fortification of salt. Mortality decreased significantly, and selenium fortification has been used since. However, other factors may have contributed to the cause of Keshan disease, because Keshan disease is not evident in other areas with similarly low intakes of selenium. It has been suggested that the low-selenium environment puts evolutionary pressure on normally harmless viruses (such as Coxsackie virus), causing them to mutate, which makes them pathogenic.[116] Evidence for such mutations in Coxsackie virus that can cause cardiomyopathy has been obtained at the molecular level,[117] but it is not yet clear whether this was a major contributing factor to Keshan disease. Selenium deficiency has been found in children receiving long-term total parenteral nutrition solutions that were not supplemented.[118] Signs of deficiency include macrocytosis and loss of skin and hair pigmentation. In severe pediatric cases, cardiomyopathy is also observed.[119] Selenium supplementation of parenteral solutions is, therefore, recommended at 2 μg/kg per day.

The selenium-dependent glutathione peroxidase found in serum and erythrocytes has been used to assess selenium status. However, the situation is complicated, because they are different gene products and, therefore, are regulated differently. To date, the concentration of serum glutathione peroxidase, which usually is closely correlated with the concentration of serum selenium, has been used as an indicator of short-term selenium status, whereas erythrocyte glutathione peroxidase concentration has been used as an indicator of long-term status. The serum selenium concentration is also used frequently to assess selenium status.

Low erythrocyte glutathione peroxidase activity and serum and hair selenium concentrations have been found in infants with low birth weight,[120] but the clinical significance of these observations is unknown. Low selenium status in pediatric HIV patients has been shown to be a predictor of more rapid disease progression and mortality,[121] and selenium supplementation of such patients may, therefore, be beneficial.

Selenium Requirements

Tissue selenium and plasma selenium concentrations are lower in preterm infants than in term infants.[122] A selenium intake of at least 1 μg/kg per day is recommended to achieve intrauterine tissue accretion. However, evaluation of the selenium status of preterm infants is difficult. When preterm infants were fed human milk (containing 24 μg/L of selenium) or formula with or without selenium fortification (34.8 and 7.8 μg/L of selenium, respectively), no differences were found in plasma selenium, erythrocyte selenium, or glutathione peroxidase concentrations.[122] However, all of these infants may have had suboptimal selenium status and selenium may have been quickly removed from the circulation and incorporated into newly synthesized tissue. A recent study in the United States showed that selenium fortification of formula improves selenium status of preterm infants,[123] possibly because the infants were not as selenium deprived as in the other study. A stable isotope study in preterm infants showed that selenite in formula was absorbed to approximately 70% and that most of it was retained.[124] It is also possible that synthesis of selenoproteins, such as glutathione peroxidase and selenoprotein P, which transport selenium in plasma, is immature in these infants. The low plasma glutathione peroxidase concentrations of infants fed preterm formula without selenium fortification decreased with age in infants in New Zealand, which may be attributable to a combination of low status at birth and a low dietary supply of selenium.[125] Concern was raised about possibly impaired antioxidant defenses, because preterm infants are at risk of oxidative diseases, such as bronchopulmonary dysplasia and retinopathy of prematurity. A study on preterm infants with respiratory distress syndrome and bronchopulmonary dysplasia showed that low plasma selenium concentration was associated with increased respiratory morbidity.[126] A recent Cochrane review showed that selenium supplementation of very preterm infants was associated with a reduction in episodes of sepsis[127]; however, 2 of the 3 trials were from countries with typically low selenium concentrations.

Dietary Sources/Bioavailability

Selenium in the diet is strongly affected by local conditions; selenium content in soil and water affect plant selenium content and the concentrations in grazing animals and their milk.[111] Similarly, selenium in human milk is affected by maternal selenium intake.[128] Thus, the selenium intake of infants and children is affected by geographic location. People in some areas of the United States have high intakes of selenium, whereas people in other areas have considerably lower intakes. The raw materials used for formulas, such as skim milk powder, whey protein, and soy protein isolate, strongly affect the selenium content of formula.

The selenium content of human milk has been shown to be as low as 3 µg/L in some areas of China, whereas the contents in other low-selenium areas, such as Finland and New Zealand, are approximately 10 µg/L.[111] Selenium content in human milk from women in the United States varies but usually is approximately 15 µg/L.[129] A lower concentration of selenium was shown in formula-fed infants than in breastfed infants in several studies.[129,130] Formulas that are not fortified with selenium often contain considerably lower amounts of selenium (2–6 µg/L) than the amount in human milk. Furthermore, the bioavailability of selenium in human milk, which is mostly in protein-bound form,[131] appears higher than that in selenium-fortified formula. A study in which the selenium status of formula-fed infants was lower than that of breastfed infants, even though the formula was fortified with selenium to an amount higher than that of human milk, supported this.[130] At least part of the difference in selenium bioavailability may be related to the form of selenium in the diet; selenite or selenate (ie, inorganic selenium) is used in formula, whereas most selenium in human milk is protein bound (organic selenium). A difference in use of selenium given in different forms was shown in a study in which lactating women were given selenium supplements. Yeast selenium (ie, organic selenium) resulted in higher selenium content in human milk than did selenite.[128] These differences were also manifested in the selenium status of breastfed infants.

Soy formula often provides even less selenium than does cow milk-based formula. Again, this depends on the soy protein source used, but several commercial soy formulas have been reported to contain only 2 to 6 µg of selenium/L.[132,133] Selenium fortification of soy formula has, therefore, recently been implemented. Both selenite[132] and selenate[133] have been studied; stable isotope studies in infants show that the latter form is better absorbed, but selenium retention is similar from both forms.[134] The amount of fortification has been chosen to provide the infant with an amount equal to the RDA of 15 to 20 µg/kg per day for infants from birth to 6 months of age. Another factor to consider is the selenium status of infants at birth. Markedly different concentrations of plasma selenium in infants in Finland and the United States may explain why increases after birth were seen in one study[130] but not in another.[135]

Selenium Toxicity

Acute selenium toxicity is very rare in humans, and such cases usually result from ingestion of selenium supplements. Signs include diarrhea and garlic-smelling breath. Chronic selenium toxicity also appears rare, with signs such as brittle nails, hair loss, and fatigue.

Iodine

Basic Science/Background

The primary biological role of iodine is synthesis of thyroid hormones, particularly thyroxine, and during iodine deficiency, circulating concentrations of thyroxine decrease. Iodine is readily absorbed and is rapidly taken up by the thyroid gland but also by other tissues. Excess iodine is excreted via the urine, and urinary iodine is often used as an indicator of iodine status.

Iodine Deficiency

Although iodine deficiency is one of the most common nutrient deficiencies worldwide, it is highly uncommon among infants and children in the United States. Common use of iodine in baked goods and in dairy cattle management, together with iodination of table salt, makes the dietary iodine intake of the US population more than sufficient to meet requirements.

It has been found that goitrous children with iron-deficiency anemia do not respond to iodine supplementation,[136] suggesting that iron may be important for some vital step in iodine metabolism. Oral iron supplementation of such children led to a significantly improved response to iodine supplementation.[137] Whether low iron status in US children can impair iodine status without precipitating goiter is not yet known.

Adequate selenium status is also vital for normal iodine metabolism, because the enzyme converting thyroxine to triiodothyronine (deiodinase) is selenium dependent (see previous section on Selenium). It may, therefore, be prudent to evaluate thyroxine/triiodothyronine status of infants and children with suspected compromised selenium status.

The RDA of iodine for preterm infants was recently increased to 30 µg/kg per day,[1] and it has been emphasized that human milk, formulas, and parenteral solutions contain insufficient iodine to meet this requirement.[138] A recent Cochrane review found only one randomized, controlled trial on iodine supplementation of preterm infants and morbidity and neurodevelopment and found insufficient data to make any conclusions.[139]

Iodine Requirement

The RDA of iodine for infants up to 6 months of age is 110 µg/day and for infants 6 to 12 months of age is 130 µg/day.[1] The concentration of iodine in human milk varies depending on maternal intake, but values of 50 to 60 µg/L were found in a multicenter study.[140] The iodine concentration in human milk of women in the United States seems higher, with a mean value of 130 µg/L[141]; maternal dietary intake strongly influences the iodine concentration.[142] Cow milk is a rich source of iodine, and cow milk-based infant formula is, therefore, a good source of iodine. Soy formula usually contains approximately 70 to 100 µg/L. Thus, it is evident that formula-fed and breastfed infants will receive adequate quantities of iodine. Children in the United States will receive an ample supply of iodine from salt, dairy products, and baked goods. For areas that are not reached by iodine fortification, low-dose oral iodized oil has been developed for children.[114]

Other Trace Elements

Chromium functions as a cofactor for insulin. Chromium deficiency is characterized by impaired growth and longevity and by impaired glucose, lipid, and protein metabolism in experimental animals. However, chromium deficiency in infants is rare and has only been reported associated with protein-calorie malnutrition. Depletion of chromium also may occur during prolonged parenteral alimentation. The only reliable indicator of chromium deficiency is the demonstration of a beneficial effect of chromium supplementation.

Cobalt is considered essential for humans only because it is a component of the vitamin B_{12} molecule. Cobalt deficiency has never been demonstrated in humans or laboratory animals, and the requirement for cobalt is considered minute.

The biochemical functions of molybdenum are the synthesis and function of xanthine oxidase, aldehyde oxidase, and sulfite oxidase. Molybdenum deficiency has not been reported under any natural conditions in humans, but it has recently been suggested that infants with low birth weight may not meet their molybdenum requirement, particularly when receiving parenteral nutrition.[143]

Arsenic, nickel, silicon, and vanadium are other trace elements considered as possibly nutritionally important. Human deficiency states have not been demonstrated, and dietary requirements have not been set because of insufficient experience.

Aluminum, although poorly absorbed, can accumulate in patients with renal insufficiency, and this accumulation has been associated with osteomalacia and encephalopathy. Care should be taken when administering aluminum-containing antacids to children with renal insufficiency. Although some soy formulas contain high amounts of aluminum, it is most likely poorly absorbed and has not been associated with negative consequences.[144]

References

1. Institute of Medicine. *Dietary Reference Intakes for Vitamin A, Vitamin K, Arsenic, Boron, Chromium, Copper, Iodine, Iron, Manganese, Molybdenum, Nickel, Silicon, Vanadium, and Zinc.* Washington, DC: National Academies Press; 2000

2. Prasad AS. Clinical and biochemical spectrum of zinc deficiency in human subjects. In: Prasad AS, ed. *Clinical, Biochemical, and Nutritional Aspects of Trace Elements*. New York, NY: Alan R Liss Inc; 1982:3–62

3. Shankar AH, Prasad AS. Zinc and immune function: the biological basis of altered resistance to infection. *Am J Clin Nutr*. 1998;68:447S–463S

4. Sazawal S, Black RE, Bhan MK, Jalla S, Sinha A, Bhandari N. Efficacy of zinc supplementation in reducing the incidence and prevalence of acute diarrhea—a community-based, double-blind, controlled trial. *Am J Clin Nutr*. 1997;66:413–418

5. Ruel MT, Rivera JA, Santizo MC, Lonnerdal B, Brown KH. Impact of zinc supplementation on morbidity from diarrhea and respiratory infections among rural Guatemalan children. *Pediatrics*. 1997;99:808–813

6. Bhutta ZA, Bird SM, Black RE, et al. Therapeutic effects of oral zinc in acute and persistent diarrhea in children in developing countries: pooled analysis of randomized controlled trials. *Am J Clin Nutr*. 2000;72:1516–1522

7. Sazawal S, Black RE, Jalla S, Mazumdar S, Sinha A, Bhan MK. Zinc supplementation reduces the incidence of acute lower respiratory infections in infants and preschool children: a double-blind, controlled trial. *Pediatrics*. 1998;102:1–5

8. Black RE. Therapeutic and preventive effects of zinc on serious childhood infectious diseases in developing countries. *Am J Clin Nutr*. 1998;68:476S–479S

9. Bhutta ZA, Black RE, Brown KH et al. Zinc Investigators Collaborative Group. Prevention of diarrhea and pneumonia by zinc supplementation in children in developing countries: pooled analysis of randomized controlled trials. *J Pediatr*. 1999;135:689–697

10. Sazawal S, Bentley P, Black RE, Dhingra P, George S, Bhan MK. Effect of zinc supplementation on observed activity in low socioeconomic Indian preschool children. *Pediatrics*. 1996;98:1132–1137

11. Sandstead HH, Penland JG, Alcock NW, et al. Effects of repletion with zinc and other micronutrients on neuropsychological performance and growth of Chinese children. *Am J Clin Nutr*. 1998;6:470S–475S

12. Castillo-Duran C, Perales CG, Hertrampf ED, Marvin VB, Rivera FA, Icaza G. Effect of zinc supplementation on development and growth of Chilean infants. *J Pediatr*. 2001;138:229–235

13. Frederickson CJ, Suh SW, Frederickson CJ, et al. Importance of zinc in the central nervous system: the zinc-containing neuron. *J Nutr*. 2000;130:1471S–1483S

14. Hambidge KM, Krebs NF, Westcott JE, Miller LV. Changes in zinc absorption during development. *J Pediatr*. 2006;149:S64–S68

15. McMahon RJ, Cousins RJ. Mammalian zinc transporters. *J Nutr*. 1998;128:667–670

16. Gaither LA, Eide DJ. The human ZIP1 transporter mediates zinc uptake in human K562 erythroleukemia cells. *J Biol Chem*. 2001;276:22258–22264

17. Eide DJ. Zinc transporters and the cellular trafficking of zinc. *Biochim Biophys Acta*. 2006;1763:711–722

18. Walravens PA. Nutritional importance of copper and zinc in neonates and infants. *Clin Chem*. 1980;26:185–189

19. Wang K, Zhou B, Kuo YM, Zemansky J, Gitschier J. A novel member of a zinc transporter family is defective in acrodermatitis enteropathica. *Am J Hum Genet*. 2002;71:66–73

20. Sandström B, Cederblad A, Lindblad BS, Lönnerdal B. Acrodermatitis enteropathica, zinc metabolism, copper status, and immune function. *Arch Pediatr Adolesc Med.* 1994;148: 980–985

21. Zimmerman AW, Hambidge KM, Lepow MI, Greenberg LD, Stover ML, Casey CE. Acrodermatitis in breast-fed premature infants: evidence for a defect of mammary zinc secretion. *Pediatrics.* 1982;69:176–183

22. Walravens PA, Hambidge KM. Growth of infants fed a zinc supplemented formula. *Am J Clin Nutr.* 1976;29:1114–1121

23. Hambidge KM, Walravens PA, Casey CE, Brown RM, Bender C. Plasma zinc concentrations of breast-fed infants. *J Pediatr.* 1979;94:607–608

24. Ruz M, Castillo-Duran C, Lara X, Codoceo J, Rebolledo A, Atalah E. A 14-mo zinc-supplementation trial in apparently healthy Chilean preschool children. *Pediatrics.* 1997;66:1406–1413

25. Rivera JA, Ruel MT, Santizo MC, Lonnerdal B, Brown KH. Zinc supplementation improves the growth of stunted rural Guatemalan infants. *J Nutr.* 1998;128:556–562

26. Umeta M, West CE, Haidar J, Deurenberg P, Hautvast JG. Zinc supplementation and stunted infants in Ethiopia: a randomized controlled trial. *Lancet.* 2000;355:2021–2026

27. Brown KH, Peerson JM, Rivera J, Allen LH. Effect of supplemental zinc on the growth and serum zinc concentrations of prepubertal children: a meta-analysis of randomized controlled trials. *Am J Clin Nutr.* 2002;75:1062–1071

28. Brown KH. Commentary: zinc and child growth. *Int J Epidemiol.* 2003;32:1103–1104

29. Diaz-Gomez NM, Domenech E, Barroso F, Castells S, Cortabarria C, Jiminez A. The effect of zinc supplementation on linear growth, body composition, and growth factors in preterm infants. *Pediatrics.* 2003;111:1002–1009

30. Jones G, Steketee RW, Black RE, Bhutta ZA, Morris SS. How many child deaths can we prevent this year? Bellagio Child Survival Study Group. *Lancet.* 2003;362:65–71

31. Brooks WA, Santosham M, Naheed A, et al. Effect of weekly zinc supplements on incidence of pneumonia and diarrhea in children younger than 2 years in an urban, low-income population in Bangladesh: randomised controlled trial. *Lancet.* 2005;366:999–1004

32. Robberstad B, Strand T, Black RE, Sommerfelt H. Cost-effectiveness of zinc as adjunct therapy for acute childhood diarrhea in developing countries. *Bull World Health Organ.* 2004;82:523–531

33. Bhatnagar S, Bahl R, Sharma PK, Kumar GT, Saxena SK, Bhan MK. Zinc with oral rehydration therapy reduces stool output and duration of diarrhea in hospitalized children: a randomized controlled trial. *J Pediatr Gastroenterol Nutr.* 2004;38:34–40

34. Fischer Walker C, Black RE. Zinc and the risk for infectious disease. *Annu Rev Nutr.* 2004;24:255–275

35. Brown KH. Effect of infections on plasma zinc concentration and implications for zinc status in low-income populations. *Am J Clin Nutr.* 1998;68:425S–429S

36. Hambidge KM. Hair analyses: worthless for vitamins, limited for minerals. *Am J Clin Nutr.* 1982;36:943–949

37. Hotz C, Brown KH. Identifying populations at risk of zinc deficiency: the use of supplementation trials. *Nutr Rev.* 2001;59:80–84

38. Greene HL, Hambidge KM, Schanler R, Tsang R. Guidelines for the use of vitamins, trace elements, calcium, magnesium, and phosphorus in infants and children receiving total parenteral nutrition. Report of Subcommittee. Committee on Clinical Practice Issues of the American Society for Clinical Nutrition. *Am J Clin Nutr*. 1988;48:1324–1342

39. Krebs NF, Westcott JE, Arnold TD, et al. Abnormalities in zinc homeostasis in young infants with cystic fibrosis. *Pediatr Res*. 2000;48:256–261

40. Solomons NW, Rosenberg IH, Sandstead HH, Vo-Khactu KP. Zinc deficiency in Crohn's disease. *Digestion*. 1977;16:87–95

41. Zemel BS, Kawchak DA, Fung EB, Ohene-Frempong K, Stallings VA. Effect of zinc supplementation on growth and body composition in children with sickle cell disease. *Am J Clin Nutr*. 2002;75:300–307

42. Krebs NF, Reidinger CJ, Robertson AD, Hambidge KM. Growth and intakes of energy and zinc in infants fed human milk. *J Pediatr*. 1994;124:32–39

43. Atkinson SA, Whelan D, Whyte RK, Lönnerdal B. Abnormal zinc content in human milk. *Am J Dis Child*. 1989;143:608–611

44. Chowanadisai W, Lönnerdal B, Kelleher SL. Identification of a mutation in SLC30A2 (ZnT-2) in women with low milk zinc concentration that results in transient neonatal zinc deficiency. *J Biol Chem*. 2006;281:39699–39707

45. Krebs NF, Hambidge KM. Zinc requirements and zinc intakes of breast-fed infants. *Am J Clin Nutr*. 1986;43:288–292

46. Sandström B, Cederblad A, Lönnerdal B. Zinc absorption from human milk, cow's milk, and infant formulas. *Am J Dis Child*. 1983;137:726–729

47. Lönnerdal B, Hoffman B, Hurley LS. Zinc and copper binding proteins in human milk. *Am J Clin Nutr*. 1982;36:1170–1176

48. Lönnerdal B. Dietary factors influencing zinc absorption. *J Nutr*. 2000;130:1378S–1383S

49. Lönnerdal B, Cederblad A, Davidsson L, Sandström B. The effect of individual components of soy formula and cow's milk formula on zinc bioavailability. *Am J Clin Nutr*. 1984;40:1064–1070

50. Lönnerdal B, Bell JG, Hendrickx AG, Burns RA, Keen CL. Effect of phytate removal on zinc absorption from soy formula. *Am J Clin Nutr*. 1988;48:1301–1306

51. Gibson RS, Yeudall F, Drost N, Mtitimuni B, Cullinan T. Dietary interventions to prevent zinc deficiency. *Am J Clin Nutr*. 1998;68:484S–487S

52. Sandström B, Davidsson L, Cederblad Å, Lönnerdal B. Oral iron, dietary ligands and zinc absorption. *J Nutr*. 1985;115:411–414

53. Lind T, Lönnerdal B, Stenlund H, et al. A community-based randomized controlled trial of iron and zinc supplementation in Indonesian infants: interactions between iron and zinc. *Am J Clin Nutr*. 2003;77:883–890

54. Krebs NF, Reidinger CJ, Hartley S, Robertson AD, Hambidge KM. Zinc supplementation during lactation: effects on maternal status and milk zinc concentrations. *Am J Clin Nutr*. 1995;61:1030–1036

55. Castillo-Duran C, Heresi G, Fisberg M, Uauy R. Controlled trial of zinc supplementation during recovery from malnutrition: effects on growth and immune function. *Am J Clin Nutr*. 1987;45:602–608

56. Brown KH. WHO/UNICEF review on complementary feeding and suggestions for future research: WHO/UNICEF guidelines on complementary feeding. *Pediatrics.* 2000;106(Suppl):S1290–S1291

57. Olivares M, Araya M, Uauy R. Copper homeostasis in infant nutrition: deficit and excess. *J Pediatr Gastroenterol Nutr.* 2000;31:102–111

58. Milne DB. Copper intake and assessment of copper status. *Am J Clin Nutr.* 1998;67: 1041S–1045S

59. Kaler SG. Diagnosis and therapy of Menkes syndrome, a genetic form of copper deficiency. *Am J Clin Nutr.* 1998;67:1029S–1034S

60. Sheela SR, Latha M, Liu P, Lem K, Kaler SG. Copper-replacement treatment for symptomatic Menkes disease: ethical considerations. *Clin Genet.* 2005; 68:278–283

61. Mercer JF, Livingston J, Hall B, et al. Isolation of a partial candidate gene for Menkes disease by positional cloning. *Nat Genet.* 1993;3:20–25

62. Camakaris J, Petris MJ, Bailey L, et al. Gene amplification of the Menkes (MNK; ATP7A) P-type ATPase gene of CHO cells is associated with copper resistance and enhanced copper efflux. *Hum Mol Genet.* 1995;4:2117–2123

63. Lönnerdal B. Copper nutrition during infancy and childhood. *Am J Clin Nutr.* 1998;67: 1046S–1053S

64. Salmenperä L, Perheentupa J, Pakarinen P, Siimes MA. Cu nutrition in infants during prolonged exclusive breast-feeding: low intake but rising serum concentrations of Cu and ceruloplasmin. *Am J Clin Nutr.* 1986;43:251–257

65. Barclay SM, Aggett PJ, Lloyd DJ, Duffty P. Reduced erythrocyte superoxide dismutase activity in low birth weight infants given iron supplements. *Pediatr Res.* 1991;29:297–301

66. Spierer A, Rabinowitz R, Pri-Chen S, Rosner M. An increase in superoxide dismutase ameliorates oxygen-induced retinopathy in transgenic mice. *Eye.* 2005;19:86–91

67. Percival SS. Copper and immunity. *Am J Clin Nutr.* 1998;67:1064S–1068S

68. Harris ZL, Takahashi Y, Miyajima H, Serizawa M, MacGillivray RT, Gitlin JD. Aceruloplasminemia: molecular characterization of this disorder of iron metabolism. *Proc Natl Acad Sci U S A.* 1995;92:2539–2543

69. Anderson GJ, Frazer DM, McKie AT, Vulpe CD. The ceruloplasmin homolog hephaestin and the control of intestinal iron absorption. *Blood Cells Mol Dis.* 2002;29:367–375

70. Salmenperä L, Siimes MA, Näntö V, Perheentupa J. Copper supplementation: failure to increase plasma copper and ceruloplasmin concentrations in healthy infants. *Am J Clin Nutr.* 1989;50:843–847

71. Sorenson AW, Butrum RR. Zinc and copper in infant diets. *J Am Diet Assoc.* 1983;83:291–297

72. Olivares M, Pizarro F, Speisky H, Lonnerdal B, Uauy R. Copper in infant nutrition: safety of World Health Organization provisional guideline value for copper content of drinking water. *J Pediatr Gastroenterol Nutr.* 1998;26:251–257

73. Olivares M, Lönnerdal B, Abrams SA, Pizarro F, Uauy R. Age and copper intake do not affect copper absorption, measured with the use of 65Cu as a tracer, in young adults. *Am J Clin Nutr.* 2002;76:641–645

74. Ehrenkranz RA, Gettner PA, Nelli CM, et al. Zinc and copper nutritional studies in very low birth weight infants: comparison of stable isotopic extrinsic tag and chemical balance methods. *Pediatr Res.* 1989;26:298–307

75. Dörner K, Dziadzka S, Hohn A, et al. Longitudinal manganese and copper balances in young infants and preterm infants fed on breast-milk and adapted cow's milk formulas. *Br J Nutr.* 1989;61:559–572

76. Lönnerdal B, Bell JG, Keen CL. Copper absorption from human milk, cow's milk and infant formulas using a suckling rat model. *Am J Clin Nutr.* 1985;42:836–844

77. Lönnerdal B, Jayawickrama L, Lien EL. Effect of reducing the phytate content and of partially hydrolyzing the protein in soy formula on zinc and copper absorption and status in infant rhesus monkeys and rat pups. *Am J Clin Nutr.* 1999;69:490–496

78. Stack T, Aggett PJ, Aitken E, Lloyd DJ. Routine L-ascorbic acid supplementation does not alter iron, copper, and zinc balance in low birthweight infants fed a cow's milk formula. *J Pediatr Gastroenterol Nutr.* 1990;10:351–356

79. Lönnerdal B, Kelleher SL, Lien EL. Extent of thermal processing of infant formula affects copper status in infant rhesus monkeys. *Am J Clin Nutr.* 2001;73:914–919

80. Pizarro F, Olivares M, Uauy R, Contreras P, Rebelo A, Gidi V. Acute gastrointestinal effects of graded levels of copper in drinking water. *Environ Health Perspect.* 1999;107:117–121

81. Tanner MS, Kantarjian AH, Bhave SA, Pandit AN. Early introduction of copper-contaminated animal milk feeds as a possible cause of Indian childhood cirrhosis. *Lancet.* 1983;2:992–995

82. Müller T, Feichtinger H, Berger H, Müller W. Endemic Tyrolean infantile cirrhosis: an ecogenetic disorder. *Lancet.* 1996;347:877–880

83. Müller T, Müller W, Feichtinger H. Idiopathic copper toxicosis. *Am J Clin Nutr.* 1998;67:1082S–1086S

84. Müller-Höcker J, Meyer U, Wiebecke B, et al. Copper storage disease of the liver and chronic dietary copper intoxication in two further German infants mimicking Indian childhood cirrhosis. *Pathol Res Pract.* 1988;183:39–45

85. Danks DM. Disorders of copper transport. In: Scriver CR, Beaudet AL, Sly WS, Valle D, eds. *The Metabolic and Molecular Bases of Inherited Disease.* Vol 1, 7th ed. New York, NY: McGraw-Hill; 1995:2211–2235

86. Brewer GJ, Hill GM, Prasad AS, Cossack ZT, Rabbani P. Oral zinc therapy for Wilson's disease. *Ann Intern Med.* 1983;99:314–319

87. Petrukhin K, Lutsenko S, Chernov I, Ross BM, Kaplan JH, Gilliam TC. Characterization of the Wilson disease gene encoding a P-type copper transporting ATPase: genomic organization, alternative splicing, and structure/function predictions. *Hum Mol Genet.* 1994;3:1647–1656

88. Panagiotataki E, Tzetis M, Manolaki N, et al. Genotype-phenotype correlations for a wide spectrum of mutations in the Wilson disease gene (ATP7B). *Am J Med Genet A.* 2004;131:168–173

89. Keen CL, Ensunsa JL, Lönnerdal B, Zidenberg-Cherr S. Manganese. In: Caballero B, Allen L, Prentice A, eds. *Encyclopedia of Human Nutrition.* 2nd ed. Amsterdam, The Netherlands: Elsevier/Academic Press; 2005:217–225

90. Doisy EA. Effects of deficiency in manganese upon plasma levels of clotting proteins and cholesterol in man. In: Hoekstra WG, Suttie JW, Ganther HE, Mertz W, eds. *Trace Element Metabolism in Animals 2*. Baltimore, MD: University Park Press; 1974:668–670

91. Stastny D, Vogel RS, Picciano MF. Manganese intake and serum manganese concentration of human milk-fed and formula-fed infants. *Am J Clin Nutr*. 1984;39:872–878

92. Vuori E. A longitudinal study of manganese in human milk. *Acta Paediatr Scand*. 1979;68:571–573

93. Lönnerdal B, Keen CL, Hurley LS. Manganese binding proteins in human and cow's milk. *Am J Clin Nutr*. 1985;41:550–559

94. Lönnerdal B. Manganese nutrition of infants. In: Klimis-Tavantzis DJ, ed. *Manganese in Health and Disease*. Boca Raton, FL: CRC Press Inc; 1994:175–191

95. Cockell KA, Bonacci G, Belonje B. Manganese content of soy or rice beverages is high in comparison to infant formulas. *J Am Coll Nutr*. 2004;23:124–130

96. Wasserman GA, Liu X, Parvez F, et al. Water manganese exposure and children's intellectual function in Araihazar, Bangladesh. *Environ Health Perspect*. 2006;114:124–129

97. USGS. National Water-Quality Assessment Program. Reston, VA: US Geological Survey. Available at: http://water.usgs.gov/nawqa. Accessed October 1, 2005

98. Davidsson L, Cederblad Å, Lönnerdal B, Sandström B. Manganese absorption from human milk, cow's milk and infant formulas in humans. *Am J Dis Child*. 1989;143:823–827

99. Keen CL, Bell JG, Lönnerdal B. The effect of age on manganese uptake and retention from milk and infant formulas in rats. *J Nutr*. 1986;116:395–402

100. Hatano S, Aihara K, Nishi Y, Usui T. Trace elements (copper, zinc, manganese, and selenium) in plasma and erythrocytes in relation to dietary intake during infancy. *J Pediatr Gastroenterol Nutr*. 1985;4:87–92

101. Mena I. Manganese. In: Bronner F, Coburn JW, eds. *Disorders of Mineral Metabolism*. New York, NY: Academic Press Inc; 1981:233–270

102. Woolf A, Wright R, Amarasiriwardena C, Bellinger D. A child with chronic manganese exposure from drinking water. *Environ Health Perspect*. 2002;110:613–616

103. Herrero Hernandez E, Discalzi G, Dassi P, Jarre L, Pira E. Manganese intoxication: the cause of an inexplicable epileptic syndrome in a 3 year old child. *Neurotoxicology*. 2003;24: 633–639

104. Tran TT, Chowanadisai W, Crinella FM, Chicz-DeMet A, Lönnerdal B. Effect of high dietary manganese intake of neonatal rats on tissue mineral accumulation, striatal dopamine levels, and neurodevelopmental status. *Neurotoxicology*. 2002;23:635–643

105. Takser L, Mergler D, Hellier G, Sahuquillo J, Huel G. Manganese, monoamine metabolite levels at birth, and child psychomotor development. *Neurotoxicology* 2003;24:667–674

106. Golub MS, Hogrefe CE, Germann SL, et al. Neurobehavioral evaluation of rhesus monkeys fed cow's milk formula, soy formula, or soy formula with added manganese. *Neurotoxicol Teratol*. 2005;27:615–627

107. Dickerson RN. Manganese intoxication and parenteral nutrition. *Nutrition*. 2001;17:689–693

108. Fell JM, Reynolds AP, Meadows N, et al. Manganese toxicity in children receiving long-term parenteral nutrition. *Lancet*. 1996;347(9010):1218–1221

109. Bayliss EA, Hambidge KM, Sokol RJ, Stewart B, Lilly JR. Hepatic concentrations of zinc, copper and manganese in infants with extrahepatic biliary atresia. *J Trace Elem Med Biol.* 1995;9:40–43

110. Sunde RA. Molecular biology of selenoproteins. *Annu Rev Nutr.* 1990;10:451–474

111. Litov RE, Combs GF Jr. Selenium in pediatric nutrition. *Pediatrics.* 1991;87:339–351

112. Thomson CD, Robinson MF. Urinary and fecal excretion and absorption of a large supplement of selenium: superiority of selenate over selenite. *Am J Clin Nutr.* 1986;44:659–663

113. Berry MJ, Banu L, Larsen PR. Type I iodothyronine deiodinase is a selenocysteine-containing enzyme. *Nature.* 1991;349:438–440

114. Zimmermann MB, Adou P, Torresani T, Zeder C, Hurell RF. Effect of oral iodized oil on thyroid size and thyroid hormone metabolism in children with concurrent selenium and iodine deficiency. *Eur J Clin Nutr.* 200;54:209–213

115. Keshan Disease Research Group of the Chinese Academy of Medical Sciences, Beijing. Observations on effect of sodium selenite in prevention of Keshan disease. *China Med J (Engl).* 1979;92:471–476

116. Nelson HK, Shi Q, Van Dael P, et al. Host nutritional status as a driving force for influenza virus. *FASEB J.* 2001;15:1846–1848

117. Peng T, Li Y, Yang Y, et al. Characterization of enterovirus isolates from patients with heart muscle disease in a selenium deficient area of China. *J Clin Microbiol.* 2000;38:3538–3543

118. Vinton NE, Dahlström KA, Strobel CT, Ament ME. Macrocytosis and pseudoalbinism: manifestations of selenium deficiency. *J Pediatr.* 1987;111:711–717

119. Lockitch G, Taylor GP, Wong LT, et al. Cardiomyopathy associated with nonendemic selenium deficiency in a Caucasian adolescent. *Am J Clin Nutr.* 1990;52:572–577

120. Lockitch G, Jacobson B, Quigley G, Dison P, Pendray M. Selenium deficiency in low birth weight neonates: an unrecognized problem. *J Pediatr.* 1989;114:865–870

121. Campa A, Shor-Posner G, Indacochea F, et al. Mortality risk in selenium-deficient HIV-positive children. *J Acquire Immune Defic Syndr Hum Retrovirol.* 1999;20:508–513

122. Smith AM, Chan GM, Moyer-Mileur LJ, Johnson CE, Gardner BR. Selenium status of preterm infants fed human milk, preterm formula, or selenium-supplemented preterm formula. *J Pediatr.* 1991;119:429–433

123. Tyrala EE, Borschel MW, Jacobs JR. Selenate fortification of infant formulas improves the selenium status of preterm infants. *Am J Clin Nutr.* 1996;64:860–865

124. Ehrenkranz RA, Gettner PA, Nelli CM, et al. Selenium absorption and retention by very-low-birth-weight infants: studies with the extrinsic stable isotope tag 74Se. *J Pediatr Gastroenterol Nutr.* 1991;13:125–133

125. Sluis KB, Darlow BA, George PM, Mogridge N, Dolamore BA, Winterbourn CC. Selenium and glutathione peroxidase levels in premature infants in a low selenium community (Christchurch, New Zealand). *Pediatr Res.* 1992;32:189–194

126. Falciglia HS, Johnson JR, Sullivan J, Hall CF, Miller JD, Riechmann GC, Falciglia GA. Role of antioxidant nutrients and lipid peroxidation in premature infants with respiratory distress syndrome and bronchopulmonary dysplasia. *Am J Perinatol.* 2003;20:97–107

127. Darlow BA, Austin NC. Selenium supplementation to prevent short-term morbidity in preterm neonates. *Cochrane Database Syst Rev.* 2003;(4):CD003312

128. Kumpulainen J, Salmenperä L, Siimes MA, Koivistoinen P, Perheentupa J. Selenium status of exclusively breast-fed infants as influenced by maternal organic or inorganic selenium supplementation. *Am J Clin Nutr.* 1985;42:829–835

129. Smith AM, Picciano MF, Milner JA. Selenium intakes and status of human milk and formula fed infants. *Am J Clin Nutr.* 1982;35:521–526

130. Kumpulainen J, Salmenperä L, Siimes MA, Koivistoinen P, Lehto J, Perheentupa J. Formula feeding results in lower selenium status than breast-feeding or selenium-supplemented formula feeding: a longitudinal study. *Am J Clin Nutr.* 1987;45:49–53

131. Milner JA, Sherman L, Picciano MF. Distribution of selenium in human milk. *Am J Clin Nutr.* 1987;45:617–624

132. Johnson CE, Smith AM, Chan GM, Moyer-Mileur LJ. Selenium status of term infants fed human milk or selenite-supplemented soy formula. *J Pediatr.* 1993;122:739–741

133. Smith AM, Chen LW, Thomas MR. Selenate fortification improves selenium status of term infants fed soy formula. *Am J Clin Nutr.* 1995;61:44–47

134. Van Dael P, Davidsson L, Ziegler EE, Fay LB, Barclay D. Comparison of selenite and selenate apparent absorption and retention in infants using stable isotope methodology. *Pediatr Res.* 2002;51:71–75

135. Litov RE, Sickles VS, Chan GM, Hargett IR, Cordano A. Selenium status in term infants fed human milk or infant formula with or without added selenium. *Nutr Res.* 1989;9:585–596

136. Zimmermann M, Adou P, Torresani T, Zeder C, Hurell R. Low dose oral iodized oil for control of iodine deficiency in children. *Br J Nutr.* 2000;84:139–141

137. Zimmermann M, Adou P, Torresani T, Zeder C, Hurell R. Persistence of goiter despite oral iodine supplementation in goitrous children with iron deficiency anemia in Côte d'Ivoire. *Am J Clin Nutr.* 2000;71:88–93

138. Ares S, Quero J, Morreale de Escobar G. Neonatal iodine deficiency: clinical aspects. *J Pediatr Endocrinol Metab.* 2005;18(Suppl 1):1257–1264

139. Ibrahim M, Sinn J, McGuire W. Iodine supplementation for the prevention of mortality and adverse neurodevelopmental outcomes in preterm infants. *Cochrane Database Syst Rev.* 2006;(2):CD005253

140. Parr RM, DeMaeyer EM, Iyengar VG, et al. Minor and trace elements in human milk from Guatemala, Hungary, Nigeria, Philippines, Sweden and Zaire. *Biol Trace Elem Res.* 1991;29:51–75

141. Bruhn JC, Franke AA. Iodine in human milk. *J Dairy Sci.* 1983;66:1396–1398

142. Gushurst CA, Mueller JA, Green JA, Sedor F. Breast milk iodide: reassessment in the1980s. *Pediatrics.* 1984;73:354–357

143. Friel JK, MacDonald AC, Mercer CN, et al. Molybdenum requirements in low-birth-weight infants receiving parenteral and enteral nutrition. *J Parenteral Enteral Nutr.* 1999;23:155–159

144. Litov RE, Sickles VS, Chan GM, Springer MA, Cordano A. Plasma aluminum measurements in term infants fed human milk or a soy-based infant formula. *Pediatrics.* 1989;84:1105-1107

Introduction

Vitamins are essential components of cofactors in a wide range of metabolic reactions. These functions are summarized in Table 20.1. Supplemental vitamins are expensive and probably unnecessary for the healthy child older than 1 year who consumes a varied diet. Milk from a well-nourished mother contains sufficient vitamins for the young, healthy, term infant except for vitamins K and D.

Recently, the Standing Committee on the Scientific Evaluation of Dietary Reference Intakes of the Institute of Medicine Food and Nutrition Board has undertaken a comprehensive expansion of the periodic reports called Recommended Dietary Allowances (RDAs) into a set of 4 nutrient-based values known as Dietary Reference Intakes (DRIs [see Appendix J for DRIs for vitamins]).[1] These reference values include the estimated average requirement (EAR), Recommended Dietary Allowance (RDA), adequate intake (AI), and the tolerable upper intake level (UL). If sufficient scientific evidence is not available to calculate an RDA, an AI is provided instead. RDAs and AIs are levels of intake recommended for individuals. They should reduce the risk of developing a condition that is associated with the nutrient in question that has a negative functional outcome. The DRIs apply to the apparently healthy general population. They are based on nutrient balance studies, the nutrient intakes of breastfed infants and healthy adults, biochemical measurement of tissue saturation or molecular function, and extrapolation from animal models. Unfortunately, only limited data are available on vitamin requirements in infants and children because of ethical, cost, and time concerns. Meeting the recommended intakes for the nutrients would not necessarily provide enough for individuals who are already malnourished, nor would they be adequate for certain disease states marked by increased nutritional requirements.

All standard commercial infant formulas contain vitamins in quantities sufficient to meet the recommended intakes if the infant consumes 750 mL of formula. Evaporated milk and pasteurized whole cow milk contain added vitamin D and sufficient vitamin A and most water-soluble vitamins except vitamin C (unless added by the processor).

Vitamin preparations available in the United States for infants and children younger than 4 years are in accord with Food and Drug Administration

(FDA) regulations.[2] These regulations (designed to minimize misuse) cover the minimum and maximum amounts allowed or required in multivitamin and multimineral supplements for infants and children younger than 4 years and for pregnant or lactating women. Preparations for older children and adults are not subject to FDA regulations, and this may increase the likelihood of the development of toxic effects from these preparations.

Vitamin and mineral products on the market for infants and children (see Table 20-II.1) consist primarily of the following:

1. Liquid drop preparations for infants that contain vitamins A, D, and C, with or without iron, or vitamins A, D, C, and E; thiamine; riboflavin; niacin; and vitamin B_6, with or without iron. One of the preparations contains vitamin B_{12} as well. It is important to note that these do not contain folate.

2. Chewable tablets for young children that contain vitamins A, D, and C, with or without iron, or vitamins A, D, E, and C; thiamine; folic acid; riboflavin; niacin; vitamin B_6; and vitamin B_{12}, with or without iron.

Infants and children who are ill or receive certain medications may require supplements of specific vitamins. Extra allowances are suggested for pregnant and lactating women. The widespread consumption of supplemental products is fostered by a combination of advertising pressure and concern about dietary adequacy. Many individuals regard vitamin and mineral supplements as a reliable method of ensuring that real or imagined dietary shortcomings are corrected. A vitamin pill containing the RDA given to the child daily, although unnecessary, probably does no harm. Like medications, these should be safely stored.

Table 20.1
Vitamins: Summary Table

Name	Characteristics	Biochemical Action	Effects of Deficiency	Effects of Excess	Food Sources
		Water-Soluble Vitamins			
Biotin	Water soluble; synthesized by intestinal bacteria; deficiency only with large intake of raw egg white (avidin irreversibly binds) or during TPN	Coenzyme: acetyl CoA carboxylase, other carboxylases	Seborrheic dermatitis, anorexia, nausea, pallor, alopecia, myalgias, paresthesias	Unknown	Liver, egg yolk, soybeans, milk, meat
Cyanocobalamin (vitamin B$_{12}$)	Slightly soluble in water, heat stable only at neutral pH, light sensitive; absorption (in ileum) depends on gastric intrinsic factor; CoA a part of the molecule	Coenzyme component; red blood cell maturation; central nervous system metabolism; methyl-malonyl-CoA mutase	Pernicious anemia; neurologic deterioration, methyl-malonicacidemia	Unknown	Animal foods only: meat, fish, poultry, cheese, milk, eggs, vitamin B$_{12}$-fortified soy milk
Folacin group of compounds containing pteridine ring, and paminobenzoic and glutamic acids	Slightly soluble in water, light sensitive, heat stable; ascorbic acid involved in interconversions; interference from oral contraceptives, antiepileptic drugs, alcohol	Tetrahydrofolic acid is the active form; synthesis of purines, pyrimidines, methylation reactions.	Megaloblastic anemia, impaired cellular immunity, irritability, paranoid behavior, neural tube defects in fetus of pregnant women	Masking of B$_{12}$ deficiency symptoms in patients with pernicious anemia not receiving cyanocobalamin	Yeast, liver, leafy green vegetables, oranges, cantaloupe, seeds, fortified breads and cereals (grains)
Niacin (nicotinic acid, amide) (vitamin B$_3$)	Water soluble, heat and light stable; availability from corn enhanced by alkali; synthesized in the body from tryptophan (60:1), some by intestinal bacteria	Component of coenzymes I and II (NAD, NADP), many enzymatic reactions	Pellagra: dermatitis, diarrhea, dementia	Nicotinic acid (not the amide): flushing, pruritus, liver abnormalities, hyperuricemia, decreased LDL and increased HDL cholesterol	Milk, eggs, poultry, meat, fish, whole grains, enriched cereals and grains

Table 20.1 (Continued)
Vitamins: Summary Table

Name	Characteristics	Biochemical Action	Effects of Deficiency	Effects of Excess	Food Sources
Pantothenic acid	Water soluble, heat stable	Component of CoA; many enzymatic reactions	Observed only with use of antagonists; depression, fatigue, hypotension, muscle weakness, abdominal pain	Unknown	Organ meats, yeast, egg yolk, fresh vegetables, whole grains, legumes
Pyridoxine (vitamin B$_6$), also pyridoxal, pyridoxamine	Water soluble, heat and light labile; interference from isoniazid; pyridoxal is the active form	Cofactor for many enzymes, (eg. transaminases, decarboxylases)	Irritability, depression, dermatitis, glossitis, cheilosis, peripheral neuritis; in infants, irritability, convulsions, microcytic anemia	Neuropathy, photosensitivity	Liver, meat, whole grains, legumes, potatoes
Riboflavin (vitamin B$_2$)	Water soluble, light labile, heat stable; synthesis by intestinal bacteria	Oxidation reduction, cofactor for many enzymes, synthesis of FMN and FAD	Pure riboflavin deficiency rare, photophobia, cheilosis, glossitis, corneal vascularization, poor growth	Unknown	Meat, dairy products, eggs, green vegetables, whole grains, enriched breads and cereals
Thiamine (vitamin B$_1$)	Water soluble, heat labile; absorption impaired by alcohol; requirements a function of carbohydrate intake	Coenzyme for decarboxylation, other reactions as thiamine pyrophosphate	Beriberi: neuritis, edema, cardiac failure, hoarseness, anorexia, restlessness, aphonia	Unknown	Enriched cereals and breads, lean pork, whole grains, legumes, in small amounts in most nutritious foods

Table 20.1 *(Continued)*
Vitamins: Summary Table

Name	Characteristics	Biochemical Action	Effects of Deficiency	Effects of Excess	Food Sources
Ascorbic acid (vitamin C)	Water soluble, easily oxidized, especially in presence of copper, iron, high pH; absorption by simple diffusion	Reversible reductant: functions in folacin metabolism, collagen biosynthesis, iron absorption and transport, tyrosine metabolism, neurotransmitter, carnitine synthesis	Osmotic diarrhea, bleeding gums, perifollicular hemorrhage, frank scurvy	Massive doses predispose to kidney stones; nausea, abdominal pain; rebound scurvy when massive doses stopped	Papaya, citrus fruits, tomatoes, cabbage, potatoes, cantaloupe, strawberries
		Fat-Soluble Vitamins			
Vitamin A (retinol) 1 µg retinol = 3.31 IU	Light sensitive, fat soluble, heat stable; bile necessary for absorption; specific plasma binding protein; stored in liver	Component of photorhodopsin; integrity of epithelial tissues, bone cell, and immune function	Night blindness, xerophthalmia, keratomalacia, poor bone growth, impaired resistance to infection, follicular hyperkeratosis	Hyperostosis, hepatomegaly, hepatic fibrosis alopecia, increased cerebrospinal fluid pressure	Fortified milk, liver, egg, cheese, yellow fruits and vegetables (carotenoid precursors)
Carotenoids (primarily carotene = 1/12 activity of retinol)	Fat soluble, converted to retinol in liver and intestinal mucosa; absorptive efficiency decreases with increased doses			Carotenemia	Dark green vegetables, yellow fruits and vegetables, tomatoes

Table 20.1 *(Continued)*
Vitamins: Summary Table

Name	Characteristics	Biochemical Action	Effects of Deficiency	Effects of Excess	Food Sources
Vitamin D (D_2, activated calciferol; D_3, activated de-hydrocholesterol) 1 µg = 40 IU	Fat-soluble D_2 from plant sources or fortification; D_3 from action of ultra-violet light on skin, animal sources, or fortification; hydroxylated sequentially in liver and kidney to form 1,25-dihydroxychole-calciferol, the active compound; regulated by dietary calcium, PTH; now called a prohor-mone; antiepileptic drugs interfere with metabolism	Maintains serum calcium via intestinal and bone effects; regulates syn-thesis of calcium-binding protein in intestinal epi-thelia cells, increasing calcium and phosphorus absorption; enhances mobilization of calcium and phosphorus from bone during deprivation	Rickets, osteomala-cia, antiepileptic drugs interfere with metabolism	Hypercalcemia, azotemia, poor growth, vomiting, nephrocal-cinosis	Fortified milk, fish, liver, egg yolk
Vitamin E (DL-alpha-tocopheryl, 1 mg = 1 IU); 8 naturally occur-ring compounds with biological activity, the most active being RRR-alpha-tocopherol, 1 mg = 1.49 IU per mg.	Fat soluble, heat labile; stored in adipose tissue, transported with lipopro-teins; absorption depends on pancreatic juice and bile (iron may interfere); tocoph-erol transport protein in liver regulates plasma levels; requirement increased by intake of large amounts of polyunsaturated fats	Free radical scavenger, antioxidant, role in red blood cell fragility; stabilizes biological membranes; prevents peroxidation of unsatu-rated fatty acids	Hemolytic anemia in preterm infants; fat malabsorption causes deficiency; hyporeflex-ia, and spinocerebellar and retinal degenera-tion; familial isolated vitamin E deficiency.	Bleeding, impaired leukocyte function	Sardines, green and leafy vegetables, vegetable oils, wheat germ, whole grains, butter, liver, egg yolk

Table 20.1 *(Continued)*
Vitamins: Summary Table

Name	Characteristics	Biochemical Action	Effects of Deficiency	Effects of Excess	Food Sources
Vitamin K (napthoquinones)	Light sensitive, fat soluble; bile necessary for absorption; synthesis by intestinal bacteria; antagonized by coumarin, salicylates, some antibiotics	Blood coagulation: factors II, VII, IX, X, proteins C, S, K, dependent bone proteins, and matrix Gla protein	Primary deficiency rare; hemorrhagic manifestations, possible effect on bone mineral density	Water-soluble analogs only: hyperbilirubinemia, hemolysis	Cow milk, green leafy vegetables, pork, liver

TPN indicates total parenteral nutrition; CoA, coenzyme A; NAD, nicotinamide adenine dinucleotide; NADP, nicotinamide-adenine dinucleotide phosphate; LDL, low-density lipoprotein; HDL, high-density lipoprotein; FMN, flavin mononucleotide; FAD, flavin adenine dinucleotide; PTH, parathyroid hormone.

Adapted from Shils ME, Olson JA, Shike M, eds. *Modern Nutrition in Health and Disease.* Philadelphia, PA: Lea and Febiger; 1994:247–448; and Forbes GB. Nutrition. In: Hoekelman RA, Blatman S, Freidman SB, Nelson NM, Seidel HM, eds. *Primary Pediatric Care.* St Louis, MO: CV Mosby; 1987:160–164

References

1. Institute of Medicine, Food and Nutrition Board. *Dietary Reference Intakes: Recommended Intakes for Individuals.* Washington, DC: National Academies Press. Available at: www.nap.edu. Accessed November 29, 2007

2. Dietary Supplement Health and Education Act (DSHEA). Pub L No. 103-417 (1994)

20-I Fat-Soluble Vitamins

Intestinal absorption of the fat-soluble vitamins (A, D, E, and K) is strongly dependent on adequate secretion of pancreatic enzymes and of bile acids from the liver into the intestinal lumen. In addition, vitamin A and vitamin E esters require hydrolysis before intestinal absorption by an intestinal esterase that is bile acid-dependent. Therefore, each of these vitamins may be poorly absorbed if any phase of fat digestion, absorption, or transport is interrupted. The fat-soluble vitamins are particularly prone to poor absorption and, therefore, deficiency in conditions associated with fat malabsorption, such as cystic fibrosis, celiac disease, and cholestatic liver diseases.[1] Deficiency in these vitamins is also associated with inadequate intake or light exposure (vitamin D) in specific clinical situations. A detailed description of each fat-soluble vitamin is given below.

Vitamin A

The term vitamin A refers to retinol and derivatives that have the same β-ionone ring and qualitatively similar biologic activities. The principal vitamin A compounds—retinol, retinal (retinaldehyde), retinoic acid, and retinyl esters—differ in the terminal C-15 group at the end of the side chain. The functions of vitamin A are maintenance of proper vision, epithelial cell integrity, and regulation of glycoprotein synthesis and cell differentiation.

Vitamin A is present in the diet as retinyl esters derived almost exclusively from animal sources (liver and fish liver oils, dairy products, kidney, and eggs) and provitamin A carotenoids (mainly beta-carotene) that are distributed widely in green and yellow vegetables. A recent report by the Institute of Medicine suggests that carotene-rich fruits and vegetables (carrots, sweet potatoes, broccoli) provide the body with half the amount of vitamin A as previously thought. Vitamin A activity is expressed as retinol activity equivalents (RAEs; 1 RAE = 3.3 IU of vitamin A activity). The Adequate Intake (AI) for vitamin A varies with age and is given in Table 20-I.1. Human milk, cow milk, and commercial infant formulas are excellent sources of vitamin A.

Deficiency

Vitamin A deficiency may occur in children receiving less than the AI and in those with fat malabsorption. Deficiency may lead to xerophthalmia, keratomalacia, and irreversible damage to the cornea as well as night blindness and pigmentary retinopathy. Deficiency may also increase morbidity and mortality from various infections, such as measles. Administration of the vitamin may be lifesaving in children with chronic deficiency and malnu-trition.[2] Additionally, routine supplementation with vitamin A during early childhood has decreased visual complications as well as overall childhood mortality in developing countries.[3] Although vitamin A supplementation dur-ing measles infection has been demonstrated to decrease overall morbidity, the role of supplementation in other infectious diseases is less clear. In several studies, vitamin A supplementation made no difference in clinical symptoms in nonmeasles infections (pneumonia, respiratory syncytial virus infection, infectious diarrhea)[4–8] and, in several instances, actually worsened clinical symptoms.[9–11]

Table 20-I.1
Vitamin A Adequate Intake by Age (See Also Appendix J, Table J-1)

Age	Vitamin A Dose (RAE)	Vitamin A Dose
0–6 mo	400 μg	1320 IU
7–12 mo	500 μg	1650 IU
1–3 y	300 μg	990 IU
4–8 y	400 μg	1320 IU
>8 y and adults	600–900 μg	1980–2970 IU

RAE indicates retinal activity equivalent; 1 RAE = 3.3 IU vitamin A.

Institute of Medicine. *Dietary Reference Intakes for Vitamin A, Vitamin K, Arsenic, Boron, Chromium, Copper, Iodine, Iron, Manganese, Molybdenum, Nickel, Silicon, Vanadium, and Zinc.* Washington, DC: National Academies Press; 2000

Assessment
Vitamin A status is monitored by serum retinol and retinol-binding protein (RBP) concentrations. In children with chronic liver disease, a modified rela-tive dose-response test may be a more specific means of assessing vitamin A deficiency,[12] although this approach should be validated in prospective stud-ies. In developing countries, screening has been performed using conjuncti-val impression cytology.[13,14]

Prevention and Treatment
The daily AI for vitamin A varies with age but is approximately 400 to 500 μg (1320–1650 IU) for infants and 600 to 1000 μg (1980–3300 IU) for older children and adults (Table 20-I.1). Children with conditions associated with fat malabsorption (cystic fibrosis, cholestatic liver disease) may require sup-plemental oral doses (2000–5000 IU daily) of a water-miscible preparation

to prevent deficiency. Treatment of frank vitamin A deficiency depends on the clinical manifestations. Significant eye findings, such as the presence of Bitot spots, xerophthalmia, or keratomalacia, should be treated with 50 000 to 100 000 IU of vitamin A administered parenterally. In patients without deficiency, supplementation with 1500 to 3000 μg (4950–9900 IU) of vitamin A during acute measles infection has been shown to be associated with lower morbidity and mortality.[15] Additionally, the World Health Organization recommends administration of an oral dose of vitamin A (100 000 IU in infants and 200 000 IU in children older than 1 year) each day for 2 consecutive days to children with measles living in areas where vitamin A deficiency may be present. A Cochrane review revealed that this approach was associated with a decrease in mortality in children younger than 2 years with measles.[16]

Toxicity

Claims that extremely high doses of vitamin A (7500–15 000 μg RAE or 24 750–49 500 IU per day) improve visual acuity in those who work in bright or dim light are unsubstantiated. As little as 6000 μg RAE daily can produce serious toxic effects in children. Vitamin A toxicity manifests as anorexia, increased intracranial pressure (vomiting and headaches), painful bone lesions, precocious bone growth, desquamative dermatitis, and hepatotoxicity.[17–19] Caffey warned that the hazards of vitamin A poisoning from the routine prophylactic use of concentrates of vitamins A to well-fed healthy infants and children in the United States are considerably greater than the hazards of vitamin A deficiency in healthy infants and children not fed vitamin concentrates.[20] Toxic effects of vitamin A were found in young children who were fed large amounts of chicken liver, which contains 90 μg RAE (297 IU) of vitamin A/g,[21] for 1 month or longer. Vitamin A excess, including vitamin A derivatives, such as retinoic acid, are teratogenic; adolescents who may become pregnant should be informed of the dangers of vitamin A or derivatives used in the treatment of acne.[22]

Assessment

To monitor for vitamin A toxicity during high-dose vitamin A therapy, serum retinyl esters, normally not present, should be monitored. Determining plasma concentrations of retinol and RBP is not always a reliable means of detecting vitamin A toxicity.[19,23]

Vitamin D

Vitamin D (calciferol) refers to 2 secosteroids, vitamin D_2 (ergocalciferol) and vitamin D_3 (cholecalciferol). Vitamin D_2 is derived from plants and fungi and is added to vitamin D-supplemented cow milk. Vitamin D_3 is synthesized in the skin from 7-dehydrocholesterol on exposure to sunlight. Vitamins D_2 and D_3 are considered prohormones and subsequently undergo 25-hydroxylation in the liver to form 25-hydroxyvitamin D (25-OH-D [calcidiol]), which is the major circulating form of vitamin D. Vitamin D_3 has greater efficiency in raising circulating 25-OH-D concentrations. From the liver, 25-OH-D is transported to the kidney for hydroxylation to form the biologically active hormone 1,25-dihydroxyvitamin D (1,25-OH_2-D [calcitriol]). Calcitriol is the biologically active form of vitamin D, which stimulates the intestinal absorption of calcium and phosphorous, renal reabsorption of filtered calcium, and mobilization of calcium and phosphorous from bone. Vitamin D is, therefore, essential for bone formation and mineral homeostasis.

Vitamin D is synthesized in the skin by the action of ultraviolet light on a cholesterol precursor (the most effective wavelengths are in the range of 290–315 nm); therefore, the requirement for dietary vitamin D depends on the amount of exposure to sunlight. The actual requirement for vitamin D in the absence of sunlight is unknown.

Deficiency

The primary manifestations of vitamin D deficiency are related to the effects on calcium metabolism. Hypocalcemia, hypophosphatemia, tetany, osteomalacia, and rickets are the most common clinical features. Deficiency occurs in those with fat malabsorption and may occur in infants not exposed to sunlight who have an inadequate dietary intake of vitamin D. The best estimate for adequate exposure to sunlight for white infants is 30 minutes per week clothed only in a diaper, or 2 hours per week fully clothed with no hat.[24]

Assessment

The best indicator of vitamin D status is serum 25-OH-D concentration, which reflects absorption from the diet and synthesis by the skin. Other potentially useful tests include 1,25-OH_2-D concentration and serum calcium, phosphorous, and alkaline phosphatase concentrations. The diagnosis of rickets is made on the basis of a history of inadequate intake and clinical findings (craniotabes, enlargement of the costochondral junctions, beading of the ribs) and is confirmed by biochemical indices and radiographic findings. Parathyroid hormone concentration is generally elevated in rickets associated with vitamin D deficiency.

Prevention and Treatment

The AI is 200 IU (5.0 µg cholecalciferol) in infants, children, and adults. The vitamin D content of human milk is low (22 IU/L), and rickets can occur in deeply pigmented breastfed infants or infants with inadequate exposure to sunlight. Consequently, vitamin D supplementation at 400 IU/day is recommended for breastfed infants. Most formulas contain 1.5 µg (62 IU) of vitamin D/100 kcal, or 10 µg/L, as do cow milk and evaporated milks.

Patients with diseases associated with fat malabsorption (cystic fibrosis, cholestatic liver disease) may require supplementation with doses 2 to 4 times the AI to prevent deficiency. During cholestasis, supplementation with either vitamin D_2 (ergocalciferol [Drisdol, sanofi aventis, Bridgewater, NJ], 10–20 µg/day; 400–800 IU/day) or vitamin D_3 (calcifediol [Calderol, Organon, West Orange, NJ], 2–4 µg/kg per day), which is better absorbed during cholestasis, should be provided.

Several approaches have been used for the treatment of nutritional or vitamin D-deficient rickets, including daily oral administration of 2000 to 5000 IU of ergocalciferol (vitamin D_2) in children with normal gastrointestinal function or oral administration of 10 000 to 25 000 IU/day in children with malabsorption for 2 to 4 weeks. In children with chronic cholestatic liver disease, parenteral administration of 0.2 µg/kg per day of 1,25-OH_2-D has been used.[25] Failure to respond to vitamin D treatment suggests a diagnosis of vitamin D-resistant rickets. Guidance on vitamin D supplementation in children with renal failure is given in chapter 41.

Toxicity

No evidence supports the claim that vitamin D, in amounts much greater than 10 µg daily, leads to improved bone mineralization. The AI provides an ample margin of safety even without exposure to sunlight. The principal manifestations of vitamin D intoxication are hypercalcemia, leading to depression of the central nervous system and ectopic calcification, and hypercalciuria, leading to nephrocalcinosis and nephrolithiasis. Overuse of vitamin D in Great Britain and Europe, with intakes between 70 and 100 µg daily, is believed to be related to the idiopathic hypercalcemia of infants, which was seen frequently during and after World War II.

AAP

The American Academy of Pediatrics states:

To prevent rickets and vitamin D deficiency in healthy infants, children, and adolescents, a vitamin D intake of at least 400 IU a day is recommended. To meet this intake, the following suggestions are made:

1. Breastfed and partially breastfed infants should be supplemented with 400 IU/day of vitamin D beginning in the first few days of life. This should be continued unless the infant is weaned to at least 1 liter or 1 quart per day of vitamin D-fortified formula or whole milk. Whole milk is not recommended before 1 year of age.
2. All nonbreastfed infants as well as older children who are ingesting less than 1000 mL per day of vitamin D-fortified formula or milk should receive a vitamin D supplement of 400 IU/day. Other dietary sources of vitamin D, such as fortified foods, may be included in the daily intake of each child.
3. Adolescents who do not obtain 400 IU of vitamin D per day through vitamin D-fortified milk (100 IU per 8-ounce serving) and vitamin D-fortified foods (such as fortified cereals and eggs [yolks]) should receive a vitamin D supplement of 400 IU/day.
4. On the basis of the available evidence, serum 25-OH-D concentrations in infants and children should be ≥50 nmol/L (20 ng/mL).
5. Children with increased risk of vitamin D deficiency, such as those with chronic fat malabsorption and those chronically taking antiseizure medications, may continue to be vitamin D deficient despite an intake of 400 IU/day. Higher doses of vitamin D supplementation may be necessary to achieve normal vitamin D status in these children, and this status should be determined with laboratory tests, such as serum 25-OH-D and PTH concentrations, and measures of bone mineral status. If a vitamin D supplement is prescribed, 25-OH-D levels should be repeated at 3-month intervals until normal levels have been achieved. PTH and bone mineral status should be monitored every 6 months until they have normalized.
6. Pediatricians and other health care professionals should strive to make vitamin D supplements readily available to all children within their community, especially for those children most at risk.

Pediatrics. 2008; in press

Vitamin E

There are 4 major forms (alpha, beta, delta, and gamma) of tocopherol and tocotrienols, the 2 main forms of vitamin E. Alpha-tocopherol has the highest biological activity and is the predominant form in foodstuffs, with the exception of soy oil, which contains high amounts of gamma-tocopherol. The major function of vitamin E is its role as an antioxidant, protecting cell membrane polyunsaturated fatty acids, thiol-rich proteins, and nucleic acids from oxidant damage initiated by free radical reactions. Vitamin E is essential for the maintenance of structure and function of the human nervous system, retina, and skeletal muscle. Common dietary sources of vitamin E are the oil-containing grains, plants, and vegetables. Vitamin E supplementation prevents severe neuropathy in infants with biliary atresia and other forms of chronic cholestatic liver disease, and it prevents muscle weakness in children with cystic fibrosis.[26] Little or no basis exists for the claim that high dietary intakes of vitamin E prolong life, increase sexual potency, and prevent cancer. Although it was suggested that vitamin E supplementation may play a role in prevention of cardiovascular disease,[27] recent large-scale prospective studies have not shown any beneficial effect.[28–30]

Deficiency

The wide distribution of vitamin E in vegetable oils and cereal grains makes deficiency in humans from industrialized nations unlikely. Vitamin E supplements are necessary for those with malabsorption (eg, pancreatic insufficiency or cystic fibrosis), biliary atresia and other biliary tract disorders, cirrhosis, and lipid transport disorders. Uncorrected vitamin E deficiency during childhood leads to a progressive neurologic disorder, including truncal and limb ataxia, hyporeflexia, depressed vibratory and position sensation, impairment in balance and coordination, peripheral neuropathy, proximal muscle weakness, ophthalmoplegia, and retinal dysfunction.[26] Significant cognitive and behavioral abnormalities have been described in association with prolonged vitamin E deficiency. Neurologic lesions may be irreversible to a substantial degree if vitamin E deficiency remains untreated. Congenital deficiency of the hepatic tocopherol transport protein also results in vitamin E deficiency and ataxia, despite normal absorption of vitamin E.[31] Deficiency of vitamin E has also been associated with hemolytic anemia in preterm infants fed a diet high in polyunsaturated fatty acids.[32]

Assessment

Vitamin E status is monitored by serum alpha-tocopherol concentrations and ratios of serum alpha-tocopherol to total lipids.

Prevention and Treatment

The AI for alpha-tocopherol is 4 mg (9.3 μmol)/day for infants 0 to 6 months of age and 5 mg (11.6 μmol)/day for infants 7 to 12 months of age (approx 0.6 mg/kg). The RDA for alpha-tocopherol is 6 mg (13.9 μmol)/ day for children 1 to 3 years of age, 7 mg (16.3 μmol)/day for children 4 to 8 years of age, and 11 to 15 mg (25.6–34.9 μmol)/day for children 9 to 18 years of age. The RDA for alpha-tocopherol for adults is 15 mg (34.9 μmol)/

day (1 mg D-alpha-tocopherol = 1 tocopherol equivalent [TE]; 1 mg of DL-alpha-tocopheryl acetate = 1 IU]).

During conditions associated with fat malabsorption (cystic fibrosis, cholestatic liver disease), supplemental doses (25 IU/kg per day) of vitamin E are required to prevent deficiency. The water-miscible form of vitamin E, alpha-tocopherol polyethylene glycol succinate, is the preferable form for oral supplementation during cholestasis and may even improve the absorption of other fat-soluble vitamins or drugs when given concurrently.[33,34]

Toxicity

Vitamin E toxicity is rare. Typical adults appear to tolerate oral doses of 100 to 800 mg/day without clinical signs or biochemical evidence of toxicity.[35] In several studies, adults who received very large doses of vitamin E (>1000–1500 IU/day) in conjunction with warfarin therapy had a significantly prolonged prothrombin time beyond that expected from the warfarin alone.[36,37] In addition, large parenteral doses of vitamin E in preterm infants, resulting in extremely high serum vitamin E concentrations (>40–50 µg/mL), were associated with an increased incidence of bacterial and fungal sepsis, presumably because of inhibition of neutrophil function.[38]

Vitamin K

Vitamin K belongs to the family of 2 methyl-1,4 naphthoquinones and exists as 3 forms.[39] Phylloquinone (vitamin K_1) is obtained from leafy vegetables, soybean oil, fruits, seeds, and cow milk. Menaquinone (vitamin K_2), which has 60% of the activity of vitamin K_1, is synthesized by intestinal bacteria. Menadione (vitamin K_3) is not a natural form but is synthesized chemically and has better water solubility than the 2 natural forms. Vitamin K is necessary for the post-translational carboxylation of glutamic acid residues of the vitamin K-dependent coagulation proteins (factors II, VII, IX, and X; protein C; and protein S). Carboxylation allows these proteins to bind calcium, thus leading to activation of the clotting factors.[40] Other proteins undergoing this carboxylation of glutamic acid residues include osteocalcin, which is involved in bone mineralization.

Deficiency

Vitamin K deficiency leads to hypoprothrombinemia and hemorrhagic disorders. Newborn infants are especially at risk of hemorrhagic disease secondary to vitamin K deficiency because of inherently poor placental transport of vitamin K, a decreased number of gut bacteria that synthesize vitamin K, and the low content of vitamin K in human milk (20 IU/L, compared with 60 IU/L in cow milk). Common sites of bleeding include the gastrointestinal tract, the umbilicus, or the site of circumcision. In older children and adults, hypoprothrombinemia associated with vitamin K deficiency is usually secondary to disorders of fat malabsorption or chronic liver disease.[41] Vitamin K deficiency may also be seen in children on highly restricted diets or after bariatric surgery. Several studies have suggested an association between low vitamin K concentrations and abnormal bone mineral density, bone turnover, and even osteoarthritis, although a causal relationship has not been definitively established.[42–44]

Assessment

Vitamin K status is monitored by prothrombin time, the measurement of vitamin K-dependent factors (factors II, VII, IX, X), plasma phylloquinone (vitamin K_1) concentration, or the analysis of proteins-induced-in-vitamin K absence.

Prevention and Treatment

The newborn infant is usually given vitamin K soon after birth for prophylaxis against hemorrhagic disease of the newborn. Vitamin K should preferentially be given as a single intramuscular dose of 1 mg (0.5 mg for preterm infants). If this is not possible, then an oral dose of 1 to 2 mg should be administered at birth, 1 to 2 weeks of age, and 4 weeks of age.[45] A recent study has suggested that maternal prenatal vitamin K administration may decrease periventricular-intraventricular hemorrhage in preterm infants.[46] After the prophylactic dose of vitamin K at birth, most formula-fed infants receive adequate vitamin K from cow milk formulas, and the formula-fed infant ordinarily does not need added vitamin K. The AI for infants is 2 μg/day of phylloquinone or menaquinone for the first 6 months of life and 2.5 μg/day for the second 6 months. The AI is 30 μg/day for children 1 to 3 years of age, 55 μg/day for children 4 to 8 years of age, and 60 to 75 μg/day for older children and adolescents.

In conditions associated with fat malabsorption (cystic fibrosis, cholestatic liver disease), supplemental doses of 2.5 to 5 mg 2 to 7 times/week may be required to prevent deficiency. Hypoprothrombinemia associated with chronic liver disease may be corrected by the administration of 5 to 10 mg of vitamin K given intramuscularly. Failure of the prothrombin time to improve after adequate administration of vitamin K suggests severe liver synthetic dysfunction. There have not been any prospective studies of vitamin K treatment for gastrointestinal bleeding in patients with liver disease, as highlighted by a recent Cochrane database review.[47] Vitamin K does not appear to be an effective treatment for the reversal of excessive anticoagulation secondary to oral anticoagulants.[48]

Toxicity

Vitamin K toxicity is rare. In newborn infants, parenteral administration of a large amount of water-soluble synthetic vitamin K (vitamin K_3) has been associated with hemolytic anemia, hyperbilirubinemia, and kernicterus. No toxicity states have been associated with administration of oral vitamin K_1.

A Note on Vitamin K and Cancer Risk

In 1990, Golding et al[49] reported a study of a 1970 birth cohort in Great Britain in which they noted an unexpected association between childhood cancer and pethidine given during labor and neonatal administration of vitamin K. Subsequently, they reported in a retrospective, case-controlled study a significant association between intramuscular vitamin K and cancer when compared with no vitamin K or oral vitamin K.[50] Draper and Stiller[51] questioned this study on the basis of other data from Great Britain and have called for large cohort studies. The American Academy of Pediatrics formed a Vitamin K Ad Hoc Task Force to study this area in greater detail.[45] The task force found no convincing links between vitamin K administration and childhood cancer. Indeed, if intramuscular vitamin K doubles the incidence of childhood leukemia, a sharp increase should have been observed after 1961, which was not the case. Golding et al suggested that sister chromatid exchanges induced by vitamin K may be responsible for the increased incidence of cancer observed in their study.[50] However, in a study of human infants, no differences in sister chromatid exchanges were observed in those who received vitamin K versus those who did not.[52] On the basis of these observations, the American Academy of Pediatrics continues to recommend the routine administration of vitamin K to newborn infants (see box).

AAP

The American Academy of Pediatrics recommendations concerning the administration of vitamin K to newborn infants:

Because parenteral vitamin K prevents a life-threatening disease of the newborn infant and the risks of cancer are unproven and unlikely, the American Academy of Pediatrics recommends:

- Vitamin K should be given to all newborn infants as a single, intramuscular dose of 0.5 to 1 mg.
- Further research on the efficacy, safety, and bioavailability of oral formulations of vitamin K is warranted.
- An oral dosage form is not currently available in the United States but should be developed and licensed. If an appropriate oral form is developed and licensed in the United States, it should be given at birth (2.0 mg) and should be administered again at 1 to 2 weeks of age and 4 weeks of age to breastfed infants. If diarrhea occurs in an exclusively breastfed infant, the dose should be repeated.
- The conflicting data of Golding et al[50] and Draper and Stiller[51] and data from the United States suggest that additional cohort studies are unlikely to be helpful.

Pediatrics 1993;91:1001–1003

References

1. Sokol RJ. Fat-soluble vitamins and their importance in patients with choleostatic liver diseases. *Gastroenterol Clin North Am.* 1994;23:673–705
2. Rahmathullah L, Underwood BA, Thulasiraj RD, et al. Reduced mortality among children in Southern India receiving a small weekly dose of vitamin A. *N Engl J Med.* 1990;323:929–935
3. Underwood BA, Arthur P. The contribution of vitamin A to public health. *FASEB J.* 1996;10:1040–1048
4. Kjolhede CL, Chew FJ, Gadomski AM, Marroquin DP. Clinical trial of vitamin A as adjuvant treatment for lower respiratory tract infections. *J Pediatr.* 1995;126:807–812
5. Quinlan K, Hayani K. Vitamin A and respiratory syncytial virus infection. Serum levels and supplementation trial. *Arch Pediatr Adolesc Med.* 1996;150:25–30
6. Bresee J, Fischer M, Dowel SF, et al. Vitamin A therapy for children with respiratory syncytial virus infection: a multicenter trial in the United States. *Pediatr Infect Dis J.* 1996;15:777–782
7. Henning B, Stewart K, Zaman K, Alam AN, Brown KH, Black RE. Lack of therapeutic efficacy of vitamin A for non-cholera, watery diarrhea in Bangladeshi children. *Eur J Clin Nutr.* 1992;46:437–443
8. Ni J, Wei J, Wu T. Vitamin A for non-measles pneumonia in children. *Cochrane Database Syst Rev.* 2005;(3):CD003700

9. Stephensen C, Franchi L, Hernandez H, Campos M, Gilman R, Alvarez JO. Adverse effects of high-dose vitamin A supplements in children hospitalized with pneumonia. *Pediatrics*. 1998;101(5):e3. Available at: http://pediatrics.aappublications.org/cgi/content/full/101/5/e3. Accessed August 24, 2007

10. Fawzi W, Mbise R, Fataki M, et al. Vitamin A supplementation and severity of pneumonia in children admitted to the hospital in Dar es Salaam, Tanzania. *Am J Clin Nutr*. 1998;68:187–192

11. Long KZ, Montoya Y, Hertzmark E, Santos JI, Rosado JL. A double-blind, randomized clinical trial of the effect of vitamin A and zinc supplementation on diarrheal disease and respiratory tract infections in children in Mexico City, Mexico. *Am J Clin Nutr*. 2006;83:693–700

12. Feranchak AP, Gralla J, King R, Ramirez RO, Corkill M, Narkewicz MR, Sokol RJ. Comparison of indices of vitamin A status in children with chronic liver disease. *Hepatology*. 2005;42:782–792

13. Tseng SC. Staging of conjunctival squamous metaplasia by impression cytology. *Ophthalmology*. 1985;92:728–733

14. Amedee-Manesme O, Luzeau R, Wittenpen JR, Hanck A, Sommer A. Impression cytology detects subclinical vitamin A deficiency. *Am J Clin Nutr*. 1988;47:875–878

15. Hussey GD, Klein M. A randomized, controlled trial of vitamin A in children with severe measles. *N Engl J Med*. 1990;323:160–164

16. Huiming Y, Chaomin W, Meng M. Vitamin A for treating measles in children. *Cochrane Database Syst Rev*. 2005;(4):CD001479

17. Rubin E, Florman AL, Degnan T, Diaz J. Hepatic injury in chronic hypervitaminosis. *Am J Dis Child*. 1970;119:132–138

18. Lippe B, Hensen L, Mendoza G, Finerman M, Welch M. Chronic vitamin A intoxication. A multisystem disease that could reach epidemic proportions. *Am J Dis Child*. 1981;135:634–636

19. Mobarhan S, Russell RM, Underwood BA, Wallingford J, Mathieson RD, Al-Midani H. Evaluation of the relative dose response test for vitamin A nurtiture in cirrhotics. *Am J Clin Nutr*. 1981;34:2264–2270

20. Caffey J. Chronic poisoning due to excess vitamin A; description of the clinical and roentgen manifestations in seven infants and young children. *Pediatrics*. 1950;5:672–688

21. Mahoney CP, Margolis MT, Knauss TA, Labbe RF. Chronic vitamin A intoxication in infants fed chicken liver. *Pediatrics*. 1980;65:893–897

22. Lammer EJ, Chen DT, Hoar RM, et al. Retinoic acid embryopathy. *N Engl J Med*. 1985;313:837–841

23. Smith FR, Goodman DS. Vitamin A transport in human vitamin A toxicity. *N Engl J Med*. 1976; 294:805–808

24. Specker BL, Valanis B, Hertzberg V, Edwards N, Tsang RC. Sunshine exposure and serum 25-hydroxyvitamin D concentrations in exclusively breast-fed infants. *J Pediatr*. 1985;107:372–376

25. Heubi JE, Tsang RC, Steichen JJ, Chan GM, Chen IW, DeLuca HF. 1,25-Dihydroxyvitamin D3 in childhood hepatic osteodystrophy. *J Pediatr*. 1979:94:977–982

26. Sokol RJ. Vitamin E and neurologic deficits. *Adv Pediatr*. 1990;37:119–148

27. Pryor WA. Vitamin E and heart disease: basic science to clinical intervention trials. *Free Radic Biol Med.* 2000;28:141–164

28. Tornwall ME, Virtamo J, Korhoen PA, et al. Effect of alpha-tocopherol and beta-carotene supplementation on coronary heart disease during the 6-year post-trial follow-up in the ATBC study. *Eur Heart J.* 2004;25:1171–1178

29. Heart Protection Study Collaborative Group. MRC/BHF Heart Protection Study of antioxidant vitamin supplementation in 20,536 high-risk individuals: a randomized placebo-controlled trial. *Lancet.* 2002;360:23–33

30. Hercberg S, Galan P, Preziosi P, et al. The SU.VI.MAX. study: a randomized placebo-controlled trial of the health effect of antioxidant vitamins and minerals. *Arch Intern Med.* 2004;164:2335–2342

31. Traber MG, Sokol RJ, Burton GW, et al. Impaired ability of patients with familial isolated vitamin E deficiency to incorporate alpha-tocopherol into lipoproteins secreted by the liver. *J Clin Invest.* 1990;85:397–407

32. Oski FA, Barness LA. Vitamin E deficiency: a primarily unrecognized cause of hemolytic anemia in the premature infant. *J Pediatr.* 1967;70:211–220

33. Sokol RJ, Butler-Simon N, Conner C, et al. Multicenter trial of d-alpha-tocopheryl polyethylene glycol 1000 succinate for treatment of vitamin E deficiency in children with chronic choleostasis. *Gastroenterology.* 1993;104:1727–1735

34. Sokol RJ, Johnson KE, Karrer FM, Narkewicz MR, Smith D, Kam I. Improvement of cycolsporin absorption in children after liver transplantation by means of water-soluble vitamin E. *Lancet.* 1991;338:212–214

35. Farrell PM, Bieri JG. Megavitamin E supplementation in man. *Am J Clin Nutr.* 1975;28:1381–1386

36. Corrigan JJ Jr, Marcus FI. Coagulopathy associated with vitamin E ingestion. *JAMA.* 1974;230:1300–1301

37. Corrigan JJ Jr. The effect of vitamin E on warfarin-induced vitamin K deficiency. *Ann N Y Acad Sci.* 1982;393:361–368

38. Johnson L, Bowen FW Jr, Abbasi S, et al. Relationship of prolonged pharmacologic serum levels of vitamin E to incidence of sepsis and necrotizing enterocolitis in infants with birth weight 1,500 grams or less. *Pediatrics.* 1985;75:619–638

39. Olson RE. The function and metabolism of vitamin K. *Annu Rev Nutr.* 1984;4:281–337

40. Suttie JW. Vitamin K responsive hemorrhagic disease of infancy. *J Pediatr Gastroenterol Nutr.* 1990;11:4–6

41. Mager DR, McGee PL, Furuya KN, Roberts EA. Prevalence of vitamin K deficiency in children with mild to moderate chronic liver disease. *J Pediatr Gastroenterol Nutr.* 2006;42:71–76

42. Conway SP, Wolfe SP, Brownlee KG, et al. Vitamin K status among children with cystic fibrosis and its relationship to bone mineral density and bone turnover. *Pediatrics.* 2005;115:1325–1331

43. Neogi T, Booth SL, Zhang YQ, et al. Low vitamin K status associated with osteoarthritis in the hand and knee. *Arthritis Rheum.* 2006;54:1255–1261

44. Nicolaidou P, Stavrinadis I, Loukou I, Papadopoulou A, Georgouli H, et al. The effect of vitamin K supplementation on biochemical markers of bone formation in children and adolescents with cystic fibrosis. *Eur J Pediatr.* 2006;165:540–545

45. American Academy of Pediatrics, Vitamin K Ad Hoc Task Force. Controversies concerning vitamin K and the newborn. *Pediatrics.* 1993;91:1001–1003

46. Liu J, Wang Q, Gao F, He JW, Zhao JH. Maternal antenatal administration of vitamin K1 results in increasing the activities of vitamin K-dependent coagulation factors in umbilical blood and in decreasing the incidence rate of periventricular-intraventricular hemorrhage in premature infants. *J Perinat Med.* 2006;34:173–176

47. Marti-Carvajal AJ, Marti-Pena AJ. Vitamin K for upper gastrointestinal bleeding in patients with liver diseases. *Cochrane Database Syst Rev.* 2005;(3):CD004792

48. Dezee KJ, Shimeall WT, Douglas KM, Shumway NM, O'Malley PG. Treatment of excessive anticoagulation with phytonadione (vitamin K): a meta-analysis. *Arch Intern Med.* 2006;166:391–397

49. Golding J, Paterson M, Kinlen LJ. Factors associated with childhood cancer in a national cohort study. *Br J Cancer.* 1990;62:304–308

50. Golding J, Greenwood R, Birmingham K, Mott M. Childhood cancer, intramuscular vitamin K, and pethidine given during labour. *Br Med J.* 1992;305:341–346

51. Draper GJ, Stiller CA. Intramuscular vitamin K and childhood cancer. *Br Med J.* 1992;305:709

52. Cornelissen EM, Smeets D, Merkx G, De Abreu R, Kollee L, Monnens L. Analysis of chromosome aberrations and sister chromatid exchanges in peripheral blood lymphocytes of newborns after vitamin K prophylaxis at birth. *Pediatr Res.* 1991;30:550–553

20-II Water-Soluble Vitamins

Deficiencies of the water-soluble vitamins are rare in formula-fed infants and in breastfed infants of mothers consuming a healthy diet. Most children and adolescents, if eating a diet consisting of fruits, vegetables, animal protein (meat, dairy, and egg), cereals, and breads, consume sufficient water-soluble vitamins to meet daily allowances. Appreciating who might be at particular risk of deficiency of water-soluble vitamins is important because of limited total body stores and lack of endogenous synthesis of most water-soluble vitamins. However, not all water-soluble vitamin deficiency states in infancy and childhood are a result of dietary deficiency. Some deficiencies result from inborn errors of metabolism. Medical conditions that may predispose one to deficiency of water-soluble vitamins include malabsorption secondary to celiac disease, Crohn disease, cystic fibrosis, food refusal, anorexia nervosa, or HIV infection or AIDS.

Health and dietary trends have the potential to influence nutritional health status in the pediatric population. The increasing use of complementary and alternative medicine (CAM) in the United States and abroad highlights this notion.[1] These practices are not limited to adults; one study reported that children and adolescents accounted for one third of visits to homeopathic and naturopathic practitioners.[2] The most common CAM product prescribed for children and adults by a naturopathic practitioner is a multivitamin. However, single-vitamin preparations, both fat soluble and water soluble, are also frequently prescribed.[3,4] It is commonly thought that water-soluble vitamins are safe if given in excess. In fact, some water-soluble vitamins have the potential for toxicity if given in excessive quantities over a prolonged period of time.

Also concerning is the rapidly increasing population of overweight children and adolescents in the United States.[5] Recent work has begun to focus on the nutritional factors leading to and consequences of this epidemic. Analysis of data from the National Health and Nutrition Examination Survey III reveals that low-nutrient density foods contribute more than 30% of the daily energy to the diets of children and adolescents. In this study, the mean reported intake of vitamins A, B_6, and folate decreased with increasing foods of low nutrient density in the diet.[6] Similarly, a study of school-aged girls demonstrated that those with a high fat intake (>30% of energy from fat) had lower intakes of vitamins A, C, B_6, folate, and riboflavin.[7]

Research from Norway in school-aged children has shown that the converse may be true. That is, a diet low in fat positively correlates with increasing intake of several water-soluble vitamins.[8] In US adolescents, a low-fat and high-fiber diet was associated with a greater likelihood of adequate intake of vitamins A, B$_6$, B$_{12}$, and C; niacin; thiamin; riboflavin; and folicin.[9] Not surprisingly, children and adolescents who eat dinner with their family regularly had substantially higher intakes of vitamins B$_6$, B$_{12}$, C, and folate.[10] Taken together, these studies demonstrate that diets high in fat and/ or with a preponderance of low-nutrient density foods place children and adolescents at risk of water-soluble vitamin deficiency.

Thiamine (Vitamin B$_1$)

Thiamine is an essential coenzyme involved in carbohydrate metabolism. Thiamine pyrophosphate (TPP) is the primary active form of thiamine. Thiamine pyrophosphate and nicotinamide adenine dinucleotide (NAD) function as coenzymes to pyruvate dehydrogenase in the oxidative decarboxylation of pyruvate to acetyl coenzyme A (CoA). Thiamine also plays an integral role with transketolase in the pentose phosphate pathway, which provides substrates for the synthesis of nucleic acids and fatty acids. In addition to functioning as a CoA, thiamine has been found to play a role in nerve impulse conduction and voluntary muscle action.[11]

Foods rich in thiamine include yeast, legumes, pork, and whole grain brown rice and cereals. Dairy products and most fruits contain little thiamine. Thiamine is lost during the processing of white flour and the milling of white rice; therefore, these foods are a poor source of thiamine. Deficiency of thiamine can result in the clinical syndromes of beriberi or Wernicke encephalopathy. Beriberi is traditionally classified in 2 forms: dry beriberi, which is characterized by a symmetrical peripheral neuropathy, and wet beriberi, in which cardiac involvement predominates.[12]

The neuropathy seen in dry beriberi is progressive, resulting in increasing weakness, muscle wasting, difficulty walking, and ataxia and is accompanied by painful paresthesias and loss of deep tendon reflexes. Edema is the hallmark symptom of wet beriberi. The cardiac involvement in wet beriberi results in a cardiomyopathy that will progress to congestive heart failure and death if untreated. Infantile beriberi generally occurs in a breastfed child whose mother has a subclinical thiamine deficiency. This form of beriberi is characterized by the sudden onset of shock in a previously well child generally between 2 and 3 months of age. These symptoms may be preceded by a hoarse, weak cry; poor feeding; and vomiting.[13] Wernicke encephalopathy is characterized by the triad of ophthalmoplegia, nystagmus, and ataxia in addition to altered consciousness. Its association with thiamine deficiency in infants and children has been reported.[14,15]

Thiamine deficiency may result from inadequate dietary intake of the vitamin, malabsorption, excessive loss, or defective transport of the vitamin. Mothers at risk of thiamine deficiency include those with a poor thiamine intake, alcohol abuse, gastrointestinal disease, hyperemesis gravidarum, and HIV infection or AIDS. Other populations at particularly high risk of developing thiamine deficiency include patients who practice food faddism, individuals with anorexia nervosa, adolescents after gastric bypass surgery, renal patients undergoing chronic dialysis, children with congenital heart disease, and potentially, those receiving long-term parenteral nutrition.[14,16–19]

The most widely used method to detect thiamine deficiency is the transketolase activation test. Transketolase is a thiamine-dependent enzyme. The transketolase activation test measures the whole blood or erythrocyte transketolase activity at baseline and then with added TPP. An increase in transketolase activity of >23% with added TPP is consistent with thiamine deficiency.[20] Symptoms of beriberi generally do not appear below an increase in enzyme activity of 40%. The direct measurement of TPP by reversed-phase high-pressure liquid chromatography (HPLC) has been optimized and correlates well with the transketolase activation test.[21] Infantile beriberi is treated with 50 to 100 mg of parenteral thiamine as a 1-time dose, often with dramatic improvement.[22] The infant should resume breastfeeding only after the mother's diet is supplemented with thiamine. Beriberi in children is treated with 10 to 25 mg of parenteral thiamine once per day for 2 weeks followed by 5 to 10 mg orally for 1 month. When mild, beriberi can be treated with 10 mg of oral thiamine per day. There is no true syndrome of thiamine toxicity.

Riboflavin (Vitamin B$_2$)

Riboflavin is a precursor of the enzyme cofactors flavin mononucleotide and flavin adenine dinucleotide (FAD). These coenzymes form the prosthetic groups of several enzymes involved in oxidation-reduction reactions integral to carbohydrate, protein, and fat metabolism. Flavin adenine dinucleotide is an essential component of the enzymes glutathione reductase and xanthine oxidase, both of which are responsible for generating anti-oxidant compounds. Riboflavin is found in abundance in animal protein (meat, dairy, and eggs) as well as green vegetables and fortified cereals. Interestingly, riboflavin deficiency is generally accompanied by deficiencies of 1 or more of the B-complex vitamins. This is likely attributable in part to riboflavin's role in the metabolism of folate, pyridoxine, and niacin.[23,24] In the mildly deficient state, the signs and symptoms of thiamine deficiency can be nonspecific. The more characteristic symptoms of severe deficiency (ariboflavinosis) include pharyngitis, cheilosis, angular stomatitis, glossitis (magenta tongue), and seborrheic dermatitis involving the nasolabial folds, flexural area of extremities, and the genital area.

Those at risk of deficiency include the economically disadvantaged with limited dietary meat or dairy, including breastfed infants after weaning. Studies have documented decreased serum riboflavin in neonates undergoing phototherapy.[25] Ariboflavinosis has been described in protein-energy malnutrition states, such as kwashiorkor and anorexia nervosa, and prolonged malabsorptive disease, such as celiac disease and short bowel syndrome. Recently, 3 cases of riboflavin deficiency in patients with cystic fibrosis have been reported.[26] Thyroid and adrenal insufficiency can impair the synthesis of riboflavin cofactors and may precipitate the deficiency state. There appear to be no adverse affects of riboflavin in excess.

Deficiency can be assessed by evaluating a 24-hour urine collection for riboflavin concentration. However, riboflavin is most commonly assessed indirectly by measuring the erythrocyte glutathione reductase activity coefficient.[27] This assay measures the stimulation of erythrocyte glutathione reductase by FAD in vitro. A higher activity coefficient represents a lack of FAD. A coefficient value of ≥1.4 is consistent with deficiency, 1.2 to <1.4 is considered marginal status, and <1.2 reflects an adequate riboflavin state.[28] The test is of limited value in patients with glutathione reductase deficiency, glucose-6-phosphate dehydrogenase deficiency, and beta-thalassemia. More recently, the direct quantification of erythrocyte riboflavin by HPLC has been demonstrated to be comparable to the erythrocyte glutathione reductase activity coefficient without the limitations.[29,30] In children, deficiency is treated with oral riboflavin, 1 mg 3 times daily until signs of deficiency resolve. Infants may respond to 0.5 mg twice weekly.

Niacin (Vitamin B$_3$)

Nicotinic acid and nicotinamide are the 2 vitamins commonly referred to as niacin. These 2 forms of niacin are chemically modified in the mitochondria to form the coenzymes NAD and NAD phosphate (NADP). Many enzymes involved in oxidation-reduction reactions require the coenzymes NAD and NADP for the purpose of accepting or donating an electron. Unlike most of the water-soluble vitamins, niacin can be synthesized in the liver and kidney by the amino acid tryptophan. This series of reactions requires adequate amounts of riboflavin and pyridoxine. Good sources of niacin include animal protein (dairy, eggs, and meat), beans, and fortified cereals; many of these are also good sources of tryptophan. The sugar molecules in nonfortified grains may bind to niacin reducing bioavailability.

Deficiency of niacin results in the clinical syndrome known as pellagra, an Italian term meaning "rough skin." It is characterized by the triad of diarrhea, dermatitis, and dementia. The gastrointestinal symptoms associated with niacin deficiency include glossitis, angular stomatitis, cheilitis, and diarrhea in one third to one half of patients.[31] The skin lesions found in pellagra are quite characteristic. The exanthem begins as painful erythema in areas of sun-exposed skin (dorsal surface of the hands, face, and neck), which can progress to an exudative phase. Re-exposure to the sun may result in vesicle or bullae formation. Affected skin eventually becomes rough, hard, and scaly, which was why it became known as pellagra.[32] This rash should not be confused with the generalized dermatitis found in kwashiorkor, which is distributed in both sun-exposed and unexposed skin. Pellagra also tends to spare the hair and nails. Early neuropsychiatric symptoms may include insomnia, fatigue, nervousness, irritability, and depression. Examination may reveal mental dullness, apathy, and memory impairment. Untreated, these symptoms may progress to dementia.[33] Left untreated, pellagra can result in death.

With few exceptions, pellagra is a disease limited to malnourished individuals in developing nations. In industrialized regions of the world, those at particular risk include homeless people and individuals with malabsorptive conditions, such as Crohn disease, and nutritional self-deprivation states, such as anorexia nervosa.[34-36] Other secondary causes of pellagra include Hartnup disease, a disorder of neutral amino acid transport that results in malabsorption of tryptophan and, as a result, niacin deficiency; patients receiving the antituberculous medication isoniazid; and patients on long-term anticonvulsants.[37-39] Adverse effects of pharmacologic niacin, generally used to treat dyslipidemia, include flushing, pruritus, nausea, vomiting, and rarely, hepatotoxicity.

Niacin status can be evaluated by urinary excretion of niacin and its metabolite N_1-methylnicotinamide by HPLC followed by fluorimetry. This technique requires a 24-hour urine collection.[40] Normal levels of urinary N_1-methylnicotinamide are between 1.5 and 5 mg/g of creatinine.[41] A more recently described method of niacin determination uses erythrocyte NAD and NADP concentrations to determine the "niacin number" (NAD/NADP × 100).[42,43] A value of <130 is consistent with niacin deficiency. This method provides a sensitive measure of niacin status without the need for a 24-hour urine collection and has been validated in carcinoid patients who are at risk of niacin deficiency.[43] The treatment for pellagra in children is oral nicotinamide (50–100 mg per dose, 3 times/day). Use of nicotinamide avoids the uncomfortable flushing associated with nicotinic acid. Therapy should be continued until resolution of acute symptoms.

Pyridoxine (Vitamin B$_6$)

There are 3 naturally occurring forms of vitamin B$_6$: pyridoxine, pyridoxal, and pyridoxamine. These pyridines are activated by phosphorylation to their coenzyme form. Pyridoxal 5'-phophate (PLP) is the most ubiquitous form of the vitamin and is integral to a multitude of enzymes in human metabolism. Vitamin B$_6$ acts as a coenzyme in amino acid and carbohydrate metabolism. It is required for the conversion of tryptophan to both niacin and the neurotransmitter serotonin. Similarly, vitamin B$_6$ is also required for the conversion of dopa to dopamine as well the synthesis of the inhibitory neurotransmitter gamma-aminobutyric acid (GABA). Hematologically, pyridoxine is a necessary cofactor in the rate-limiting step of heme biosynthesis. Foods rich in pyridoxine include banana, fish, milk, yeast, eggs, and fortified cereals.

Isolated deficiency of pyridoxine is rare, because its metabolism is dependent on adequate levels of riboflavin, niacin, and zinc. Further, sufficient pyridoxine is necessary for the biosynthesis and metabolism of niacin and folate. In the early 1950s, seizures were observed in infants as a result of severe vitamin B$_6$ deficiency resulting from an error in the manufacture of infant formula. As with other water-soluble vitamins, children in developing countries with marginal nutrition are at risk of deficiency.[44] Other conditions in which deficiency has been described include childhood leukemia and chronic renal failure.[45,46] Deficiency of vitamin B$_6$ can result from the covalent binding of certain drugs to PLP.[47] The manifestations of pyridoxine deficiency are nonspecific and include glossitis, angular stomatitis, cheilosis, irritability, depression, and confusion.

There are several rare vitamin B$_6$-dependency syndromes. Pyridoxine-dependent seizure is an autosomal recessive disorder presenting with intractable seizures that result from a reduced pyridoxine-dependent synthesis of the inhibitory neurotransmitter GABA. Despite a normal serum vitamin B$_6$

concentration, the seizures in these infants respond to a rather large paren-teral dose of vitamin B_6 (10–500 mg). Maintenance therapy with pyridoxine (0.2–3 mg/kg per day) is required indefinitely.[48] Other vitamin B_6-dependency syndromes include vitamin B_6-responsive anemia (microcytic and hypochromic), xanthurenic aciduria, cystathionuria, and homocystinuria.

Vitamin B_6 has been used at pharmacologic doses with little proof of efficacy to remedy the symptoms of autism, carpal tunnel syndrome, depression, hyperoxaluria, and dysmenorrhea, among others.[49–54] Despite the lack of evidence, vitamin B_6 continues to be used for many of the aforementioned conditions. However, vitamin B_6 has the potential for toxicity when given in excess. When administered in excess on a chronic basis, vitamin B_6 can cause a peripheral sensory neuropathy characterized by bilateral paresthesias, hyperesthesia, limb pain, ataxia, and poor coordination. No motor deficit or central nervous system involvement is usually observed.[47]

Various methods have been used to assess vitamin B_6 status, including 24-hour urine assay for the pyridoxine metabolic product 4-pyridoxic acid and the more current practice of functional (enzymatic) assay or HPLC. The predominant B_6 vitamer present in the plasma is PLP and, as such, is the most commonly assayed.[55] A recent direct comparison of these 2 methods between 10 laboratories in North America, Europe, and Asia has demonstrated greater precision of the HPLC method over enzymatic assay. There were, however, large differences in laboratory proficiency, highlighting the need for a true reference method and reference materials.[56] A PLP concentration of >30 nmol/L reflects adequate vitamin B_6, whereas a level of <20 nmol/L indicates deficiency. Children deficient in vitamin B_6 without neuritis should receive 5 to 25 mg of pyridoxine per day for 3 weeks orally followed by 1.5 to 2.5 mg/day in a multivitamin product. If a peripheral neuropathy is present, the dosing is increased to 10 to 50 mg of pyridoxine per day orally for 3 weeks, then 1 to 2 mg/day.

Cobalamin (Vitamin B₁₂)

Cobalamin functions as a coenzyme of a number of enzymes involved in red blood cell maturation and development of the central nervous system. Cobalamin and folate are necessary for the remethylation of homocysteine to methionine by methionine synthase. Higher concentrations of cobalamin are found in colostrum than during the third month of lactation. There are, however, no significant differences in cobalamin and its binding protein among the various categories of human milk (foremilk, mid-feed milk, and hindmilk) or among and morning, afternoon, and evening samples. Thus, representative samples of human milk for cobalamin analysis can be obtained for population studies regardless of time of day or moment within the feed.[57] Cobalamin is found only in animal foods, including meat, fish, poultry, cheese, milk, and eggs, and vitamin B_{12}-fortified soy milk. Signs and symptoms of deficiency include macrocytic megaloblastic anemia and neurologic problems (ataxia, muscle weakness, spasticity, incontinence, hypotension, vision problems, dementia, psychoses, and mood disturbances). Vitamin B_{12} deficiency is accompanied by hyperhomocysteinemia, which is thought to be a risk factor for cardiovascular disease.[58]

Breastfed infants of strict vegan mothers are at risk of vitamin B_{12} deficiency. Maternal vitamin B_{12} deficiency has also been associated with neural tube defects.[59] Plasma methylmalonic acid and total homocysteine concentrations are useful indicators of functional cobalamin deficiency in infants on macrobiotic diets, and administration of oral or intramuscular vitamin B_{12} normalized urinary values of methylmalonic acid in vitamin B_{12}-deficient infants.[60,61] Abnormalities can often, but not always, be reversed by administration of parenteral or oral vitamin B_{12}. Megaloblastic anemia secondary to vitamin B_{12} deficiency in children consuming alternative diets has also been reported.[62]

Other subjects at risk of B_{12} deficiency include those having undergone resection of stomach and/or ileum, because gastric intrinsic factor is necessary for absorption of B_{12}, which occurs in the ileum. Pernicious anemia is an autoimmune disease characterized by megaloblastic anemia secondary to absence of gastric intrinsic factor. Patients with phenylketonuria on an unrestricted or relaxed diet are at risk of vitamin B_{12} deficiency.[63] There are a number of vitamin B_{12}-responsive inborn errors of metabolism, including transcobalamin II deficiency, homocystinuria, and hereditary juvenile cobalamin deficiency caused by mutations in gastric intrinsic factor.[64–66] Imerslund-Grasbeck syndrome, which is familial selective vitamin B_{12} malabsorption, can be successfully treated by intramuscular administration of vitamin B_{12}.

The diagnosis of cobalamin deficiency is made by determination of the serum concentration of cobalamin. If serum concentrations are borderline low and the diagnosis of deficiency is uncertain, then increased plasma homocysteine and urinary methylmalonic acid concentrations would be confirmatory. Deficiency is treated by administration of large doses of cobalamin given orally or, in the case of malabsorption syndromes, by periodic administration via the intramuscular or intranasal route. The dose for treatment of vitamin B_{12} deficiency in children is 30 to 50 µg, intramuscularly or deep subcutaneously, daily for 2 weeks followed by maintenance doses of 100 µg monthly.

Folate

Folic acid carries hydroxymethyl and formyl groups necessary for the synthesis of purines and thymine, which are required for DNA formation.[67] The vitamin is necessary for the maturation of red blood cells and promotes cellular growth in general. Total serum homocysteine is increased in the presence of folate deficiency in neonates.[68] Supplemental folate, taken alone or added to food, is better absorbed than folate that is a normal constituent in a food. Cereals, grains, and breads are now fortified with folate. Natural sources include fresh green vegetables, liver, yeast, and some fruits. Megaloblastic anemia is the primary sign of deficiency.

It is now well established that low serum and red blood cell concentrations of folic acid in women of childbearing potential increase the risk of fetal birth defects, particularly neural tube defects, such as anencephaly and spina bifida. There is some evidence that maternal deficiency of either folic acid or vitamin B_{12} are independent risk factors for this phenomenon.[69] 5,10–Methylenetetrahydrofolate reductase is involved in folate metabolism. It is located on chromosome 1, and 2 common alleles have been described: C677T and A1298C. In infants, C677T homozygosity is associated with a moderately increased risk of spina bifida.[70] Maternal C677T homozygosity appears to be a moderate risk factor for spina bifida in the fetus as well. There are some data to suggest that decreased periconceptual intake of folate by pregnant women is associated with orofacial clefts and congenital heart disease.[71,72] It has also been reported that the prevalence of the C677T allele may be doubled in children with stroke compared with controls of the same age group.[73] Thus, systematic studies are indicated to determine whether folate supplementation of children with this polymorphism would prevent recurrent stroke.

In contrast to most of the other water-soluble vitamins, potentially inadequate intake of folate in children is not rare. In one study of white preschool children of middle and upper socioeconomic status 2 to 5 years of age, the mean folate intake was consistently below recommended amounts.[74] Foods most commonly eaten were fruit drinks, carbonated beverages, 2% milk, and French fries. Picciano et al also noted that folate intakes at 12 months of age were 79% of recommended amounts, with an increase to 100% by

18 months of age.[75] There have been fairly dramatic changes in US adolescent food choices over the last 30 years, with increased consumption of soft drinks and noncitrus juices. The intake of fruits and vegetables is below the recommended 5 servings per day, and intakes of folate by girls have consistently been below recommended amounts.[76]

Patients with malabsorption syndromes, including Crohn disease, are at risk of folate deficiency, as are patients with HIV infection.[77,78] In addition, folate deficiency has been shown to play a role in erythropoietin resistance in pediatric and adolescent patients on chronic dialysis.[79] Methylenetetrahydrofolate reductase deficiency has been described in 4 siblings; clinical manifestations included retarded psychomotor development, poor social contact, and seizures. Folate concentrations in serum and red blood cells were low.[80] Cerebral folate deficiency is a newly described disorder in which autoantibodies prevent the transfer of folate from the plasma to the cerebrospinal fluid. 5-Methyltetrahydrofolate concentrations in the cerebrospinal fluid are low, but serum and erythrocyte folate concentrations are normal.[81] Folinic acid supplements can reverse the characteristic neurologic abnormalities.

The diagnosis of folate deficiency is made by assessment of serum or plasma folate (which reflects short-term deficiency) and red blood cell folate, which is a better index of chronic folate deficiency. A recently developed method for 5-methyltetrahydrofolate, the principal circulating form of plasma folates, may prove to be clinically useful in the future for diagnosis of folic acid deficiency.[82] Folic acid deficiency is associated with increased serum concentration of homocysteine. Folic acid deficiency is treated with daily administration of oral supplements.

Vitamin C

Vitamin C is a reversible reductant and functions in folacin metabolism, collagen biosynthesis, and iron absorption and transport. Dietary sources include papaya, citrus fruits, tomatoes, cabbage, potatoes, cantaloupe, and strawberries. In the Dietary Reference Intakes recommended by the Institute of Medicine, the Recommended Dietary Allowance (RDA) for vitamin C for adults was established on the basis of the vitamin C intake to maintain near-maximal neutrophil concentration with minimal urinary excretion of ascorbate.[83] Because similar data in infants were not available, the adequate intake for vitamin C in infants was based on mean vitamin C intake of breastfed infants. RDAs for children and adolescents were estimated on the basis of relative body weight. Signs and symptoms of deficiency include osmotic diarrhea, bleeding gums, perifollicular hemorrhage, and frank scurvy with painful bones and arthropathy.[84]

The intake of vitamin C by school-aged children has been studied extensively in the 1994–1996 Continuing Survey of Food Intakes by Individuals. Among 7- to 12-year-olds, 12% of boys and 13% of girls had mean vitamin C intakes that were less than 30 mg/day.[85] Among 13- to 18-year-olds, 14% of boys and 20% of girls had low vitamin C intakes. Children with low vitamin C intake tended to have greater energy-adjusted intakes of fat and saturated fat. Children with desirable vitamin C intakes consumed more high-vitamin C-containing fruit juice, high-vitamin C-containing vegetables and whole milk, and more citrus fruits than did children with low vitamin C intake. In a group of children receiving long-term dialysis, dietary intake of vitamin C (and, in fact, all water-soluble vitamins) was <100% of RDA in most; supplementation was necessary to reach the RDA.[86] Although scurvy is increasingly rare in children, it is still reported, particularly among children who ingest only well-cooked foods and few fruits or vegetables.[87]

Low periconceptual intake of vitamin C has been associated with low birth weight.[88] A new form of hereditary methemoglobinemia in infants that is responsive to vitamin C has been described.[89] Vitamin C deficiency may play a role in oxidant stress in children with chronic renal disease and in children with sickle cell anemia.[90,91] Vitamin C status is best assessed by measuring the concentration of ascorbate in blood leukocytes, considered a better measure of tissue reserves than plasma ascorbate concentration.[92] In children, scurvy is treated with 100 mg of ascorbic acid given 3 times daily for 1 week, then 100 mg daily for several weeks until tissue saturation is normal. The regimen may be administered intramuscularly, intravenously, or orally.

Other

Information on human needs for pantothenic acid is limited. Pantothenic acid is a component of CoA and is involved in many enzymatic reactions. It is found in organ meats, yeast, egg yolk, fresh vegetables, whole grains, and legumes. Deficiency symptoms have not been characterized. In one survey, 49% of female adolescents and 25% of male adolescents consumed less than 4 mg/day, the amount recommended by the Institute of Medicine.[93] However, average blood concentrations for both groups were in the normal range. Biotin is the coenzyme for 5 mammalian carboxylases. Dietary sources include liver, egg yolk, soybeans, milk, and meat. Clinical biotin deficiency is characterized by hypotonia and severe exfoliative dermatitis. To date, symptomatic deficiency has been described only in infants given total parenteral nutrition that was free of biotin and in children given undercooked eggs containing large amounts of avidin, a biotin-binding protein. However, children given long-term anticonvulsant therapy exhibit impaired biotin status.[94] The growing list of inborn errors of metabolism that exhibit biotin dependency and various degrees of neurologic and dermatologic abnormalities include holocarboxylase synthetase deficiency, biotinidase deficiency, and a defect in biotin transport.[95] Diagnosis of deficiency is by urinary biotin, urinary 3-hydroxyisovaleric acid, and lymphocyte propionyl-CoA carboxylase concentrations. Expression of SLC19A3, a potential biotin transporter, in leukocytes may prove to be a useful indicator of marginal biotin deficiency.[96]

Conclusion

Some vitamin-dependency states are the result of inborn errors of metabolism, in which pharmacologic doses of vitamins may ameliorate signs of disease. These states have been described for thiamin, pyridoxine, folic acid, vitamin B_{12}, biotin, niacin, riboflavin, vitamin C, and vitamin D. The genetic polymorphisms responsible for some of these diseases have been delineated. In the era of the human genome project, it can be predicted that many more such diseases will be described in the future.

In conclusion, supplemental vitamins are probably unnecessary for the healthy child older than 1 year who consumes a varied diet. However, some at-risk children may benefit from supplemental multivitamin preparations providing the RDA. Research priorities for the future include investigation of the global prevalence of micronutrient deficiencies, the role of vitamins in cognitive development, the importance of nutrient-nutrient interactions, and the effects of age, gender, genetics, and other conditions, such as infection, on micronutrient status in the pediatric age group.[97,98]

Table 20-II.1
Multivitamin Preparations

Formulation	Content Given Per	A (IU)	C (mg)	D (IU)	E (IU)	B$_1$ (mg)	B$_2$ (mg)	B$_3$ (mg)	B$_5$ (mg)	B$_6$ (mg)	Folate (µg)	B$_{12}$ (µg)	Elemental Iron (Fe) (mg)	Fluoride (mg)	Other
Drops															
Poly-Vi-Sol*	1 mL	1500	35	400	5	0.5	0.6	8		0.4		2			
Poly-Vi-Sol with Iron*	1 mL	1500	35	400	5	0.5	0.6	8		0.4			10		
Tri-Vi-Sol*	1mL	1500	35	400											
Tri-Vi-Flor*	1 mL	1500	35	400										Two strengths: 0.25 and 0.5	
ADEKs†	1 mL	1500	45	400	40	0.5	0.6	6	3	0.6		4			Vitamin K 100 µg, biotin 15 µg, Zn 5 mg, beta-carotene 1 mg
Tablets															
Flintstones Complete‡	1 tablet	3000	60	400	30	1.5	1.7	15	10	2	400	6	18		Biotin 40 µg, Ca 100 mg, P 100 mg, I 150 µg, Mg 20 mg, Zn 12 mg, Cu 2 mg, Na 10 mg, choline 38 mg

Table 20-II.1 *(Continued)*
Multivitamin Preparations

Formulation	Content Given Per	A (IU)	C (mg)	D (IU)	E (IU)	B₁ (mg)	B₂ (mg)	B₃ (mg)	B₅ (mg)	B₆ (mg)	Folate (µg)	B₁₂ (µg)	Elemental Iron (Fe) (mg)	Fluoride (mg)	Other
Centrum Kids§	1 tablet	3500	60	400	30	1.5	1.7	20	10	2	400	6	18		Vitamin K 10 µg, biotin 45 µg, Zn 15 mg, Ca 108 mg, I 150 µg, Mg 40 mg, Mn 1 mg, P 50 mg, Cu 2 mg, Cr 20 µg, Mo 20 µg
One-A-Day Kids Complete‡	1 tablet	3000	60	400	30	1.5	1.7	15	10	2	400	6	18		Biotin 40 µg, Ca 100 mg, P 100 mg, I 150 µg, Mg 20 mg, Zn 12 mg, Cu 2 mg, Na 10 mg
Poly-Vi-Sol w/Iron*	1 tablet	2500	60	400	15	1.05	1.2	13.5		1.05	300	4.5	12		Zn 8 mg, Cu‖
ADEKs†	1 tablet	4000	60	400	150	1.2	1.3	10	10	1.5	200	12			Vitamin K 150 µg, biotin 50 µg, Zn 7.5 mg, beta-carotene 3 mg

Table 20-II.1 *(Continued)*
Multivitamin Preparations

Formulation	Content Given Per	A (IU)	C (mg)	D (IU)	E (IU)	B₁ (mg)	B₂ (mg)	B₃ (mg)	B₅ (mg)	B₆ (mg)	Folate (µg)	B₁₂ (µg)	Elemental Iron (Fe) (mg)	Fluoride (mg)	Other
Gummies															
Flintstones Complete‡	2 gummies	2000	30	200	20				5	1	200	5			Biotin 75 µg, Zn 2.5 mg, choline 30 µg, inositol 20 µg
L'il Critters¶	2 gummies	2500	18	50	15				5	0.7	204	4			Biotin 60 µg, Zn 2.2 mg, choline 10 µg, inositol 10 µg
Disney Gummies#	2 gummies	1500	15	200	15				2.5	0.5	200	3			Biotin 45 µg, Ca 3 mg, Mg 2 mg, Zn 2 mg, inositol 10 µg

Zn indicates zinc; Ca, calcium; P, phosphorous; I, iodine; Mg, magnesium; Cu, copper; Na, sodium; Mn, manganese; Cr, chromium; Mo, molybdenum.

* Mead Johnson, Evansville, IN.

† Axcan Scandipharm, Birmingham, AL.

‡ Bayer Consumer Care Products, Morristown, NJ.

§ Wyeth Consumer Healthcare, Richmond, VA.

‖ The amount of Cu in Poly-Vi-Sol with Iron is not available.

¶ Northwest Natural Products, Vancouver, WA.

NBTY, Bohemia, NY.

Sources: Nutritional combination products. In: *Drug Facts and Comparisons.* St Louis, MO: Wolters Kluwer Health Inc; 2007 and Lexi-Comp. Multivitamin Formulations table. Available at: http://www.crlonline.com.

REFERENCES

1. Eisenberg DM, Davis RB, Ettner SL, et al. Trends in alternative medicine use in the United States, 1990–1997: results of a follow-up national survey. *JAMA*. 1998;280:1569–1575

2. Lee AC, Kemper KJ. Homeopathy and naturopathy: practice characteristics and pediatric care. *Arch Pediatr Adolesc Med*. 2000;154:75–80

3. Wilson K, Busse JW, Gilchrist A, Vohra S, Boon H, Mills E. Characteristics of pediatric and adolescent patients attending a naturopathic college clinic in Canada. *Pediatrics*. 2005;115(3):e338. Available at: http://pediatrics.aappublications.org/cgi/content/full/115/3/e338. Accessed August 30, 2007

4. Boon HS, Cherkin DC, Erro J, et al. Practice patterns of naturopathic physicians: results from a random survey of licensed practitioners in two US states. *BMC Complement Altern Med*. 2004;4:14

5. Ogden CJ, Flegal KM, Carroll MD, Johnson CL. Prevalence and trends in overweight among US children and adolescents, 1999–2000. *JAMA*. 2002;288:1728–1732

6. Kant AK. Reported consumption of low-nutrient-density foods by American children and adolescents: nutritional and health correlates, NHANES III, 1988–1994. *Arch Pediatr Adolesc Med*. 2003;157:789–796

7. Lee Y, Mitchell DC, Smiciklas-Wright H, Birch LL. Diet quality, nutrient intake, weight status, and feeding environments of girls meeting or exceeding recommendations for total dietary fat of the American Academy of Pediatrics. *Pediatrics*. 2001;107(6):e95. Available at: http://pediatrics.aappublications.org/cgi/content/full/107/6/e95. Accessed August 30, 2007

8. Tonstad S, Sivertsen M. Relation between dietary fat and energy and micronutrient intakes. *Arch Dis Child*. 1997;76:416–420

9. Niklas TA, Myers L, O'Neil C, Gustafson N. Impact of dietary fat and fiber on nutrient intake of adolescents. *Pediatrics*. 2000;105(2):e21. Available at: http://pediatrics.aappublications.org/cgi/content/full/105/2/e21. Accessed August 30, 2007

10. Gilman MW, Rifas-Shiman SL, Frazier AL, et al. Family dinner and diet quality among older children and adolescents. *Arch Fam Med*. 2000;9:235–240

11. Ishibashi S, Yokota T, Shiojiri T, et al. Reversible acute axonal polyneuropathy associated with Wernicke-Korsakoff syndrome: impaired physiological nerve conduction due to thiamine deficiency? *J Neurol Neurosurg Psychiatry*. 2003;74:674–676

12. Carpenter KJ. Studies in colonies: a Dutchman's chickens 1803–1896. In: *Beriberi, White Rice, and Vitamin B: A Disease, a Cause, and a Cure*. Berkeley, CA: University of California Press; 2000:24–51

13. Luxemberger C, White NJ, ter Kuile F, et al. Beri-beri: the major cause of infant mortality in Karen refugees. *Trans R Soc Trop Med Hyg*. 2003;97:251–255

14. Hahn JS, Berquist W, Alcorn DM, Chamberlain L, Bass D. Wernicke encephalopathy and beriberi during total parenteral nutrition attributable to multivitamin infusion shortage. *Pediatrics*. 1998;101(1):e10. Available at: http://pediatrics.aappublications.org/cgi/content/full/101/1/e10. Accessed August 30, 2007

15. Davis RA, Wolf A. Infantile beriberi associated with Wernike's encephalopathy. *Pediatrics*. 1958;21:409–420

16. Towbin A, Inge TH, Garcia VF, et al. Beriberi after gastric bypass surgery in adolescence. *J Pediatr.* 2004;145:263–267

17. Hung SC, Hung SH, Tarng DC, Yang WC, Chen TW, Huang TP. Thiamine deficiency and unexplained encephaolopathy in hemodialysis and peritoneal dialysis patients. *Am J Kidney Dis.* 2001;38:941–947

18. Shamir R, Dagan O, Abramovitch D, Abramovitch T, Vidne BA, Dinari G. Thiamine deficiency in children with congenital heart disease before and after corrective surgery. *JPEN J Parenter Enteral Nutr.* 2000;24:154–158

19. Winston AP, Jamieson CP, Madira W, Gatward NM, Palmer RL. Prevalence of thiamin deficiency in anorexia nervosa. *Int J Eat Disord.* 2000;28:451–454

20. Bayoumi RA, Rosalki SB. Evaluation of methods of coenzyme activation of erythrocyte enzymes for detection of deficiency of vitamins B1, B2, and B6. *Clin Chem.* 1976;22:327–335

21. Talwar D, Davidson H, Cooney J, St O'Reilly D. Vitamin B(1) status assessed by direct measurement of thiamine pyrophosphate in erythrocytes and whole blood by HPLC: comparison with erythrocyte transketolase activation assay. *Clin Chem.* 2000;46:704–710

22. Reid DH. Acute infantile beriberi. *J Pediatr.* 1961;58:858–863

23. Powers HJ. Riboflavin (vitamin B-2) and health. *Am J Clin Nutr.* 2003;77:1352–1360

24. McCormick DB. Two interconnected B vitamins riboflavin and pyridoxine. *Physiol Rev.* 1989;69:1170–1198

25. Amin HJ, Shukla AK, Snyder F, Fung E, Anderson NM, Parsons HG. Significance of phototherapy-induced riboflavin deficiency in the full-term neonate. *Biol Neonate.* 1992;61:76–81

26. McCabe H Riboflavin deficiency in cystic fibrosis: three case reports. *J Hum Nutr Diet.* 2001;14:365–370

27. Tillotson JA, Baker EM. An enzymatic measurement of the riboflavin status in man. *Am J Clin Nutr.* 1972;25:425–431

28. Sauberlich HE, Judd JH Jr, Nichoalds GE, Broquist HP, Darby WJ. Application of the erythrocyte glutathione reductase assay in evaluating riboflavin nutritional status in a high school student population. *Am J Clin Nutr.* 1972;25:756–762

29. Floridi A, Palmerini CA, Fini C, Pupita M, Fidanza F. High performance liquid chromatographic analysis of flavin adenine dinucleotide in whole blood. *Int J Vitam Nutr Res.* 1985;55:187–191

30. Graham JM, Peerson JM, Haskel MJ, Shrestha RK, Brown KH, Allen LH. Erythrocyte riboflavin for the detection of riboflavin deficiency in pregnant Nepali women. *Clin Chem.* 2005;51:2162–2165

31. Spivak JL, Jackson DL, Pellagra: an analysis of 18 patients and a review of the literature. *Johns Hopkins Med J.* 1977;140:295–309

32. Hegyi J, Schwartz RA, Hegyi V. Pellagra: Dermatitis, dementia, and diarrhea. *Int J Dermatol.* 2004;43:1–5

33. Adams RD, Victor M, Ropper AH. Diseases of the nervous system due to nutritional deficiency. In: *Principles of Neurology.* 6th ed. New York, NY: McGraw-Hill; 1997:1138–1165

34. Kertesz SG. Pellagra in 2 homeless men. *Mayo Clin Proc.* 2001;76:315–318

35. Pollack S, Enat R, Haim S, Zinder O, Barzilai D. Pellagra as the presenting manifestation of Crohn's disease. *Gastroenterology*. 1982;82:948–952

36. Prousky JE. Pellagra may be a rare secondary complication of anorexia nervosa: a systematic review of the literature. *Altern Med Rev*. 2003;8:180–185

37. Darvay A, Basarab T, McGregor JM, Russel-Jones R. Isoniazid induced pellagra despite pyridoxine supplementation. *Clin Exp Dermatol*. 1999;24:167–169

38. Kaur S, Goraya JS, Thami GP, Kanwar AJ. Pellagrous dermatitis induced by phenytoin. *Pediatr Dermatol*. 2002;19:93

39. Lyon VB, Fairley JA Anticonvulsant-induced pellagra. *J Am Acad Dermatol*. 2002;46:597–599

40. Carpenter KJ, Kodieck E. The fluorometric estimation of N_1-methylnictotinamide and its differentiation from coenzyme. *Biochemistry*. 1950;46:421

41. Fu CS, Swendseid ME, Jacob RA, et al. Biochemical markers for assessment of niacin status in young men: Levels of erythrocyte niacin coenzymes and plasma tryptophan. *J Nutr*. 1989;119:1949–1955

42. Jacobson EL, Jacobson MK. Tissue NAD as a biochemical measure of niacin status in humans. *Methods Enzymol*. 1997;280:221–230

43. Shah GM, Shah RG, Veillette MD, Kirkland JB, Pasieka JL, Warner RR. Biochemical assessment of niacin deficiency among carcinoid patients. *Am J Gastroenterol*. 2005;100:2307–2314

44. Setiawan B, Giraud DW, Driskell JA. Vitamin B-6 inadequacy in rural and urban Indonesian children. *J Nutr*. 2000;130:553–558

45. Pais RC, Vanous E, Hollins B, et al. Abnormal vitamin B6 in childhood leukemia. *Cancer*. 1990;66:2421–2428

46. Mydlik M, Derzsiova K, Guman M, Hrehorovsky M. Vitamin B6 requirements in chronic renal failure. *Int Urol Nephrol*. 1992;24:453–457

47. Lheureux P, Penaloza A, Gris M. Pyridoxine in clinical toxicology: a review. *Eur J Emerg Med*. 2005;12:78–85

48. Baxter P. Pyridoxine-dependent seizures: a clinical and biochemical conundrum. *Biochem Biophys Acta*. 2003;1647:36–41

49. Findling RL, Maxwell K, Scotese-Wojtila L, Huang J, Yamashita T, Wiznitzer M. High-dose pyridoxine and magnesium administration in children with autistic disorder: an absence of salutary effects in a double-blind placebo-controlled study. *J Autism Dev Disord*. 1997;27:467–478

50. Aufier E, Stitik TP, Foye PM, Chen B. Pyridoxine hydrochloride treatment of carpal tunnel syndrome: a review. *Nutr Rev*. 2004;62:96–104

51. Williams AL, Cotter A, Sabina A, Girard C, Goodman J, Katz DL. The role of vitamin B-6 as treatment for depression: a systematic review. *Fam Pract*. 2005;22:532–537

52. Malouf R, Grimley Evans J. The effect of vitamin B6 for cognition. *Cochrane Database Syst Rev*. 2003;(4):CD004393

53. Kaelin A, Casez JP, Jaeger P. Vitamin B6 metabolism in idiopathic calcium stone formers: no evidence for a link to hyperoxaluria. *Urol Res*. 2004;32:61–68

54. Proctor ML, Murphy PA. Herbal and dietary treatment of primary and secondary dysmenorrhea. *Cochrane Database Syst Rev.* 2001;(3):CD002124

55. Bor MV, Refsum H, Bisp MR, et al. Plasma vitamin B6 vitamers before and after oral vitamin B6 treatment: a randomized placebo-controlled study. *Clin Chem.* 2003;49:155–161

56. Rybak ME, Jain RB, Pfeiffer CM. Clinical vitamin B6 analysis: an interlaboratory comparison of pyridoxal 5'-phosphate measurements in serum. *Clin Chem.* 2005;51:1223–1231

57. Trugo N, Sardinha F. Cobalamin and cobalamin-binding capacity in human milk. *Nutr Res.* 1994;14:23–33

58. Chambers JC, Seddon MD, Shah S, Kooner JS. Homocysteine—a novel risk factor for vascular disease. *J R Soc Med.* 2001;94:10–13

59. Steen MT, Boddie AM, Fisher AJ, et al. Neural-tube defects are associated with low concentrations of cobalamin (vitamin B12) in amniotic fluid. *Prenat Diagn.* 1998;18:545–555

60. Schneede J, Dagnelie PC, van Staveren WA, Vollset SE, Refsum H, Ueland PM. Methylmalonic acid and homocysteine in plasma as indicators of functional cobalamine deficiency in infants on macrobiotic diets. *Pediatr Res.* 1994;36:194–201

61. Specker BL, Miller D, Norman EJ, Greene H, Hayes KC. Increased urinary methylmalonic acid excretion in breast-fed infants of vegetarian mothers and identification of an acceptable dietary source of vitamin B-12. *Am J Clin Nutr.* 1988;47:89–92

62. Dagnelie PC, van Staveren WA, Hautvast JG. Stunting and nutrient deficiencies in children on alternative diets. *Acta Paediatr Scand Suppl.* 1991;374:111–118

63. Robinson M, White FJ, Cleary MA, Wraith E, Lam WK, Walter JH. Increased risk of vitamin B12 deficiency in patients with phenylketonuria on an unrestricted or relaxed diet. *J Pediatr.* 2000;136:545–547

64. Bibi H, Gelman-Kohan Z, Baumgartner ER, Rosenblatt DS. Transcobalamin II deficiency with methylmalonic aciduria in three sisters. *J Inherit Metab Dis.* 1999;22:765–772

65. Wilcken DE, Wilcken B. The natural history of vascular disease in homocystinuria and the effects of treatment. *J Inherit Metab Dis.* 1997;20:295–300

66. Tanner SM, Li Z, Perko JD, et al. Hereditary juvenile cobalamin deficiency caused by mutations in gastric intrinsic factor gene. *Proc Natl Acad Sci U S A.* 2005;102:4130–4133

67. Morrell MJ Folic acid and epilepsy. *Epilepsy Curr.* 2002;2:31–34

68. Minet JC, Bisse E, Aebischer CP, Wieland H, Lutschg J. Assessment of vitamin B-12, folate, and vitamin B-6 status and relation to sulfur amino acid metabolism in neonates. *Am J Clin Nutr.* 2000;72:751–757

69. Kirke PN, Molloy AM, Daly LE, Burk H, Weir DG, Scott JM. Maternal plasma folate and vitamin B12 are independent risk factors for neural tube defects. *Q J Med.* 1993;86:703–708

70. Botto LD, Yang Q. 5,10-Methylenetetrahydrofolate reductase gene variants and congenital anomalies: a HuGE review. *Am J Epidemiol.* 2000;151:862–877

71. Rouget F, Monfort C, Bahuau M, et al. [Periconceptional folates and the prevention of orofacial clefts: role of dietary intakes in France.] [Article in French.] *Rev Epidemiol Sante Publique.* 2005;53:351–360

72. Pei L, Zhu H, Zhu J, et al. Genetic variation of infant reduced folate carrier (A80G) and risk of orofacial defects and congenital heart defects in China. *Ann Epidemiol.* 2006;16:352–356

73. Cardo E, Monros E, Colome C, et al. Children with stroke: polymorphism of the MTHFR gene, mild hyperhomocysteinemia, and vitamin status. *J Child Neurol.* 2000;15:295–298

74. Skinner JD, Carruth BR, Houck KS, et al. Longitudinal study of nutrient and food intakes of white preschool children aged 24 to 60 months. *J Am Diet Assoc.* 1999;99:1514–1521

75. Picciano MF, Smiciklas-Wright H, Birch LL, Mitchell DC, Murray-Kolb L, Mc-Conahy KL. Nutritional guidance is needed during dietary transition in early childhood. *Pediatrics.* 2000;106:109–114

76. Cavadini C, Siega-Riz AM, Popkin BM. US adolescent food intake trends from 1965 to 1996. *Arch Dis Child.* 2000;83:18–24

77. Jeejeebhoy KN. Clinical nutrition: 6. Management of nutritional problems of patients with Crohn's disease. *CMAJ.* 2002;166:913–918

78. Meira DG, Lorand-Metz I, Toro AD, Silva MT, Vilela MM. Bone marrow features in children with HIV infection and peripheral blood cytopenias. *J Trop Pediatr.* 2005;51:114–19

79. Bamgbola OF, Kaskel F. Role of folate deficiency on erythropoietin resistance in pediatric and adolescent patients on chronic dialysis. *Pediatr Nephrol.* 2005;20:1622–1629

80. Tonetti C, Burtscher A, Bories D, Tulliez M, Zittoun J. Methylenetetrahydrofolate reductase deficiency in four siblings: a clinical, biochemical, and molecular study of the family. *Am J Med Genet.* 2000;91:363–367

81. Ramaekers VT, Rothenberg SP, Sequeira JM, et al. Autoantibodies to folate receptors in the cerebral folate deficiency syndrome. *N Engl J Med.* 2005;352:1985–1991

82. Opladen T, Ramaekers VT, Heimann G, Blau N. Analysis of 5-methyltetrahydrofolate in serum of healthy children. *Mol Genet Metab.* 2005;87:61–65

83. Institute of Medicine. *Dietary Reference Intakes for Vitamin C, Vitamin E, Selenium, and Carotenoids.* Washington, DC: National Academies Press; 2000

84. Fain O. Musculoskeletal manifestations of scurvy. *Joint Bone Spine.* 2005 ;72:124–128

85. Hampl JS, Taylor CA, Johnston CS. Intakes of vitamin C, vegetables and fruits: which schoolchildren are at risk? *J Am Coll Nutr.* 1999;18:582–590

86. Pereira AM, Hamani N, Nogueira PC, Carvalhaes JT. Oral vitamin intake in children receiving long-term dialysis. *J Ren Nutr.* 2000;10:24–29

87. Ratanachu-Ek S, Sukswai P, Jeerathayasakun Y, Wongtapradit L. Scurvy in pediatric patients: a review of 28 cases. *J Med Assoc Thai.* 2003;86(Suppl 3):S734–S740

88. Matthews F, Yudkin P, Neil A. Influence of maternal nutrition on outcome of pregnancy: prospective cohort study. *BMJ.* 199;319:339–343

89. Jamal A. Hereditary methemoglobinemia. *J Coll Physicians Surg Pak.* 2006;16:157–159

90. Zwolinska D, Grzeszczak W, Szczepanska M, Kilis-Pstrusinska K, Szprynger K. Vitamins A, E, and C as non-enzymatic antioxidants and their relation to lipid peroxidation in children with chronic renal failure. *Nephron Clin Pract.* 2005;103:c12–c18

91. Amer J, Ghoti H, Rachnileqitz E, Koren A, Levin C, Fibach E. Red blood cells, platelets and polymorphonuclear neutrophils of patients with sickle cell disease exhibit oxidative stress that can be ameliorated by antioxidants. *Br J Haematol.* 2006;132:108–113

92. Thurnham DI. Micronutrients and immune function: some recent developments. *J Clin Pathol.* 1997;50:887–891

93. Eissenstat BR, Wyse BW, Hansen RG. Pantothenic acid status of adolescents. *Am J Clin Nutr.* 1986;44:931–937

94. Krause KH, Bonjour JP, Berlit P, Kynast G, Schmidt-Gayk H, Schellenberg B. Effect of long-term treatment with antiepileptic drugs on the vitamin status. *Drug Nutr Interact.* 1988;5:317–343

95. Mardach R, Zempleni J, Wolf B, et al. Biotin dependency due to a defect in biotin transport. *J Clin Invest.* 2002;109:1617–1623

96. Vlasova TI, Stratton SL, Wells AM, Mock NI, Mock DM. Biotin deficiency reduces expression of slc19a3, a potential biotin transporter, in leukocytes from human blood. *J Nutr.* 2005;135:42–47

97. Bryan J, Osendarp S, Hughes D, Calvaresi E, Bayhurst K, van Klinken JW. Nutrients for cognitive development in school-aged children. *Nutr Rev.* 2004;62:295–306

98. Viteri FE, Gonzalez H. Adverse outcomes of poor micronutrient status in childhood and adolescence. *Nutr Rev.* 2002;60:S77–S83

New Food Ingredients

The nature of the food we eat evolves in response to new knowledge in health and nutrition, to changing consumer demands, and to changes designed to improve the production, shelf-life, or sensory characteristics of foods. These changes in foods and food ingredients are developed through a variety of traditional methods (eg, plant and animal breeding, fermentation), addition of new ingredients designed for specific food functional or health benefits, and newer technologies (eg, biotechnology).

Biotechnology

New methods of bioengineering foods through genetic modification of plants and animals, including recombinant DNA (rDNA) and transgenic techniques, represent a continuum from the more traditional plant and animal breeding techniques.[1-4] Traditional breeding typically consists of hybridization between varieties of the same species and screening for progeny with desired characteristics. Such hybridization can only introduce traits found in close relatives. These techniques require extensive back-crossing with the parent line to eliminate mutations linked to that responsible for the desired phenotype and undesirable traits in extraneous genetic material introduced along with that encoding the desired trait. Biotechnology involves the isolation and subsequent introduction of discrete DNA segments containing the gene(s) of interest into recipient (host) plants or animals. The DNA segments can come from any organism (microbial, animal, or plant). These techniques are more precise (although not necessarily safer) than traditional cross-breeding approaches, because they introduce only the gene or genes of interest with little or no extraneous DNA materials. Therefore, they increase the potential for better-characterized and more predictable foods. However, because of the wider variety of potential source organisms for the DNA segments, substances may be introduced into bioengineered foods that cannot be introduced by traditional breeding. Thus, there is a greater likelihood that some of the new substances will be significantly different from substances that have a history of safe use in food.

For purposes of this chapter, the terms "foods derived from biotechnology," "genetically modified (GM) foods," or "bioengineered foods" will be used interchangeably to describe foods or food ingredients that are, or are derived from, plants and animals that have been modified (engineered) through the use of rDNA techniques.

Regulation

When consumed by humans, GM products are regulated as foods and food additives.[1-5] As such, they must meet the same types of safety and labeling regulations as foods and food ingredients produced under more traditional means. Use of biotechnology to transfer genes that encode pharmaceutical proteins, oral vaccines, and enzymes for human or animal use will require that these products meet regulatory requirements for biologicals, drugs, or veterinary drugs, even when foods are used as the delivery vehicle (eg, bananas containing vaccines). In some cases, residual substances from a GM drug- or vaccine-producing plant or animal may enter the food supply (eg, recombinant bovine somatotropin [rbST] in milk as a consequence of its use as an animal drug). In these cases, regulatory evaluations must include considerations of human food exposures and safety. Plant products bioengineered to contain substances with pesticidal properties to improve agronomic properties must meet requirements of both the US Environmental Protection Agency (EPA) and the US Food and Drug Administration (FDA).

Safety

All plant and animal breeding techniques have the potential for unintentionally introducing undesired new characteristics into foods.[1-4,6,7] This may occur either from bringing extraneous genetic material encoding trait(s) in addition to the desired trait(s) or from introducing mutations (such as deletions, amplifications, insertions, rearrangements, or DNA base-pair changes) into the native genetic material. Newly introduced DNA may physically insert into a transcriptionally active site on the chromosome and may, thereby, inactivate a host gene or alter control of its expression. The introduced gene product or a metabolic product affected by the genetic change may interact with other cellular processes. Pleiotropic effects (multiple effects resulting from a single genetic change) may also occur. Altered expression of an enzyme at high levels may lead to secondary biochemical effects (eg, altered metabolic flux resulting in changing metabolic patterns). Products of biotechnology have the additional potential to introduce substances into foods that cannot be introduced by traditional breeding. These techniques can, therefore, present more complex and novel safety issues than are seen with more conventional processes and often require nontraditional approaches to evaluating safety.

Safety concerns with GM foods can be categorized as relatively low or relatively high. A recent expert consultation of the Food and Agriculture Organization of the United Nations (FAO) and the World Health Organization (WHO) concluded that the concept of "substantial equivalence" is a practical, science-based approach for evaluating the safety of many GM foods.[6,7] The goal of this approach is to ensure that the GM food and any substances that have been introduced into the food as a result of GM is "as safe as its traditional counterpart" when such a counterpart exists. This approach is deemed useful because of the practical difficulties in obtaining meaningful information from conventional toxicologic studies on the safety of whole foods. For example, use of whole foods as a test substance in animal studies is difficult, because (1) the bulkiness of the food dilutes the nutritional value of the diet, causing adverse effects unrelated to the genetic modification; (2) the satiety of the diet is adversely affected, resulting in reduced food intake; and (3) the bulk and satiety effects limit the dose-response range to low multiples of the amounts that might be present in the human diet. However, the FAO/WHO expert panel also recognized that the "substantial equivalence" approach is not always sufficient and that animal testing is needed for cases in which: (1) the genetically modified food is expected to make a significant dietary contribution; (2) there is an absence of history of consumption of the novel gene product; or (3) the genetic modification affects several metabolic pathways. In these cases, animal testing is recommended, starting with appropriate isolated substances and also including testing of the whole food in a form that reflects the food as it will be consumed by humans.

Safety concerns are least likely to be raised in GM foods if the proteins or other substances produced by the transferred genetic material do not differ significantly from other substances commonly found in food and are already present at generally comparable or greater levels in currently consumed foods.[1,2,6] An example would be insertion of the GmFad2-1 gene into the soybean genome to produce a high-oleic acid soybean oil. Comparability to historic uses of foods will include such factors as the content of significant nutrients, naturally occurring toxicants, antinutrients, and previous safe use.

Transferred genetic material (ie, DNA) is generally not considered to raise safety concerns.[1,2,6] All food, rDNA-derived or otherwise, contains large amounts of DNA. Individuals consume approximately 0.1 to 1.0 g/day of DNA when eating conventional foods.[7] The added DNA from genetically modified foods is estimated to contribute <1/250 000 of this ingested quantity of DNA. Normally, ingested DNA is rapidly digested in the gastrointestinal tract. Thus, evaluating the digestibility of the DNA in a GM food provides useful insight into the possibility of a gene transfer. In general, the FAO/WHO concluded that horizontal gene transfer from genetically modified foods to gut micro-organisms or human cells is a possibility. A few recent reports have shown antibiotic resistance genes transferring in human mouth and gut from animal microbial sources to human gut bacteria. This genetic material has not been shown to incorporate into human DNA. For gene transfer from a GM food to gut microflora or human cells to occur, all of the following events need to occur: (1) the relevant gene would need to be released; (2) the gene would need to survive plant and gastrointestinal tract nucleases; (3) the gene would have to compete for uptake with dietary DNA; (4) the recipient or mammalian cells would have to be competent for transformation; (5) the gene would have to survive their restrictive enzymes; and (6) the gene would have to be inserted into the host DNA by rare repair or recombination events.

Safety concerns are more likely to be raised if the GM food will contain substances that are significantly different from, or are present in food at a significantly higher level than, counterpart substances historically consumed in food.[1,2,6] Examples of these types of safety concerns include the potential for: (1) introducing a food allergen that would not be expected to be in a particular food; (2) an expression of allergens at higher concentrations than they would otherwise be expressed; (3) compositional changes that would affect the nutritional quality of the food by altering nutrient levels, bioavailability, or stability of relied-on nutrients; (4) increasing the level of naturally occurring toxicants; or (5) producing new metabolic pathways that would result in the synthesis of toxicants not normally found in a food.

A potential consequence of transferring genetic material from one source into another is the possibility of introducing a food allergen that would not be expected to be in a particular food.[1,2,4,6,7] This is because genes code for proteins, and virtually all allergens are proteins (although only a small subset of proteins are allergens). Thus, by increasing the range of potential proteins that can be introduced into food over that possible by traditional breeding, there is an increased potential for introducing an allergen into a GM food that could have an allergenic characteristic completely different from that of its conventional counterpart. Also, bioengineering can be used to express proteins at higher concentrations than they would otherwise be expressed, and these higher concentrations may increase the potential for such proteins to be allergenic. If the allergen were moved into a food product that never before produced that allergen, the susceptible consumer population would not know to avoid that food. For example, a gene from a Brazil nut plant was introduced into a soy plant to improve the protein content of soybeans for use in animal feed. The seed was never commercialized, however, because when the company tested the soybeans for allergenicity, they found that people allergic to Brazil nuts were also allergic to the GM soy.

Most common allergic reactions are mediated by allergen-specific immunoglobulin E antibodies. The FAO/WHO recommends that the potential for allergenicity be evaluated if: (1) the source of transferred material contains known allergens or an amino acid sequence homology similar to known allergens; (2) there is immunoreactivity to the immunoglobulin E of blood serum of humans with known allergenicity to the source material; and (3) the substance is resistant to the effect of pH and digestion (unlike other dietary proteins, most allergens are resistant to gastric acidity and digestive proteases). Additionally, allergens that are labile to heat and processing should be allowed only if the GM food is always eaten in cooked or processed food.[7]

Genetic modifications have the potential to activate cryptic pathways synthesizing unknown or unexpected toxicants or to increase expression from active pathways that ordinarily produce low or undetectable amounts of toxicants.[1,2,6,7] Plants are known to naturally produce a number of toxicants and antinutritional factors (eg, protease inhibitors, hemolytic agents, and neurotoxins), which often serve the plant as natural defense compounds against pests or pathogens. Additionally, plants, like other organisms, have metabolic pathways that no longer function as a result of mutations that occurred during evolution. Such silent pathways may be activated by mutations, chromosomal rearrangements, or new regulatory regions introduced during breeding, and toxicants not associated with a plant species may be produced. Many of these toxicants are present in today's foods in amounts that do not cause acute toxicity. Others require proper preparation to make them safe. To be considered safe and approved, new GM foods should not have significantly higher amounts of toxicants than present in other edible varieties of the counterpart food.

The safety of selectable markers for antibiotic resistance has been the focus of considerable discussion.[1,4,6-9] For research purposes, scientists enhance their ability to isolate plant cells that have taken up and stably incorporated the desired genes by physically linking the desired gene to a selectable marker gene, such as a gene that specifies the production of a substance that inactivates antibiotics. By linking the selectable marker gene to another gene that specifies a desired trait, scientists can identify and select plants that have taken up and express the desired genes. Selectable marker genes that produce enzymes that inactivate clinically useful antibiotic agents have the potential of reducing the therapeutic efficacy of the antibiotic when taken orally if the enzyme in the food inactivates the antibiotic. These genes may be expressed in the transgenic plant.

The kanamycin resistance gene is one of the most widely used selectable plant marker genes in GM foods. The kanamycin resistance gene specifies the information for the production of the enzyme, aminoglycoside 3'-phosphotransferase II. The common name for this enzyme is kanamycin (or neomycin) phosphotransferase II. The kanamycin phosphotransferase II enzyme modifies aminoglycoside antibiotics, including kanamycin, neomycin, and geneticin (G418), chemically inactivating the antibiotic and rendering the cells that produce the kanamycin resistance gene refractory or resistant to the antibiotic. Plant cells that have received and stably express the kanamycin resistance gene survive and replicate on laboratory media in the presence of the antibiotic, kanamycin. Plant cells that did not take up and express the introduced kanamycin resistance gene will be killed by the antibiotic. Both the kanamycin resistance gene and its product, the kanamycin phosphotransferase II enzyme protein, are in foods derived from plants in which the marker gene has been used unless removed through special techniques.

The WHO (1993)[9] and the FDA[8] reviewed safety issues associated with the use of selective antibiotic resistance genes in GM plants. They found no evidence that markers currently in use pose a health risk, but they recommended that genes that confer resistance to drugs with specific medical use or limited alternative therapies should not be used in widely disseminated rDNA biotechnology foods. They concluded that safety assessments for the presence of these genes in food products should include such factors as: (1) an assessment of the potential toxicity of the protein; (2) an assessment of whether the protein has the potential to elicit allergenic reactions; and (3) an assessment of whether the presence in food of the enzyme or protein encoded by the antibiotic resistance marker gene would compromise the therapeutic efficiency of orally administered antibiotic. Safety evaluations should also consider whether the antibiotic is an important medication, frequently used, orally administered, or unique; whether the antibiotic has selective pressure for transformation to occur; the background level of resistance to the antibiotic in bacterial populations; and the availability of alternative effective therapies. If the information suggests that the presence of the marker gene or gene in the GM food could compromise the use of the relevant antibiotic(s), the marker gene or gene product should not be present in finished food. For example, in certain cases, there is only 1 antibiotic available to treat an infection (eg, vancomycin for treating certain staphylococcal infections). Marker genes that encode resistance to such antibiotics should not be used in GM foods.

It should be noted also that antibiotic resistance is increasing rapidly and drugs that are currently not important to humans may become important.

Thus, it may come to pass that all marker genes for antibiotic resistance should not be incorporated into GM foods.

Because of the novel safety concerns raised by the use of the kanamycin resistance gene in such products as the Flavr Savr tomato (Monsanto, St Louis, MO), the FDA reviewed evidence on the safety of this gene via the food-additive petition process.[10] The evidence showed that, like other dietary proteins, the marker gene used to confer kanamycin resistance is rapidly degraded when subjected to conditions that simulate mammalian digestion. On the basis of this evidence, the FDA concluded that DNA for kanamycin resistance was not different from other rDNA in its digestibility. A food-additive regulation authorized the use of kanamycin phosphotransferase II in canola, cotton, and tomatoes (see Table 21.1).

Table 21.1
Examples of Marketed Foods or Food Products Developed Through Biotechnology[3,11]

Food(s)	Intended Effects of Genetic Modification	Gene, Gene Product, or Gene Fragments	Source
Corn, rice, cotton, canola, flax, soybean, sugar beet, radicchio	Herbicide resistance to glufosinate	Phosphinothricin acetyltransferase	*Streptomyces viridochromogenes* or *hygroscopicus*
Corn, cotton, sugar beet, canola, soybean	Herbicide resistance to glyphosate	5-Enolpyruvylshikimate-3-phosphate synthase; or glyphosate oxidoreductase	*Agrobacterium* species strain CP4; *Ochrobactrum anthropi; Achromobacter* strain BAA
Canola, cotton	Herbicide resistance to bromoxynil	Nitrilase	*Klebsiella ozaenae* or *pneumoniae* subspecies *Ozaenae*
Flax, cotton	Herbicide resistance to sulfonylurea	Acetolactate synthase (csr-1)	*Arabidopsis; Nicotiana tabacum* cv *Xanthi*
Corn, tomato, potato, cotton	Insect resistance*	CryIF, CryIAb, CryIAc, CryIIIA, Cry9C proteins	*Bacillus thuringiensis*
Potato, squash, papaya	Virus resistance*	Plant virus coat proteins or mosaic viruses; potato leafroll virus replicase	Potato virus Y, potato leafroll virus, cucumber mosaic virus, zucchini yellow mosaic virus, watermelon mosaic virus 2, papaya ringspot virus
Cantaloupe, tomato	Delayed fruit ripening	S-adenosylmethionine hydrolase	*Escherichia coli* bacteriophage T3

Table 21.1 *(Continued)*
Examples of Marketed Foods or Food Products Developed Through Biotechnology[3,11]

Food(s)	Intended Effects of Genetic Modification	Gene, Gene Product, or Gene Fragments	Source
Tomato	Delayed fruit ripening	Gene fragment for amino cyclopropane carboxylic acid synthase; polyga-lacturonase (PG) or the antisense PG gene	Tomato
Tomato	Delayed fruit ripening	1-aminocyclopropane-1-carboxylic acid deaminase	*Pseudomonas chlororaphis*
Tomato, cotton, canola	Antibiotic resistance marker that inacti-vates aminoglycosides (kanamycin, neomycin, geneticin)	Amino glycoside 3'-phosphotransferase II encoded *kanr* gene from the transposon Tn5	*E coli*
Corn, canola, radicchio, canola	Male sterility; fertility restorer	Barnase; Barstar	*Bacillus amyloliquefaciens*
Corn	Male sterility	DNA adenine methylase	*E coli*
Canola	Degradation of phytate in animal feed	Phytase	*Aspergillus niger* van Tieghem
Dairy products	Increase milk production in dairy animals		Recombinant bovine growth hormone (rbGH) or somatotro-pin (rbST)[†]
Soybean	To produce a high-oleic acid soybean oil)	GmFad2-1 gene (to suppress endogenous GmFad2-1 gene which encodes delta-12 desaturase)	Soybean
Canola	To produce high-laurate canola oil	12:0 acyl carrier protein thioesterase	*Umbellularia californica* (California Bay)

*Foods that contain an introduced pesticidal substance are regulated by both the Environmental Protection Agency (EPA) and the Food and Drug Administration (FDA).

† Regulated as an animal drug, taking into account safety for humans when dairy products from treated cows are consumed as foods.

Purpose of Biotechnology Changes

To date, the use of bioengineering applications for food products has primarily been for agronomic purposes (Table 21.1).[3,11,12] Increasingly, however, there is also interest in using biotechnology to improve benefits to consumers.

Agronomic uses of biotechnology include those uses that (1) increase crop productivity through increased resistance to herbicides, insects, or viruses; (2) increase shelf life through delayed fruit ripening; (3) affect fertility to control against cross-fertilization in field conditions or alter seed viability; (4) increase milk production in dairy cows; or (5) increase the bioavailability of phosphates in animal feeds (see Table 21.1).[11,12]

The use of recombinant bovine growth hormone (rbGH) or rbST to increase milk production in dairy animals was approved in 1993 for use as an animal drug.[13] rbGH is essentially the same as bovine growth hormone (bGH [pituitary derived]). To grant approval of this product as an animal drug, the FDA determined, among other things, that food products from cows treated with rbGH are safe for consumption by humans. This conclusion, however, is controversial. Subsequent to approval by the FDA, Canada's Health Department concluded that results of a 90-day oral rat toxicity study and the report of an antibody response to oral rbGH suggested possible adverse health effects of this product.[14] Therefore, Canada did not approve the use of rbGH or rbST as an animal drug. After the Canadian decision, the FDA conducted a comprehensive audit of the human food safety used to support the 1993 rbGH approval, including the studies that Canada relied on in making its finding of safety concerns. On the basis of this audit, the FDA concluded that the Canadian reviewers did not interpret the study results correctly and that there were no new scientific concerns regarding the safety of milk from cows treated with rbGH. The FDA, therefore, reconfirmed its determination that safety had been established and that long-term studies were not necessary for assessing the safety of rbGH. The decision of the FDA was made on the basis of evidence that showed that bGH is biologically inactive in humans even if ingested, rbGH is orally inactive, and bGH and rbGH are biologically indistinguishable.

The use of the Cry9C gene to produce toxicity to certain insects (ie, StarLink Corn [Aventis CropScience, Morrisville, NC]) has also been considerably controversial.[15] Before October 2001, plants containing the Cry9C proteins had been approved by the EPA only for corn earmarked for animal feed and industrial uses. Approval had not been given for human consumption because of unresolved questions about the potential of Cry9C to cause allergic reactions. In approving this product for animal feed use, the EPA required StarLink's developer to ensure that the GM corn did not enter the food supply. However, some of the GM corn became mingled with corn destined for human consumption (eg, taco shells). The presence of

an unapproved pesticide in food means that the food is adulterated. Therefore, the manufacturer recalled contaminated products from the market. On
October 16, 2001, the EPA, on the basis of a review of scientific evidence
demonstrating that *Bacillus thuringiensis* is not toxic to humans or other animals, approved corn genetically modified with *B thuringiensis* for 7 years for
use in human food.

Although not yet approved for human use, scientists have created a
genetically engineered variety of Atlantic salmon that grows to market
weight in approximately 18 months, compared with the 24 to 30 months
that it normally takes for the fish to reach that size.[16,17] The idea for the fast-
growing salmon was discovered by accident 20 years ago when a researcher
in Canada accidentally froze a tank filled with flounder. When the tank was
thawed out, the flounder were still alive. This species has a gene that produces a protein that works like antifreeze. Researchers isolated and copied
the part of the flounder DNA that works like a genetic switch to turn on the
production of the antifreeze protein. They then attached the flounder's gene
to a previously isolated gene from Chinook salmon that produces a growth-
stimulating hormone and inserted the new combination into fertilized
salmon eggs. In the resulting salmon, the founder's genetic switch produces
a continuous supply of salmon growth hormone that accelerates the fish's
development. The resulting fish do not become larger than conventional
salmon; they simply grow faster. If approved, these salmon products will be
regulated similarly to rbST in that they will need to meet regulatory requirements for safety and efficacy as a veterinary drug and also establish safety
for use as human food.

Consumer Benefits

Bioengineering can also be used to develop foods that are designed to
provide direct benefits to consumers (eg, improved quality or nutritional
and health benefits of foods).[7,11,12] For example, rDNA techniques have been
used to modify the nutrient composition of plants (eg, increase carotenoid
content of rice), improve the healthfulness of foods (eg, decaffeinated coffee
beans fresh off the tree), and increase characteristics desired by consumers
(eg, fruit solids, fruit sweetness, prolonged shelf life). Transgenic animals
may also be modified to produce GM foods. Examples include fish that
produce more omega-3 fatty acids or trout with pink muscle tissue.

Two plants that serve as sources of food oils have been modified to
change their fatty acid composition (see Table 21.1). Soybeans have been
modified to produce soybean oil higher in oleic acid and lower in linoleic

and linolenic acids so that use of these oils in margarines and shortenings will not require hydrogenation and the resultant production of trans fatty acids. This will also reduce the potential for oxidation during shelf life. The canola (rapeseed) is genetically modified to increase the content of lauric and myristic fatty acids in their oils to make them functionally useful as a replacement for lauric oils, such as palm kernel oil. These modified oil-producing plants were determined by manufacturers not to be different from their traditional counterparts in antinutritional factors, allergen content, and other components with potential safety concerns (eg, isoflavones in soy). To avoid confusion with the traditional plants, these plants were given distinctive names, such as "high-oleic acid soybean oil" and "laurate canola oil."

Macronutrient Substitutes

Macronutrient substitutes are added to foods in place of their usual macronutrients (eg, fat or sugars) to provide a potential health benefit.[18] The primary functions of these ingredients are to provide calorie, fat, or sugar reduction in familiar foods. Macronutrient substitutes can also add bulk to food, provide texture, and serve as carriers for the flavors in the product. The use of these substitutes to provide health benefits for children and adolescents has been inadequately studied. As such, they should not form a significant part of a child's diet.

Carbohydrate Replacements

Carbohydrate replacements include materials that reduce carbohydrate calories without loss of sweetness, reduce the cariogenic potential of a food, and add bulking or sensory properties to compensate for reductions in sugar content. These ingredients include a range of ingredients, such as artificial sweeteners, sugar alcohols, and complex carbohydrates that serve as bulking agents.

Artificial Sweeteners

Artificial sweeteners are many times sweeter than sugar. Therefore, it takes a smaller amount of them to create the same sweetness as sugar, resulting in negligible calories to achieve the same sweetening effect. To date, several sugar substitutes have been approved for use in a variety of foods (ie, saccharin, aspartame, acesulfame K, and sucralose). Several other sweeteners are under FDA review (eg, cyclamate and Alitame [Pfizer, New York, NY]).[19]

Saccharin was discovered in 1879 and was used to help compensate for sugar rationing during both world wars. Saccharin is the chemical 1,2-

benzisothiazolin-3-one 1,1-dioxide ($C_7H_5NO_3S$) and specified salts. It is 300 times sweeter than sugar. Because of animal studies suggesting saccharin caused bladder cancer in rats, the FDA proposed in 1977 to ban the use of saccharin as a food additive. Congress responded by passing the Saccharin Study and Labeling Act that placed a moratorium on any ban of the sweetener while additional safety studies were conducted. Also, the law originally required that any foods containing saccharin must carry a label that stated, "Use of this product may be hazardous to your health. This product contains saccharin which has been determined to cause cancer in laboratory animals." Congress has extended the moratorium against banning the use of saccharin several times, most recently renewing it until 2002. However, in 2001, Congress repealed the requirement for the warning label, and subsequent studies have not demonstrated any increased risk of cancer with the consumption of saccharin.

Aspartame is the chemical 1-methyl N-L-alpha-aspartyl-L-phenylalanine ($C_{14}H_{18}N_2O_5$). Aspartame is sold under trade names such as NutraSweet (The NutraSweet Company, Chicago, IL) and Equal (Merisant Company, Chicago, IL). Aspartame is 180 times sweeter than sugar. Because aspartame contains phenylalanine, its use is potentially harmful to people with phenylketonuria. Therefore, all products containing aspartame are required to bear a warning that the product contains phenylalanine.

Acesulfame potassium, also called acesulfame K, is also known by its trade name Sunett (Nutrinova, Celanese, Dallas, TX). It is about 200 times sweeter than sugar. Acesulfame K is the potassium salt of 6-methyl-1,2,3-oxathiazine-4(3H)-one-2,2-dioxide.

Sucralose is the chemical 1,6-dichloro-1,6-beta-D-fructofuranosyl-4-chloro-4-deoxy-alpha-D-galactopyranoside. Sucralose is 600 times sweeter than sugar. It is also known by its trade name, Splenda (McNeil Nutritionals, Washington, PA). Sucralose tastes and looks like sugar because it is made from table sugar. Because it cannot be digested, it adds no calories.

Sugar Alcohols

Sugar alcohols are used as anti- or reduced-cariogenic substitutes for sugars, as reduced-calorie substitutes for starch or sugar, and as bulking agents when starch or sugar is removed from foods.[18] Sugar alcohols are naturally present in fruits and vegetables. For commercial food ingredient purposes, they are generally prepared by the catalytic hydrogenation of the parent sugars.

The digestion, absorption, and metabolism of the sugar alcohols differ among the alcohols and are generally less complete that that of the parent sugars. Bioavailability in the upper gastrointestinal tract varies significantly among the alcohols. The portion of the ingested sugar alcohols that reaches the colon undergoes anaerobic fermentation by the colonic microflora to product methane, hydrogen, and short-chain fatty acids. Fermentation in the colon generates some usable energy but generally less than would be obtained from the parent sugar. The production of short-chain fatty acids and lactic acid also lowers the pH of colonic material and may change the species distribution of colonic microorganisms. The reduced- and anticariogenic properties of sugar alcohols, as compared with the caloric sweeteners, is related to their resistance to fermentation by the oral microflora and production of reduced quantities of plaque.

Mannitol
Approximately 25% of ingested D-mannitol is absorbed via passive diffusion.[18] Once absorbed, it is oxidized by mannitol dehydrogenase or L-iditol 2-dehydrogenase to fructose and undergoes normal fructose metabolism. The net energy value of mannitol may be as low as 1.5 kcal/g.

Sorbitol
Approximately 50% of ingested sorbitol is absorbed through passive diffusion in the small intestine and up to 85% of this is metabolized.[18] Sorbitol is absorbed more slowly than glucose. When consumed in large quantities, a laxative effect may be observed. Approximately 50% of ingested sorbitol reaches the colon, where it is rapidly fermented to short-chain fatty acids, hydrogen, and methane. Estimates of the caloric value of sorbitol range from 2.0 to 3.9 kcal/g.

Xylitol
The absorption of xylitol occurs by simple diffusion and ranges from 13% to 95%.[18] The unabsorbed xylitol is completely fermented in the colon. Most of the absorbed xylitol is metabolized in the liver. The metabolizable energy from xylitol is approximately 2.5 to 2.9 kcal/g.

Erythritol
Erythritol has a unique metabolic fate in animals, presumably because of its low molecular weight. The sugar alcohol is almost completely absorbed in the small intestine and quantitatively excreted unchanged in the urine.[18] The result is a bulking agent with no caloric value.

Isomalt

Isomalt is an equimolar mixture of alpha-D-glucopyranosyl-1-6-D-sorbitol and alpha-D-glucopyranosyl-1,5-mannitol.[18] Although both components are slowly hydrolyzed by various glucan 1,4-alpha-glucosidases, including jejunal mucosal enzymes, most of the energy derived from them is a result of fermentation in the colon. The energy value is approximately 3 kcal/g.

Lactitol

Lactitol is rapidly hydrolyzed to D-galactose and D-sorbitol by microbial enzymes; however, hydrolysis in the gastrointestinal tract is slow.[18] Lactitol undergoes little or no absorption in the stomach or small intestine. Lactitol in the colon is readily fermented. Lactitol is estimated to provide approximately 2 kcal/g.

Maltitol

In the stomach, maltitol is hydrolyzed to glucose and sorbitol, both of which are readily absorbed.[18] A substantial portion of maltitol reaches the large intestine and is fermented to short-chain fatty acids. The net energy value for maltitol is approximately 3 kcal/g.

Other Carbohydrate Bulking Agents

Carbohydrate-based bulking agents can be used to replace sugar, starch, or fat in foods. Low-molecular weight materials (eg, polydextrose) are used as sucrose replacements in syrup confections and baked product applications.[18] Some complex mixtures of carbohydrate polymers can function as low-calorie bulking agents because of their ability to hold several times their weight and, thus, reduce the amount of carbohydrate or fat in a food (eg, gums). Some of these complex carbohydrate polymer mixtures also are measured analytically as dietary fibers (eg, cellulose, hemicelluloses, pectins, gums, mucilages, and lignins). The bulk provided by some of these polymers reduces transit time in the bowel. The complex carbohydrate bulking agents are poorly digested by normal gastrointestinal enzymes in the upper gastrointestinal tract, but many are fermented by the colonic microflora to shorter-chain fatty acids.

Reduced starch hydrolysates are mixtures of monomeric, dimeric, and oligomeric polyols.[18] They are prepared by partial hydrolysis of starch followed by hydrogenation. On ingestion, they are hydrolyzed to glucose, sorbitol, and maltitol, with insignificant portions of the hydrolysis products reaching the colon. Their rate of absorption and metabolism is similar to maltitol but slower than sorbitol. Where the hydrogenated starch hydrolysates reach the colon, they are completely fermented to short-chain fatty acids. The net energy value of the hydrolysates is approximately 3 to 4 kcal/g.

Polydextrose is a low-molecular weight, randomly-bonded polymer of glucose, sorbitol, and citric or phosphoric acid.[18,20] Polydextrose is only partially metabolized by humans and is not fermented by the colonic micro-flora. The caloric availability of polydextrose in humans is 1 kcal/g. Laxation can occur when high amounts of polydextrose are consumed; thus, food products delivering more than 15 g per serving must be labeled accordingly.

Pectins are complex galacturono glycans composed primarily of polymers of D-galacturonic acid. Frequently, the polymers include arabinans, arabinoga-lactan, and galactans. Pectins are found primarily in the cell walls of plants. Pectins are slowly degraded and fermented by microflora in the large intestine and colon.

Beta-glucans are complex carbohydrate materials composed of glucose polymers containing both beta (1→3) and beta (1→4) linkages.[18] Barley and oats are both excellent sources of beta-glucans. Concentrated amounts of beta-glucans in oats have been marketed commercially as oatrim.[18,20] The mouth feel of this ingredient mimics that of triglycerides, thus serving as a lower-calorie alternative to fats.

Galactomannans are complex carbohydrate bulking agents composed of beta (1→4)-D-mannopyranosyl chains with beta (1→6)-D galactopyranosyl units attached at carbon 6 of the mannoses.[18] Major sources of galactoman-nan are guar gum and carob gum. These are frequently used in low-calorie foods to emulate the texture of the fat that has been removed.

Cellulose refers to a group of complex carbohydrates whose primary structure is a beta (1→4) glucan.[18] It also includes a number of chemically modified celluloses (eg, carboxymethylcellulose, microcrystalline cellulose, and methylcellulose). The derivatized celluloses can be used in foods as functional bulking agents, binders, stabilizers in frozen food systems, and thickeners. Cellulose acts as a noncaloric insoluble bulking agent and fat mimetic in a variety of food applications.

Resistant starch is indigestible.[18] Its "resistance" occurs in several ways. The cell wall of the plant may make the starch inaccessible for digestive enzymes (eg, milled grains and seeds). Differences in the crystalline patterns of starch in the granule can affect its susceptibility to enzymatic digestion (eg, raw bananas and potato starch). Finally, cooking or processing resistant starch-containing foods may initially make the resistant starch digestible (eg, potatoes, cereals, legumes). However, on cooling, the starch can re-crystallize to an indigestible form. Resistant starch content is high in food products processed under relatively high moisture contents, such as boiling, baking, or autoclaving. Significant amounts of resistant starch may escape digestion in the small intestine and pass into the colon, where it is fermented. Resistant starch in the large intestine may share some of the health benefits attributed to dietary fiber.

Fat Replacers

Three types of substitutes have been developed to replace fat.[18,20] Fat mimetics are proteins or carbohydrates that imitate the organoleptic or physical properties of fat. Therefore, they provide 4 kcal/g rather than the 9 kcal/g provided by food fats. Fat substitutes are synthetic or enzymatically modified lipids that chemically resemble conventional fats. They can replace food fat on a gram-for-gram basis while providing no, or significantly fewer, calories than food fat. Structured triglycerides are similar to conventional fats in that they contain fatty acids attached to a glycerol backbone. However, they are designed to provide fewer calories than normal (<9 kcal/g) by substituting poorly absorbed fatty acids and short-chain fatty acids with lower caloric value than the usual fatty acids found in foods.[18,20]

Fat Mimetics

The typical constituents of fat mimetics are carbohydrates (eg, starch, cellulose, pectin, protein, hydrophilic colloids, dextrins, and polydextrose [see previous discussions on carbohydrate ingredients]) and proteins (eg, egg, milk, whey, soy, gelatin, and wheat gluten).[18,20] These materials are frequently microparticulated to emulate the particle size and mouth feel of emulsified fats. Most of the fat mimetic materials are fully digestible, providing 4 kcal/g as compared with the 9 kcal/g for the food fats they replace. However, some mimetics are not digested (eg, cellulose, seaweed, some gums), so they contribute no calories. Many fat mimetics are highly hydrated; thus, part of the caloric advantage comes from the replacement of fat with water. One of the mimetics, Simplesse (CP Kelco, Chicago, IL), is manufactured from whey protein concentrate by a patented microparticulation process. It retains any antigenic/allergenic properties of the parent protein.

Fat Substitutes

Fat substitutes are macromolecules that can replace food fat on a one-to-one basis.[18,20] Olestra is one example of a fat substitute. Olestra contains a mixture of octa-, hepta-, and hexa-esters of sucrose with fatty acids derived from edible fats and oils. It is formed by chemical transesterification or interesterification of sucrose with 6 to 8 conventional food fatty acids. Because humans lack enzymes to break the sucrose/fatty acid bonds, olestra is not absorbed or metabolized. Therefore, olestra provides no calories. However, because this is a nonabsorbed lipid, products containing olestra are required to add vitamins A, D, E, and K to compensate for any interference with the absorption of these fat-soluble vitamins. These added nutrients, because they are unlikely to be physiologically available, will not be considered in nutrient declarations in the food label nutrition facts box but will be listed in the ingredient list. Products are also required to carry a warning label for potential gastrointestinal effects.

Structured Lipids

Structured lipids are triglycerides that are designed to provide fewer than 9 kcal/g.[18,20] Examples of structured lipids include caprenin, salatrim, and medium-chain triglycerides (MCTs).

Caprenin is a reduced-calorie fat. Its caloric reduction is achieved by esterifying 2 MCTs (caprylic and capric acids) and behenic acid to a glycerol backbone. Because behenic acid is only partially absorbed and caprylic and capric acids are more readily metabolized than other longer-chain fatty acids, caprenin provides only 5 kcal/g.

Salatrim represents a family of low-calorie fats comprising a mixture containing at least one short-chain fatty acid (eg, C2:0, C3:0, C4:0) and at least one long-chain fatty acid (predominately C18:0) attached to the glycerol backbone.[18,20] Because short-chain fatty acids have a lower caloric value than do long-chain fatty acids and because stearic acid is incompletely absorbed, the caloric value of salatrim is about 5/9 the value of conventional fats.

Medium-chain triglycerides predominately contain saturated fatty acids of chain length C8:0 (caprylic acid) and C11:0 (capric acid), with traces of C6:0 and C12:0 fatty acids.[18,20] MCTs are absorbed intact into the intestine as free fatty acids without the need for enzymes or bile salts. They bind to serum albumin and are transported to the liver via the portal system. They are oxidized to ketone bodies in the liver. They are less likely to be stored in adipose tissue. They have been used clinically in enteral and parenteral diets for individuals with lipid absorption, digestion, or transport disorders. They provide approximately 8.3 kcal/g.

References

1. US Food and Drug Administration. Statement of policy: foods derived from new plant varieties. *Fed Regist.* 1992;57(104):22964–23001

2. US Food and Drug Administration. Premarket Notice Concerning Bioengineered Foods; Proposed Rule. *Fed Regist.* 2001;66:4706–4738

3. IFT expert report on biotechnology and foods. Introduction. *Food Technol.* 2000;54(8): 124–136

4. National Research Council. *Genetically Modified Pest-Protected Plants: Science and Regulation.* National Academies Press, Washington, DC. 2000

5. Formanek R Jr. Proposed rules issued for bioengineered foods. *FDA Consumer.* 2001; Mar–Apr. Available at: http://www.fda.gov/fdac/features/2001/201_food.html. Accessed August 30, 2007

6. IFT Expert Report on Biotechnology and Foods. Human Food Safety Evaluation of rDNA Biotechnology-Derived Foods. *Food Technol.* 2000;54(9):53–61

7. Food and Agricultural Organization of the United Nations and World Health Organization. Safety aspects of genetically modified foods of plant origin. Joint FAO/WHO Expert Consultation on Foods Derived from Biotechnology; Geneva, Switzerland; May 29–June 2, 2000. Available at: http://www.who.int/foodsafety/publications/biotech/ec_june2000/en/index.html. Accessed August 30, 2007

8. US Food and Drug Administration. Guidance for Industry: Use of Antibiotic Resistance Marker Genes in Transgenic Plants; Report and Guidance for Industry; Availability. *Federal Register.* 1998;63:47505–47506. Available at: http://www.fda.gov/ohrms/dockets/98fr/090898d.txt. Accessed August 30, 2007

9. World Health Organization, Food Safety Unit. Health aspects of marker genes in genetically modified plants: report of WHO workshop. Geneva, Switzerland: World Health Organization; 1993. Publication No. WHO/FNU/FOS/93.6

10. Modified polyacrylamide resin. 21CFR§173.170 (2007)

11. US Food and Drug Administration. List of Completed Consultations on Bioengineered Foods. Available at: http://www.cfsan.fda.gov/~lrd/biocon.html. Accessed August 30, 2007

12. IFT Expert Report on Biotechnology and Foods. Benefits and concerns associated with recombinant DNA biotechnology-derived foods. *Food Technol.* 2000;54(11):61–80

13. US Food and Drug Administration. Report on the Food and Drug Administration's Review of the Safety of Recombinant Bovine Somatotropin. http://www.fda.gov/cvm/RBRPTFNL.htm. Accessed August 30, 2007

14. US Food and Drug Administration. Update on Human Food Safety of BST. Rockville, MD: US Food and Drug Administration; 1999. Available at: http://www.fda.gov/cvm/CVM_Updates/BSTSAFUP.html. Accessed August 30, 2007

15. US Environmental Protection Agency. Biotechnology Corn Approved for Continued Use. October 16, 2001. Available at: http://yosemite.epa.gov/opa/admpress.nsf/b0789fb70f8ff03285257029006e3880/8db7a83e66e0f7d085256ae7005d6ec2!OpenDocument. Accessed August 30, 2007

16. US Food and Drug Administration. Questions and Answers About Transgenic Fish. Available at: http://www.fda.gov/cvm/transgen.htm. Accessed August 30, 2007

17. Lewis C. A New Kind of Fish Story: The Coming of Biotech Animals. FDA Consumer Magazine. 2001;Jan–Feb. Available at: http://www.fda.gov/fdac/features/2001/101_fish.html. Accessed August 30, 2007

18. Finley JW, Leveille GA. Macronutrient substitutes. In: Ziegler EE, Filer LJ Jr, eds. *Present Knowledge in Nutrition.* 7th ed. Washington, DC: International Life Sciences Institute Press; 1996:581–595

19. Henken J. Sugar substitutes: Americans opt for sweetness and lite. *FDA Consum.* 1999;33(6):12–16

20. Akoh CC. Fat replacers. *Food Technol.* 1998;52:47–53

Nutrient Delivery Systems   IV

Clinical experience has demonstrated the value of optimal nutritional status in resisting the effects of trauma and disease and in improving the response to medical and surgical therapy. The metabolic demands of rapid growth and the low nutritional reserves in infancy make the potential benefit of appropriate nutrition to critically ill pediatric patients even greater.

Parenteral nutrition has become an integral part of the care of any neonate, infant, or child who cannot be supported by enteral nutrition alone. This may occur in children who suffer from malnutrition (failure to thrive) or are at high risk of developing malnutrition as a result of acute or prolonged medical or surgical illnesses. This commonly includes (1) preterm infants with severe respiratory disease, congenital anomalies of the gastrointestinal tract, or inflammatory disease of the intestinal mucosa (eg, necrotizing enterocolitis); (2) infants and children in whom prolonged starvation is anticipated (eg, pancreatitis, graft-versus-host disease, after surgery); (3) pediatric patients with inadequate intestinal nutrient absorption (eg, short-bowel syndrome, after chemotherapy). Extensive body-surface burns, malignancies (especially after bone marrow transplantation), cardiac failure, and renal failure are examples of extraintestinal disorders in which parenteral nutrition has been useful. Specific formulations and procedures are available for such situations in adults,[1] but each of these regimens must be specifically tailored for infants and children. The therapeutic goal of parenteral nutrition is to maintain nutritional status and achieve or maintain appropriate somatic growth. Parenteral nutrition and its components may induce major metabolic disturbances, end-organ dysfunction, and nutrient-drug interactions that mandate periodic monitoring and surveillance.[2]

A nutritional support team is beneficial in providing care for all patients requiring parenteral nutrition. An interdisciplinary team consisting of medical, nursing, dietary, pharmaceutical, and surgical staff with expertise in parenteral nutrition provides invaluable consultative services, helps to decrease costs, and potentially shortens the length of hospital stays and occurrence of complications associated with parenteral nutrition. However, problems with providing supplemental nutrition support still remain, as evidenced by errors reported in the literature.[3,4] These sorts of issues led to a comprehensive review resulting in the publication of guidelines by the American Society of Parenteral and Enteral Nutrition.[5] These guidelines include critical elements of screening, establishing nutrition care plans, and practice guidelines for enteral and parenteral nutritional support, including home specialized nutritional support.

Catheters

Parenteral nutrition can be administered through peripheral veins using standard peripheral intravenous catheters and solutions (dextrose concentrations less than 12.5%). When solutions of higher osmolarity are used, larger veins with a high blood flow must be used to avoid sclerosis and inflammation of the wall of the vein. Several commercially available central venous catheters can be used when long-term access is needed. Strict asepsis is mandatory during catheter placement. Peripheral parenteral nutrition regimens maintain existing body composition and are a reasonable choice for a normally nourished infant or child without significant fluid restrictions who is likely to tolerate an adequate enteral regimen in fewer than 2 weeks. Use of central parenteral nutrition can result in normal and catch-up growth and is a more reasonable choice for infants or older children, regardless of initial nutritional status, who will be intolerant of enteral feedings for more than 2 weeks. Percutaneously inserted catheters advanced into the superior vena cava are now becoming the route of choice for delivery of parenteral nutrition.

Central venous catheters are made of a flexible material, such as silicone elastomer or polyurethane. Anesthesia is usually required for their placement in the subclavian or internal jugular vein, from which they are advanced to the junction of the superior vena cava and the right atrium. Internal jugular venous catheters are associated with a higher rate of local hematoma formation, arterial injury, and catheter-related bloodstream infections (CRBSIs) than are subclavian venous catheters.[6,7] Some of these catheters can be introduced percutaneously into the subclavian vein. The more flexible catheters (eg, Hickman and Broviac) can be introduced through a hollow needle or can be placed by incising the skin and subcutaneous tissue to expose the vein. For long-term use, a subcutaneous tunnel can be created to provide some protection from the migration of skin bacteria into the vein. A subcutaneous tunnel is not created for a temporary catheter. Some catheters are impregnated with silver salts to prevent infection at the site of insertion of the catheter. A randomized controlled trial and meta-analysis indicated that central venous catheters impregnated with an antiseptic combination of chlorhexidine and silver sulfadiazine are efficacious in reducing the incidence of CRBSIs. Subsequently, these catheters have been shown to decrease the incidence of CRBSIs and death and provide significant savings in cost.[8] Full barrier precautions should be used during insertion of catheters. Low-dose anticoagulant therapy is also recommended in high-risk patients, including neonates. There is a fair amount of research-based evidence to recommend that specialized nursing teams should care for venous access devices in patients receiving parenteral nutrition. Other special catheters and infusion ports are available. Polymeric silicone (Silastic [Dow Corning, Midland, MI] catheters in preterm infants have a lower incidence of vein perforation and thrombosis than do stiffer catheters. Occasionally, when jugular or subclavian sites are unavailable, veins that course toward the inferior vena cava, such as the inferior epigastric veins, can be used. Peripherally inserted central catheters (PICCs) are becoming increasingly popular as an alternative for patients needing intermediate to long-term access.[9] Regardless of the site, radiographic confirmation of the intravascular placement of the catheter is mandatory before parenteral nutrition solutions are infused.

A number of complications directly related to the catheter may occur. Malposition of a central venous catheter outside the vein, with infusion of hypertonic solutions into the pleural or pericardial space, may be life threatening. A rapid decrease in serum glucose concentration or the acute onset of circulatory or respiratory compromise should signal malposition of the catheter. Hemorrhage, associated with erosion of central veins or of the wall of the right atrium, has been reported. Pneumothorax and brachial plexus injuries may complicate the placement of percutaneous subclavian line insertion in infants and small children. Air embolus may occur, but air-eliminating filters and properly secured tubing junctions help prevent this complication. Catheter emboli have occurred from the rupture of silicone elastomer catheters perfused under a high pressure or from the tips of polyethylene catheters sheared off when the catheter was withdrawn through the hub of the needle used to insert it. Thrombophlebitis may be observed in peripheral veins receiving hypertonic solutions. Skin slough is a rare but serious complication of extravasation of the parenteral solution into the interstitial space, particularly if the solution is of high osmolality or contains calcium. A prospective randomized study contrasting centrally inserted catheters versus PICCs demonstrated a significantly higher rate of thrombophlebitis and malposition with the central venous catheters but no differences in overall rates of infection.[10] Hyaluronidase is injected locally by the subcutaneous or intradermal route for suspected and known extravasations caused by dextrose, total parenteral nutrition, calcium solutions, aminophylline, and nafcillin to prevent possible tissue damage from the extravasation. Best results occur if the hyaluronidase is administered within the first few minutes to 1 hour after the extravasation is recognized.

IV

Table 22.1

Suggested Clinical and Laboratory Monitoring Schedule During Total Parenteral Nutrition in the Hospitalized Patient*†

Variable Monitored	Initial Period‡	Later Period§
Serum electrolytes (and carbon dioxide)	3–4 times/wk	Weekly
Serum urea nitrogen	3 times/wk	Weekly
Serum calcium, magnesium, phosphorous	3 times/wk	Weekly
Serum glucose		
Serum protein or albumin		Weekly
Liver function studies	Weekly	Weekly
Hematocrit	Weekly	Weekly
Urine glucose	Daily	Daily
Clinical observations (eg, activity, temperature)	Daily	Daily
Complete blood cell count and differential count	As indicated	As indicated
Cultures	As indicated	As indicated
Serum triglyceride	4 hours after an increase in dose	Weekly

* Schedule may vary with age and underlying medical condition of the patient.

† In several institutions, the frequency of monitoring after the initial period has been significantly prolonged. It should be noted that prealbumin/transferrin are short term indicators of nutritional status, whereas albumin has a longer half life and therefore, more indicative of stable nutritional status. The usefulness of weekly liver function tests needs to be reexamined, because direct hyperbilirubinemia, the most specific indicator of cholestasis, takes several weeks to develop.

‡ Initial period is the period before full glucose, protein, and lipid intake is achieved or any period of metabolic instability.

§ Later period is the period during which patient is in a metabolic steady state.

Blood glucose should be monitored closely during a period of glucosuria and for 2 to 3 days after cessation of parenteral nutrition to determine the degree of hypoglycemia. In the latter instance, frequent determination of blood glucose levels in fingertip venous blood constitutes adequate screening. After a month or more of receiving total parenteral nutrition, measurements can be made once a week or less frequently.

Catheter-related sepsis is a major complication of an indwelling central venous catheter. Fever alone is not an indication for removal of a parenteral nutrition catheter. Other sources of infection should be sought; if none are found, removal of the catheter should be considered. Some episodes of sepsis may be treated with the catheter in place. Fungal sepsis almost always necessitates removal of the catheter. Signs of sepsis in the neonate include lethargy, hyperbilirubinemia, temperature instability, and nutrient intolerance (eg, hyperglycemia or hypertriglyceridemia in response to previously tolerated glucose and lipid loads). Careful placement of the central catheter and strict adherence to established guidelines for catheter care and maintenance considerably decrease the incidence of catheter-related complications.[11] Catheter occlusion may be caused by a clot or thrombus, fat deposition, calcium-phosphorus precipitation, or drug precipitation. Currently, alteplase is recommended for catheter-related thrombosis; it has been proven to be an effective and well-tolerated alternative to urokinase.[12]

Metabolic complications caused by the composition and administration of the infusate are discussed in the next section. A schedule for monitoring of parenteral nutrition is shown in Table 22.1.

Composition of Solutions for Infants and Children

For the preterm neonate, various investigators have provided estimated nutrient requirements for infants with birth weight from 500 to 1800 g. Required intakes have been estimated to be 3.2 to 3.5g/kg per day of protein via the parenteral route and 3.6 to 4g/kg per day by the enteral route.[13] Energy intakes have been estimated to be 89 to 109 kcal/kg per day by the parenteral route and 105 to 128 kcal/kg per day by the enteral route. The consensus from the literature about parenteral requirements by age is shown in Tables 22.2 through 22.4.[14]

IV

Table 22.2
Components of Maintenance Parenteral Nutrition in Infants and Children*

	Weight		
Base Components	<10 kg	10–20 kg	>20 kg
Fluid	100–150 mL/kg	1000 mL + 50 mL/ kg >10 kg	1500 mL + 20 mL/kg >20 kg
Calories, kcal/kg[†] Dextrose, g/kg (3.4 kcal/g)	80–130 10–30	60–90 8–28	30–75 5–20
Protein, g/kg[†] (1 g protein = 0.16 g nitrogen)	1.5–3	1–2.5	0.8–2.0
Fat, g/kg	0.5–4	1–3	1–3
Additive	Infants and Toddlers	Children	Adolescents
Sodium	2–4 mEq/kg	2–4 mEq/kg	60–150 mEq
Potassium	2–4 mEq/kg	2–4 mEq/kg	70–180 mEq
Chloride	2–4 mEq/kg	2–4 mEq/kg	60–150 mEq

Table 22.2 (*Continued*)
Components of Maintenance Parenteral Nutrition in Infants and Children*

	Weight		
Magnesium (125 mg/mEq)	0.25–1 mEq/kg	0.25–1 mEq/kg	8–32 mEq
Calcium[‡] (20 mg/mEq)	0.45–4 mEq/kg	0.45–3.15 mEq/kg	10–40 mEq
Phosphorus (31 mg/mmol)	0.5–2 mmol/kg	0.5–2 mmol/kg	9–30 mmol/kg
Heparin (optional)	0.5–1 U/mL	0.5–1 U/mL	0.5–1 U/mL
Trace elements	0.2 mL/kg (pediatric trace elements)[§]	0.2 mL/kg (pediatric trace elements)[§]	5 mL (adult trace elements)[§]
Selenium (maximum 30 µg/day)	2 µg/kg	2 µg/kg	2 µg/kg
Molybdenum (maximum 5 µg/day)	0.25 µg/kg	0.25 µg/kg	0.25 µg/kg
Adult multivitamin (maximum 10 mL/day)[¶]	NA	NA	10 mL[#]
Pediatric multivitamin (maximum 5 mL/day)[¶]	<2.5 kg: 2 mL/kg	2.5–40 kg: 5 mL	>40 kg: NA

NA indicates not applicable.
* See Chapter 4 for preterm infants.
[†] Ideal weight (50th percentile for length or height).
[‡] If given as calcium gluconate: 1 mL of a 10% solution of calcium gluconate provides 9.3 mg of elemental calcium.
[§] See Table 22.3. If patient receives parenteral nutrition for more than 30 days with no significant enteral intake, the addition of trace elements is advisable.
Omit copper and manganese in patients with obstructive jaundice; omit selenium, chromium, and molybdenum in patients with renal dysfunction. Maximum pediatric trace elements: 5 mL/day.
[¶] See Table 22.4.
[#] Add 200 µg of vitamin K (phytonadione).

Table 22.3
Parenteral Trace Element Solutions*

Ingredient	Adult Trace/mL	Pediatric Trace/mL
Zinc	1 mg	0.5 mg
Copper	0.4 mg	0.1 mg
Manganese	100 µg	30 µg
Chromium	4 µg	1 µg

*Trace Elements Injection 4, USP Pediatric, American Regent Laboratories Inc, Shirley, NY.

Carbohydrate

Glucose (dextrose), fructose, galactose, sorbitol, glycerol, and ethanol all have been used as sources of carbohydrate calories in infants. The small amount of glycerol present in lipid emulsions contributes to carbohydrate calories. The other carbohydrate sources have no advantage over glucose and can produce serious complications in preterm infants.

Table 22.4
Parenteral Vitamin Solutions

Ingredient	Adult MVI/10 mL*	Pediatric MVI/5 mL*
Vitamin A	1.0 mg (3300 U)	0.7 mg (2300 U)
Vitamin D	5 μg (200 U)	10 μg (400 U)
Vitamin E	10 mg (10 U)	7 mg (7 U)
Vitamin B$_1$	6 mg	1.2 mg
Vitamin B$_2$	3.6 mg	1.4 mg
Vitamin B$_6$	6 mg	1 mg
Niacin	40 mg	17 mg
Dexpanthenol	15 mg	5 mg
Folic acid	600 μg	140 μg
Vitamin B$_{12}$	5 μg	1 μg
Biotin	60 μg	20 μg
Ascorbic acid	200 mg	80 mg
Vitamin K$_1$	150 μg	200 μg

*AstraZeneca LP, Westborough, MA.

The quantity of infused glucose that preterm infants tolerate varies. Infusing glucose at 5 mg/kg per minute and advancing gradually to 15 mg/kg per minute over several days may reduce intolerance. This is best accomplished by increasing the concentration of glucose in the solution while keeping the volume of infusate constant at between 80 and 150 mL/kg per day, depending on the infant's fluid requirements. Gradual increases of 2.5% to 5% dextrose per day are usually well tolerated. The consequences of acute intolerance to glucose are serum hyperosmolarity and osmotic diuresis, which can be avoided by careful monitoring. Hypoglycemia is usually related to the sudden cessation of the parenteral nutrition solution. In adult postsurgical patients, an increase in the glucose infusion rate from 4 to 7 mg/kg per minute is associated with an increased rate of glucose oxidation; at higher infusion rates, fat is synthesized from the glucose without a further increase in oxidation.[15] Higher glucose loads delivered by solutions containing more than 25% dextrose at 150 mL/kg per day (>26 mg/kg per minute) may not be beneficial to infants and may contribute to the fatty infiltration of the liver.

Continuous insulin infusion (0.01–0.1 unit/kg per hour) has been shown to be safe and effective in managing hyperglycemia in the neonate[16,17] and in promoting greater weight gain.[18,19] However, little is known about its effects on quality of weight gain and counter-regulatory hormone concentrations. One study demonstrated a significant increase in plasma lactate as a result of insulin therapy.[20] Further study of the effects of insulin in infants is suggested before it is recommended for routine use.[21]

Protein

Current solutions supply nitrogen requirements as crystalline amino acids. Infants have demonstrated adequate growth with this source of protein. Commercial products available as 6% or 10% solutions (eg, TrophAmine [B. Braun Medical Inc, Bethlehem, PA], Aminosyn PF [Hospira, Lake Forest, IL], Premasol [Baxter, Deerfield, IL]) have been specially formulated to meet the special requirements of neonates (see Appendix T). The latter solution was approved by the US Food and Drug Administration (FDA) as a sulfite-free product. These solutions contain taurine, tyrosine, histidine, aspartic acid, and glutamic acid, all of which are found in human milk. They contain lower concentrations of methionine, glycine, and phenylalanine than are found in amino-acid solutions intended for older patients. The plasma amino acid profile of infants receiving these solutions for nutritional maintenance is similar to that of term breastfed infants. In addition, greater weight gain and positive nitrogen balance are achieved by infants receiving these formulations than by infants receiving standard adult amino-acid solutions. These solutions may reduce the incidence of parenteral nutrition-induced cholestasis in neonates who receive parenteral nutrition for long periods.[22,23] Two studies demonstrate a significantly lower incidence of cholestasis with TrophAmine compared with Aminosyn PF.[24,25]

The commercial solutions do not contain cysteine, although separate preparations of cysteine can be added to the solutions. Cysteine must be added during compounding, because it converts to its dimeric form and precipitates over time in solution. Cysteine may be an essential amino acid in infants with low activity of hepatic cystathionine gamma-lyase, which converts methionine to cysteine. Taurine, which is formed from cysteine and is present in human milk, may also be important in preterm infants. Tyrosine is provided as N-acetyl-L-tyrosine (0.24%).[26] Albumin at a dose of 0.5 to 1.0 g/kg per day may be administered to patients receiving parenteral nutrition who have hypoalbuminemia from nonnutritive causes. Such infusions are for oncotic—never nutritive—benefits, because albumin has a long half-life and is not useful nutritionally. Albumin should be infused separately via a "Y" connector and not placed in the parenteral nutrition solution, because (1) albumin is a blood product and should not be hung for more than 8 hours; (2) recent concerns exist about flocculation of albumin in parenteral nutrition solutions; and (3) albumin in parenteral nutrition solutions increases the risk of sepsis.[2,21] Because albumin contains a significant amount of aluminum, caution should be exercised with the routine use of exogenous albumin in parenteral nutrition for neonates (see Chapter 19).

No commercially available parenteral nutrition amino-acid solution currently contains glutamine (primarily because of its short shelf life when placed in solution), the most abundant amino acid in both plasma and human milk.[27] Glutamine is a primary fuel for enterocytes, lymphocytes, and macrophages and is a precursor for nucleotide synthesis and glutathione, an important antioxidant. Previous studies in animals and critically ill adults have suggested that parenteral nutrition supplemented with glutamine reduces the risk of sepsis and mortality.[28,29] However, in a large, multicentered, randomized, double-masked clinical trial, glutamine supplementation of infants between 401 and 1000 g did not decrease the mortality rate or incidence of late-onset sepsis. Although well tolerated, routine supplementation was not recommended.[30] Glutamine supplementation may be of value in infants with very low birth weight and pediatric patients with short-bowel syndrome.[31] A small, randomized trial conducted by Lacey and colleagues showed no adverse effects of parenteral glutamine supplementation in preterm infants.[32] In the subgroup of infants with birth weight <800 g, they also found that infants receiving glutamine required fewer days on parenteral nutrition (13 vs 21 days) had shorter length of time to full enteral feeds (8 vs 14 days) and needed less time on the ventilator (38 vs 47 days). In addition, the <800-g subgroup receiving glutamine supplementation had a significantly higher lymphocyte count and fewer infants with episodes of neutropenia versus the control group. No significant toxicities were seen in infants who received 20% of their protein intake as glutamine.

Despite the recognized potential deficiencies, infants have tolerated the available solutions and have grown well while using them. Most metabolic

IV

complications related to amino acids, such as azotemia and acidosis, have occurred when infants received more than 4 g of protein equivalent/kg per day and from earlier total parenteral nutrition preparations. Complications are rarely encountered with the recommended intake of 1.5 to 3 g of protein equivalent/kg per day.

Lipids

The composition, use, and complications of intravenous fat emulsions have been discussed previously.[21,33] They are a concentrated source of energy, provide essential fatty acids, and are iso-osmolar. When lipid and amino-acid/glucose solutions are infused simultaneously into the same vein, the patient receives a higher-energy and lower-osmolar solution (which helps spare peripheral veins) than with a glucose and amino-acid solution alone. The use of "Y" connector tubing after the in-line filter (Micropore [Micropore Technologies Ltd, Leicestershire, United Kingdom]) to infuse lipids simultaneously with, but separately from, the amino-acid/glucose solution has greatly improved the effectiveness of peripheral intravenous nutrition and increased substantially its use in nutritional support.

Some centers are using a 3-in-1 solution (also called a total nutrient admixture), in which the lipid emulsion is mixed with the amino-acid/glucose solution and administered through a single line. This method of delivery has certain advantages: (1) simplified administration, which may prove to be a cost savings; (2) less manipulation of the delivery system (reduced opportunity for contamination); (3) lessened loss of vitamin A; and (4) continuous infusion of all nutrients. One retrospective study of 3-in-1 solutions in infants found such use safe, efficacious, and cost-effective for infants younger than 1 year.[34] If these infusates are administered without an in-line filter, the presence of lipid in the infusate will obscure any visual precipitation that may occur on removal from refrigeration (4°C) and warming before or during administration. However, a 1.2-Tm (maximal tubular transport rate) in-line filter is available that can be used with lipids. The use of 3-in-1 solutions in infants with low birth weight may compromise efforts to maximize calcium and phosphate intakes to meet their high requirements. The addition of lipid emulsion to the amino-acid/glucose solution increases the pH of the solution, which may result in a decrease in solubility of calcium and phosphorus; therefore, a lower concentration of these nutrients is available to the infant. On April 18, 1994, a safety alert was issued by the FDA about 3-in-1 solutions, because one institution reported 2 deaths and 2 cases of respiratory distress using such solutions. The solutions may have contained a precipitate of calcium phosphate. Autopsies revealed diffuse microvascular pulmonary emboli containing calcium phosphate.[21] However, the precipitates were caused by improper preparation of the solution, and 3-in-1 solutions are widely and safely used in pediatrics. Iron is not compatible with 3-in-1 solutions. This is particularly a problem for home administration of total parenteral nutrition solutions, because 3-in-1 formulations simplify administration, and patients who receive long-term total parenteral nutrition are most likely to need iron supplementation.[2]

The requirement for alpha-linoleic acid (an essential fatty acid) can be achieved by supplying 0.5 to 1 g/kg per day of intravenous lipid. Small amounts of alpha-linolenic acid should also be included, perhaps one tenth the amount of linoleic acid. Preterm infants younger than 32 weeks' gestation may be unable to clear lipid doses in excess of 2 g/kg per day. Nephelometry results and visual inspection of serum for turbidity correlate well with serum chylomicron concentration but not well with triglyceride or free fatty acid concentrations; therefore, serum lipid monitoring is required. Serum triglyceride concentrations can be determined by microtechnique by most laboratories, which allows for frequent triglyceride monitoring as the intravenous lipid doses are advanced (Table 22.1). Continuous infusion of up to 3 g/kg per day of intravenous lipid should minimize the chance of lipid intolerance. Under certain circumstances (eg, sepsis), the lowest dose that meets essential fatty acid requirements should be used to avoid potential complications.

The lipid preparation of choice is 20% intravenous fat, because it is cleared more efficiently than 10% fat emulsions. The phospholipid-triglyceride ratio is 0.12 in 10% intravenous fat and 0.06 in 20% intravenous fat. Phospholipid is believed to inhibit lipoprotein lipase, the main enzyme for intravenous fat clearance; therefore, using a fat emulsion with the lowest ratio of phospholipid to triglyceride (eg, 20% fat emulsions) is preferable. Recently, concerns have been raised about the safety of using fat emulsions during the first week of life in the preterm infant.[35] Toxic lipid peroxidation products in fat emulsions may lead to the development of chronic lung disease, and ambient and phototherapy light increases this lipid oxidation.[36] Data to date are conflicting but disturbing. This adds to the previously known photo-oxidation of amino acids and has implications for the development of hepatic dysfunction.[37] No available parenteral nutrition solutions contain carnitine, which is required for the optimal metabolism of fatty acids. Infants have a poorly developed capacity to synthesize and store carnitine. Some experts recommend supplementation (2.4 to 10 mg/kg per day in preterm and term infants),[38,39] but the lack of carnitine in parenteral

IV

nutrition formulations has not been associated with any clinical deficiency syndrome, and the results of clinical studies of its addition to parenteral nutrition formulations have been contradictory.

Vitamins, Minerals, and Trace Elements

Vitamins, minerals, and trace elements must be supplied in parenteral solutions. Metabolic complications have been described for deficiencies and excesses of some of these nutrients. Intravenous dose requirements are not fully known. Guidelines from an expert panel[40] for multivitamin and trace element preparations for parenteral use are shown in Tables 22.5 and 22.6.

Table 22.5
Suggested Daily Intakes of Parenteral Vitamins in Infants and Children

Vitamin	Term Infants and Children ≥2.5 kg	Infants <2.5 kg*
Lipid soluble†		
A, µg	700	280
E, mg	7	2.80
K, µg	200	80
D, IU‡	400	160
Water soluble		
Ascorbic acid, mg	80	32
Thiamine, mg	1.2	0.48
Riboflavin, mg	1.4	0.56
Pyridoxine, mg	1.0	0.40
Niacin, mg	17	6.80
Pantothenate, mg	5	2
Biotin, µg	20	8
Folic acid, µg	140	56
Vitamin B_{12}, µg	1	0.40

* Dose/kg of body weight per day for preterm infants, not to exceed daily dose for term (≥2.5 kg) infants.

† 700 µg retinol equivalents = 2300 IU; 7 mg alpha-tocopherol = 7 IU; 10 µg vitamin D = 400 IU.

‡ Recent data indicate that 40 IU/kg per day of vitamin D (maximum of 400 IU/day) is adequate for term and preterm infants. The higher dose of 160 IU/kg per day has not been associated with complications and maintains blood concentrations within the reference range for term infants fed orally. This dosage, therefore, appears acceptable until further studies using the lower-dose formulation indicate its superiority.

A higher, more physiologic calcium-phosphorus ratio of 1.7:1 by weight (1.3:1 by molar ratio, similar to the fetal mineral accretion ratio) allows for the highest absolute retention of both minerals. This ratio provides 76 mg/kg per day of elemental calcium and 45 mg/kg per day of phosphorus.[41] Dunham et al[42] have generated calcium and phosphorus precipitation curves for parenteral nutrition using TrophAmine (its low pH allows for the maximum possible calcium and phosphorous in solution) to help pharmacists and clinicians avoid compounding total parenteral nutrition solutions that will precipitate. Different precipitation curves for parenteral nutrition should be used if Aminosyn PF is used or cysteine is added to the base amino-acid solution. Precipitation information can also be found in the package inserts of the amino-acid solutions.

Table 22.6
Suggested Parenteral Intakes of Trace Minerals in Infants and Children

Element	Preterm, µg/kg per day	Term, µg/kg per day	Children, µg/kg per day (Maximum, µg/day)
Zinc*	400	250 <3 mo	50 (5000) 100 ≥3 mo
Copper[†]	20	20	20 (300)
Selenium[‡]	2	2	2 (30)
Chromium[‡]	0.20	0.20	0.20 (5.0)
Manganese[†]	1	1	1 (50)
Molybdenum[‡§]	0.25	0.25	0.25 (5.0)
Iodide	1	1	1 (1.0)

* When total parenteral nutrition is supplemental only or is limited to less than 4 weeks, only zinc need be added. Thereafter, addition of the remaining elements is advisable.

[†] Omit in patients with obstructive jaundice. (Manganese and copper are excreted primarily in bile.)

[‡] Omit in patients with renal dysfunction.

[§] Available concentrations of molybdenum and manganese are such that dilution of the manufacturer's product may be necessary. Neotrace (Lyphomed Co, Rosemont, IL) contains a higher ratio of manganese to zinc than suggested in this table (ie, zinc: 1.5 mg, and manganese: 25 µg in each mL).

Vitamin A supplementation for infants with very low birth weight has been used to decrease the risk of bronchopulmonary dysplasia.[43,44] This must be delivered intramuscularly, not in parenteral nutrition solutions and is discussed in Chapter 4.

A number of substances commonly administered intravenously, including calcium and phosphorus salts and albumin, have high concentrations of aluminum. Preterm infants receiving intravenous fluid therapy may accumulate aluminum and show evidence of aluminum toxicity.[45] Calcium gluconate can contribute up to 80% of the total aluminum load from parenteral nutrition. The FDA has proposed labeling requirements concerning aluminum contents on parenteral nutrition additives, establishing an upper limit permitted in parenteral nutrition additives, and has suggested that manufacturers develop validated assay methods.[46] Bishop and others demonstrated developmental delay in preterm infants on parenteral nutrition solutions receiving aluminum at a rate of 45 µg/kg per day.[47] Aluminum intake should be determined in children at high risk of toxicity, including preterm infants, infants, or children with impaired renal function, as well as patients receiving prolonged parenteral nutrition.[21]

Ordering Parenteral Nutrition

Preprinted parenteral nutrition order sheets or computerized, commercially available total parenteral nutrition ordering programs save time for the house staff, nutritionists, and pharmacy personnel. In addition, order sheets helps to avoid errors of omission, ensuring that all necessary nutrients are ordered. However, order sheets have limitations; they require manual calculations at times, and they do not provide nutrition education, just generic reminders. Computerized programs have the potential of providing nutrition education as well as minimizing errors of commission and omission. Required data for some of these programs include the patient's weight (in kg), total fluid intake for the day (mL/kg per day), the amount of fat emulsion (g/kg per day), fat concentration (10% or 20%), fluid volumes contributed by other parenteral solutions or enteral feedings, desired protein intake via amino acids (g/kg per day), and the percentage concentration of dextrose. The doses of trace elements, vitamins, and electrolytes are ordered in amounts per day or amounts per kg per day. The computer performs all necessary calculations. The output of the computer program includes:

1. Total parenteral nutrition and fat emulsion bottle labels;
2. Mixing instructions for the pharmacy with calcium phosphate precipitation curve data; and
3. A detailed nutritional summary including calories, nitrogen ratio, kcal/kg per day, and percentage of total calories to be given as fat.

The American Academy of Pediatrics recommends the following:

1. Aluminum-containing phosphate binders should not be administered to infants and children with renal failure.
2. Continued efforts should be made to reduce the amount of aluminum in products that are added to intravenous solutions that are used for preterm infants and infants and children with renal failure.
3. Continued efforts should be made to reduce the aluminum content of all formulas used for infants, but especially soy formulas and formulas tailored specifically for preterm infants.
4. In infants at risk of developing aluminum toxicity (renal failure and prematurity), attention should be paid to the aluminum content of the water used in reconstitution of infant formulas.

Table 22.7
Complications Associated With Parenteral Nutrition

Type	Complication
Metabolic	Hypo- or hyperglycemia Electrolyte imbalance Metabolic bone disease Hepatic dysfunction
Infectious	Bacterial sepsis Fungal sepsis
Mechanical	Extravasation Pericardial effusion, pleural effusion Diaphragmatic palsy

Adapted from Bhatia J, Bucher C, Bunyapen C. Feeding the premature infant. In: Berdanier CD, ed. *Handbook of Nutrition and Food.* Boca Raton, FL: CRC Press; 2002:203–218

IV

Metabolic complications (Table 22.7) can be avoided by careful assessment of tolerance to the macronutrients as nutrition delivery is advanced. Early recognition of metabolic effects (by a pharmacist or nutritionist) or catheter-related effects (by nursing staff) could help minimize the potential complications of parenteral nutrition. The most common complications observed are hepatic dysfunction and metabolic bone disease.

Gastrointestinal and Hepatic Effects of Parenteral Nutrition

Hepatic disease is the major complication of parenteral nutrition. When the liver is examined histologically, cholestasis, hepatocellular necrosis, and in advanced cases, cirrhosis may be found.[48] The hepatic response to total parenteral nutrition depends on the age of the patient. A cholestatic response predominates in infants; steatosis and steatohepatitis develop in older children and adults. In either case, end-stage liver disease may result. Biliary sludge and cholelithiasis occur in both groups. In infants, the first clinical indication of parenteral nutrition-induced injury is mild hepatomegaly followed by biochemical evidence of cholestasis. The first biochemical abnormality is an increase in serum bile salts (not available for clinical use), followed by an increase in conjugated bilirubin concentration with other enzymes demonstrating late increases. Serum conjugated bilirubin concentration increases are the most specific but least sensitive indicator of cholestasis. These changes may develop any time after 2 to 3 weeks of total parenteral nutrition. Serum alkaline phosphatase and transaminase concentrations increase days to weeks later. Steatosis is the result of excess energy infusions, usually in the form of glucose.[49]

Enteral starvation is a critical factor in the pathogenesis of total parenteral nutrition-related hepatic disease. The most severe hepatic pathologic changes are noted in patients with the poorest enteral intake. Significantly fewer cases of serious hepatic disease have been documented in recent years because of more appropriate amino acids (especially for neonates) and the earlier initiation of enteral feeding (stimulating bile flow and increasing secretion of gastrointestinal hormones). In all patients receiving parenteral nutrition, enteral feedings should be initiated as soon as possible, even if only in minimal amounts (trophic feedings), to minimize the risk of hepatic dysfunction.

Less is known about the long-term effects of total parenteral nutrition on the stomach, pancreas, and small bowel. Studies in animals have documented decreased pancreatic secretion and intestinal mucosal atrophy, which are reversible on resumption of enteric feeding. A few studies in humans suggest that exocrine pancreatic secretion and gastric parietal cell mass are decreased and that the small intestine atrophies during total parenteral nutrition, although the observed changes are minor. Amino acids infused intravenously stimulate gastric acid secretion, but much less so than if these solutions are infused into the stomach. Gastrointestinal effects disappear over a variable period after return to enteral nutrition. Although similar studies have not been performed in preterm infants, clinical experience suggests that enteric function in preterm infants also returns to normal with time.

Preterm infants are at high risk of the development of metabolic bone disease, most commonly attributable to inadequate intakes of calcium and phosphorus during parenteral nutrition. In general, both calcium and phosphorus concentrations are maintained in serum, whereas the bones appear more osteopenic on radiographs, and ultimately, hypophosphatemia with increasing alkaline phosphatase concentration is observed. An increasing alkaline phosphatase concentration in the absence of increased liver enzymes is a strong indicator of metabolic bone disease. Incidence of rickets or metabolic bone disease is inversely proportional to birth weight and has been reported to be as high as 50% to 60% in infants with very low birth weight.

Compatibilities

The approach to interrupting parenteral nutrition therapy for drug administration differs from institution to institution and should be carefully discussed with pharmacy staff and the institution's parenteral nutrition committee. Acyclovir, amphotericin B, metronidazole, and trimethoprim-sulfamethoxazole cannot be given with the parenteral nutrition solution. They may be given in 10% dextrose with the parenteral nutrition turned off. Bicarbonate also should not be given with the parenteral nutrition solution. Ranitidine is compatible with parenteral nutrition solutions. However, the association of the use of ranitidine and sepsis in neonates should be considered before a decision to use ranitidine routinely is made. Information about the compatibility of individual drugs with parenteral nutrition is available in the pharmacy of all major hospitals.

IV

Transition to Enteral Feedings

Initiation of enteral feedings should begin as soon as the gastrointestinal tract is functional. Initially, enteral feedings may supplement parenteral nutrition. Parenteral nutrition should not be discontinued until the patient tolerates enteral feedings well enough to meet nutritional requirements. The central catheter may be kept in place until the patient tolerates full enteral feedings. Enteral feedings provide less risk of infection, are less expensive, are associated with fewer metabolic abnormalities, and facilitate recovery of intestinal morphology and enzymes. See Chapter 23 for further details.

Conclusion

The nutritional requirements of young infants, preterm and term, can be met better by recognizing their limitations in absorption and digestion. When gastrointestinal disease is superimposed on an immature digestive system, special nutrition support is needed to maintain adequate growth. This support can be given with parenteral or specialized enteral feeding techniques and formulations. Because parenteral solutions can provide complete nutrition support, they may be used for extended periods. Recommendations for use include the following:

1. Catheters should be placed carefully, and position should be confirmed by radiography; aseptic techniques and established guidelines of catheter care should be followed strictly; and patients should be monitored, clinically and by laboratory testing, for intolerance to components of the parenteral nutrition solution.

Table 22.8
Parenteral Nutrition Advancing Guidelines

Guideline by Age	Dextrose	Fat, g/kg per day	Amino Acids, g/kg per day
Preterm infant			
Initial	4–6 mg/kg per min	0.5	2.5–3.5[†]
Advance*	1–2 mg/kg per min	05	0.5
Term neonate			
Initial	5%	0.5–1.0	2.5
Advance*	2.5%	0.5	0.5
Older infant/child			
Initial	10%	1.0	1.5
Advance*	5%	0.5–1.0	1.0
Adolescent and older			
Initial	10%	1.0	1.5
Advance*	5%–10%	1.0	1.0

* Rate of advancement may be limited by metabolic tolerance (eg, hyperglycemia, hypertriglyceridemia, azotemia).

† When given parenteral glucose alone, an infant will lose 1% of body protein stores per day.[50] A number of studies over the past 12 years indicate that most preterm infants will tolerate 2.5 to 3.5 g/kg per day of parenteral amino acid intake on the first day of life.[51–53]

2. Protein should be provided in the form of crystalline amino acids at a rate of 1.5 to 3 g/kg per day. The concentration of glucose should be advanced methodically to ensure tolerance. Essential fatty acid requirements can be met by infusing 0.5 to 1 g/kg per day of intravenous lipid.

The continuous infusion (over 24 hours) of up to 3 g/kg per day of intravenous lipid should maximize tolerance. Vitamins, minerals, and trace elements are essential nutrients and should be contained in parenteral nutrition solutions. See Table 22.8 for suggested advancing guidelines for macronutrients.

3. The transition to enteral nutrition should begin as soon as possible, with continuation of parenteral nutrition until full nutritional support is achieved via the gastrointestinal tract.

4. Nutritional status should be monitored continuously to ensure the adequacy of nutritional support. A nutrition support team with expertise in parenteral nutrition can help to provide optimal care, decrease costs and complications, and potentially, shorten the length of hospitalization.

References

1. Fischer JE. *Total Parenteral Nutrition.* 2nd ed. Boston, MA: Little Brown & Co Inc; 1991

2. Acra SA, Rollins C. Principles and guidelines for parenteral nutrition in children. *Pediatr Ann.* 1999;28:113–120

3. Lumpkin MM. Safety alert: hazards of precipitation associated with parenteral nutrition. *Am J Hosp Pharm.* 1994;51:1427–1428

4. Cobel MR. Compounding pediatric dextrose solutions. Medications error alert. *ASHP Newsletter.* 1995;August

5. ASPEN Board of Directors and the Clinical Guidelines Task Force. Guidelines for the use of parenteral and enteral nutrition in adult and pediatric patients. *JPEN J Parenter Enteral Nutr.* 2002;26(1 Suppl):1SA–138SA

6. Sznajder JI, Zveibil FR, Bitterman H, Weiner P, Bursztein S. Central vein catheterization, failure and complication rates by three percutaneous approaches. *Arch Intern Med.* 1986;146:259–261

7. Mermel L: Central venous catheter-related infections and their prevention: is there enough evidence to recommend tunneling for short-term use? *Crit Care Med.* 1998;26:1315–1316

8. Veenstra DL, Saint S, Sullivan SD. Cost effectiveness of the antiseptic-impregnated central venous catheters for the prevention of catheter-related bloodstream infection. *JAMA.* 1999;282:554–560

9. Loughran SC, Borzatta M. Peripherally inserted central catheters: a report of 2506 catheter days. *JPEN J Parenter Enteral Nutr.* 1995;19:133–136

10. Cowl CT, Weinstock JV, Al-Jurf A, Ephgrave K, Murray JA, Dillon K. Complications and cost associated with parenteral nutrition delivered to hospitalized patients through either subclavian or peripherally-inserted central catheters *Clin Nutr.* 2000;19:237–243

11. Maki DG, ed. *Improving Catheter Site Care.* London, England: Royal Society of Medicine; 1991

IV

12. Haire WD, Herbst SL. Use of Alteplase (t-PA) for the management of thrombotic catheter dysfunction: guidelines from a consensus conference of the National Association of Vascular Access Networks (NAVAN). *Nutr Clin Pract.* 2000;15:265–275

13. Adamkin DH. Feeding the preterm infant. In: Bhatia J, ed. *Perinatal Nutrition: Optimizing Infant Health and Development.* New York, NY: Marcel Dekker; 2005:165–190

14. Chan DS. Recommended daily allowance of maintenance parenteral nutrition in infants and children. *Am J Health Syst Pharm.* 1995;52:651–653

15. Wolfe RR, Allsop JR, Burke JF. Glucose metabolism in man: responses to intravenous glucose infusion. *Metabolism.* 1979;28:210–220

16. Heron P, Bourchier D. Insulin infusions in infants of birthweight less than 1250 g and with glucose intolerance. *Aust Pediatr J.* 1988;24:362–365

17. Kanarek KS, Santeiro ML, Malone JI. Continuous infusion of insulin in hyperglycemic low-birth-weight infants receiving parenteral nutrition with and without lipids. *JPEN J Parenter Enteral Nutr.* 1991;15:417–420

18. Collins JW Jr, Hoppe M, Brown L, Edidin DV, Padbury J, Ogata ES. A controlled trial of insulin infusion and parenteral nutrition in extremely low birth weight infants with glucose intolerance. *J Pediatr.* 1991;118:921–927

19. Ostertag SG, Javanovic L, Lewis B, Auld PA. Insulin pump therapy in the very low birth weight infant. *Pediatrics.* 1986;78:625–630

20. Poindexter BB, Karn CA, Denne SC. Exogenous insulin reduces proteolysis and protein synthesis in extremely low birth weight infants. *J Pediatr.* 1998;132:948–953

21. Mascarenhas MR, Kerner JA Jr, Stallings VA. Parenteral and enteral nutrition. In: Walker WA, Durie PR, Hamilton JR, Walker-Smith JA, Watkins JB, eds. *Pediatric Gastrointestinal Disease.* 3rd ed. Toronto, Ontario: BC Decker Inc; 2000;1705–1752

22. Heird WC, Dell RB, Helms RA, et al. Amino acid mixture designed to maintain normal plasma amino acid patterns in infants and children requiring parenteral nutrition. *Pediatrics.* 1987;80:401–408

23. Heird WC, Hay W, Helms RA, Storm MC, Kashyap S, Dell RB. Pediatric parenteral amino acid mixtures in low birth weight infants. *Pediatrics.* 1988;81:41–50

24. Ernst K, Gaylord M, Burnette T, et al. Aminosyn PF associated with doubled incidence of neonatal cholestasis (abstr). *Pediatr Res (Suppl).* 2000;47:286A

25. Cloney DB, Bouthillier MJ, Staublin SA, et al. Total parenteral nutrition-associated cholestasis in neonates receiving two different pediatric amino acid formulations (abstr). *Pharmacotherapy.* 1996:16:66

26. Zlotkin SH, Bryan MH, Anderson GH. Intravenous nitrogen and energy intakes required to duplicate in utero nitrogen accretion in prematurely born human infants. *J Pediatr.* 1981;99:115–120

27. Bulus N, Cerosimo E, Gishan F, Abumrad N. Physiologic importance of glutamine. *Metabolism.* 1989;38(8 Suppl 1):1–5

28. Griffiths RD, Jones C, Palmer TE. Six-month outcome of critically ill patients given glutamine-supplemented parenteral nutrition. *Nutrition.* 1997;13:295–302

29. Ziegler TR, Young LS, Benfell K, et al. Clinical and metabolic efficacy of glutamine-supplemented parenteral nutrition after bone marrow transplantation. A randomized, double-blind, controlled study. *Ann Intern Med.* 1992;116:821–828

30. Poindexter BB, Erenkranz RA, Stoll BJ, et al. Parenteral glutamine supplementation does not reduce the risk of mortality or late-onset sepsis in extremely low birth weight infants. National Institute of Child Health and Human Development Neonatal Research Network. *Pediatrics.* 2004;113:1209–1215

31. LeLeiko NS, Walsh MJ. The role of glutamine, short chain fatty acids, and nucleotides in intestinal adaptation to gastrointestinal disease. *Pediatr Clin North Am.* 1996;43:451–470

32. Lacey JM, Crouch JB, Benfell K, et al. The effects of glutamine-supplemented parenteral nutrition in premature infants. *JPEN J Parenter Enteral Nutr.* 1996; 20:74–80

33. American Academy of Pediatrics, Committee on Nutrition. Use of intravenous fat emulsions in pediatric patients. *Pediatrics.* 1981;68:738–743

34. Rollins CJ, Elsberry VA, Pollack KA, Pollack PF, Udall JN Jr. Three-in-one parenteral nutrition: a safe and economical method of nutritional support for infants *JPEN J Parenter Enteral Nutr.* 1990;14:290–294

35. Sosenko IR. Intravenous lipids and the management of chronic lung injury: helpful or harmful? *Semin Neonatal Nutr Metab.* 1995;3:3–5

36. Neuzil J, Darlow BA, Inder TE, Sluis KB, Winterbourn CC, Stocker R. Oxidation of parenteral lipid emulsion by ambient and phototherapy lights: potential toxicity of routine parenteral feeding. *J Pediatr.* 1995;126:785–790

37. Bhatia J, Moslen MT, Haque AK, McCleery R, Rassin DK. Total parenteral nutrition-associated alterations in hepatobiliary function and histology in rats; is light exposure a clue? *Pediatr Res.* 1993;33:487–492

38. Koo WWK, Cepeda EE. Parenteral nutrition in neonates. In: Rombeau JL, Rolandelli RH, eds. *Clinical Nutrition: Parenteral Nutrition.* 3rd ed. Philadelphia, PA: W.B. Saunders Co; 2001;463–475

39. Falcone RA Jr, Warner BW. Pediatric parenteral nutrition. In: Rombeau JL, Rolandelli, RH, eds. *Clinical Nutrition: Parenteral Nutrition.* 3rd ed. Philadelphia, PA: W.B. Saunders Co; 2001;476–496

40. Greene HL, Hambidge KM, Schanler R, Tsang RC. Guidelines for the use of vitamins, trace elements, calcium, magnesium, and phosphorous in infants and children receiving total parenteral nutrition: report of the Subcommittee of Pediatric Parenteral Nutrient Requirements from the Committee on Clinical Practice Issues of the American Society for Clinical Nutrition. *Am J Clin Nutr.* 1988;48:1324–1342

41. Pelegano JF, Rowe JC, Carey DE, et al. Effect of calcium/phosphorous ratio on mineral retention in parenterally fed premature infants. *J Pediatr Gastroenterol Nutr.* 1991;12:351–355

42. Dunham B, Marcuard S, Khazanie PG, Meade G, Craft T, Nichols K. The solubility of calcium and phosphorus in neonatal total parenteral nutrition solutions. *JPEN J Parenter Enteral Nutr.* 1991;15:608–611

43. Hazinski TA. Vitamin A treatment for the infant at risk for bronchopulmonary dysplasia. *NeoReviews.* 2000;1:e11–e15

IV

44. Tyson JE, Wright LL, Oh W, et al. Vitamin A supplementation for extremely-low-birth-weight infants. National Institute of Child Health and Human Development Neonatal Research Network. *N Engl J Med.* 1999;340:1962–1968

45. American Academy of Pediatrics, Committee on Nutrition. Aluminum toxicity in infants and children. *Pediatrics.* 1996;97:413–416

46. Klein GL, Leichtner AM, Heyman MB. Aluminum in large and small volume parenterals used in total parenteral nutrition: response to the food and drug administration notice of proposed rule by the North American Society for Pediatric Gastroenterology and Nutrition. *J Pediatr Gastroenterol Nutr.* 1998;27:457–460

47. Bishop NJ, Morley R, Day JP, Lucas A. Aluminum neurotoxicity in preterm infants receiving intravenous-feeding solutions. *N Engl J Med.* 1997;29:1557–1561

48. Whitington PF. Cholestasis associated with total parenteral nutrition in infants. *Hepatology.* 1985;5:693–696

49. Quigley EM, Marsh MN, Shaffer JL, Markin RS. Hepatobiliary complications of total parenteral nutrition. *Gastroenterology.* 1993;104:286–301

50. Heird WC. The importance of early nutritional management of low-birthweight infants. *Pediatr Rev.* 1999;20(9):e43–e44

51. Thureen PJ. Early aggressive nutrition in the neonate. *Pediatr Rev.* 1999;20(9):e45–e55

52. te Braak FW, van den Akker CH, Wattimena DJ, Huijmans JG, van Goudoever JB. Amino acid administration to premature infants directly after birth. *J Pediatr.* 2005;147:457–461

53. Ibrahim HM, Jeroudi MA, Baier RJ, Dhanireddy R, Krouskop RW. Aggressive early total parental nutrition in low-birth-weight infants. *J Perinatol.* 2004;24:482–486

Enteral Nutrition

Pediatric patients who do not have adequate growth on oral intake may be given enteral nutrition for nutritional management. Commonly used enteral tube feeding routes include nasogastric, gastrostomy, nasojejunal, gastrojejunal, and jejunostomy. Although enteral and parenteral routes can be used to provide nutritional support to pediatric patients, enteral nutritional support is preferred because it is more "physiological" and economical and is easier and safer than parenteral feedings. Enteral nutrition produces fewer metabolic and infectious complications and better supports the integrity of the barrier function of the gastrointestinal tract. Enteral nutrition also allows for better physiological control of electrolyte concentrations and serves as effective prophylaxis against stress-induced gastropathy and gastrointestinal hemorrhage. Enteral nutrition also can provide a more complete range of nutrients, including glutamine, long-chain polyunsaturated fatty acids, short-chain fatty acids, and fiber. Finally, enteral nutrition provides a trophic effect on the gut by promoting pancreatic and biliary secretions as well as endocrine, paracrine, and neural factors that help promote the physiologic and immunologic integrity of the intestine. Timely initiation of enteral nutrition is also important, with the greatest metabolic benefits resulting from initiating early enteral nutrition within less than 72 hours of injury or admission. Within the setting of critical illness, however, enteral nutrition should not be initiated until the child achieves hemodynamic stability, thus minimizing the risk of bowel ischemia.[1]

IV

Indications for Enteral Tube Feedings: Management of Nutrition-Related Disorders (see Table 23.1)

Preterm Birth
A feeding method for preterm infants should be individualized to gestational age, birth weight, and medical status. Preterm infants present a unique nutritional challenge because of their gastrointestinal immaturity, limited fluid tolerance, high nutrient requirements, limited renal function, and predisposition to specific metabolic and clinical complications, such as hypoglycemia and necrotizing enterocolitis. Because the coordination of sucking and swallowing appears at approximately 34 weeks of gestation, intragastric or jejunal feedings are often used before this time. These techniques may be useful beyond 34 weeks in selected infants who are unable to achieve and/or tolerate adequate oral feedings. Studies in preterm infants suggest that minimal

enteral feedings (2–8 mL/kg per day) administered soon after birth promote a gastrointestinal hormonal response and, thus, mediate intestinal adaptation.[2] These small-volume, hypocaloric enteral feedings, in conjunction with parenteral nutrition, are used to prime the gut and are thought to promote maturation of gastrointestinal motor patterns, increase general growth and feeding tolerance, and encourage earlier progression to full enteral feedings and discharge from the hospital. For further information about feeding the preterm infant, see Chapter 4 (Nutritional Needs of the Preterm Infant).

Table 23.1
Conditions in Which Enteral Tube Feeding May Be Warranted*

Preterm birth	Protracted diarrhea of infancy
Cardiorespiratory illness	Chronic nonspecific diarrhea
Chronic lung disease	Renal disease
Cystic fibrosis	Hypermetabolic states
Congenital heart disease	Burn injury
Gastrointestinal tract disease and dysfunction	Severe trauma or closed head injury
Inflammatory bowel disease	Cancer
Short-bowel syndrome	Neurologic disease or cerebral palsy
Biliary atresia	Oral motor dysfunction
Gastroesophageal reflux	Inadequate spontaneous oral intake

* Adapted from Walker AW, Kleinman RE, Sherman PM, Sanderson IR, Goulet O, Shneider BL, eds. *Pediatric Gastrointestinal Disease.* 2nd ed. Burlington, Ontario: BC Decker Inc; 1995

Cardiorespiratory Illness

Infants and children with pulmonary disease often require enteral nutritional support during acute exacerbations of their primary disease and for nutritional rehabilitation of chronic secondary malnutrition. Growth failure in patients with neonatal chronic lung disease can be caused by hypoxia, hypercapnia, elevated metabolic rates, inefficient suck and swallow mechanisms, poor appetite, decreased intake, and recurrent emesis with decreased gastric motility. Children with cystic fibrosis (see also Chapter 46: Nutrition in Cystic Fibrosis) also have increased energy needs and poor intake, which results from their lung disease, malabsorption, chronic infection, debilitation, and fatigue. Nocturnal nasogastric feedings using elemental or polymeric nutrient formulas supplemented with pancreatic enzymes have been promoted for use with children and adolescents with cystic fibrosis in whom conservative nutritional supplement measures have failed. Short-term nasogastric feedings have resulted in increased caloric intake and significant weight gain for patients with cystic fibrosis, but long-term effectiveness may be limited by noncompliance. Gastrostomy tube feedings are more appropriate when long-term (beyond 3 months) infusions are required.

Infants with congenital heart disease (see also Chapter 45: Cardiac Disease) are also at significant nutritional risk. Growth failure resulting from inadequate intake and elevated energy expenditure may be caused by labored and rapid respiration, increased metabolic needs, decreased peripheral blood flow, tissue hypoxia, impaired absorption, and protein-losing enteropathy. Because of their elevated nutritional needs and limited fluid tolerance, infants with congenital heart disease often require formulas with high caloric density achieved through formula concentration (Appendix F, Table F-1). Concentration beyond 24 kcal/oz, although not absolutely contraindicated, may not allow enough free water for excretion of the renal osmotic load. When necessary, additional calories can be provided through carbohydrate (eg, Polycose [Abbot Laboratories, Abbott Park, IL]) or fat supplementation (eg, Microlipid [Novartis Medical Nutrition, Freemont, MI]) or supplementation with powdered infant formula. Infants with congenital heart disease often experience delayed gastric emptying that may result in early satiety or promote gastroesophageal reflux (GER).[3] Continuous nocturnal nasogastric feedings or 24-hour enteral feedings of infants with congenital heart disease may result in significant catch-up growth. Alternatively, providing intermittent oral feedings with nasogastric supplementation of the remainder of the required volume may also facilitate achievement of the nutritional goals.[4]

Gastrointestinal Disease and Dysfunction

Pediatric patients with acute and chronic gastrointestinal disease and dysfunction often benefit from enteral feeding regimens (see also Chapter 43: Inflammatory Bowel Disease). Growth failure in children with Crohn disease is multifactorial in origin but is most often related to inadequate nutrient intake. Elemental diets administered orally and nasogastrically have been demonstrated to produce a clinically significant improvement in nutritional status. Clinical remission of Crohn disease of the small bowel by the use of elemental diets alone has been reported, but this effect remains controversial.[5]

The nutritional management of short-bowel syndrome is particularly challenging and involves the artful implementation of enteral and parenteral nutrition. It inevitably involves the initial use of total parenteral nutrition. As soon as possible after recovery from surgery, enteral feedings should begin at a slow rate and should be advanced as tolerated. The period of transition to

IV

complete enteral feedings may take weeks to years, depending on the length of intestinal resection. If the ileocecal valve is preserved, the outcome may be improved, but overall length of the remaining intestine is the most important consideration determinant of ultimate recovery. Polymeric nutrients are usually not well tolerated in the initial stages of the enteral feeding progression, whereas glucose and glucose polymers, medium-chain triglycerides, and hydrolyzed protein and dipeptides, which require less digestion, are more easily tolerated.[6] Long-term parenteral nutrition for infants with short-bowel syndrome can lead to hepatic disease, including total parenteral nutrition-associated cholestasis, which is a significant cause of morbidity in infants and children with short-bowel syndrome. In fact, end-stage total parenteral nutrition cirrhosis is the most dire consequence of short-bowel syndrome and may be fatal unless a combined liver-intestine transplantation can be performed. Sepsis, bacterial overgrowth, and absence of enteral intake are factors that increase the probability of cholestasis. Enteral nutrition helps prevent hepatic disease in this situation. Cyclic (10–12 hours) total parenteral nutrition with continuous and intermittent enteral feedings plus oral intake as tolerated are usually the most successful strategies to avoid liver disease.[7]

When children with short-bowel syndrome are fed enterally, they will inevitably have diarrhea, and in general, it should be ignored as long as there is adequate weight gain and positive electrolyte and fluid balance. In particular, extra sodium should be provided if the serum sodium concentration is not well into the normal range. Prevention of diaper rashes is critical in this situation, because the diarrhea can be extreme. It is useful to monitor the number of diapers that have urine alone without fecal material as measure of the adequacy of fluid balance. As the concentration or volume of formula is advanced, ultimately, the maximum absorptive capability of the intestine will be exceeded and an abrupt increase in stool output will occur or the maximum rate of gastric emptying will be exceeded and emesis will occur. At that point, the feedings should be decreased and a variable amount of time should be allowed for the intestine to adapt to the increased intake. Judicious, often empirical treatment of bacterial overgrowth periodically will facilitate the advance of formula. It is not uncommon to need a few days of metronidazole every 2 to 3 weeks to help with the advance in feedings.

Continuous feedings may provide the best nutrient absorption, but it is important to allow a break of a few hours in both enteral and parenteral feedings. During this time, oral intake, especially in infants, should be encouraged to maintain oral motor function.

Several other illnesses affecting gastrointestinal function and nutritional status can be managed successfully with enteral tube feedings. Infants with biliary atresia frequently experience reduced intake associated with hepatic disease and infection. Nutritional support with nasogastric feedings using an elemental or semi-elemental formula rich in medium-chain triglycerides can promote energy and nitrogen balance in preparation for and after hepatic transplantation. Once the clinical condition of the infant or child is stable after transplantation, transition to an intact nutrient formula or an oral diet should be made. Infants with GER and poor weight gain may benefit from continuous nasogastric feedings with improved weight gain, reduction or cessation of vomiting, and catch-up growth.[8] However, one should be cautious in attributing poor weight gain to GER alone, and other underlying diseases, such as cystic fibrosis, should be ruled out with appropriate tests before embarking on aggressive enteral feeding programs. Children with chronic nonspecific or protracted diarrhea and malnutrition can also benefit from continuous enteral tube feedings.

Perioperative Malnutrition
Postoperative feeding via the gut can hasten recovery by reducing sepsis and enhancing immune function. Clinical studies have demonstrated that gastrointestinal function can be adequately maintained with improved nitrogen balance and nutritional status in the postsurgical trauma patient. Postsurgical pediatric patients may be treated with oral, enteral, or parenteral nutrition or a combination of these, depending on the affected portion of the gastrointestinal tract and the extent of the operative procedure.

Renal Disease
Chronic renal failure in infants and children commonly results in growth failure and developmental delay, particularly in patients with congenital renal disease early in life.[9] The cause of growth failure is thought to be related to protein-energy malnutrition, renal osteodystrophy, chronic metabolic acidosis, and endocrine dysfunction. Despite aggressive medical management and specialized formulas with high caloric density, inadequate weight gain often persists. Early nutritional intervention can augment the effect of dialysis by improving anabolism and reducing nitrogen losses.

Critical Illness and Hypermetabolic States
Patients who have extensive trauma, head or spinal cord injury, or burn injury and children with hypermetabolic states, such as cancer (see Chapter 42: Nutritional Management of Children With Cancer, HIV infection, or

IV

AIDS (see Chapter 39: Nutrition of Children With HIV-1 Infection), often require specialized nutritional support. Children with advanced cancer who are at high nutritional risk and who have minimal gastrointestinal symptoms may be enterally fed via nocturnal or 24-hour nasogastric or gastrostomy feedings, depending on the extent of oral intake.[10] Enteral nutrition is the preferred method for the nutritional support of children with uncomplicated trauma, such as severe head and spinal cord injuries, who have a significant increase in their basal metabolic rates in the initial days following injury.[11] Given the disordered nutrient metabolism that occurs in critical illness, permissive underfeeding of calories to meet the initial basal energy needs within the first week after injury or acute illness will help to prevent the negative outcomes associated with overfeeding of calories, including hypercapnia, difficulty weaning from the ventilator, hepatotoxicity, hyperglycemia, and increased infection rates.[11] Metabolic effects associated with burn wounds that can lead to malnutrition include accelerated rate of energy expenditure, increased urine and wound nitrogen losses, and abnormal protein and glucose metabolism. Pediatric patients with >20% total body surface area burns usually require enteral nutrition using continuous tube feedings.[12]

Neurologic Disease or Impairment

The specific nutritional requirements and feeding approach for neurologically impaired children are highly variable and depend on the degree of impairment, oral motor function, mobility, and muscle control. Children with Down syndrome, Prader-Willi syndrome, or myelomeningocele have decreased energy needs, growth rates, and motor activity compared with typical children.[13] Children with cerebral palsy are generally underweight for height and may have increased energy needs, particularly if they have severe contractures or choreoathetoid movements. The nutritional goals for feeding the child with devastating neurologic disease may be less than those predicted by standard growth charts. Excessive intake may place the child at risk of aspiration. Obesity can compromise neuromuscular and respiratory function. The concerns of primary caregivers about lifting heavy children must also be considered. Often, a general children's multivitamin, preferably in liquid form, as well a calcium and phosphorous supplement, may need to be given to children with restricted volume intake to ensure their vitamin and mineral requirements are being met.

Finally, but perhaps most important, one must remember to provide adequate water for children with neuromuscular disease. These children may not be able to communicate thirst to the caregiver. Often in an attempt to decrease risk of aspiration, more concentrated formulas are used with a resultant decrease in water intake. Fluid balance is important in the pediatric patient who is fed via tube, because several metabolic complications can be related to inadequate intake. Fluid requirements can be calculated by estimating normal water requirements adjusted for specific disease-related factors. Special consideration must be given to monitoring the fluid balance of children receiving high-calorie, high-protein formulas and children with excess water loss resulting from emesis, diarrhea, fever, or polyuria.[14]

Enteral Formula Selection for Children 1 to 10 Years of Age

When children are older, they are more capable of expressing their own preferences for favorite foods. It is important to remember that few of them spontaneously decide that they prefer nutritional supplements to other favorite foods that they see other children eating and/or see advertised in the media. Before one embarks on a control struggle to force or tube feed an unappetizing supplement to a thin child who does not want to eat, it is useful to try commonly available high-calorie foods that are appetizing. There is no lethal dose for ice cream, pizza, potato chips, French fries, and similar dietary items. If these diet items lead to adequate weight gain and early discharge from the hospital, they can be very helpful. After nutritional status improves, more "prudent" dietary options may be provided. Indeed, obese individuals seldom curl up in front of the television with a case of their favorite dietary supplement—instead, they prefer an appetizing variety of foods consumed at frequent intervals.

If it is not possible for a child to gain weight on his or her favorite energy-dense foods and enteral feedings are necessary, they should be started in a timely manner, optimally within the first 48 to 72 hours after injury or hospitalization, depending on the child's clinical status.[9] They should be offered by mouth, preferably by a trusted caregiver. If they are refused by the child, enteral tube feedings can be used. Formula selections for infants are discussed in Chapter 3. Until fairly recently, adult formulas had been used for the enteral nutrition support of children older than 1 year, because a tube-feeding formula for young children had not been available. The primary disadvantages of using adult tube-feeding formulas for young children are increased renal solute load and insufficient vitamin and mineral intakes. Dilution of the formulas to reduce the renal solute load may decrease the vitamin and mineral intake.

A variety of formulas are now available to meet the specialized nutritional needs of the 1- to 10-year-old child (PediaSure [Abbott Laboratories, Abbott Park, IL], Peptamen Jr [Nestlé Nutrition, Glendale, CA], Nutren Jr [Nestlé Nutrition, Glendale, CA], Kindercal [Mead Johnson, Evansville, IN], Pepdite One + [Nutricia North America, Rockville, MD], EleCare [Abbott Laboratories, Abbott Park, IL], Neocate One + [Nutricia North America, Rockville, MD]). These products can be used for enteral tube feedings and as an oral supplement. The energy distribution of protein, carbohydrate, and fat is between that of infant and adult formulas (Appendix U). The vitamin and mineral concentrations in 950 to 1200 mL of formula meet or exceed 100% of the Recommended Dietary Allowances (RDAs) for children 1 to 10 years of age. At a caloric density of approximately 1 kcal/mL, the formulas are useful for children with increased metabolic needs or for those with fluid restrictions. The 1-kcal/mL caloric density permits some flexibility in dilution; 1100 mL of 24-kcal/oz formula meets 100% of the RDAs. Children 10 years or older or those with highly specialized nutrient and metabolic needs can generally be adequately fed adult formulas. It is important to remember that "predigested" or elemental formulas are only necessary when there is a deficiency in the digestive process. They have no advantage for the child with normal digestive function.

Formulas for Use in Children Older Than 10 Years of Age: Standard Tube-Feeding Formulas

Standard tube-feeding formulas are presented in Appendix U. These formulas, most of which are lactose free and low residue, vary in osmolality from 300 to 650 mOsm/kg and in caloric density from 1.0 to 2.0 kcal/mL. Isotonic formulas (Osmolite [Abbott Laboratories, Abbott Park, IL] and Isocal [Nestlé Nutrition, Glendale, CA]), which contain medium-chain triglyceride oil, are often useful for people with a history of delayed gastric emptying, dumping syndrome, or osmotic diarrhea. Tube-feeding formulas with added fiber, such as Jevity (Abbott Laboratories, Abbott Park, IL) and Ultracal (Nestlé Nutrition, Glendale, CA) are often useful in the management of patients with chronic constipation and diarrhea. Because of their low osmolality, caloric density, and moderate protein content, isotonic tube feedings, including those with added fiber, are the formulas of choice for general use with pediatric patients older than 10 years.

Although high-calorie, high-nitrogen, hypertonic formulations are often well tolerated by adults with increased metabolic needs, they are usually not

tolerated by children and may lead to diarrhea, emesis, abdominal distention, and delayed gastric emptying. Children and adolescents with markedly
increased calorie and protein requirements resulting from severe trauma or
burn injury are best managed with high-calorie formulations such as Jevity
1.5 (17.1% protein) and Nutren 1.5 (16% protein). Because of the elevated
protein contents in these formulas, however, hydration status must be
closely monitored.

Peptide-Based and Elemental Formulas

Peptide-based and elemental formulas with predigested nutrients can be
used for the nutritional support of pediatric patients with short-bowel
syndrome, inflammatory bowel disease, and/or food protein sensitivity
(Appendices G and U). Peptide-based formulas may be used in the enteral
nutritional support of patients with cystic fibrosis, although the use of intact
protein formulas with appropriate pancreatic enzyme administration may
be just as effective. Amino acid-based formulas offer further protection from
food protein sensitivity over protein hydrolysates (peptide-based) formulas.
However, there is a quantum leap in cost between hydrolysates and
elemental amino acid formulas. Additionally, recent data suggest a possible
small additional benefit from supplementation with the amino acid glutamine. Before considering newer products fortified with glutamine, however, consideration of intact whole protein foods as a less expensive and more
palatable alternative is prudent. On the basis of the most recent meta-analysis on the topic of the clinical efficacy of immunonutrition, these products
may be beneficial in trauma patients or malnourished patients undergoing
surgery.[15] It is important to note, however, that there are no published data
or guidelines established for the use of immunonutrition products in pediatric patients or adolescents. The added cost and minimal increased benefit
often preclude their use in many hospitals.

Oral Supplements

Various flavored milk-based and polymeric formulas may be used as oral
supplements for pediatric patients. As noted previously, high-calorie commercially available snack foods may be more palatable and economical
than specialized supplements for most children. The constant supervision
required to enforce frequent intake of commercial supplements can be a
source of considerable family conflict. Oral supplements mixed with milk,
such as Carnation Instant Breakfast (Nestlé, Glendale, CA), are often better

IV

accepted by children than are the lactose-free commercial supplements. Flavored polymeric formulas that contain intact proteins, long-chain fatty acids, and simple carbohydrates are usually marketed as oral supplements because of their palatability. These products, which have osmolalities ranging from 450 to 600 mOsm/kg, are often not sufficiently palatable for long-term voluntary supplementation for children. Some examples of milk-based and polymeric oral supplements include Boost (Nestlé Nutrition, Glendale, CA), Ensure Plus (Abbott Laboratories, Abbott Park, IL), and Resource Plus (Nestlé Nutrition, Glendale, CA). It is useful to remember that salt is an appetite stimulant and that the combination of salty foods accompanied by sugary fluids to slake the resultant thirst can stimulate oral intake and initiate insulin surges that may be useful in further increasing appetite.

It may be preferable to use commonly available energy-dense foods and supplements to increase energy intake (see Tables 23.2 and 23.3). These have the advantage of improved taste and lower cost. Plus, the child may see siblings consuming similar foods and be encouraged by example.

Table 23.2
Increasing the Nutrient Density of Foods

Use cream, whole milk, or evaporated whole milk instead of water for baking whenever possible.
Use liberal portions of butter, margarine, oil, and cheeses on vegetables and breads and in soups and hot cereals. Add sauces and gravies to foods.
Add sugar, jelly, or honey to toast and cereals. Use fruits canned in heavy syrup, or sweeten fresh fruits with added sugar.
Add skim milk powder or instant breakfast powder to regular whole milk for use as a beverage or for cooking. Add powdered milk to puddings, potatoes, soups, and cooked cereals.
Use peanut butter (after 3 years of age) or cheese on fruit or crackers. Make finger sandwiches for meals or snacks.
Provide a variety of high-calorie salad dressings for addition to vegetables or other foods to increase caloric density.
Emphasize variety with all high-calorie foods to decrease flavor fatigue and increase exploratory behavior with foods.

Blenderized Formulas

Commercially available blenderized diets consist of beef, eggs, milk, cereal, fruits and vegetables, and vegetable oils. These formulas, which contain a moderate to high level of residue, usually have osmolalities ranging from 300 to 500 mOsm/kg. Blenderized feedings are beneficial for chronically ill patients who have normal digestive function and require long-term enteral nutrition; however, they may not be well tolerated by the malnourished pediatric patient with compromised gastrointestinal function. Often, these products are expensive. Their high viscosity may predispose to obstruction of pediatric feeding tubes.

Blenderized feedings can be prepared at home from milk, juices, cereals, and baby food. Parents of neurologically impaired children who require long-term nutritional management through a feeding gastrostomy are often interested in learning how to prepare blenderized feedings at home because of the economic and psychosocial advantages. The help of a registered dietitian is important to ensure that adequate free water, macronutrient, and micronutrient concentrations are appropriate with these mixtures.

Table 23.3
Energy and Protein Content of Selected Energy-Dense Foods*

	Energy, Kcal	Protein, g
Instant breakfast powder (1 packet)	130	7
Mixed with 1 cup whole milk	280	15
Powdered milk (1 tbsp)	33	3
Evaporated milk (1 tbsp)	25	1
Cheese (1 oz)	100	7
Peanut butter (1 tbsp)	95	4
Butter or margarine[†] (1 tsp)	45	0

* See also Appendix V.
[†] Not the "spreads," which have a lot of air and water added and, therefore, are lower in kcal.

Formula Concentration and Supplementation With Use of Modular Components

Because of the unique and often elevated nutritional requirements of the enterally fed pediatric patient, modification of enteral formulas through either formula concentration or supplementation with modular components is often necessary. Formula concentration with the use of formula concentrates and sterile water or supplementation with liquid modular products is usually the preferred modality for increasing formula concentration to ensure safe formula preparation and minimize the risk of formula contamination with nonsterile powdered products. Infant formula powder may also be used as a convenient and economical way to increase the caloric density of human milk and infant formulas. However, within the hospital setting, use of liquid formula concentrates and liquid modular components is the preferred method to minimize the risk of formula contamination (see Appendix U, Table U-2). It is important to remember that formula concentration may lead to decreased intake in patients who are voluntarily drinking the formula and may lead to vomiting because of their tendency to prolong gastric emptying in patients who are being fed via tube. Therefore, fluid and electrolyte balance must be monitored.

Tube Feeding

When the requirement for enteral nutritional support has been established, the optimal route of delivering nutrients must be determined. Many health care professionals recommend the placement of nasogastric or nasoduodenal feeding tubes when the estimated course of therapy will not exceed 3 months (size 5 or 6 French tubes are usually adequate). These tubes should be changed from one nostril to the other every 1 to 3 weeks to decrease associated sinus and ear disease. During upper respiratory infections, extra care should be taken to avoid airway compromise. Tube placement should be verified after episodes of emesis before restarting feedings. If the risk of aspiration is not significant, gastric feedings are preferable because of ease of management. Tubes made of polyurethane and silicone rubber are soft and pliable and may be left in place for indefinite periods. Polyvinyl chloride tubes become stiff and nonpliable when left in place for more than a few days; however, they are useful for intestinal decompression or short-term feeding. They should be changed every 2 to 3 days to avoid skin necrosis or intestinal perforation.

Some feeding tubes made of polyurethane or silicone rubber have a tungsten or mercury weight at the tip that makes them useful for duodenal or jejunal feedings. Placement of transpyloric tubes can be greatly facilitated by the use of an intravenous prokinetic drug, such as metoclopramide. Children who require long-term tube feeding are candidates for placement of a gastrostomy tube. Gastroesophageal reflux, which may occur in children with neurologic disabilities or healthy infants after gastrostomy tube placement, may necessitate an operative antireflux procedure (eg, Nissen fundoplication).[16] Although the procedure is effective in reducing GER, postoperative complications can be troublesome. Intractable retching episodes, dumping syndrome, continued problems with swallowing, impaired esophageal emptying, slow feeding, and gas bloating have all been reported. Controversy exists over the necessity of an antireflux procedure in neurologically impaired children who require a feeding gastrostomy tube. A trial of nasogastric feedings to determine whether they are well tolerated without significant GER before the placement of the gastrostomy tube can help the health care professional determine the need for a simultaneous Nissen fundoplication. During the trial nasogastric feed, documented pulmonary disease associated with GER in the face of maximal medical therapy is an indication for a Nissen fundoplication when a subsequent gastrostomy tube placement is performed.

A common problem with all gastrostomy tubes is migration of the tube through the ostomy site. Ultimately, the tip of the catheter contacts the pylorus, where it occasionally induces retching as it passes in and out of the gastric outlet. These problems may be minimized by firmly attaching the tube and placing a mark on the tube to detect inward migration. When a urinary catheter is used as a temporary gastrostomy tube, migration (resulting from lack of an effective external bolster) remains a common problem. The gastrostomy button is a feeding device that can be used to form an effective 1-way valve at the gastrostomy site. The button fits flush with the skin and attaches to commercial feeding tubes that lock onto the button in a variety of ways. Gastrostomy buttons generally do not migrate through the pylorus and cause retching and are also less prone to accidental removal. Buttons may be placed in percutaneous gastrostomies after the site has matured by healing for at least 8 weeks.

To overcome problems related to gastric emptying and frequent GER, transpyloric feedings offer potential benefit. Feeding jejunostomy tubes can be placed through existing gastrostomy sites. If a modified (eg, urinary catheter) tube is used to convert a gastrostomy site to a jejunostomy site, extreme care must be exercised to be certain that retching or emesis has not moved the tip of the tube into the esophagus. Even commercial gastrojejunostomy feeding tubes can be accidentally moved into an esophageal position when persistent emesis occurs. Retrograde continuous delivery of formula into the esophagus presents an extreme risk for aspiration. Nasal transpyloric tubes may be easily displaced and are uncomfortable as a long-term approach to enteral nutritional support. Operative feeding jejunostomy tubes overcome these difficulties and may be indicated for a select few patients. Patients with feeding jejunostomy tubes generally do not tolerate large bolus feeding over short intervals without experiencing dumping syndrome. Also, button adapters by virtue of the large internal bolster are often precluded for feeding jejunostomy tubes.

IV

The transition from enteral feeding to full oral feeding can be prolonged. If infants and children are completely deprived of oral feeding during critical maturation phases, feeding refusal often occurs when oral feedings are resumed.[17] Reinstituting oral feedings in children who have been fed by means of a gastrostomy tube can evoke a resistant response, such as gagging, choking, or vomiting. To preserve oral motor function during prolonged tube feedings, it is important to continue to offer oral intake whenever possible. This may require interrupting the infusion to allow a sufficient amount of hunger to develop to facilitate oral intake. Generally, this may require several hours. Speech pathologists and occupational therapists can help provide oral motor stimulation exercises for such children. Without continuous oral stimulation, within a few weeks, infants can lose the suckle reflex, which severely limits their ability to control oral intake and also compromises language and oral motor development. They may also develop oral defensiveness as a result of failure of oral stimulation.

Continuous Versus Intermittent Feeding

Two methods are used for delivery of enteral feedings. Intermittent bolus feedings deliver the formula over a period similar to that for an oral feeding (ie, 10–20 minutes). This technique is simple, requires minimal supplies, and may facilitate the transition to home care. Generally, bolus feedings are used during the day and are not used at night because of the greater tendency for GER with the bolus feed. Gastric distension by bolus feeding can lead to a better gastrocolic reflex and aid in the prevention of constipation, which is a common problem in tube-fed patients. When intermittent bolus feeding is not tolerated, a continuous infusion using an infusion pump may be effective. To improve patient mobility, a backpack pump may be of considerable benefit. Continuous feeding may be particularly beneficial when used for patients who have impaired absorption, as with chronic diarrhea or short-bowel syndrome.

One Final Note

Specialized formulas are very expensive, and their cost can easily exceed the food budget of an entire family. Many patients have discovered that it is possible to buy large quantities of expensive elemental and other specialized formulas over the Internet from people who have "left-over" quantities that were prescribed for them. Although this can represent an enormous savings, it is important to remember that the bidder is depending on the integrity of the seller in Internet purchases from private individuals. Counterfeit nutritional products are almost certainly occasionally sold in a manner similar to the well-recognized problem with counterfeit medications.

References

1. Canete A, Duggan C. Nutritional support of the pediatric intensive care unit patient. *Curr Opin Pediatr.* 1996;8:248–255

2. Meetze W, Valentine C, McGuigan JE, Conlon M, Sacks N, Neu J. Gastrointestinal priming prior to full enteral nutrition in very low birth weight infants. *J Pediatr Gastroenterol Nutr.* 1992;15:163–170

3. Cavell B. Effect of feeding an infant formula with high energy density on gastric emptying in infants with congenital heart disease. *Acta Paediatr Scand.* 1981;70:513–516

4. Abad-Sinden A, Sutphen A. Growth and nutrition. In: Allen HD, Clark EB, Gutgessell HP, Driscoll DJ, eds. *Moss and Adams' Heart Diseases in Infants, Children and Adolescents, Including the Fetus and Young Adult.* 6th ed. Philadelphia, PA: Williams & Wilkins; 2001;325–332

5. Bernstein CN, Shanahan F. Braving the elementals in Crohn's disease. *Gastroenterology.* 1992;103:1363–1364

6. Vanderhoof JA, Langnas AN, Pinch LW, Thompson JS, Kaufman SS. Short bowel syndrome. *J Pediatr Gastroenterol Nutr.* 1992;14:359–370

7. Weber TR, Tracy T Jr, Connors RH. Short bowel syndrome in children: quality of life in an era of improved survival. *Arch Surg.* 1991;126:841–846

8. Ferry GD, Selby M, Pietro TJ. Clinical response to short-term nasogastric feeding in infants with gastroesophageal reflux and growth failure. *J Pediatr Gastroenterol Nutr.* 1983;2:57–61

9. Spinozzi NS. Chronic renal disease. In: Queen Samour P, King Helm K, Lang CE, eds. *Handbook of Pediatric Nutrition.* 2nd ed. Gaithersburg, MD: Aspen Publishers Inc; 1999:385–394

10 Barale KV, Charuhas PM. Oncology and bone marrow transplantation. In: Queen Samour P, King Helm K, Lang CE, eds. *Handbook of Pediatric Nutrition.* 2nd ed. Gaithersburg, MD: Aspen Publishers Inc; 1999:465–492

11. Chwals WJ. Overfeeding the critically ill child: fact or fantasy? *New Horiz.* 1994;2:147–155

12. Trocki O, Michelini JA, Robbins ST, Eichelberger MR. Evaluation of early enteral feeding in children less than 3 years old with smaller burns (8–25 per cent TBSA). *Burns.* 1995;21:17–23

13. Cloud HH. Developmental disabilities. In: Queen Samour P, King Helm K, Lang CE, eds. *Handbook of Pediatric Nutrition.* Gaithersburg, MD: Aspen Publishers Inc, 1999:293–314

14. Schwenk WF, Olson D. Pediatrics. In: Gottschlich MM, ed. *The Science and Practice of Nutrition Support: A Case-Based Core Curriculum.* Dubuque, IA: Kendall/Hunt Publishing Company; 2001:347–372

15. Heyland DK, Novak F, Drover JW, Jain M, Su X, Suchner U. Should immunonutrition become routine in critically ill patients? A systematic review of the evidence. *JAMA.* 2001;286:944–953

16. Albanese CT, Towbin RB, Ulman I, Lewis J, Smith SD. Percutaneous gastrojejunostomy versus Nissen fundoplication for enteral feeding of the neurologically impaired child with gastroesophageal reflux. *J Pediatr.* 1993;123:371–375

IV

17. Illingworth RS, Lister J. The critical or sensitive period, with special reference to certain feeding problems in infants and children. *J Pediatr*. 1964;65:839–848

18. Sutphen JL, Dillard VL. Effect of feeding volume on early postcibal gastroesophageal reflux in infants. *J Pediatr Gastroenterol Nutr*. 1988;7:185–188

Nutrition in Acute and Chronic Illness

Assessment of nutritional status is the primary step in the evaluation of all children whose growth differs from the norm and should be an integral part of the evaluation and management of all children with acute and chronic disease.[1] During a prolonged hospital stay, nutritional disturbances can occur, particularly when oral intake is suspended or limited. This chapter discusses nutritional assessment methods and their practical application. For most patients, a dietary history, physical examination, and longitudinal changes in height, weight, and body mass index are sufficient to assess nutritional status.

Assessment by History

Because an assumption cannot be made that all children eat normally, a detailed diet history is important. Children on a strict vegetarian diet may ingest inadequate amounts of protein, vitamin B_{12}, iron, or pyridoxine if their meals are not properly planned. Adolescents often skip meals, and athletic children may not ingest adequate calories, or they may become involved in fad diets associated with some sports. Older children and adolescents may attempt weight loss by starvation, or anorexia nervosa or bulimia may develop. On the other hand, children may be snacking continuously and ingesting large amounts of sugar-containing beverages and have sedentary behavior, all of which leads to obesity.

The most accurate method of dietary assessment is a 3- to 5-day "diet diary" to account for most of the daily variation in diet and eliminate the subjectiveness of diet recall records. Dietary analysis is best performed by a registered dietitian. Some medications can cause nutritional disturbances (see Appendix N: Food-Drug Interactions).

Clinical Assessment

Careful inspection of the patient remains a valid method of nutritional assessment.[2] The current epidemic of childhood obesity has begun to distort perceptions of what is the normal appearance of children. Distinguishing wasting from stunting in the young child is also difficult. Obesity and wasting are not necessarily obvious and need to be confirmed by weight-for-height or BMI reference charts. Observation is a useful screening test for gross changes in body composition, and edema, dehydration, excess or inadequate subcutaneous fat, and increase or decrease of the muscle mass can be detected. Some of the findings of vitamin and mineral deficiencies are listed in Tables 24.1 and 24.2. Deficiency of any trace substance can result in growth failure. The clinical signs and symptoms of specific vitamin or mineral deficiencies or toxic effects are usually not pathognomonic.

Table 24.1
Signs and Symptoms of Vitamin Deficiency or Excess

Vitamin	Deficiency	Excess
A	Night blindness, xerophthalmia, keratomalacia, follicular hyperkeratosis	Scaly skin, bone pain, pseudotumor cerebri, hepatomegaly
C	Scurvy: capillary hemorrhage of gingiva, skin, bone, poor wound healing	"Rebound" deficiency after high intake
D	Rickets, osteomalacia	Constipation, renal stones, myositis ossificans, hypercalcemia
E	Hemolysis (in preterm infant), peripheral neuropathy	Suppresses hematologic response to iron in anemia
K	Bruising, bleeding	Jaundice
Thiamine	Beriberi: cardiomyopathy, peripheral neuropathy, and encephalopathy	None known
Riboflavin	Cheilosis, glossitis, angular stomatitis	None known
Niacin	Pellagra: dementia, diarrhea, and dermatitis	Flushing
Pyridoxine	Seizures, anemia, irritability	Neuropathy
Biotin	Dermatitis, alopecia, muscle pain	None known
Folate	Macrocytic anemia, stomatitis paresthesia, glossitis, neural tube defects of fetus	Masking of B_{12} deficiency symptoms in patients with pernicious anemia
B_{12}	Megaloblastic anemia, neuropathy, paresthesia, glossitis	None known

Anthropometry

Anthropometric measurements can assess growth cross-sectionally or longitudinally. If children are measured once, their growth status for age can be assessed by comparing this measurement with the appropriate reference chart. If children are measured more than once, growth velocity data are obtained that can be more valuable, because they reflect change. The intervals between measurements that are necessary to develop meaningful incremental data are listed in Table 24.3. Particular care should be taken to use appropriate equipment and techniques for measuring stature or length and weight. This can significantly improve the assessments that need to be performed and may preclude the need to evaluate aspects of body composition, such as body fatness.

Table 24.2
Signs and Symptoms of Mineral Deficiency or Excess

Mineral	Deficiency	Excess
Aluminum	None known	Central nervous system disorder
Boron	Calcification abnormalities	None known
Calcium	Osteomalacia, tetany	Constipation, heart block, vomiting
Chloride	Alkalosis	Acidosis
Chromium	Diabetes (in animals)	None known
Cobalt	Vitamin B_{12} deficiency	Cardiomyopathy
Copper	Anemia, neutropenia, osteoporosis, neuropathy, depigmentation of hair and skin	Cirrhosis, central nervous system effects, Fanconi nephropathy, corneal pigmentation
Fluoride	Dental caries	Fluorosis
Iodine	Goiter, cretinism	Goiter
Iron	Anemia, behavioral abnormalities	Hemosiderosis
Lead	None known	Encephalopathy, neuropathy, stippled red blood cells
Magnesium	Hypocalcemia, hypokalemia, tremor, weakness, arrhythmia	Weakness, sedation, hypotension, nausea, vomiting
Molybdenum	Growth retardation (in animals)	None known
Phosphorus	Rickets, neuropathy	Calcium deficiency
Potassium	Muscle weakness, cardiac abnormalities	Heart block
Selenium	Cardiomyopathy, anemia, myositis	Nail and hair changes, garlic odor
Sodium	Hypotension	Edema
Sulfur	Growth failure	None known
Zinc	Growth failure, dermatitis, hypogeusia, hypogonadism, alopecia, impaired wound healing	Gastroenteritis

V

Table 24.3
Minimal Time Intervals to Detect Changes in Growth

Measurement	Interval
Weight	7 days
Length	4 weeks
Stature	8 weeks
Head circumference	7 days, infants 4 weeks, up to 4 years of age
Mid-arm circumference	4 weeks

Length or Stature

Length or stature is the most useful indicator of growth status. Unfortunately, in infants and small children, it is also the most difficult measurement to obtain accurately. In infants and children younger than 2 years, recumbent length is measured. Two people are required to accomplish this measurement. The measuring table or board should consist of a fixed headboard, a movable footboard, and a rule attached at one side. One of the measurers should hold the crown of the infant's head against the headboard so the external auditory meatus and the lower margin of the eye orbit are aligned perpendicular to the table. The second measurer grips both ankles of the infant with one hand and positions the heels firmly against the footboard, which is manipulated with the other hand. The knees, which are slightly flexed, are then pressed down on the table with the lateral edge of the hand. The recumbent length should be recorded to the nearest 0.1 cm (according to recommendations of the National Center for Health Statistics of the Centers for Disease Control and Prevention [CDC]).

Stature, or standing height, is measured in children older than 2 years. Several apparatuses are available that can be affixed to a wall. Measurements are made with the child's feet bare. The child should stand erect, and if possible, the heels, buttocks, shoulders, and head all should touch the measuring board or wall. The feet should be positioned at a 90-degree angle. The child's axis of vision should be horizontal, with the child looking ahead and the external auditory meatus and lower margin of the orbit aligned horizontally. Children should be told to make themselves "as tall as possible with their heels on the ground." The head projection of the measuring apparatus is then slid down firmly onto the crown of the head and the stature is recorded to the nearest 0.1 cm. The use of the measuring device attached to a beam balance scale is discouraged, because a standard posture cannot be achieved without standing against a hard surface.

Reference and standard values for length, stature, and growth velocity are shown in Appendix D.[3-6] Reference values for length and stature are also available for children with Down syndrome (Appendix D) and many other conditions. Preterm infants can be compared with reference values derived from intrauterine lengths for various gestational ages as shown in Appendix D. The reference charts used should be appropriate for the population segment.

When possible, the parents' stature should be obtained to determine the influence of genetics on growth). If only one parent is available, the maternal stature is more valuable for comparison.

Weight

Various types of apparatuses, such as infant scales, beam-balance scales, and readout scales, are available to measure body weight. The type used needs to be regularly calibrated to maintain accuracy. Weight should always be recorded as nude weight, particularly with infants, for whom clothing can represent a large proportion of total weight. If the subject is not weighed nude, then the estimated weight of the clothing should be subtracted from the total weight. Reference and standard values for body weight are included in Appendix D, as are reference values for children with Down syndrome. Weight reference values for preterm infants are shown in Appendix D.

Weight for Height

The ratio of actual weight to ideal weight for height (usually referred to as weight for height) can be used to differentiate stunted growth from wasting and is independent of age. Stunting frequently is constitutional but can be caused by genetic or endocrine abnormalities as well as by chronic illness and/or chronic malnutrition. This results in a child who is small for age but has a body weight proportional to the length. Wasting results from acute or subacute nutritional deprivation and can be caused by medical conditions, such as diarrhea or malabsorption, in which body weight is depleted out of proportion to length, making the weight-for-height ratio low. The current internationally accepted index is the weight-for-height z-score or percentile based on the CDC or WHO growth references or standards. Reference values that reflect the normal distribution of weight in relation to height for healthy prepubescent children are shown in Appendix D.

BMI

Body mass index (weight/height^2) is the best anthropometric indicator of adiposity in children and adolescents (Appendix D). To calculate BMI, divide the weight in kg by the square of the height in meters (kg/m^2). It can also be calculated by dividing the weight in lb by the height in in^2, multiplied by 703 (lb/in^2 × 703). BMI is an important tool to determine overweight in children. By consensus, any child with BMI greater the 85th percentile is "overweight," and any child with BMI greater than the 95th percentile is considered "obese." Some confusion regarding the nomenclature of childhood obesity exists because the Institute of Medicine uses the terms overweight and obese as defined here, whereas the CDC uses the terms "at risk of overweight" instead of "overweight" and the term "overweight" instead of "obese." All children followed by a physician should have their BMI calculated periodically. If the child begins to cross percentile lines on the BMI chart, the family can be counseled early about prevention of obesity.

Head Circumference

Head circumference is a useful measurement until approximately 3 years of age, when head growth slows. It must be measured with a narrow and non-stretchable measuring tape. To obtain an accurate measurement, the tape must cross the forehead just above the supraorbital ridges, passing around the head at the same level on both sides to the occiput. It is then moved up or down slightly to obtain the maximum circumference. The tape should have sufficient tension to press the hair against the skull. Normal reference values from birth to 3 years are shown in Appendix D. Reference values for preterm infants are shown in Appendix D.

Mid-arm Circumference

The mid-upper-arm circumference is an indicator of muscle growth in all ages. The left arm is usually measured by convention. The tape to be used should be the same as that used to measure the head circumference. A point is marked midway between the acromion (shoulder) and the olecranon (elbow) on the vertical axis of the upper arm with the arm bent at a right angle and between the lateral and medial surface of the arm. The child should then stand or sit with the arm hanging loose at the side. The tape is passed around the arm at the level marked and is tightened so it touches but does not compress the skin or alter the contour of the arm. Because the arm on cross section is not an exact circle, some difficulty is usually met in ensuring that the tape touches the arm on the medial surface. To accomplish this, the middle finger of the examiner's left hand can be used to gently press the tape to the skin. Normal reference values for children 1 year and older and are shown in Appendices D and W, Table W-1.[7]

Mid-Arm Circumference-to-Head Circumference Ratio

The ratio of mid-arm circumference to head circumference was developed by Kanawati and McLaren[8] as a method to estimate nutritional status when the proper apparatus for measuring weight or height is not available, although this is rarely the case in clinical practice today. The mid-arm circumference is substantially influenced by subcutaneous fat and, therefore, fluctuates with total body weight. The head circumference in an infant and young child parallels the child's linear growth. Therefore, the mid-arm circumference-to-head circumference ratio varies directly with the weight-for-height ratio and can be used as a substitute until head growth slows at approximately 3 years of age. A ratio greater than 0.31 is considered normal, and a ratio less than 0.25 indicates severe malnutrition. Various degrees of undernutrition lie between.

Nutritional Assessment Through the Measurement of Body Composition

The major form of stored energy in the body is fat. A small amount of carbohydrate in the form of glycogen is present, but this can be depleted after only 1 or 2 days of starvation. Protein can also be used for energy, but all protein in the body is present as functional tissue, so its utilization results in a decrease in the functional body mass. Because fat is used preferentially by the body as an energy source during starvation or periods of metabolic stress, the accurate measurement of this body compartment would be the ideal method to assess a child's nutritional status. Longitudinal measurements would allow estimates of nutritional sufficiency during periods of recovery from disease. Many methods of measurement of the fat and fat-free compartments of the body exist; however, most are not applicable to the child, because they are too inaccurate or too cumbersome for use in children.[9] New methods that offer easy measurement of fat and fat-free mass have been developed.[10,11] As these methods prove more practical and as reference standards for body fat for children are developed,[12] they can enhance the accuracy of surveillance of the nutritional status of children.

V

Table 24.4 shows the average amount of lean body mass and body fat in nonobese healthy individuals from birth to 22 years of age.

Table 24.4
Lean Body Mass and Body Fat*

	Males			Females		
Age[†]	LBM, kg	Fat, kg	% Fat	LBM, kg	Fat, kg	% Fat
Birth	3.06	0.49	14	2.83	0.49	15
6 mo	6.0	2.0	25	5.3	1.9	26
12 mo	7.9	2.3	22	7.0	2.2	24
2 y	10.1	2.5	20	9.5	2.4	20
4 y	14.0	2.7	16	13.2	2.8	18
6 y	17.9	2.8	14	16.3	3.2	16
8 y	22.0	3.3	13	20.5	4.3	17
10 y	27.1	4.3	14	26.2	6.4	20
12 y	34	8	19	32	10	24
14 y	45	10	18	38	13	25
16 y	57	9	14	42	13	24
18 y	61	9	13	43	13	23
20 y	62	9	13	43	14	25
22 y	62	10	14	43	14	25

LBM indicates lean body mass.

* Data are given as normative means.

† At nearest birthday.

Fat-Fold Measurements

The most frequently used method to estimate body fatness in the hospitalized patient is the skin fat-fold measurement. This method is limited because of 2 assumptions: (1) that the subcutaneous fat mantle reflects the total amount of fat in the body; and (2) that the measurement sites selected represent the average thickness of the entire mantle. Neither assumption is true. Two studies of humans address the first assumption. Forbes et al[13] showed that only 42% of the total body fat of a full-term neonate resides in the subcutaneous compartment. Moore et al[14] found the value to be 32% in an adult woman. The second assumption can be discredited simply by observing the regional variation of subcutaneous fat among individual people.

In the infant and young child, the use of skin fat-fold measurements as an index of total body fat has not been fully validated by an alternative method.[15] Accurately and reproducibly measuring a skin fat fold is difficult and, in edematous or obese individuals, perhaps impossible. These problems limit the usefulness of this measurement as a tool for nutritional assessment. It is sometimes useful, however, for the longitudinal assessment of a patient's response to nutritional therapy. The calipers recommended for fat-fold measurements include the Holtain caliper (Pfister Imports [Carlstadt, NJ]) and the Lange caliper (Cambridge Instruments [Silver Spring, MD]). All measurements are taken on the left side of the child. The most frequent sites of skinfold measurements are the triceps and the suprailiac crest. The level for the triceps skinfold is the same level of the upper arm as marked for a circumference measurement (midway between the acromion and the olecranon with the arm bent at a right angle). With the arm dropped and hanging loosely, the skinfold is lifted away from the underlying muscle fascia with a sweeping motion of the fingers with the observer gripping the "neck" of the fold between middle finger and thumb. The skinfold caliper is then applied to the fold. The point of measurement for the suprailiac skinfold is 1 cm above and 2 cm medial to the anterior superior iliac spine. This position is best palpated with the subject standing facing the observer and is marked with a pen. The skinfold is picked up as a vertical skinfold, and the caliper is applied below the fingers.[7,16]

Hydrodensitometry
The oldest method of estimating the relative proportion of lean and fat compartments in the human body is densitometry, which was introduced in 1942 by Albert Behnke.[17] This method uses the Archimedes principle to determine the density of a person by dividing actual weight by the amount of weight lost when the person is completely submerged in water and air in the lungs is maximally expired. Because the density of fat and the lean compartments of the body are assumed to be constants, calculation of the proportion of each is possible when the density of the whole body is known. This method is widely used to measure body fat in adults. Its use in children, however, is limited, because young children cannot be submerged under water. Even in older children, the method is limited by the change in density of lean body mass during maturation, thus, invalidating one of the basic assumptions of the method.[18] In the hospitalized patient, this method is useless, because neither sick children nor adults can be submerged in

water, even if problems such as intravenous lines and dressings could be managed. Newer methods using this principle with air rather than water displacement have been developed.

Air-Displacement Plethysmography

A more recent method developed for the purpose of measuring body composition in both adults and children is air-displacement plethysmography.[19] In air-displacement plethysmography, the volume of air displaced by an individual sitting in a sealed chamber of known volume is determined. Because the individual's weight is known and volume is measured, density can be calculated, and the proportions of fat and lean compartments can be determined as in hydrodensitometry. Only 2 versions of this instrument exist at the present time. One dedicated to the measurement of adults is called the Bod Pod (Life Measurement Inc [Concord, CA]), and another for the measurement of smaller children is called the Pea Pod. Both machines consist of 2 chambers of known volume. An individual is sealed into 1 of the chambers, and a diaphragm oscillates between the chambers, producing very small pressure changes in both. These pressure changes are accurately measured and displaced volume determined by invoking Boyle's Law, which states that volume and pressure are inversely related. Corrections are made for lung volume and for noncompressible regions around the body, such as hair and skin surface. These instruments are more user friendly than underwater weighing but are still limited in diseased individuals, because they require the individual to be sealed into a chamber.

Total Body Potassium

Another method that has become a standard for the measurement of lean body mass and body fat is the measurement of total body potassium.[20-21] This method is based on the fixed proportion (0.0118%) of the radioactive isotope ^{40}K contained in the naturally occurring potassium ^{39}K. In determining lean body mass, the subject is placed in a specially designed scintillation chamber, and the number of radioactive emissions from ^{40}K is recorded during a 30- to 60-minute period. Total body potassium is then calculated from the amount of ^{40}K present. Because potassium resides in a relatively fixed concentration only in the lean body mass and not in fat, an estimate of the total amount of lean body mass can be derived. Fat can then be calculated by the subtraction of lean body mass from total body weight. This technique is noninvasive but has several limitations, particularly for the hospitalized patient. The counting time is long and requires isolation in a special chamber, which may not be possible for a child or a person who is seriously ill. Few machines have sufficient sensitivity to measure infants or small children who have little lean body mass and relatively fewer radioactive disintegrations per unit of time than do adults.

Total Body Water

Because neutral fat does not bind water, the measurement of total body water offers a means of estimating the nonfat compartment of the body.[22] This can be accomplished in a fairly noninvasive manner by oral administration of water labeled with a known amount of radioactive tritium (^{3}H) or the stable isotopes, deuterium (^{2}H) or oxygen 18. Total body water then can be estimated by determining the dilution of the isotope within a body fluid, such as serum, urine, or saliva, after a suitable period of equilibration. Because the water content of lean body mass is relatively constant in adults (72.3%), this compartment can be estimated. Although this method is simple, its application for clinical problems is limited, because the assays for deuterium and oxygen 18 are cumbersome, and radioactive tritium is not suitable for use in children. A basic methodologic problem also exists, because the water content of lean body mass changes with age and may also vary slightly among people of the same age. Isotopes of hydrogen also appear to exchange with nonaqueous hydrogen, resulting in an overestimation of body water content. Oxygen 18 does not seem to have the same problem, but it is expensive.

Neutron Activation

Many elements can be made radioactive by bombarding them with neutrons. The neutron-activation method of total body analysis uses this principle by activating the body with a known amount of neutron energy and counting the induced radioactivity in a whole-body counting chamber. A given dose of neutrons will generate a known amount of activity within a defined mass of substance. The total activity will, therefore, reflect the total mass of the substance. A particular element can be identified by the characteristic energy of the electromagnetic radiation it emits. This method can be used to determine the amount of a number of elements in the body, including calcium, sodium, chlorine, phosphorus, magnesium, and nitrogen. Total body nitrogen can be used to estimate lean body mass. This method has allowed a much better understanding of human body composition through its use as a research tool; however, its clinical use is limited by the great expense of a neutron-activation facility. Also, although the radiation exposure by this method is small (approximately 30 mrad), any radiation exposure limits its use in children.

Photon and X-ray Absorptiometry

Abnormalities in bone mineralization as a complication of preterm birth or disease (such as renal or hepatic disease) are being recognized with increasing frequency. The traditional method to assess this parameter has been radiography, but radiographs are not a sensitive indicator of bone density. The development of photon absorptiometry and, more recently, x-ray absorptiometry may provide tools for the assessment of this parameter. In x-ray absorptiometry, the bone is scanned transversely by a low-energy photon beam generated by ^{125}I or an x-ray beam, and the transmission is monitored by a scintillation detector. The change in transmission of the beam as it is moved across the bone is a function of the bone density in the region. Evidence exists that the bone density of the distal radius can be related to the total skeletal mass, at least in adults. Dual-energy x-ray absorptiometry of the spine provides an index of the density of trabecular bone, and total body scans can generate an estimate of total body calcium. Total body scans can also give an estimate of fat mass, because fat also has differential absorption of x-rays relative to lean body mass. Even though this method of determining percent body fat is not as accurate as other methods, the noninvasive methodology and the relative inexpense of the apparatus has made this a relatively popular tool.

Bioelectrical Impedance Analysis

Bioelectrical impedance analysis[23–26] has become somewhat popular as a research tool. This method is based on the principle that a weak electrical current passes through the body by way of the lean compartment rather than through fat. The impedance to electrical flow is directly proportional to the amount of lean tissue present. This method has been validated with hydrodensitometry and total body water measurement by isotope dilution in adults. It is noninvasive, portable, and relatively inexpensive; however, it appears to be imprecise. Small changes in body water, such as normal diurnal variation, appear to make significant differences in the estimate of lean body mass. Placement of the electrodes (on the wrist and ankle) that inject and record the electrical current is critical. As a result, the standard error of the estimate is rather high (2–2.5 kg in adults). Bioelectrical impedance analysis has not yet been accurately applied to infants. The changing water content and distribution of the lean body mass of growing children should cause the impedance to change progressively with age, making this method extremely difficult to calibrate for children. Various modifications are being made to these instruments in an attempt to enhance their precision.

Total Body Electrical Conductivity

Another electrical method that can be very useful in the clinical setting is total body electrical conductivity,[27–29] which is based on the principle that organisms placed in an electromagnetic field perturb the field. The degree of perturbation depends on the amount and volume of distribution of electrolytes present within the body. Electrolytes reside exclusively in the lean body mass, thus, allowing estimation of this body compartment. Fat is then estimated by subtracting lean body mass from total body weight. This method is safe. The total energy dissipated in a subject measured is at least 100 times less than what has been established as a safety standard for exposure to electromagnetic energy. The instrument consists of a hollow chamber, open at both ends, the walls of which contain transducer coils that generate the appropriate electromagnetic field. To obtain a reading, the subject is passed through the chamber and current is applied for less than 1 minute in the machine for older children and adults and approximately 1 second in the machine for infants. The machine for infants has been calibrated against the fat-free mass of infant miniature pigs as determined by chemical analysis. The machine for older children and adults has been calibrated against hydrodensitometry, total body water measurement by isotope dilution, and total body potassium measurement. The standard error of the estimate of lean body mass for this method is approximately 70 g for infants and 930 g for adults. The total body electrical conductivity method allows rapid, safe, noninvasive, and accurate determination of body composition. Its major limitation is its lack of portability and the cost of the instrument. Very few of these instruments exist in the United States.

Laboratory Assessment

The initial laboratory assessment of nutritional status includes the measurement of hematologic status and protein nutrition. The absence of anemia may not exclude nutritional deficiencies, such as iron, folate, and vitamin B_{12} deficiencies. Red blood cell size is valuable in the differential diagnosis of anemias. The total serum protein determination is interpretable only if the globulins can be assumed to be normal. Albumin concentration is a better measure of protein nutrition than is serum globulin concentration, because its biologic half-life is shorter. A low concentration occurs when albumin is lost from the body in large amounts, as in nephrosis, exudative enteropathy, burns, or surgical drains. The so-called visceral proteins synthesized by the liver (such as retinol-binding protein with a half-life of 12 hours, transthyretin [prealbumin] with a half-life of 1.9 days, and transferrin with a half-life of 8 days) have shorter half-lives than does albumin, and their concentrations are better indicators of protein status than is the serum albumin concentration. Serum concentrations of essential amino acids may be lower than those of nonessential amino acids, and 3-methyl histidine excretion is increased during states of protein insufficiency. Other abnormalities of protein depletion include a decreased creatinine concentration and decreased hydroxyproline excretion. Values for protein status may or may not reflect the degree of nutritional deficiency. In simple starvation (marasmus), a tendency to maintain the circulatory pool of visceral proteins at the expense of somatic protein is evident. The blood urea nitrogen concentration tends to decrease during starvation; however, in patients in whom water intake is restricted, such as those with anorexia nervosa, the serum concentration may be elevated.

The serum sodium concentration is frequently decreased in malnutrition as the result of dilution, because total body water is physiologically increased during starvation. This value is seldom lower than 133 mEq/L, however. The dilution effect can also be seen with hematologic parameters, such as hematocrit and hemoglobin concentrations. Immunologic abnormalities, such as loss of delayed hypersensitivity, fewer T-lymphocytes, and changes in lymphocyte response to in vitro stimulation by phytohemagglutinin, are sometimes helpful clinical measurements of nutritional status.

Assays of specific nutrients can be helpful in the assessment of the nutritional status of an individual, but their usefulness is limited by their wide variation within normal groups and the lack of easy availability of many of the vitamin assays. Normal values for some of these biochemical measurements are shown in Table 24.5. Other vitamins, such as biotin and niacin, as well as essential fatty acids can be measured. These measurements are seldom clinically indicated. Assessment of the concentrations of minerals, such as calcium, magnesium, phosphorus, iodine, copper, and selenium, is readily available in most laboratories and sometimes is important to measure as part of the nutritional assessment.

Table 24.5

Normal Values: Biochemical Measurement of Specific Nutritional Parameters

Test	Normal Value	Exceptions
Protein, Blood		
Serum albumin, g/dL	3.7–5.5	Infant, 2.9–5.5
Retinol binding protein, mg/dL	1.3–9.9	Children <9 y, 1–7.8
Blood urea nitrogen, mg/dL	7–22	
Thyroxine binding protein, mg/dL	20–50	
Transferrin, mg/dL	170–440	
Fibronectin, mg/dL	30–40	
Prealbumin, mg/dL	17–42	Preterm infant, 4–14; term infant, 4–20; 6- to 12-mo-old child, 8–24; 1- to 6-y-old child, 17–30
Protein, Urine		
Creatinine/height index	>0.9	
3-methyl histidine, μmol/kg	3.2±0.6 male, 2.1±0.4 female, 4.2±1.3 neonate	
3-methyl histidine, μmol/g	126±32 male, 92±23 female,	
creatinine	253±78 neonate	
Hydroxyproline index	>2	
Vitamin A		
Plasma retinol, μg/dL	20–72	Infant, 13–50
Vitamin D		
25-OH-D_3, μg/L	2–30	…
1-25-OH-D_3, μg/L	15–60	
Riboflavin		
Red blood cell glutathione reductase stimulation, %	<20	…
Vitamin B$_6$		
Red blood cell transaminases, plasma pyridoxal phosphate, xanthurenic acid excretion	Feasible and useful in all age groups, but not readily available and not practical in children <9 y	…
Folic acid		
Serum folate, ng/mL	>6	…
Red blood cell folate, ng/mL	>160	

V

Table 24.5 *(Continued)*
Normal Values: Biochemical Measurement of Specific Nutritional Parameters

Test	Normal Value	Exceptions
Vitamin K		
Prothrombin time, sec	11–15	11–15
Vitamin E		
Plasma alphatocopherol, mg/dL	0.7–10	Preterm infant, 0.5–3.5
Red blood cell hemolysis test, %	10	
Vitamin C		
Plasma level, mg/dL	0.2–2.0	…
Leukocyte level, mg/100 cells	Difficult to perform on children because of sample requirements	
Thiamine		
Red blood cell transketolase stimulation, %	<15	…
Vitamin B$_{12}$		
Serum vitamin B$_{12}$, pg/mL	200–900	…
Absorption test	Excretion of more than 7.5% of ingested labeled vitamin B$_{12}$	
Iron		
Hematocrit, %	39	Neonate, 31; infant, 33; child and menstruating females, 36
Hemoglobin, g/dL	14	Neonate, 11; infant, 12; child and menstruating females, 13
Serum ferritin, ng/mL	>15	Neonate, <60
Serum iron, µg/dL	>60	Neonate, >30; infant, >40; child <4 y, >50
Serum total iron binding capacity, µg/dL	350–400	
Serum transferrin saturation, %	>16	Infant, >12; child <9 y, >14-15
Serum transferrin, mg/dL	170–250	Neonate, <80; infant, <75
Erythrocyte protoporphyrin, µg/dL red blood cells	<70	

Table 24.5 *(Continued)*
Normal Values: Biochemical Measurement of Specific Nutritional Parameters

Test	Normal Value	Exceptions
Zinc		
Serum level, μg/dL	60–120	...
Erythrocyte level	Erythrocytes contain approximately 10 times more zinc than does plasma	
Phosphorus		
Serum phosphate, mg/dL	2.9–5.6	Newborn, 4.0–8.0; 1-y-old child, 3.8–6.2; 2- to 5-y-old child, 3.5–6.8
Calcium		
Serum total calcium, mg/dL	8.5–10.5	Preterm infant, 6–10; term infant, 7–12; child, 8–10.5
Serum ionized calcium, mg/dL	4.48–4.92	
Magnesium		
Serum magnesium, mEq/L	1.5–2.0	...

References

1. Fomon SM. *Nutritional Disorders of Children: Prevention, Screening, and Followup.* Bethesda, MD: Department of Health and Human Services; 1977. US Dept of Health Education and Welfare; 1997. DHEW Publication No. HSA 77–5104

2. Baker JP, Detsky AS, Wesson DE, et al. Nutritional assessment: a comparison of clinical judgment and objective measurements. *N Engl J Med.* 1982;306:969–972

3. Hamill PV, Drizd TA, Johnson CL, Reed RB, Roche AF, Moore WM. Physical growth: National Center for Health Statistics percentiles. *Am J Clin Nutr.* 1979;32:607–629

4. Roche AF, Himes JH. Incremental growth charts. *Am J Clin Nutr.* 1980;33:2041–2052

5. Tanner JM, Davies PS. Clinical longitudinal standards for height and height velocity for North American children. *J Pediatr.* 1985;107:317–329

6. Himes JH, Roche AF, Thissen D, Moore WM. Parent-specific adjustments for evaluation of recumbent length and stature of children. *Pediatrics.* 1985;75:304–313

7. Frisancho AR. New norms of upper limb fat and muscle areas for assessment of nutritional status. *Am J Clin Nutr.* 1981;34:2540–2545

8. Kanawati AA, McLaren DS. Assessment of marginal malnutrition. *Nature.* 1970; 228:573–575

9. Kagan BM, Stanincova V, Felix NS, Hodgman J, Kalman D. Body composition of premature infants: relation to nutrition. *Am J Clin Nutr.* 1972;25:1153–1164

10. Lohman TG. Research progress in validation of laboratory methods of assessing body composition. *Med Sci Sports Exerc.* 1984;16:596–605

V

11. Lohman TG. Applicability of body composition techniques and constants for children and youths. *Exerc Sport Sci Rev.* 1986;14:325–357

12. McCarthy HD, Cole TJ, Fry T, Jebb SA, Prentice AM. Body fat reference curves for children. *Int J Obes (Lond).* 2006;30: 598–602

13. Forbes RM, Cooper AR, Mitchell HH. The composition of the adult human body as determined by chemical analysis. *J Biol Chem.* 1953;203:359–366

14. Moore FD, Lister J, Boyden CM, Ball MR, Sullivan N, Dagher FJ. The skeleton as a feature of body composition: values predicted by isotope dilution and observed by cadaver dissection in an adult human female. *Hum Biol.* 1968;40:135–188

15. Infant body composition by skinfold measurements. *Nutr Rev.* 1975;33:7–9

16. Karlberg P, Engstrom I, Lichtenstein H, Svennberg I. The development of children in a Swedish urban community. A prospective longitudinal study. III. Physical growth during the first three years of life. *Acta Paediatr Scand Suppl.* 1968;187:48–66

17. Lohman TG. Skinfolds and body density and their relation to body fatness: a review. *Hum Biol.* 1981;53:181–225

18. Forbes GB. Body composition in adolescence. *Prog Clin Biol Res.* 1981;61:55–72

19. Fields DA Goran MI, McCrory MA. Body-composition assessment via air-displacement plethysmography in adults and children: a review. *Am J Clin Nutr.* 2002;75:453–467

20. Forbes GB, Schultz F, Cafarelli C, Amirhakimi GH. Effects of body size on potassium-40 measurement in the whole body counter (tilt-chair technique). *Health Phys.* 1968;15:435–442

21. Remenchik AP, Miller CE, Kessler WV. Body composition estimates derived from potassium measurements. ANL-7461. *ANL Rep.* 1968;Jul:73–90

22. Lukaski HC, Johnson PE. A simple inexpensive method of determining total body water using a tracer dose of D_2O and infrared absorption of biological fluids. *Am J Clin Nutr.* 1985;41:363–370

23. Katch FI, Solomon RT, Shayevitz M, Shayevitz B. Validity of bioelectrical impedance to estimate body composition in cardiac and pulmonary patients. *Am J Clin Nutr.* 1986;43: 972–973

24. Lukaski HC, Bolonchuk WW, Hall CB, Siders WA. Validation of tetrapolar bioelectrical impedance method to assess human body composition. *J Appl Physiol.* 1986;60:1327–1332

25. Lukaski HC, Johnson PE, Bolonchuk WW, Lykken GI. Assessment of fat-free mass using bioelectrical impedance measurements of the human body. *Am J Clin Nutr.* 1985;41:810–817

26. Rinke WJ. Electrical impedance: a new technique to assess human body composition. *Mil Med.* 1986;151:338–341

27. Cochran WJ, Klish WJ, Wong WW, Klein PD. Total body electrical conductivity used to determine body composition in infants. *Pediatr Res.* 1986;20:561–564

28. Fiorotto ML, Cochran WJ, Funk RC, Sheng HP, Klish WJ. Total body electrical conductivity measurements: effects of body composition and geometry. *Am J Physiol.* 1987;252: R794–R800

29. Fiorotto ML, Klish WJ. Total body electrical conductivity measurements in the neonate. *Clin Perinatol.* 1991;18:611–627

Introduction

Compromised health or nutrition in children related to feeding and/or swallowing difficulties is a common concern for pediatricians and parents. Failure to thrive, aspiration pneumonia, and food refusal are some of the common issues reported in this at-risk group of children. Because pediatric swallowing dysfunction may result in substantial morbidity, timely recognition, evaluation, and intervention are essential. Swallowing is a complex sequence of motor events requiring coordination of muscles in the oral cavity, pharynx, larynx, and esophagus. Thus, swallowing problems may occur if function at any level of the upper aerodigestive tract is compromised. Common etiologies in pediatric dysphagia include neurologic disease, gastrointestinal issues (eg, food allergies, reflux), respiratory compromise, and anatomical anomalies.[1–3] Intact sensation from areas of the mouth, pharynx, and larynx is essential to normal swallowing, because initiation of swallowing and protection of the airway rely on adequate sensory input to the swallowing control centers in the brain. Anatomic defects of the oropharynx, larynx, or esophagus, as well as disease processes that alter motor or sensory function, may lead to swallowing abnormalities.[3–7]

Swallowing is generally described in 3 phases: oral, pharyngeal, and esophageal. Changes occur in these phases during the progression of normal development.[8,9] Therefore, swallowing problems in children can be either congenital or acquired. Dysfunction in the oral phase of swallowing with children is often characterized as a feeding problem unless the problem compromises the safety of the swallow. Feeding problems can be developmental in nature in which there is a delay in acquiring developmental feeding skills, such as mature sucking, chewing, or cup drinking.[7,10]

Common Conditions Associated With Feeding and Swallowing Disorders

The prevalence of feeding and swallowing disorders in the general pediatric population is largely unknown; however, among certain pediatric disease states, it is quite high. The causes of dysphagia are numerous. Dysphagia among children and adults with neuromuscular disease has been well documented.[11–15] The problem may be in the muscles, nerves, neuromuscular junction, or central nervous system. Central nervous system disease is a common cause of pediatric dysphagia. Of all children with cerebral palsy, 27% to 40% are believed to have a swallowing abnormality.[16] Also, behavioral components are often interwoven with biologic or organic causes related to feeding and swallowing problems and can be difficult to distinguish as separate etiologies.[1,17] Burklow and colleagues[2] found that 80% of their study cohort (n = 103) had behavioral and biologic components to their feeding disorders and, thus, they proposed a biobehavioral classification system of pediatric feeding issues. Other common etiologies of pediatric dysphagia or swallowing dysfunction include gastrointestinal, psychosocial, cardiorespiratory, metabolic, and anatomical problems.[2,5,15] Less common issues that may affect feeding and swallowing include chronic illness, organ transplantation, and immune-suppressant diseases.[9,18,19] Medication requirements in the latter group may lead to disruption in hunger drive.

Finally, anatomic abnormalities leading to dysphagia may be congenital or acquired and located in the nasopharynx, oral cavity, oropharynx, larynx, or esophagus. Cleft lip and cleft palate represent some of the more common anatomic defects that interfere with swallowing. The incidence is believed to be between 0.8 and 2.7 cases per 1000 live births.[20] Other anatomic anomalies associated with dysphagia include esophageal atresia, tracheoesophageal fistula, and type III and IV laryngeal clefts. These are generally identified and surgically corrected at birth to prevent aspiration. In addition, choanal atresia, severe micrognathia, subglottic stenosis, type I and II laryngeal clefts, and tracheal or laryngomalacia can lend to respiratory problems that compromise coordination of respiration with swallowing.[4-5,21]

Differential Diagnosis of Feeding Versus Swallowing Disorders

Dysphagia is usually indicated by a history of unsuccessful feeding (eg, gagging or vomiting during feeding, nasopharyngeal regurgitation, malnutrition, or failure to thrive); or a history of aspiration, evidenced by choking or coughing during feeding, recurrent pneumonia, or upper respiratory tract infections.[5,22,23] Feeding problems generally refer to the oral stage of feeding and can be sensory and/or motor-based. The swallow function is intact without risk of aspiration. Deficits in the mechanics of eating (chewing, drinking), development of feeding skills, and controlling the food or drink in the mouth can be involved. Feeding problems are different from swallowing disorders involving the pharyngeal stage of the swallow, in which there is a risk of aspiration. There can be difficulty in differentiating feeding and swallowing problems when children with oral sensitivity gag on textured foods.

Parents can sometimes describe gagging on textures as choking. Observing the onset of gagging is critical to note whether the gagging begins before the swallow. Most often, the gagging will start as the textured food contacts the back of the tongue or hypopharynx before swallowing. Solid food dysphagia (swallowing disorder) is uncommon in children unless there is pharyngeal/esophageal motility issues, esophageal stenosis, or previous tracheoesophageal fistula repair. If the child can consume liquids and smooth foods without difficulty but chokes on textured foods, this is a feeding disorder, not a swallowing problem. Issues of drooling, behavioral feeding problems, long-term deprivation of oral feeding as infants, or abnormal posture (eg, hyperextension of the neck with scapular retraction and shoulder girdle elevation) are also risk factors for swallowing abnormalities.[22,24] Dysphagia should also be suspected in children who have diseases that have been associated with swallowing dysfunction. Table 25.1 provides key differences between feeding and swallowing problems.

Table 25.1
Signs and Symptoms of Swallowing and Feeding-Based Issues

Swallowing	Feeding
Greater difficulty with liquids, especially water or juice	Strong preference for either smooth or crunchy foods
A gurgly vocal quality after eating	No problems with taking liquids or smooth foods
Difficulty swallowing solids related to dysmotility of pharynx or upper esophageal sphincter dysfunction	Gag on foods that require chewing
Respiratory compromise, including pneumonia	Will separate textures from smooth food and pocket them or spit them out
Coughing or choking during or immediately after eating	Difficulty with chewing; prolonged mealtimes

Feeding Disorders

Etiologies

Feeding disorders are oral stage issues that can be motor or sensory based.[25] Motor-based feeding problems can involve difficulty moving the food from the front to the back of the mouth before swallowing. For example, children with low muscle tone may have weak or uncoordinated tongue movements resulting in prolonged mealtimes or even choking with liquids because food spills in the airway before the swallow has been initiated. They may have difficulty chewing because of weak chewing muscles. Also, the child may present with developmental feeding delays, such as slow onset of chewing skills, related to lack of experience or compromise from chronic illness. In contrast with motor-based swallowing problems, difficulties with eating can also stem from dysfunction with the sensory system. This includes difficulty integrating sensory information related to the taste and texture of food. It is not uncommon to find sensory-based feeding problems when there is a history of reflux, slow gastric emptying, and sensitivity to touch. A common feeding history may include difficulty transitioning to textured foods or gagging and vomiting either at the smell of foods or when the food is placed on the tongue. These children may also present with additional sensory problems, such as sensitivity to touch, loud noises, and light. Parent reports may include not tolerating going barefoot on the carpet or grass; preferring not to be "messy" while eating; and dislike of tags in their clothing or seams in their socks. Thus, these "sensitive" infants and children may have more pronounced reactions to reflux or bodily discomfort that result in feeding disruption. Neurologic-based sensory issues, as seen in autism spectrum disorders, can result in long-term feeding issues, including high food selectivity and oral aversion behaviors.[26] Gastrointestinal issues occur commonly in children with autism spectrum disorders.[27]

Symptoms

Parents often pose questions regarding whether or when their child's feeding issues will resolve. Once early reflux and food allergy symptoms begin to subside by 1 to 2 years of age, feeding difficulties related to gastrointestinal issues generally begin to resolve as well. However, do these otherwise healthy children then establish typical or normal eating habits? Lefton-Grief[28] reported on retrospective findings from an 8-year follow-up of 19 otherwise healthy children with early respiratory problems of unexplained etiology. Aspiration of liquids was found in approximately 58% of the cases, and most of these resolved at an average age of 3 years. Approximately 30% of the children had persistent coughing issues in grade school. This longevity finding may not be unexpected; Hawdon et al[29] reported persistent feeding issues for approximately 50% of 35 preterm infants with an average gestational age of 34 weeks as the babies reached 6 and 12 months of age. Certainly, children with developmental disability and neurologic deficits may have lifelong feeding difficulties. However, this milder subgroup of persistent feeding problems may require our attention as well. Subsequently, some school programs are formally addressing feeding and swallowing issues within the school setting. Homer[30] described the challenge of more medically fragile children with feeding issues attending school. School therapists, including speech-language pathologists and occupational and physical therapists, may be involved in feeding programs. Homer[30] emphasized the importance of systematic written documentation to document feeding procedures and performance outcomes as well as training teaching staff or classroom aides to implement feeding techniques at meal or snack times. Educational statutes, such as Section 504 of the Rehabilitation Act of 1973 and the Individuals with Disabilities Education Act (IDEA), have mandated that schools provide health-related services.

Management

Intervening with sensory-based feeding issues can be a long process. Patel et al[31] have offered some feeding approaches. When children demonstrate frequent food packing or retaining textured foods in the mouth, this can lead to a low intake of food volume. A better volume and caloric intake may be achieved with offering less-textured foods during meal times. Also, high-texture foods can increase oral aversion responses in children with high oral sensitivity. Thus, starting with low-texture foods and graduating texture as tolerated can be a better feeding approach. Children can also be overwhelmed with large amounts per spoon, so smaller spoonfuls can be better accepted. Praise and encouragement are a good model for shaping positive feeding behavior versus critical statements and negative reinforcement.[32,33]

Summary of Feeding Disorders

- Etiologies: Developmental delay, lack of experience, chronic illness, autism spectrum disorder, neuromuscular, craniofacial, sensory integration disorder, behavioral, food allergies, gastroesophageal reflux disease (GERD).

- Symptoms: Difficulty chewing, drooling, food spilling from mouth, gagging and/or choking on chewable foods, prolonged time to finish meal or manage single bite, food refusal, poor progression with textures, selective eating or limited food repertoire, nausea or vomiting with smell of food, disrupted family dynamics, feeding best when partly asleep.

- Management of problem: Feeding or sensory treatment, multidisciplinary assessment, and treatment that may include: services of a speech-language pathologist, occupational therapist, physical therapist, dietitian, nurse, pediatrician, social services agent, or medical subspecialist, such as a neurologist, gastroenterologist, pulmonologist, otorhinolaryngologist, psychologist, or developmental/behavioral pediatrician. Often, feeding teams have a core of these individuals and additional referrals are made as needed. Adequate management of gastrointestinal symptoms can be critical for developmental or behavioral treatment approaches to be effective. Sometimes, reflux medications are discontinued too early when mild symptoms persist and eating regression can occur. Intensive, short-term multidisciplinary treatment options are available primarily at hospital-based venues for severe feeding issues, such as inability to wean from nonoral tube feeding or dysfunctional behavioral feeding dynamics that lend to persistent feeding difficulties.

Swallowing Disorders

Etiologies

Swallowing disorders involve pharyngeal and esophageal dysfunction that create aspiration risks. Primary aspiration risks during the act of swallowing occur when there is disruption of the complex nature of the pharyngeal stage of swallowing while the larynx is elevating, the vocal cords are closing to protect the airway, and the pharyngeal muscles are moving in a wave-like motion to move food into the esophagus. Vocal cord paralysis, especially bilateral paralysis, is an important cause of dysphagia and choking disorders, especially in the presence of other airway anomalies or neuromotor involvement. Abnormal muscle tone can also affect the muscles in the pharynx (pharyngeal constrictors), creating weak peristalsis, smooth muscle dysmotility, or muscle spasm, such as cricopharyngeal dysfunction. Medical problems that affect the respiratory system (eg, chronic lung disease, laryngo- or tracheomalacia, significant tachypnea) can also disrupt swallowing coordination and create risks of choking or even aspiration.[10]
In addition, children with significant gastroesophageal reflux can develop reduced sensitivity in the hypopharynx from inflammation, which can result in compromise of swallow coordination. These motor and sensory-based swallowing problems can lead to serious medical compromise and, because of concern for aspiration, may warrant further radiologic assessment with imaging techniques that examine the oral/pharyngeal stages of swallowing, such as the videofluoroscopic swallowing study (VFSS) or fiberoptic endoscopic examination of swallowing (FEES).[34–36]

Symptoms

Aerodigestive disorders are often paired with swallowing issues. Airway problems that may affect swallowing include vocal fold paralysis or paresis, significant subglottic stenosis, laryngomalacia, tracheoesophageal fistula, moderate to severe laryngeal clefts, neck or airway tumors such as a teratoma, or inflammation with reduced sensation. Such issues can create risks of laryngeal aspiration. Digestive issues such as reflux more commonly lead to feeding problems with food refusal and gagging symptoms. Reflux can also be the cause of secondary aspiration. Upper airway issues and subsequent swallowing problems are more frequently being managed with a team approach, often called "airway teams."[37] Such teams may include otolaryngology, pulmonology, gastroenterology, nursing, and speech-language pathology services. Reasons for referral often include chronic cough, asthma, persistent pulmonary issues with unclear etiology, and upper airway anomalies. The most common swallowing complaints include chronic cough during drinking and gagging on chewable foods. Consequences of feeding and swallowing issues may include inadequate volume or caloric intake and subsequent inadequate growth. When chronic cough is reported, it may or may not be the result of a swallowing problem. Therefore, it is important to determine whether the cough occurs in tandem with the act of swallowing or as a delayed symptom after eating, such as with gastroesophageal reflux. Chronic cough is a common initial symptom of mild laryngeal cleft.[38,39] Chronic cough can also be unrelated to feeding, such as with asthma and upper airway irritation.

Aspiration pneumonia in children is another concerning symptom. How much aspiration can a child tolerate and when should concerns be raised? Aspiration without pulmonary symptoms occurs in both healthy and disabled populations. This has been documented in both adult and pediatric literature.[6,40,41] Ramsey et al[40] reviewed several studies that indicated silent aspiration occurred in 20% to 30% of dysphagic cases in adult populations. Silent aspiration of saliva also was noted in normal sleeping adults. The presence of aspiration does not necessarily result in pulmonary compromise. Newman et al[6] examined swallow studies of 43 infants referred for dysphagia. Laryngeal penetration, aspiration, and nasal backflow occurred in almost half of the infants. Interestingly, these symptoms generally emerged after multiple normal swallows, with an average of almost 1 minute from the onset of the first swallow. Laryngeal penetration and aspiration occurred most frequently from material pooled in the pyriform sinus (above the upper esophageal opening). In addition, unlike adults, the infants cleared laryngeal penetration during the swallow without coughing. Newman et al[6] indicated that half of the infants developed 1 episode of pneumonia. However, the study did not find a strong correlation between timing of identified aspiration on the modified barium swallow (MBS) examination and the episodes of pneumonia. How accurate is an MBS examination? It is a limited time frame and may provide false-positive information.[42] Newman et al[6] recommended evaluating at least 1 minute of swallowing performance when performing a VFSS, because dysphagic episodes may not occur during the first several swallows.

When children experience aspiration on thin liquids, a common recommendation is for thickened fluids. This can lead to concerns with hydration, especially when children refuse thickened liquids. The question arises: can children with thin-liquid dysphagia have water? Wier and colleagues[43] reviewed multiple studies and found no randomized controlled studies that adequately examined the safety for children with thin-liquid dysphagia to consume water. They found no data to support full restriction of water intake for children who demonstrated primary aspiration of thin liquids. There are no current consistent guidelines on water restriction for thin-liquid aspiration with children.

Management

Evaluation of swallowing problems may include nasoendoscopy, bronchoscopy, pH probe, VFSS (or modified MBS), and/or FEES. The gold standard for swallow assessment continues to be the MBS or VFSS. The MBS examination provides information on the dynamics of all 3 swallowing phases, presence or absence of aspiration, and pharyngeal function issues. If the MBS result is negative but aspiration is suspected, FEES can be helpful in detecting mild dysphagia issues, such as intermittent microaspiration as sometimes seen with type I laryngeal clefts.[38] In addition, FEES provides information on the anatomy of the upper airway, including vocal fold function, edema, or anatomical anomalies. Therefore, FEES and the MBS examination can complement one another. Successful use of FEES with children can be age dependent for tolerance.

Summary of Swallowing Problems

- Etiologies: Respiratory, neuromuscular, anatomical, airway anomalies, pharyngeal or esophageal dysmotility, abnormal muscle tone, poor tongue control, laryngeal cleft, tracheoesophageal fistula, chronic lung disease, tachypnea.

- Symptoms: Choking associated with swallowing, especially on thin liquids; pneumonia; vocal quality change after swallowing; frequent upper respiratory infections.

- Management: Swallow assessment with MBS examination and/or FEES; medical management of gastroesophageal reflux, respiratory issues, and airway problems; and swallowing therapy when indicated with a speech-language pathologist. The World Health Organization has outlined 4 parameters to examine the effects of swallow problems: (1) impairment of structure/function; (2) degree of limiting activity; (3) ability to participate in daily routines; and (4) degree of distress to the child.[44] Progress in swallow function can be monitored across these parameters.

Evaluation of Pediatric Dysphagia

Multidisciplinary Process

The complex nature of feeding and swallowing problems requires multidisciplinary involvement to address the multifaceted issues that affect the feeding and swallowing process. The evaluation process can involve both a clinical evaluation of feeding behavior as well as instrumental assessment when swallowing concerns are present. Clinical evaluations may include a feeding team to manage feeding concerns or an airway clinic for upper airway and swallowing concerns. A comprehensive history and physical examination are important in the evaluation of the child with dysphagia; during this evaluation, emphasis should be placed on the feeding history and neurologic, pulmonary, and gastrointestinal function. If a risk of aspiration or oropharyngeal stage dysfunction is suspected, then a VFSS or FEES is indicated to further assess the swallow function and safety for oral eating. This examination is generally conducted by a speech-language pathologist in conjunction with a pediatric radiologist. If concerns related to feeding and growth occur, a referral should be made to a multidisciplinary feeding team.[45,46] Core members of such a team usually include a speech-language pathologist or an occupational therapist, nurse, dietitian, and perhaps, a gastroenterologist, developmental pediatrician, or physical therapist. Table 25.2 provides referral guidelines for further evaluation of feeding and swallowing problems. Despite these general guidelines, the referral process continues to need better standards of care for consistency in management of dysphagia problems. Sheppard[47] has expressed support for early referral of children

V

with developmental delay or medically complex issues that affect feeding and swallowing.

Table 25.2

Referral Guidelines for Feeding and Swallowing Problems

Feeding Team Evaluation	Modified Barium Swallow and/or FEES
Concerns with feeding:	Concerns with swallowing safety:
Taking liquids and smooth foods but choking on chewable food	Choking on liquids
Falling off growth curve	Fevers; congested breathing or other signs of respiratory infection
Refusing bottle/food	Does better with solid foods
Not progressing with age-appropriate diet	Neurologic involvement (abnormal muscle tone)
Behind in age-expected feeding skills	Poor head control
Prolonged time to complete a meal	Anatomical anomaly interfering with swallowing (repaired tracheoesophageal fistula; cleft palate; laryngeal/tracheal stenosis; laryngeal cleft)
Developmental delays (eg, poor chewing)	Wet vocal quality immediately after eating or during eating
Gastrointestinal/respiratory/neurologic/cardiac medical history	

Clinical Evaluation

Clinical evaluation of pediatric feeding and swallowing involves assessment of how effectively the child performs the oral, pharyngeal, and esophageal phases of swallowing along with several other factors.[6,10,48,49] The child's feeding history is important to the clinical evaluation. Elements of the history include: (1) how the child received nutrients and fluids; (2) the duration of nonoral nutrition; and (3) the child's ability to swallow effectively when first given oral feedings. Children who have been ill and have been fed by alternative methods have often not had normal oral experiences and, therefore, may not seek oral input.

Once the medical status, medication use, and feeding history of the child have been ascertained, examination of the oral-peripheral structures is performed. In addition, respiratory status at baseline and during eating should be monitored along with developmental feeding skills. Observing how the child manages oral secretions provides information about swallowing function, airway protection, and oral-motor control. Swallow function can be screened with observation of secretion management, laryngeal movement, and vocal quality during and after swallowing. When problems with the pharyngeal or esophageal phase of the swallow are suspected and the reason is unclear, radiographic or instrumental evaluation is indicated.

Instrumental Evaluation of Dysphagia

Videofluoroscopy

The current procedures of choice for the assessment of infants and children with swallowing disorders are the VFSS and MBS examination. These are generally performed under the direction of a radiologist and a speech-language pathologist. During a swallow, the oral cavity, pharynx, and cervical esophagus are visualized first in the lateral view to assess aspiration, and an anter-posterior view is later taken to study symmetry. Therapeutic techniques may be evaluated at this time to monitor their effectiveness. The study is videotaped or recorded digitally for later review.[50] In the detection of aspiration,[23,51] a pharyngeal-phase swallowing abnormality defined as the passage of food below the true vocal cords, the VFSS has proved superior to bedside clinical assessment[21,50] and has also effectively determined which patients are at risk of pneumonia.[12,23] Other radiologic methods to evaluate dysphagia include ultrasonography and scintigraphy.[52-55] Ultrasonography is a noninvasive approach that provides information regarding tongue, hyoid, and soft-palate movement during swallowing but does not allow direct viewing of aspiration or penetration. Advancing technology in ultrasonography has allowed more detailed and effective swallow assessment for both oral stage function (eg, tongue dynamics) and pharyngeal swallowing development (eg, in utero).[56]

Pharyngeal Manometry

Pharyngeal manometry is the best method for evaluating pharyngeal and esophageal motor function. Manometry requires the transnasal insertion of a catheter housing a series of intraluminal pressure transducers.[43] In the evaluation of dysphagia, it is best used as a complementary diagnostic procedure to endoscopy, VFSS, or electromyography.[57-60] In children, manometry has been used mainly to investigate gastroesophageal reflux, esophageal motor, and pharyngeal motor disorders. Videomanometry has been reported as a useful means to further examine manometry findings in children by looking at concurrent fluoroscopic images.[61]

Fiberoptic Endoscopic Evaluation of Swallowing
Instrumental evaluation of dysphagia includes FEES. It has been used primarily in the evaluation of adults for whom a VFSS is unsuitable, but the use in the pediatric population is now increasing. An endoscope is passed transnasally through the nasopharynx and hypopharynx and positioned just above the false vocal folds. This technique is particularly useful to directly assess laryngeal function for adduction and airway protection. Children with reflux and upper airway issues in addition to swallowing concerns can benefit from FEES. Other indications for FEES include assessment of possible anatomic contributing factors, assessment of pharyngeal or laryngeal sensitivity, and a risk of aspiration of even minute amounts of material.[35] Other reported advantages include detection of pooling in the pharynx and training the child to use compensatory swallowing techniques. The age of the child is a factor for tolerance of the procedure.[35,36,39]

Treatment

Treatment of pediatric feeding and swallowing disorders varies greatly depending on the symptoms, the cause of the problem, and the child's feeding history. However, treatment can generally be categorized into 6 areas: positioning, oral sensory normalization, modification of food consistency, swallowing maneuvers, adaptive feeding devices, and oral feeding exercises.[62,63] Providers of pediatric feeding therapy are typically speech-language pathologists or occupational therapists. Children with neuromotor involvement require secure positional support while maintaining head and spine alignment. Collaboration with a physical therapist and a feeding specialist for proper seating and positional needs can be helpful.[64] Children with motor impairment may also require simplification of food choices (smooth vs chewable foods), the use of swallow maneuvers for older children (eg, effortful swallow, breath hold and cough after swallowing) and thickened liquids in cases of aspiration risk. Children with behavioral and sensory-related eating issues can benefit from regulation of sensory modulation, food texture modification, and fostering developmental feeding skills.[65] In general, thinner consistencies (eg, thin liquids) are indicated for children with problems with bolus transport and children who are weak or fatigue easily. Thicker consistencies (eg, purees and soft solids) are indicated when the problem is oral containment of the bolus, poor tongue control, delayed swallow initiation, or decreased laryngeal closure during the swallow. Bottles and cups with varying flow rate can be selected as well.[21]

Behavioral Approaches

Behavioral approaches may include following the child's lead, feeding the child when hunger signs begin, gaining the child's attention but not overarousing, and watching for the child's signals for satiation.[32] Also, some general rules to follow may include maintaining a regular mealtime schedule, providing a neutral atmosphere with avoidance of force feeding, and offering small portions with solids first and fluids last. In the interim to achieving a normal eating pattern, parents are encouraged to maintain mealtime routines when possible, not to have the child "grazing" on food continuously, and to provide a high-calorie diet to reduce episodes of forced feeding to meet caloric intake goals. Nutritional supplements can provide an entire meal for children who are averse to solid foods. Evaluation by a dietitian is critical when determining the child's caloric and growth needs and the optimal nutrition plan to meet those needs.[18,66]

Enteral Feeding: How It Affects the Feeding Process

When children require supplemental alternative nutrition for prolonged periods, gastrostomy tubes are preferred over nasogastric tubes to minimize issues of oral aversion, discomfort with oral feeding, irritation of the upper aerodigestive tract, and increasing gastroesophageal reflux episodes.[67] For children with marked developmental disability or severe failure to thrive who require a gastrostomy tube, enteral feedings can assuage mealtime pressures on parents for nutrition and growth. Caloric needs that are not met at mealtimes can be given later by gastrostomy tube until the child is ready to begin weaning from the tube feedings. However, along with these benefits, parents of children who receive all their nutrition by enteral feeds experience other stress situations, such as coping with a child who does not eat by mouth, social stigmata, and medical complications with tube function.[68] Burklow and colleagues[68] reported that families of children with developmental problems and feeding issues experienced an equal amount of stress as did families of children who were totally dependent on gastrostomy tubes. One concerning population is children without oral motor or swallow dysfunction who require gastrostomy tubes for poor growth and frequent refusal of oral feeding. These children can be at risk of future difficulties transitioning to full oral feeding once tube feedings are introduced. This is an area that requires further investigation for long-term implications.[69] Most health care professionals who treat patients with dysphagia believe that the best exercise for swallowing is swallowing. Therefore, the goal for all children with dysphagia is safe eating, even if only in small amounts.

V

Weaning From Nonoral Feedings

Weaning from nonoral feedings should be a slow and gradual process.[70] The approach requires attention to establishing adequate hunger cues, adequate feeding and oral motor skills, maximizing caregiver interactions, and many times, behavioral therapy.[71] Children who have received chronic tube feedings often miss critical transition periods for eating, such as beginning solid foods. Subsequently, these children can demonstrate significant oral aversion to eating, especially textured foods. Senz and colleagues[72] discussed the effects of nonoral feeding during the first year of life, intimating that cortical development can be affected from reduced input to the motor and sensory pathways between the oropharynx and cortex. A methodical process to wean from tube feedings is required for children who meet the appropriate criteria.[69] One method is to first transition patients on continuous feedings to bolus feedings. Next, offer food by mouth before each daytime bolus feeding to simulate a mealtime schedule. The eventual plan is to eliminate nighttime tube feedings. As the child consumes more calories by mouth, then the tube feedings can be decreased accordingly. This process will be most successful when performed in conjunction with an oral sensory treatment program and close monitoring by a dietitian and pediatrician. Assessment scales, such as the *Pediatric Assessment Scale for Severe Feeding Problems*, can be helpful to measure and monitor the tube-weaning process.[73] Currently, there are multiple approaches to the tube-weaning process, including intensive inpatient and outpatient hospital-based programs. Components to consider when selecting a weaning approach may include medical diagnosis, developmental feeding skill level, child temperament, duration and method of tube feeding, and family psychosocial dynamics.[69]

Current Trends and Perspectives in Pediatric Feeding and Swallowing Disorders

Changes in Referrals: Whom Are We Treating?

The children that frequent multidisciplinary feeding teams and primary care offices with feeding and swallowing difficulties have gradually changed over the past decade. There is an apparent trend of increasing gastrointestinal-related feeding difficulties versus previously more common referrals for neuromuscular disorders. Referral intakes are, thus, frequently peppered with key phrases, such as sensory-based feeding difficulties, food allergies, inadequate nutrition intake, and gagging and vomiting with solid foods.[1,3,74,75] The bases for this trend are not clearly identified. Perhaps the increasing survival rate of preterm infants, food allergies, and possibly environmental influences are factors to consider. Garcia-Careaga and Kerner[76] reported a food allergy incidence of 2% to 8% in young infants. They further described issues of irritability, food refusal, and dysphagia in cases of allergic eosinophilic esophagitis. Rommel and colleagues[75] reported that of 700 children younger than 10 years presenting to a tertiary care center with feeding and nutrition problems, 50% were younger than 1 year, more than 50% had gastrointestinal issues (especially GERD), and almost 50% had medical (gastrointestinal) and neurologic (most commonly autism spectrum disorders) problems and oral feeding issues (3 most common: sucking, oral sensory, experience delay because of illness). Of note, 18% of cases were suspected to be Munchausen by proxy, and most children with oral feeding issues were younger than 2 years. Behavioral problems were more common in children older than 2 years. Thus, it appears that the longer feeding issues persist, behavioral problems are more likely to occur as part of the feeding problem milieu. Often, health care professionals will find a continuum of organic-based versus functional-based feeding problems that cannot be easily separated. For example, Rommel and colleagues[75] found that sensory-based feeding problems were associated with a history of nasogastric tube feeding and a history of aspiration or ventilation in first 6 months of life. They described their study population as overrepresented with preterm infants with a gestational age of <34 weeks.

Overall, children born preterm or those who present with developmental delays are more likely to have persistent feeding issues.[1,3,29] Manikam and Perman[1] indicated that up to 80% of this population may demonstrate feeding difficulties. Gastrointestinal issues were most common, with various accompanying problems: behavior/sensory issues, airway compromise, or oral motor problems. As extremely preterm infants filter more into feeding clinics, results of their feeding issues are being described. Wood and colleagues[77] examined 283 preterm infants of less than 25 weeks' gestation for more than 30 months. It was found that 33% had persistent feeding issues after 2 years of age. Swallowing problems and food refusal were the most common issues reported. The authors described increased risk of poor growth that was more often associated with developmental delay and neurologic problems compared with respiratory issues.

Approaches for Long-Term Feeding Difficulties

Many support early initiation of feeding treatment and close follow-up on discharge home from the neonatal intensive care unit.[3,75] It is important with preterm infants to advance their solid food diet according to developmental readiness versus corrected age. Burklow and colleagues[3] found that preterm infants who were fed solid foods too early were likely to have food texture aversion, including gagging/vomiting. This is important to monitor, given the tendency for preterm infants or neonates with feeding problems to later develop gagging and vomiting on textured foods.[29] It will require multidisciplinary efforts to identify the complex nature of contributors to feeding behaviors that disrupt adequate nutrition and growth, including reflux, esophagitis, neuromotor immaturity, irritability, food refusal, and gagging/vomiting. Issues of reflux and esophagitis may be managed with H-2 blockers, proton pump inhibitors, thickened feeds, or surgery (eg, fundoplication).[78–80] In recent years, medication has been favored over fundoplication for management of reflux with the exception of severe reflux cases.[81] For preterm infants with persistent pulmonary problems and subsequent growth failure, supplemental nutrition via gastrostomy tube feedings has been shown to be beneficial.[82] In addition to medical management concerns, family dynamics and mealtime routines also influence feeding success. Therefore, it is important to query parents about how they are feeding their children, including whether they are force feeding, chasing their child room to room, offering inappropriate textures, having prolonged mealtimes, or acting as short-order cooks for their children. All of these scenarios do not foster a positive or helpful feeding environment for children with feeding difficulties. Community support services and family education are vital components of the intervention process for children with feeding problems.

Assessment and Treatment Updates

Fiberoptic Endoscopic Examination of Swallowing With Sensory Testing
A helpful tool for assessing laryngeal sensory function is laryngopharyngeal sensory threshold testing via FEES with sensory threshold testing (FEESST).[83] Signs of extraesophageal reflux can be detected with evidence of edema and irritation at the laryngeal entrance, including the arytenoids. Subsequent altered sensation may be present. Upper airway sensation is critical for maintaining airway protection from aspiration or penetration.[35,36] Additional information to FEES is provided by FEESST on sensation levels of the upper airway. A small puff of air is delivered from the flexible endoscope to the aryepiglottic folds to elicit a laryngeal adductor response (LAR). Delivery intensity can range from 4 to 10 mm. Link and colleagues[84] reported in a study with 100 pediatric patients that a LAR of less than 4 was rarely associated with laryngeal penetration or aspiration. Elevated LARs (>10)

were positively associated with aspiration pneumonia, neurologic problems, and GERD. This threshold may be reduced in the presence of GERD, and subsequently, an increased risk of laryngeal penetration and aspiration has been reported.[83] Willging and Thompson[85] found no adverse reactions using FEESST with children. Further, FEEST was reported to be as accurate in detecting aspiration risk as is a VFSS.

Functional Magnetic Resonance Imaging Assessment of Swallowing
Functional magnetic resonance imaging (FMRI) studies of swallowing have provided insight with regard to specific areas of the brain involved in normal swallowing. The primary work to date has been completed with an adult population. It has been shown that both central brain activation and brainstem control are involved, as are the basal ganglia and cerebellum.[86] Hartnick and colleagues[87] examined children 3 children with dysphagia to examine cortical and brainstem mapping. They found preliminary differences in mapping between types of swallowing problems. However, the use of dry swallows was noted as a likely limiting factor in examining true swallow function. The research designs continue to evolve for optimal use of FMRI to examine normal swallowing.[88,89] There is future potential for examining pediatric dysphagia with FMRI, including sensory-based swallowing problems.

Drooling and Saliva Management
Children with marked saliva management issues can have social acceptability issues as well as risks of choking, reduced cough function, and aspiration. Airway safety issues with excessive saliva are primarily present in profound neurologic cases. Conservative management may include medication, behavioral or oral motor therapy, and sometimes, surgery to close or excise 1 or more of the saliva glands. One alternative to surgery in severe cases, such as with quadriplegic cerebral palsy, is botulinum toxin type A injection to the salivary glands.[90] This must be done cautiously to avoid trauma to the facial nerve and nearby muscles and arteries. Ultrasonography and electromyographic assistance can guide accurate location of glands during the procedure. Kim and colleagues[90] reported reduced saliva production and improved pulmonary problems in 2 cases of neurologically involved children.

External Electrical Stimulation for Swallowing Treatment
Electrical stimulation therapy for swallowing is a form of neuromuscular electrical stimulation to affect the cranial nerves. The reported concept is that the stimulation causes the muscles for swallowing to contract and, thus, results in muscle strengthening or improved motor control. Research is

currently underway to examine the efficacy of this procedure with children and adults. Limited supportive data are currently available, although there are numerous positive anecdotal reports of swallowing improvement using electrical stimulation. Placement of the surface electrodes is critical, because results opposite of what is desired have been achieved, such as the larynx descending versus ascending during the swallow.[91] Further research is needed to verify validity and efficacy of electrical stimulation therapy for swallowing disorders.

Conclusion

Dysphagia is commonly associated with certain pediatric disorders and can result in substantial morbidity. Further, the type of medical condition or developmental problems a child demonstrates can often be a strong predictor of specific feeding and swallowing symptoms.[65] The timely identification of pediatric feeding and swallowing disorders is important for initiating evaluation and treatment when indicated. This can prevent or reduce future medical and/or nutritional compromise for the at-risk child. Differentiating between feeding and swallowing problems helps to guide proper evaluation and treatment approaches and streamline health care. Finally, a multidisciplinary team approach is the most effective means for managing pediatric feeding and swallowing problems.

References

1. Manikam R, Perman, JA. Pediatric feeding disorders. *J Clin Gastroenterol.* 2000;30:34–46
2. Burklow KA, Phelps AN, Schultz JR, McConnell K, Rudolph C. Classifying complex pediatric feeding disorders. *J Pediatr Gastroenterology Nutr.* 1998;27:143–147
3. Burklow KA, McGrath AM, Valerius KS, Rudolph C. Relationship between feeding difficulties, medical complexity, and gestational age. *Nutr Clin Pract.* 2002;17:373–378
4. Derkay CS, Schechter GL. Anatomy and physiology of pediatric swallowing disorders. *Otolaryngol Clin North Am.* 1998;31:397–404
5. Kosko JR, Moser JD, Erhart N, Tunkel DE. Differential diagnosis of dysphagia in children. *Otolaryngol Clin North Am.* 1998;31:435–451
6. Newman LA, Keckley C, Petersen MC, Hamner A. Swallowing function and medical diagnoses in infants suspected of dysphagia. *Pediatrics.* 2001;108(6):e106. Available at: http://pediatrics. aappublications.org/cgi/content/full/108/6/e106. Accessed September 5, 2007
7. Rudolph CD, Link DT. Feeding disorders in infants and children. *Pediatr Clin North Am.* 2002;49:97–112, vi
8. Bosma JF. Postnatal ontogeny of performances of the pharynx, larynx, and mouth. *Am Rev Respir Dis.* 1985;131:S10–S15

9. Diamant NE. Development of esophageal function. *Am Rev Respir Dis.* 1985;131:S29–S32

10. Miller CK, Willging JP. Advances in the evaluation and management of pediatric dysphagia. *Curr Opin Otolaryngol Head Neck Surg.* 2003;11:442–446

11. Griggs CA, Jones PM, Lee RE. Videofluoroscopic investigation of feeding disorders of children with multiple handicap. *Dev Med Child Neurol.* 1989;31:303–308

12. Taniguchi MH, Moyer RS. Assessment of risk factors for pneumonia in dysphagic children: significance of videofluoroscopic swallowing evaluation. *Dev Med Child Neurol.* 1994;36:495–502

13. Waterman ET, Koltai PJ, Downey JC, Cacace AT. Swallowing disorders in a population of children with cerebral palsy. *Int J Pediatr Otorhinolaryngol.* 1992;24:63–71

14. Weiss MH. Dysphagia in infants and children. *Otolaryngol Clin North Am.* 1998;21:727–735

15. Arvedson JC. Dysphagia in pediatric patients with neurologic damage. *Semin Neurol.* 1996;16:371–386

16. Love RJ, Hagerman EL, Taimi EG. Speech performance, dysphagia and oral reflexes in cerebral palsy. *J Speech Hear Disord.* 1980;45:59–75

17. Arvedson, JC. Behavioral issues and implications with pediatric feeding disorders. *Semin Speech Lang.* 1997;18:51–69

18. Baer MT, Bradford Harris A. Pediatric nutrition assessment identifying children at risk. *J Am Diet Assoc.* 1997;97(Suppl 2):S107–S115

19. Douglas JE, Hulson B, Trompeter RS. Psycho-social outcomes of parents and young children after renal transplantation. *Child Care Health Dev.* 1998;24:73–83

20. Vanderas AP. Incidence of cleft lip, cleft palate, and cleft lip and palate among races: a review. *Cleft Palate J.* 1987;24:216–225

21. Arvedson JC, Brodsky L. *Pediatric Swallowing and Feeding: Assessment and Management.* San Diego, CA: Singular Publishing; 1993

22. Lespargot A, Langevin MF, Muller S, Guillemont S. Swallowing disturbances associated with drooling in cerebral-palsied children. *Dev Med Child Neurol.* 1993;35:298–304

23. Friedman B, Frazier JB. Deep laryngeal penetration as a predictor of aspiration. *Dysphagia.* 2000;15:153–158

24. Tuchman DN. Cough, choke, sputter: the evaluation of the child with dysfunctional swallowing. *Dysphagia.* 1989;3:111–116

25. Palmer MM, Heyman MB. Assessment and treatment of sensory-versus motor-based feeding problems in very young children. *Infant Young Child.* 1993;6:67–73

26. Whiteley P. Developmental, behavioural and somatic factors in pervasive developmental disorders: preliminary analysis. *Child Care Health Dev.* 2004;30:5–11

27. Horvath K, Papadimitriou JC, Rabsztyn A, Drachenberg C, Tildon TJ. Gastrointestinal abnormalities in children with autistic disorder. *J Pediatr.* 1999;135:559–563

28. Lefton-Greif M. Long-term follow-up of oropharyngeal dysphagia in children without apparent risk factors. *Pediatr Pulmonol.* 2006;41:1040–1048

29. Hawdon JM, Beauregard N, Slattery J, Kennedy G. Identification of neonates at risk of developing feeding problems in infancy. *Dev Med Child Neurol.* 2000;42:235–239

30. Homer EM. An interdisciplinary team approach to providing dysphagia treatment in the schools. *Semin Speech Lang.* 2003;24:215–234

31. Patel MR, Piazza CC, Layer SA, Coleman R, Swartzwelder DM. A systematic evaluation of food textures to decrease packing and increase oral intake in children with pediatric feeding disorders. *J Appl Behav Anal.* 2005;38:89–100

32. Satter E. Feeding dynamics: helping children to eat well. *J Pediatric Health Care.* 1995;9:178–184

33. Satter E. *How to Get Your Kid to Eat...But Not Too Much.* Palo Alto, CA: Bull Publishing; 1987

34. Sonies BC. Instrumental procedures for dysphagia diagnosis. *Semin Speech Lang.* 1991;12:185–198

35. Hartnick CJ, Hartley BE, Miller C, Willging P. Pediatric fiberoptic endoscopic evaluation of swallowing. *Ann Otol Rhinol Laryngol.* 2000;109:996–999

36. Leder SB, Karas DE. Fiberoptic endoscopic evaluation of swallowing in the pediatric population. *Laryngoscope.* 2000;110:1132–1136

37. Wiatrak BJ, Hood J, Lackey P. Paediatric airway clinic: an 18 month experience. *J Otolaryngol.* 1997;26:149–154

38. Ashland J, Haver K, Hardy S, Hartnick CJ. Type I laryngeal clefts in children: dysphagia assessment and outcomes. Paper presented at the Dysphagia Research Society Annual Meeting; March 23–26, 2006; Scottsdale AZ

39. Boseley ME, Ashland J, Hartnick CJ. The utility of the fiberoptic evaluation of swallowing (FEES) in diagnosing and treating children with Type I laryngeal clefts. *Int J Pediatr Otorhinolaryngol.* 2006;70:339–343

40. Ramsey D, Smithard D, Kalra L. Silent aspiration: what do we know? *Dysphagia.* 2005;20:218–225

41. Shiekh S, Allen E, Shell R, et al. Chronic aspiration without gastroesophageal reflux as a cause of chronic respiratory symptoms in neurologically normal infants. *Chest.* 2001;120:1190–1195

42. Hill M, Hughes T, Milford C. Treatment for swallowing difficulties (dysphagia) in chronic muscle disease. *Cochrane Database Syst Rev.* 2004;(2):CD004303

43. Weir K, McMahon S, Chang AB. Restriction of oral intake of water for aspiration lung disease in children. *Cochrane Database Syst Rev.* 2005(4):CD005303

44. Skeat J, Perry A. Outcome measurement in dysphagia: not so hard to swallow. *Dysphagia.* 2005;20:113–122

45. Lane SL, Cloud HH. Feeding problems and intervention: an interdisciplinary approach. *Top Clin Nutr.* 1988;3:23–32

46. Lefton-Greif MA, Arvedson JC. Pediatric feeding/swallowing teams. *Semin Speech Lang.* 1997;18:5–11

47. Sheppard JJ. Case management challenges in pediatric dysphagia. *Dysphagia.* 2001;16:74

48. Darrow DH, Harley CM. Evaluation of swallowing disorders in children. *Otolaryngol Clin North Am.* 1998;31:405–418

49. Newman L. Optimal care patterns in pediatric patients with dysphagia. *Semin Speech Lang.* 2000;21:281–291

50. Arvedson JC, Lefton-Grief MA. *Pediatric Videofluoroscopic Swallow Studies: A Professional Manual with Caregiver Guidelines*. San Antonio, TX: Communication Skill Builders/ Psychological Corporation; 1998

51. Arvedson JC, Rogers B, Buck G, Smart P, Msall M. Silent aspiration prominent in children with dysphagia. *Int J Ped Otorhinolaryngol*. 1994;28:173–181

52. Weber F, Woolridge MW, Baum JD. An ultrasonographic study of the organization of sucking and swallowing by newborn infants. *Dev Med Child Neurol*. 1986;28:19–24

53. Guillet J, Basse-Cathalinat B, Christophe E, Ducassou D, Blanquet P, Wynchank S. Routine studies of swallowed radionuclide transit in paediatrics: experience with 400 patients. *Eur J Nucl Med*. 1984;9:86–90

54. Muz J, Mathog RH, Rosen R, Miller PR, Borrero G. Detection and quantification of laryngotracheopulmonary aspiration with scintigraphy. *Laryngoscope*. 1987;97:1180–1185

55. Baikie G, South MJ, Reddihough DS, et al. Agreement of aspiration tests using barium videofluoroscopy, salivagram, and milk scan in children with cerebral palsy. *Dev Med Child Neurol*. 2005;47:86–93

56. Miller JL. Ultrasound and the aerodigestive system: The research past, the imaging present, and the clinical future. Paper presented at the Dysphagia Research Society Annual Meeting; March 23–26, 2006; Scottsdale, AZ

57. Feussner H, Kauer W, Siewert JR. The place of esophageal manometry in the diagnosis of dysphagia. *Dysphagia*. 1993;8:98–104

58. Elidan J, Shochina M, Gonen B, Gay I. Manometry and electromyography of the pharyngeal muscles in patients with dysphagia. *Arch Otolaryngol Head Neck Surg*. 1990;116:910–913

59. Palmer JB. Electromyography of the muscles of oropharyngeal swallowing: basic concepts. *Dysphagia*. 1989;3:192–198

60. Elidan J, Gonen B, Shochiana M, Gay I. Electromyography of the inferior constrictor and cricopharyngeal muscles during swallowing. *Ann Otol Rhinol Laryngol*. 1990;99:466–469

61. Kawahara H, Kubota A, Okuyama H, Oue T, Tazue Y, Okada A. The usefulness of videomanometry for studying pediatric esophageal motor disease. *J Pediatr Surg*. 2004;39:1754–1757

62. Rudolf MC, Logan S. What is the long-term outcome for children who fail to thrive? A systematic review. *Arch Dis Child*. 2005;90:925–931

63. Morris SE, Klein MD. *Pre-Feeding Skills: A Comprehensive Resource for Mealtime Development*. 2nd ed. San Antonio, TX: TBS/Harcourt; 2000

64. Redstone F, West JF. The importance of postural control for feeding. *Pediatr Nurs*. 2004;30:97–100

65. Field D, Garland M, Williams K. Correlates of specific childhood feeding problems. *J Paediatr Child Health*. 2003;39:299–304

66. Kovar AJ. Nutrition assessment and management in pediatric dysphagia. *Semin Speech Lang*. 1997;18:39–49

67. Bazyk S. Factors associated with the transition to oral feeding in infants fed by nasogastric tubes. *Am J Occup Ther*. 1990;44:1070–1078

68. Burklow KA, McGrath AM, Allred KE, Rudolph C. Parent perceptions of mealtime behaviors in children fed enterally. *Nutr Clin Pract.* 2002;17:291–295

69. Mason SJ, Harris G, Blissett J. Tube feeding in infancy: implications for the development of normal eating and drinking skills. *Dysphagia.* 2005;20:46–61

70. Palmer MM. Weaning from gastrostomy tube feeding: commentary on oral aversion. *Pediatr Nurs.* 1995;24:475–478

71. Benoit D, Wang EE, Zlotkin SH. Discontinuation of enterostomy tube feeding by behavioral treatment in early childhood: a randomized controlled study. *J Pediatr.* 2000;137:498–503

72. Senz C, Guys JM, Mancini J, Paz Peredes A, Lena G, Choux M. Weaning children from tube to oral feeding. *Childs Nerv Syst.* 1996;12:590–594

73. Crist W, Dobbelsteyn C, Brousseau AM, Napier-Phillips A. Pediatric assessment scale for severe feeding problems: validity and reliability of a new scale for tube-fed children. *Nutr Clin Pract.* 2004;19:403–408

74. Terres N, Ashland J. Tracking patterns of children's feeding problems in hospital-based feeding team [abstr]. *J Pediatr Nurs.* 2005;20:228

75. Rommel N, De Meyer AM, Feenstra L, Veereman-Wauters G. The complexity of feeding problems in 700 infants and young children presenting to a tertiary care institution. *J Pediatr Gastroenterol Nutr.* 2003;37:75–84

76. Garcia-Careaga M Jr, Kerner JA Jr. Gastrointestinal manifestations of food allergies in pediatric patients. *Nutr Clin Pract.* 2005;20:526–535

77. Wood NS, Costeloe K, Gibson AT, et al. The EPICure study: growth and associated problems in children born at 25 weeks of gestational age or less. *Arch Dis Child Fetal Neonatal Ed.* 2003;88: F492–F500

78. McPherson V, Wright ST, Bell AD. What is the best treatment for gastroesophageal reflux and vomiting in infants? *J Fam Pract.* 2005;54:372–375

79. Jones NL, Wine E. Pediatric gastrointestinal diseases: are drugs the answer? *Curr Opin Pharmacol.* 2005;5:604–609

80. Hassall E. Decisions in diagnosing and managing chronic gastroesophageal reflux disease in children. *J Pediatr.* 2005;146:S3–S12

81. Hassall E. Outcomes of fundoplication: causes for concern, newer options. *Arch Dis Child.* 2005;90:1047–1052

82. Guimber D, Michaud L, Storme L, Deschildre A, Turck D, Gottrand F. Gastrostomy in infants with neonatal pulmonary disease. *J Ped Gastroenterol Nutr.* 2003;36:459–463

83. Thompson DM. Laryngopharyngeal sensory testing and assessment of airway protection in pediatric patients. *Am J Med.* 2003;115:166S–168S

84. Link DT, Willging JP, Miller CK, Cotton RT, Rudolph CD. Pediatric laryngopharyngeal sensory testing during flexible endoscopic evaluation of swallowing: feasible and correlative. *Ann Otol Rhinol Laryngol.* 2000;109:899–905

85. Willging JP, Thompson DM. Pediatric FEEST: fiberoptic endoscopic evaluation of swallowing with sensory testing. *Curr Gastroentrol Rep.* 2005;7:240–243

86. Suzuki M, Asad Y, Ito J, Hayashi K, Inoue H, Kitano H. Activation of cerebellum and basal ganglia on volitional swallowing detected by functional magnetic resonance imaging. *Dysphagia.* 2003;18:71–77

87. Hartnick CJ, Rudolph C, Willging JP, Holland SK. Functional magnetic resonance imaging of the pediatric swallow: imaging the cortex and brainstem. *Larygnoscope.* 2001;111:1183–1191

88. Toogood JA, Barr AM, Stevens TK, Gati JS, Menon RS, Martin RE. Discrete functional contributions of cerebral cortical foci in voluntary swallowing: a functional magnetic resonance imaging (fMRI) "Go, No-Go" study. *Exp Brain Res.* 2005;161:81–90

89. Malandraki GA, Perlman AL. The use of MRI and FMRI in swallowing: Present and future applications. Paper presented at the Dysphagia Research Society Annual Meeting; March 23–26, 2006; Scottsdale, AZ

90. Kim H, Lee Y, Weiner D, Kaye R, Cahill AM, Yudkoff M. Botulinum toxin type A injections to salivary glands: combination with single event multilevel chemoneurolysis in 2 children with severe spastic quadriplegic cerebral palsy. *Arch Phys Med Rehabil.* 2006;87:141–144

91. Humbert I, Poletts C, Saxon K, et al. The effects of surface electrical stimulation on hyo-laryngeal movement at rest and during swallowing in normal volunteers. Paper presented at the Dysphagia Research Society Annual Meeting; March 23–26, 2006; Scottsdale AZ

V

26 Failure to Thrive

Failure to thrive (FTT) is an imprecise, archaic term that refers to children whose growth is significantly lower than the norms for their age and gender.[1] Less pejorative terms, such as "growth faltering," have been suggested[2] but have never come into widespread clinical use. Traditionally, FTT was characterized as "organic failure to thrive," in which the child's growth failure was ascribed to a major medical illness, and "nonorganic failure to thrive," which was attributed primarily to psychological neglect or "maternal deprivation."[3] This simplistic dichotomous conceptualization of FTT is obsolete.[4] We now recognize that in all cases of "nonorganic" FTT and in many cases of "organic" FTT, the proximate cause of growth failure is malnutrition, whether primary or secondary.[4-6] Malnutrition not only jeopardizes the child's growth but also impairs immunocompetence and contributes to concurrent and long-term deficits in cognition and socioaffective competence.[7,8] The modern diagnosis and treatment of FTT focus on the assessment of and therapy for malnutrition and its complications as well as the social and medical context in which they occur.[1,4,6,8] The needs of each child who is not thriving and his or her family should be assessed along 4 parameters: medical, nutritional, developmental, and social. Before addressing the clinical care of any individual child and family, however, it is important to understand the ecologic context in which childhood malnutrition occurs in an industrialized nation.

Ecologic Context

Although not all children with FTT come from food-insecure families, poverty remains the most significant social risk factor for developing FTT. Many additional children experience food insecurity, defined as a household's inability to provide all its members consistently with enough food for an active and healthy life. Nearly 19% of households in the United States with children younger than 6 years were food insecure in 2004 (http://www.ers.usda.gov/publications/err11).

The cumulative effects of days and weeks of inadequate diets are reflected in higher rates of short stature among low-income children participating in various national and state surveys in the United States and the United Kingdom, with rates approaching 10% of children with heights below the National Center for Health Statistics (NCHS) 5th percentile norms in most settings.[9,10] Thus, children clinically identified as "failing to thrive," who are drawn disproportionately from low-income families, represent the extreme end of a spectrum of nutritional deprivation of children in or near poverty that often goes unrecognized by health care professionals in less obvious cases.[11]

By definition, the federal poverty level ($20 000/year for a family of 4 in 2006) is set at 3 times the annual cost of a minimally nutritious diet. In addition to an insufficient budget for food purchases, economically disadvantaged families often lack access to supermarkets and live in homes lacking adequate food storage and preparation facilities.[12,13] National programs designed to protect the health and nutritional status of low-income children have not been adequately funded to meet the needs of American children. For example, only 66% of income-eligible urban families across the nation receive food stamps.[14] In 2006, food stamps provided maximal benefits of less than $1.40 per meal per person on average. Most families do not receive even this inadequate maximum benefit, so many families relying on the program routinely run out of food near the end of the month.[13] The US Department of Agriculture estimates that the Special Supplemental Food Program for Women, Infants, and Children (WIC) reaches only 81% of all eligible women participants, but the Committee on National Statistics has stated that the actual number is "substantially lower" than that estimate.[15] Although the WIC program food packages have been updated and improved over recent years, they are intended as only a supplement to the other food provided in the household and, thus, provide less than 100% of the Recommended Dietary Allowances (RDAs) for a number of nutrients.[16] For some children in certain age groups receiving WIC benefits and many pregnant and postpartum women, the combination of WIC food and other food available in the household is insufficient to provide adequate nutrients.[16] School breakfast is available to only about 1 in 4 children who receive school lunch.[17] Even with simultaneous participation in multiple programs (food stamps, WIC, school meals), many low-income families are unable to obtain enough food to avoid frequent episodes of food insecurity and hunger and the chronic mild-to-moderate undernutrition that may ensue (see also Chapter 49: Community Nutrition Services).[13,18]

To minimize the temptation to scapegoat families in clinical assessment and intervention, it is important to recognize that FTT often reflects economic conditions and changes in social policy that are far beyond the control of individual parents or health care professionals.[19] Children also fail to thrive in homes of any social class in cases of severe parent-child interactive disorders, parental psychopathology, family dysfunction, organic pathology, or developmental impairment. The effect of such problems on children's health increases dramatically in the context of poverty; lack of economic means to provide adequate care for a child with increased or unusual nutritional requirements is often a major factor in the development of FTT.[12,13,19] Clinicians must always consider that FTT most often occurs in financial and social circumstances that would make it difficult for any parent to address a child's physical and emotional needs successfully. For this reason, true primary prevention of FTT, which is beyond the scope of this chapter, requires a concerted effort to decrease or eliminate family poverty.[13,19]

Medical Issues in Evaluation and Treatment

Family History

The assessment of FTT begins with a family history, focusing on issues such as consanguinity, recurrent miscarriage or stillbirth, developmental delay, atopy, human immunodeficiency virus (HIV) infection, alcoholism and other substance use, psychiatric diagnoses, and potentially growth-retarding familial illnesses, such as cystic fibrosis, celiac disease, or inflammatory bowel disease (see Chapters 46, 27, and 43, respectively). The height of both parents should be ascertained, as should their history of growth delay in childhood and timing of puberty. A familial pattern of short stature or constitutional delay of growth may obviate the need for extensive workup if the child is short but not underweight for height.[20] It is critical, however, to assess whether the parents themselves were malnourished as children, as is often the case among immigrant and low-income families. In such cases, parents' stature does not provide an accurate indication of the child's genetic growth potential.[21] Moreover, an experience of severe childhood deprivation may influence the parents' caregiving practices.[22]

Perinatal Factors

After ascertaining family history, the medical assessment of a child who is not thriving should proceed to a detailed assessment of the child's prenatal and perinatal history by interview and, when possible, by review of neonatal records. This approach not only elucidates potential biologic risks to growth but also may be helpful in identifying ongoing psychosocial risk factors that are concurrently influencing postnatal growth. Low birth weight is a major predictor of later referral for FTT. In several clinical series, 10% to 40% of children hospitalized for FTT without a major medical diagnosis had a birth weight less than 2500 g, compared with 7% of the general population.[4] To evaluate the effects of perinatal risk factors on later growth accurately, a detailed history should be obtained covering the issues summarized in Table 26.1. It is critical to ascertain not only the child's birth weight but also gestational age, length, and head circumference at birth. Such data will identify prematurity as well as various patterns of intrauterine growth retardation that have prognostic implications for later growth.

Table 26.1
Pregnancy and Delivery

Mother's reproductive history
Age Gravidity/parity/abortions (spontaneous or induced), stillbirths History of pregnancy with identified patient

Conception planned or unplanned
    Difficulties with fertility
    Conceived while mother using contraception
    Was abortion considered?
Mother's nutritional status during pregnancy
    Weight at conception
    Pregnancy weight gain
    WIC status
    Hyperemesis
Mother's health habits during pregnancy
    Cigarettes, packs per day
    Alcohol
    Prescribed drug use (particularly anticonvulsants and antidepressants)
    Illicit drug use
    X-rays
    Occupational exposures
Complications of pregnancy
    Infections/high fevers
    Bleeding
    Toxemia
    Violence or trauma
Labor and delivery

Vaginal or cesarean
Anesthesia
Maternal complications
Neonatal status

Table 26.1 *(Continued)*
Pregnancy and Delivery

Gestational age
Apgar scores
Birth weight, length, head circumference (parameters and percentiles for gestational age)
Neonatal course
Mother and child separation
Need for neonatal intensive care
Duration of hospitalization for mother and child
Complications: jaundice, respiratory, central nervous system, sepsis, necrotizing enterocolitis
Early feeding difficulties
Transfusions
Eye examination
Hearing examination

Prematurity

Children born preterm may be inappropriately labeled as FTT if the percentiles used for assessing growth parameters are not corrected for gestational age by subtracting the number of weeks the child was preterm from the child's postnatal age at time of assessment. A statistically significant difference in growth percentiles will be found without such correction in head circumference until 18 months' postnatal age, in weight until 24 months' postnatal age, and in length until 40 months' postnatal age.[23] Even after such correction, infants with a very low birth weight (less than 1501 g) may remain smaller than infants born at term for at least the first 3 years of life.[24] In these children, the distribution of mean weight, height, and head circumference is shifted downward relative to the NCHS norms so that the proportion of children with attained weight or height below the NCHS 5th percentile is increased.[24] The rate of growth of such infants, however, should be the same as that of term infants of the same corrected age.[24,25] Moreover, weight for length should be proportional despite somewhat lower fat stores.[26]

Although the field lacks clear guidelines, preterm infants born before 34 weeks' gestation generally should receive a preterm formula until they weigh at least 2000 g. The benefits of a "postdischarge formula" that is higher in calories and micronutrients per ounce than formula designed for term infants remain controversial. Such enriched formulas are more expensive than term formulas and may be difficult for economically stressed families to afford unless the family receives a physician's prescription for WIC. In general, if they are used, postdischarge formulas are often continued until 9 to 12 months' corrected age or until the baby's weight for length is maintained above the 25th percentile (see also Chapter 4: Nutritional Needs of the Preterm Infant).

Children who were born preterm and show depressed weight for height or whose growth progressively deviates from a channel parallel to NCHS norms should be assessed carefully for potentially correctable (and sometimes iatrogenic) causes of growth failure, starting with inappropriate feeding practices for corrected age, such as early discontinuation of postdischarge formula or initiation of solid feedings at 6 months' postnatal age for an infant born at 28 weeks whose corrected age is only 3 months. In addition, the neurologic, gastrointestinal, and cardiorespiratory sequelae of preterm birth as well as the behavioral disorganization characteristic of some preterm infants may contribute to postnatal malnutrition. Growth difficulties should not be discounted in such children on the grounds that they were "born small." In addition to affecting the infant's behavior or physical growth potential directly, preterm birth and low birth weight also may act indirectly to increase the risk of growth failure by intensifying family stress and requiring early separation between parents and child for neonatal intensive care.

Intrauterine Growth Retardation

Size at birth reflects both the duration and the rate of growth during gestation. Infants whose rate of intrauterine growth is depressed are at risk of postnatal growth failure, regardless of gestational age. Intrauterine growth retardation (IUGR) is conventionally defined as birth weight less than the 10th percentile for gestational age. The degree of risk of postnatal growth failure after IUGR is not uniform, varying with both the cause of the IUGR and the pattern of relative deficit in length, weight, or head circumference at birth.

The best prognosis for postnatal growth pertains to infants with asymmetric IUGR whose weight at birth is disproportionately more depressed than their length or head circumference. Such infants are at risk of FTT, because they are often behaviorally difficult.[27] With enhanced postnatal nutrition, however, they can manifest significant catch-up growth in the first 6 to 8 months of life so that later growth trajectories may be within the normal range.[27,28] For such infants, early identification of growth failure and intensive nutritional and environmental intervention is critical, because the potential for catch-up growth to repair the intrauterine deficit is maximal in the first 6 months of life.[29]

Infants with severe symmetric IUGR whose weight, length, and head circumference are proportionately depressed at birth carry a relatively poor prognosis for later growth and development. A symmetric pattern of IUGR should alert the clinician to the possibility of chromosomal abnormalities, intrauterine infections, or prenatal teratogen exposure. For this reason, children with symmetrical growth retardation should be scrutinized carefully for dysmorphic features that may provide clues to syndrome diagnosis. Exposure to anticonvulsants, including hydantoin and valproate, may be associated with symmetric IUGR and dysmorphic features.[30] Prenatal exposure to legal and illegal psychoactive substances during pregnancy often contributes to symmetric IUGR, but the prognostic implications for later growth, particularly somatic growth, are variable.[31]

Prenatal Exposure to Legal Psychoactive Substances and Later Growth

Although heavy use of caffeine prenatally is associated in some studies with depressed intrauterine growth, such use has no detectable effects on the later size of exposed infants.[32] Some, but not all, investigators have noted correlations between heavy cigarette exposure during pregnancy and statistically significant decrements in stature at school age, but the magnitude of the deficit (1–2 cm) usually is not large enough to trigger referral for FTT.[33,34] Postnatal use of fluoxetine in breastfeeding women was associated with some reduction in infant weight gain between 2 weeks and 6 months of age.[35] The effects of prenatal alcohol exposure are variable. Growth deficits persist from infancy to school age in children with dysmorphic features consistent with fetal alcohol syndrome and in children from lower-income (but not higher-income) families who were exposed yet are not dysmorphic.[34,36,37] Length and head circumference are more depressed than weight in such cases.[34]

Although fetal alcohol syndrome, and perhaps fetal alcohol spectrum disorder, constrains postneonatal growth, clinicians also must remain alert to potentially treatable postneonatal medical and psychosocial factors that may be preventing children with fetal alcohol syndrome or other intrauterine exposures from attaining even their limited growth potential. As with infants with very low birth weight, children with fetal alcohol syndrome in whom rate of growth deviates from their own previously established patterns should be evaluated meticulously.[38] Neurologically based oral-motor difficulties are often associated with fetal alcohol syndrome and may limit caloric intake, unless gastrostomy tubes are placed.[39] Even more commonly, the growth of children with fetal alcohol syndrome who remain in the care of mothers with active untreated alcoholism shows effects of inadequate care and nutrition. Such children should not remain in conditions of profound deprivation on the grounds that they have fetal alcohol syndrome and "cannot grow." Clinical experience shows that with appropriate nutritional, neurodevelopmental, and psychosocial intervention, children with fetal alcohol syndrome and fetal alcohol spectrum disorder can be brought into the normal range of weight for height, but they may remain short and microcephalic despite intervention.

Prenatal Exposure to Illicit Psychoactive Substances and Later Growth

Until recently, the 3 most frequently used illicit drugs during pregnancy were marijuana, cocaine, and opiates. Increasing concern is focusing on methamphetamine exposure during pregnancy. Unfortunately, few follow-up studies of the growth of infants exposed to marijuana, cocaine, or opiates beyond the neonatal period have been performed, and none have been published regarding children with intrauterine exposure to methamphetamines. Newborn infants exposed to marijuana during pregnancy have been reported as having a decreased weight and length and sometimes head circumference, compared with unexposed infants, presumably because smoking marijuana, like smoking tobacco, increases maternal carbon monoxide concentrations and decreases fetal oxygenation.[40–42] In a long-term follow-up study, children 6 years of age were found to have decreased height correlated with prenatal marijuana exposure.[42] However, in a similar study of prenatal marijuana exposure, children with a history of prenatal marijuana exposure had weights and lengths significantly greater than their nonexposed peers, even after controlling for confounding variables.[43] Therefore, it is unclear whether prenatal marijuana exposure is a biologic risk factor for later FTT, and clinicians should not dismiss FTT in these children by attributing it to prenatal marijuana exposure.

Intrauterine cocaine exposure is independently associated with decrements in gestational age and with consistently lower birth weight, length, and head circumference.[41] At 7 to 16 weeks of age, no difference was found in feeding behaviors between infants who were exposed prenatally to cocaine and those who were not exposed.[44] If levels of exposure to cigarettes and alcohol are not controlled statistically, researchers have noted small but statistically significant decrements in head circumference, and in weight in one cohort, among intrauterine cocaine-exposed children followed until 3 years of age.[45,46] However, in 2 studies that controlled statistically for the level of prenatal exposure to tobacco and alcohol, no incremental negative effect of prenatal cocaine exposure was noted on weight, height, or head circumference.[47,48] Accelerated rates of postneonatal weight gain have been noted after prenatal cocaine exposure.[45,47,49] Therefore, clinicians should not accept prenatal exposure to cocaine as a sufficient explanation for postnatal failure to gain weight.

Intrauterine exposure to heroin or methadone also has been linked to depressed birth weight, length, and head circumference, but follow-up studies of the growth patterns of these infants are not entirely consistent. Wilson et al[50] reported that 3- to 6-year-old children with intrauterine exposure to heroin were smaller in all growth parameters than were nonexposed social class controls. In most studies, however, smaller head circumference but few differences in somatic growth were noted when opiate-exposed infants were compared with children of the same social class without opiate exposure.[51]

The quality of care the child is receiving at the time of referral also must be evaluated, because continued parental substance abuse may be contributing to concurrent nutritional deprivation of the child. Even though intrauterine exposure to psychoactive substances may cause a decrease in birth weight, length, and head circumference, most such substances do not inhibit a child from showing postnatal somatic catch-up growth in response to adequate nutrition.[31] Heavy prenatal exposure to alcohol or opiates may be associated with relative microcephaly, and fetal alcohol syndrome is characterized by persistent short stature. However, intrauterine exposure to the most commonly used psychoactive substances does not adequately explain a child who is underweight for height or one whose growth progressively deviates from a previously established trajectory.

Postnatal Medical Issues

Almost all severe and chronic childhood illnesses can cause growth failure. The mechanisms of such failure can be multiple—enzymatic, metabolic, and endocrinologic—in some cases but can also nutritional and psychosocial.[52,53] Chronic physical problems that necessitate procedures such as gastrostomy or nasogastric feedings may impede the development of normal patterns of feeding (see also Chapter 23: Enteral Nutrition).

Hospitalization of children with FTT should not be regarded as a diagnostic test for chronic illness.[54] According to an old myth, environmentally deprived children (nonorganic FTT) grow in the hospital, whereas children with serious medical illnesses (organic FTT) will not. In fact, a positive growth response to hospitalization is a poor indicator of major organic

V

illness, because both children with such illness and children with primary malnutrition will grow if given adequate caloric intake.[55] Chronically ill children who do well in the hospital usually have complex technical, psychosocial, and nutritional needs that can be met by multiple shifts of highly trained medical personnel but overwhelm parents who are not receiving adequate caregiving support at home. Conversely, unless the hospital provides specialized milieu therapy, usually not available on acute care wards, children with severe interactive feeding disorders or depression may deteriorate nutritionally in the hospital, because separation from primary attachment figures and interaction with multiple caregivers may exacerbate their affective and behavioral feeding difficulties. Children who are simply underfed do well either in the hospital or in any setting when adequate calories are offered. Thus, response to hospitalization in itself does not necessarily contribute to identifying the cause of FTT.

Whether in inpatient or outpatient settings, chronic illnesses severe enough to jeopardize growth usually can be ascertained from a meticulous history and physical examination (Tables 26.2 and 26.3). The list of occult medical conditions presenting as FTT is relatively circumscribed, and often these are identified during the review of systems (outlined in Table 26.2), focusing on infections and conditions that interfere with caloric intake or utilization. In reported series of children hospitalized for FTT of unknown origin, the most common previously undiagnosed illnesses are gastrointestinal, including chronic nonspecific diarrhea, celiac disease, food allergies, gastroesophageal reflux, and cystic fibrosis.[3,56–58] Immigrant children, those who have recently traveled abroad, and children attending congregate child care or living in homeless shelters should be evaluated for giardiasis and enteric pathogens if they have gastrointestinal symptoms, such as diarrhea or abdominal pain, because these infections are treatable causes of malabsorption and growth failure.[59]

Outside the gastrointestinal system, clinicians should consider urinary tract infections and renal tubular acidosis as potentially clinically silent contributors to FTT. Subtle neurologic dysfunction manifested as fine and oral motor dysfunction also should be considered and evaluated by direct observation.[60] Poor appetite, observed sometimes as early as the first 6 weeks of life,[2] delayed or dysfunctional oral-motor development with unusually prolonged feedings,[61] and deficient signaling of needs during mealtimes may contribute to FTT by decreasing nutrient intake (see also Chapter 25: Pediatric Feeding and Swallowing Disorders; and Chapter 36: Nutritional Support for Children With Developmental Disabilities).

Table 26.2
Child's Postneonatal Health History

Immunizations	(continued)
Allergies	Dysphagia
Surgeries	Snoring, difficulty with tonsils or adenoids
Hospitalizations	Recurring pneumonia, otitis, or sinusitis
Current medications	Painful teeth
Midparental height	Loss of previously acquired milestones, seizures
Consanguinity	Thrush/recurrent monilial rash
Heritable conditions	Atopic dermatitis, hives
Review of systems	Pets
Timing of onset of growth faltering	Travel
Weight loss	Passive tobacco exposure
Diarrhea/vomiting	Congregate child care

Overdiagnosis and underdiagnosis of "food allergy" or food sensitivities, such as lactose or gluten intolerance, can contribute to FTT. Only those reactions that are the consequence of an immune response to a food or food additive are clinically considered to be food allergies, which are a subgroup of adverse reactions to foods.[62]

An exceedingly restrictive diet based on an imprecise or factitious diagnosis of food allergy may present as FTT. It is crucial that the cause of an apparent adverse reaction to a food be aggressively sought. Whereas negative skin test results are 95% accurate, positive test results are only 50% accurate and must be confirmed by history or a food challenge.[62] Conversely, 30% of atopic dermatitis in young children is triggered by food allergy, so evaluation for food allergy should be considered in any child with FTT and eczema. It may take as long as 14 days to see a clinical response to an elimination diet. A double-blind, placebo-controlled food challenge is the "gold standard" for food allergy diagnosis but is often not practical in primary care settings.[63] Skin or serum tests for immunoglobulin (Ig) E anti-food allergens are more commonly used in this setting. Because children often "outgrow" their adverse reaction to cow milk, soy, and egg white by 3 years of age, such evaluations should be repeated periodically so that the child's diet does not remain unnecessarily restricted (see also Chapter 34: Food Sensitivity).[63]

Table 26.3
Physical Examination

Vital signs: blood pressure if over 3 years of age, temperature, pulse, respirations Anthropometry (see Table 26.5)
General appearance: activity, affect, posture
Skin: hygiene, rashes, trauma (bruises, burns, scars)
Head: hair whorls, color and pluckability of hair, occipital alopecia, fontanel size and patency, frontal bossing, sutures, shape, facial dysmorphisms, philtrum
Eyes: ptosis, strabismus, fundoscopic where possible, palpebral fissures, conjunctival pallor
Ears: external form, rotation, tympanic membranes
Mouth, nose, throat: thinness of lip, hydration, dental eruption and hygiene caries, glossitis, cheilosis, gum bleeding
Neck: hairline, masses, lymphadenopathy
Abdomen: protuberance, hepatosplenomegaly, masses
Genitalia: Malformations, hygiene, trauma
Rectum: fissures, trauma, hemorrhoids
Extremities: edema, dysmorphisms, rachitic changes, nails and nail beds
Neurologic: cranial nerves, reflexes, tone, retention of primitive reflexes, quality of voluntary movement

In addition to primary illnesses that may be associated with secondary malnutrition and growth failure, the clinician must be alert to the medical complications of primary malnutrition, particularly recurring infections and lead poisoning. Malnutrition severe enough to produce growth failure also impairs immunocompetence, particularly cell-mediated immunity and the production of complement and secretory IgA.[64,65] Recurring otitis media and gastrointestinal and respiratory illnesses are more common among children who fail to thrive than among well-nourished children of the same age.[10,66]

In recent years, the differential diagnosis of FTT with recurring infections has expanded to include HIV infection, usually acquired perinatally (see Chapter 39). During the same period, the diagnosis has become more difficult, because known maternal risk factors are changing. Women of childbearing age in the United States acquire HIV primarily via heterosexual contact, making risk factors more difficult to discern. However, the diagnosis must also be ruled out in children of immigrants from areas where HIV is endemic. For information on HIV risk factors, refer to the guidelines provided by the Centers for Disease Control and Prevention (www.cdc.gov/HIV/resources/factsheets/perinatl.htm).

Even among the majority who are not HIV infected, children with FTT are often trapped in an infection-malnutrition cycle. With each illness, the child's appetite and nutrient intake decrease while nutrient requirements increase as a result of fever, diarrhea, and vomiting. In settings in which nutrient intake is already marginal, even when the child is well, cumulative nutritional deficits occur, leaving the child increasingly vulnerable to more severe and prolonged infections and even less adequate growth. Commonly in developing countries and occasionally in industrialized countries, malnourished children succumb to fulminating infections (see also Chapter 35: Nutrition and Immunity).

Elevated lead concentrations correlate with impaired growth, even in the 5- to 35-mg/dL range.[67] Here, too, a negative cycle develops. Nutritional deficiencies of iron and calcium enhance the absorption of lead and other heavy metals.[68] As lead concentrations increase, constipation, abdominal pain, and anorexia occur, leading to even less adequate dietary intake.[69] In one study, 16% of children with FTT had lead concentrations high enough to warrant chelation.[70]

Physical Examination and Laboratory Evaluation

The physical examination of the child who fails to thrive, summarized in Table 26.3, has 3 goals: (1) identification of chronic illness; (2) recognition of syndromes that alter growth; and (3) documentation of the effects of malnutrition. Some findings may be nonspecific and require elucidation by laboratory assessment; for example, hepatic enlargement may be seen with primary malnutrition, acquired immunodeficiency syndrome, or primary liver disease.

Laboratory evaluation should be restrained and guided by history and the findings of the physical examination. For example, a child who has no symptoms of cardiorespiratory distress or heart murmur does not need electrocardiography. Basic laboratory studies should be used to identify derangements caused by malnutrition and to rule out the potentially occult diseases just described. All children with FTT should have a complete blood cell count, assessment of lead and free erythrocyte protoporphyrin concentrations, urinalysis, and a tuberculin test. Iron deficiency is a common finding. If the child does not respond promptly to nutritional intervention, blood urea nitrogen and creatinine and serum electrolyte concentrations should be measured. These tests also are mandatory in children with vomiting or diarrhea, clinically obvious dehydration, or severe malnutrition, which is often associated with hypokalemia. In children with severe anthropometric deficits, it is useful to obtain albumin and prealbumin concentrations to assess protein status and to determine serum alkaline phosphatase, calcium, and phosphorus concentrations. A depressed alkaline phosphatase concentration suggests zinc deficiency; an elevated concentration, especially if associated with a depressed phosphorous concentration, is suggestive of rickets.[71] Testing for HIV infection, sweat tests, and stool assessments for *Giardia* infection should be performed in epidemiologically at-risk populations.[65] Serum IgA anti-tissue transglutaminase and antiendomysial antibodies screen for celiac disease.[72] Serum or skin testing for food allergies should be considered in children with FTT and atopic dermatitis as well as for those with a history of rash, urticaria, or recurring vomiting and diarrhea after ingestion of selected foods. In a child with FTT and vomiting not explained by food allergies and unresponsive to empiric management, radiographic, pH probe, or endoscopic studies may be indicated to rule out anatomic abnormalities, gastroesophageal reflux, and esophagitis, particularly among children with neurologic impairments and unexplained respiratory symptoms.[73] For short children with weight proportionate to height, bone-age radiographic studies of the wrists and knees are helpful in discriminating those who are constitutionally short (bone age equals chronologic age and is greater than height age) from those with growth hormone or thyroid deficiencies or chronic malnutrition (bone age equals height age and is less than chronologic age).[53] Children with enlarged livers should have liver functions evaluated.

Careful physical examination will usually identify untreated dental cavities and abscesses that make eating and chewing painful and lead to inadequate caloric intake.[74] Large tonsils or a history of chronic snoring warrant ear, nose, and throat evaluation and possibly a sleep study, because tonsillar-adenoidal hypertrophy and sleep-disordered breathing may contribute to growth failure. Furthermore, it is important to observe a feeding, because subtle oral-motor difficulties may interfere with dietary intake in children with otherwise subclinical neurologic abnormalities.[60]

Medical Management

The pediatric health care professional should play an ongoing role in the management of children who fail to thrive. Children must be seen more frequently than is dictated by routine health management schedules to monitor their growth and development in response to interventions. Weekly visits are often necessary at the beginning of the diagnosis and treatment. Meticulous management of concurrent chronic illness is essential, enlisting and coordinating assessments in as many disciplines as necessary. Lead poisoning, if identified, should be treated according to standard protocols.

The health care professional must take an aggressive stance to interrupt the infection-malnutrition cycle. In addition to all immunizations routinely recommended by the American Academy of Pediatrics (AAP), influenza vaccine is indicated in children with FTT even after 24 months of age because of their nutritional depletion.[65] Families should be instructed to seek care at the first signs of infection so that immediate workup and treatment are provided. Recurring otitis or sinusitis are indications for otolaryngologic referral. In addition, for each episode of acute illness, the clinician should provide specific instruction about appropriate diet during and after the illness to try to maintain and repair nutritional status. In general, children should never receive a clear liquid diet for more than 24 hours.[59]

Hospitalization should be considered for severely malnourished children, for children with serious intercurrent infections, for those whose safety is in question, or if the specialized coordination of disciplines or diagnostic procedures is necessary and can be assembled most efficiently inside the hospital. In many centers, the availability of interdisciplinary outpatient clinics for the diagnosis and management of FTT has greatly reduced the need for hospitalization.[75] Referral for specialized inpatient or outpatient assessment should be considered, however, for any child who has not responded to 2 or 3 months of intensive management in a primary care setting.

Nutritional Evaluation and Treatment

The major components of a nutritional history for a child who is failing to thrive are summarized in Table 26.4. The assessment should focus not only on current feeding practices but also on the development of feeding since birth. Often, a child's growth failure is triggered by a shift in feeding practices. For example, the shift from soy formula to whole milk at age 12 months, as mandated by the WIC program, may trigger FTT in a child with severe lactose intolerance or milk protein allergy.[76] In many children, feeding struggles and growth failure begin with the introduction of solid foods at age 5 to 7 months. In rare instances, the introduction of gluten-containing cereals triggers celiac disease and growth failure. Nutritional rickets occurs almost exclusively in breastfed infants who have not received vitamin D supplementation. Thus, comparison of the lifelong feeding history with the growth curve can provide diagnostic clues to the nutritional risk factors in FTT.

Table 26.4
Nutritional Evaluation Protocol

Interview
Feeding history adjusted for age
Breastfed or formula fed
Age solids introduced
Age switched to whole milk
Food allergy or intolerance
Vitamin or mineral supplements
Current feeding behaviors
Difficulties with sucking, chewing, or swallowing
Frequency of feeding
Duration of feeding episodes
Who feeds?
Where fed (alone or held, with or separate from family, lap or high chair)?
Finicky? Negative?
Perceived appetite
Pica
Caregivers' nutrition knowledge
Difficulties with English or literacy
Adequacy of developmentally appropriate nutrition information
Unusual dietary belief (religious or food fad constraints on permitted foods): are some foods perceived as dangerous?
Adequacy of financial resources for food purchase
Food stamps: how much/month for how many people
WIC status
Adequacy of earned income
Benefits: Transitional Aid to Needy Families, SSI
Recent change in food budget (cuts or increases in benefits, new mouths to feed, job gain or loss)
Family's knowledge of how to budget food purchasing
Material resources for food preparation and storage
Refrigeration
Cooking facilities
Running water
24-hour dietary recall: was yesterday typical?
Food frequency

In assessing current feeding practices of the child who fails to thrive, the clinician should ascertain when, where, how, and by whom the child is fed as well as what the child is fed and why. Comprehensive assessment of feeding problems requires a combination of methods, such as structured interviews with primary caregivers and direct observation of the child's response to feeding in multiple situations. Breastfeeding difficulties should be managed by a pediatric health care professional experienced in such issues, perhaps with input from an experienced certified lactation consultant. Overdilution of formula is a readily treatable contributor to failure to thrive in infancy.[77] A licensed dietitian should ask caregivers to fill out a checklist of possible behavioral feeding problems (eg, spitting out food, tantrums during meals, food refusal), to supply a few days of food-intake records, and to indicate how the parents have tried to manage the child's problems.[78] Ideally, the history should be supplemented by a home-based feeding observation that will elucidate not only interactive or mechanical feeding difficulties but also the material conditions of the home and family routines.[79]

Heptinstall et al[80] found that inconsistent timing of the presentation of meals and dysfunctional mealtime procedures, such as solitary meals without supervision, occurred more frequently in growth-deficient children than in normal controls. Common sources of difficulty in the timing of feedings include infrequent feedings (restricting a toddler to 3 meals a day), constant feedings (grazing), and lack of a consistent feeding schedule. Children are often fed in inappropriate settings, which may or may not be under the parents' control. For example, children in welfare motels or homeless shelters may have to be fed sitting on the floor or the bed, because there is nowhere else to sit. Many parents can be encouraged to put the child in a high chair when one is available and not to position the child in front of the television or other distractions during feeding. A hammerlock hold in a parent's lap is usually ineffective and uncomfortable for both parent and child. A home observation also will elucidate the affective tone of the feeding process and identify dysfunctional interactions, such as interrupting the feeding too often to clean the child, struggles over the child's efforts to feed independently, or inappropriate coaxing or threatening of the child. Efforts should be made to identify all the different caregivers (relatives, neighbors, siblings, child care providers, etc) involved in feeding the child to enlist these individuals in improving the child's nutritional intake.

In addition to how the child is fed, the clinician must ascertain what the child is fed and why. The family's level of nutritional knowledge and dietary beliefs should be assessed. Parents and children are continually bombarded with nutritional misinformation from television and other commercial sources, urging them to spend their scarce food resources on expensive heavily sweetened or salted foods of low nutritional quality.[81,82] Certain groups of parents, particularly adolescents, and those who are intellectually limited, illiterate or, in the United States, unable to speak English, are particularly likely to lack adequate information regarding nutritionally sound feeding practices. Immigrants are at risk unless they are able to obtain culturally appropriate foods. Most ethnic diets are adequate, but when traditional foods are unavailable, immigrants may not know what to select from the foods available in US markets. Even privileged parents sometimes offer children an inadequate, strictly vegan, or other overly restricted diet because of adherence to unusual dietary practices prescribed by a nontraditional religion or food fads, such as macrobiotics.[83] Parents seeking to prevent obesity or cardiovascular disease also may inadvertently cause their toddlers to fail to thrive by overzealous enforcement of a low-fat "prudent diet" appropriate for adults but not for growing children.[84] Restricted diets imposed because of actual or presumed food allergies or gluten intolerance often are not adequately supplemented with alternate sources of calories and micronutrients, with consequent nutritional deficiencies.[62]

As discussed in the introduction to this chapter, the family's economic resources for food purchase, food storage, and food preparation must be tactfully ascertained. Finally, a 24-hour dietary recall and 7-day food frequency are essential in determining the quality and quantity of the child's diet. Common findings among children with FTT include excessive intake of juice, water, tea, or carbonated and sweetened beverages, which depress appetite but provide few nutrients. In addition, fruit juices high in fructose or sorbitol have been associated with malabsorption and osmotic diarrhea in some cases of FTT.[85] Low-income families may have particular difficulties in meeting the needs of children with increased nutritional needs (such as children born preterm or children with significant heart or lung disease) or those with medically restricted and, therefore, more expensive diets, as in the cases of multiple food allergies, lactose intolerance, or gluten-sensitive enteropathy.[86]

Anthropometric Assessment

Serial anthropometric assessments are critical to the management of FTT. Initial measurements of the growth trajectory form the basis for triage and calculation of caloric needs (see subsequent discussion) and provide some prognostic information for later developmental potential. Frequent follow-up assessments also provide the clearest indication of the effectiveness of intervention.

Children referred for FTT must be measured in a standard fashion by trained personnel using the same scale and linear measuring instrument at each visit, according to published protocols for obtaining accurate and reproducible anthropometric measurements (www.cdc.gov/nccdphp/dnpa/growthcharts/guide). Infants should be weighed naked, and young children should wear underwear only.

The relationship of the child's weight and height to each other and to reference norms is used to identify both the chronicity and the severity of nutritional deficit. The NCHS growth charts (www.cdc.gov/nchs/data/nhanes/growthcharts and Appendix D) should be used to evaluate the growth of infants and preschool children. By international consensus, the NCHS growth charts serve currently as the references for evaluating growth in young children regardless of ethnic or racial background.[87] These revised growth charts eliminate the discontinuity between recumbent length and standing height (both for simplicity termed in subsequent sections as "height") and provide percentile measurements between the 5th and 95th percentiles.[88] It is important to note that, despite their accepted use, these references include an unknown number of ill and deprived children and many formula-fed infants and, thus, may be imprecise tools for identifying aberrant growth.[87] The World Health Organization recently developed and published prescriptive standards for expected growth from a multiethnic, multinational sample restricted to healthy, initially breastfed children. These new growth charts are available at www.who.int/childgrowth/standards/en (see also Appendix D). Weight for age, the most powerful predictor of mortality, provides a composite measure of past and present nutrition and growth, reflecting both current and previous insults.[89] When constitutional, endocrine, and genetic factors can be ruled out, depressed length or height for age is considered a manifestation of the cumulative effects of chronic malnutrition.[90] In contrast, depressed weight for height indicates acute and recent nutritional deprivation.[90] The NCHS norms provide weight-for-height graphs for children up to 6 years of age as well as body mass index norms for children older than 2 years. Children at highest risk are those for whom both weight for height and height for age are depressed, indicating acute malnutrition superimposed on a chronic problem.

By definition, most children diagnosed with FTT have weights or heights at or below the lower percentiles on NCHS charts, so additional calculations are necessary to quantify the severity of nutritional risk. A useful clinical technique initially devised by Waterlow et al[91,92] is to categorize the child's malnutrition as first (mild), second (moderate), or third (severe) degree. This is done by dividing the child's current weight for corrected age by the median value ("the standard") for that parameter on NCHS grids. To assess the severity of chronic malnutrition, height for age is assessed in the same way. Table 26.5 provides translation of these "percent standards" into malnutrition categories. Children with third-degree malnutrition (weight for age less than 60% of standard, or weight for height less than 70% of standard) are in acute danger of severe morbidity and possible mortality from their malnutrition and should be hospitalized. Calculating a patient's z-score will reflect how far from the mean a child's parameters veer, thus giving a more accurate calculation of how malnourished the child is in comparison with a healthy child of that gestational age. Z-scores already used in academic settings, research publications, and clinical settings with widely available computer resources are now shown in the new World Health Organization reference grids (www.who.int/childgrowth/standards/en).

Table 26.5
Percent Median Values as Indicator of Severity of Nutritional Deficit

Grade of Malnutrition	Weight for Age	Height for Age	Weight for Height
Normal	90–110	>95	>90
First degree (mild)	75–89	90–94	80–90
Second degree (moderate)	60–74	85–89	70–79
Third degree (severe)	<60	<85	<70

The goal of nutritional intervention in FTT is to achieve catch-up growth—that is, growth at a faster-than-normal rate for age so that the child's relative deficit of body size is restored. If the child with an established growth deficit simply resumes growth at the normal rate for age, relative deficits persist compared with children of the same age who have always grown normally. To assess whether catch-up growth is occurring, the clinician must be aware of age-specific changes in normal growth rates, as summarized by Guo et al[88]; these are not altered by the new edition of the NCHS norms.[88] In the first 3 months of life, median weight gain averages 26 to 31 g/day; from 3 to 6 months of age, it averages 17–18 g/day; from 6 to 9 months of age, it averages 12 to 13 g/day; from 9 to 12 months of age, it averages 9 g/day; and from 12 months of age onward, it averages 7 to 9 g/day. A minimal goal for catch-up growth is 2 to 3 times the average rate of weight gain for corrected age. Thus a 1-year-old child who is gaining

30 g/day is showing excellent catch-up growth, whereas a 1-month-old child who also is gaining 30 g/day is growing at only the normal rate for age and will not repair existing deficits. The goal for catch-up growth must be continually revised as the child matures and gradually decreased as the child's weight for height approaches the target level.

Principles of Nutritional Treatment

To achieve catch-up growth, the underweight child must receive nutrients in excess of the normal age-specific requirements of the RDAs for age.[92] One commonly used formula based on the RDA for weight age (age at which child's current weight would be 50th percentile) is:

$$\text{kcal/kg required} = \frac{\text{RDA for weight age (kcal/kg)} \times \text{Ideal weight for height}}{\text{Actual weight}}$$

in which ideal weight for height is the median weight for the patient's height (as read from the NCHS weight-for-height curves).

For example, a 6.5-month-old male term infant with a weight of 6.1 kg and length of 64.5 cm has the following anthropometric measures: weight for age z-score: −2.52; height for age z-score: −1.35; weight for height z-score: −1.96. Weight age is approximately 3 months. By Gomez criteria, the child's current weight is 72% of the median (second-degree malnutrition). In addition, assessment via the Waterlow classification shows that he is suffering from mild acute malnutrition (weight for height = 87% of the median) and mild chronic malnutrition (height for age = 94% of the median). Because his RDA for calories for a weight age of 3 months is 108 kcal/kg per day and his ideal weight for length is 7.05 kg, his estimated caloric requirement for catch-up growth is (108 × 7.05)/6.1 = 125 kcal/kg per day. Similarly, because his RDA for protein is 2.2 g/kg per day, his protein requirement for catch-up growth is closer to (2.2 × 7.05)/6.1 = 2.54 g/kg per day.

Nutritional rehabilitation must address the child's needs for micronutrients as well as calories and protein. Iron deficiency, with or without associated anemia, is seen in as many as one half of all children presenting with FTT.[1] Vitamin D-deficiency rickets also has been described.[71] Even among children whose micronutrient stores are adequate at initial presentation with FTT, the demand of rapid tissue synthesis during catch-up growth may produce nutritional deficiencies. Whether or not zinc status can be measured, zinc supplementation should be provided to meet the RDA, but not in excess, because appropriate zinc supplementation has been shown to decrease the energy cost of weight gain.[93,94] A multivitamin supplement containing the RDA for all vitamins and for iron and zinc should, therefore, be prescribed routinely for children with FTT during nutritional rehabilitation, with additional supplementation of iron or vitamin D to therapeutic amounts in children with iron deficiency or rickets. Use of a once-a-day vitamin supplement also is useful to reduce pressure on caregivers to ensure that the child is receiving a completely balanced diet. Caregivers no longer have to worry whether their child is eating green beans or other low-calorie vegetables as a source of vitamins and can focus on ensuring adequate intake of minerals, fiber, calories, and protein.

In general, it is not possible for a child to eat twice the normal volume of food to obtain the nutrient amounts necessary for catch-up growth. Instead, the child's usual diet must be fortified to increase nutrient density—for example, by providing formula of 24 to 30 kcal/oz rather than the standard 20 kcal/oz. A prepackaged 30-kcal/oz preparation for children 1 to 6 years of age is now commercially available. This preparation appears to be well accepted, well tolerated for rapid weight gain, and effective when its cost can be subsidized by health insurance or other mechanisms.[92] Because the formula does not require parental preparation and is often perceived by families as "medicine" exclusively for the use of the child with FTT, it can be used effectively in high-risk families who otherwise have difficulties in preparing appropriately enriched diets for their children. Detailed protocols for other methods of dietary supplementation have been published elsewhere.[95] The participation of an experienced pediatric nutritionist is critical in developing a dietary regimen appropriate for each child.

The process of refeeding to promote catch-up growth must be undertaken with care in children with third- and severe second-degree malnutrition. If high food intakes are provided at the beginning of nutritional resuscitation, these children may develop vomiting, diarrhea, electrolyte imbalance, pancreatitis, and circulatory decompensation (refeeding syndrome).[96] To minimize these complications, such children should, for the first 7 to 10 days of treatment, be restricted to the normal dietary intake for age, offered as frequent small feedings. During a hospitalization, clinicians need to be aware that this may not coincide with cafeteria schedules and may require scheduling of additional feedings. Intake may then be gradually advanced over the next week to a diet that meets the calculated requirements for catch-up growth. Moderately and mildly malnourished children may be offered food ad libitum, while calorie counts are maintained. Once a baseline of spontaneous intake is established, preferred foods may be enriched to bring dietary intake to catch-up amounts.

Depending on the severity of the initial deficit, 2 days to 2 weeks may be required to initiate catch-up growth.[5] Less severely malnourished children who are not hospitalized should be monitored at least weekly as outpatients during this phase. Accelerated growth must then be maintained for 4 to 9 months to restore a child's weight for height.[5,92] Biweekly to monthly outpatient visits for weight checks, adjustment of diet, and treatment of intercurrent medical problems are essential during this period. Intake and rates of growth spontaneously decelerate toward normal levels for age as deficits are repleted. Because weight is restored more rapidly than height, caregivers may become alarmed that the child is becoming obese. They should be reassured that the catch-up growth in height lags behind that in weight by several months, but balance will occur if dietary treatment is not prematurely terminated.[97] Although no firm guidelines exist, a criterion for discharge from a specialized outpatient program is often when the child is able to maintain weight for height above the 10th percentile and a normal rate of weight gain for age on at least 2 assessments, 1 month apart, on a normal diet for age (ie, the weight-for-height deficit is repaired and the child no longer requires a specially enriched diet to sustain normal growth).

Psychosocial Issues in Evaluation and Treatment

Intellectual Development

Children who experience prolonged malnutrition and/or chronic FTT appear to be at risk of intellectual deficits severe enough to affect their learning potential.[98,99] The severity of developmental impairments varies substantially, however, among preschool and school-aged children with histories of early FTT.[100–104] Studies have underscored the central importance of a history of serious malnutrition as well as the quality of the home environment and educational experience in predicting the cognitive development of affected children later in life.[102,103,105–109]

Intellectual assessment can be a productive means of involving the parents of children with FTT in their child's treatment planning.[110] Observing their child's assessment helps parents to appreciate the nature of their children's intellectual strengths and weaknesses. When parents have observed developmental testing, it is also easier and more productive to discuss the pattern of their child's intellectual strengths and deficits with them. If parents are invited to discuss their child's development and participate in the evaluation, they are also less defensive about the overall evaluative process.

In evaluating the child's development, the clinician should pay careful attention to the potential effects of the child's nutritional state on his or her response to test items. Infants who have experienced nutritional and/ or stimulus deprivation are often withdrawn, which may severely limit their capacity to respond, at least initially.[111] For this reason, intellectual tests given early during the hospitalization, when the child is apathetic from undernutrition, may underestimate intellectual potential. Conducting the assessment soon after the hospital admission and repeating it once nutritional recovery is well underway (taking into account practice effects) should provide a more predictive estimate of intellectual potential than one assessment.[112] In addition, just as the child's progress in physical growth can be evaluated through the use of the growth grid, the child's intellectual progress can be monitored through the use of repeated assessments; however, assessment of the child's current intellectual level does not shed light on the causes of deficits or on developmental prognosis, with the exception that extremely low scores are more predictive than are those within the normal range.[113]

Socioemotional Development

Children with FTT are at risk of suboptimal socioemotional development. Although no one pattern of behavioral disturbance is associated with FTT, deficits in social responsiveness, affect, activity level, and avoidance of social contact have been noted by many observers.[114-116] Polan[117] found that children with FTT consistently demonstrated less positive affect in a range of situations than did normally growing children and that acute and chronic malnutrition were associated with heightened negative affect.

Because multiple areas of psychological development may be affected, a comprehensive assessment of several behavioral domains, including social responsiveness, affect, and response to feeding, is generally necessary for children with FTT.[118] A comprehensive assessment of the child's behavior and emotional development can be used to generate a profile of behavioral strengths and deficits to guide treatment planning and evaluation of the child's progress. Ordinarily, one would expect improvement in social responsiveness and affect of a child with FTT after nutritional treatment. Some children, however, continue to demonstrate significant deficits in responsiveness and/or problems in feeding that pose a salient burden to their caregivers and, hence, should be addressed in specialized intervention.

Assessment of the Family Environment

In addition to assessing the effects of FTT and associated risk factors on the child's psychological development, it also is necessary to assess aspects of the family environment (relationships, resources, and parent-child interaction) that would be expected to influence the child's response to medical and psychological intervention. Given the effect of parent-child relationships on child development, observations of the parents' interactions with the child in a range of situations (feeding, teaching the child a skill, or free play) provides a useful method of assessment.[119] The patterns of parent-child relationships associated with FTT are complex and heterogeneous.[78,120–122] Deficient or excessive but insensitive stimulation are some typical patterns; conflict and parental reinforcement of deviant behavior are others.[78,122] Several methods of assessment are available.[78,120]

One of the difficulties in assessing parent-child interaction in a hospital or clinic situation is that the child is removed from his or her home environment, and it is difficult to create a naturalistic setting for assessment. It may be possible, however, to use play or feeding situations to approximate important interactions. To make effective judgments about strengths and problem areas in parent-child relationships, clinicians must have extensive experience with a wide range of infants with FTT and their parents.

Intervention

Failure to thrive should be approached as a chronic condition requiring long-term multidisciplinary follow-up, with exacerbations and remissions expected. Successful intervention from the time of diagnosis requires active team involvement of a pediatric health care professional, a pediatric nutritionist, a social worker, and professionals with expertise in behavior, development, and family function. The initial focus of interdisciplinary management is assessment of the child and family for purposes of planning treatment. Subsequently, the focus concerns intervention and ongoing monitoring of the child's progress. In an optimal team approach, professionals interact frequently and directly with the family and with each other, ideally in the context of scheduled weekly to monthly clinic visits and periodic case conferences. In addition, regular home visits by one or several of these professionals are effective to gather diagnostic information and to provide ongoing support and guidance for the family.[4,123]

The first priority must be to stabilize the child's acute medical problems and nutritional deficits and to enhance, as much as possible, the material

V

conditions of the home and family resources by helping parents to use federal feeding programs, referring to local emergency relief programs, and providing advocacy around housing, heat, and other survival issues. Certainly, medical care and nutritional resuscitation alone are not sufficient to deal with the developmental and emotional deficits that constitute the major long-term morbidity in children who have had malnutrition in early life. For this reason, it is often useful to distinguish between (1) a core intervention plan, which includes identification and treatment of the child's medical problems, nutritional treatment, advice to parents about nutrition, pediatric follow-up, and attempts to stabilize issues such as heating and housing; and (2) specialized interventions, such as parent training, family counseling, or behavioral treatment of feeding problems, which may be necessary to address specific problems.[112]

Once care of medical and nutritional problems has been initiated and is well in place, the assessment refocuses on the ongoing developmental needs of the child and the quality of interaction between family and child. Referral to early intervention or HeadStart programs is often indicated to enhance the child's level of cognitive development and to reduce the risk of developmental problems in later life.[124] Children who fail to thrive may be eligible, on the basis of their deficits in growth and development, for Supplemental Security Income (SSI) payments, which are frequently higher than those usually provided by Transitional Assistance to Needy Families. However, SSI standards for disability are strict and can be difficult to meet. Impoverished families should receive help in applying for these benefits. Moreover, whenever possible, services that supplement and structure the efforts of the primary caregiver, such as visiting nurses, trained homemakers, or respite child care, can be helpful and should be used. Various forms of mental health intervention, ranging from behavior modification of feeding problems, to medication for a severely depressed parent, to multigenerational family therapy, should be provided as indicated by the clinical assessment. Even after nutritional resuscitation has been achieved, families and children should be offered periodic reassessment as the child reaches school age to ensure early identification of behavioral or psychoeducational problems, which may require specialized educational services.

Indications for Protective Service Involvement
Although the AAP recently published a clinical report titled "Failure to Thrive as a Manifestation of Child Neglect,"[125] it is important to recognize that

abuse or neglect are clear precursors of FTT in a relatively small proportion of children. Many of the risk factors for neglect as a cause of FTT listed in the AAP statement, including social isolation, lack of knowledge of normal growth and development, and parental psychopathology, are common psychosocial correlates of living in poverty, the overriding context that puts children at higher risk of developing FTT, and do not necessarily suggest neglect or abuse on part of the child's caregivers. Nonetheless, health care professionals inevitably encounter families of children with FTT who are both highly dysfunctional and resistant to recommended interventions. In a minority of children, FTT may result from diagnosable neglect by caregivers. One study found increased risk of subsequent involvement with child protective service agencies in children diagnosed with FTT during the first year of life.[126] For this reason, the health care professional must clearly and carefully document the family's response to intervention as well as the child's physical, nutritional, and developmental progress.

Children with FTT who are referred to protective agencies fall into 2 broad categories: those whose safety, in the judgment of clinical personnel, requires placement away from their current caregivers, and those in less severe jeopardy, whose current caregivers require protective monitoring and support to obtain or comply with necessary services for the health and growth of the child. Placement of a child with FTT outside of the home should not be considered a routine diagnostic strategy but is the only safe intervention in certain situations, particularly when caregivers are out-of-control substance abusers, have inflicted injury on the child, have intentionally withheld available food from the child, or are profoundly psychiatrically or cognitively impaired and when no other competent caregivers are available within the existing family system.[127–130] School-aged children with psychosocial dwarfism (more recently termed "hyperphagic short stature") are systematically physically abused, often confined in small spaces, and given only periodic access to food and water. To this treatment, they often respond by binge eating when food is available and by developing bizarre behaviors, such as drinking from toilets. These children present as stunted and behaviorally disturbed with transient deficiencies of growth hormone. Unlike most infants with FTT, children with psychosocial dwarfism should immediately be treated by removal from the home or institution in which the maltreatment occurred. [126,131,132]

Placement must be undertaken with great care, because suboptimal foster care only worsens FTT.[133] Because children who fail to thrive usually have multiple special needs requiring visits to many different professionals as well as special dietary, developmental, and medical management at home, foster parents must not be overburdened with the care of many other young children or children with special needs. Foster parents (whether professional or kinship) require the same intensive multidisciplinary support as biologic parents to provide adequate care for a child who is failing to thrive. To avoid deterioration of the child with FTT who is placed in foster care, health care professionals should meet face to face with prospective alternate caregivers and educate them regarding the child's dietary and behavioral regimen, medical problems, and emotional needs. Professional foster parents and kinship caregivers should have a WIC referral, appropriate nutritional supplements, child care equipment, and a health insurance card before children are placed in their homes. The professional or kinship foster family must be willing to commit to close cooperation with clinic visits and home-based treatment for the child who fails to thrive.

Protective service intervention without placement out of the home may be useful when the family is seriously noncompliant with health and nutritional care of the child despite multiple efforts at voluntary outreach and the child continues to grow poorly. Close communication between the protective agency and the health care professionals usually enhances parental compliance. In addition, in some jurisdictions, the only way to obtain needed multidisciplinary services, such as home visits or developmentally appropriate child care, for a child who is failing to thrive, even from relatively compliant families, may be through a child protective services referral. Ideally, such services should be available through other community agencies without the stigma of child protective services involvement, but in today's fiscal climate, this is often not the case.

Conclusion

Failure to thrive is a chronic condition that is the final common pathway of the interaction of diverse medical, nutritional, developmental, and social stresses. Effective care is multidisciplinary, respectful of parents, and sustained beyond the time of acute nutritional and medical crises. Ultimately, the goal of sustained interdisciplinary management is a thriving child in a thriving family.

References

1. Bithoney WG, Rathbun JM. Failure to thrive. In: Levine M, Carey W, Crocker A, Gross RT, eds. *Developmental-Behavioral Pediatrics*. Philadelphia, PA: WB Saunders; 1983:557–572

2. Wright CM, Parkinson KN, Drewett DF. How does maternal and child feeding behavior relate to weight gain and failure to thrive? *Pediatrics*. 2006;117:1262–1269

3. Sills RH. Failure to thrive. The role of clinical and laboratory evaluation. *Am J Dis Child*. 1978;132:967–969

4. Frank DA, Zeisel SH. Failure to thrive. *Pediatr Clin North Am*. 1988;35:1187–1206

5. Casey PH, Arnold WC. Compensatory growth in infants with severe failure to thrive. *South Med J*. 1985;78:1057–1060

6. Whitten CF, Pettit MG, Fischoff J. Evidence that growth failure from maternal deprivation is secondary to undereating. *JAMA*. 1969;209:1675–1682

7. Barrett DE, Frank DA. *The Effects of Undernutrition on Children's Behavior*. New York, NY: Gordon & Breach Science Publishers; 1987

8. Drotar D. Failure to thrive. In: Routh D, ed. *Handbook of Pediatric Psychology*. New York, NY: Guilford; 1988:71–107

9. Dowdney L, Skuse D, Morris K, Pickles A. Short normal children and environmental disadvantage: a longitudinal study of growth and cognitive development from 4 to 11 years. *J Child Psychol Psychiatry*. 1998;39:1017–1029

10. Mitchell WG, Gorrell RW, Greenberg RA. Failure to thrive: a study in a primary care setting. Epidemiology and follow-up. *Pediatrics*. 1980;65:971–977

11. Bithoney WG, Newberger EH. Child and family attributes of failure-to-thrive. *J Dev Behav Pediatr*. 1987;8:32–36

12. Bickel G, Carlson S, Nord M. *Household Food Security in the United States, 1995–1998 (Advance Report)*. Washington, DC: USDA Food and Nutrition Services and Economic Research Service; 1999. Available at: http://www.fns.usda.gov/oane/MENU/Published/FoodSecurity/foodsec98.pdf. Accessed November 1, 2007

13. Castner L, Anderson J. *Characteristics of Food Stamp Households: Fiscal Year 1998 (Advance report)*. Alexandria, VA: 1999

14. Powers S. *Food Stamp Access in Urban America: A City-by-City Snapshot*. Washington, DC: Food Research and Action Center; 2006

15. Institute of Medicine. *Estimating Eligibility and Participation for the WIC Program: Final Report*. Ver Ploeg M, Betson DM, eds. Washington, DC: National Academies Press; 2003

16. Kramer-LeBlanc CS, Mardis A, Gerrior S, et al. *Review of the Nutritional Status of WIC Participants*. Washington, DC: Center for Nutrition Policy and Promotion, US Department of Agriculture; 1999

17. Nord M, Bickel G. Estimating the prevalence of children's hunger from the current population survey food security supplement. In: Andrews MS, Prell MA, eds. *Second Food Security Measurement and Research Conference, Volume II: Papers*. Washington, DC: Economic Research Service, US Department of Agriculture; 2001:31–49

18. Neault N, Cook JT, Morris V, Frank DA. *The Real Cost of a Healthy Diet: Healthful Foods Are Out of Reach for Low-Income Families in Boston, Massachusetts*. Boston, MA: Boston Medical Center, Department of Pediatrics; 2005. Available at: http://dcc2.bumc.bu.edu/csnappublic/HealthyDiet_Aug2005.pdf. Accessed November 1, 2007

19. Huston A, McLoyd V, Cull C. Children and poverty: issues in contemporary research. *Child Dev.* 1994;65:275–282

20. Kaplowitz P, Webb J. Diagnostic evaluation of short children with height 3 SD or more below the mean. *Clin Pediatr (Phila).* 1994;33:530–535

21. Frisancho AR, Cole PE, Klayman JE. Greater contribution to secular trend among offspring of short parents. *Hum Biol.* 1977;49:51–60

22. Fraiberg S, Adelson E, Shapiro B. Ghosts in the nursery. *J Am Acad Child Psychiatry.* 1975;14:387–421

23. Brandt I. Growth dynamics of low birthweight infants with emphasis on the prenatal period. In: Falkner F, Tanner JM, eds. *Human Growth, Postnatal Growth*. New York, NY: Plenum Press; 1979:557–617

24. Casey PH, Kraemer HC, Bernbaum J, Yogman MW, Sells JC. Growth status and growth rates of a varied sample of low birth weight preterm infants: a longitudinal cohort from birth to three years of age. *J Pediatr.* 1991;119:599–605

25. Karniski W, Blair C, Vitucci JS. The illusion of catch-up growth in premature infants. Use of the growth index and age correction. *Am J Dis Child.* 1987;141:520–526

26. Georgieff MK, Mills MM, Zempel CE, Chang PN. Catch-up growth, muscle and fat accretion, and body proportionality of infants one year after neonatal intensive care. *J Pediatr.* 1989;114:288–292

27. Als H, Tronick E, Adamson L, Brazelton B. The behavior of the full-term but underweight infant. *Dev Med Child Neurol.* 1976;18:590–602

28. Villar J, Smeriglio V, Martorell R, Brown CH, Klein RE. Heterogeneous growth and mental development of intrauterine growth-retarded infants during the first 3 years of life. *Pediatrics.* 1984;74:783–791

29. Hediger M, Overpeck MD, Mauer KR, Kuczmarski RJ, McGlynn A, Davis WW. Growth of infants and young children born small or large for gestational age: finding from the Third National Health and Nutrition Examination Survey. *Arch Pediatr Adolesc Med.* 1998;152:1225–1231

30. Hanson J, Smith D. The fetal hydantoin syndrome. *J Pediatr.* 1975;87:285–290

31. Frank DA, Wong F. Effects of prenatal exposures to alcohol, tobacco, and other drugs. In: Kessler D, Dawson P, eds. *Failure to Thrive and Pediatric Undernutrition: A Transdisciplinary Approach*. Baltimore, MD: Paul H. Brookes Publishing; 1999:275–280

32. Fried PA, O'Connell CM. A comparison of the effects of prenatal exposure to tobacco, alcohol, cannabis and caffeine on birth size and subsequent growth. *Neurotoxicol Teratol.* 1987;9:79–85

33. Lassen K, Oei TPS. Effects of maternal cigarette smoking during pregnancy on long-term physical and cognitive parameters of child development. *Addict Behav.* 1998;23:635–653

34. Nordstrom-Klee B, Delaney-Black V, Covington C, Ager J, Sokol R. Growth from birth onwards of children prenatally exposed to drugs: a literature review. *Neurotoxicol Teratol.* 2002;24:481–488

35. Chambers CD, Anderson PO, Thomas RG, et al. Weight gain in infants breastfed by mothers who take fluoxetine. *Pediatrics.* 1999;104(5):e61. Available at: http://pediatrics. aappublications.org/cgi/content/full/104/5/e61. Accessed September 5, 2007

36. Coles CD, Brown RT, Smith IE, Platzman KA, Erickson S, Falek A. Effects of prenatal alcohol exposure at school age. I. Physical and cognitive development. *Neurotoxicol Teratol.* 1991;13:357–367

37. Fried PA, Watkinson B. 36- and 48-month neurobehavioral follow-up on children prenatally exposed to marijuana, cigarettes, and alcohol. *J Dev Behav Pediatr.* 1990;11:49–58

38. Hanson JW, Jones KL, Smith DW. Fetal alcohol syndrome. Experience with 41 patients. *JAMA.* 1976;235:1458–1460

39. Van Dyke DC, Mackay L, Ziaylek E. Management of severe feeding dysfunction in children with fetal alcohol syndrome. *Clin Pediatr (Phila).* 1982;21:336–339

40. Frank DA, Bauchner H, Parker S, et al. Neonatal body proportionality and body composition following in utero exposure to cocaine and marijuana. *J Pediatr.* 1990;116:622–626

41. Zuckerman B, Frank DA, Hingson R, et al. Effects of maternal marijuana and cocaine use on fetal growth. *N Engl J Med.* 1989;320:762–768

42. Cornelius MD, Goldschmidt L, Day NL, Larkby C. Alcohol, tobacco and marijuana use among pregnant teenagers: 6-year follow-up of offspring growth effects. *Neurotoxicol Teratol.* 2002;24(6):703–710

43. Fried PA, Watkinson B, Gray R. Differential effects on cognitive functioning in 9- to12-year olds prenatally exposed to cigarettes and marijuana. *Neurotoxicol Teratol.* 1998;20:293–306

44. Neuspiel DR, Hamel C, Hochberg E, Greene J, Campbell D. Maternal cocaine use and infant behavior. *Neurotoxicol Teratol.* 1991;13:229–233

45. Chasnoff IJ, Griffith DR, Freier C, Murray J. Cocaine/polydrug use in pregnancy: two-year follow-up. *Pediatrics.* 1992;89:284–289

46. Hurt H, Brodsky NL, Betancourt L, Braitman LE, Malmud E, Gianetta J. Cocaine-exposed children: follow-up through 30 months. *J Dev Behav Pediatr.* 1995;16:29–35

47. Jacobson JL, Jacobson SW, Sokol RJ. Effects of prenatal exposure to alcohol, smoking, and illicit drugs on postpartum somatic growth. *Alcohol Clin Exp Res.* 1994;18:317–323

48. Richardson GA, Conroy ML, Day NL. Prenatal cocaine exposure: effects on the development of school-age children. *Neurotoxicol Teratol.* 1996;18:627–634

49. Harsham J, Hayden-Keller J, Disbrow D. Growth patterns of infants exposed to cocaine and other drugs in utero. *J Am Diet Assoc.* 1994;94:999–1007

50. Wilson GS, McCreary R, Kean J, Baxter JC. The development of preschool children of heroin-addicted mothers: a controlled study. *Pediatrics.* 1979;63:135–141

51. Deren S. Children of substance abusers: a review of the literature. *J Subst Abuse Treat.* 1986;3:77–94

52. Kappy MS. Regulation of growth in children with chronic illness. Therapeutic implications for the year 2000. *Am J Dis Child.* 1987;141:489–193

53. Phillip M, Hershkovitz E, Rosenblum H, et al. Serum insulin-like growth factors I and II are not affected by undernutrition in children with nonorganic failure to thrive. *Horm Res.* 1998;49:76–79

54. Fryer GE Jr. The efficacy of hospitalization of nonorganic failure-to-thrive children: a meta-analysis. *Child Abuse Negl.* 1988;12:375–381

55. Bithoney WG, McJunkin J, Michalek J, Ega H, Snyder J, Munier A. Prospective evaluation of weight gain in both nonorganic and organic failure-to-thrive children: an outpatient trial of a multidisciplinary team strategy. *J Dev Behav Pediatr.* 1989;10:27–31

56. Berwick DM, Levy JD, Kleinerman R. Failure to thrive: diagnostic yield of hospitalisation. *Arch Dis Child.* 1982;57:347–351

57. Homer C, Ludwig S. Categorization of etiology of failure to thrive. *Am J Dis Child.* 1981;135:848–851

58. Fleisher DR. Comprehensive management of infants with gastroesophageal reflux and failure to thrive. *Curr Probl Pediatr.* 1995;25:247–253

59. Sullivan PB. Nutritional management of acute diarrhea. *Nutrition.* 1998;14:758–762

60. Reilly S, Skuse DH, Wolke D, Stevenson J. Oral-motor dysfunction in children who fail to thrive: organic or non-organic? *Dev Med Child Neurol.* 1999;41:115–122

61. Mathisen B, Skuse D, Wolke D, Reilly S. Oral-motor dysfunction and failure to thrive among inner-city infants. *Dev Med Child Neurol.* 1989;31:293–302

62. James JM, Burks AW. Food hypersensitivity in children. *Curr Opin Pediatr.* 1994;6:661–667

63. Niggeman B, Sielaff B, Beyer K, Binder C, Wahn U. Outcome of double-blind, placebo-controlled food challenge tests in 107 children with atopic dermatitis. *Clin Exp Allergy.* 1999;29:91–96

64. Chevalier P, Sevilla R, Sejas R, Zalles L, Belmonte G, Parent G. Immune recovery of malnourished children takes longer than nutritional recovery: implications for treatment and discharge. *J Trop Pediatr.* 1998;44:304–307

65. American Academy of Pediatrics. *Red Book: 2006 Report of the Committee on Infectious Diseases.* Pickering LK, Baker CJ, Long SS, eds. 27th ed. Elk Grove Village, IL: American Academy of Pediatrics; 2006

66. Cunningham-Rundles S, McNeeley DF, Moon A. Mechanisms of nutrient modulation of the immune response. *J Allergy Clin Immunol.* 2005;115:1119–1128

67. Schwartz J, Angle C, Pitcher H. Relationship between childhood blood lead levels and stature. *Pediatrics.* 1986;77:281–288

68. Mahaffey KR, Amnest JL, Roberts J, Murphy RS. National estimates of blood lead levels: United States, 1976–1980: association with selected demographic and socioeconomic factors. *N Engl J Med.* 1982;307:573–579

69. Centers for Disease Control and Prevention. *Preventing Lead Poisoning in Young Children: A Statement by the Centers for Disease Control.* Atlanta, GA: US Centers for Disease Control; 1991. Available at: http://www.cdc.gov/nceh/lead/publications/books/plpyc/contents.htm. Accessed November 1, 2007

70. Bithoney WG. Elevated lead levels in children with nonorganic failure to thrive. *Pediatrics.* 1986;78:891–895

71. Bergstrom WH. Twenty ways to get rickets in the 1990s. *Contemp Pediatr.* 1991;December:88–93

72. Catassi C, Farsano A. Celiac disease as a cause of growth retardation in childhood. *Curr Opin Pediatr.* 2004;16:445–449

73. Hillemeier AC. Gastroesophageal reflux: diagnostic and therapeutic approaches. *Pediatr Clin North Am.* 1996;43:197–212

74. Acs G, Shulman R, Ng MW, Chussid S. The effect of dental rehabilitation on the body weight of children with early childhood caries. *Pediatr Dent.* 1999;21:109–113

75. Peterson KE, Washington J, Rathbun JM. Team management of failure to thrive. *J Am Diet Assoc.* 1984;84:810–815

76. Zeiger RS, Sampson HA, Bock SA, et al. Soy allergy in infants and children with IgE-associated cow's milk allergy. *J Pediatr.* 1999;134:614–622

77. McJunkin JE, Bithoney WG, McCormick MC. Errors in formula concentration in an outpatient population. *J Pediatr.* 1987;111:848–850

78. Linscheid TR, Rasnake LK. Behavioral approaches to the treatment of failure to thrive. In: Drotar D, ed. *New Directions in Failure to Thrive: Implications for Research and Practice.* New York, NY: Plenum Press; 1985:279–294

79. Pollitt E. Failure to thrive: socioeconomic, dietary intake and mother-child interaction. *Fed Proc.* 1975;34:1593–1597

80. Heptinstall G, Puckering C, Skuse D, Start K, Zur-Szpiro S, Dowdney L. Nutrition and meal-time behavior in families of growth retarded children. *Hum Nutr Appl Nutr.* 1987;41:390–402

81. Faine MP, Oberg D. Snacking and oral health habits of Washington state WIC children and their caregivers. *ASDC J Dent Child.* 1994;61:350–355

82. Siener K, Rothman D, Farrar J. Soft drink logos on baby bottles: do they influence what is fed to children? *ASDC J Dent Child.* 1997;64:55–60

83. Zmora E, Gorodicher R, Bar-Ziv J. Multiple nutritional deficiencies in infants from a strict vegetarian community. *Am J Dis Child.* 1979;133:141–144

84. Pugliese MT, Weyman-Daum M, Moses N, Lifshitz F. Parental health beliefs as a cause of nonorganic failure to thrive. *Pediatrics.* 1987;80:175–182

85. American Academy of Pediatrics, Committee on Nutrition. The use and misuse of fruit juice in pediatrics. *Pediatrics.* 2001;107:1210–1213

86. Maldonado J, Gil A, Narbona E, Molina JA. Special formulas in infant nutrition: a review. *Early Hum Dev.* 1998;53(Suppl):S23–S32

87. Garza C, de Onis M. Rationale for developing a new international growth reference. *Food Nutr Bull.* 2004;25:S5–S14

88. Guo S, Roche AF, Fomon SJ, et al. Reference data on gains in weight and length during the first two years of life. *J Pediatr.* 1991;119:355–362

89. Kielman AA, McCord C. Weight-for-age as an index of risk of death in children. *Lancet.* 1978;1:1247–1250

90. Waterlow JC. Classification and definition of protein-calorie malnutrition. *Br Med J.* 1972;3:566–569

91. Gomez F, Ramos Galvan R, Freak S, Craviato Munoz J, Chavez R, Vazquez J. Mortality in second and third degree malnutrition. 1956. *Bull World Health Organ.* 2000;78:1275–1280

92. Morales E, Craig LD, MacLean WC Jr. Dietary management of malnourished children with a new enteral feeding. *J Am Diet Assoc.* 1991;91:1233–1238

93. Doherty CP, Sarkar MA, Shakur MS, Ling SC, Elton RA, Cutting WA. Zinc and rehabilitation from severe protein-energy malnutrition: higher-dose regimens are associated with increased mortality. *Am J Clin Nutr.* 1998;68:742–748

94. Black MM. Zinc deficiency and child development. *Am J Clin Nutr.* 1998;68:464S–469S

95. Rathbun JM, Peterson KE. Nutrition in failure to thrive. In: Grand RJ, Sutphen JL, Dietz WH, eds. *Pediatric Nutrition: Theory and Practice.* Boston, MA: Butterworths; 1987:627–643

96. Waterlow J. Treatment of children with malnutrition and diarrhoea. *Lancet.* 1999;354(9185):1142

97. Black MM, Krishnakumar A. Predicting longitudinal growth curves of height and weight using ecological factors for children with and without early growth deficiency. *J Nutr.* 1999;129(Suppl 2):539S–543S

98. Galler JR, Ramsey F, Solimano G, Lowell WE, Mason E. The influence of early malnutrition on subsequent behavioral development. I. Degree of impairment in intellectual performance. *J Am Acad Child Psychiatry.* 1983;22:8–15

99. Silver J, DiLorenzo P, Zukoski M, Ross PE, Amster BJ, Schlegel D. Starting young: Improving the health and developmental outcomes of infants and toddlers in the child welfare system. *Child Welfare.* 1999;78:148–165

100. Drewett RF, Corbett SS, Wright CM. Cognitive and educational attainments at school age of children who failed to thrive in infancy: a population-based study. *J Child Psychol Psychiatry.* 1999;40:551–561

101. Galler JR, Ramsey F, Solimano G. The influence of early malnutrition on subsequent behavioral development. III. Learning disabilities as a sequelae to malnutrition. *Pediatr Res.* 1984;18:309–313

102. Galler JR, Ramsey F, Solimano G. A follow-up study of the effects of early malnutrition on subsequent development. II. Fine motor skills in adolescence. *Pediatr Res.* 1985;19:524–527

103. Mendez MA, Adair LS. Severity and timing of stunting in the first two years of life affect performance on cognitive tests in late childhood. *J Nutr.* 1999;129:1555–1562

104. Skuse DH, Pickles A, Wolke D, Reilly S. Postnatal growth and mental development evidence for a "sensitive period." *J Child Psychol Psychiatry.* 1994;35:521–545

105. Black MM, Hutchenson JJ, Dubowitz H, Berenson-Howard J. Parenting style and developmental status among children with nonorganic failure to thrive. *J Pediatr Pscyhol.* 1994;19:689–707

106. Drotar D, Eckerle D. Family environment in nonorganic failure to thrive: a controlled study. *J Pediatr Pscyhol.* 1989;14:245–257

107. Galler JR, Ramsey F, Solimano G. The influence of early malnutrition on subsequent behavioral development. V. Child's behavior at home. *J Am Acad Child Psychiatry.* 1985;24:58–64

108. McKay H, Sinisterra L, McKay A, Gomez H, Lloreda P. Improving cognitive ability in chronically deprived children. *Science.* 1978;200:270–278

109. Zeskind PS, Ramey CT. Fetal malnutrition: an experimental study of its consequences on infant development in the caregiving environments. *Child Dev.* 1978;49:1155–1162

110. Drotar D, Wilson F, Sturm L. Parent intervention in failure to thrive. In: Schaefer CE, Briesmeister JM, eds. *Handbook of Parent Training: Parents as Co-Therapists for Children's Behavioral Problems.* New York, NY: John Wiley & Sons; 1989:364–391

111. Dobbing J. Infant nutrition and later achievement. *Nutr Rev.* 1984;42:1–7

112. Drotar D, Sturm L. Failure to thrive: psychological issues. In: Olson RA, Mullins LL, Chaney JM, eds. *The Sourcebook of Pediatric Psychology.* Needham Heights, MA: Allyn & Bacon; 1994:29–41

113. VandeVeer B, Schweid W. Infant assessment: stability of mental functioning in young retarded children. *Am J Ment Retard.* 1979;79:1–4

114. Drotar D, Sturm LA. Behavioral symptoms, problem solving, and personality development of preschool children with early histories of nonorganic failure to thrive. *J Dev Behav Pediatr.* 1992;13:226–273

115. Powell GF, Low JL. Behavior in non-organic failure to thrive. *J Dev Behav Pediatr.* 1983;8:18–24

116. Ramey CT, Yeates KO, Short EJ. The plasticity of intellectual development: insights from preventive intervention. *Child Dev.* 1984;55:1913–1925

117. Polan HJ, Leon A, Kaplan MD, Kessler DB, Stern DN, Ward MJ. Disturbances of affect expression in failure to thrive. *J Am Acad Child Adolesc Psychiatry.* 1991;30:897–903

118. Wolke D, Skuse D, Mathisen B. Behavioral style in failure to thrive: a preliminary communication. *J Pediatr Pscyhol.* 1990;15:237–254

119. Richards CA, Andrews PL, Spitz L, et al. Role of the mother's touch in failure to thrive: a preliminary investigation. *J Am Acad Child Adolesc Psychiatry.* 1994;33:1098–1105

120. Casey PH. Failure to thrive: a reconceptualization. *J Dev Behav Pediatr.* 1983;4:63–66

121. Ramey CT, Heiger L, Klisz D. Synchronous reinforcement of vocal responses in failure-to-thrive in infants. *Child Dev.* 1972;43:1449–1455

122. Ramey CT, et al. Nutrition, response-contingent stimulation and the maternal deprivation syndrome: Results of an early intervention program. *Mer Palm Q.* 1975;21:45–53

123. Black MM, Dubowitz H, Hutchenson J, Berenson-Howard J, Starr HJ Jr. A randomized clinical trial of home intervention for children with failure to thrive. *Pediatrics.* 1995;95:807–814

124. Grantham-McGregor S, Schofield W, Powell C. Development of severely malnourished children who received psychosocial stimulation: six-year follow-up. *Pediatrics.* 1987;79:247–254

125. Block RW, Krebs NF. American Academy of Pediatrics, Committee on Child Abuse and Neglect and Committee on Nutrition. Failure to thrive as a manifestation of child neglect. *Pediatrics.* 2005;116:1234–1237

126. Skuse DH, Gill D, Reilly S, Wolke D, Lynch MA. Failure to thrive and the risk of child abuse: a prospective population study. *J Med Screen.* 1995;2:145–149

127. Bullard DM Jr, Glaser HH, Heagarty MC, Pivchik EC. Failure to thrive in the "neglected" child. *Am J Orthopsychiatry.* 1966;37:680–690

128. Goldson E, Cadol RV, Fitch MJ, Umlauf HJ Jr. Nonaccidental trauma and failure to thrive. *Am J Dis Child.* 1976;130:490–492

129. Koel BS. Failure to thrive and fatal injury as a continuum. *Am J Dis Child.* 1969;118:565–567

130. Mackner LM, Starr RH Jr, Black MM. The cumulative effect of neglect and failure to thrive on cognitive functioning. *Child Abuse Negl.* 1997;21:691–700

131. Gilmour J, Skuse D. A case-comparison study of the characteristics of children with a short stature syndrome induced by stress (Hyperphagic Short Stature) and a consecutive series of unaffected "stressed" children. *J Child Psychol Psychiatry.* 1999;40:969–978

132. Kreiger I. Food restriction as a form of child abuse in ten cases of psychosocial deprivation dwarfism. *Clin Pediatr (Phila).* 1974;13:127–133

133. Wyatt DT, Simms MD, Horwitz SM. Widespread growth retardation and variable growth recovery in foster children in the first year after initial placement. *Arch Pediatr Adolesc Med.* 1997;151:813–816

Chronic Diarrheal Disease

Introduction and Pathophysiology

Infants and children with chronic or persistent diarrhea often pose a continuous significant medical challenge. Aggressive oral rehydration programs have reduced the frequency of hospitalization and death from acute diarrhea but have not yet demonstrated any influence on the morbidity and mortality from chronic diarrhea in developing countries. Chronic or persistent diarrhea still accounts for 30% to 40% of diarrhea-associated deaths worldwide.

The World Health Organization defines persistent diarrhea as "diarrheal episodes of presumed infectious etiology that begin acutely but last at least 14 days."[1] To the physician, diarrhea is often best defined on the basis of volume rather than frequency or consistency. Thus, diarrhea in infants and toddlers is defined as a volume of more than 10 g of stool/kg per day and in older children and adults is defined as a volume of more than 200 g/day.[2] To the parents, it is one more dirty diaper than they wish to change each day.

The etiologies of chronic diarrhea can be divided by pathophysiology into 4 often overlapping mechanisms. The first is osmotic diarrhea, secondary to the failure to absorb a solute that creates an osmotic load in the distal bowel, producing increased fluid losses. This can result from either congenital or acquired disease and is most evident in the failure to absorb a carbohydrate, such as lactose. Excessive carbohydrate intake, as seen with juices in early childhood, also contributes to this form of diarrhea.[3] By definition, the diarrhea ceases with elimination of the offending solute from the diet.

The second form, secretory diarrhea, occurs when there is a net secretion of electrolyte and fluid from the intestine, relative to the degree of absorption. This includes disorders such as congenital chloridorrhea and neural crest tumors. This form of diarrhea persists even with cessation of oral intake.

The third form of diarrhea is associated with dysmotility. Children with this form usually have intact absorptive ability, even in the face of rapid transit. The most common form of "benign" dysmotility in childhood causing diarrhea is toddler's or chronic nonspecific diarrhea (although this may also be a result of nonabsorbed solute in the diet or excessive fluid intake) and irritable bowel syndrome (IBS) in the older child and adolescent.

The fourth pathophysiologic form of diarrhea is inflammatory diarrhea. This often encompasses components of all of the previous 3 forms as well. The etiologies range from acute viral enteritis, to chronic villus or colonic inflammation from celiac disease, to inflammatory bowel diseases. Increased enteric loss of protein, mucus, and blood may also be noted in the stool.

Evaluation of the Infant and Child With Persistent Diarrhea

History and Physical Examination

It is very important initially to define the character of the diarrhea using criteria such as frequency, volume, duration, characteristics of the stool, and relationship to feeding or dietary intake. A prospective 3- to 5-day history of dietary intake, stool pattern, and associated symptoms is very helpful. Important historical features include family history, cultural influences on feeding, travel, and preschool exposures.

The physical examination begins with the documentation of weight, height, and head circumference, plotted on a standardized reference growth chart. The examination should focus on evidence of chronic disease; features of nutrient deficiency, such as rickets (eg, vitamin D deficiency) or hypotonia (eg, vitamin E deficiency); or abdominal distension with loss of subcutaneous tissue (eg, malabsorption characteristic of celiac disease) and should include a rectal examination.

Examination of a Stool Sample

Confirmation of the cause of persistent diarrhea requires evaluation of a fresh stool sample.[4] This begins with the macroscopic inspection of the stool for consistency and color. The stool should be tested for the presence of blood and polymorphonuclear leukocytes. The presence of leukocytes is expected with invasive bacterial disease and inflammatory colitis and argues against viral or malabsorptive diarrheas. Techniques for analysis of the stool for malabsorbed fat using Sudan black stains are available in clinical laboratories but are too cumbersome and dependent on an experienced observer for routine office use. Unabsorbed carbohydrates in the stool can be detected by reagent tablets (eg, Clinitest [Bayer Diagnostics, Tarrytown, NY]) for reducing sugars or test-tape analysis for glucose. Breastfed healthy infants will often have traces of reducing sugar in the stool. Sucrose is not a reducing sugar; thus, stool samples from infants who are fed sucrose-containing formulas will need to be hydrolyzed with hydrochloric acid solution and heated before testing for reducing sugars.

In patients with high-volume ostomy losses, it is often helpful to quantify the volume, osmolarity, and electrolyte content of the ostomy effluent. An osmotic diarrhea is present if the gap between measured and calculated osmolarity is >50 mOsm, and secretory diarrhea needs to be strongly considered if the gap is <50 mOsm. Alternatively, if the patient is stable and well-hydrated or receiving intravenous fluids, food and drink can be withheld for 24 hours to see if the volume of the diarrhea is affected. In a purely secretory diarrhea, a liquid stool output continues, even when the patient is not consuming any food or liquid orally. The measurement of stool volume and electrolytes also allows documentation of the child's ongoing electrolyte needs and the effect of malabsorbed carbohydrates in the feedings. Suspected loss of protein from the mucosal surface can be confirmed by determining the fecal content of alpha-1-antitrypsin, a large molecular weight serum protein that is resistant to proteolytic degradation in the gastrointestinal tract.

To exclude ongoing infection as a factor that is contributing to persistent diarrhea, it is appropriate to culture the stool for enteric pathogens and analyze for parasites, including *Giardia* species, *Cryptosporidium* species, and *Cyclospora* species. Fecal analysis for *Giardia* and *Cryptosporidia* antigens is now readily available and highly sensitive. Persistent infection lasting more than 14 days, or recurrent infection, is common in preschoolers and children with immune deficiencies. Diarrhea caused by viral agents rarely continues for more than 2 weeks. Although most relevant after use of antibiotic agents, analysis for the toxin of *Clostridium difficile* should be performed routinely with persistent diarrhea, especially in the presence of fecal leukocytes and/or blood.

For children with diarrhea in the context of failure to thrive or suspected steatorrhea, a formal documentation of quantitative fecal fat can be performed on a 72-hour collection of stool. This is coupled with a 4-day history of dietary fat intake, which is optimized to be >30 g/day in infants and >50 g/day in school-aged children. A coefficient of fat malabsorption of more than 5% is generally abnormal after early infancy. Fecal elastase concentrations can be assayed as a measure of pancreatic function.

Sweat Test

The analysis of sweat sodium and/or chloride by iontophoresis should be performed in all infants and toddlers with growth failure and diarrhea as well as any child with suspected or documented steatorrhea, to rule out cystic fibrosis. A genotypic analysis for the known mutations in cystic fibrosis can also be performed (and in many states is part of the newborn screening process). The nutritional support of children with cystic fibrosis is discussed in detail in Chapter 46.

Screening Laboratory Blood Studies

An analysis of blood or serum constituents is individualized according to the clinical situation and degree of concern for malabsorption, malnutrition, and inflammatory disease. A routine complete blood cell count with indices addresses issues of anemia and the status of iron, vitamin B_{12}, and folate sufficiency. An elevated platelet count may indicate vitamin E deficiency or inflammation, because platelets are acute phase reactants. Characteristic alterations of red blood cell morphology are seen in abetalipoproteinemia. Although they are nonspecific, erythrocyte sedimentation rate and C-reactive protein concentration will usually be elevated with chronic inflammatory bowel disease.

Serum immunoglobulin concentrations are measured specifically, with special emphasis on immunoglobulin (Ig)A. To screen for celiac disease or gluten-sensitive enteropathy, the specific IgA antitissue transglutaminase antibody has replaced less specific antigliadin antibodies. However, these cannot be interpreted in individuals with IgA deficiency. Low serum albumin and prealbumin concentrations reflect low dietary protein intake.

To evaluate the status of vitamin D, serum calcium, phosphorus, and alkaline phosphatase concentrations are determined. When fat-soluble vitamin malabsorption or deficiency is suspected, serum concentrations of 25-OH vitamin D, vitamin A, and vitamin E can be measured. Prothrombin time can be measured as an indirect measure of vitamin K sufficiency in the absence of liver disease. Serum vasoactive intestinal peptide concentration and/or urinary concentrations of the catecholamines homovanilmandelic and vanilmandelic acids should be obtained when diarrhea appears to be secretory.

Imaging

The value of radiologic studies for the evaluation of chronic diarrhea is limited. A plain film of the abdomen may reveal constipation, dilated blind loops of bowel, or calcifications of the biliary or pancreatic system. Oral contrast studies and computed tomographic scans with contrast are routine for the evaluation of inflammatory bowel disease.

Breath Hydrogen Analysis

The hydrogen breath test is a noninvasive test that can be used to examine for carbohydrate malabsorption. The test requires commensal, hydrogen-generating enteric bacterial flora, and generally is not valid after recent antibiotic use. When an oral carbohydrate is given, it is either digested and absorbed normally or it reaches the bacterial flora (normally found in the cecum and colon) intact and is metabolized to produce hydrogen gas that is absorbed and excreted in the breath. Analysis of breath hydrogen that reveals an increase of >20 ppm suggests carbohydrate malabsorption or bacterial overgrowth. The test is performed with oral lactose (for lactase deficiency), sucrose (for sucrase-isomaltase deficiency), or lactulose (for small-bowel bacterial overgrowth).

Endoscopic Procedures

When persistent diarrhea appears to be related to an inflammatory process of the small bowel or colon, invasive endoscopic visualization of the bowel with biopsy is indicated. Even grossly normal bowel specimens are routinely biopsied, because the diagnostic features may only be seen on histologic examination. Routine staining of tissue samples may be supplemented by electron microscopy, which might reveal microvillus inclusion disease, or biochemical analysis of the biopsy sample, which might reveal the lack of a digestive enzyme.

Differential Diagnosis of Persistent Diarrhea

A review of the many disorders capable of inducing persistent or chronic diarrhea is beyond the scope of this chapter. In Table 27.1, the major conditions are listed according to those commonly associated with normal growth or those expected to be complicated by growth failure or failure to thrive. Inappropriate nutritional management of any of these disorders, however, can lead to weight loss and growth failure.[5]

Table 27.1
Chronic Diarrhea in Childhood

Diarrhea Without Failure to Thrive
Chronic nonspecific (toddler's) diarrhea
Dietary-induced diarrhea • Excessive juice, tea • Prolonged low-fat diet • Disaccharide intolerance: lactose, sucrose
Persistent enteritis • Parasitic: *Giardia, Strongyloides, Cryptosporidium, Cyclospora* organisms • Immunodeficient: IgA deficiency, HIV infection • Small-bowel bacterial overgrowth
Factitious diarrhea • Laxative abuse • Encopresis • Munchausen by proxy

Table 27.1 *(Continued)*
Chronic Diarrhea in Childhood

Secretory diarrhea
• Neural crest tumors
• Congenital chloride diarrhea
• Congenital sodium diarrhea

Diarrhea With Failure to Thrive

Pancreatic insufficiency
- Cystic fibrosis
- Shwachman-Diamond syndrome

Disorders of lipid digestion, absorption, or transport
- Primary bile acid (micelle) deficiency
- abetalipoproteinemia
- Intestinal lymphangiectasia
- Chylomicron retention disease

Disorders of the mucosal villus
- Congenital
  - Microvillus inclusion disease
  - Tufting disease
- Reduced mucosal surface area
  - Short-bowel syndrome
  - Malnutrition
  - Ischemic, radiation enteropathy
  - Graft-versus-host disease

Disorders of ion transport
    Congenital chloride diarrhea
    Glucose-galactose malabsorption
    Congenital sodium diarrhea
    Absence of enteric hormones
    Congenital bile-acid diarrhea
    Congenital lactase deficiency
- Inflammatory villus injury
  - Postgastroenteritis diarrhea with malabsorption
  - Acute infectious diarrhea
  - Gluten-sensitive enteropathy
  - Dietary protein induced enteropathy: milk, soy, egg, fish
  - Eosinophilic gastroenteropathy
  - Autoimmune enteritis
  - Crohn disease
  - Blind loop/pseudo-obstruction
  - Whipple enteropathy
  - Intractable diarrhea

Diarrhea Without Failure to Thrive

Chronic Nonspecific (Toddler's) Diarrhea

This is the most common form of persistent diarrhea in the first 3 years of life.[6] It may begin acutely before 1 year of age but settles into a pattern of 2 to 5 loose to watery stools daily. There is an occasional day with formed stool, and there is almost never stooling during sleep. Multiple dietary manipulations may produce transient improvement but usually contribute to the problem by removing higher-fat foods and increasing ingestion of fruit juices ("juiceorrhea"). This is especially true with the intake of high-sorbitol-containing noncitrus juices, such as prune, pear, cherry, or apple (Appendix M). The American Academy of Pediatrics policy statement on the use and misuse of fruit juice discourages fruit juice in infants younger than 6 months and recommends against the use of fruit juice in the treatment of dehydration or the management of diarrhea.[7]

By definition, infants with chronic nonspecific diarrhea are clinically well with normal intestinal digestive and absorptive ability. Toddlers will do best on a normal diet that includes approximately 30% of total calories from fat and less than 4 to 6 oz of juice per day. The diarrhea often resolves with the acquisition of successful bowel toilet training, which allows greater duration of rectal retention.

Irritable Bowel Syndrome

The symptoms of IBS often start in adolescence. The history often suggests the diagnosis, with abdominal pain relieved with defecation and an associated change in stool frequency without evidence of a structural or metabolic abnormality. No consistent food or food group has been implicated as a cause of IBS. Probiotics have been used with some degree of success for IBS in adults, but the one randomized controlled trial in children with IBS showed no effect of *Lactobacillus rhamnosus* GG over placebo in the relief of pain.[8]

Disaccharide Intolerance

Lactose is a major dietary constituent for most children, because it is the primary carbohydrate of all mammalian milks other than the sea lion. Lactose is both a major source of calories and a facilitator for the intestinal absorption of calcium, magnesium, and manganese. It is digested by an intestinal mucosal brush-border oligosaccharidase, lactase, to glucose and galactose. Lactase activity decreases, in many species, under genetic control after weaning. In humans, there are ethnic variations in this decrease, with some groups becoming lactase deficient at a relatively early age. The lactase enzyme is especially sensitive to intestinal mucosal injury. Congenital lactase deficiency is very rare.[9]

As lactase activity decreases, dietary lactose is incompletely digested and induces an osmotic secretion of electrolytes and fluid in the distal small bowel. As the lactose reaches the bacterial flora of the distal bowel, it is fermented to hydrogen, methane, and carbon dioxide. This allows the diagnosis by breath hydrogen and methane analysis and also contributes to the child's sense of discomfort from gas and increased flatus. The fermentation of lactose also produces volatile fatty acids that are absorbed across the colonic epithelium as a calorie source.

The first step in the treatment of lactose malabsorption involves eliminating lactose from the diet to see whether diarrhea resolves. A gradual reintroduction of lactose-containing foods can help determine the threshold for tolerance of lactose in the diet. Lactose-reduced milks are commonly available, as are lactase tablets, which are taken before ingesting lactose-containing foods. A number of probiotics to enhance lactose tolerance are under investigation, but the commonly marketed *Lactobacillus acidophilus* has minimal lactase activity. The heating and fermentation of many cheeses reduce lactose content, and yogurt is also lower in lactose than is fluid milk. The major risk of lactose-restricted diets is the reduction in dietary calcium intake, particularly in the age group of 9 to 20 years, during which desired daily intakes of 1300 mg of calcium are difficult to achieve in the absence of dairy products in the diet.

Infants with diarrhea on sucrose or glucose polymer-containing formulas may have congenital sucrase-isomaltase deficiency. This diagnosis is confirmed by sucrose breath hydrogen testing, and sucrase deficiency can be treated with a recently produced baker's yeast (*Saccharomyces cerevisiae*) processed to a high content of a yeast invertase that cleaves sucrose. In normal children, sucrase-isomaltase activity reaches near-adult levels by 1 month of age and is highly resistant to mucosal injury.[10]

Small-Bowel Bacterial Overgrowth

There is an increasing awareness of bacterial overgrowth as a cause of persistent diarrhea and abdominal discomfort, especially in children younger than 2 years of age.[11] The diagnosis is established by a breath hydrogen test using lactulose as the carbohydrate; because there is no mucosal enzyme for lactulose hydrolysis, it is fermented by the bacteria in the proximal small bowel and in the large intestine. Thus, both an early and a late rise of breath hydrogen after ingestion may indicate bacterial overgrowth in the small intestine. As well, a high fasting baseline breath hydrogen level (>40 ppm) has been invoked as indicative of bacterial overgrowth. Treatment with a brief course of an antibiotic agent, such as metronidazole or the non-absorbable rifaximin, often followed by the use of a probiotic, may be very effective in relieving symptoms.[12,13]

Diarrhea With Failure to Thrive

Postgastroenteritis Diarrhea With Malabsorption

Persistent diarrhea after an acute episode of infectious diarrhea (intractable diarrhea of infancy) remains a major clinical issue in developing countries but has decreased dramatically in the industrialized world with the increased attention paid to the nutritional management of the child with acute diarrhea. In contrast with toddler's diarrhea, the intestinal morphology is not normal, even after the infectious cause has been cleared. Small-bowel biopsies reveal patchy villus atrophy with increased inflammatory infiltrates, featuring intraepithelial lymphocytes with increased plasma cells and macrophages in the lamina propria and adherent bacteria on the mucosal surface.[14] Nutrient malabsorption may occur in the jejunum and ileum. Disaccharide intolerance is common, contributing to osmotic diarrhea and increased fluid needs.

Although persistent infection requires exclusion, because there are differences in the duration of diarrhea resulting from common infectious agents,[15] the characteristics most commonly associated with persistent inflammation after an episode of infectious diarrhea include young age, relative malnutrition, and an altered immune response.[5] In developing countries, lack of breastfeeding is a major risk factor. Infants younger than 6 months are particularly susceptible. The diagnosis of protracted diarrhea of infancy is made on the basis of the practitioner's awareness and the exclusion of alternative explanations. Intestinal biopsy should be deferred until the infant fails to respond to nutritional intervention with a lactose-free, sucrose-free diet with medium-chain triglycerides. Although a subgroup will require amino acid-based or elemental diets, most can be managed on traditional diets or mixed-protein diets.[5,16,17] Breastfeeding of infants is encouraged, unless lactose malabsorption is clinically significant. Both macronutrient and micronutrient deficiencies may occur from reduced intake and increased fecal loss. Total caloric needs for enteric recovery and catch-up growth often exceed 120 kcal/kg per day.

Enteric feedings are encouraged, either by continuous tube feeding or frequent small-volume bolus feedings. Initial caloric intake is attempted at

50 to 75 kcal/kg per day, increasing over 5 to 7 days to 130 to 150 kcal/kg per day. Protein is initiated at 1 to 2 g/kg per day, increasing to 3 to 4 g/kg per day as caloric intake is maximized. The requirements for potassium, calcium, phosphorus, magnesium, and trace minerals are usually increased and must be monitored closely in severely affected children. Although renal and cardiac function are usually normal, rapid increases in fluid and electrolytes must be monitored closely. Aggressive refeeding may rarely precipitate acute pancreatitis. The tolerance of normal feedings and clinical improvement are usually noted in 2 to 3 weeks.

Gluten-Sensitive Enteropathy (Celiac Disease)

This enteropathy is characterized by severe villus injury and loss of mucosal surface area. It is the result of a T-lymphocyte-mediated immune response against gluten protein in wheat and related proteins in barley and rye. Oat proteins are generally tolerated, although this remains somewhat controversial. The protein-induced injury triggers a release of tissue transglutaminase, a highly specific endomysial antigen. The IgA antibody to this transglutaminase is detected in serum of affected children and serves as a highly specific screening test. The diagnosis is confirmed by small-bowel biopsy, obtained by esophagogastroduodenoscopy. Treatment consists of complete elimination of foods containing wheat (gluten), barley and rye. Gluten-free foods are now readily marketed, and parents are instructed to read the labels of processed foods carefully. Antitissue transglutaminase antibody testing is repeated 6 to 8 months after the start of the gluten-free diet, and a decrease in serum concentrations is usually seen if the patient is adhering to the diet. Recent reports suggest that the incidence of celiac disease is significantly higher than earlier reports, with an incidence of approximately 1:100 to 1:200 in most industrialized countries.[18] It is also now recognized that chronic diarrhea is only one of the many possible presenting symptoms of the disease. The risk of developing celiac disease is even higher in children with diabetes, trisomy 21, and thyroid-related autoimmune disorders.

Short-Bowel Syndrome

Short-bowel syndrome is the consequence of massive small-bowel resection and the resulting severe nutrient malabsorption that occurs with loss of mucosal surface area. It is seen after surgical intervention for long-segment necrotizing enterocolitis, midgut volvulus, acute ischemic injury, small-bowel aganglionosis, gastroschisis, and diffuse Crohn disease of the small bowel. The best prognosis is for children in whom the duodenum, distal ileum, and ileocecal valve can be preserved.

In the initial postoperative period after loss of a significant length of small bowel, total parenteral nutrition is universally used. The early initiation of enteral feedings maximizes the enteric hormonal stimulation and adaptation of the residual bowel by elongation, hypertrophy, and reduction in peristaltic rate.

The greatest potential for recovery is in infancy. The normal absorptive surface area at birth is approximately 950 cm,[2] increasing to 7500 cm^2 in the adult. As noted earlier, enteral feedings are begun as soon as possible to minimize the mucosal atrophy that occurs with prolonged total parenteral nutrition. The initial feedings usually contain protein as a hydrolysate or amino acids, lipid with a combination of medium- and long-chain triglycerides, and carbohydrate as glucose polymer. As with postgastroenteritis malabsorption, calories are gradually increased by 5 to 15 kcal/kg per day by intragastric infusion to full oral intake.

Inflammatory Bowel Disease

The nutritional consequences of diffuse small-bowel inflammatory bowel disease (Crohn disease) can be devastating. Affected children present with abdominal pain and diarrhea that is minimized by reduced caloric intake. Combined with increased enteric loss of protein, zinc, and blood across the inflamed mucosa, the result is weight loss, reduced growth rate, delayed puberty, and anemia unresponsive to dietary iron. This is further complicated when active disease occurs during puberty, when nutritional needs for growth are increased, and by the use of anti-inflammatory and growth-inhibiting corticosteroid therapy. For further discussion of nutritional support in patients with inflammatory bowel disease, see chapter 43.

Allergic Enteropathy

Food-sensitive enteropathies, along with postgastroenteritis enteropathies, account for the majority of patients with chronic diarrhea. Enteropathy induced by food protein is often diagnosed in infancy and presents with profuse vomiting and/or diarrhea. When severe, these symptoms may lead to lethargy, dehydration, and hypotension (often mimicking sepsis). Alternatively, this may present at 1 year of age, when breastfeeding is commonly discontinued and the ingestion of cow milk is begun. The enteropathy resolves with elimination of the responsible protein, most often cow milk or soy. Protein hydrolysate and, sometimes, amino acid-based formulas, are used as nutritional sources for these children.

Probiotics and Chronic Diarrhea

Probiotics, as defined by the Food and Agriculture Organization of the United Nations,[19] are live microorganisms that confer a beneficial health effect on the host when administered in adequate amounts. Although probiotics have been shown to be of benefit in the management of acute diarrheal disorders, especially secondary to rotavirus, their advantage in chronic diarrhea is more variable, depending on the probiotic and the disease entity. Probiotics have been shown to be effective in the prevention of pouchitis and its attendant diarrhea in patients with ulcerative colitis after colectomy and ileoanal pull through as well as in the prevention of antibiotic-associated diarrhea. *Lactobacillus rhamnosus* GG and *Saccharomyces boulardii* have been effective in treating severe recurrent *C difficile* diarrhea, and some probiotics have shown efficacy in the management of IBS and in bacterial overgrowth syndromes.

Summary

Chronic diarrhea in childhood can result from many different causes that often must be defined before definitive treatment can be initiated. Nutrition support is the mainstay of treatment in children with an undefined cause of chronic diarrhea. Throughout the evaluation process, appropriate nutrition must be provided to meet the child's needs, either enterally or parentally if necessary, to facilitate healing and good health.

References

1. Snyder JD, Merson MH. The magnitude of the global problem of acute diarrheal disease: a review of active surveillance data. *Bull World Health Organ.* 1982;60:605–613

2. Vanderhoof JA. Chronic diarrhea. *Pediatr Rev.* 1998;19:418–422

3. Hyams JS, Etienne NL, Leichtner AM, Theuer RC. Carbohydrate malabsorption following fruit juice ingestion in young children. *Pediatrics.* 1988;82:64–68

4. Sondheimer JM. Office stool examination: a practical guide. *Contemp Pediatr.* 1990;Feb:63–82

5. Bhutta ZA, Hendricks KM. Nutritional management of persistent diarrhea in childhood: A perspective from the developing world. *J Pediatr Gastroenterol Nutr.* 1996;22:17–37

6. Cohen SA, Hendricks KM, Eastham EJ, Mathis RK, Walker WA. Chronic nonspecific diarrhea: a complication of dietary fat restriction. *Am J Dis Child.* 1979;133:490–492

7. American Academy of Pediatrics, Committee on Nutrition. The use and misuse of juice in pediatrics. *Pediatrics.* 2001;107:1210–1213

8. Bausserman M, Michail S. The use of Lactobacillus GG in irritable bowel syndrome in children: a double-blind randomized control trial. *J Pediatr.* 2005;147:197–201

9. Heyman MB, American Academy of Pediatrics, Committee on Nutrition. Lactose intolerance in infants, children, and adolescents. *Pediatrics.* 2006;118:1279–1286

10. Treem WR. Clinical heterogeneity in congenital sucrase-isomaltase deficiency. *J Pediatr.* 1996;128:727–729

11. deBoissieu D, Chaussain M, Badoual J, Raymond J, Dupont C. Small-bowel bacterial overgrowth in children with chronic diarrhea, abdominal pain, or both. *J Pediatr.* 1996;128:203–207

12. Vanderhoof JA. Probiotics and intestinal inflammatory disorders in infants and children. *J Pediatr Gastroenterol Nutr.* 1995;21:125–129

13. Lauritano EC, Gabrielli M, Lupascu A, et al. Rifaximin dose-finding study for the treatment of small intestinal bacterial overgrowth. *Aliment Pharmacol Ther.* 2005;22:31–35

14. Shiner M, Putman M, Nichols VN, Nichols BL. Pathogenesis of small-intestinal mucosal lesions in chronic diarrhea of infancy: I. A light microscopic study. *J Pediatr Gastroenterol Nutr.* 1990;11:455–463

15. Keating JP. Chronic diarrhea. *Pediatr Rev.* 2005;26:5–14

16. Kleinman RE, Galeano NF, Ghishan F, Lebenthal E, Sutphen J, Ulshen MH. Nutritional management of chronic diarrhea and/or malabsorption. *J Pediatr Gastroenterol Nutr.* 1989;9:407–415

17. Bhatnagar S, Bhan MK, Singh KD, Saxena SK, Shariff M. Efficacy of milk-based diets in persistent diarrhea: a randomized, controlled trial. *Pediatrics.* 1996;98:1122–1126

18. Fasano A, Berti I, Gerarduzi T, et al. Prevalence of celiac disease in at-risk and not-at-risk groups in the United States: a large multicenter study. *Arch Intern Med.* 2003;163:286–292

19. Food and Agriculture Organization of the United Nations, World Health Organization. FAO/WHO Expert Consultation. Health and Nutritional Properties of Probiotics in Food Including Powder Milk with Live Lactic Acid Bacteria; 2001; Cordoba, Argentina. Available at: http://www.who.int/foodsafety/publications/fs_management/en/probiotics.pdf. Accessed November 2, 2007

28 Oral Therapy for Acute Diarrhea

Diarrheal illness and accompanying acute dehydration remains a major cause of childhood deaths in the world.[1] Reduction of the morbidity and mortality from diarrhea through the use of an oral rehydration salt or solution (ORS) continues to be one of the major strategies of the United Nations Children's Fund (UNICEF) and the World Health Organization (WHO) for saving children's lives.[1-3] Because of its simplicity, great effectiveness, and low expense, ORS is an ideal treatment for use in the developing world and in industrialized nations.[2-4] In developing countries, ORS has played a major role in reducing the estimated number of deaths from diarrhea in children younger than 5 years by more than half.[1,5,6] Although the death rate from diarrheal illness in industrialized nations like the United States is low, diarrheal illness still accounts for a substantial proportion of preventable childhood deaths worldwide and a large proportion of the morbidity and the expense associated with pediatric care.[7] For example, in the United States alone, roughly $1.5 billion is spent annually to provide evaluation and care for approximately 16 million episodes of diarrheal illness in children younger than 5 years.[8]

Physiological Principles

The physiological basis of ORS is at the same time simple and extraordinarily elegant. A combination of sodium with simple organic molecules, such as glucose, in the lumen of the small intestine can promote the absorption of water.[9] This system, discovered and characterized in the 1960s,[10] is now referred to as the glucose-sodium cotransport system.[9,11] Molecular details of the system are now reasonably well understood. In the cotransport mechanism, a single molecule of glucose or other simple organic substrate is transported across the luminal membrane of the villus crypt cells of the small intestine.[9,11] In concert with the transport of a glucose molecule, a sodium molecule is also brought from the luminal side of the membrane to the interior of the cell. This sodium ion is subsequently transferred into the adjacent capillaries and, thus, into the circulation. Water follows the movement of sodium along a concentration gradient, with the net result being absorption of sodium and water. The earliest clinical studies of solutions that take advantage of the cotransport system were performed in patients with cholera diarrhea.[12] We now know that the glucose-sodium cotransport system remains intact in virtually all kinds of infectious diarrhea. This fact makes oral therapy appropriate for use in any kind of enteric infection in which dehydration is an end result.[4,9] The other components of ORS include potassium and chloride to replace stool losses and base, usually in the form of citrate, to replace stool losses and to combat acidosis.[9,11]

Many fluids that have traditionally been recommended for the treatment of diarrhea and dehydration are inappropriate and nonphysiological and may worsen the condition.[3,4,9] For example, juices such as apple or white grape juice have a high osmolality related to their high sugar content and contain virtually no sodium and very little potassium. Table 28.1 lists the composition of some currently available rehydration solutions. Some of the frequently used inappropriate fluids are listed for comparison. Particular attention should be paid to the osmolality of the fluids. In general, solutions with osmolality lower than serum (approximately 310 mOsm/L) make the

Table 28.1
Composition of Fluids Frequently Used in Oral Rehydration*

Solution	Glucose/ CHO, g/L	Sodium, mEq/L	HCO$_3^-$, mEq/L	Potassium mEq/L	Osmolality, mmol/L	CHO/ Sodium
Pedialyte (Abbott Laboratories, Columbus, OH)	25	45	30	20	250	3.1
Pediatric Electrolyte (PendoPharm, Montreal, Quebec)	25	45	20	30	250	3.1
Kaolectrolyte (Pfizer, New York, NY)	20	48	28	20	240	2.4
Rehydralyte (Abbott Laboratories, Columbus, OH)	25	75	30	20	310	1.9
WHO ORS, 2002 (reduced osmolarity)	75	75	10[†]	30	224	1.0
WHO ORS, 1975, (original formulation)	111	90	10[†]	20	311	1.2
Cola*	126	2	13	0.1	750	1944
Apple juice*	125	3	0	32	730	1278
Gatorade* (Gatorade, Chicago, IL)	45	20	3	3	330	62.5

CHO indicates carbohydrate; HCO$_3^-$, bicarbonate; WHO, World Health Organization.

* Cola, juice, and Gatorade are shown for comparison only; they are not recommended for use.

Mainly for maintenance therapy; may be used for rehydration therapy in mildly dehydrated patients.

† Citrate.

most effective ORSs if the ratio of glucose to sodium is maintained near one.[9] Solutions containing less sodium than the standard WHO/UNICEF formulation and having glucose-to-sodium ratios of approximately 3 have also proven effective in maintaining hydration in noncholera diarrhea.[4]

The Search for a More Effective ORS

Although ORSs have an impressive record of success, they remain underused.[13] Perhaps the most important factor limiting the use of ORSs has been the lack of antidiarrheal properties.[13] The original ORSs were very effective at replacing fluid and electrolyte losses but had no effect on the volume or duration of diarrhea.[9,13]

The initial efforts to create an ORS that would decrease stool volume and output focused on the addition of other sodium cotransport molecules, such as the amino acids glycine, alanine, and glutamine.[9,14] However, these solutions proved to be no more effective than ORS and were more expensive and had some potentially dangerous adverse effects.[2,15] At about the same time, studies of complex carbohydrates (starches) from cereals were undertaken.[9] Starches do not contribute significantly to the osmotic content of the solution and yield individual glucose molecules at the brush border of the small intestine.[9] This allows the delivery of large numbers of glucose molecules to the cotransport system without causing osmotic diarrhea. Numerous studies demonstrated that cereal-based ORSs can reduce the volume of stools and the duration of diarrheal illness.[16] However, these solutions have not been well received, because the precooked dry cereal forms were more expensive than standard ORSs and the home-cooked cereal forms were time-consuming to prepare and required often-expensive cooking fuel. In addition, when cereal-based solutions were compared with the combination of glucose-based solutions and the early reinstitution of feeding, the differences between the 2 approaches disappeared so that cereal-based ORSs have not replaced the easier-to-prepare glucose ORSs.[16,17]

The search for more effective ORSs was greatly aided by the discovery that reduced-osmolarity glucose-electrolyte solutions can result in improved water and electrolyte transport from the intestinal lumen.[18] This discovery led to a series of studies that have demonstrated that reduced-osmolarity ORSs are more effective in replacing fluid and electrolyte losses compared with the standard WHO-formulation ORS.[19,20] A meta-analysis of clinical trials in children in developing countries showed that these solutions resulted in less need for supplemental intravenous fluids, less vomiting, and a slight reduction in stool output compared with the standard WHO-formulation ORS.[21] On the basis of these findings, WHO and UNICEF have recommended that a single reduced-osmolarity ORS be used to treat all cases of diarrhea.[22]

The main concern raised about the reduced-osmolarity ORSs is that they would lead to hyponatremia, especially when used for treatment of patients with high-purging diarrheas, such as cholera, because the sodium content is only approximately two thirds that of the standard WHO-formulation ORS.[23] Data from initial trials indicate that hyponatremia occurs more commonly with these solutions, but symptomatic hyponatremia has been very uncommon.[2,22]

Early, Appropriate Feeding

For more than 15 years, clinicians have recognized that return to an age-appropriate and healthy diet early in the course of diarrheal illness is superior to the outdated practice of "resting the gut" by providing only clear liquids or dilute milks.[4,9,24] Appropriate feeding is the component of oral therapy that has the greatest potential for effect on stool volume and duration.[3,4] In addition, the appetite of the infant and child is generally better maintained, and intestinal repair can occur.[4]

Successful feeding trials have been carried out using human milk, dilute or full-strength animal milk or animal milk formulas, dilute and full-strength lactose-free formulas, and mixed diets of staple foods with milk.[4,24,25] Recent data support the use of lactose-containing milks during diarrhea, especially if given with complex carbohydrates.[26] In general, changes to a lactose-free formula should be made only if the stool output increases on a milk-based diet.[4] Semi-solid and solid foods that have proven to be effective in controlled trials include: rice, wheat, peas, potatoes, chicken, and eggs.[4,24]

Oral Therapy for Diarrhea

In addition to the use of a physiologically sound ORS solution and early, appropriate feeding, effective oral therapy requires a thoughtful parental education component. When possible, explaining to the parent that the child's diarrhea is likely to continue, regardless of therapy, for between 3 and 7 days can be extremely helpful. Parents who understand that hydration is the primary concern, not the duration of the diarrheal stool, will generally be more comfortable managing the child's illness at home. By emphasizing to the parents that the ORS replaces fluid and electrolyte losses but does not stop diarrhea, less disappointment and discouragement should develop. A positive approach to teaching parents includes pointing out the degree of control that parents retain when the child receives an ORS compared with the loss of that control that results when intravenous solutions are used. In addition, pointing out that an ORS is less painful and has fewer complications than intravenous therapy is useful. Finally, most parents greatly desire to feed their child, particularly when the child appears to be hungry and thirsty, and this should be encouraged.

The following management guidelines are based on the severity of the child's condition.[3,4]

Children With Diarrhea and No Dehydration

If no dehydration develops, which is the case in the great majority of diarrhea cases in the United States, continued age-appropriate feeding is the only therapy required.[3] Infants should continue to be breastfed or fed regular formula. Formula does not require dilution if the diarrhea remains mild. If a diluted formula is used, the concentration should be increased rapidly if the diarrhea does not worsen. Weaned infants and children should have their regular nutritionally balanced diet continued, emphasizing complex carbohydrates (such as rice, wheat, and potatoes), meats (especially chicken), and the child's regular milk or formula. Diets high in simple sugars and fats should be avoided.[3,4] The "BRATT" diet (bananas, rice, applesauce, tea, and toast) should be avoided, because it is not a balanced diet and is low in calories.[4]

Children With Mild or Moderate Dehydration

After dehydration is corrected (Table 28.2), appropriate feeding is begun, using the guidelines above. The most convenient method for carrying out rehydration is to divide the total volume deficit by 4 and aim to deliver this volume of fluid during each of the 4 hours of the rehydration phase. A teaspoon or 5-mL syringe can be used for the initial administration of fluid, especially if the child is vomiting. The parent is instructed to administer at least 1 teaspoon (5 mL) of solution each minute. Having a clock with a sweep second hand available is useful. Although this rate of fluid delivery may appear slow, 5 mL/minute results in an hourly intake of 300 mL. In an infant weighing 10 kg, this is equivalent to 30 mL/kg. Children weighing more than 15 to 20 kg can receive 2 teaspoons (10 mL)/minute and achieve a similar volume of fluid intake. In general, this rate of fluid administration is more than adequate to replace the entire calculated volume deficit within a 4-hour period.

V

Table 28.2
Fluid Therapy Chart

Degree of Dehydration	Signs	Fluids	Feeding
Mild*	Slightly dry mucous membranes, increased thirst	ORS, 50–60 mL/kg[†]	Breastfeeding, undiluted lactose-free formula, full-strength cow milk, or lactose-containing formula
Moderate	Sunken eyes, sunken fontanelle, loss of skin turgor, dry mucous membranes	ORS, 80–100 mL/kg[†]	Same as above
Severe	Signs of moderate dehydration plus one or more of the following: rapid thready pulse, cyanosis, rapid breathing, delayed capillary refill time, lethargy, coma	Intravenous or intraosseous isotonic Fluids (0.9% saline or Ringer lactate), 40 mL/kg per hour until pulse and state of consciousness return to normal, then 50–100 mL/kg of ORS based on remaining degree of dehydration[‡]	Begin after clinically improved and ORS has begun

* If no signs of dehydration are present, rehydration phase may be omitted. Proceed with maintenance therapy and replacement of ongoing losses.

[†] First 4 hours, repeat until no signs of dehydration remain. Replace ongoing stool losses and vomitus with ORS, 10 mL/kg for each diarrheal stool and 5 mL/kg for each episode of vomiting.

[‡] Although parenteral access is being sought, nasogastric infusion of ORS may be begun at 30 mL/kg per hour, provided airway protective reflexes remain intact.

During rehydration, the volume of stool and emesis should be carefully recorded and added to the hourly quantity of fluid to be administered. After 1 or 2 hours of successful rehydration using a syringe or teaspoon, most infants and children will be able to take the fluid ad libitum. On rare occasions, a child will not cooperate in taking the solution from a syringe (this is most often the case with toddlers) or may be too exhausted to remain awake during the administration of fluid. In these cases and after carefully establishing that airway protective reflexes are intact, a soft 5F polymeric silicone nasogastric tube may be placed into the lumen of the stomach. The ORS may then be administered via the nasogastric tube at approximately 5 to 10 mL/kg per minute. This method has been widely used in the developing world and has also proved quite successful in industrialized countries.

Children With Severe Dehydration

Severe dehydration in children, which is a shock or a near shock-like condition, should be treated as an emergency.[3,4] A large-bore intravenous catheter should be used for the infusion of lactated Ringer solution, normal saline solution, or a similar solution and boluses of 20 to 40 mL/kg should be administered until signs of shock resolve. Fluid and electrolyte resuscitation may require more than one intravenous site, and the use of alternate access sites including venous cutdown or femoral vein or interosseous locations may be needed. As the level of consciousness improves, oral rehydration therapy can be instituted. The hydration status must be frequently reassessed to monitor the effectiveness of the therapy. When rehydration is complete, feeding is continued as described previously.

Common Concerns About ORSs in the United States

Refusal to Take ORS

One of the most common complaints about ORSs from children and their parents in the United States is the salty taste.[13] However, children who are dehydrated rarely refuse an ORS, because they usually crave salt and water. By recognizing that ORS may not be required in children with mild diarrhea and no dehydration, the problem of refusal could be greatly reduced.[4] Methods to try to increase ORS intake have included the use of a flavored ORS, which does not alter the composition of fluid and electrolytes but improves taste.[4] These flavored solutions are now the most popular forms of ORSs sold in North America. Another effective technique to increase intake is to freeze the ORS in an ice-pop form.

Vomiting

Vomiting, which is commonly associated with acute diarrhea, can make oral therapy more challenging, but almost all children with vomiting can be treated successfully with an ORS.[3,4] Correction of fluid and electrolyte deficits by use of a balanced-electrolyte ORS can help speed recovery from vomiting. As vomiting decreases, the ORS can be given in larger volumes. Because vomiting can signal bowel obstruction, efforts should be made to eliminate the possible diagnosis of bowel obstruction on a clinical basis before proceeding with an ORS. In a patient who may have an obstructive or other acute process, immediate vascular access must be gained, a surgical consultation must be obtained, and the child should be kept without oral fluids or food.

Hypernatremia

Oral rehydration solutions were originally developed to treat the dehydration resulting from cholera, in which stool losses of sodium are substantial. In industrialized nations like the United States, concerns have been expressed about the risk of hypernatremia with the use of solutions containing 90 mEq/L of sodium in infants and children whose diarrhea results from noncholera organisms.[3,4,13] In the presence of mature, functioning kidneys, the use of a 90-mEq sodium solution is safe and extremely effective in children with a wide range of initial serum sodium concentrations and is an effective treatment for hypernatremia.[3,4] In contrast, when solutions with little sodium, such as juices, sodas, or water (Table 28.1), are used, the risk of hyponatremia is very real.[3,4] Of greater importance than the sodium concentration is the ratio of sodium to glucose (or other cotransport molecule), which should be close to one.[2,9]

Failure of Therapy

Failure of oral rehydration therapy occurs when the net output over a 4- to 8-hour period exceeds net intake or when clinical indicators of dehydration are worsening rather than improving. Before determining that oral rehydration therapy has failed in a child, a review of the treatment guidelines should be made with the parents or other caregiver. Often, treatment failures and unnecessary intravenous line placement can result from lack of understanding or encouragement to staff or parents to continue to administer the ORS.

References

1. Black RE, Morris SS, Bryce J. Where and why are 10 million children dying every year? *Lancet.* 2003;361:2226–2234

2. Duggan C, Fontaine O, Pierce NF, et al. Scientific rationale for a change in the composition of oral rehydration solution. *JAMA.* 2004;291:2628–2631

3. King CK, Glass R, Breese JS, Duggan C. Management of acute gastroenteritis among children: oral rehydration, maintenance and nutritional therapy. *MMWR Morb Mortal Wkly Rep.* 2003;52:1–16

4. American Academy of Pediatrics, Provisional Committee on Quality Improvement, Subcommittee on Acute Gastroenteritis. Practice parameter: the management of acute gastroenteritis in young children. *Pediatrics.* 1996;97:424–435

5. Parashar U, Hummelman E, Bresee JS, Miller M, Glass R. Global illness and death caused by diarrheal disease in children. *Emerg Infect Dis.* 2003;9:565–572

6. Snyder JD, Merson MH. The magniturde of the global problem of acute diarrhoeal disease: a review of active surveillance data. *Bull World Health Organ.* 1982;60:605–613

7. Ho MS, Glass RI, Pinsky PF. Diarrheal deaths in American children: are they preventable? *JAMA*. 1988;260:3281

8. Glass RI, Lew JF, Gangarosa RE, LeBaron CW, Ho MS. Estimates of morbidity and mortality rates for diarrheal diseases in American children. *J Pediatr*. 1991;118:S27–S33

9. Hirschhorn N, Greenough W. Progress in oral rehydration therapy. *Sci Am*. 1991;264:50–56

10. Sladen GE, Dawson AM. Interrelationships between the absorptions of glucose, sodium and water by the normal human jejunum. *Clin Sci (Colch)*. 1969;36:119–132

11. Field M. Intestinal ion transport and the pathophysiology of diarrhea. *J Clin Invest*. 2003;11:943

12. Hirschhorn N. The treatment of acute diarrhea in children: an historical and physiological perspective. *Am J Clin Nutr*. 1980;33:637–663

13. Avery ME, Snyder JD. Oral therapy for acute diarrhea: The underused simple solution. *N Engl J Med*. 1990;323:891

14. Bhan MK, Mahalanabis D, Fontaine O, Pierce NF. Clinical trials of improved oral rehydration solution formulations: a review. *Bull World Health Organ*. 1994;72:945–955

15. Santosham M, Burns BA, Reid R, et al. Glycine-based oral rehydration solution: reassessment of safety and efficacy. *J Pediatr*. 1986;109:795–801

16. Gore SM, Fontaine O, Pierce NF. Impact of rice based oral rehydration solution of stool output and duration of diarrhoea: meta-analysis of 13 clinical trials. *BMJ*. 1992;304:287–291

17. Fayad IM, Hashem M, Duggan C, et al. Comparative efficacy of rice-based and glucose-based oral rehydration salts plus early reintroduction of food. *Lancet*. 1993;342:772–775

18. Thillainayagam AV, Hunt JB, Farthing MJG. Enhancing clinical efficacy of oral rehydration therapy. Is low osmolality the key? *Gastroenterology*. 1998;114:197–210

19. Santosham M, Fayad I, Abu Zikri M, et al. A double-blind clinical trial comparing World Health Organization oral rehydration solution with a reduced osmolarity solution containing equal amounts of sodium and glucose. *J Pediatr*. 1996;128:45–51

20. CHOICE Study Group. Multicentre, randomized, double-blind clinical trial to evaluate the efficacy and safety of a reduced osmolarity oral rehydration salts solution in children with acute watery diarrhea. *Pediatrics*. 2001;107:613–618

21. Hahn S, Kim Y, Garner P. Reduced osmolarity oral rehydration solution for treating dehydrating diarrhea in children: systematic review. *BMJ*. 2001;323:81–85

22. World Health Organization. Reduced Osmolarity Oral Rehydration Salts (ORS) Formulation. New York, NY: UNICEF House; July 18, 2001. Report No. WHO/FCH/CAH/01.22. Available at: http://www.who.int/child-adolescent-health/New_Publications/NEWS/Expert_consultation.htm. Accessed November 2, 2007

23. Nalin DR, Hirschhorn N, Greenough W, Fuchs GJ, Cash RA. Clinical concerns about reduced-osmolarity oral rehydration solution. *JAMA*. 2004;291:2632–2635

24. Brown KH. Dietary management of acute childhood diarrhea: optimal timing of feeding and appropriate use of milks and mixed diets. *J Pediatr*. 1991;118:S92–S98

25. Brown KH. Appropriate diets for the rehabilitation of malnourished children in the community setting. *Acta Paediatr Scand*. 1991;374S:151–159

26. Brown KH, Peerson JM, Fontaine O. Use of non-human milks in the dietary management of young children with acute diarrhea: a meta-analysis of clinical trials. *Pediatrics*. 1994;93:17–27

V

Definitions

Metabolism may be defined as the sum of chemical processes through which food is converted into smaller molecules and energy. An inborn error of metabolism (IEM), therefore, may be defined as an inherited defect in the structure or function of a key protein in a metabolic pathway. These diseases involve processes of energy production; the anabolism and catabolism of fats, carbohydrates, or amino acids; the synthesis and degradation of complex macromolecules; the transport of substances across cell membranes; and the detoxification of cellular wastes. The spectrum of cardinal features, age of clinically apparent symptoms, morbidity, mortality, and types of currently used therapies vary widely across this diverse group of disorders.

Inheritance

Each IEM occurs only rarely, with population incidences ranging from 1:2500 births for hemochromatosis to only a few single case reports for other disorders. Collectively, the total incidence of IEMs in the population is approximately 1:1000 births. Many IEMs are known or considered to be autosomal-recessive diseases attributable to single-gene defects encoded by nuclear DNA. A few IEMs are inherited in an autosomal-dominant pattern, and a small proportion of IEMs are X-linked disorders, exhibiting a more severe phenotype in hemizygous males than in heterozygous females. Still other IEMs are caused by alterations in the mitochondrial DNA and are inherited only through a maternal lineage.

Newborn Screening

Although a few IEMs, such as fructokinase deficiency (essential fructosuria), do not cause any clinical disease, most cause organ dysfunction. With some disorders, signs and symptoms may not be present in the immediate neonatal period, although deleterious compounds are accumulating in the brain, other organs, and body fluids. Because recognition of the disease and early institution of therapy can significantly alter the morbidity and mortality of these initially occult disorders, screening methods have been developed. As of August 2006, all states require neonatal blood screening for phenylketonuria, hypothyroidism, galactosemia, and hemoglobinopathies.

Many states mandate additional screening for congenital adrenal hyperplasia, biotinidase deficiency, and a variety of other aminoacidopathies. Adaptation of tandem mass spectrometry for mass population testing has allowed a major expansion of the screening repertoire to include a range of fatty acid oxidation disorders and organic acidemias. A recent report from the American College of Medical Genetics advocates for a nationwide uniform screening panel to include tandem mass spectrometry,[1] but this ideal not yet been reached. The National Newborn Screening Resource Center (http://genes-r-us.uthscsa.edu) maintains an up-to-date database listing the disorders for which individual states perform screening. The American Academy of Pediatrics has published a policy statement containing newborn screening fact sheets.[2] Key elements to a successful screening program are rapid transit of specimens to the newborn screening laboratory, timely specimen testing and identification of abnormal results, notification of health care professionals, follow-up with a definitive confirmatory assay, and the initiation of effective treatment to be conducted in consultation with a multidisciplinary center specializing in IEM therapy. Patients with abnormal results, especially when the disease in question may have acute manifestations, should be referred promptly to a metabolic disease center that can further evaluate the potential disorder. If the patient is at risk of acute or severe illness, immediate consultation with a metabolic specialist by telephone for diagnosis and treatment options is advised. Precise and early diagnosis is essential so effective therapies are instituted safely and the family receives proper counseling.

Signs and Symptoms of an IEM

Inborn errors of metabolism should be suspected whenever a newborn infant has an acute catastrophic illness after a period of normal behavior and feeding or when a child of any age has unexplained lethargy or coma, recurrent seizures, persistent or recurrent vomiting, jaundice, failure to thrive, unusual body odor, developmental delay, hyperammonemia, hypoglycemia, metabolic acidosis, or a family history of recurrent illness or unexplained deaths in siblings. The steps and timing of the evaluation are tempered in part by the acuity of the problem and by the presentation. Algorithms for evaluation of patients with these signs and symptoms have been published.[3,4] If an IEM is suspected, early consultation with a metabolic specialist for advice regarding the appropriate diagnostic evaluation is advised.

Emergency Therapy for a Suspected IEM

Once an IEM is diagnosed, or in the case of infants in an acutely decompensated state, as soon as the suspicion of such a disorder occurs, therapy should be instituted. After appropriate blood, urine, and cerebrospinal fluid samples have been obtained for diagnostic evaluation, but before a definitive diagnosis is made, immediate nonspecific therapy should include restriction of dietary protein and fat intake with vigorous administration of intravenous fluids containing dextrose. Although this initial approach is not ideal for every known IEM, it is appropriate for the most common IEMs, which are usually the result of urea cycle defects or abnormalities of amino, organic, or fatty acid metabolism. The key to acute nonspecific therapy is the reversal of catabolism and the promotion of anabolism. Intravenous fluids should contain at least 10% dextrose and appropriate electrolytes and be given at 1.5 to 2 times the usual maintenance rate to provide calories and to promote urinary excretion of toxic metabolites. Severe acidosis (pH <7.1) should be treated with sodium bicarbonate infusion. Hyperammonemia, if not immediately responsive to intravenous fluid therapy and alternative pathway therapy, when appropriate, should be treated by hemodialysis. Insulin infusions have been used to prevent hyperglycemia when giving large amounts of glucose for metabolic decompensation in such disorders as maple sugar urine disease, disorders of fatty acid oxidation, and organic acidemias and may also promote anabolism.[5] Enteral feedings will also promote anabolism and may be given safely if the protein content is restricted to 0.5 gm/kg per day and the fat content is limited to less than 30% of total energy intake. Multivitamins should also be provided in this situation.

Once the diagnosis of a specific IEM has been made, therapy should be tailored to the specific disorder. Therapy for IEM is rapidly evolving, and metabolic specialists and contemporary medical literature should be consulted for new advances. Well-organized treatment guides for many IEMs have been published.[6] Therapy for any inherited metabolic disease is based on the pathophysiologic effects of the disease. For many IEMs attributable to a single enzyme defect, disease-associated abnormalities are caused by accumulation of an immediate or remote precursor of the impaired reaction. The accumulated substrate may have direct toxic effects or may secondarily impair other critical biochemical reactions. For instance, the accumulation of phenylalanine in phenylalanine hydroxylase deficiency is the primary cause of the pathologic changes associated with untreated phenylketonuria (PKU). For other disorders, symptoms may be caused by a deficiency of a critical reaction product. Finally, the substrate of the deficient reaction may be converted to an alternative product via little-used pathways. These secondary metabolites may, in themselves, be toxic. For example, succinylacetone, a product of alternative metabolism of fumarylacetoacetic acid, accumulates in the disease tyrosinemia type I, inhibits certain steps in heme synthesis, and causes symptoms mimicking porphyria. Disease-specific therapy may, therefore, include attempts to limit the accumulation of substrate, enhance the excretion of toxic substrate or secondary metabolites, restore the supply of an essential product, or inhibit alternative metabolism of the substrate. Other therapeutic approaches may include stabilization of the impaired enzyme to improve residual activity, replacement of deficient enzymatic cofactors, induction of enzyme production, enzyme replacement, or even correcting the defect at the level of the abnormal gene (gene therapy).

Nutritional Therapy Using Synthetic Medical Foods

Manipulation of precursors and limitation of substrates that lead to toxic metabolites form a major portion of the available therapies for many IEMs. Special diets have been devised to limit the amount of precursor nutrients, balancing the requirements for those nutrients to support appropriate growth and homeostasis with their potential toxicities. For some disorders, commercially available medical foods are the mainstay of diet therapy (see Table 29.1 and Appendix U, Table U-3). Medical foods are, by design, incomplete nutrition and should be used only under the supervision of a physician. In addition to the commercial synthetic diet components, low-protein foods available from several vendors are used to complete a nutritionally appropriate diet.

Education of the patient and family regarding the pathophysiology of and the dietary therapy for the disorder in question is essential. Families must be taught to measure and mix special medical food powders, prepare meals with special food products, and determine the protein or fat content and serving size of table foods. Systems of food exchanges based on protein and caloric content are useful in assisting families to provide a varied diet that is compliant with the required dietary restrictions. For some IEMs, families must also be taught to recognize the signs and symptoms of impending metabolic decompensation and to institute emergency procedures, including administration of a generally more restrictive "sick" diet (see next section). Education of the family and patient at regular intervals is a critical component to a successful therapy plan.

Table 29.1

Select IEMs Treated With Commercially Available Medical Foods

IEM	Modify or Restrict	Vitamin or Cofactor Responsive	Other Therapies
Phenylketonuria	Phenylalanine	10% of cases attributable to classic phenylalanine hydroxylase deficiency are responsive to biopterin supplementation	Supplemental tyrosine
Tyrosinemia type I	Phenylalanine, tyrosine, methionine	No	Nitisinone, a 4-hydroxyphenyl-pyruvate dioxygenase inhibitor
Tyrosinemia type II	Phenylalanine, tyrosine	No	
Maple syrup urine disease	Leucine, valine, isoleucine	Some cases are thiamine responsive	
Isovaleric acidemia	Leucine	No	Supplemental carnitine and glycine
Methylmalonic acidemia	Isoleucine, valine, methionine, threonine	Some cases attributable to defect in cobalamin metabolism	Supplemental carnitine
Propionic acidemia	Isoleucine, valine, methionine, threonine	Possible role for biotin	Supplemental carnitine
Homocystinuria	Methionine	50% pyridoxine responsive	Supplemental folate, betaine
Defects of cobalamin (vitamin B_{12}) processing (methylmalonic acidemia and/or homocystinuria)	Isoleucine, valine, methionine, threonine	Hydroxycobalamin intramuscular injections	Supplemental carnitine, folate, or betaine
Ornithine transcarbamylase deficiency	Protein	No	Supplemental citrulline, benzoate, phenylacetate, phenylbutyrate
Citrullinemia	Protein	No	Supplemental arginine, benzoate, phenylacetate, phenylbutyrate
Argininosuccinic aciduria	Protein	No	Supplemental arginine, benzoate, phenylacetate, phenylbutyrate
Glutaric aciduria type I	Lysine, tryptophan	Possible role for riboflavin	Supplemental carnitine

V

Other Nutritional Therapies

Some IEMs are or may be vitamin or cofactor responsive. Cofactor supplementation may be an adjunct to therapy with medical foods for some of the IEMs listed in Table 29.1. For other IEMs, cofactor administration may be the mainstay of treatment. Cofactor responsiveness can be determined empirically through controlled trials of vitamin supplementation with monitoring of laboratory studies and clinical response. For some IEMs, such as maple syrup urine disease, cofactor dependency may be assessed through in vitro assays of enzyme function in the presence and absence of cofactor. The goal of cofactor therapy may be to stabilize a poorly functional enzyme, to overcome a block in cofactor binding, or to correct a block in cofactor metabolism that results in secondary metabolic derangement.

Therapy for other select IEMs is presented in Table 29.2. The treatment of several of these IEMs is based on dietary avoidance of substrate, but for these disorders, dietary supplement with a synthetic medical food is not required. For instance, the treatment of galactosemia includes avoidance of dietary galactose, which is primarily found as lactose (milk sugar) in dairy products. In infancy, this dietary restriction is easy to accomplish, because the affected infant may be fed lactose-free or soy-based formula. As the child ages, however, avoidance of dairy products, especially in baked goods and processed foods, is more difficult. Parents and patients must be taught to read food labels and to contact manufacturers of prepared foods to determine whether foodstuffs contain galactose. They should assume that all new foods contain galactose until proven otherwise and should be encouraged to seek other hidden sources of galactose in over-the-counter and prescription medications.

Fructose ingestion must be strictly avoided by individuals with either hereditary fructose intolerance or fructose 1,6-bisphosphatase deficiency. Ingestion of fruit, fruit juices, or any food product sweetened with a fructose-containing sweetener (eg, high-fructose corn syrup in baked goods and soda) can trigger potentially life-threatening episodes of abdominal pain, vomiting, metabolic acidosis, and electrolyte disturbance. Individuals with fructose 1,6-bisphosphatase deficiency are also intolerant of fasting, because this enzyme participates in gluconeogenesis. In mannose phosphate isomerase deficiency (congenital disorder of glycosylation type 1b), a rare disease that impairs glycosylation of cellular proteins and lipids, potentially fatal liver dysfunction is completely prevented by addition of mannose to the diet.

Table 29.2
Therapy of Other Select IEMs

IEM	Modify or Restrict	Vitamin or Cofactor Responsive	Other Therapies
Biotinidase	None	Biotin	
Familial hypophos-phatemic rickets	None	1,25-dihydroxyvitamin D	Phosphorus
Acrodermatitis entero-pathica	None	Zinc	
Pyruvate dehydroge-nase deficiency	Low-carbohydrate, high-fat diet	Possibly thiamine responsive	Alkali therapy
Galactosemia (trans-ferase deficiency)	Galactose, lactose		Lactose-free infant formula
Glycogen storage diseases	Lactose, fructose, sucrose		Frequent feedings, complex starches, high-protein diet
Fructosemia (fructose-1,6-bisphosphatase or aldolase deficiency)	Fructose		Frequent glucose feedings in bisphos-phatase deficiency
Congenital disorder of glycosylation type 1b (mannose phosphate isomerase deficiency)			Mannose supplementation
Medium-chain acyl-CoA dehydrogenase deficiency			Avoid fasting; supplemental carnitine
Long-chain fatty acid oxidation disorders	Dietary long-chain fatty acids		Avoid fasting; supple-ment with medium-chain triglyceride oil and carnitine
Barth syndrome (X-linked 3-methyl-glutaconic aciduria)	None	Pantothenic acid	
Cystinosis	None	None	Cysteamine, phos-phate, potassium, vitamin D, alkali
Methylene tetrahy-drofolate reductase deficiency	None	Folate	Pyridoxine
Alcaptonuria	None	Vitamin C	
Pyridoxine-responsive seizures	None	Pyridoxine	
Cerebral folate deficiency	None	Folinic acid	

V

Table 29.2 *(Continued)*
Therapy of Other Select IEMs

IEM	Modify or Restrict	Vitamin or Cofactor Responsive	Other Therapies
Creatine synthesis disorders		Creatine	
Thiamine-responsive megaloblastic anemia syndrome	None	Thiamine	

In type 1 glycogen storage disease, glycogenolysis during fasting is impaired, because glucose-6-phosphate cannot be converted to glucose. Consumption of nonglucose carbohydrates (fructose, galactose) leads to excessive glycogen storage or shunting down alternative pathways to form lactate, uric acid, or triglycerides. Frequent feedings during infancy, overnight enteral tube feedings, and after 1 year of age, the administration of uncooked cornstarch as a slowly released source of glucose, are key to the prevention of hypoglycemia and preservation of liver function. In the other forms of glucose-6-phosphate deficiency involving the liver, gluconeogenesis is intact. Amino acids can serve as precursors for endogenous glucose production, and a high-protein diet (3 g/kg per day) is recommended.

In medium-chain acyl-coenzyme A (CoA) dehydrogenase deficiency, the most common disorder of fatty acid oxidation, prevention of fasting eliminates the body's need to metabolize fat for energy, reduces the accumulation of toxic partially oxidized fatty acids, and reduces the risk of hypoglycemia. Infants with disorders of long-chain fatty acid oxidation, such as very long-chain acyl-CoA dehydrogenase deficiency or long-chain 3-hydroxyacyl-CoA dehydrogenase deficiency, and others are more sensitive to fasting, with associated hypoglycemia, metabolic acidosis, liver dysfunction, or cardiomyopathy. Dietary long-chain fatty acid intake must be restricted; supplementation with medium-chain triglyceride oil provides a fuel source that bypasses the block in fatty acid oxidation.

Prevention of micronutrient deficiencies is another important aspect of nutritional therapy for IEMs. These deficiencies may be direct effects of certain IEMs or may be a consequence of dietary restrictions. For instance, the elimination of dairy products in low-protein diets or in the therapy of galactosemia increases the risk of calcium deficiency and osteoporosis. The lack of meat in low-protein diets also raises the risk of iron-deficiency anemia and vitamin B_{12} deficiency. Zinc and selenium deficiencies are also potential problems in organic acidemias. Severe dietary fat restriction for disorders of fatty acid metabolism or the administration of nutritionally incomplete synthetic medical foods may lead to deficiencies of essential polyunsaturated fatty acids. Multivitamin preparations with minerals should be prescribed to all patients on altered diets who are not receiving most of their nutrition from vitamin-fortified medical foods. All patients on nutritional therapy must be periodically assessed for micronutrient deficiencies.

The successful implementation of a satisfactory diet during a period of relative health does not ensure that the diet is appropriate during periods of metabolic decompensation. Further restriction or even elimination of protein intake and increasing energy intake from other sources are used in many of the organic acidemias and aminoacidemias during minor illnesses. Such manipulations are designed to compensate for the metabolic stress of illness with the attendant increased energy demands and propensity for muscle catabolism leading to an increased endogenous protein load. Families must be encouraged to contact health care professionals during these minor illnesses, because the additionally restricted diet is nutritionally incomplete and may not be adequate to prevent further metabolic derangement. Illnesses that would normally be manageable at home in typical children may trigger the need for hospitalization in patients with an IEM. Intravenous hydration, nutrition, and in some IEMs, administration of special medications play major roles in correcting the acutely decompensated state.

Other Therapeutic Modalities

Nutritional therapy, although important, is only one modality used for many of the IEMs. Pharmacologic agents, such as alkali to reduce metabolic acidosis, sodium benzoate and phenylacetate to provide alternative metabolic sinks and to enhance alternative pathways for ammonia excretion in urea cycle disorders, vitamin D and phosphorus supplementation in hypophosphatemic rickets, and cysteamine to enhance cellular cystine release in the lysosomal storage disease cystinosis, form another class of therapies. Ascorbic acid (vitamin C) administration greatly reduces the potential for degenerative arthritis in alcaptonuria. Folate and pyridoxine supplementation have been shown to reduce blood homocysteine concentrations and, probably, cardiovascular disease risk in individuals with deficiency of methylene tetrahydrofolate reductase. A rare form of congenital megaloblastic anemia is completely corrected with thiamine supplementation. Treatment with pyridoxine or folinic acid is critical to the prevention of convulsions in pyridoxine-responsive seizure disorder or cerebral folate deficiency, respectively. Rare disorders of creatine synthesis present with seizures and abnormal involuntary movements; creatine supplementation may improve the symptoms drastically.

For a few disorders, enzyme replacement therapies are available. In cystic fibrosis, exogenous digestive enzymes are given as enteral supplements to replace the deficient secretion of the exocrine pancreas. In Gaucher disease, a lysosomal storage disorder, repetitive intravenous infusions of purified enzyme are used to gradually reduce the amount of stored glucocerebroside, reversing some of the pathophysiologic changes and improving the quality of life. Similar enzyme replacement strategies are now clinically available or are under development for a variety of lysosomal storage disorder, including Pompe disease, Fabry disease, and several mucopolysaccharidoses.

Organ transplantation has been attempted in several IEMs. The most commonly transplanted organs are bone marrow and liver. Bone marrow or stem cell transplantation has been employed in many lysosomal storage disorders, such as the mucopolysaccharidoses, in attempts to provide tissue that is capable of metabolizing the stored material. The efficacy of this therapy is highest when the procedure is carried out in young children (typically younger than 2 years, even better in infancy) in disorders associated with accumulation of storage material in brain because of the inability to populate the central nervous system with enzyme-producing cells derived from the bone marrow graft. Liver transplantation has been performed in tyrosinemia type I to prevent hepatocellular carcinoma, a known complication of the disease, and to correct the primary defect. With the use of nitisinone, liver transplantation is now required only for a small minority of patients with tyrosinemia, although long-term (lifelong) monitoring for hepatocellular carcinoma is recommended. Recent evidence suggests that by 10 years of age, less than 5% of children placed on nitisinone before 2 years of age will develop hepatocellular carcinoma.[7] Liver transplantation has also been used to successfully cure urea cycle disorders and maple syrup urine disease. Thus, a successful graft may have a profound effect on the health of an individual with an IEM. The infusion of hepatocytes into the portal vein for engraftment into the liver may also hold promise as a treatment for ornithine transcarbamylase deficiency and other IEMs.

Permanent replacement of the mutant gene with the correct DNA sequence in the somatic cells of an individual with an IEM is a very attractive potential treatment modality for the future. Several research centers around the world are actively investigating gene therapy as a treatment for a wide variety of IEMs. Using contemporary DNA transfer methods, achieving stable, physiologically significant gene expression continues to be the major limiting factor in clinical gene therapy trials. Issues of treatment toxicity using certain gene transfer technologies have also slowed the progress of moving gene therapy from the laboratory to the clinical bedside. However, recent limited success using gene therapy to treat hemophilia and severe combined immunodeficiency in humans has provided renewed promise that gene therapy may be a viable treatment option for IEMs in the future.

Conclusion

Regardless of the specific therapy plan, successful treatment of IEMs requires a multidisciplinary approach to include the expertise of the metabolic physician, clinic nurse, nutritionist, genetic counselor, and social worker backed up by a full complement of medical specialists and ancillary services. Education of the family, genetic counseling, and family support are all essential components. Genetic counseling teaches the family about the risks associated with future offspring and demystifies the concepts of defective genes being passed from asymptomatic carrier to affected child. The availability and implications of prenatal diagnosis for IEMs are also explained. Heterozygote detection and the ethical issues of sharing that information within a family or with future mates are other issues that may be addressed by counseling. Support for the family should ensure the availability of coping mechanisms for dealing with a member who may have significant restrictions in developmental capacity or who has extraordinary needs for care. Educational goals include the successful implementation of the diet and the need for immediate intervention during metabolic crises.

Nutritional therapies will continue to be the cornerstone of the treatment for most IEMs in the foreseeable future. The lessons learned with several IEMs, especially PKU, emphasize the need for lifelong therapy in all these disorders. The necessity of "diet for life" has recently been affirmed by a National Institutes of Health consensus development conference on the treatment of PKU.[8] This necessity, therefore, requires a long-term commitment from parents, patients, and health care professionals to implement and maintain appropriate dietary therapies. The needs of an individual for energy, protein, and cofactors change with age and body mass. Therapeutic diets must be established and reevaluated at regular intervals to allow for the most normal growth and development possible. The adequacy of nutritional therapy must be assessed periodically through combinations of diet diary review, food list recollection, anthropometric measurement, and laboratory testing. Cooperation of the patient, family, and the metabolic clinic as a dedicated team throughout the life of the patient is essential for successful treatment of an IEM.

> ## AAP
>
> ### American Academy of Pediatrics recommendations:
>
> It is the position of the American Academy of Pediatrics that special medical foods that are used in the treatment of amino acid and urea cycle disorders are medical expenses that should be reimbursed.
>
> *Pediatrics.* 2003;111:1117–1119 (Reaffirmed January 2006)

References

1. Watson MS, Mano MY, Lloyd-Puryear MA, Rinaldo P, Howell RR. Newborn screening: toward a uniform screening panel and system. *Genet Med.* 2006;8:1S–11S

2. Kaye CE, American Academy of Pediatrics, Committee on Genetics. Newborn screening fact sheets. *Pediatrics.* 2006;118(3):e934–e963. Available at: http://aappolicy.aappublications.org/cgi/content/full/pediatrics;118/3/e934. Accessed September 14, 2007

3. Saudubray J, Charpentier C. Clinical phenotypes: diagnosis/algorithms. In: Scriver CR, Beaudet AL, Sly WS, Valle D, eds. *The Metabolic & Molecular Bases of Inherited Disease.* Vol 1. 8th ed. New York, NY: McGraw-Hill, 2001:1327–1406

4. Gilbert-Barness E, Barness LA. Approach to diagnosis of metabolic diseases. In: Metabolic Disease. Foundations of Clinical Management, Genetics, and Pathology. Vol I. Natick, MA: Eaton Publishing, 2000:1–14

5. Prietsch V, Linder M, Zschocke J, Nyhan WL, Hoffmann GF. Emergency management of inherited metabolic diseases. *J Inherit Metab Dis.* 2002;25:531–546

6. Blau N, Hoffman GF, Leonard J, Clarke JTR, eds. Physician's Guide to the Treatment and Follow-Up of Metabolic Diseases. Berlin, Germany: Springer-Verlag; 2006

7. Scott CR. The genetic tyrosinemias. *Am J Med Genet C Semin Med Genet.* 2006;142:121–126

8. National Institutes of Health, Consensus Development Conference on Phenylketonuria. Phenylketonuria (PKU): screening and management. *NIH Consens Statement.* 2000;17:1–27

Type 1 Diabetes Mellitus

Introduction

Type 1 diabetes mellitus is a disorder caused by autoimmune destruction of beta cells resulting in hyperglycemia and, with complete absence of insulin, ketoacidosis. Treatment consists of insulin administration, diet, exercise, and blood glucose monitoring, which is essential to maintaining near-normal glycemia. Teaching the patient to adjust all the components of the diabetes regimen is essential to attainment and maintenance of good metabolic control. It is recommended that children with diabetes who are receiving fixed doses of insulin eat at consistent times to coincide with peak action of the insulin preparation used and to adjust insulin doses on the basis of food intake, physical activity, and blood glucose concentrations. Children using the insulin pump or basal-bolus regimens using the long-acting basal insulin preparations (glargine, detemir) have more flexibility in timing of meals, because there are no significant peaks in the basal insulins. The Diabetes Control and Complications Trial (DCCT), a 5- to 9-year prospective, randomized multicenter trial of 1441 patients with type 1 diabetes mellitus, found that a combination of intensive therapy, defined as 3 or more insulin injections daily or the insulin pump; 4 or more blood glucose readings per day; frequent contact with the diabetes care team; and education in self-management was superior to conventional treatment (1–2 blood glucose tests daily, 1–2 insulin injections daily, quarterly clinic visits) in improving metabolic control. This improvement in metabolic control was associated with reduced onset and progression of microvascular disease.[1] Patients were predominantly young adults, but children 13 years and older were included. Because the study conclusively showed that any improvement in glycemic control conferred a reduced risk of retinopathy and nephropathy, pediatric endocrinologists have intensified the care of children with diabetes to improve metabolic control. Subsequently, the United Kingdom Prospective Diabetes Study of more than 5000 patients with type 2 diabetes mellitus followed prospectively for up to 16 years showed that normalizing blood pressure and serum lipid concentrations also reduced the risk of both microvascular and macrovascular disease.[2-4] The Epidemiology of Diabetes Intervention and Complications study was initiated in 1994 to continue observation of the participants of the DCCT. More than 90% of the original

DCCT participants have maintained involvement in the subsequent study, which has demonstrated that the benefits of improved control during the DCCT study persisted for the 9 years of follow-up, even though the hemoglobin (Hb)A1c values of the 2 groups converged by 1 year after discontinuation of the DCCT.[5,6]

Metabolic control is monitored by HbA1c concentrations, a measure of average glycemia over a 2- to 3-month period of time, and home blood glucose monitoring. It is important to remember, however, that widely fluctuating blood sugar concentrations may result in reasonable HbA1c values but are not indicative of good metabolic control. Also, a rapid turnover of red blood cells can result in misleadingly low HbA1c concentrations. Erratic glucose values most often indicate inconsistent timing and amount of food, inconsistent insulin coverage for meals, or lack of blood glucose monitoring to allow for determination of insulin dose.

In addition, weight and blood pressure should be checked every 3 months and hypertension should be treated aggressively. Treatment of prehypertension in children with diabetes should include dietary intervention. If the child is overweight, dietary intervention should also include strategies for weight control.[7]

Lipid concentrations and renal status should be assessed annually; persistent microalbuminuria and hyperlipidemia require treatment and close monitoring.

Insulin

In an individual without diabetes, insulin is secreted into the portal vein in a continuous low-dose basal pattern to inhibit hepatic gluconeogenesis with a 7- to 10-fold increased amount secreted in response to meals. Insulin regimens have attempted to duplicate these patterns with the use of insulin analogues. By substituting amino acids on the beta chain of the insulin molecule, these insulin analogues have a more rapid onset (15–30 minutes) and shorter duration of action (2–4 hours) than the previous short-acting regular insulin and are designed to time the action of each insulin dose to cover the expected increase in blood glucose after ingestion of food.[8] Attempts to mimic basal and postprandial physiologic insulin secretion are made by various combinations of the aforementioned insulin analogues. However, not all children are able or willing to check blood glucose concentrations, calculate insulin doses before meals, and give insulin injections before every meal. These children are usually treated with a short-acting insulin and the intermediate-acting isophane insulin suspension (neutral protamine Hagedorn

[NPH]) to provide coverage throughout the day. Because a single daily injection is inadequate to cover glucose excursions with the normal pattern of meals and snacks, children taking NPH insulin receive 2, 3, or more daily insulin injections, with variable amounts of an insulin analogue and/or regular insulin mixed with the NPH before breakfast and, commonly, before dinner as well. Many children are also taking short-acting insulins before lunch or before mid-afternoon snacks and many are splitting their evening dose with short-acting insulin given before dinner and an intermediate-acting insulin given before bed. Studies have shown that there is a reduced risk of nocturnal hypoglycemia if an insulin analogue rather than regular insulin is used for the evening injection.[9] The average daily insulin dose for prepubertal children is approximately 0.6 to 1.0 U/kg of body weight. Increased doses of up to 1.5 U/kg may be needed during puberty because of the insulin resistance caused by increased growth hormone concentrations present during that time. Higher reported insulin requirements together with inadequate glycemic control, especially if accompanied by weight loss, strongly suggest missed injections. Overeating, as evidenced by excessive weight gain, may be another cause of high insulin doses and poor metabolic control.

Insulin glargine and insulin detemir, long-lasting insulin analogues with minimal peak of action, have a duration of action of 24 hours in most children, although increasing numbers of children are requiring 2 daily doses, indicating a shorter-lived effect. Young children most often require 2 injections of the glargine/detemir insulin. They serve as basal insulins and can be given with short-acting insulin analogues injected before meals to cover the glycemic excursion of the meal. This regimen allows for flexibility in timing of meals and avoids the need for snacks. By obtaining blood glucose concentrations before and after injection of the rapid-acting insulin analogue, the insulin-to-carbohydrate ratio (number of units of insulin given for a given amount of carbohydrates) and insulin sensitivity (number of units of insulin required to adequately treat hyperglycemia) can be determined. This method of basal/bolus insulin treatment requires at least 4 injections of insulin daily and monitoring of blood glucose concentrations before all meals, thus requiring more diabetes management to be performed in the school setting. Increasing numbers of children are choosing to use this insulin regimen because of the increased flexibility in lifestyle it confers and ability to tailor administration to amount of food consumed.

Continuous subcutaneous infusion using an insulin pump is also becoming increasingly common in the pediatric age group. Children receiving insulin using an insulin pump base their meal insulin bolus on the amount of carbohydrates consumed as well as ambient blood glucose concentrations, using the insulin-to-carbohydrate ratio and insulin sensitivity as described above. Thus, the bolus is often given after the meal when the actual consumption of carbohydrates is known.

Nutrition Overview

The philosophical approach to the nutrition component of diabetes treatment in children has varied widely from the "free diet," in which intake is unrestricted except for avoidance of foods rich in concentrated sweets or refined sugars, to a system in which all food is measured. The overriding principle, however, is that children with diabetes should eat the same nutritious food that the entire family should eat.

The overall goals of dietary treatment for children with diabetes are the provision of adequate nutrition and balanced calories for (1) normal growth and development; (2) prevention of hyperglycemia and hypoglycemia; (3) achievement of optimal serum lipid concentrations; and (4) for youth with type 2 diabetes, facilitating changes in eating and physical activity habits that reduce insulin resistance and improve metabolic control.[10] The dietary management of diabetes is one of the most challenging aspects of the diabetes regimen for both patients and physicians. Teaching dietary principles and meal planning is an important part of the education and ongoing care of a child with diabetes and is essential for effective home management.

Optimal glycemic control is achieved only if patients and their families can adequately balance food, insulin, and physical activity. Consistent timing, portion sizes, and relative content of food are important for good glycemic control in patients using NPH insulin. The DCCT identified key nutritional behaviors that are associated with significantly improved blood glucose control. These behaviors include adherence to the recommended meal and snack plan, adjustment of insulin dose in response to meal size, adjustment of food or insulin in response to hyperglycemia, and avoidance of overtreatment of hypoglycemia.[11–13] Nutrition counseling, therefore, should emphasize these effective behaviors.

A team consisting of physicians, nurse educators, dietitians, and mental health professionals is optimal for effective disease management. Although not all children require the services of a mental health professional, psychological counseling is invaluable for dealing with children who are having difficulty coping with their disease or families that require behavior modification. Nutrition education of the child and family should be provided by a registered dietitian trained and experienced in childhood diabetes. As with all health care professionals involved in the care of this age group, dietitians must also be able to implement goal plans based on the behavioral, emotional, and psychological factors that interfere with the individual's and/or family's ability to resolve problems.[7]

The dietitian must perform a thorough initial assessment of the nutritional needs of the child and the family to provide adequate nutrition education. This assessment includes the pattern of growth plotted on a standard growth curve, body mass index (BMI), and pattern of activity and food intake including meals and snacks.[14]

The family's living style and pattern of eating should be considered, and, as far as possible, a schedule of meals and snacks should be created to fit the child's usual times of eating and pattern of activity. In addition, the meal plans should take into account food preferences on the basis of the family's ethnicity, religious beliefs, vegetarian eating habits, etc. After diagnosis, several sessions with the dietitian are usually needed for a full nutritional assessment, basic nutrition education, setting goals, and teaching the skills the family will need to plan appropriate meals and snacks. In addition, continued follow-up visits with a thorough review of dietary intake should occur annually and when there is:

- Unexplained failure to grow;
- Unexplained recurrent hypoglycemia;
- Unexplained recurrent hyperglycemia;
- Excessive weight gain or loss;
- Elevated glycohemoglobin concentration;
- Hypertension;
- Hyperlipidemia;
- Nephropathy; or
- Pregnancy or lactation.

Meal Plans

To allow for changes in growth rate, activity, and development of different food preferences, the meal plans and patient's nutritional knowledge should be reviewed at least twice a year.[12] At each visit, growth increments in height and weight should be plotted on the appropriate standard curves.

The percentages of calories from fat, protein, and carbohydrate recommended for the diabetic meal plan differ from those currently found in the average American diet,[15-17] which tends to be higher in total fat than recommended. The 2001 American Diabetes Association position statement for nutrition recommendations provides dietary guidelines for people with diabetes.[18] Fat should provide up to 30% of the total calories with no more than one third as saturated fat. A protein intake of 10% to 20% of the total calories is recommended. Carbohydrates should contribute the remaining 50% of the total calories; the majority should be provided by sugars, starch, and fiber. These guidelines promote a healthy diet and are identical to those recommended for the population as a whole.[19] Nutrition guidelines are provided in Table 30.1.

Table 30.1
Nutrition Guidelines

Calories
The caloric needs of the patient should be sufficient to attain and/or maintain a reasonable body weight to support normal growth and development for children and adolescents.
Estimating Needs for Calories in Youth

1. Base calories on nutrition assessment
2. Validate calorie needs
  • Method 1: National Academy of Sciences/Recommended Dietary Allowance (RDA) guidelines
  • Method 2: 1000 kcal for first y
    – Toddlers 1–3 y of age, 40 kcal/in of body length
    – Add 100 kcal/y up to age 11
    – Girls 11–15 y, add 100 kcal or less/y after age 10
    – Girls >15 y, calculate as an adult
    – Boys 11–15 y, add 200 kcal/y after age 10
    – Boys >15 y, 23 kcal/lb very active
  • 18 kcal/lb usual
  • 16 kcal/lb sedentary
  • Method 3: 1000 kcal for first y
    – Add 125 kcal × age for boys
    – Add 100 kcal × age for girls
    – Up 20% more kcal for activity

Protein
10%–20% of kcal. Should not exceed the RDA (0.8 g of high-quality protein/kg of body weight per day for all children of all ages.)[20]

Table 30.1 *(Continued)*
Nutrition Guidelines

Fat
Saturated fat <10% of daily kcal, <7% with elevated LDL.
Polyunsaturated fat up to 10% of total kcal.
Remaining total fat varies with treatment goals.
30% for normal lipids.
<Step 2 American Heart Association diet if elevated LDL cholesterol.
Predominately monounsaturated fat.
Cholesterol <300 mg/day.

Carbohydrate
Difference after protein and fat goals have been met.
Percentages varies with treatment goals.

Sweeteners
Sucrose need not be restricted and must be counted in the meal plan as carbohydrate.
Nutritive sweeteners have no advantage over sucrose and must be substituted as carbohydrate.
Nonnutritive sweeteners approved by the Food and Drug Administration include saccharin, aspartame, acesulfame potassium, sucralose.

Fiber
20–35 g/day

Sodium
<3000 mg/day
<2400 mg/day with mild to moderate hypertension

Vitamins/Minerals
Same as general population

Adapted from American Diabetes Association. *Maximizing the Role of Nutrition in Diabetes Management.* Alexandria, VA: American Diabetes Association; 1994

Low-carbohydrate diets are not recommended for children with diabetes. The American Diabetes Association, in agreement with the National Academy of Sciences Food and Nutrition Board, recommends a minimum daily carbohydrate intake of 130 grams for children older than 1 year. This is the absolute glucose requirement for normal functioning of the brain and nervous system. The ideal caloric percentages of protein, carbohydrate, and fat may vary depending on individual circumstances.[20]

In school, snacks should be provided to cover the peak action of insulin and vigorous activities, such as physical education. The older child may manage without a morning snack as long as the lunch break is not late. A less-active older child may not need an afternoon snack if dinner is relatively early. More dietary flexibility is gained with basal/bolus insulin regimens using the newer insulin analogues.

All children with diabetes require assistance in managing their blood glucose at school and child care settings, with older children largely independent in their diabetes care and elementary students dependent on their school nurse and, perhaps, other school personnel to supervise blood glucose monitoring, insulin administration, and treatment of hypoglycemia. Two guides that should be reviewed by families and school administration are:

- American Diabetes Association. The care of children with diabetes in the school and day care setting. *Diabetes Care.* 2005;28:S43–S49; and

- National Diabetes Education Program. *Helping the Student with Diabetes Succeed: A Guide for School Personnel.* Bethesda, MD: National Diabetes Education Program; 2003. Available at: www.ndep.nih.gov.

Medical Nutrition Therapy Education

The approach to nutrition education is dependent on the education level and motivation of the family. Other factors that need consideration when designing the meal plan are school routines, weekend routines, who does the food shopping, who takes care of the child after school, and whether the family has any formal education in nutrition. Basic nutrition education focuses on providing basic information and goal setting in a manner that is simple, easy to understand, and adaptable to individual needs. Several excellent publications can help in this endeavor (Table 30.2).

Table 30.2
Resources for Nutrition Education and Intervention

General Diabetes Nutrition Information
The following recently updated pamphlets and booklets are available from the American Diabetes Association (http://store.diabetes.org) or the American Dietetic Association (www.eatright.org): • *Basic Carbohydrate Counting* • *Advanced Carbohydrate Counting* • *Exchange Lists for Meal Planning* • *The First Step in Meal Planning* • *Eating Healthy With Diabetes* • *Healthy Food Choices*

Table 30.2 *(Continued)*
Resources for Nutrition Education and Intervention

Diabetes Education Resources for Health Care Professionals

- *Pediatric Diabetes* (journal from the International Society for Pediatric and Adolescent Diabetes)
- American Dietetic Association: 26 different diabetes nutrition and diabetes education handouts on CD-ROM with accompanying tips and resources for the health care professional on each topic. Handouts written at the sixth-grade level. Available at www.eatright.org.

Nutrition Information for Children With Type 2 Diabetes or Prediabetes

- *Eating Healthy Rocks*, published by the International Diabetes Center (www.internationaldiabetescenter.org)
- *Helping Your Overweight Child and Take Charge of Your Health! A Teenager's Guide to Better Health*, published by the Weight Control Information Network (WIN), a service of the National Institute of Diabetes and Digestive and Kidney Diseases. The WIN assembles and disseminates to health care professionals and the general public information on weight control, obesity, and nutritional disorders (www.niddk.nih.gov/health/nutrit/nutrit.htm).
- New Tip Sheet Series for Kids With Type 2 Diabetes and Their Families, from the National Diabetes Education Program's Diabetes in Children and Adolescents Work Group. Six fact sheets: "Eat Healthy Foods," "Stay at a Healthy Weight," "Be Active," "What Is Diabetes?" "Lower Your Risk for Type 2 Diabetes," and "Ups and Downs of Diabetes." The facts sheets focus on key components of a personal diabetes plan. Written at the sixth-grade reading level and field-tested with a variety of ethnic groups, they are bright, colorful, and geared toward school-aged children. Download at www.ndep.nih.gov or call to order tip sheets: 1-800-438-5383.

Education

General Nutrition: Dietary Guidelines for Americans
                    Guide to Good Eating
                    Food Guide Pyramid
National Institutes of Health/National Institute of Diabetes and Digestive and Kidney Diseases
Diabetes Nutrition: First Step in Diabetes Meal Planning
                    Healthy Food Choices
                    Healthy Eating
                    Single-Topic Diabetes Resources
American Diabetes Association (www.diabetes.org)
American Dietetic Association (www.eatright.org)

Medical Nutrition Therapy Intervention

Menu-based: Month of Meals 1, 2, 3, 4, and 5 (American Diabetes Association)
Exchange lists (American Diabetes Association, American Dietetic Association):
    Healthy Food Choices
    Exchange Lists for Meal Planning
Counting (American Diabetes Association, American Dietetic Association):
    Carbohydrate Counting Levels 1, 2, and 3
    Calorie Counting and Fat Gram Counting

V

Nutrition Intervention

Nutrition intervention is defined as offering structure to the process of meal planning with information on specific nutrition or calorie content. This allows for more individualized meal planning. There are 3 recommended approaches: menu based, exchange list, and carbohydrate counting.

Table 30.3

Four-Step Process of Medical Nutrition Therapy: Illustration of Carbohydrate Counting

Step 1	Assessment
	Calculate usual eating habits by evaluating 24-h recall and food history.
	Determine usual carbohydrate intake for each meal and snack.
	Evaluate other factors that may affect diabetes and nutritional health (eg, timing of meals, timing and amount of exercise, frequency and treatment of hypoglycemia, dining out.
	Assess readiness to change.
Step 2	**Goal setting**
	Determine the diet and lifestyle changes patient is willing to make.
	Determine clinical or metabolic outcomes (target HbA1c, fasting BG, target lipids).
Step 3	**Intervention**
	Level 1: Practice identifying carbohydrate foods.
	Recognize 15-g carbohydrate portion of foods.
	Demonstrate measuring skills using scale, cups, and spoons.
	Discuss plan for keeping protein consistent and fat intake low to moderate.
	Practice label-reading skills to obtain nutrition information.
	Plan a sample meal.
	Level 2: Practice reading food records, blood glucose readings, and physical activity log to interpret blood glucose patterns.
	Determine appropriate actions or strategies, including adjustment of carbo-hydrates to achieve blood glucose goals.
	Level 3: Calculate carbohydrate/insulin ratio by dividing the total grams of carbohy-drate usually consumed for each meal by the number of units of rapid-acting insulin analogue taken before that meal. (This is appropriate for patients being treated with insulin pumps or multiple daily injections.)
	Demonstrate how both carbohydrate intake and insulin can be adjusted to fine-tune blood glucose levels.
Step 4	**Evaluation**
	Assess effect of intervention by conducting process, outcome and impact evaluations. Continuously collect data on progress towards behavioral goals and changes in medical status (HbA1c, weight, blood pressure, lipids) risk factor reduction (decrease in hypoglycemia, increase in exercise).

Reprinted with permission from Maryniuk MD. *Medical Nutrition Therapy in Diabetes: Clinical Guidelines for Primary Care Physicians.* New York, NY: Dekker, 2000.

The exchange list offers a structure on which to base food choices for consistent caloric intake and quantities of carbohydrate, fat, and protein.[21] The foods in each of 6 food groups (ie, starch, fruit, vegetable, milk, meat, and fat) have relatively consistent amounts of carbohydrate, fat, and protein. This approach serves as an excellent educational tool.

Carbohydrate counting has received renewed attention since it was used in the DCCT trials. Patients enjoy the flexibility it provides and it has become the preferred nutrition intervention for determining insulin dosing at mealtimes. This simple approach focuses on determining the number of grams of carbohydrate in the diet (ie, starch, fruit, starchy vegetables, and milk).[22] The rationale for carbohydrate counting is that postprandial hyperglycemia is largely attributable to the amount of carbohydrate in a given meal. Meals containing more than the usual amount of carbohydrate can be covered by using extra insulin. For example, if a child is going to attend a class party and will eat more carbohydrate than usual, he or she could administer additional rapid-acting insulin to prevent postprandial hyperglycemia (Table 30.3).

When used in conjunction with postprandial blood glucose monitoring, carbohydrate counting offers patients more freedom to choose the type and amount of food they eat. If the postprandial readings are out of range, patients can choose to (1) increase the dose of insulin analogue for a given carbohydrate consumption, or (2) increase exercise. Carbohydrate counting does not take into account the protein and fat content of meals, making it easy to ignore good nutrition if only carbohydrate counting is emphasized during nutritional counseling. It is essential to discuss the importance of a healthy, well-balanced diet in any discussion of nutrition.

The Nutrition Facts label now available on packaged foods has made the carbohydrate counting approach to nutrition therapy more practical and allows the patient to have more flexibility in food choices. Because all carbohydrates are broken down to simple sugars, families are taught to ignore the sugar content per serving. Label reading should concentrate on serving size, calories, and total carbohydrates. "Sugar" is defined as the sum of all monosaccharides and disaccharides contained in a defined serving (glucose, fructose, lactose, and maltose) and added sucrose, high fructose, corn syrup, honey, and fruit-juice concentrate. Many times, patients and families will read the sugar content and not total carbohydrate and wonder why their blood sugars are so high after a meal. For example, Fritos (Frito Lay, Dallas, TX) have no "sugar" on the label but contain 29 g of carbohydrate in a serving. The expanded food choices available with carbohydrate counting eliminate the "forbidden food" philosophy of the past. However, serving sizes are very important. A cup of raisin bran cereal has 29 g of carbohydrate, whereas a cup of Cheerios (General Mills, Minneapolis, MN) has only 13 g. Both serving sizes are the same, but the carbohydrate content is quite different and will have an effect on postprandial blood sugar concentrations. Further, many of the packaged snack foods contain 2 or more servings; patients must be taught to look at numbers of servings as well as serving size.

Glycemic index refers to the degree blood glucose increases after ingestion of a single food. A number of factors influence glycemic responses to food, including the amount of carbohydrate, type of sugar (glucose, fructose, sucrose, lactose), nature of starch (amylase, amylopectin, resistant starch), cooking and food processing (degree of starch gelatinization, particle size, cellular form), food form, and other food components such as fat and natural substances that slow digestion (lectins, phytates, tannins, and starch-protein and starch-lipid combinations). Fasting and preprandial glucose concentrations, the severity of glucose intolerance, and second-meal or "lente" effect of carbohydrate are other factors affecting glycemic response to foods.

Studies in patients with both type 1 and type 2 diabetes mellitus indicate that ingestion of a variety of starches or sucrose, both acutely and for up to 6 weeks, produced no significant difference in glycemic response if the amount of carbohydrate was similar. Therefore, the total amount of carbohydrate in meals and snacks will be more important than the source.[11] The use of the glycemic index is controversial; classification of carbohydrates as "simple" or "complex" is of little use in predicting glycemic index, because foods are rarely eaten alone. The glycemic index is influenced by starch structure (amylose vs amylopectin), fiber content, food processing, physical structure of the food, and other macronutrients in the meal.[21,22] In a recent analysis of research on glycemic index, however, it has been shown that there may be a benefit in using this technique along with total carbohydrate consumed in evaluating the glycemic response of a meal or snack.[20] Researchers suggest that fat or protein in combination with carbohydrate reduces the postprandial glycemic increase because of delayed food absorption. Thus, although carbohydrates have different glycemic responses, the data reveal no clear benefits from low- versus high-glycemic-index diets consumed by individuals with diabetes. More research is needed in this area, because the number of studies is limited and results are conflicting.[10,11,23,24]

A more appropriate use of the glycemic index is assessing the individual response to specific carbohydrates using pre- and postprandial blood glucose measurements. Blood glucose testing before and 2 hours after a meal is essential in adjusting insulin dose and/or diet no mater what method of meal planning is used. This was confirmed by the Dose Adjusted for Normal Eating Study (DAFNE).[14]

Carbohydrate

For children receiving NPH insulin twice daily, carbohydrate intake should be distributed throughout the day, considering the child's pattern of activity. For example, a younger child might have a meal plan with 20% of carbohydrates given at breakfast, 20%, at lunch, 30% at dinner, and 10% for mid-morning, mid-afternoon, and bedtime snacks. Consistency in the timing and amount of ingested carbohydrate for each meal and snack allows for a more predictable glycemic response to injected insulin. Children using insulin pumps or basal/bolus insulin regimens have more flexibility in timing and content of meals, because the amount of rapid-acting insulin given immediately before a meal or snack is dependent on the carbohydrate content of that meal.

Once the family becomes comfortable knowing which foods contain carbohydrates and the effect of that particular food on the child's blood sugars, the multiple special events in a child's life (school picnics, birthday parties, eating outside the home, holidays) can proceed smoothly with adjustment of insulin dose to cover the extra carbohydrate intake. The more the family is able to determine how to maintain glycemic control by knowledge of how to match food choices with adjustments of insulin and activity, the less the child will be limited by diabetes.

Fat

Dietary fat intake requires attention because of the increased risk of cardiovascular disease in people with diabetes.[25,26] The United Kingdom Prospective Diabetes Study trial showed that a decrease in total cholesterol or low-density lipoprotein (LDL) of 1 mmol/L reduced the risk of any diabetes-related endpoint (myocardial infarction, angina, heart failure, stroke, renal failure, amputation, or retinopathy requiring photocoagulation) by 15% and 18% respectively. An increase in high-density lipoprotein of 0.1 mmol/L reduced the risk by 5%. The Bogalusa Heart Study, a long-term longitudinal study of individuals in a small county in Louisiana, found that 8% of children who died from an accident or violence between the ages of 2 and 15 years already have fibrous plaques in their coronary arteries, and 50% had fatty streaks in their coronary arteries. The atherosclerotic lesions correlated with triglyceride, LDL, and total cholesterol concentrations.[26] Thus, fat intake and lipid concentrations must be monitored throughout childhood. For infants and children younger than 2 years, dietary fat should not be restricted. For those older than 2 years, the guidelines from the pediatric panel of the National Cholesterol Education Program should be followed.

No more than 30% of total calories should come from fat and no more than 10% of that should be saturated fat. Monitoring of blood lipid concentrations should follow the American Diabetes Association guidelines, in which it is recommended that LDL be maintained at a concentration less than 100 mg/dl.[27] If LDL concentration is high, the diabetes regimen and dietary intake should be reevaluated. Inadequate metabolic control is the predominant cause of hyperlipidemia in type 1 diabetes mellitus. However, if attempts at dietary modification, increase in exercise, and intensification of the diabetes regimen fail to normalize serum lipid concentrations, pharmacologic therapy may be indicated. Autoimmune hypothyroidism occurs more commonly in children with diabetes and should be excluded as a cause of an elevated blood cholesterol concentration.

Protein

Protein consumption by Americans generally exceeds the recommended dietary allowance. Protein intake should be similar to that recommended for the general population (10%–20% of daily caloric intake). Lower intakes of protein should be considered in patients with overt nephropathy, because several small studies have shown that a protein diet of 0.7 g/kg per day slows the decrease in glomerular filtration rate. However, the Modified Diet in a Renal Disease study failed to show a benefit of protein restriction. Only a minority (3%) of patients in that study, however, had diabetes and none had type 1 diabetes mellitus.[28] Although there is a lack of clear-cut evidence on which to base a recommendation, the American Diabetes Association has issued a consensus recommendation that patients with nephropathy be prescribed a protein intake of 0.8 mg/kg per day. They further suggest that when the glomerular filtration rate begins to decrease, further restriction of protein to 0.6 mg/kg per day be initiated in selected patients.[29]

- Approximately 50% to 60% of dietary protein is converted to glucose and released into the bloodstream. This process occurs between 2 and 5 hours after the meal/snack.

- Protein-rich foods include meat, fish, poultry, eggs, peanut butter, cheese, and meat alternatives.

- A protein-rich food is recommended at lunch.

Sweeteners

Sucrose is the most widely used sweetener, but its use had been limited in children with diabetes because of concern it would cause elevated blood glucose concentrations. Recent studies, however, do not show an adverse effect of usual amounts of dietary sucrose on glycemic control in type 1 or type 2 diabetes mellitus.[30] Sucrose is present in many prepared foods and must be counted in the tally of carbohydrates. The nutritive sweeteners, fructose, and other sugars have no significant advantage over sucrose. Recent data suggests that high fructose intake may adversely affect the lipid profile. Sorbitol and other sugar alcohols have lower glycemic response than sucrose but may have a laxative effect when large amounts are ingested. Sugar alcohols may be indicated on the food label as a specific sugar alcohol or as a generic "sugar alcohol." They provide approximately 2 kcal/g, or about half the amount of calories provided by sucrose. The carbohydrate content of foods that contain sugar alcohols can be calculated by subtracting one half of the sugar alcohol grams from the total carbohydrate grams.[20]

The nonnutritive sweeteners, aspartame, saccharine, and acesulfame potassium, do not affect blood glucose concentrations and are acceptable alternatives for children with diabetes.

Fiber

The addition of fiber to reduce the glycemic effect of food does not appear to be significant enough to recommend intake beyond that recommended for the general population. The average daily fiber intake among children ranges from 11.2 g (3–5 years old) to 14.0 g (6–11 years old). These levels have remained unchanged since 1976. The most recent recommendation from the Food and Nutrition Board of the National Institutes of Medicine (www.nap.edu) for total fiber intake (the Adequate Intake) is 19 g/day for children 1 to 3 years of age, 25 g/day for children 4 to 8 years of age, and 26 to 38 g/day for boys and girls 9 to 18 years of age (see also Chapter 15: Carbohydrate and Dietary Fiber and Appendix J, Table J-1: Dietary Reference Intakes). Adequate dietary fiber intake may be achieved by increasing consumption of fruits, vegetables, cereal, and other whole-grain products. On a Nutrition Facts food label, the grams of fiber are included in the total grams of carbohydrate. On a practical basis, only cereals containing 5 g or more of insoluble fiber per serving need to have fiber grams subtracted from the total carbohydrates.[31]

Sugar alcohols are also included in the total grams of carbohydrate on the Nutrition Facts panel. Sugar alcohols are calculated as having half the calories (2 kcal/g) of most other carbohydrates (4 kcal/g). Specific sugar alcohol values approved by the Food and Drug Administration include:

- Hydrogenated starch hydrolysate: 3 g
- Isomalt: 2 g
- Maltitol: 3 g
- Mannitol: 1.6 g
- Sorbitol: 2.6 g
- Xylitol: 2.4 g

Exercise
Children with diabetes are encouraged to exercise regularly. However, to avoid hypoglycemia, families must be taught to monitor blood glucose concentrations before exercise and to give appropriate snacks on the basis of blood glucose value and intensity of exercise (Table 30.4).

Different Stages for Different Phases
The age and developmental stage of the child should be considered when determining which meal plan to use. It is much easier to design the insulin regimen around the patient's typical lifestyle than it is to change behaviors to match the insulin. Children in elementary school are more likely to have predictable lifestyles, whereas middle- and high-school adolescents will not. Most pediatric diabetes educators prefer to start with a structured meal plan and later teach a more flexible approach that is dependent on active decision making. Continuous assessment with frequent contact should be made. Changes in growth and development, school routines, seasonal sports, and child care arrangements may necessitate a change in meal plans.

Preschool children often have inconsistent food intake and activity. If the child has eaten poorly or activity is prolonged, small snacks may be offered. Food battles should be avoided, and parents may need assistance in developing the skills needed to deal with instances in which the child will not cooperate. Children who have erratic eating patterns may receive the rapidly acting insulin analogues after the meal to decrease the fear of acute hypoglycemia if the child refuses to eat. The dose of insulin to be given is based on the amount of food consumed.

Table 30.4
Sample Nutrition Guidelines for Exercise

Type of Activity	If Blood Sugar Before Activity Is (mg/dL):	Then Eat the Following Carbohydrates Before Activity
Short duration (<30 min)	<100 ≥100	15 g No carbohydrate necessary
Moderate duration (1 h)	<100 100–180 180–240	25–50 g plus protein source 15 g No carbohydrate necessary
Strenuous (1–2 h)	<100 100–180 180–240	50 g plus protein source 15 g No carbohydrate necessary
Snack Choices for Physical Activity		
15 g carbohydrates	4-oz juice box 1 cup Gatorade 1 sliced orange or apple 1 small box raisins	6 saltines 1 cup light yogurt 3/4 cup dry cereal
30 g carbohydrates	1 cereal bar 8-oz juice box	2 slices bread 1 small bagel
45–50 g carbohydrates plus protein	1 sports nutrition bar 1 package (6) cheese or peanut butter sandwich crackers plus 4 oz juice	
Protein Sources	Peanut butter Sliced or string cheese Lunch meat	Egg Peanuts, walnuts, or almonds

Carbohydrate should always be ingested if blood glucose is less than 100 mg/dL before exercise.

Children in the early grades of school need constructive supervision of meal and snack times until they are able to understand food groups and select appropriate foods and portion sizes. As adolescents become increasingly independent, education should be geared toward teaching them to take responsibility for label reading and choosing appropriate foods.[3] They should be taught that extra food (eg, pizza parties) can be handled with extra rapid-acting insulin. During the early adolescent years, compliance is often challenged by youngsters wanting to fit in and be like everybody else, not wanting people to know they have special needs, and not wanting to snack for fear of gaining weight.

V

Issues of Weight Loss and Weight Gain

Weight loss, poor growth, and delayed sexual maturation in children with type 1 diabetes mellitus is most often associated with poor metabolic control. Inadequate insulin dose results in excessive glycosuria with caloric loss. However, poor weight gain may also be associated with inadequate energy intake attributable to rigorous adherence to an outgrown meal plan or inappropriate fat restriction in a young child. Delayed linear growth is associated with prolonged inadequate control of diabetes, but hypothyroidism should be excluded.

Eating disorders are more common in adolescents with diabetes mellitus than in the general population.[32,33] Bulimia is most common and may be associated with deliberate limitation of the insulin dose resulting in weight loss and glycosuria ("insulin purging"), erratic blood glucose concentrations, diabetes, fluctuating weight, and a very high concentration of glycosylated hemoglobin. Anorexia nervosa, with limitation of food intake and insulin, may manifest as recurrent episodes of severe and unexplained hypoglycemia, with the unstable management of diabetes masked by acceptable glycosylated hemoglobin concentrations. Clinicians should be aware of the manifestations of eating disorders in adolescents with type 1 diabetes mellitus.

"Overweight" occurs more readily in children with diabetes. Rapid weight gain is normal just after starting treatment for diabetes, but it should slow to a normal rate after the appropriate weight for the child is regained. Children may receive excess insulin if repeated increases in the insulin dose are made in response to hyperglycemia without investigating the cause or modifying the food intake. Increased weight gain was noted during intensified insulin management in young adults during the DCCT study, but weight gain may be controlled by careful attention to dietary management.[34] Many children with a history of low blood sugar gain weight because they eat in an attempt to prevent hypoglycemia. When weight reduction is necessary, the treatment program for a child with diabetes must include closely integrated efforts of the physician, dietitian, diabetes educator, and mental health professional to balance decreased food and insulin needs.

Treatment of Hypoglycemia

Hypoglycemia commonly occurs with decreased food intake or with increased physical activity. The goal of treatment is to achieve rapid normalization of blood sugar concentration without use of excess food and resultant hyperglycemia.

Low blood sugar concentrations should initially be treated with simple sugar (juice, glucose tablets). This will be rapidly absorbed and raise the blood glucose concentration in 10 to 15 minutes. In general, 15 g of carbohydrate will raise the blood glucose concentration approximately 30 mg/dL. The blood glucose concentration should again be checked 10 to 15 minutes after treatment. If the glucose concentration is less than 80 mg/dL, another 15 g of carbohydrate should be given and blood glucose concentration should again be checked 15 minutes later. Once the blood glucose concentration is greater than 80 mg/dL, the child should be given 15 g of carbohydrate in a protein snack (Table 30.5) or fed a meal or snack if it is scheduled to be given within 30 to 60 minutes. This regimen allows for more rapid correction of hypoglycemia and avoids the overfeeding that usually occurs because of persistence of symptoms despite normalization of blood glucose concentration.

Table 30.5
Sources of 15 g of Carbohydrate

Fluids containing 10–15 g of carbohydrates
1 cup Gatorade (Gatorade, Chicago, IL)
1 cup milk (any kind)
½ cup fruit juice
½ cup regular soft drink
Foods containing 10–15 g of carbohydrates
½ cup regular Jello (Kraft foods, Northfield, IL)
½ cup cooked cereal
½ cup mashed potatoes
½ cup regular ice cream
1 ice pop
6 saltines
6 vanilla wafers
3 graham crackers
1 slice bread or toast

Treatment of Hyperglycemia

The insulin analogues have made treatment of acute hyperglycemia feasible. Administration of an insulin analogue according to a predetermined formula with measurement of blood glucose concentration before and 2 hours after insulin injection will allow for assessment of adequacy of dosing. The postinjection blood glucose should be in the range of 100 to 150 mg/dL.

Cow Milk And Type 1 Diabetes Mellitus

Type 1 diabetes mellitus occurs in genetically susceptible individuals as the endpoint of an immunologically mediated attack on pancreatic beta cells. The autoimmune process is thought to be triggered by environmental factors. Once immune destruction of the beta cells has begun, there is release of pancreatic beta cell antigens associated with antibody production to these islet antigens. These antibodies (islet cell antibodies, insulin autoantibodies, antibodies to glutamic acid decarboxylase, and tyrosine decarboxylase) are present for months to several years before clinical onset of disease and have been used to predict disease in both high- and low-risk populations. In children especially, the presence of these autoantibodies is predictive of later onset of diabetes. Cow milk protein contains a 17-amino acid fragment of bovine serum albumin (ABBOS), which has structural similarities to an islet autoantigen protein (islet cell antibody 69). Because of this structural similarity, some investigators have hypothesized that early introduction of cow milk would result in absorption of the intact protein before gut maturation, thus immunizing the infant and directing an immune response to the islets through molecular mimicry. In both the BB rat and NOD mice, animal models for type 1 diabetes mellitus, semipurified diets composed of simple sugars and hydrolyzed casein routinely retards the development of diabetes mellitus.[35] Over the past 17 years, there has been a plethora of articles, mainly case-controlled epidemiologic surveys, either supporting or challenging the cow milk hypothesis. The extensive meta-analysis of 13 such studies demonstrated a weak but statistically significant association (odds ratio, 1.5) between type 1 diabetes mellitus and both the shortened period of breast-feeding and cow milk exposure before 3 to 4 months of age.[36] Others found no difference in exposure to milk or foods containing cow milk up to 6 months of age in 18 children who had positive test results for beta cell autoimmunity compared with children who had no evidence of autoimmunity.[33] Cow milk consumption has been shown to be correlated with type 1 diabetes in some countries, but this is not consistent. Sardinia has the second-highest incidence rates of diabetes in Europe, after Finland, yet cow milk ingestion is less than half that in Finland. Serum samples from patients with childhood- and adult-onset type 1 diabetes mellitus do not have an increased incidence of antibodies to bovine serum albumin at diagnosis, and bovine serum albumin antibodies are not increased in high-risk patients who later developed type 1 diabetes mellitus.[37,38] Because of these conflicting data, the relationship between type 1 diabetes mellitus and early ingestion of cow milk formula is unclear. Long-term, prospective, double-blind clinical trials, such as those currently being performed in Finland and Canada, are necessary for resolution of this issue. Current data are too preliminary and not conclusive.

Type 2 Diabetes Mellitus

Since 1979, when type 2 diabetes mellitus was first reported in the Pima Indian population, the prevalence of type 2 diabetes mellitus in the pediatric age group has increased markedly. In the initial report, 9 of 1000 individuals 15 to 24 years old had type 2 diabetes mellitus. No cases in children younger than 15 years were reported.[39] By the 1990s, the prevalence of type 2 diabetes mellitus in the 15- to 19-year age group had increased to 51 of 1000, with a prevalence rate of 22 of 1000 in the 10- to 14-year-old Pima Indian population. Thirteen of 3000 American children 12 to 19 years of age studied between 1988 and 1994 were identified as having diabetes mellitus. This provided a national prevalence estimate for all types of diabetes of 4.1 per 1000 and suggested that approximately 30% of people with the disease in this age group have type 2 diabetes mellitus.[40] This is comparable with the experience of many pediatric diabetes clinics and is borne out by the recent publication of the incidence of type 2 diabetes mellitus in adolescents in the 1999–2002 National Health and Nutrition Examination Survey database. Of those with the disease, 70.9% had type 1 diabetes mellitus and 29.1% had type 2 diabetes mellitus. The overall prevalence of diabetes was 0.5%, and the prevalence of impaired fasting glucose was 11%. Using population-based sample weights, the authors extrapolated this to be 39 005 adolescents with type 2 diabetes mellitus and 2 769 736 with impaired fasting glucose.[40]

The increased incidence of type 2 diabetes mellitus in childhood parallels the increased incidence of obesity. Since 1980, the incidence of type 2 diabetes mellitus has increased by 33% in black adults and by 11% in white adults. During the same period, the incidence of overweight has increased from 25% to 48% in adults.[41] Since 1970, the rate of obesity in childhood has doubled, with 22% of children being obese in 1990.

The initial problem in children with type 2 diabetes mellitus is insulin resistance. This is influenced by (1) pubertal stage—insulin sensitivity of adolescents in general is approximately 30% lower than that of either preadolescents or adults, likely because of increased activity of the growth hormone axis[42]; (2) family history—prepubertal children with a family history of type 2 diabetes mellitus are more insulin resistant than prepubertal children without a family history when data are controlled for body mass index[43]; (3) ethnicity—insulin sensitivity is approximately 35% to 40% lower in black adolescents than in white peers matched for age, sex, weight, and body composition,[44] and American Indian/Alaska Native and Hispanic individuals are also at high risk; and (4) adiposity—total adiposity explains 55% of the variance in insulin sensitivity.[45] Obese children have hyperinsulinism and a 40% decrease in insulin-stimulated glucose metabolism compared with children who are not obese. The inverse relationship between insulin sensitivity and abdominal fat is greater for visceral than for abdominal subcutaneous fat.[39] The insulin resistance is reflected by elevated fasting insulin concentrations followed by impaired insulin secretion with inadequate first phase-stimulated insulin release, resulting in postprandial hyperglycemia. Subsequent blunting of second phase insulin release causes fasting hyperglycemia.[46] Because pediatric endocrinologist are relative newcomers to dealing with type 2 diabetes mellitus, there are no longitudinal studies on the management of this disease in children. Guidelines have, therefore, been extrapolated from those for adults.[47] As with type 2 diabetes mellitus in adults, the cornerstone of treatment is lifestyle modification including dietary changes and increased exercise. Implementation of such measures is extremely challenging and requires involvement of the whole family. Longstanding habits and attitudes toward eating and exercise must be recognized and changed. Dietary modifications are most likely to be effective when kept simple and attainable. It is recommended that patients make 2 to 3 basic changes that are not too demanding. Examples include switching from regular to diet soda and decreasing the amount of high-calorie juices and whole milk in the diet. It is important to stress to patients that incremental weight loss could result in significantly improved insulin sensitivity and blood pressure. A reasonable weight-loss goal is 3 to 4 lb per month. Increased exercise and a diet with moderate caloric restriction (eg, 500–1000 kcal below usual daily intake) should be adequate to produce gradual weight loss. Exercise, too, must be easily incorporated into the patient's and family's lifestyle. Physical activity need not involve organized sports. It may involve walking or bicycling to school and using the stairs instead of the elevator. It has been recommended that patients exercise for at least 60 minutes daily. All family members should adopt the same healthy eating patterns and exercise together or individually.

Children and adolescents at high risk of developing or who have already developed type 2 diabetes mellitus should be involved in programs that emphasize behavior changes that improve lifestyle habits that result in achieving and maintaining a healthy weight. These programs must provide education and support to promote regular physical activity and healthy eating habits. Weight loss medications are not commonly used in children but may be beneficial in youth with inability to achieve adequate weight loss despite good attempts at lifestyle change and who have comorbidities (eg, hypertension, dyslipidemia). The only weight loss medications approved for children are sibutramine (for children older than 16 years) and orlistat. Both have significant adverse effects and limited efficacy, with regain of weight after discontinuation of the medication in most cases.[48] Bariatric surgery is rarely performed but has a role for children with BMI ≥40 with significant comorbidities (eg, sleep apnea, type 2 diabetes mellitus, or pseudotumor cerebri) or BMI ≥50 with skeletal maturity in whom lifestyle modification has failed despite good effort by the patient and family. The surgery may be performed laparoscopically but involves a rate of significant complications of approximately 20%.[49]

Treatment of type 2 diabetes mellitus in children is based on symptoms at diagnosis. Asymptomatic children who are diagnosed following a routine examination or family testing and who have an initial HbA1c concentration less than 8% can be treated with nonpharmacologic means. These children are instructed to monitor their blood glucose concentrations at least twice per day (before breakfast and 2 hours after dinner). If dietary modification and lifestyle changes are unsuccessful in achieving fasting plasma glucose concentrations of 120 mg/dL and HbA1c concentrations of 7% or less, pharmacotherapy is necessary. In addition, monitoring and aggressive treatment of blood pressure and hyperlipidemia, comorbidities associated with insulin resistance, are an essential part of the care of patients with type 2 diabetes mellitus. Children with slightly higher HbA1c concentrations and mild symptoms may initially be treated with oral hypoglycemic agents, most commonly metformin, and those with ketosis or high HbA1c concentrations require initial treatment with insulin.

Prevention

Although the nonmodifiable factors that predispose to type 2 diabetes mellitus (ethnicity, sex, and family history) cannot be prevented, it is essential that all children and parents are educated about the need for physical activity and healthy diet so that we can improve factors that are modifiable in high-risk children. Lifestyle modification is essential for prevention of type 2 diabetes mellitus. The Diabetes Prevention Program showed that exercise of 25 minutes for 6 days per week combined with decreased caloric intake was more effective in preventing development of type 2 diabetes mellitus in adults with impaired glucose tolerance than was use of metformin. Both were more effective than placebo or routine care. Thus, it is important to involve the entire family in modifying behavior to increase exercise and encourage healthy eating habits as soon as a trend toward overweight is detected on the child's growth curve.[50] If the increasing incidence of obesity and, thus, of insulin resistance and type 2 diabetes mellitus in children is not curbed, it will become a tremendous public health problem.

References

1. The Diabetes Control and Complications Trial Research Group. The effect of intensive treatment of diabetes on the development and progression of long-term complications in insulin-dependent diabetes mellitus. *N Engl J Med.* 1993;329:977–986

2. UKPDS Prospective Diabetes Study group: Tight blood pressure control and risk of macrovascular and microvascular complication in type 2 diabetes: UK Prospective Diabetes Study Group 38. *BMJ.* 1998;317:703–713

3. Cull CA, Mehta Z, Stratton IM, et al. Association of lipid levels over time with clinical outcomes in patients with type 2 diabetes in the UKPDS [abstr]. *Diabetes.* 2000;49(Suppl 1): A267

4. Haffner SM, Alexander CM, Cook TJ, et al. Reduced coronary events in simvastatin treated patients with coronary heart disease and diabetes of impaired fasting glucose levels: subgroup analysis in the Scandinavian Simvastatin Survival Study. *Arch Intern Med.* 1999;159:2661–2667

5. National Institute of Diabetes and Digestive and Kidney Diseases. Epidemiology of diabetes interventions and complications study (EDIC). Available at: www.niddk.nih.gov/patient/edic/edic-public.htm. Accessed September 17, 2007

6. The Diabetes Control and Complications Trial/Epidemiology of Diabetes Interventions and Complications (DCCT/EDIC) Study Research Group. Intensive diabetes treatment and cardiovascular disease in patients with type 1 diabetes. *N Engl J Med.* 2005;353:2643–2653

7. Silverstein J, Klingensmith G, Copeland K, et al. Care of children and adolescents with type 1 diabetes mellitus: a statement of the American Diabetes Association. *Diabetes Care.* 2005;28:186–212

8. Lebovitz HE. Insulin secretagogues, old and new. *Diabetes Rev.* 1999;7:139–152

9. Stewart C, Ferguson M, Strachan WJ, et al. Insulin lispro lowers the incidence of severe hypoglycemia, without a detrimental effect on glycemic control, in those individuals with type 1 diabetes at high risk of severe hypoglycemia [abstr]. *Diabetes.* 1999;48(Suppl):A526

10. Delahanty LM, Halford BN. The role of diet behaviors in achieving improved glycemic control in intensely treated patients in the Diabetes Control and Complications Trial. *Diabetes Care.* 1993;16:1453–1458

11. American Diabetes Association, Task Force for Writing Nutrition Principles and Recommendations for the Management of Diabetes and Related Complications. American Diabetes Association position statement: evidence based nutrition principles and recommendations for the treatment and prevention of diabetes and related complications. *J Am Diet Assoc.* 2002;102:109–118

12. Maryniuk MD. Carbohydrate counting: a return to basics. *Diabetes Spectrum.* 2000;13(3):149

13. Anderson EJ, Richardson M, Castle G, et al. Nutrition interventions for intensive therapy in the Diabetes Control and Complications Trial. The DCCT Research Group. *J Am Diet Assoc.* 1993;93:768–772

14. DAFNE Study Group. Training in flexible, intensive insulin management to enable dietary freedom in people with type 1 diabetes: dose adjustment for normal eating (DAFNE) randomised controlled trial. *BMJ.* 2002;325:746

15. American Dietetic Association. Position of the American Dietetic Association: child and adolescent food and nutrition programs. *J Am Diet Assoc.* 1996;96:913–917

16. Wildey MB, Pampalone SZ, Pelletier RL, Zive MM, Elder JP, Sallis JF. Fat and sugar levels are high in snacks purchased from student stores in middle schools. *J Am Diet Assoc.* 2000;100:319–322

17. The obesity epidemic: a mandate for a multidisciplinary approach. Proceedings of a roundtable. Boston, Massachusetts, USA. October 27, 1997. *J Am Diet Assoc.* 1998;98(10 Suppl 2):S1–S61

18. American Diabetes Association. Nutrition recommendations and principles for people with diabetes mellitus. *Diabetes Care.* 2001;24:S44–S47

19. US Department of Agriculture. *Nutrition and Your Health: Dietary Guidelines for Americans.* 3rd ed. Washington, DC: US Department of Agriculture, Human Nutrition Information Service; 1990. Available at: http://www.health.gov/dietaryguidelines/1990thin.pdf. Accessed November 2, 2007

20. American Diabetes Association. Position statement: standards of medical care in diabetes. *Diabetes Care.* 2005;28(Suppl):S4–S36

21. American Diabetes Association, American Dietetic Association. *Exchange Lists for Meal Planning.* Alexandria, VA: American Diabetes Association; and Chicago, IL: American Dietetic Association; 1986

22. Maryniuk MD. *Medical Nutrition Therapy in Diabetes: Clinical Guidelines for Primary Care Physicians.* New York, NY: Dekker; 2000

23. Morris KL, Zemel MB. Glycemic index, cardiovascular disease, and obesity. *Nutr Rev.* 1999;57:273–276

24. Brand Miller J, Colagiuri S, Foster-Powell K. The glycemic index is easy and works in practice [lett]. *Diabetes Care.* 1997;20:1628–1629

25. Manley SE, Stratton IM, Cull CA, et al. Effects of three months' diet after diagnosis of type 2 diabetes on plasma lipids and lipoproteins. (UKPDS 45.) *Diabet Med.* 2000;17:518–523

26. Berenson GS, Srinivasin SR, Bao W, Newman WP III, Tracy RE, Wattigney WA. Association between multiple cardiovascular risk factors and atherosclerosis in children and young adults. The Bogalusa Heart Study. *N Engl J Med.* 1998;338:1650–1656

V

27. American Diabetes Association. Management of dyslipidemia in adults with diabetes. *Diabetes Care*. 2002;25(Suppl 1):574–577

28. Levey AS, Adler S, Caggiula AW, et al. Effects of dietary protein restriction of the progression of advanced renal disease in the Modification of Diet in Renal Disease Study. *Am J Kidney Dis*. 1996;27:652–663

29. American Diabetes Association. Diabetic nephropathy (position statement). *Diabetes Care*. 2002;25(Supp 1):S88–S89

30. American Diabetes Association. Evidence-based nutrition principles and recommendations for the treatment and prevention of diabetes and related complications. *Diabetes Care*. 2002;25(Suppl 1):S50–S60

31. Williams CL. Importance of dietary fiber in childhood. *J Am Diet Assoc*. 1995;95:1140–1146

32. Rodin GM, Daneman D. Eating disorders and IDDM. A problematic association. *Diabetes Care*. 1992;15:1402–1412

33. Meltzer LJ, Johnson SB, Prine JM, Banks RA, Desrosiers PM, Silverstein JH. Disordered eating, body mass, and glycemic control in adolescents with type I diabetes. *Diabetes Care*. 2001;24:678–682

34. DCCT Research Group. Weight gain associated with intensive therapy in the Diabetes Control and Complications Trial. *Diabetes Care*. 1988;11:567–573

35. Schatz DA, Maclaren NK. Cow's milk and insulin-dependent diabetes mellitus: innocent until proven guilty. *JAMA*. 1996;276:647–648

36. Gerstein H. Cow's milk exposure and type 1 diabetes mellitus. A critical overview of the clinical literature. *Diabetes Care*. 1994;17:13–19

37. Norris JM, Beaty B, Klingensmith G, et al. Lack of association between early exposure to cow's milk protein and beta-cell autoimmunity. Diabetes Autoimmunity Study in the Young (DAISY). *JAMA*. 1996;276:609–614

38. Atkinson MA, Bowman MA, Kao KJ, et al. Lack of immune responsiveness to bovine serum albumin in insulin-dependent diabetes. *N Engl J Med*. 1993;329:1853–1858

39. Savage PJ, Bennett PH, Senter RG, Miller M. High prevalence of diabetes in young Pima Indians: evidence of phenotypic variation in a genetically isolated population. *Diabetes*. 1979;28:937–942

40. Fagot-Campagna A, Pettitt DJ, Engelgau MM, et al. Type 2 diabetes among North American children in adolescence: an epidemiological review in a public health perspective. *J Pediatr*. 2000;136:664–672

41. Duncan GE. Prevalence of diabetes and impaired fasting glucose levels among US adolescents: National Health and Nutrition Examination Survey, 1999–2002. *Arch Pediatr Adolesc Med*. 2006;160:523–528

42. Troiano RP, Flegal KM. Overweight children and adolescents: description, epidemiology, and demographics. *Pediatrics*. 1998;101(3 Suppl):497–504

43. Arslanian SA, Kalhan SC. Correlations between fatty acid and glucose metabolism. Potential explanation of insulin resistance of puberty. *Diabetes*. 1994;43:908–914

44. Danadian K, Balasekaran G, Lewy V, Meza MP, Robertson R, Arslanian SA. Insulin sensitivity in African-American children with and without a family history of type 2 diabetes. *Diabetes Care*. 1999;22:1325–1329

45. Arslanian SA. Insulin secretion and sensitivity in healthy African American vs American white children. *Clin Pediatr (Phila)*. 1998;37:81–88

46. Caprio S, Tamberlane WV. Metabolic impact of obesity in childhood. *Endocrinol Metab Clin North Am*. 1999;28:731–747

47. Martin MM, Martin LA. Obesity, hyperinsulinism, and diabetes mellitus in childhood. *General Pediatr*. 1973;82:192–201

48. Dean H. Treatment of type 2 diabetes in youth: an argument for randomized controlled studies. *Pediatr Child Health*. 1992;4:265–269

49. Berkowitz RI, Wadden TA, Tershakovec AM, Cronquist JL. Behavior therapy and sibutramine for the treatment of adolescent obesity: a randomized controlled trial. *JAMA*. 2003;289:1805–1812

50. Inge TH, Zeller MH, Lawson ML, Daniels SR. A critical appraisal of evidence supporting a bariatric surgical approach to weight management for adolescents. *J Pediatr*. 2005;147:10–19

51. Knowler WC, Barrett-Connor E, Fowler SE, et al. Reduction in the incidence of type 2 diabetes with lifestyle intervention or metformin. *N Engl J Med*. 2002;346:393–403

Hypoglycemia in Infants and Children

Introduction and Definition of Hypoglycemia

Hypoglycemia can be considered only a surrogate marker for harmfully low levels of energy in the central nervous system. Therefore, the degree and duration of low plasma glucose that can cause central nervous system damage in infants and children are uncertain. Important determinants of central nervous system energy sufficiency include the efficiency of the transport of glucose into the brain, the need of brain cells for energy, and the availability of alternative energy sources. Serum glucose concentrations do not accurately measure any of these processes.[1] Glucose is transported from the circulation across the blood-brain barrier, and such transport may vary depending on the availability and efficiency of specific glucose transporters (GLUT-1 is the major transporter of the blood-brain barrier, but other transporters are important for the entry of glucose into neurons and glial cells).[2] Children with a defective copy of one GLUT-1 gene may have severe symptomatic central nervous system glucose deficiency with normal circulating serum glucose concentrations.[3] Energy utilization in the central nervous system varies depending on the activation state of neural tissues. Seizure activity, for instance, rapidly depletes neurons of energy even when peripheral plasma glucose concentration is normal.[4] Alternative substrates, such as ketones, lactate, and perhaps free fatty acids and amino acids, also support the energy needs of the brain.[1,5,6] These substrates circulate in the plasma in concentrations that are dependent on the metabolic state of the child and, in general, cross the blood-brain barrier assisted by specific transporters.[7] Because of the potential differences in glucose transport to the brain, the utilization rate by neural tissues, and the availability of alternative energy substrates, plasma glucose is not a precise measure of central nervous system cellular energy supply.

Variation in measurement of circulating glucose can further confound this problem. Early studies used whole-blood glucose measures. Human red blood cell concentrations of glucose are about half those of the plasma. Therefore, measures of whole-blood glucose are 10% to 15% lower than the plasma or serum glucose measurement commonly obtained in automated analyzers. If the hematocrit concentration is higher than adult norms, as occurs in ill neonates, whole-blood glucose measures may be even lower. In addition, blood samples obtained for the assay of glucose must be maintained on ice, analyzed rapidly, and/or protected from glycolysis by the addition of fluoride. Glycolytic degradation of glucose is more rapid in the neonate than in adult blood and can markedly decrease measured blood glucose in unprotected samples stored at room temperature.[8]

Acceptable plasma glucose concentrations in the neonate may be defined statistically or by examination of acute or chronic outcomes. A recent systematic review of this issue suggests that no adequate data exist to define the concentration of peripheral glucose in the neonate that is associated with a poor developmental outcome.[9] However, there is a reasonable correlation among these statistical, epidemiologic, and acute experimental approaches, which gives some assurance that for most infants, the plasma glucose concentrations commonly accepted as normal are clinically sound. Lower limits in term newborn infants have been defined epidemiologically as a plasma glucose concentration less than 45 mg/dL (2.5 mmol/L) in the first 48 hours.[10,11] A plasma glucose concentration less than 47 mg/dL (2.6 mmol/L) was the lower limit of normal for venous cord blood in term newborn infants.[12] A plasma glucose less than 47 mg/dL (2.6 mmol/L) was associated with abnormal auditory evoked responses in older infants.[13] Blood glucose concentrations between 30 and 45 were associated with increased cerebral blood flow in preterm neonates.[14] In addition, a single plasma glucose concentration less than 47 mg/dL (2.6 mmol/L) in newborn infants was associated with a worse neurodevelopmental outcome at 18 months of age.[15] In another study, recurrent neonatal hypoglycemia in preterm neonates who were small for gestational age correlated better with worse neurodevelopmental outcomes at 5 years of age than did the severity of a single episode.[16] In adults, hypoglycemic symptoms are generally reported below plasma glucose concentrations of 60 mg/dL (3.3 mmol/L),[17,18] and this number is often taken as the lower limit of normal in children and adolescents. However, the set point for physiologic counter regulation seems higher in children than in adults.[19]

Operational thresholds for neonates (plasma glucose concentrations at which clinical interventions should be considered) were determined by a consensus conference and were based on available data (Table 31.1).[20] The participants of the consensus conference determined that routine monitoring of plasma glucose concentration is not necessary in a term infant with a normal pregnancy and delivery. However, low plasma glucose concentrations were considered sufficient for intervention if drawn because of symptoms of hypoglycemia or risk factors for hypoglycemia.[12] Previous data suggesting that preterm infants have lower plasma glucose concentrations seem to reflect deficient nutritional management. The same operational thresholds were suggested for term and preterm neonates.

Table 31.1
Operational Thresholds for Hypoglycemia in Neonates, Including Preterm Infants*

• Plasma glucose <45 mg/dL (2.5 mmol/L) and symptoms of hypoglycemia
• Plasma glucose <36 mg/dL (2.0 mmol/L) in a neonate with risk factors†
• Plasma glucose <60 mg/dL (3.3 mmol/L) in a neonate with persistent hyperinsulinemic hypoglycemia

* Breastfed term infants were not included; it was felt that they may tolerate lower plasma glucose concentrations, because they have more ketogenesis and higher ketone concentrations than formula-fed infants.

† Risk factors include: those associated with maternal metabolism (intrapartum administration of glucose, terbutaline, ritodrine, propranolol, oral hypoglycemic agents, infant of a mother with diabetes); those associated with neonatal problems (perinatal hypoxia-ischemia, infection, hypothermia, hyperviscosity, erythroblastosis fetalis, congenital cardiac disease, preterm birth); intrauterine growth restriction, hyperinsulinism, endocrine disorders, inborn errors of metabolism.

Clinical Manifestations of Hypoglycemia

Signs and symptoms of hypoglycemia can be broadly divided into those resulting from neuroglycopenia and those from autonomic responses to hypoglycemia. The early symptoms and signs of hypoglycemia are usually autonomic and include sweating, weakness, tachycardia, tremor, hunger, paresthesias, pallor, anxiety or nervousness, nausea, and palpitations. Prolonged hypoglycemia may lead to more signs and symptoms of neuroglycopenia, including lethargy, dizziness, irritability, mental confusion, behavior that is out of character, blurred vision, difficulty speaking, loss of coordination, and in its extreme, seizures, coma, and death.

These signs and symptoms are less obvious or absent in infants and young children. The nonspecific signs of hypoglycemia in newborn and young infants may be manifested by irritability, jitteriness, feeding difficulties, lethargy, apnea, cyanosis, bradycardia, tachypnea, abnormal cry, hypothermia, hypotonia, lethargy, apathy, and seizures. These signs are not specific of hypoglycemia and are also the early manifestations of other severe disorders (sepsis, congenital heart disease, ventricular hemorrhage, respiratory distress syndrome, and aspiration).

With repeated or prolonged episodes of hypoglycemia, the threshold for autonomic symptoms increases to that of neuroglycopenic symptoms. As a result, the individual develops severe hypoglycemia with little or no warning, a condition termed "hypoglycemia unawareness."[21]

Etiology of Hypoglycemia

Neonate

In newborn infants, the differential diagnosis of hypoglycemia can initially be guided but not limited by the birth weight (Table 31.2).

Table 31.2
Causes of Hypoglycemia in Newborn Infants

Small for Gestational Age (SGA)
Primary failure to produce and store glycogen
Appropriate for Gestational Age (AGA)
Endocrine deficiency: • Hypopituitarism/growth hormone deficiency • Cortisol/adrenocorticotropic hormone (ACTH) deficiency • ACTH unresponsiveness
Increased rate of glucose utilization: • Perinatal stress/hypoxia • Cold stress • Sepsis
Depletion of glycogen stores in congenital heart failure/congenital heart disease
Inborn errors of carbohydrate, protein, and lipid metabolism
Hyperinsulinism attributable to: • Rh incompatibility • Exchange transfusion • Malposition of an umbilical catheter
Large for Gestational Age (LGA): Hyperinsulinism
Infant of a diabetic mother
Beckwith-Wiedemann syndrome
Beta-cell gene mutations causing congenital hyperinsulinism (persistent hyperinsulinemic hypoglycemia of infancy)* • Sulphonylurea receptor type 1-inactivating gene mutation • KIR 6.2 (inward-rectifying potassium channel)-inactivating gene mutation • Short-chain L-3-hydroxyacyl-coenzyme A dehydrogenase enzyme-inactivating gene mutation • Glucokinase-activating gene mutation • Glutamate dehydrogenase-activating gene mutation

* Because these disorders can be of variable severity and may not always present at birth, they are not invariably associated with fetal overgrowth.

Children

The most common cause of hypoglycemia in children is insulin-induced hypoglycemia in individuals with type 1 diabetes mellitus. In other children, hypoglycemia can be categorized as ketotic fasting hypoglycemia, non-ketotic fasting hypoglycemia, and reactive or postprandial hypoglycemia (Table 31.3). This categorization generally aids in diagnosis but should not limit clinical judgment. Mild reactive hypoglycemia is very common in the otherwise healthy population and is not considered a disease.

Table 31.3
Causes of Hypoglycemia in Children

Ketotic Fasting Hypoglycemia
"Accelerated starvation" (ketotic hypoglycemia)
Endocrine deficiencies: growth hormone, ACTH/cortisol, hypopituitarism (ACTH/cortisol and growth hormone)

Metabolic defects:
  Disorders of carbohydrate metabolism:
    Glycogen synthase deficiency
        Type III glycogen storage disease (amylo-1,6-glucosidase deficiency)
        Type VI glycogen storage disease (phosphorylase deficiency)
        Type IX glycogen storage disease (phosphorylase kinase deficiency)
        Defects in gluconeogenesis: pyruvate carboxylase deficiency, fructose 1-6-biphosphatase deficiency
  Disorders of protein metabolism (organic acidemias) examples:
        Maple syrup urine disease (branched-chain ketoacid decarboxylase deficiency)
        Methylmalonic acidemia

Miscellaneous:
  Salicylate intoxication
  Reye syndrome
  Ethanol intoxication
  Malaria
  Diarrhea
  Malnutrition
  Jamaican vomiting sickness (ingestion of unripe ackee)

Table 31.3 *(Continued)*
Causes of Hypoglycemia in Children

Nonketotic Fasting Hypoglycemia
Glycogen storage disease type 1 (glucose-6-phosphate dehydrogenase deficiency) Tyrosinemia
Disorders of fatty oxidation and ketone synthesis: Carnitine transport and metabolism   Beta-oxidation cycle
Electron transfer
3-Hydroxy-3-methylglutaryl coenzyme A (HMG-CoA) synthase or lyase deficiency
Insulin-like growth factor (IGF)-1, IGF-2 excess
Insulinoma
Sulfonylurea or other insulin secretogogue ingestion
Exogenous insulin administration
Persistent hyperinsulinemic hypoglycemia of infancy
Reactive or postprandial hypoglycemia: "Metabolic dumping syndrome"   Galactosemia
Fructose intolerance (fructose-1-phosphate aldolase deficiency)

Evaluation of Hypoglycemia

Neonates

The history and physical examination can often be revealing. Gestational age and birth weight; maternal health, including history of diabetes or glucose intolerance; and medications may guide diagnosis, prognosis, and therapy. Most hypoglycemic infants who are large for gestational age are hyperinsulinemic. Most have mothers with diabetes, and the hypoglycemia and hyperinsulinemia are of relatively short duration (24 hours to a few days).[22] Other rare transient causes of hyperinsulinism include Beckwith-Wiedemann syndrome, characterized by macrosomia, large tongue, omphalocele/umbilical hernia, visceromegaly, and horizontal grooves on ear lobes.[23] Persistent hyperinsulinism and hypoglycemia require careful genetic and physiologic evaluation and management planning. Most infants born preterm or small for gestational age are unable to produce enough glucose through glycogenolysis and gluconeogenesis to meet the needs of their relatively large brains. These babies usually will respond with increased glucose when sufficient fat is included in their diet to alter the hepatocellular ratio of nicotinamide adenine dinucleotide to NADH in favor of gluconeogenesis.[24] However, some of these infants may also have prolonged hyperinsulinism, and the etiology is, as yet, unclear.[25] Normal-weight babies are most likely to have an endocrine deficiency disorder or an inborn error of carbohydrate or fatty acid metabolism. Prolonged neonatal jaundice, microphallus in a boy, or facial midline anomalies might suggest hypopituitarism. Hepatomegaly might suggest a storage disorder or an abnormality of glycogen synthesis or release. Metabolic disorders may present in the immediate neonatal period or somewhat later. Those that cause acidosis may manifest as hyperventilation that is misdiagnosed as pneumonia or reactive airway disease or may be misdiagnosed as overwhelming sepsis in the first months of life. A history of unusual odors may be a clue in maple syrup urine disease, isovaleric academia, 3-methylcrotonyl coenzyme A carboxylase deficiency, and glutaric acidemia type II. Many regions now perform neonatal screening for these disorders so that diagnosis is made early, often before the infants are symptomatic.[26]

Children

Birth weight, history of neonatal complications, age of onset, and frequency of symptoms can aid in diagnosis. Symptoms of hypoglycemia at birth or during the neonatal period might point to hypopituitarism or hyperinsulinism; prolonged neonatal jaundice might suggest cortisol and/or thyroid deficiency. The temporal relationship of symptoms to food intake may aid in diagnosis. Hypoglycemia that occurs within about 2 hours of eating is considered reactive. It may be seen in dumping syndrome, in obese individuals with overactive insulin response to carbohydrate, and in rare individuals with galactosemia or fructose intolerance. The specific content of feedings and relationship to onset of symptoms as well as food intolerance or aversion may guide the diagnosis, as may the usual laboratory evaluation. Complete dumping syndrome is characterized by postprandial irritability, diaphoresis, abdominal pain, and diarrhea. It may follow a fundoplication. However, many individuals may manifest metabolic dumping syndrome with hypoglycemia without other systemic symptoms.[27]

Symptomatic hypoglycemia that appears approximately 4 hours after eating more commonly occurs in defects of glycogenolysis or in hyperinsulinism. Hypoglycemia that occurs 10 to 12 hours after feedings suggests a defect of gluconeogenesis or fatty acid oxidation but may also represent hyperinsulinism.

A potential drug exposure should be sought in all children with hypoglycemia. Insulin, hypoglycemic agents, and alcohol are often implicated. Erratic episodes of hypoglycemia may be a warning of Munchausen syndrome by proxy.[28]

Findings from the physical examination suggestive of growth hormone deficiency or hypopituitarism are short stature or growth failure, microphallus, midline defects (cleft lip and palate, single central incisor), and optic nerve hypoplasia (in septo-optic dysplasia). Hepatomegaly is usually present in glycogen storage diseases, disorders of gluconeogenesis, galactosemia, hereditary fructose intolerance, disorders of fatty acid oxidation and carnitine metabolism, and tyrosinemia type 1. Increased pigmentation may be present in Addison disease. Disorders of carnitine transport or metabolism may cause cardiomyopathy.

Laboratory Investigation of Unexplained Hypoglycemia

Glucose meters for self-plasma glucose monitoring are calibrated to normal blood or plasma glucose ranges and adult ranges for hypoglycemia (50 mg/dL or less plasma glucose concentration). Readings may be influenced by hematocrit, because meters are calibrated to read plasma glucose concentration within an adult range of hematocrit, and plasma glucose concentration is higher than blood cell glucose concentration. Even the best meters are not consistently reliable at low blood glucose concentrations. Hence, a glucose meter value below 45 mg/dL should be confirmed by a laboratory glucose value. If appropriate additional laboratory studies are obtained at the same time, this laboratory plasma glucose value may serve as a "critical" or diagnostic sample. It may be necessary to perform a monitored fast of 8 to 24 hours, depending on the age of the child. Fasting may induce cerebral edema in a child with a fatty-acid oxidation defect. This should be ruled out before performing the fast by determination of nonfasting plasma acylcarnitines and urinary acylglycines.[29] The protocol outlined in Table 31.5 can be used for the monitored fasting evaluation and contains a list of the laboratory tests to send with the "critical blood sample."

Differential Diagnosis of Hypoglycemia

Newborn Infant

Hyperinsulinism
In the neonate, the diagnostic challenge is to ensure that the child does not have persistent hyperinsulinism. This disorder carries a worse prognosis

than other causes of hypoglycemia for several reasons. First, high insulin concentrations will make alternative brain fuels like ketones, lactate, and free fatty acids unavailable so that the central nervous system need for glucose will be greater than in other types of hypoglycemia.[30] Second, some of the disorders associated with hyperinsulinism involve metabolic pathways common to the brain so that the underlying disorder may separately interfere with neuronal function and development.[31] Last, hypoglycemia from hyperinsulinism is often quite difficult to control, requiring large quantities of glucose (>12 µg/kg per minute, intravenously) and additional therapeutic agents like diazoxide and octreotide, which have their own toxicities.[30,32] In many children, either partial or total pancreatectomy is necessary for control of blood glucose concentration. The decision about surgery and the type of surgery requires sophisticated techniques to assess the etiology of the hyperinsulinism and the nature of the pancreatic involvement. Once congenital hyperinsulinism is confirmed or suspected, transfer to a specialist is prudent. Diagnosis should be suspected if need for glucose is greater than 12 µg/ kg per minute and the child's hypoglycemia is not relieved by physiologic cortisol supplementation. It is imperative that the plasma insulin concentration be determined at the same time as the glucose concentration. Insulin concentrations obtained at the time of hypoglycemia are generally higher than anticipated for hypoglycemia (>2 µU/mL), but many assays designed to measure adult insulin concentrations will not be able to detect concentrations this low and will report unmeasurable insulin in plasma even in infants suffering from hyperinsulinism.

Other Etiologies of Hypoglycemia

Cortisol deficiency can be difficult to diagnose in neonates who often do not respond to hypoglycemia with elevations in cortisol but can respond to adrenocorticotropic hormone (ACTH) testing. However, treatment with cortisol should rapidly ameliorate the hypoglycemia. Absence of ketosis is indicative of hyperinsulinism, except in rare disorders of ketogenesis. Neonates have a high renal threshold for ketones and may have normal ketogenesis with hypoglycemia without measurable ketonuria.[33] Ketonuria in a newborn infant with hypoglycemia suggests either glycogen storage disease type III or a metabolic disorder with production of large quantities of ketoacids. Urinary organic acid determination is critical to determine the presence of abnormal ketoacids.

V

Children

The laboratory differential diagnosis can be initially guided by the presence or absence of ketonuria or ketonemia.

Ketotic Hypoglycemia

Ketoacids in normal fasting individuals include beta-hydroxybutyrate, measured in plasma with specific reagent strips or (preferred) by a reference laboratory, and acetoacetate, measured in urine as "ketones" on a test strip. Acetoacetate is quite labile and will not persist in a stored plasma sample unless handled very carefully. In the presence of adequate ketosis, if the urine organic acids do not show an abnormal diagnostic pattern and there is no suspicion of hepatomegaly, the following diagnoses should be considered: accelerated starvation, growth hormone or cortisol deficiency, and glycogen synthase deficiency. "Accelerated starvation" (previously termed ketotic hypoglycemia) is a diagnosis of exclusion and should be made when the other causes of ketotic hypoglycemia have been ruled out. Children with this disorder are typically underweight for height. Hypoglycemia usually occurs after 12 to 24 hours of fasting and is associated with a normal metabolic response to hypoglycemia with ketonuria, low plasma alanine concentration, normal lactate and pyruvate concentrations, suppressed insulin, and elevated growth hormone and cortisol concentrations. The response to glucagon administration is blunted at the time of hypoglycemia, because hepatic and other glycogen stores have been used for energy.[26]

The presence of a large liver should guide to the diagnosis of glycogen storage disease and disorders of gluconeogenesis. The diagnosis of glycogen synthase deficiency can be confirmed at the molecular level after an oral glucose tolerance test demonstrates initial hyperglycemia followed by hypoglycemia at 3 to 4 hours.[34] The urine organic or amino acid pattern should give the diagnosis in the case of disorders of protein metabolism. A plasma cortisol concentration less than 10 µg/dL during hypoglycemia suggests cortisol/ACTH deficiency. A low plasma growth hormone concentration should raise the question of growth hormone deficiency/hypopituitarism, but low growth hormone and cortisol levels are sometimes found in normal individuals following persistent or frequent hypoglycemia.

Nonketotic Hypoglycemia

Insulin should be undetectable during hypoglycemia. In hyperinsulinism, insulin inhibits ketone production and lipolysis, and ketone and free fatty acid concentrations are inappropriately low during hypoglycemia. The plasma insulin concentration will be inappropriately high during hypoglycemia

(>2 µU/mL). A positive response to glucagon (30 µg/kg, subcutaneously or intravenously) with an increment in plasma glucose of at least 30 mg/dL (1.7 mmol/L), despite severe hypoglycemia, is also diagnostic of hyperinsulinism.[35] Typically, the intravenous glucose rate required to maintain normoglycemia is 2 or 4 times greater than the glucose production rate (6–8 mg/kg per minute in a newborn infant, 4–6 mg/kg per minute in a slightly older child, and 1–2 mg/kg per minute in an adult). The reason for the differences in glucose production rate is evident in Fig 31.1, which demonstrates that to maintain euglycemia, glucose production rate must equal glucose utilization rate. As the relative brain size compared with body weight decreases with age, the relative glucose utilization rate per kg of body weight also decreases.[36]

In hyperinsulinism, plasma cortisol and growth hormone concentrations may be normal or inappropriately low if the hypoglycemia occurs gradually or is recurrent (blunted counter-regulatory response). A low C-peptide concentration associated with elevated insulin concentrations suggests exogenous insulin administration.

Imaging of the pancreas with computerized axial tomography or ultrasonography is not often sensitive enough to differentiate between an adenoma, focal adenomatous hyperplasia, and diffuse beta-cell hyperplasia. The type and location of the pancreatic lesion (diffuse versus focal) can be determined by preoperative pancreatic catheterization and intraoperative histopathologic studies, which should be performed at a center experienced in these studies. Preoperative positron emission tomography may have additional utility in this diagnostic distinction.[30,37]

If the plasma insulin concentration is adequately suppressed with non-ketotic hypoglycemia, a fatty acid oxidation defect should be suspected. A diagnostic pattern is seen in the concentrations of urine organic acids and acylglycine and plasma acylcarnitine.[29]

Treatment

Neonatal Hypoglycemia

A pragmatic management plan is not based on outcome measures but, rather, the clinical picture, including laboratory-determined plasma glucose concentration and symptomatology.

If the plasma glucose concentration is between 35 and 45 mg/dL (1.9–2.5 mmol/L) and the neonate is able to feed, then breastfeeding or formula or 5% dextrose administration by nipple is appropriate. If the neonate is very symptomatic and unable to feed, intravenous glucose with 5% to 12.5% dextrose at a rate of 4 to 6 mg/kg per min should be initiated. If the plasma glucose is between 25 and 34 mg/dL (1.4–1.9 mmol/L), intravenous glucose with 5% to 12.5% dextrose at a rate of 6 to 8 mg/kg per min[-1] should be started regardless of symptoms, and oral feedings should be allowed as tolerated.[38]

Fig 31.1

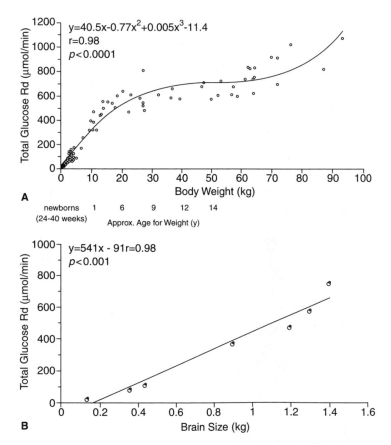

A. Total glucose rate of disappearance (Rd) (μmol/min) as a function of body weight from infancy to adulthood (n = 141; body weights range from 0.6 to 94 kg).

B. Relationship between total glucose Rd (μmol/min) and estimated brain weight from infancy to adulthood (n = 141). The data points represent mean values for subjects with brain sizes in kg of 0.14 (0.070–0.20); 0.37 (0.22–0.40); 0.44 (0.40–0.57); 0.0, 1.2, 1.3, and 1.4, respectively. Reprinted with permission. Haymond MW, Sunehag A. Controlling the sugar bowl. Regulation of glucose homeostasis in children. *Endocrinol Metab Clin North Am.* 1999;28:663–694

If the plasma glucose concentration is less than 25 mg/dL (1.4 mmol/L), it is appropriate to administer a mini bolus of 2 mL/kg of 10% dextrose (200 mg/kg) over 5 to 10 minutes, followed by an infusion rate of 6 to 8 mg/kg per min[-1]. It has been argued that a mini bolus given over 1 minute could cause hyperosmolar cerebral edema, because it exceeds glucose uptake capacity and might, if the dose is large enough, induce excessive insulin secretion, worsening the hypoglycemia.[39–41] The glucose infusion rate can be calculated with the following formula:

$$\text{glucose (mg/kg/min}^{-1}) = (\%\text{glucose in solution} \times 10) \times (\text{rate of infusion per hour}) / (60 \times \text{weight [kg]})$$

The glucose concentration should be monitored every 30 minutes. Therapy should be intensified if hypoglycemia is not corrected by the initial measures. The glucose infusion rate should be increased gradually to achieve euglycemia with the minimal concentration of glucose required. Infusion rates greater than 15 mg/kg per min[-1] should be given by a central venous catheter, except in emergency situations. The glucose infusion rate should be gradually reduced rather than abruptly terminated to avoid reactive hypoglycemia.

If euglycemia is not maintained with a dextrose infusion rate above 15 mg/kg per min, the use of corticosteroids should be considered. Hydrocortisone can be administered at a dose of 5 mg/kg per day, given intravenously or orally, divided every 12 hours, or prednisone at a dose of 2 mg/kg per day[-1], orally. Gradual decrease should be attempted once euglycemia is achieved.

Glucagon may be given in a dose of 30 μg/kg at the time of hypoglycemia to assess glycogenolysis. A response of more than 30 mg/dL at 30 minutes is confirmatory of hyperinsulinism.[35] Infants of women with diabetes may be somewhat resistant to glucagon and require a higher dose initially.

Plasma glucose concentrations should be maintained above 50 mg/dL (2.8 mmol/L) in children with persistent hyperinsulinism. This may require glucose infusion rates of higher than 20 mg/kg per min[-1] in addition to frequent enteral feedings. A central venous catheter and a nasogastric tube or gastrostomy tube may be necessary. Pharmacologic agents should be added to normalize the carbohydrate intake and decrease insulin secretion.[30,32] Diazoxide (10–20 mg/kg per day in 2–3 divided oral doses) and chlorothiazide (7–10 mg/kg per day in 2 divided oral doses) are recommended for the initial treatment and should usually be given together to enhance the response to diazoxide and decrease the risk of fluid retention. The response is variable depending on the underlying etiology of the hyperinsulinism. If the response is suboptimal or the adverse effects of fluid retention and cardiac failure from diazoxide are significant, nifedipine could be the next choice in management, at a dose of 0.25 to 2.5 mg/kg per day orally, given every 8 hours. A limited number of hyperinsulinemic children have responded to nifedipine. Monitoring of blood pressure is mandatory.

Second-line agents given by infusion or injection include octreotide, a somatostatin analogue, and glucagon. Both can cause tachyphylaxis at high doses. They should be used when the orally administered drugs have not been effective and if the child remains glucose-infusion dependent. Some argue to use both concurrently, because glucagon may stimulate insulin secretion. Glucagon has specific benefit in neonates who are hyperinsulinemic and may be infused at a rate of approximately 5 to 10 µg/kg per hour. This may be a useful adjunct as a child is being prepared for management in an experienced referral center. Prolonged glucagon usage in this manner would be associated with proteolysis and skin rashes, as seen in the glucagonoma syndrome. Octreotide can be given at a rate of 5 to 20 µg/kg per day in an intravenous or subcutaneous infusion. If octreotide is effective as an infusion, it can be converted to a chronic parenteral therapy, administered by subcutaneous injection 3 times a day.

The criterion for successful medical management of hyperinsulinism is a feeding regimen acceptable to the family with normal plasma glucose concentrations after reasonable periods of fasting (at least 6 hours in newborn infants). Failure of pharmacologic therapy in a period of a few weeks should lead to surgical treatment with either a localized or a near-total (95%–99%) pancreatectomy.[30] Recurrent hypoglycemia is to be avoided as much as possible because of its long-term deleterious effects on neurologic functioning.

Older Children

Acute hypoglycemia associated with a mismatch between insulin administration and insulin need in children with diabetes should be treated on the basis of the severity of the hypoglycemia. If the child is alert and able to drink or eat safely, treatment with 10 to 20 g of rapidly available carbohydrate in the form of fruit juice, sweetened drink, candy, or specially prepared glucose tablets is adequate for initial therapy. The response usually lasts less than 2 hours, so it should be followed by a mixed snack containing carbohydrate, fat, and protein or a scheduled meal. In children who require the assistance of another person to treat hypoglycemia, gel preparations of carbohydrates are available that can be administered orally and are effective as long as swallowing is preserved. Buccal absorption of carbohydrate is minimal. Children who are unable to eat or drink by mouth or are comatose or seizing should immediately receive a subcutaneous or intramuscular injection of glucagon of 0.02 to 0.03 mg/kg to a maximum of 1 mg. Families should be taught how much glucagon to prepare and administer for such emergencies, and the dosage should be changed as the child gains weight. Children respond within 15 minutes and then should be encouraged to eat, because the effect of the glucagon is relatively short lived and nausea and vomiting are common adverse effects of both hypoglycemia and glucagon administration.

In the emergency department or hospital, regardless of the cause of hypoglycemia, if the child is unable drink or eat, 25% dextrose (2–3 mL/kg) should be administered intravenously. This should be followed by a continued infusion of 10% dextrose, initially at a rate of 6 to 8 mg/kg per min^{-1}, to avoid rebound hypoglycemia and maintain normoglycemia. The plasma glucose concentration should be monitored and the infusion rate should be adjusted to maintain a concentration above 80 mg/dL (4.5 mmol/L). Children with hyperinsulinism will require higher rates of infusion. Long-term treatment is similar to that in the neonate (see previous section).

In disorders of fatty acid oxidation, an infusion rate of 10 mg/kg per min^{-1}, by stimulating insulin release and inhibiting lipolysis, reverses the acute metabolic disorder over days.[29] Long-term treatment of endocrine deficiency disorders and genetic metabolic disorders should be specific for the disorder.

Treatment and prevention of the ketotic hypoglycemia of accelerated starvation consists of educating parents to avoid prolonged periods of fasting and offer a bedtime snack consisting of both carbohydrate and protein. During an intercurrent illness, carbohydrate-rich drinks at frequent intervals should be given. Parents are instructed to test urine for ketones. Ketonuria precedes hypoglycemia by several hours.

Frequent feedings with glucose protect children with types I and III glycogen storage diseases from hypoglycemia and reduces hepatomegaly. Intermittent or continuous glucose can be provided during the day, and continuous glucose can be provided during the night by a nasogastric or gastrostomy tube. After 6 to 8 months of age, the infantile gut has matured to the point that it can slowly digest uncooked cornstarch. Feedings of uncooked starch (1.75–2.5 g) can be given intermittently, because it is slowly absorbed into the circulation, acting like a continuous source of glucose. It is given in water or artificially flavored drinks. Carbohydrate sources should only be glucose or glucose polymers. Blood glucose monitoring allows the creation of a successful feeding regimen.[42] Uncooked cornstarch at bedtime may help to prevent hypoglycemia in other groups of children, including children receiving insulin for diabetes.[43]

Children with metabolic dumping syndrome causing reactive hypoglycemia can be treated with an alpha-glucosidase inhibitor like acarbose (12.5–50 mg) before each feeding to slow carbohydrate absorption.[27]

Hereditary fructose intolerance is treated with elimination of fructose and sucrose. Fructose 1,6-diphosphatase deficiency is treated by elimination of fructose and sucrose and avoidance of prolonged fasting. During intercurrent illness, intravenous glucose may be necessary to arrest catabolism. Galactosemia is treated by elimination of galactose from the diet.

Hypoglycemia is the result of an alteration in the metabolic and hormonal interrelationships that balance glucose absorption, release, and production with glucose utilization. Symptomatic hypoglycemia is caused by decreased central nervous system energy levels and is reflected somewhat imperfectly in measures of blood sugar. It is the health care professional's task to recognize the signs and symptoms of hypoglycemia, document hypoglycemia in the laboratory, and obtain appropriate studies to identify the etiology. Initial symptomatic treatment of hypoglycemia will preserve brain function, but long-term management depends on identification of the cause of the energy imbalance.

References

1. McCall AL. Cerebral glucose metabolism in diabetes mellitus. *Eur J Pharmacol*. 2004;490:147–158

2. McEwen BS, Reagan LP. Glucose transporter expression in the central nervous system: relationship to synaptic function. *Eur J Pharmacol*. 2004;490:13–24

3. Wang D, Pascual J, Yang H, et al. Glut-1 deficiency syndrome: clinical and therapeutic aspects. *Ann Neurol*. 2005;57:111–118

4. Fujikawa DG, Vannucci RC, Dwyer BE, Wasterlain CE. Generalized seizures deplete brain energy reserves in normoxemic newborn monkeys. *Brain Res*. 1988;454:51–59

5. Settergren G, Lindblad BS, Persson B. Cerebral blood flow and exchange of oxygen, glucose, ketone bodies, lactate, pyruvate and amino acids in infants. *Acta Paediatr Scand*. 1976;65:343–353

6. Vannucci RC, Vannucci SJ. Hypoglycemic brain injury. *Semin Neonatol*. 2001;6:147–155

7. Mason GF, Peterson KF, Lebon V, Rothman DL, Shulman GI. Increased brain monocarboxylic acid transport and utilization in type 1 diabetes. *Diabetes*. 2006;55:929–934

8. Cornblath M, Schwartz R. Factors influencing glucose in the neonate. In: *Disorders of Carbohydrate Metabolism in Infancy*. 3rd ed. Boston, MA: Blackwell Scientific; 1991:55–86

9. Boluyt N, van Kempen A, Offringa M. Neurodevelopment after neonatal hypoglycemia: A systematic review and design of an optimal future study. *Pediatrics*. 2006;117:2231–2243

10. Heck LJ, Erenberg A. Serum glucose levels in term neonates during the first 48 hours of life. *J Pediatr.* 1987;110:119–122

11. Srinivasan G, Pildes RS, Cattamanchi G, Voora S, Lilien LD. Plasma glucose values in normal neonates: a new look. *J Pediatr.* 1986;109:114–117

12. Hawdon JM, Ward Platt MP, Aynsley-Green A. Patterns of metabolic adaptation for preterm and term infants in the first neonatal week. *Arch Dis Child.* 1992;67:357–365

13. Koh TH, Aynsley-Green A, Tarbit M, Eyre JA. Neural dysfunction during hypoglycaemia. *Arch Dis Child.* 1988;63:1353–1358

14. Pryds O, Christensen NJ, Friis-Hansen B. Increased cerebral blood flow and plasma epinephrine in hypoglycemic, preterm neonates. *Pediatrics.* 1990;85:172–176

15. Lucas A, Morley R, Cole TJ. Adverse neurodevelopmental outcome of moderate neonatal hypoglycaemia. *BMJ.* 1988;297:1304–1308

16. Duvanel CB, Fawer CL, Cotting J, Hohlfeld P, Matthieu JM. Long-term effects of neonatal hypoglycemia on brain growth and psychomotor development in small-for-gestational-age preterm infants. *J Pediatr.* 1999;134:492–498

17. Schwartz NS, Clutter WE, Shah SD, Cryer PE. Glycemic thresholds for activation of glucose counterregulatory systems are higher than the threshold for symptoms. *J Clin Invest.* 1987;79:777–781

18. Mitrakou A, Ryan C, Veneman T, et al. Hierarchy of glycemic thresholds for counterregulatory hormone secretion, symptoms, and cerebral dysfunction. *Am J Physiol.* 1991;260 (1 Pt 1):e67–e74

19. Jones TW, Boulware SD, Kraemer DT, Caprio S, Sherwin RS, Tamborlane WV. Independent effects of youth and poor diabetes control on responses to hypoglycemia in children. *Diabetes.* 1991;40:358–363

20. Cornblath M, Hawdon JM, Williams AF, et al. Controversies regarding definition of neonatal hypoglycemia: suggested operational thresholds. *Pediatrics.* 2000;105:1141–1145

21. Cryer PE. Mechanisms of hypoglycemia-associated autonomic failure and its component syndromes in diabetes. *Diabetes.* 2005;54:3592–3601

22. Nold JL, Georgieff MK. Infants of diabetic mothers. *Pediatr Clin North Am.* 2004;51: 619–637, vii

23. Weksberg R, Shuman C, Smith A. Beckwith-Wiedemann syndrome. *Am J Med Genet C Semin Med Genet.* 2005;137:12–23

24. Sabel KG, Olegard R, Mellander M, Hildingsson K. Interrelation between fatty acid oxidation and control of gluconeogenic substrates in small-for-gestational-age (SGA) infants with hypoglycemia and with normoglycemia. *Acta Paediatr Scand.* 1982;71:53–61

25. Hoe FM, Thorton PS, Wanner LA, Steinkrauss L, Simmons RA, Stanley CA. Clinical features and insulin regulation in infants with a syndrome of prolonged neonatal hyperinsulinism. *J Pediatr.* 2006;148:207–212

26. Bodamer OA, Hussein K, Morris AA, et al. Glucose and leucine kinetics in idiopathic ketotic hypoglycemia. *Arch Dis Child.* 2006;91:483–486

27. Ng DD, Ferry RJ Jr, Kelly A, Weinzimer SA, Stanley CA, Katz LE. Acarbose treatment of postprandial hypoglycemia in children after Nissen fundoplication. *J Pediatr.* 2001;139: 877–879

28. de Lonlay P, Giurgea I, Sempoux C, Touati G, Jabert F, Rahier J, et al. Dominantly inherited hyperinsulinaemic hypoglycaemia. *J Inherit Metab Dis*. 2005;28:267–276

29. Vianey-Liaud C, Divry P, Gregersen N, Mathieu M. The inborn errors of mitochondrial fatty acid oxidation. *J Inherit Metab Dis*. 1987;10:159–200

30. Aynsley-Green A, Hussain K, Hall J, et al. Practical management of hyperinsulinism in infancy. *Arch Dis Child Fetal Neonatal Ed*. 2000;82:F98–F107

31. Raizen DM, Brooks-Kayal A, Steinkrauss L, Tennekoon GI, Stanley CA, Kelly A. Central nervous system hyperexcitability associated with glutamate dehydrogenase gain of function mutations. *J Pediatr*. 2005;146:388–394

32. Hussain K, Aynsley-Green A, Stanley C. Medications used in the treatment of hypoglycemia due to congenital hyperinsulinism of infancy (HI). *Pediatr Endocrinol Rev*. 2004;2:163–167

33. Warshaw JB, Curry E. Comparison of serum carnitine and ketone body concentrations in breast- and formula-fed newborn infants. *J Pediatr*. 1980;97:122–125

34. Bachrach BE, Weinstein DA, Orho-Melander M, Burgess A, Wolfsdorf JI. Glycogen synthase deficiency (glycogen storage disease type 0) presenting with hyperglycemia and glycosuria: report of three new mutations. *J Pediatr*. 2002;140:781–783

35. Finegold DN, Stanley CA, Baker L. Glycemic response to glucagon during fasting hypoglycemia: an aid in the diagnosis of hyperinsulinism. *J Pediatr*. 1980;96:257–259

36. Haymond MW, Sunehag A. Controlling the sugar bowl. Regulation of glucose homeostasis in children. *Endocrinol Metab Clin North Am*. 1999;28:663–694

37. Hussain K, Seppanen M, Nanto-Salonen K, et al. The diagnosis of ectopic focal hyperinsulinism of infancy with (^{18}F)-dopa positron emission tomography. *J Clin Endocrinol Metab*. 2006;91:2839–2842

38. Cornblath M. Neonatal hypoglycemia. In: Donn SM, Fisher CW, eds. *Risk Management Techniques in Perinatal and Neonatal Practice*. Armonk, NY: Futura Publishing; 1996:437–448

39. Cowett RM, Farrag HM. Neonatal glucose metabolism. In: Cowett RM, ed. *Principles of Perinatal-Neonatal Metabolism*. 2nd ed. New York, NY: Springer-Verlag; 1998:683–722

40. Farrag HM, Cowett RM. Hypoglycemia in the newborn, including infant of a diabetic mother. In: Lifshitz F, ed. *Pediatric Endocrinology*. 4th rev exp ed. New York, NY: Marcel Dekker; 2003:541–574

41. Mehta A. Prevention and management of neonatal hypoglycaemia. *Arch Dis Child Fetal Neonatal Ed*. 1994;70:F54–59

42. Wolfsdorf JI, Crigler JF Jr. Cornstarch regimens for nocturnal treatment of young adults with type 1 glycogen storage disease. *Am J Clin Nutr*. 1997;65:1507–1511

43. Kaufman FR, Devgan S. Use of uncooked cornstarch to avert nocturnal hypoglycemia in children and adolescents with type 1 diabetes. *J Diabetes Complications*. 1996;10:84–87

32 Hyperlipidemia and Prevention of Cardiovascular Disease

Coronary artery disease and blood cholesterol concentrations are statistically related. Although the incidence of coronary artery disease is now decreasing in the United States, it remains the leading cause of death for adults in the United States and most industrialized countries. Experts have known about the familial occurrence of coronary heart disease since the 19th century; however, the familial risk factors have been delineated only in recent decades. The Framingham study[1] and subsequent studies have identified the following risk factors for coronary heart disease:

1. Family history
2. Male gender
3. Low serum concentration of high-density lipoprotein (HDL)
4. High concentrations of serum total cholesterol and low-density lipoprotein (LDL)
5. Hypertension
6. Cigarette smoking
7. Impairment of carbohydrate tolerance
8. Lack of physical activity
9. High serum triglyceride concentration

Not all investigators agree that a high concentration of plasma triglycerides is an independent risk factor for coronary heart disease. Although a direct correlation is evident in univariate analysis, this effect is lost when the influences of obesity, diabetes mellitus, and total cholesterol and HDL concentrations are removed.[1]

In 1992, and again most recently in 1998, the American Academy of Pediatrics (AAP) endorsed the findings and recommendations of the Expert Panel on Blood Cholesterol in Children and Adolescents of the National Cholesterol Education Program (NCEP).[2-4] The AAP and the NCEP found that:

1. Certain inborn or acquired diseases accompanied by hypercholesterolemia are associated with premature atherosclerosis.
2. Serum cholesterol concentrations are higher than usual in people with coronary heart disease.
3. People with high serum cholesterol concentrations develop coronary heart disease more often than those with normal concentrations.

4. The mortality rate from coronary heart disease in different countries varies in relation to the average blood cholesterol concentrations (and with dietary fat and animal protein intake).
5. Experimentally induced hypercholesterolemia in animals is associated with atherosclerotic deposits.
6. Atherosclerotic plaques contain lipids similar in composition to those in the blood.

Evidence that atherosclerosis begins in childhood includes the following:

1. In autopsies of black and white males and females between 15 and 19 years of age, the coronary arteries showed fatty streaks in 71% to 83% and raised atherosclerotic lesions in 7% to 22%.[5]
2. When bodies of US soldiers killed at a mean age of 22 years were examined, 77% of those from the Korean Conflict[6] and 45% of those from the Vietnam War[7] showed evidence of coronary vessel atherosclerosis.
3. American adolescents who died of nonatherosclerotic causes show atherosclerotic changes of a magnitude directly related to postmortem LDL and very low-density lipoprotein (VLDL) concentrations inversely related to HDL concentrations.[8]

Lipoproteins

Lipoproteins are necessary to make fats soluble so they can be transported in the plasma. All lipoproteins contain an outer polar layer of phospholipid, unesterified cholesterol, and protein (called apoprotein). The inner, nonpolar core contains cholesterol ester and triglyceride in varying proportions. The types of lipoproteins are:

1. Chylomicrons, which are formed from dietary fat and enter the plasma via the thoracic duct and are removed from the blood by the activity of lipoprotein lipase (LPL) with the fatty acids, stored in adipose tissue as triglyceride, or catabolized by the liver. They do not form other lipoproteins.
2. Very low-density lipoproteins (also called prelipoproteins) are formed from dietary glucose and nonesterified fatty acids in the liver and are then secreted into the plasma. The outer surface of VLDLs contains apoproteins B-100 and E. The LPL on the capillary endothelium of adipose tissue and cardiac and skeletal muscle partially metabolizes VLDLs to nonesterified fatty acids for storage or for energy, with a remnant remaining. The apoprotein E allows the remnant to be taken up by the liver. Several types of hyperlipoproteinemia have been identified.[9]

3. If the remnant also contains apoprotein B-100, it can be used for synthesis of LDL in the liver.
4. Low-density lipoprotein is formed in the liver from VLDL remnants containing apoprotein B-100; LDL is an important source of cholesterol for peripheral tissues. An important step in the regulation of cholesterol metabolism is the attachment of LDL to receptor sites on cell surfaces.
5. High-density lipoprotein is secreted by the liver and small intestine and is important in helping to remove cholesterol from cells (high concentrations are protective; low concentrations are a strong risk factor for coronary heart disease).

Types of Hyperlipidemia

The hereditary types of hyperlipidemias are sometimes difficult to distinguish from the hyperlipidemias related to diabetes and other conditions, but an attempt should be made to do so by family studies and other tests.[9,10]

Type I

Type I hyperlipoproteinemia is found in children and is usually associated with pancreatitis and abdominal pain. The triglycerides in this disorder are primarily chylomicron triglycerides. The activity of LPL is diminished or absent. This enzyme is responsible for hydrolysis and removal of chylomicrons from the blood. Thus, the pathophysiologic mechanism is decreased triglyceride catabolism. Type I hyperlipoproteinemia is relatively rare; it may occur secondarily in children with lupus erythematosus, pancreatitis, or immunologic disorders.

Type II-a

Type II-a hyperlipoproteinemia, characterized by high serum concentrations of total cholesterol and LDL, is probably the most common of the 5 lipoprotein disorders to manifest in childhood. The homozygous form can be seen during the first year of life, and the differential diagnosis can be made on the basis of the following:

1. Serum total cholesterol concentration higher than 12.95 mmol/L (500 mg/dL)
2. Concentrations of LDL about twice that of heterozygotes in the same kindred
3. Both parents with high serum total cholesterol concentration
4. Xanthomas appearing before 10 years of age
5. Vascular disease before 20 years of age
6. Exclusion of clinically similar secondary hyperlipidemias

In the heterozygous condition, usually no skin xanthomas are present, and the serum cholesterol concentration is lower than 12.95 mmol/L (500 mg/dL); yet, these individuals have a definite predisposition to coronary heart disease during early adulthood. The basic metabolic defect is a lack of functional LDL receptors on the cell membrane, with 3 different classes of mutations.[11] As a result of the LDL not attaching to the cell membrane, cholesterol is not released to suppress the rate-limiting enzyme in cholesterol synthesis, hydroxymethylglutaryl-coenzyme A (CoA) reductase.

Type II-b

Type II-b hyperlipoproteinemia, which includes familial combined hyperlipidemia, is defined as high serum triglyceride and total cholesterol concentrations, with concomitant increased LDL and VLDL. This is the third most frequent of the types with onset during childhood, but the situation frequently is confusing, because the parents may have other types of hyperlipoproteinemia and because of the variations in the cholesterol and triglyceride concentrations caused by changes in diet and exercise.

Type III

Type III hyperlipoproteinemia, "floating beta," with the LDL having an abnormal density and consisting of an abnormal protein, is rare. The onset is usually after 20 years of age. The basic defect is thought to be in the conversion of VLDL to LDL (abnormal remnant catabolism) because of an abnormal apoprotein E. Increased remnants, VLDL, chylomicrons, and apoprotein E are all present. Xanthomas may occur, and early coronary and peripheral vascular disease have been reported.

Type IV

Type IV hyperlipoproteinemia, "familial hypertriglyceridemia," is associated with high concentrations of serum triglycerides and is the second most common of the disorders found in children, although the increase in serum triglyceride concentration may not occur in some patients until a later age. This condition is a monogenic autosomally inherited disorder. It involves an increase in production and secretion of triglyceride-rich VLDL. High triglyceride concentrations can occur in relation to other factors, such as infrequent exercise, stress, an inadequate period of fasting before obtaining blood samples, diabetes, and obesity. Establishing that the patient has the genetic disease and excluding another cause for the elevation is important. This is best accomplished by studying parents and other family members as well as the patient.

Type V

Type V hyperlipoproteinemia is rare in childhood and is associated with high triglyceride concentrations related to increased chylomicrons and high VLDL concentration. This condition may be primarily familial or it may be secondary to diabetes, nephrotic syndrome, or hypothyroidism. The onset may be similar to that of type I, although it occurs in adulthood rather than childhood.

Prevention of Atherosclerosis and Prudent Lifestyle and Diet

In 1983, 1986, 1992, and 1998,[2,3,11,12] the AAP made recommendations about the risks of atherosclerosis and, when possible, the avoidance of risks. Of these, avoiding smoking, increasing physical activity, and receiving treatment for hypertension and diabetes are emphasized. After 1 year of age, it was recommended that a varied diet be followed to ensure nutritional adequacy. Decreased consumption of saturated fats, cholesterol, and sodium and increased intake of monounsaturated and polyunsaturated fats were recommended (see Appendices X and Y). In these statements, no restriction of fat or cholesterol intake was recommended for infants younger than 2 years, because this is a period of rapid growth and neurologic development with high requirements for energy. Early recognition and treatment of obesity and hypertension, a regular exercise program, and counseling about the dangers of smoking were recommended for all children older than 2 years. Intake of skim or partly skimmed milk still is not recommended during the first year of life because of the high protein and electrolyte concentrations. Furthermore, the low caloric density of these milks increases the volume necessary to satisfy caloric requirements. For children between the ages of 12 months and 2 years, low-fat dairy products should be considered if the child's body mass index is at the 85th percentile or greater or if there is a strong family history of obesity. It is recommended that less than 10% of calories in the diet come from saturated fat. The optimal total fat intake was suggested to be approximately 30% of calories for children older than 2 years.

Although some studies have shown safety in lowering fat intakes in infants,[13] the transition to a lower-fat diet beginning at the age of 2 years requires special consideration. Approximately half of the calories in the diet of the exclusively breastfed infant come from the fat content of the milk. As solids are introduced during the first and second years of life, the percentage of calories in the diet contributed by fat decreases. At 2 to 3 years of age, if only 30% of total calories are derived from fat, for some infants, the protein

V

content would have to provide 15% or more of calories for the diet to meet the recommended dietary allowances for minerals. Early childhood, then, should be considered a transition period during which the fat and cholesterol content of the diet should gradually decrease to recommended amounts. Particular care should be taken to avoid excessive restriction of dietary fat. Care should also be taken to avoid intake of excess calories, which may lead to obesity. The consumption of lower-fat dairy products and lean meats, which are critical sources of protein, iron, and calcium, as well as grains, cereals, fruits, and vegetables should be encouraged throughout childhood and adolescence.

The NCEP Expert Panel on Blood Cholesterol Levels in Children and Adolescents and the AAP offer the following specific recommendations for the population older than 2 years[3,4]:

1. Nutritional adequacy should be achieved by eating a wide variety of foods.
2. Energy (calories) should be adequate to support growth and to reach or maintain desirable body weight and avoid development of obesity.
3. The following intake pattern is recommended: saturated fatty acids, less than 10% of total energy intake (serum total cholesterol concentration appears most responsive to dietary saturated fatty acids); total fat (averaged over several days), no less than 20% of total calories and no more than 30% of calories; and dietary cholesterol, less than 300 mg/day.

Carbohydrate content of the diet should be 55% to 60% of the calories, of which the majority should be complex carbohydrates. Fiber is an important dietary constituent that can affect blood cholesterol concentrations. Current recommendations for fiber intake in children range from 0.5 g/kg to approximately 12 g/1000 kcal. Protein should provide 10% to 15% of dietary calories.

This diet is similar to the diet recommended by the American Heart Association for moderate reduction of serum cholesterol concentrations. Similarly composed diets may be useful in controlling obesity.

Screening for Hyperlipidemia

The AAP endorses an individualized approach to screening and treating children (older than 2 years) and adolescents whose risk of developing coronary vascular disease as adults can be identified through family history. The family history should be updated periodically to include information on family members who had heart attack, stroke, hypertension, hyperlipidemia, diabetes, or obesity. If a positive family history is present, then cholesterol screening is indicated for children. If the family history cannot be ascertained and other risk factors are present, screening should be performed at the discretion of the physician.

AAP

The American Academy of Pediatrics states:

1. The population approach to a healthful diet should be recommended to all children older than 2 years according to the Dietary Guidelines for Americans. This includes the use of low-fat dairy products. For children between 12 months and 2 years of age with a BMI the ≥85th percentile or a family history of obesity, dyslipidemia, or CVD, the use of reduced-fat milk should be considered.

2. The individual approach for children and adolescents at higher risk of CVD and with a high concentration of LDL includes recommended changes in diet with nutritional counseling and other lifestyle interventions, such as increased physical activity.

3. The most current recommendation is to screen children and adolescents with a positive family history of dyslipidemia or premature (≤55 years of age for men and ≤65 years of age for women) CVD or dyslipidemia. It is also recommended that pediatric patients for whom family history is not known or those with other CVD risk factors, such as overweight (BMI ≥85th percentile, <95th percentile), obesity (BMI ≥95th percentile), hypertension (blood pressure ≥95th percentile), cigarette smoking, or diabetes mellitus, be screened with a fasting lipid profile.

4. For these children, the first screening should take place after 2 years of age but no later than 10 years of age. Screening before 2 years of age is not recommended.

5. A fasting lipid profile is the recommended approach to screening, because there is no currently available noninvasive method to assess atherosclerotic cardiovascular disease in children. This screening should occur in the context of well-child and health maintenance visits. If values are within reference range on initial screening, the patient should be retested in 3 to 5 years.

6. In pediatric patients who are overweight or obese and have a high triglyceride concentration or a low HDL concentration, weight management is the primary treatment. This includes improvement of diet with nutritional counseling and increased physical activity to produce improved energy balance.

7. For patients 10 years and older with an LDL concentration ≥190 mg/dL (or ≥160 mg/dL with a family history of early heart disease or 2 or more additional risk factors present or ≥130 mg/dL if diabetes mellitus is present), pharmacologic intervention should be considered. The initial goal is to lower LDL concentration to <160 mg/dL. However, targets as low as 130 mg/dL or even 110 mg/dL maybe warranted when there is a strong family history of CVD, especially with other risk factors including obesity, diabetes mellitus, the metabolic syndrome, and other higher-risk situations.

Pediatrics. 2008;122:198–208

The poor predictive value of a total cholesterol concentration for a high LDL concentration[14] (high LDL concentrations in childhood have better predictive value for adult cardiovascular events, but are still imperfect) and the imperfect tracking of blood cholesterol concentrations from childhood to adulthood[15,16] are among the factors that weigh against a recommendation for universal cholesterol testing. Universal screening by any method other than family history will continue to be inadvisable until tests become available that better predict later coronary vascular disease. A high total blood cholesterol concentration in childhood is only a risk factor for high blood cholesterol concentration as an adult, which in turn is a risk factor for coronary vascular disease.[17]

Children with high blood cholesterol concentrations undoubtedly will be missed by selective screening.[18–20] Family history may be unavailable or unknown. However, a universal (population-based) approach to dietary modification of fat and cholesterol intake and the potential reversibility of coronary vascular lesions when diet and drug therapy are used at older ages suggests that selective screening of children is an appropriate recommendation. Children whose parents or grandparents had a documented myocardial infarction, positive results on a coronary angiogram, or cerebrovascular or peripheral vascular disease before the age of 55 years qualify for screening blood tests. Children (older than 2 years) whose parents have a serum total cholesterol concentration greater than or equal to 6.2 mmol/L (240 mg/dL) should also be screened. For these children, the initial test should be determination of blood lipoprotein concentrations, obtained after a 12-hour fast (or 8 hours for children who cannot fast for 12 hours). Cholesterol values alone (without triglycerides) can be determined without a fast. Fig 32.1 presents an algorithm for screening and initiating therapy.

For a youth at risk, blood determinations are recommended. For initial screening of those whose parents have high concentrations of serum total cholesterol or children with a family history of cardiovascular disease, the child should fast for 12 hours. Blood is drawn with the patient in the sitting position. Concentrations of total cholesterol, HDL, and triglycerides are determined; the LDL concentration is estimated from these. Some laboratories can measure LDL concentration directly. Interpretations are provided in Table 32.1 for children and adolescents. Appropriate examinations or tests for secondary causes of hypercholesterolemia should be performed (Table 32.2) before treatment. To accomplish the more restrictive diet, the meat serving size should be decreased and the calories from the other food groups should be increased (see Table 32.3).

Fig 32.1
Classification, education, and follow-up based on LDL concentration (from the NCEP[4]).
To convert mg/dL to mmol/L, multiply by 0.02586.

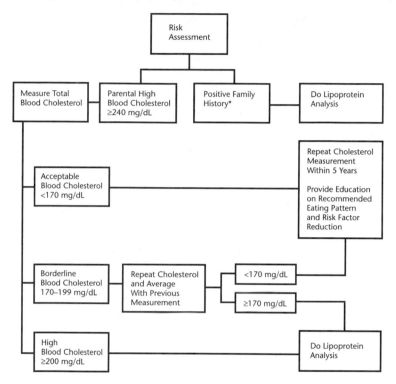

* Cardiovascular risk reduction in high-risk pediatric patients: a scientific statement from the American Heart Association Expert Panel on Population and Prevention Science; the Councils on Cardiovascular Disease in the Young, Epidemiology and Prevention, Nutrition, Physical Activity and Metabolism, High Blood Pressure Research, Cardiovascular Nursing, and the Kidney in Heart Disease; and the Interdisciplinary Working Group on Quality of Care and Outcomes Research. *Circulation.* 2006;114:2710–2738

V

Table 32.1
Interpretation of Cholesterol Concentrations for Children and Adolescents*

Term	Total Cholesterol, mg/dL	LDL, mg/dL
Acceptable	<170	<110
Borderline	170–199	110–129
High	>200	>130

* From the NCEP.[4] To convert mg/dL to mmol/L, multiply by 0.02586.

Table 32.2
Causes of Secondary Hypercholesterolemia

Exogenous
Drugs
  Oral contraceptives, corticosteroids,
  isotretinoin, thiazides, anticonvulsants,
  beta-blockers, anabolic steroids
Alcohol
Obesity
	Storage Diseases
	Glycogen storage diseases
	Sphingolipidoses

	Obstructive Liver Diseases Biliary atresia Biliary cirrhosis
Endocrine and Metabolic Hypothyroidism Diabetes mellitus Lipodystrophy Pregnancy Idiopathic hypercalcemia	Chronic Renal Diseases Nephrotic syndrome
	Others Anorexia nervosa Progeria Collagen vascular disease Klinefelter syndrome

Table 32.3
Serving Sizes in Food Groups

Bread, Cereal, Rice, and Pasta Group (Grains Group)—Whole Grain and Refined
- 1 slice of bread
- About 1 cup of ready-to-eat cereal
- 1 cup of cooked cereal, rice, or pasta

Vegetable Group
- 1 cup of raw leafy vegetables
- ½ cup of other vegetables—cooked or raw
- 1 cup of vegetable juice

Fruit Group
- 1 medium apple, banana, orange, pear
- 1 cup of chopped, cooked, or canned fruit
- 1 cup of fruit juice

Milk, Yogurt, and Cheese Group (Milk Group)
- 2 cups of fat-free milk or yogurt
- 1 oz of natural cheese (such as cheddar)
- 2 oz of processed cheese (such as American)

Meat, Poultry, Fish, Dry Beans, Eggs, and Nuts Group (Meat and Beans Group)
- 2–3 oz of cooked lean meat, poultry, or fish
- ½ cup of cooked dry beans or ½ cup of tofu (count as 1 oz of lean meat)
- 2 oz of soy burger or 1 egg (count as 1 oz of lean meat)
- 2 tbsp of peanut butter or ⅓ cup of nuts (count as 1 oz of meat)

Treatment

Treatment should be initiated after the diagnosis of hyperlipidemia is confirmed by 2 separate blood tests performed at least 2 weeks apart. Reference distributions of serum lipoprotein concentrations by age and gender for older children and adolescents have recently been published.[21] Dietary therapy is the first mode of treatment in almost all instances, whether or not elevations are attributable to a genetic cause. A 3-day diet record is extremely helpful for suggesting changes; this record should be as typical as possible of the child's usual intake. Consultation with a dietitian or nutritionist is helpful.

The population diet (Table 32.4) suggests an average intake of saturated fatty acids less than 10% of total calories, total fat no more than 30% of calories, and cholesterol less than 300 mg/day. The polyunsaturated fatty acids constitute up to 10% and the monounsaturated fatty acids constitute 10% to 15% of the total calories.

Avoidance of smoking, the value of exercise, attaining weight appropriate for age and body build, and correction or treatments of other risk factors are emphasized. If, after 3 months, desired lipid concentrations are not achieved, a more restrictive diet is initiated. Saturated fatty acids are reduced to approximately 7% of the caloric intake, and intake of cholesterol is reduced to less than 200 mg/day. Dietary fat must be even further restricted in patients with type I hyperlipoproteinemia to achieve lower plasma triglyceride concentrations.

Table 32.4
Diets for Control of Cholesterol*

Nutrient	Recommended Intake	
	Population Diet	More Restrictive Diet
Total fat	Average of no more than 30% of total calories and no less than 20%	Same as step I diet[†]
Saturated fatty acids	Less than 10% of total calories	Less than 7% of total calories
Polyunsaturated fatty acids	Up to 10% of total calories	Same as step I diet[†]
Monounsaturated fatty acids	Remaining dietary fat calories	Same as step I diet[†]
Cholesterol	Less than 300 mg/day	Less than 200 mg/day
Carbohydrates	About 55% of total calories	Same as step I diet[†]
Protein	About 15% of total calories	Same as step I diet[†]
Calories	To promote growth and development	Same as step I diet[†]

* Adapted from the NCEP[4] and AAP.[3]
[†] For an explanation of the step I diet, see Table 32.5.

The NCEP Panel for Children and Adolescents recommends that after an adequate trial of diet therapy has been completed (6 months to 1 year), drug therapy should be considered in children 10 years or older under the following conditions:

1. If LDL concentration remains above 4.9 mmol/L (190 mg/dL); or
2. If LDL concentration remains above 4.1 mmol/L (160 mg/dL) **and** there is a positive family history of cardiovascular disease before age 55; **or** 2 or more other risk factors for cardiovascular disease are present.

The goal of drug therapy is to achieve an LDL concentration to approach 2.85 mmol/L (110 mg/dL). Drugs recommended for children and adolescents are the bile acid sequestrants because of their apparent safety. Hydroxymethylglutaryl-CoA reductase inhibitors (statins) are also recommended for routine use in children and adolescents, because clinical trials of these agents in children have now been completed.[22–25] Several short-term studies of the use of hydroxymethylglutaryl-CoA reductase inhibitors in adolescents have shown their efficacy, acceptability, and safety.[26,27] However, because the long-term effects of these drugs have not been evaluated, careful monitoring of liver function and the presence of skeletal myolysis should be regularly assessed throughout childhood and adolescence. In addition, ezetimibe, which blocks cholesterol absorption in the gastrointestinal tract, can also be used in children and adolescents. Niacin, which is most effective for raising HDL concentrations, is not generally recommended for use in children because of adverse effects of flushing.

Table 32.5

Number of Servings From Each of the Food Groups for the Step I Diet*

Food Groups	Children 2 to 6 y, Women, Some Older Adults (approx 1600 kcal)	Older Children, Teen Girls, Active Women, Most Men, (approx 2200 kcal)	Teen Boys, Active Men (approx 2800 kcal)
Bread, cereal, rice, and pasta group (grains group)—especially whole grain	6	9	11
Vegetable group	3	4	5
Fruit group	2 or 3	2 or 3	2 or 3
Meat, poultry, fish, dry beans, eggs, and nut group, (meat and beans group—preferably lean or low fat)	2, for a total of 5 oz	2, for a total of 6 oz	3, for a total of 7 oz

* Adapted from *Dietary Guidelines for Americans.*[28]

References

1. Kannel WB, Castelli WP, Gordon T. Cholesterol in the prediction of atherosclerotic disease. New perspectives based on the Framingham study. *Ann Intern Med.* 1979;90:85–91

2. American Academy of Pediatrics, Committee on Nutrition. Statement on cholesterol. *Pediatrics.* 1992;90:469–473

3. American Academy of Pediatrics, Committee on Nutrition. Cholesterol in childhood. *Pediatrics.* 1998;101:141–147

4. National Cholesterol Education Program (NCEP): highlights of the report of the Expert Panel on Blood Cholesterol Levels in Children and Adolescents. *Pediatrics.* 1992;89:495–501

5. Strong JP, McGill HC Jr. The pediatric aspects of atherosclerosis. *J Atherosclerosis Res.* 1969;9:251–265

6. Enos WF Jr, Beyer JC, Holmes RH. Pathogenesis of coronary disease in American soldiers killed in Korea. *JAMA.* 1955;158:912–914

7. McNamara JJ, Molot MA, Stremple JF, Cutting RT. Coronary artery disease in combat casualties in Vietnam. *JAMA.* 1971;216:1185–1187

8. Strong JP, Malcom GT, McMahan CA, et al. Prevalence and extent of atherosclerosis in adolescents and young adults: implications for prevention from the Pathobiological Determinants of Atherosclerosis in Youth Study. *JAMA.* 1999;281:727–735

9. Fredrickson DS, Goldstein JL, Brown MS. The familial hyperlipoproteinemias. In: Stanbury JB, Wyngaarden JB, Fredrickson DS, eds. *The Metabolic Basis of Inherited Disease.* 4th ed. New York, NY: McGraw-Hill Book Co; 1978:604–655

10. Havel RJ, Kane JP. Introduction: structure and metabolism of plasma lipoproteins. In: Scriver CR, Beaudet AL, Sly WS, Valle D, eds. *The Metabolic Basis of Inherited Disease.* Vol 1. 6th ed. New York, NY: McGraw-Hill Book Co; 1989:1129–1138

11. Goldstein JL, Brown MS. The LDL receptor defect in familial hypercholesterolemia. Implications for pathogenesis and therapy. *Med Clin North Am.* 1982; 66:335–362

12. American Academy of Pediatrics, Committee on Nutrition. Toward a prudent diet for children. *Pediatrics.* 1983;71:78–80

13. Simell O, Niinikoski H, Viikari J, Rask-Nissila L, Tammi A, Ronnemaa T. Cardiovascular disease risk factors in young children in the STRIP baby project. Special Turku Coronary Risk Factor Intervention Project for Children. *Ann Med.* 1999;31(suppl 1):55–61

14. American Academy of Pediatrics, Committee on Nutrition. Prudent life-style for children: dietary fat and cholesterol. *Pediatrics.* 1986;78:521–525

15. Dennison BA, Kikuchi DA, Srinivasan SR, Webber LS, Berenson GS. Serum total cholesterol screening for the detection of elevated low-density lipoprotein in children and adolescents: the Bogalusa Heart Study. *Pediatrics.* 1990;85:472–479

16. Lauer RM, Clarke WR. Use of cholesterol measurements in childhood for the prediction of adult hypercholesterolemia. The Muscatine Study. *JAMA.* 1990;264:3034–3038

17. Stuhldreher WL, Orchard TJ, Donahue RP, Kuller LH, Gloninger MF, Drash AL. Cholesterol screening in childhood: sixteen-year Beaver County Lipid Study experience. *J Pediatr.* 1991;119:551–556

18. Newman TB, Browner WS, Hulley SB. The case against childhood cholesterol screening. *JAMA*. 1990;264:3039–3043

19. Griffin TC, Christoffel KK, Binns HJ, McGuire PA. Family history evaluation as a predictive screen for childhood hypercholesteremia. Pediatric Practice Research Group. *Pediatrics*. 1989;84:365–373

20. Dennison BA, Kikuchi DA, Srinivasan SR, Webber LS, Berenson GS. Parental history of cardiovascular disease as an indication for screening for lipoprotein abnormalities in children. *J Pediatr*. 1989;115:186–194

21. Joliffe C, Janssen I. Distribution of lipoproteins by age and gender in adolescents. *Circulation*. 2006;114:1056–1062

22. Stein EA, Illingworth DR, Kwiterovich PO Jr, et al. Efficacy and safety of lovastatin in adolescent males with heterozygous familial hypercholesterolemia: a randomized controlled trial. *JAMA*. 1999;281:137–144

23. Lambert M, Lupien PJ, Gagne C, et al. Treatment of familial hypercholesterolemia in children and adolescents: effect of lovastatin. Canadian Lovastatin in Children Study Group. *J Pediatr*. 2003;143:74–80

24. deJongh S, Ose L, Szamosi T, et al. Efficacy and safety of statin therapy in children with familial hypercholesterolemia: a randomized, double-blind, placebo-controlled trial with simvastatin. *Circulation*. 2002;106:2231–2237

25. Belay B, Belamarich PF, Tom-Revzon C. The use of statins in pediatrics: knowledge base, limitations, and future directions. *Pediatrics*. 2007;119:370–380

26. McCrindle BW, Ose L, Marais AD. Efficacy and safety of atorvastatin in children and adolescents with familial hypercholesterolaemia or severe hyperlipidemia: a multicenter, randomized, placebo-controlled trial. *J Pediatr*. 2003;143:74–80

27. Wiegman A, Hutten BA, deGroot E, et al. Efficacy and safety of statin therapy in children with familial hypercholesterolemia: a randomized controlled trial. *JAMA*. 2004;292:331–337

28. US Department of Agriculture, US Department of Health and Human Services. *Nutrition and Your Health: Dietary Guidelines for Americans*. 5th ed. Washington, DC: US Government Printing Office; 2000

Pediatric Obesity

Definition and Epidemiology

Definition

Obesity may be defined functionally as a maladaptive increase in the mass of somatic fat stores. An ideal medical definition of obesity in children will reflect both the likelihood that the child will become an obese adult and the present and future risk of adiposity-related morbidity. In evaluating diagnostic criteria for obesity, the following should be considered:

1. The risk of persistence of pediatric obesity into adulthood increases with age, independent of the length of time that the child has been obese.[1-3]
2. The risks of adiposity-related morbidities, such as cardiovascular disease, type 2 diabetes mellitus, asthma, orthopedic disease, and certain cancers, are strongly influenced by family history of such morbidities, regardless of whether affected family members are obese.[4-7]
3. Growth patterns are familial. A mildly overweight child with a family history of excessive weight gain in adulthood may be at greater risk of subsequent obesity than a more severely overweight child with a negative family history of obesity in adulthood.[4,8,9]

Direct assessment of body fatness by hydrodensitometry (underwater weighing) or various radiologic methods (dual-energy x-ray absorptiometry) is not feasible in the pediatrician's office. Plots of weight, height, and weight-for-height measures versus normative "standards" are the indices of body fatness that are generally used by clinicians to assess body fatness in children. However, these standards are neither sufficiently sensitive to identify all children at risk of adiposity-related morbidity nor sufficiently specific to identify only children at such risk. Interpretation of these weight and height measures must be highly individualized for each child, and the morbidity risk should be assessed within the context of family history and other risk factors for disease.

Body mass index (BMI, weight [kg]/[height {m}]^2) is a surrogate measure of body fatness that correlates quite well with direct measures of body fatness within a population.[10,11] An American Medical Association expert panel on obesity has suggested that adults with a BMI >25 be defined as overweight or "at risk" of adiposity-related morbidity and those with BMI >30 be defined as obese.[12] Because normative values for BMI are highly age dependent and BMI values in children are significantly lower than in adults at the same level of adiposity[13] (see Table 33.1), these adult definitions based on BMI cannot be used in children.

Table 33.1
Mean BMI of Children Enrolled in NHES II or III (1963–1970) or NHANES III (1988–1994)[13]

| Age (y) | BMI | | | |
| | Males | | Females | |
	NHES II or III	NHANES III	NHES II or III	NHANES III
6	15.6	16.3	15.4	16.1
7	15.9	16.5	15.8	16.9
8	16.3	17.3	15.4	17.3
9	16.9	18.0	17.0	18.2
10	17.1	18.4	17.6	18.4
11	17.9	19.4	18.2	19.4
12	18.4	20.1	19.2	20.2
13	19.4	20.5	19.9	21.8
14	20.2	22.3	20.8	22.4
15	20.9	22.3	21.4	21.9
16	21.3	22.3	21.9	23.0
17	22.1	23.4	21.7	23.3

Expert panels from the International Life Sciences Institute and American Academy of Pediatrics have suggested a classification system for overweight in children similar to that described above in adults.[12] Children with BMI between the 85th and 95th percentile for age and gender based on National Health and Nutrition Examination Survey I (NHANES I, 1971–1974) data are defined as "at risk" of overweight, and those with BMI greater than the 95th percentile are defined as overweight.[14] It should also be noted that BMI may incorrectly label individuals at the extremes of body composition as nonoverweight in the case of someone with a high percentage of body fat but low body weight or as overweight in the case of the extremely muscular individual with a low percentage of body fat but high body weight.[15] However, in most cases, the clinician should be able to visually distinguish the obese child from the extremely muscular child. If this distinction cannot readily be made (ie, the clinician is uncertain whether a child with an elevated BMI has an elevated body weight predominantly attributable to an abnormally large adipose tissue or lean body mass), then body fat can be evaluated further by triceps skinfold thickness. Growth charts of age- and sex-specific BMI percentiles are now available and can be downloaded directly from the Centers for Disease Control and Prevention Web site (http://www.cdc.gov/nchs/data/ad/ad314.pdf) (see also Appendix D). It should also be noted that body fat distribution at any given level of body fatness may constitute an independent risk factor for adiposity-related morbidity.[16,17]

Epidemiology

Sociodemographic Data

In the United States, obesity is more prevalent among children raised in urban communities and in smaller families. The prevalence of obesity also varies among different ethnic groups (more prevalent among black and Hispanic individuals), geographic regions (more prevalent in the northeast than in the Midwest, in the Midwest than in the south, and in the south than in the west; more prevalent in urban areas than in rural areas) and socioeconomic classes (more prevalent in poorer, less-educated families, families with less access to recreational areas or single-parent/older-parent families; less prevalent in large families).[18-28] These strong demographic trends demonstrate that there is potent environmental biasing of whatever genetic predispositions toward obesity may exist.

Prenatal and Postnatal Influences on Adiposity and Comorbidities

Obesity and adiposity-related comorbidities, such as type 2 diabetes mellitus, are the result of the interactions of genetic susceptibility to store excess calories as fat as well as heritable predilection toward insulin resistance, impaired beta-cell function, dyslipidemia, hypertension, etc, with an environment that favors the expression of these susceptibilities. The intrauterine environment and the patterns of energy intake and expenditure that are established in childhood influence later patterns of energy storage, feeding behavior, and morbidity risk. As discussed below, it is clear that the infrastructure underlying the susceptibility to adult diseases is established through gene x environment interactions beginning at the moment of conception, if not before.

Prenatal Undernutrition

Low birth weight, defined in various studies as full term newborn infants weighing less than 2500–3000 g, or small for gestational age (SGA), defined as birthweight >2 standard deviations below the mean for gestational age, is associated with an increased risk of obesity. Birth weight is negatively correlated with waist-to-hip ratio[29] (r = –0.42, P<.05) and visceral adipose tissue volume.[30] Low birth weight has been reported to increase the risk of developing the metabolic syndrome (defined as 3 of the following[31–33]: waist circumference >90th percentile for age and gender,[29,30,34] hypertension,[29,35] hypertriglyceridemia,[30,36–43] low concentration of high-density lipoprotein,[36–40] or hyperglycemia[40,44–49]) by twofold to threefold.[34,50] In the San Antonio Heart Study, being at the lowest tercile for birth weight was associated with an odds ratio of 1.72 for insulin-resistance syndrome (defined as diabetes or impaired glucose tolerance with dyslipidemia or hypertension). In contrast, Byberg et al[51] reported that the odds ratio for insulin-resistance syndrome was increased by 0.66 per kg increase in birth weight in Swedish men at 50 years of age and 0.71 per kg increase in birth weight in Swedish men at 70 years of age.

Ravelli et al[39,52] examined adults conceived during the Nazi-imposed Dutch famine (the "Winter Hunger," 1944–1945) versus those conceived before or after the famine and found that the prevalence of impaired glucose tolerance was highest in infants with low birth weight who were in utero while mothers were exposed to the famine during the last 2 trimesters of pregnancy.

The hypothesized mechanisms for the association of low birth weight and metabolic syndrome phenotypes have included the "thrifty phenotype" hypothesis and the "catch-up growth" hypothesis. In the thrifty phenotype view,[53] intrauterine undernutrition results in endocrine changes (insulin resistance and beta-cell dysfunction) that would tend to divert a limited nutrient supply to nourish vital organs, such as the heart and brain, at the expense of somatic growth. In a nutrient-rich extrauterine environment, this tendency to optimize the efficiency of caloric storage coupled with insulin resistance results in obesity, increased diabetes risk, and dyslipidemia (ie, the canonical features of the metabolic syndrome).[54] In the catch-up growth view,[55] intrauterine undernutrition leads to a decrease in insulin and insulin-like growth factor production. As insulin and insulin-like growth factor production increase substantially during the postnatal catch-up growth phase when nutrients are readily available, tissues respond by becoming resistant to insulin and insulin-like growth factor to protect against hypoglycemia.[56]

Both of these hypotheses are probably correct. As discussed below, low birth weight is associated with an increased risk of multiple metabolic syndrome phenotypes, independent of whether or not catch-up growth occurs. However, the risk of abdominal obesity[57,58] and insulin resistance,[59,60] but not dyslipidemia,[38] was further increased if infants experienced earlier catch-up growth. Frayling and Hattersley[61] have suggested that impaired fetal growth and type 2 diabetes mellitus may represent 2 distinct phenotypes of a single "thrifty genotype"[62] in which resistance to the auxotrophic actions of insulin and other growth-promoting factors (eg, insulin-like growth factors) on somatic and organ growth act to maximize energy storage at the expense of growth in the setting of an unstable food supply and in which genes that reduce insulin secretion or increase insulin resistance also predispose infants to low birth weight. Once adequate nutrients are available, these phenotypes that minimized energy expenditure in growth now predispose to obesity and type 2 diabetes mellitus. Although these formulations focus on somatic effects of intrauterine dysnutrition, it is certainly possible—even likely—that such effects also influence brain development in a manner that could also predispose to neuroendocrine and behavioral phenotypes favoring increased adiposity and its comorbidities.

Alternatively, or in addition, a nutritionally adverse intrauterine environment has been shown to induce long-term changes in gene expression in both terminally differentiated (eg, pancreatic beta-cells) and pluripotential (eg, mitochondria in multiple cell lines) cells in a manner that perpetuates phenotypes associated with the metabolic syndrome, especially among those already genetically predisposed to these phenotypes.[63–65] Intrauterine growth retardation in rats results in abnormalities of multiple genes involved in beta-cell differentiation and function, lipogenesis, and hepatic function that are evident in the adult animal.[54] On the basis of observations of lower mitochondrial density in various tissues from adult rodents and humans subjected to intrauterine growth retardation, Lee et al[66] have recently proposed a mitochondria-based hypothesis. They propose that fetal undernutriton leads to increased oxidative stress (which is damaging to the developing pancreatic beta-cell in particular) and depletion of taurine, nucleotides, and methyl donors, which have been shown in animal studies to limit mitochondrial DNA content. When mitochondrial stress is increased in the setting of aging and a westernized lifestyle, the individual is, by virtue of an inability to generate adequate mitochondrial DNA, predisposed to mitochondrial dysfunction in liver, muscle, and pancreas resulting in both insulin resistance and insufficiency.

Associations of low birth weight with type 2 diabetes mellitus and impaired glucose tolerance have been reported in adults through the seventh and eighth decades of life.[46,67,68] Attempts to separate the effects of low birth weight on insulin sensitivity and secretory capacity have yielded varied results. Studies of insulin sensitivity in 7-year-olds[69] found a significant negative correlation of insulin sensitivity and birth weight, even corrected for age, sex, gestational age at delivery, and current weight. Veening et al[59] found that insulin sensitivity was significantly lower in prepubertal children who were SGA, but no significant differences were noted in insulin secretory capacity or glucose disposition compared with controls who were appropriate size for gestational age. Li et al[30] reported that acute insulin response and glucose disposal, but not insulin sensitivity, were impaired in 8- to 14-year-old black and white US children who had low birth weight. Postnatal factors obviously also exert strong influences on glucose homeostasis. Regardless of the mechanisms, the clinician should be alert to an increased risk of adiposity-related comorbidities at lower levels of body fatness in individuals with a history of low birth weight.

Prenatal Overnutrition

Macrosomia at birth, indicative of fetal overnutrition, is associated with increased deposition of body fat in childhood and increased risk of obesity in adulthood[70–73] and, as for the baby who is SGA, with all of the phenotypes associated with the metabolic syndrome.[74] The infant of a mother with diabetes is a model for the influences of fetal overnutrition on postnatal adiposity. Exposure of the fetus to high ambient glucose concentrations stimulates fetal hyperinsulinism, increased fat deposition, and macrosomia. Because women with gestational diabetes are often obese, it is difficult to separate the metabolic effects of gestational diabetes on subsequent adiposity of the infant of a mother with diabetes from the possibility that the mother has transmitted a genetic tendency toward obesity to her offspring. In studies controlled for the effects of maternal adiposity, being an infant of a mother with diabetes is still associated with an increased risk of obesity, independent of pre- and perigravid maternal adiposity.[75–78] Exposure of the fetal pancreas to high glucose concentrations results in prenatal hyperinsulinism leading to macrosomia and also alters the developing neuroendocrine systems in a manner that favors deposition of stored calories as fat (increased cortisol, resistance to insulin-mediated glucose transport but not lipogenesis) as well as insulin resistance.[79]

More recently, maternal smoking in the first trimester of pregnancy has been associated with increased body fatness and blood pressure in childhood.[80,81]

Postnatal Nutrition

A number of recent well-designed studies have suggested that predominantly breastfeeding for at least 4 months is associated with an approximately 20% to 30% reduction in the prevalence of obesity (defined as BMI >95th percentile for age and sex) through early adolescence,[82,83] even when controlled for other adiposity-risk variables, such as socioeconomic status and maternal adiposity. However, although associations have been reported between breastfeeding and diminution of some risk factors for adult cardiovascular disease, there does not appear to be a reduction in adult adiposity in those who were breastfed as infants.[39] Furthermore, it is unclear whether breastfeeding causes a reduction in early obesity or is merely reflective of other factors in the environment in which the child is raised[84,85] that may influence subsequent adiposity.

Neither the age at which specific foods are introduced into the diet nor the proportions of fat, carbohydrate, or protein in the diet significantly influence subsequent adult adiposity.[86,87] The lack of association of diet composition per se with subsequent adiposity is also relevant to adiposity-related morbidities. In the Women's Health Initiative Randomized Controlled Dietary Modification Trial, prospective analyses of diet found no statistically significant associations between consumption of a low-fat diet and the incidence of cardiovascular disease,[88] colorectal cancer,[89] or breast cancer,[90] although trends toward beneficial effects on some of these morbidities were noted. That said, the institution of a well-balanced diet in childhood may form the basis for long-term healthy dietary habits that will persist into adulthood and, over time, may translate into significant reductions in body fat. Physical activity is equally important and exerts an independent effect on risks of adiposity-related morbidities (including cardiovascular disease, dyslipidemia, and type 2 diabetes mellitus) even if body fatness is not reduced.[91-94] Significant negative correlations have been reported between physical activity and body fatness in preschool children, and positive correlations have been noted between adiposity and the amount of time spent watching television in adolescence.[95-99] More than 60% of television commercials during children's programs are food-related, and television watching promotes both inactivity and increased caloric intake.[100] Both early physical activity and dietary patterns track into adolescence and correlate with adolescent adiposity, emphasizing the potential benefits of early encouragement of regular exercise and a healthful diet.

V

Demographic Trends in the Prevalence of Pediatric Obesity

In a study of US adolescents conducted between 1988 and 1991, the prevalence of obesity (defined as BMI >85th percentile on the basis of data obtained in the 1976 to 1980 survey) increased from 15% (by definition) to 21%.[101] Using the criteria of BMI described previously (defining obesity in children as BMI >95th percentile on the basis of data from the National Health Examination Survey [NHES] II and III data), the prevalence of obesity among children 6 to 17 years of age has increased from approximately 3.7% in NHANES I (1971–1974) to 6% in NHANES II (1976–1980) and to 10.5% in NHANES III (1998–1994).[24,102,103] Changes in the mean BMI of children 6 to 17 years of age from NHES II or III to NHANES III are indicated in Table 33.1.

Although there are clearly genetic influences on susceptibility to obesity (see "The Molecular Biology of Body Fatness"), the current demographics of obesity and the large increases in the prevalence of obesity over a single decade must reflect major changes in nongenetic factors. The interaction of genetic factors favoring storage of calories as fat and an environment that is permissive to the clinical expression of this genetic tendency is, thus, evident in the increasing prevalence of pediatric (and adult) obesity. Such secular trends may also be taken as tacit evidence that some instances/aspects of obesity are responsive to and, therefore, preventable by environmental manipulation (eg, diet, physical activity, improved prenatal and perinatal care). However, the resistance of obesity to current therapies (including a variety of environmental and behavioral manipulations) is reflected in an overall 75% to 95% reported recidivism rate to obesity among formerly-obese adults and children.[104–109]

Pathophysiology

The first law of thermodynamics dictates that the accumulation of stored energy (fat) must be attributable to caloric intake in excess of energy expenditure. A small excess of energy intake relative to expenditure will, over time, lead to a substantial increase in body weight. For example, an individual increasing daily caloric intake by 150 kcal (8 oz of whole milk) above daily energy expenditure would consume a caloric excess of 55 000 kcal per year and could gain approximately 27 lb per year. Despite the potentially large effects of small imbalances in energy intake versus expenditure, adults maintain a relatively constant body weight and most children tend to grow steadily along individualized weight percentile isobars for age, with little conscious effort to regulate energy intake or expenditure. The high rate of recidivism to previous levels of fatness of weight-reduced obese children and adults who were previously obese and lost weight[104–109] and the tendency for individuals to maintain a relatively stable body weight over long periods of time despite wide variations in caloric intake[110] provide empirical evidence that body weight is regulated and that energy intake and expenditure are not independent processes but rather are regulated by complex interlocking control mechanisms. Data generated from studies of energy homeostasis in adults must be applied cautiously to children. Unlike adults, children accrete both fat mass and fat-free mass as they grow, and the magnitude and composition of this weight gain is more age and gender dependent.[10,111,112]

Energy Intake

No a priori judgments of caloric requirements can be made for any child without detailed knowledge of individual growth rate (as discussed previously), body size, and level of physical activity (see next paragraph). Feeding behavior consists of "decisions" regarding initiation, composition, and termination of meals; these decisions are influenced by many internal and external factors. Voluntary food intake is increased in rodents and humans after intentional undernutrition relative to the same person or animal before food restriction.[113] The observed hyperphagia after caloric restriction ceases once "usual" body weight or, in the case of rodents, body weight similar to nonrestricted littermates is reached. Reciprocal changes are seen after imposed weight gain by overfeeding. Once the overfeeding is terminated, relative hypophagia ensues until the individual has returned to usual weight.[114–119] These transient changes in spontaneous food ingestion support the view that systems regulating energy intake are directly responsive to changes in stored calories.

Energy Expenditure

Total energy expenditure (TEE) is the sum of the energy expended at rest in cardiorespiratory work and the maintenance of transmembrane ion gradients (resting energy expenditure, approx 50%–60% of TEE), the work of digestion and absorption of nutrients (thermic effect of feeding, approx 5%–10% of TEE), and energy expended as physical activity (nonresting energy expenditure, approx 20%–40% of total) and, to a small extent in the growing child beyond infancy, energy expended in the process of storing fat and nonfat mass in growth.[120] Energy costs of growth reflect both net rates of growth (highest in infancy and adolescence) and the proportion of calories being stored as high-caloric-density fat (higher in females, especially during adolescence) versus carbohydrate (glycogen) or protein.[111,112] A number of studies have demonstrated that the maintenance of a reduced body weight and/or the process of weight loss are associated with significant decreases in 24-hour energy expenditure (weight-maintenance caloric requirements) beyond those expected solely on the basis of weight loss[121–133] and that, in adults, the maintenance of a reduced body weight is associated with a decrease in weight maintenance caloric requirements that is significantly (approx 300 kcal/day) greater than would be predicted solely on the basis of the mass and composition of the weight lost or compared with body composition-matched control subjects. Fewer studies have reported that 24-hour energy expenditure does not remain suppressed during maintenance of a reduced body weight[134–137] and that weight-maintenance caloric need, corrected for changes in body composition after weight loss, is unchanged. However, as the many studies cited here suggest, this is an active area of research with discordant results often arising from methodologic differences between studies. Although carefully controlled studies of the effects of weight loss on energy expenditure in children are not yet available, the high rate of recidivism to previous levels of fatness among children who were previously obese and lost weight suggests that these same systems are operant.[105,138–141]

Systems Integrating Energy Intake and Energy Expenditure: Physiology and Molecular Genetics

Overview

The relative long-term constancy of body weight in humans, their lack of success in sustaining therapeutic weight loss, and the metabolic/behavioral alterations that accompany weight change provide strong evidence that weight (fat) is biologically regulated. The amount of energy stored in the body as fat exerts potent effects on growth, pubescence, fertility, and autonomic nervous system and thyroid function, suggesting that humoral "signals" reflecting adipose tissue mass interact directly or indirectly with many neuroendocrine systems.[113,142–146] Weight loss and maintenance of a reduced body weight are accompanied by changes in autonomic nervous system function (increased parasympathetic and decreased sympathetic nervous system tone), circulating concentrations of thyroid hormones (decreased triiodothyronine [T_3] and thyroxine [T_4] without a compensatory increase in thyroid-stimulating hormone [TSH]), and circulating concentrations of glucocorticoids (increased cortisol)[142,147,148] that are consistent with a homeostatic resistance to altered body weight acting, in part, through effectors that mediate energy expenditure. In addition, states of low energy stores (low fat mass) are associated with suppression of activity of the hypothalamic-pituitary-gonadal axis in males[149] and females.[150] Such a neurohumoral system to protect body energy stores would convey clear evolutionary advantages. During periods of undernutrition, the perceived reduction in energy stores would result in hyperphagia, hypometabolism, and decreased fertility (protecting females from the increased metabolic demands of pregnancy and lactation and the delivery of progeny into inhospitable environments).

Any alteration in this system that is associated with obesity must increase energy intake, decrease energy expenditure, and/or increase the partitioning of stored calories as fat. Rodent and human single-gene mutations that cause obesity have been identified. As discussed in the section "The Molecular Biology of Body Fatness," many of these mutations have been shown to alter specific biochemical and physiological aspects of the neurohumoral system that regulates body weight, but the precise mechanistic effects of other mutations remain unknown.

The Hypothalamus and Energy Homeostasis

The hypothalamus is part of a complex system of energy homeostasis through which signals regarding the nutritional state of the organism, as well as hedonic signals regarding the palatability of available food, are integrated by a number of neuronal tracts. As schematized in Fig 33.1, this system is particularly sensitive to perturbations in energy stores (adipose tissue mass) below usual amounts. Reduction in stored energy appears to provoke a cascade of metabolic, neuroendocrine, and autonomic changes that act coordinately to oppose the maintenance of a reduced body weight.

Within the hypothalamus, the arcuate nucleus responds to signals regarding energy stores emanating from the gut, adipose tissue, pancreas, and nervous system by increasing or decreasing the expression of the potent orexigens neuropeptide Y (NPY) and agouti-related peptide (AgRP) in response to decreasing or increasing energy stores, respectively. Also within the arcuate nucleus are pro-opiomelanocortin (POMC)-expressing neurons that, when activity is decreased as in a weight-reduced state, will project to other tracts with the net result of decreasing energy expenditure and increasing food intake.[143,151–153] Pro-opiomelanocortin is processed posttranslationally in the hypothalamus to yield multiple neuropeptides including alpha-melanocyte-stimulating hormone (MSH), beta-MSH, gamma-3-MSH, and beta-endorphin.

Fig 33.1A
The role of the hypothalamus in systems regulating energy homeostasis.

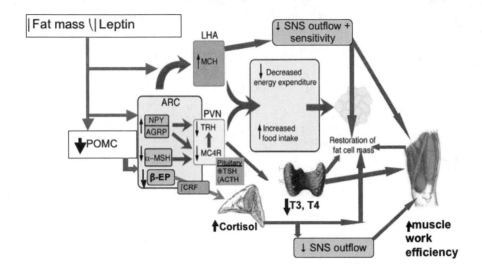

Fig 33.1B

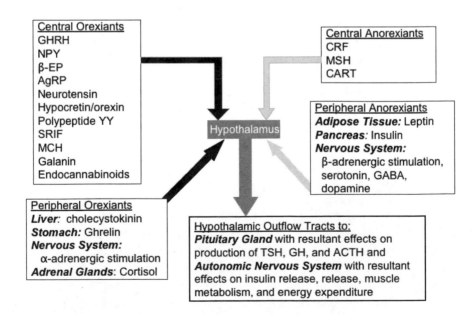

A. Schematic of model of effects of weight loss on hypothalamic neuropeptides, neuroendocrine function, autonomic function, and energy homeostasis. Decreased leptin leads to decreased POMC, increased NPY, and increased MCH. Decreased POMC leads to decreased α-MSH, decreasing pro-TRH release with resultant declines in pituitary TSH release and circulating concentration of thyroid hormones, and β-EP, disinhibiting CRF release and increasing pituitary ACTH and adrenal cortisol production. CRF has also been shown to have an anorexiant effect when administered directly into the hypothalamus. Increased NPY and AGRP expression and decreased α-MSH lead to decreased activation of melanocortin receptors. Increased MCH inhibits SNS outflow and sensitivity. The net result of these leptin-mediated actions in the hypothalamus are decreased sympathetic nervous system tone and hypothalamus-pituitary-thyroid axis activation, increased hypothalamus-pituitary-adrenal axis activation, decreased energy expenditure, and increased hunger. Adapted from Korner J, Aronne LJ. *J Clin Invest*. 2003;111:565–570. LHA indicates lateral hypothalamus area; SNS, sympathetic nervous system; ARC, arcuate nucleus; AGRP, agouti-related peptide; β-EP, beta-endorphin; PVN, paraventricularis nucleus; TRH, thyrotropin-releasing hormone; MC4R, melanocortin-4 receptor; CRF, corticotropin-releasing factor.

B. Major molecules affecting food intake by primary site of secretion and the human chromosome encoding them. All of these molecules directly or indirectly input to the hypothalamus, for which outflow tracts affect energy expenditure. GHRH indicates growth hormone-releasing hormone; SRIF, somatotropin release-inhibiting factor; CART, cocaine-amphetamine-related transcript; GABA, gamma-aminobutyric acid; GH, growth hormone.

Beta-endorphin inhibits corticotropin-releasing factor.[154] This signaling system is schematized in Fig 33.1 and comprises neurotransmitters, peptide hormones, and other hormonal signals from the gastrointestinal, central nervous, peripheral nervous, and endocrine systems, as well as adipose tissue itself. The importance of POMC is emphasized by the observations that human autosomal mutations leading to defects in POMC production result in central hypoadrenalism (as a result of lack of pituitary adrenocorticotropic hormone [ACTH] production), red hair (as a result of lack of alpha-MSH production), hyperphagia, and obesity[153] and that heterozygous mutations in the gene for the melanocortin-4 receptor have been identified in 5% of individuals with BMI >40.[153,155–157] The pivotal role of the hypothalamus in regulating multiple systems relevant to energy homeostasis (energy intake and output, autonomic function, and neuroendocrine function) is schematized in Fig 33.1.

Major chemical mediators of ingestive behavior and energy expenditure are reviewed briefly as follows.

Neurotransmitters
The mixed alpha- and beta-adrenergic agonists norepinephrine and epinephrine are secreted predominantly from nerve endings and by the adrenal medulla, respectively. Central alpha-adrenergic stimulation results in increased food intake and decreased energy expenditure, whereas beta-adrenergic and dopaminergic stimulation have anorectic effects and increase energy expenditure. In addition, peripheral alpha-adrenergic stimulation inhibits lipolysis,

whereas peripheral beta-adrenergic stimulation is lipolytic. Injections of gamma-amino butyric acid (GABA) or opioid agonists or of glutamate antagonists have been shown to increase energy consumption and may modulate signaling by some of the hypothalamic peptide hormones described in the next paragraph.[158,159] More specifically, opioid, glutamate, and GABAergic receptors are present in high concentrations in the nucleus accumbens, which projects to the ventral palladium and the lateral hypothalamus to disinhibit or inhibit feeding by increasing or decreasing expression of melanocyte concentrating hormone (MCH [see next paragraph]).[159]

Peptides

Peptides of central and peripheral origin exert potent effects on feeding behavior. Peptides that increase food intake include MCH, NPY, AgRP, galanin, orexigens, and growth hormone-releasing hormone (GHRH), which are synthesized in the hypothalamus, and insulin, somatostatin, neurotensin, ghrelin, and polypeptide Y, which are synthesized in the pancreas and gut.[160–162] Peptide anorexiants include centrally synthesized corticotropin-releasing hormone, melanocortin, proctoring, and cocaine-amphetamine related transcript (CART); leptin which is synthesized in adipose tissue; and peptide YY, pancreatic polypeptide, cholecystokinin, glucagon, and glucagon-like peptides, which are synthesized in the gut, as well as oxyntomodulin, which is synthesized from preproglucagon in the gut and the brain.[160–162] The variety of these molecules and the multiple tissues from which they originate reflects the intricacy and redundancy of systems regulating energy homeostasis. This redundancy is evident throughout energy homeostatic systems and illustrates the basis of the difficulty in finding a single pharmacological agent that will sustain weight reduction.

Neuropeptide Y is a potent orexigen and also acts to decrease production of thyrotropin-releasing hormone, resulting in increased hunger and decreased energy expenditure by virtue of decreases in bioactive thyroid hormones.[151,163] In rodents, food restriction is associated with a significant increase in NPY production and release, and intraventricular administration of NPY is a highly potent stimulus of feeding behavior. In addition, injection of NPY into the periventricular nucleus has been shown to increase adipogenesis and to decrease thermogenesis, indicating that NPY has coordinate effects on energy intake and output, which favor weight gain. Agouti-related peptide is a hypothalamic neuropeptide coexpressed with NPY in arcuate neurons and acts as an inverse agonist (ie, it stabilizes the melanocortin-4 receptor in an inactive state rather than antagonizing the binding of an agonist to the receptor).[151]

Leptin is secreted from adipose tissue and provides a signal linking fat mass to food intake and energy expenditure. Mice homozygous for the *ob* mutation (leptin deficient) are obese as a result of increased food intake and reduced energy expenditure. Administration of leptin in the region of the hypothalamus or peripherally to *Lep*^{ob} mice decreases food intake and increases energy expenditure. Rare families have been identified in which hypoleptinemia (leptin gene mutation)[164,165] or leptin nonresponsiveness (leptin receptor mutation)[166] is inherited as an autosomal-recessive disorder associated with obesity. Administration of physiological leptin doses to leptin-deficient individuals promotes weight loss as well as normalization of thyroid and immune function.[167] Although examination of the phenotypes of humans with such rare mutations can be extremely useful in elucidating the molecular physiology of human weight regulation, gross deficiency of leptin or its receptor are not common causes of human obesity.

Leptin does play a central role in fasting-mediated and weight-reduced neuroendocrine responses[152,168] but a lesser role in response to overfeeding. Short-term leptin administration to weight-reduced lean and obese individuals reverses many of the metabolic, neuroendocrine, and autonomic phenotypes associated with attempts to sustain weight loss,[169] and much larger doses are needed to induce even moderate weight loss in individuals at their usual weights.[170] Consistent with view that leptin acts primarily to defend energy stores rather than to oppose weight gain is the observation that diet-induced obesity in rodents promotes leptin insensitivity in the arcuate nucleus of the hypothalamus.[171,172]

Whereas hormones like leptin reflect long-term energy stores, gut peptides provide a link between short-term energy intake and systems regulating food intake and energy homeostasis.[160,173] Obvious examples of this include insulin and glucagon (and its derivatives glucagon-like peptides and oxyntomodulin) which reflect not only the quantity of food ingested but also its carbohydrate content; ghrelin, which is inhibited by gastric distention; and cholecystokinin, which is secreted from the intestines in response to fat and protein in the chyme.

Steroids

Corticosterone, and other glucocorticoids, may also play a potent role in the regulation of feeding behavior and energy expenditure. Surgical or pharmacologic adrenalectomy of many genetically obese rodent mutations results in marked amelioration of obesity, and intraventricular injection of corticosterone increases food intake. Corticosterone also increases brain concentrations of norepinephrine and the affinity of alpha-adrenoreceptors for their agonists, and the orexigenic effects of central norepinephrine are blocked by adrenalectomy. Hyperglucocorticoidemia (whether endogenous, as in Cushing syndrome, or iatrogenic) is associated with increased food intake and increased partitioning of stored calories to fat in specific depots (reduction of lean body and deposition of fat in a centripetal pattern).

Endocannabinoids

More recently, a group of endogenous tricyclic terpenoids known as endo-cannabinoids have been identified as having potent orexiant effects. The most studied endocannabinoids are anandamide and 2-arachidonoylglycer-ol. These phospholipids are synthesized within neurons. Cannabinoid $(CB)_1$ receptors, and endocannabinoids to activate them, have been detected in all brain and peripheral tissues involved in the control of energy intake, processing, and storage, including the hypothalamus, the nucleus acumbens, the vagus nerve and the nodose ganglion, myenteric neurons and epithelial cells of the gastrointestinal tract, the adipocytes, and the liver. Although the highest expression rate of CB_1 receptors is in the brain, CB_2 receptors are present almost exclusively in immune and blood cells, where they may participate in regulating immune responses by suppressing chemotaxis and other immune functions and increasing endogenous secretion of beta-endorphins to dull pain. Antagonists of the CB_1 receptor, most notably rimonabant, are currently being studied as possible pharmacotherapeutic agents for obesity and the metabolic syndrome.[174-176]

Outflow Tracts

The autonomic nervous system (both parasympathetic and sympathetic) and thyroid gland secretions of T_4 and T_3 probably constitute the major outflow tracts linking afferent biochemical signals regarding energy stores to efferent systems regulating energy expenditure via the central nervous systems regulating body weight. Obese and never-obese adults studied at their usual body weight, during weight loss, and during the maintenance of a reduced body weight demonstrate significant decreases in sympathetic nervous system activity and in circulating concentrations of thyroid hormone compared with usual weight both during weight loss and during maintenance of a reduced body weight.[142]

Adiponectin is an adipose-specific plasma protein that improves insulin sensitivity, inhibits the expression of adhesion molecules in endothelial cells and the secretion of tumor necrosis factor-alpha from monocyte-macrophages—that is, adiponectin inhibits atherogenesis and increases the rate of the oxidation of fatty acids as fuel. Unlike the adipose-specific protein leptin (see "Peptides"), circulating concentrations of adiponectin are significantly lower in states of obesity and insulin resistance, including type 2 diabetes.[177,178]

The Molecular Biology of Body Fatness

Heritability of Body Fatness

The ability to store calories as fat would presumably have conferred a survival advantage to our progenitors by enabling them to survive periods of prolonged caloric restriction, providing greater energy stores to nourish mother and fetus during pregnancy, and enhancing the ability of women to breastfeed their offspring. Thus, it is likely that the human genome would be enriched with genes favoring the storage of calories as adipose tissue.[153,179]

The calculation of heritability in twin studies is based on the assumption that each member of a monozygotic or dizygotic pair is gestated and reared in the same environment and that the degree to which body fatness is more similar within mono- than dizygotic twin pairs is attributable to the greater genetic similarity of identical versus nonidentical twins. Studies comparing adopted children with their adoptive and their biologic parents assume that each child shares 50% of his or her genotype (but little or none of the immediate environment) with each biologic parent and that the degree to which body fatness is more similar between children and their biologic versus adoptive parents is primarily attributable to genetic effects. Twin and adoption studies indicate that the heritability of body fatness and of body fat distribution in adulthood is 30% to 70%.[180] Recent studies have also identified significant genetic influences (heritability greater than 30%) on resting metabolic rate, feeding behavior, food preferences, and changes in energy expenditure that occur in response to overfeeding. Genetic influences on resting energy expenditure are suggested by studies demonstrating that black children in the United States tend to have lower resting energy expenditures than do white children, even when adjusted for body composition, gender, age, and pubertal status.[181]

Single Gene Mutations Producing Obesity

The pivotal role of genetics in the control of body weight is confirmed by the existence of single gene mutations capable of producing profound increases in body fat content. As shown in Fig 33.2 and Table 33.2, any of these single gene mutations affect specific aspects of the signaling system described above (see Fig 33.1). Some are "syndromic" (eg Prader-Willi, Bardet-Biedl, Alström, Cohen syndromes) in association with characteristic phenotypes in addition to obesity.[182] However, as indicated earlier, in most humans, body fatness is a continuous quantitative trait reflecting the interaction of development and environment with genotype.

Fig 33.2
Control of food intake by peripheral signaling to the central nervous system.

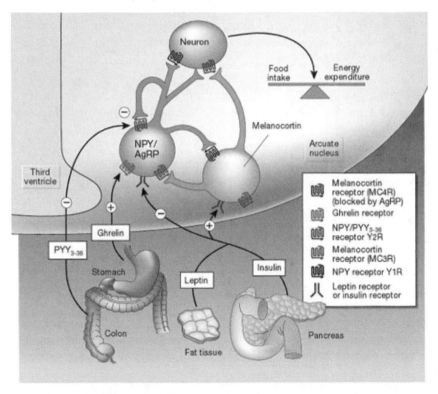

NPY indicates neuropeptide Y; PYY, polypeptide YY; MC3R, melanocortin 3 receptor; MC4R, melanocortin 4 receptor; AgRP, agouti-related protein.

Schwartz MW, Morton GJ. Obesity: keeping hunger at bay. *Nature.* 2002;418:595–597

Table 33.2
Human Single Gene Mutations* Associated With Obesity[182]

Syndrome	Chromosome	Phenotype
Prader-Willi	15q11–q13 (uniparental maternal disomy)	Short stature, small hands and feet, mental retardation, neonatal hypotonia, failure to thrive, cryptorchidism, almond-shaped eyes, and fish-like mouth.
Alström	2p13 (autosomal recessive)	Childhood blindness attributable to retinal degeneration, nerve deafness, acanthosis nigricans, chronic nephropathy, primary hypogonadism in males only, type 2 diabetes mellitus, infantile obesity that may diminish in adulthood. This gene has been cloned.
Bardet-Biedl	11q13,16q21, 3p12–13, 15q22–23, 2q31, 20p12, 4q27 (2 mutations), 14q32	At least 8 different forms of varying severity. Most common phenotypes are retinitis pigmentosa, mental retardation, polydactyly, hypothalamic hypogonadism, rarely glucose intolerance, deafness, and cystic renal disease. Known genes are in pathway(s) affecting ciliary motor function.
Borjeson-Forssman-Lehmann	Xq26 (X-linked dominant)	Truncal obesity, mental retardation, coarse facies, microcephaly, short stature, gynecomastia. Infants show poor feeding, hypotonia, failure to thrive, large ears, and hypogonadism. Females may be asymptomatic because of selective lyonization of carrier X-chromosome.
Carpenter	unknown (autosomal recessive)	Acrocephaly, syndactyly, polydactyly, congenital heart disease, mental retardation, hypogonadism (males only), obesity, umbilical hernia, and bony abnormalities.
Cohen	8q22–q23 (autosomal recessive)	Mental retardation, microcephaly, short stature, dysmorphic facies.
Prohormone convertase	5q15–q21 (autosomal recessive)	Abnormal glucose homeostasis, hypogonadotropic hypogonadism, hypocortisolism, and elevated plasma proinsulin.
Beckwith-Wiedemann	11p15.5 (autosomal recessive)	Hyperinsulinism, hypoglycemia, neonatal hemihypertrophy, intolerance of fasting.
Nesidioblastosis	11p15.1 (autosomal recessive or dominant)	Hyperinsulinism, hypoglycemia, intolerance of fasting This gene has been cloned.
Pseudohypoparathyroidism (type IA)	20q13.2 (autosomal recessive)	Mental retardation, short stature, short metacarpals and metatarsals, short thick neck, round facies, subcutaneous calcifications, increased frequency of other endocrinopathies (hypothyroidism, hypogonadism).
Leptin	7q31.3 (autosomal recessive)	Hypometabolic rate, hyperphagia, pubertal delay, infertility, impaired glucose tolerance attributable to leptin deficiency.

Table 33.2 *(Continued)*
Human Single Gene Mutations* Associated With Obesity[182]

Syndrome	Chromosome	Phenotype
Leptin receptor	1p31–p32 (autosomal recessive)	Hypometabolic rate, hyperphagia, pubertal delay attributable to deranged leptin signal transduction.
POMC	2p23.3 (autosomal recessive)	Red hair, hyperphagia, adrenal insufficiency attributable to impaired POMC production in individuals unable to make POMC.
Melanocortin-4 receptor defects	multiple auto-somal recessive and dominant mutations	Obesity, tall stature, increased bone density, eating disorders.

* The primary physiological sites of the derangements in some of the human mutations can be seen in Fig 33.2.

Clinical and Laboratory Correlates of Obesity in Children

As summarized in Table 33.3, obesity adversely affects virtually every organ system. Obesity in childhood constitutes a risk factor for adiposity-related adult morbidity and mortality, even if childhood obesity does not persist. In 40- to 50-year follow-up studies of obese and lean adolescents (defined on the basis of weight-for-height indices), adolescent fatness was a powerful predictor of mortality, cardiovascular disease, colorectal cancer, gout, and arthritis irrespective of body fatness at the time that the morbidity was diagnosed.[183] Also, adiposity-related morbidities, such as hyperlipidemia, which are evident in childhood, track well into adulthood,[184] as do the precursors of coronary artery disease, including elevated circulating concentrations of inflammatory markers and hypertension.[185]

Some morbidities, such as slipped capital-femoral epiphyses, are physical consequences of excessive body weight. Other morbidities, cardiovascular disease in particular, are more closely correlated with the centrality of body fat distribution than absolute body fatness per se. Although certain endocrinopathies, such as hypothyroidism, may precipitate weight gain, most endocrine disorders associated with obesity are secondary to excess body fat and will correct with weight loss. There are rare endocrine or genetic syndromes associated with obesity (see Tables 33.2 and 33.4). Assessment of the presence or absence of age-appropriate secondary sexual characteristics as well as syndrome-specific morphology or symptomatology (eg, hypotension, constipation in hypothyroidism, centripetal distribution of fat in hypercortisolism) can usually rule out these syndromes as causes of obesity.

Table 33.3
Potential Effects of Increased Adiposity on Organ Systems in Children[3,186]

Organ System	Effects
Nonendocrine	
Cardiovascular	Most common identifiable cause of pediatric hypertension, increased total cholesterol, increased low-density lipoproteins, decreased high-density lipoproteins, metabolic syndrome
Respiratory	Abnormal respiratory muscle function and central respiratory regulation, difficulty with ventilation during surgery, lower arterial oxygenation, sleep apnea, pickwickian syndrome, more frequent and severe upper respiratory infections, asthma
Orthopedic	Coxa vara, slipped capital femoral epiphyses, Blount disease, Legg-Calve-Perthe disease, degenerative arthritis
Dermatologic	Intertrigo, furunculosis, acanthosis nigricans (HAIR-AN syndrome)
Digestive	Fatty liver, transaminitis
Immunologic	Impaired cell-mediated immunity
Endocrine	
Somatotroph	Decreased basal and stimulated growth hormone release, normal concentration of insulin-like growth factor-I, accelerated linear growth and bone age
Lactotroph	Increased basal serum prolactin but decreased prolactin release in response to provocative stimuli
Gonadotroph	Early entrance into puberty with normal circulating gonadotropin concentrations
Thyroid	Normal serum T_4 and reverse T_3, normal or increased serum T_3, decreased TSH-stimulated T_4 release
Adrenal	Normal serum cortisol but increased cortisol production and excretion, early adrenarche, increased adrenal androgens and dehydroepiandrosterone, normal serum catecholamines and 24-hour urinary catecholamine excretion
Gonads	Decreased circulating gonadal androgens attributable to decreased sex-hormone binding globulin, dysmenorrhea, dysfunctional uterine bleeding, polycystic ovarian syndrome, increased aromatization of androgens to estrogens by adipose tissue
Pancreas	Increased fasting plasma insulin, increased insulin and glucagon release, increased resistance to insulin-mediated glucose transport

Type 2 diabetes mellitus has emerged over the past decade in almost epidemic proportions among obese adolescents, and the clinician must now consider type 2 diabetes mellitus as a pediatric illness. Until recently, type 2 diabetes mellitus was thought of as an "adult" disease and constituted fewer than 2% of the new cases of diabetes in children as recently as a decade ago. Now, however, between 25% and 60% of children with new onset of diabetes have type 2 diabetes mellitus. Thus, over the last decade and along with the increasing prevalence of obesity among children, type 2 diabetes mellitus has also become a "pediatric" disease, and children with type 2 diabetes mellitus suffer the same morbidities as do adults with the disease.[187]

Obesity is the major risk factor for type 2 diabetes mellitus in adolescents,[187] and adiposity accounts for approximately 55% of the variance in insulin sensitivity in children.[188] As in adults, 50% to 90% of children with type 2 diabetes mellitus have a BMI greater than the 85th percentile.[187] This is especially true in black and Hispanic adolescents, who have experienced the greatest increase in the prevalence of adolescent obesity over the past generation.[13,25,189] The prevalence of obesity in black individuals relative to other ethnic groups increases specifically during puberty.[190,191] Insulin sensitivity has been shown to be approximately 35% lower in black than in white adolescents in the United States[192] and approximately 40% lower in prepubertal children than in adolescents after controlling for adiposity and body fat distribution[193,194] in most but not all[195] studies.

The association of obesity with insulin resistance is related not only to the degree of body fatness but also to the centrality of body fat distribution. Body fat distribution is usually defined on the basis of waist circumference or the ratio of waist-to-hip circumference or by magnetic resonance imaging of visceral versus subcutaneous adipose tissue. Central distribution of body fat, by various measures, is an independent predictor of insulin resistance and dyslipidemia in prepubertal and pubertal children[193,195–197] and of type 2 diabetes mellitus, cardiovascular disease, stroke, and death in adults.[16,17,198] Free fatty acids from omental fat drain directly into the portal circulation. Bjorntorp[17] first suggested that the direct exposure of the liver to higher circulating free fatty acid concentrations in individuals with a higher visceral adipose tissue volume results in increased hepatic glucose production and decreased insulin clearance, which in turn lead to insulin resistance and dyslipidemia. In addition to central body fat distribution, intramyocellular lipid content has recently been identified as a strong correlate of insulin resistance in adults and children and a possible cause of the impaired glucose transport resulting in lipodystrophy-associated type 2 diabetes mellitus.[199–201]

The psychological stress of social stigmatization imposed on obese children may be just as damaging to some children as the medical morbidities. These negative images of the obese are so strong that growth failure and pubertal delay have been reported in children as a result of self-imposed caloric restriction arising from fears of becoming obese.[202]

Identification of the Obese Child and Decisions Regarding Therapeutic Intervention

The rapid increase in prevalence of obesity in the United States pediatric population during the last 25 years demonstrates the potent effect of environment on adiposity, especially in genetically susceptible individuals and populations[203] (see Fig 33.3). The environment has changed progressively to favor the consumption of calorically dense foods (through availability of fast foods, "supersizing," lower prices per calorie for less healthful foods, and increased advertising of these same foods) and an increasingly sedentary lifestyle (through increased media and computer availability as well as decreased availability of safe recreational areas in many neighborhoods). In addition, improvements in prenatal and postnatal care have resulted in improved survival of infants suffering from intrauterine growth retardation who are, as discussed earlier, more prone to obesity and its comorbidities. Other putative explanations (ie, changes in relevant factors that are known to affect body fatness and that may contribute to the increasing prevalence of obesity) include less sleep, disruption of endocrine function through the addition of artificial aromatase inhibitors and other "endocrine disruptors" to the environment, increased time spent in thermoneutral environments because of exogenous heaters and air conditioners, decreased smoking, increased use of pharmaceuticals (antidepressants, antipsychotics, antidiabetics, antihistamines, and protease inhibitors) that promote weight gain, increased representation of ethnic groups more predisposed to obesity (eg, Hispanic and black individuals) in the US population, and increasing gravida age.[204]

The pediatrician should seek to identify the child at risk of adiposity-related morbidity, as well as the already-obese child, with the goal of encouraging a lifestyle (environment) that will minimize obesity and its comorbidities. A detailed history and physical examination should be performed to assess each child for current obesity-related morbidities and for birth history or family history that suggests risk of such morbidities. Anthropometric data should be plotted on height and weight velocity charts as well as standard curves for BMI (see Appendix D), with the aim of detecting increased weight gain velocity before actual obesity occurs. It is not unlikely that this list will expand to include some measure of the centrality of body fat in the near future. Any child, regardless of body weight, with a history of first-degree relatives with obesity, type 2 diabetes mellitus, hypertension, hyperlipidemia, or premature myocardial infarction and any child with BMI greater than the 85th percentile should be considered to be "at risk" of adiposity-related morbidity.

Fig 33.3
Overweight trends in children and adolescents.[203,228]

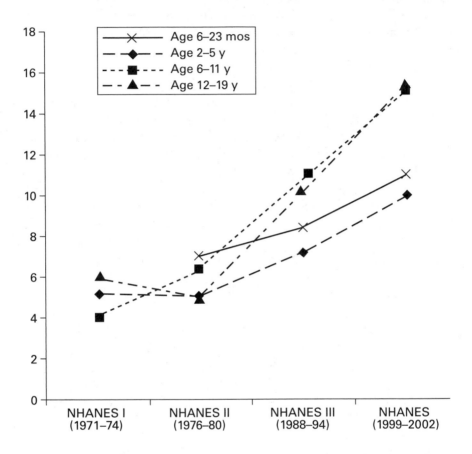

Not every obese child requires or will benefit from treatment. The likelihood of persistence of pediatric obesity into adulthood increases with age. The obese 2-year-old is approximately twice as likely as a nonobese 2-year-old to become an obese adult. In contrast, that risk increases to sixfold or sevenfold by adolescence, independent of the duration of the obesity. In large epidemiologic studies, if neither of a child's parents is obese, the likelihood of childhood obesity persisting into adulthood may be less than the risk for a nonobese child of the same age with 1 or 2 obese parents.[4]

Because risk of persistence is lower and risk of treatment-associated impairment of statural or brain growth is higher, caloric restriction to decrease weight should not be used for children younger than 2 years. Although hypothyroidism is an unusual cause of obesity in infants, the profound neurologic sequelae of untreated hypothyroidism in infancy justify heightened attention to this possibility. Similarly, children younger than 2 years who are severely obese, especially if they have concurrent adiposity-related morbidities, evidence of developmental delay, or other phenotypic features associated with obesity syndromes (such as Prader-Willi syndrome) discussed previously (see Table 33.4) should be referred to a physician who specializes in the treatment and evaluation of pediatric obesity.[205]

Table 33.4
Other Diseases and Injuries Associated With Obesity[153]

Disease	Structural/Biochemical Lesion	Clinical Features
Acquired hypothalamic lesions	Infectious (sarcoid, tuberculosis, arachnoiditis, encephalitis), vascular malformations, neoplasms, trauma	Headache and visual disturbance, hyperphagia, hypodipsia, hypersomnolence, convulsions, central hypogonadism-hypothyroidism-hypoadrenalism, diabetes insipidus, hyperprolactinemia, hyperinsulinism, hyperlipidemia
Cushing disease	Hypercortisolism	Moon facies, central obesity, decreased lean body mass, glucose intolerance, short stature
Hypothyroidism	Hypothalamic, pituitary, or thyroidal	Hypometabolic state (constipation, hypotension, bradycardia, cold intolerance), cretinism (if congenital)

The decision whether or not to initiate therapy in the toddler or young child (2–9 years of age) should be strongly influenced by family history of obesity and adiposity-related morbidities. For the preadolescent or adolescent child with obesity-related morbidity (eg, hypertension), the child with central obesity, and/or the child with a strong family history of adiposity-related morbidity (eg, hyperlipidemia, hypertension, diabetes mellitus), medical evaluation might also include screening for hyperlipidemia (fasting cardiovascular disease risk profile) and an oral glucose tolerance test.

Before beginning any type of therapy, it is essential to have the cooperation of the child and his or her family. Clinicians should not assume that the obese child is necessarily depressed or that every obese child is significantly

V

motivated to lose weight. Beginning weight-loss therapy if the overweight child and his or her family are not motivated to do so is likely to be unsuccessful and may have negative influences on the child's self-esteem and likelihood of future successful weight loss. The clinician should assess the family's therapeutic readiness by asking the entire family how concerned they are about the patient's overweight. The clinician should make these inquiries in a supportive manner designed to elicit cooperation from the family and patient. Questions such as "Do you feel that weight is a problem?" or "What do you think that you could change to help you lose weight?" rather than "Why can't you control your eating?" are suggested. If family members are not concerned or feel they cannot change, initiation of therapy should be delayed. Depending on the degree of obesity and adiposity-related morbidity, noncooperative families may benefit from further counseling to improve motivation.[205] Issues that should be addressed in such counseling include:

1. The risk of persistence of obesity into adulthood increases with age.
2. There are medical risks of obesity, some of which may already be evident in other family members.
3. The cooperation of the entire family (including all caregivers) in any therapeutic regimen is essential.
4. There are potential benefits to the entire family of adopting a healthier lifestyle, regardless of whether any individual family member is obese.
5. The major goal is long-term maintenance of reduced body fatness, not just short-term weight reduction.
6. The increased likelihood that good health habits (diet and exercise) that are started early will persist into adulthood.

The importance of family-based therapy and of the setting of realistic weight-loss goals is illustrated by the work of Epstein et al,[206] who followed 55 obese children and their families over a 10-year study period. At the start of the study, children and their families received a total of 14 therapy sessions. Subjects were randomly assigned to receive either therapy positively reinforcing weight loss plus behavior modification that was directed at the parent and child, similar therapy directed at the child alone, or a control group in which emphasis was placed on attendance at meetings rather than weight loss or behavioral modification relevant to obesity. All 3 treatment groups received identical information on diet, exercise, and behavioral principles. On entrance into the study, the parent- and child-targeted group, child alone-targeted group, and control group were, respectively 42%, 44%, and 46% above ideal body weight. During the initial treatment period, all children were placed on weight-reduction diets of 1200 to 1500 kcal/day and lost weight to within 25% of ideal body weight. At 10-year follow-up examinations, the parent- and child-targeted group, child alone-targeted group, and control group were, respectively 34%, 48%, and 60% above ideal body weight. Thus, although the family-oriented therapeutic approach did not result in children maintaining their maximally reduced level of body fatness outside of the 6-month treatment period, it did result in a modest sustained level of weight loss well beyond the initial 6-month therapeutic trial and maintenance of a significantly lower level of body fatness than subjects in other treatment groups.

Obesity is only one of many possible risk factors for cardiovascular disease. Because the adverse effects of cardiovascular disease, hyperlipidemia, diabetes, and hypertension are often cumulative, a combination of a cholesterol-lowering diet and program of regular exercise may be sufficient to reduce cardiovascular morbidity even if body weight is not significantly altered.[91,92,207–209] Children with a strong family history of any morbidity that can be exacerbated by obesity should be firmly and repeatedly counseled regarding good dietary and exercise habits, regardless of whether or not there is a family history of obesity per se.

Treatment of the Obese Child

Overview of Therapy (See Fig 33.4 and 33.5)

Initial evaluation should include a dietary history of the child's and family's typical eating habits (including snacks and the frequency with which they eat foods prepared outside of the home). A physical activity history should also be obtained, including school physical education, after-school activities, activities of daily living (such as walking to school), family activities, and sedentary activities (such as television watching and computer use). Treatment of the overweight child must, of necessity, be individualized, and the clinician should remain sensitive to issues such as ability of the parents to prepare meals for the child and neighborhood safety or availability of adult supervision that may affect access to physical activity after school. A complete physical examination should also be performed with special attention to the possibility of adiposity-related morbidities (hypertension, dyslipidemia, acanthosis nigricans [indicative of insulin resistance], etc; see Table 33.3).

Fig 33.4
Evaluation of the overweight child.

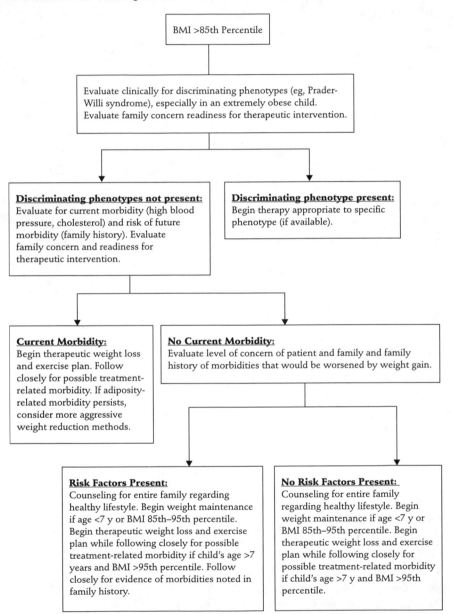

Fig 33.5
Therapeutic approach to obesity: roles of physician, parents, and patient.

Physician:
1. Identify child at risk of adiposity-related morbidity and initiate therapy early.
2. Educate families regarding the complications of obesity and benefits of therapy.
3. Assess factors in the child's environment that increase the risk of adiposity-related morbidity and can be modified.
4. Recommend gradual lifestyle changes that are not disruptive.
5. Involve the entire family in the treatment plan, including nonparent caregivers.
6. Educate parents to monitor child's eating behavior and activity.
7. Set reasonable and achievable weight goals from visit to visit.
8. Emphasize need for long-term lifestyle changes rather than just loss of body fatness.
9. Be supportive, not critical of child and family.
10. Be alert to therapy-associated morbidities.

Parent:
1. Encourage your child and give positive reinforcement for healthy lifestyle changes. Be consistent.
2. Never use food as a reward or punishment.
3. Adopt similar lifestyle changes to those that the child is being asked to make. Ask for nonfood rewards from children for good parental behavior.
4. Establish a regular schedule of meals, snacks, and exercise.
5. Remove calorically dense foods from the home for everyone.
6. Offer only healthy meals.
7. Discourage television watching.
8. Encourage physical activity.
9. Be a role model to the child.
10. Stay in close contact with the physician, even if compliance with the recommended lifestyle changes is incomplete. Discuss the recommendations with the physician.

Child:
1. Realize that being overweight is not the same as being lazy and greedy.
2. Realize that losing weight takes time and that someone who is overweight is not less of a person.
3. Realize that small changes in diet and exercise over time will produce big changes in fatness.
4. Remind the entire family that everyone benefits from a healthier lifestyle.
5. Do not hesitate to discuss fears, frustrations, and any other feelings about weight, diet, and exercise with your family and your doctor.
6. Be patient.
7. Be honest.
8. Do your best.
9. Respect your best.
10. Respect yourself.

The major goal of obesity therapy should be to diminish morbidity and risk of morbidity rather than to achieve a "societally endorsed" body weight. The severity of obesity should be assessed by degree of overweight and presence of current morbidities. Any child with BMI greater than the 95th percentile for age and sex or with BMI greater than the 85th percentile for age and gender and current adiposity-related morbidity should be considered severely obese, especially if there is a family history of comorbidities.[205]

In the otherwise healthy overweight child with no evidence of adiposity-related morbidity, clinicians and parents are generally concerned that the child will become an obese adult. Initial therapy in such instances should be directed toward decreasing or eliminating weight growth while allowing height growth to continue at age- and gender-appropriate velocity so that height eventually becomes appropriate for weight. Avoidance of calorically dense foods and substitution of fruit and vegetable snacks for sugared sodas, juices, and cookies without restricting access to such snacks will, in most cases, result in significant slowing of weight velocity.[210] The time required to significantly reduce adiposity can be estimated. One to 2 years of weight maintenance (1 year during normally rapid weight gain periods, such as adolescence, and 2 years during periods of slower weight gain) compensates for approximately 20% of excess weight-for-height.

If gradual statural growth into the child's weight is not possible because weight is already obese by adult standards (ie, body mass is so great that BMI will still be greater than the 85th percentile even if weight remains stable until adult stature is achieved), then a weight-loss regimen, as outlined below, should be considered. Therapeutic weight reduction is usually indicated for the child with evidence of current adiposity-related morbidity. The child with hypertension or diabetes mellitus should endeavor to reduce weight or alter body composition within 1 year to the point that the morbidity is no longer evident. Needless to say, if the morbidity is more severe (eg, pickwickian syndrome), then more rapid weight-reduction, even in an inpatient setting, may be necessary. The obese child with poor self-image, feelings of isolation from peers, and depression should also attempt weight reduction, perhaps with adjunctive psychotherapy. The initial therapeutic approach for children with predominantly psychiatric obesity-related morbidities should combine exercise and a closely supervised dietary plan, preferably with the involvement of a dietitian. Studies of compliance with weight-reduction plans have emphasized the importance of a family-oriented approach. Any therapeutic regimen should involve the entire family as well as the child's school. Frequent physical examination of the child and monitoring of school performance should be included. Patients and their families should be made aware that the treatment period does not end once the prescribed reduction in body fatness has been achieved and that caloric restriction must continue beyond the period of weight reduction to maintain reduced body weight.

AAP

The American Academy of Pediatrics states:

1. Prevalence of overweight and its significant comorbidities in pediatric populations has rapidly increased and reached epidemic proportions.
2. Prevention of overweight is critical, because long-term outcome data for successful treatment approaches are limited.
3. Genetic, environmental, or combinations of risk factors predisposing children to obesity can and should be identified.
4. Early recognition of excessive weight gain relative to linear growth should become routine in pediatric ambulatory care settings. BMI (kg/m2 [see Appendix D]) should be calculated and plotted periodically.
5. Families should be educated and empowered through anticipatory guidance to recognize the impact they have on their children's development of lifelong habits of physical activity and nutritious eating.
6. Dietary practices should be fostered that encourage moderation rather than overconsumption, emphasizing healthful choices rather than restrictive eating patterns.
7. Regular physical activity should be consciously promoted, prioritized, and protected within families, schools, and communities.
8. Optimal approaches to prevention need to combine dietary and physical activity interventions.
9. Advocacy is needed in the areas of physical activity and food policy for children; research into pathophysiology, risk factors, and early recognition and management of overweight and obesity; and improved insurance coverage and third-party reimbursement for obesity care.

Pediatrics. 2003;112:424-430 (reaffirmed October 2006)

Diet

Dietary restriction should never be presented in a punitive manner and, if possible, the obese child and the entire family should adhere to a similar diet to minimize feelings of isolation by the obese child. Parents, pediatricians, and patients (especially adolescents) will be frustrated by the need for prolonged attention to diet and exercise that is required to achieve and maintain a reduced level of body fatness. Encouragement can be provided by examining growth and growth velocity curves with patients and their families to illustrate progress. If appropriate, the significance of any evident reduction in morbidity (eg, lowering of blood pressure or cholesterol) can be reinforced. Reasonable goals in the form of a "target" body weight at the next visit should be set at each office visit so that the patient and parents are aware of what is expected. These goals should be modest and attainable even if patients are only moderately compliant with their diet and exercise regimens since achievement of an interval "target weight" will also encourage the patient.

Dietary Intervention

The prescribed diet should initially provide 300 to 400 kcal/day below weight-maintenance requirements as assessed by dietary history or as calculated on the basis of a formula relating anthropometry to energy expenditure (eg, the Harris-Benedict equation).[211] Self-reported caloric intake is generally very inaccurate and tends to underestimate actual intake. A 300- to 400-kcal/day energy deficit should result in weight loss of approximately 1 lb per week. Weight reduction per se causes decreased energy expenditure. This phenomenon, plus the ongoing loss of metabolic mass, necessitates periodic downward adjustments of energy intake to sustain ongoing weight loss. The family should be instructed in long-term monitoring of caloric intake within and outside of the home and cautioned not to become overly critical or punitive toward the child if weight loss is slow or compliance is suboptimal.

The composition of the diet should be in accordance with the American Heart Association "heart healthy" recommendations and contain at least the minimal recommended amounts of protein, essential fatty acids, vitamins, and minerals and be low in saturated fats.[212] Diets consisting of drastically altered proportions of nutrients may be dangerous and yield no better results than a limited intake of a nutritionally balanced diet. Nutritional counseling should encourage decreasing the use of calorically dense (high-fat or fried) foods and adding more fruits and vegetables to the diet. The substitution of water for nonnutritious high-calorie sugar-containing drinks (juices, iced teas, and sodas) may be very helpful.[210] In some cases, reductions in calorically dense foods and sugar-containing drinks through substitution and/or elimination alone can decrease calories and weight without changing the general pattern of food consumption in the family. When families eat at restaurants and fast food establishments, they have less control over food choices than they do at home. Thus, reduction in the number of meals prepared outside the home may also be an effective weight-loss strategy.

Parents and adult caregivers should understand the important role they play in the development of proper eating habits in their young children. The parents' food preferences, the quantities and variety of foods in the home, and the parents' eating behavior and physical activity patterns all determine how supportive the home environment is to the obese child.

Therapeutic Exercise

Regular aerobic exercise will allow the patient to ingest more calories and, hopefully, encourage the long-term continuation of such a regimen. Exercise will promote increased muscle mass, thereby raising total metabolic rate, and the putative effect of exercise to reduce visceral adipose tissue mass may independently lower the risk of hyperlipidemia and diabetes mellitus. However, the energy cost of even vigorous exercise is low when compared with the caloric content of many fast foods or other snacks, and exercise should not be viewed as a "license to eat." For example, walking at 3 miles/hour for 1 hour consumes approximately 200 kcal, approximately the same amount contained in a 1¾-oz bag of potato chips. Obviously, treats, such as ice cream or potato chips, should not be used as incentives to exercise.

Although no specific aspect of the sedentary lifestyle has been shown to directly cause obesity, behaviors such as television viewing, reading, working at a computer, or driving a car or commuting do exert effects on health. Television viewing appears to be directly associated with the incidence of obesity and inversely associated with the remission of obesity. The effect of television viewing on obesity seems to be attributable to both displacing more vigorous activities and its effect on diet. Not only is television viewing a sedentary behavior, but also, food constitutes the most heavily advertised product on children's television in the United States. In Hispanic children in the United States, adiposity was significantly correlated with time spent watching television but not with time spent watching videos,[213] suggesting that the bulk of the positive association of television watching and adiposity is attributable to the approximately 60% of advertising that is devoted to food.[100] Children and adolescents should be encouraged to view as little television as possible. Limitation of television, video games, and Internet surfing will encourage greater physical activity. Clinicians should encourage children to participate in organized or individual sports (stressing participation, not watching from the bench) and advocate for better community- and school-based activity programs.

If the patient is unable to lose weight and/or comorbid conditions persist, consideration should be given to referral of the child to a physician specializing in the treatment of pediatric obesity. Weight-loss programs, weight-reduction camps, etc are often not covered by medical insurance and should be considered for the morbidly obese child with some caution. Enrollment in a highly supervised environment may demonstrate to an overweight child that weight loss is possible and encourage the child to continue. However, rapid weight loss may precipitate cholelithiasis or eating disorders. A child may become overly preoccupied with his or her weight and lose self-esteem, even if a moderate degree of weight loss is achieved. Obsession with weight on the part of the child or their family may lead to serious deterioration of intrafamily relationships.

Surgical Intervention

In obese adults, surgery is usually recommended only for individuals with severe obesity (BMI >40), or those with BMI values between 35 and 40 who have significant comorbid conditions. Gastroplasty with gastroduodenal bypass can initially lead to a great deal of weight loss, and approximately 80% of patients remain at least 10% below their preoperative body weight for 10 years after surgery. Patients who have such procedures must be carefully followed. It is possible to consume excess calories or volume on liquid or semisolid diets or to develop intestinal obstruction and electrolyte disturbances.

The most common procedures are gastric bypass surgery, vertical banded gastroplasty, and adjustable gastric banding. There is extensive experience with adult gastric bypass surgery. Briefly, a 15- to 30-mL gastric pouch is created surgically just below the gastroesophageal junction and is then anastomosed to the jejunum. In vertical banded gastroplasty, a pouch just below the gastroesophageal junction is created by a vertical closure and a band is placed at the inferior outlet of the pouch allowing it to empty slowly into the more distal stomach. The least invasive and most reversible procedure is an adjustable gastric banding in which a prosthetic band with an adjustable inner diameter is placed around the proximal stomach restricting food entry to the volume of a small proximal gastric pouch. The band is connected to a subcutaneous port into which saline can be injected to alter the inner diameter of the band, thus requiring close follow-up with a physician and perhaps resulting in earlier detection of any complications.

There have been some recent short-term studies of gastroplasty and bypass surgery in small groups of adolescents (n = 30–40).[214] Early complications observed among adolescent patients undergoing bariatric surgery have been similar to those observed among adults, including pulmonary embolism, wound infections, stomal stenoses, dehydration, and marginal ulcers.

Late complications in small studies have included small-bowel obstruction, incisional hernias, and late weight regain in up to 15% of cases. Longer-term complications are also similar to adults and include inadequate vitamin and micronutrient intake.[215] In a recent review of 39 adolescent patients undergoing gastric bypass surgery, there was a 36% mean reduction in BMI as well as significant improvements in insulin sensitivity and total cholesterol and triglyceride concentrations postoperatively. Fifteen patients (39%) experienced complications requiring rehospitalization. Of these complications, 9 were classified as minor, requiring hospitalization of fewer than 7 days; 4 were classified as moderate, requiring 7 to 30 days of rehospitalization; and 2 were classified as severe, requiring more than 30 days of hospitalization and, in one case, resulting in death. There are no similar studies of examining only gastroplasty procedures in adolescents, but a significantly lower incidence of complications have been reported in adults undergoing gastroplasty as opposed to gastric bypass surgery.[216]

It is appropriate to consider bariatric surgery in some extremely obese children with serious morbidity (eg, pickwickian syndrome) in whom all other interventions have failed, with the caveat that long-term follow-up and monitoring is needed. Adolescents may be especially prone to vitamin and micronutrient deficiencies because of difficulty complying with postoperative dietary restrictions. In adults, adjustable gastric banding appears to result in less dramatic weight loss than does gastric bypass. However, in most, if not all children, the lower morbidity associated with the less invasive, adjustable, and reversible nature of banding probably outweighs the potentially greater weight loss associated with the riskier gastric bypass.

Pharmacotherapy

Drug therapy in children is not recommended, and there are currently no weight-loss medications approved by the Food and Drug Administration for use in children younger than 16 years. However, in some extremely obese adolescent patients with life-threatening morbidities, this approach may be necessary with the caveat that studies of the effectiveness of these drugs in children have not yet been reported.

Current pharmacotherapies can be subdivided into those that are designed primarily to (1) increase energy expenditure; (2) decrease caloric intake; or (3) decrease nutrient absorption. Catecholaminergic agonists, such as the schedule IV (low abuse potential) drug phentermine (Adipex-P [Gate Pharmaceuticals, Ambler, PA], Ionamin [Medeva Pharmaceuticals, Rochester, NY]), have been shown to decrease food intake and to increase energy expenditure in short-term studies. Adverse effects include insomnia, nervousness, dry mouth, and increased heart rate and blood pressure.[217-219] In many patients, these symptoms are transient and not clinically significant. Sibutramine (Meridia [Abbott Laboratories, North Chicago, IL]) has been available in the United States since November 1997 and acts by inhibiting the neuronal reuptake of both norepinephrine and serotonin. Sibutramine suppresses appetite and, to a lesser degree, increases energy expenditure. Adverse effects include increase in blood pressure, increase in heart rate, insomnia, constipation, increased sweating, headache, and dry mouth.[220,221] A long-acting pancreatic lipase inhibitor, Orlistat (Xenical [Roche Pharmaceuticals, Nutley, NJ]) was approved in 1999 for use in adults. Decreased lipase activity results in decreased hydrolysis of dietary fat and, thus, allows approximately 30% of the fat ingested to pass through the gut undigested. The most common adverse effects are loose stools, flatulence, and oily discharge leading to soiling of underwear. Inhibition of pancreatic lipase also causes loss of fat-soluble vitamins (A, D, E, and K) in the stool, and vitamin supplementation is recommended.[222,223] The use of lipase inhibitors has not been well studied in adolescents. Because of the possible effects of impaired vitamin D absorption on the extensive bone mineralization that occurs in adolescence, the use of any therapy that inhibits such absorption should be thoroughly investigated before it is prescribed for teenagers. Initial studies of lipase inhibitors as part of weight-reduction therapy in obese adolescents have reported that all patients experienced some gastrointestinal adverse effects and that 1 in 3 found them intolerable.[224] In addition, lipase inhibitor therapy in adolescents provoked significant reductions in circulating concentrations of vitamin D even when they were provided vitamin supplements.[225] Combinations of caffeine and ephedrine (derived from ephedra in the commonly available herb ma huang) are available as thermogenic agents but have not been approved for the treatment of obesity. The combination of ephedrine and caffeine may precipitate serious cardiac arrhythmias.[218]

More recently, CB_1 antagonists have been studied as possible weight loss drugs.[174] A number of studies of rodents and humans have indicated that CB_1 receptor antagonists act centrally as anorexiants and decrease activity of the hypothalamic-pituitary-adrenal axis. Peripherally, CB_1 receptor antagonists release other anorexiant signals as well de novo lipogenesis and gluconeogenesis.[226] Initial trials in adults have been promising, resulting in weight loss similar to that observed with sibutramine,[227] but no studies have yet been reported in children.

Overview of Therapeutic Options

Before prescribing any type of treatment for obesity, the clinician should assess the risk-benefit ratio for any treatment in an individual patient. In the older and otherwise healthy overweight child without family history of adiposity-related morbidity, the fact that adolescent obesity may constitute an independent risk factor for adult mortality and morbidity must be weighed against the possible morbidities associated with therapeutic weight reduction (poor statural growth, precipitation of eating disorders, etc). Long-term studies of weight-reduced children and adults have shown that 80% to 90% return to their previous weight percentiles. Obese children and their families must recognize that maintenance of a reduced degree of body fatness will probably require a lifetime of attention to energy intake and expenditure. The cautions emphasized in previous sections in deciding which patients should undergo a therapeutic weight reduction and the relatively slow rate at which weight should be lost reflect the significant morbidities associated with these processes. Diets extremely low in caloric content or with unusual distributions of calories as fat, protein, and carbohydrate may precipitate cardiac arrhythmias, severe electrolyte disturbances, or other morbidities. As many as 80% of children using unsupervised diets obtained from popular magazines have been found to suffer from weakness, headaches, fatigue, nausea, constipation, nervousness, dizziness, poor concentration, dysmenorrhea, and/or fainting. Children on a supervised diet must also be closely monitored for treatment-associated psychological morbidities.

Therapeutic intervention should emphasize the need for participation of the entire family and lifelong attention to, and benefits of, a healthy lifestyle as well as positive reinforcement for even small degrees of compliance. Preparation of the family and child for therapeutic intervention is as important as the intervention itself (see Fig 33.5).

References

1. Freedman DS, Kahn LK, Serdula MK, Dietz WH, Srinivasan SR, Berenson GS. The relation of childhood BMI to adult adiposity: The Bogalusa Heart Study. *Pediatrics*. 2005;115:22–27
2. Guo SS, Wu W, Chumlea WC, Roche AF. Predicting overweight and obesity in adulthood from body mass index values in childhood and adolescence. *Am J Clin Nutr*. 2002;76:653–658
3. Whitlock EP, Williams SB, Gold R, Smith PR, Shipman SA. Screening and interventions for childhood overweight: a summary of evidence for the US Preventive Services Task Force. *Pediatrics*. 2005;116(1):e125–e144. Available at: http://pediatrics.aappublications.org/cgi/content/full/116/1/e125. Accessed September 25, 2007

4. Whitaker RC, Wright JA, Pepe MS, Seidel KD, Dietz WH. Predicting obesity in young adulthood from childhood and parental obesity. *N Engl J Med*. 1997;337:869–873

5. Rosenbaum M, Nonas C, Horlick M, et al. Beta-cell function and insulin sensitivity in early adolescence: association with body fatness and family history of type 2 diabetes mellitus. El Camino Diabetes Prevention Group. *J Clin Endocrinol Metab*. 2004;89:5469–5476

6. Mora S, Yanek LR, Moy TF, Fallin MD, Becker LC, Becker DM. Interaction of body mass index and Framingham risk score in predicting incident coronary disease in families. *Circulation*. 2005;111:1871–1876

7. Snieder H, Harshfield GA, Trieber FA. Heritability of blood pressure and hemodynamics in African- and European-American youth. *Hypertension*. 2003;41:1196–1201

8. Treuth MS, Butte NF, Sorkin JD. Predictors of body fat gain in nonobese girls with a familial predisposition to obesity. *Am J Clin Nutr*. 2003;78:1212–1218

9. Davison KK, Birch LL. Child and parent characteristics as predictors of change in girl's body mass index. *Int J Obes Relat Metab Disord*. 2001;25:1834–1842

10. Pietrobelli A, Faith MS, Allison DB, Gallagher D, Chiumello G, Heymsfield SB. Body mass index as a measure of adiposity among children and adolescents: a validation study. *J Pediatr*. 1998;132:204–210

11. Reilly JJ, Dorosty AR, Emmet PM. Identification of the obese child: adequacy of the body mass index for clinical practice and epidemiology. Avon Longitudinal Study of Pregnancy and Childhood Study Team. *Int J Obes Relat Metab Disord*. 2000;24:1623–1627

12. Expert Panel on the Identification, Evaluation, and Treatment of Overweight in Adults. Clinical guidelines on the identification, evaluation, and treatment of overweight and obesity in adults: executive summary. *Am J Clin Nutr*. 1998;68:899–917

13. Troiano RP, Flegal KM. Overweight children and adolescents: description, epidemiology, and demographics. *Pediatrics*. 1998;101(Suppl):497–504

14. Must A, Dallal G, Dietz W. Reference data for obesity: 85th and 95th percentiles of body mass index (wt/ht^2) and triceps skinfold thickness. *Am J Clin Nutr*. 1991;53:839–846

15. Himes JH, Bouchard C, Pheley AM. Lack of correspondence among measures identifying the obese. *Am J Prev Med*. 1991;7:107–111

16. Bjorntorp P. Classification of obese patients and complications related to the distribution of surplus fat. *Am J Clin Nutr*. 1987;45:1120–1125

17. Bjorntorp P. Possible mechanisms relating fat distribution and metabolism. In: Bouchard C, Johnston FE, eds. *Fat Distribution During Growth and Later Health Outcomes*. New York, NY: Alan R. Liss Inc.; 1988:175–191

18. Ford ES, Mokdad AH, Giles WH, Galuska DA, Serdula MK. Geographic variation in the prevalence of obesity, diabetes, and obesity-related behaviors. *Obes Res*. 2005;13:118–122

19. Schoenborn CA, Adams PF, Barnes PM. Body weight status of adults: United States, 1997–98. *Adv Data*. 2002;(330):1–15

20. Gordon-Larsen P, Nelson M, Page P, Popkin B. Inequality in the built environment underlies key health disparities in physical activity and obesity. *Pediatrics*. 2006;117:417–424

21. Stettler N. Environmental factors in the etiology of obesity in adolescents. *Ethn Dis*. 2002;12:S1-41–S1-45

22. Strauss RS, Knight J. Influence of the home environment on the development of obesity in children. *Pediatrics*. 1999;103(6):e85. Available at: http://pediatrics.aappublications.org/cgi/content/full/103/6/e85. Accessed September 25, 2007

23. Stettler N, Tershakovec AM, Zemel BS, et al. Early risk factors for increased adiposity: a cohort study of African American subjects followed from birth to young adulthood. *Am J Clin Nutr*. 2000;72:378–383

24. Troiano RP, Flegal KM, Kuczmarski RJ, Campbell SM, Johnson CL. Overweight prevalence and trends for children and adolescents. *Arch Pediatr Adolesc Med*. 1995;149:1085–1091

25. Flegal K, Troiano P. Changes in the distribution of body mass index of adults and children in the US population. *Int J Obes Relat Metab Disord*. 2000;24:807–818

26. Kuczmarski RJ, Flegal KM, Campbell SM, Johnson CL. Increasing prevalence of overweight among US adults. The National Health and Nutrition Examination Survey, 1960 to 1991. *JAMA*. 1994;272:205–211

27. Overpeck MD, Hedger ML, Ruan WJ, et al. Stature, weight, and body mass among US children born at term with appropriate birth weights. *J Pediatr*. 2000;137:205–213

28. Rosner B, Prineas R, Loggie J, Daniels SR. Percentiles for body mass index in U.S. children 5 to 17 years of age. *J Pediatr*. 1998;132:211–222

29. Serne EH, Stehouwer CD, Maaten JC, ter Wee PM, Donker AJ, Gans RO. Birth weight relates to blood pressure and microvascular function in normal subjects. *J Hypertens*. 2000;18:1421–1427

30. Li C, Johnson MS, Goran MI. Effects of low birth weight on insulin resistance syndrome in Caucasian and African-American children. *Diabetes Care*. 2001;24:2035–2042

31. Lipsy RJ. The National Cholesterol Education Program Adult Treatment Panel III guidelines. *J Manag Care Pharm*. 2003;9:2–5

32. Cook S, Weitzman M, Auinger P, Nguyen M, Dietz WH. Prevalence of a metabolic syndrome phenotype in adolescents: findings from the third National Health and Nutrition Examination Survey,1988–1994. *Arch Pediatr Adolesc Med*. 2003;157:821–827

33. Ford ES, Giles WH, Dietz WH. Prevalence of the metabolic syndrome among US adults: findings From the Third National Health and Nutrition Examination Survey. *JAMA*. 2002;287:356–359

34. Yarborough DE, Barrett-Connor E, Kritz-Silverstein D, Wingard DL. Birth weight, adult weight, and girth as predictors of the metabolic syndrome in postmenopausal women: the Rancho Bernardo Study. *Diabetes Care*. 1998;21:1652–1658

35. Law CM, Shiell AW. Is blood pressure inversely related to birth weight? The strength of evidence from a systematic review of the literature. *J Hypertens*. 1996;14:935–941

36. Owen CG, Whincup PH, Odoki K, Gilg JA, Cook DG. Birth weight and blood cholesterol level: a study in adolescents and systematic review. *Pediatrics*. 2003;111:1081–1089

37. Barker DJ. Fetal origins of cardiovascular disease. *Ann Med*. 1999;31(Suppl 1):3–6

38. Tenhola S, Martikainen A, Rahiala E, Herrgard E, Halonen P, Voutilainen R. Serum lipid concentrations and growth characteristics in 12-year-old children born small for gestational age. *Pediatr Res*. 2000;48:623–628

39. Ravelli A, van der Meullen J, Osmond C, Barker DJ, Bleker OP. Infant feeding and adult glucose tolerance, lipid profile, blood pressure, and obesity. *Arch Dis Child*. 2000;82:248–252

40. Godfrey KM, Barker DJ. Fetal nutrition and adult disease. *Am J Clin Nutr.* 2000;71: 1344S–1352S

41. Donker GA, Labarthe DR, Harrist RB, et al. Low birth weight and serum lipid concentrations at age 7–11 years in a biracial sample. *Am J Epidemiol.* 1997;145:398–407

42. Pulzer F, Haase U, Kratzch J, et al. Lipoprotein(a) levels in formerly small-for-gestational-age children. *Horm Res.* 1999;52:241–246

43. Okosun IS, Dever GE, Choi ST. Low birth weight is associated with elevated serum lipoprotein(a) in white and black American children ages 5–11 y. *Public Health.* 2002; 116:33–38

44. Newsome CA, Shiell AW, Fall CH, Phillips DI, Shier R, Law CM. Is birth weight related to later glucose and insulin metabolism? — a systematic review. *Diabet Med.* 2003;20: 339–348

45. Forsen T, Eriksson J, Tuomilehto J, Reunanen A, Osmond C, Barker D. The fetal and childhood growth of persons who develop type 2 diabetes. *Ann Intern Med.* 2000;133:176–182

46. Eriksson M, Wallander M, Krakau I, Wedel H, Svarsudd K. Birth weight and cardiovascular risk factors in a cohort followed until 80 years of age: the study of men born in 1913. *J Intern Med.* 2004;255:236–246

47. Curhan GC, Willett WC, Rimm EB, Spiegelman D, Ascherio AL, Stampfer MJ. Birth weight and adult hypertension, diabetes mellitus, and obesity in US Men. *Circulation.* 1996;94:3246–3250

48. Rich-Edwards JW, Colditz GA, Stampfer MJ, et al. Birthweight and the risk for type II diabetes mellitus in adult women. *Ann Intern Med.* 1999;130:278–284

49. Wei JN, Sung FC, Li CY, et al. Low birth weight and high birth weight infants are both at an increased risk to have type 2 diabetes among schoolchildren in Taiwan. *Diabetes Care.* 2003;26:343–348

50. Barker DJ, Hales CN, Fall CH, Osmond C, Phipps K, Clark PM. Type 2 (non-insulin-dependent) diabetes mellitus, hypertension, and hyperlipidaemia (syndrome X): relation to reduced fetal growth. *Diabetologia.* 1993;36:62–67

51. Byberg L, McKeigue PM, Zethelius B, Lithell HO. Birth weight and the insulin resistance syndrome: association of low birth weight with truncal obesity and raised plasminogen activator inhibitor-1 but not with abdominal obesity or plasma lipid disturbances. *Diabetologia.* 2000;43:54–60

52. Ravelli A, van der Meulen JH, Michels RP, et al. Glucose tolerance in adults after prenatal exposure to famine. *Lancet.* 1998;351:173–177

53. Hales CN, Barker DJ. Type 2 (non-insulin-dependent) diabetes mellitus: the thrifty phenotype hypothesis. *Diabetologia.* 1992;35:595–601

54. Simmons R. Developmental origins of adult metabolic disease: concepts and controversies. *Trends Endocrinol Metab.* 2005;16:390–394

55. Bhargava S, Sachdev HS, Fall CH, et al. Relation of serial changes in childhood body mass index to impaired glucose tolerance in young adulthood. *N Engl J Med.* 2004;350:865–875

56. Cianfarani S, Germani D, Branca F. Low birthweight and adult insulin resistance: the "catch-up growth" hypothesis. *Arch Dis Child Fetal Neonatal Ed.* 1991;81:F71–F73

57. Whitaker RC, Pepe MS, Wright JA, Seidel KD, Dietz WH. Early adiposity rebound and the risk of adult obesity. *Pediatrics.* 1998;101(3):e5. Available at: http://pediatrics. aappublications.org/cgi/content/full/101/3/e5. Accessed September 25, 2007

58. Ong KK, Ahmed ML, Emmett PM, Preece MA, Dunger DB. Association between postnatal catch-up growth and obesity in childhood: prospective cohort study. *BMJ.* 2000;320:967–971

59. Veening MA, van Weissenbruch MM, Heine RJ, Delemarre-van de Waal HA. Beta-cell capacity and insulin sensitivity in prepubertal children born small for gestational age: influence of body size during childhood. *Diabetes.* 2003;52:1756–1760

60. Colle E, Schiff D, Andrews G, Bauer CB, Fitzhardinge P. Insulin responses during catch-up growth of infants who were small for gestational age. *Pediatrics.* 1976;57:363–371

61. Frayling TT, Hattersley AT. The role of genetic susceptibility in the association of low birth weight with type 2 diabetes. *Br Med Bull.* 2001;60:89–101

62. Neel JV. Diabetes mellitus: a "thrifty" genotype rendered detrimental by "progress"? *Am J Hum Genet.* 1962;14:353–362

63. Sattar N, McConnachie A, O'Reilly D, et al. Inverse association between birth weight and C-reactive protein concentrations in the MIDSPAN Family Study. *Arterioscler Thromb Vasc Biol.* 2004;24:583–587

64. Levin B. Metabolic imprinting on genetically predisposed neural circuits perpetuates obesity. *Nutrition.* 2000;16:909–915

65. Martin RJ, Hausman GH, Hausman DB. Regulation of adipose cell development in utero. *Proc Soc Exp Biol Med.* 1998;219:200–210

66. Lee H, Park K, Cho Y, Lee Y, Pay Y. Mitochondria-based model for fetal origin of adult disease and insulin resistance. *Ann N Y Acad Sci.* 1999;104:1–18

67. Phillips DI, Barker DJ, Hales CN, Hirst S, Osmond C. Thinness at birth and insulin resistance in adult life. *Diabetologia.* 1994;37:150–154

68. Hales C, Barker D, Clark PM, et al. Fetal and infant growth and impaired glucose tolerance at age 64. *BMJ.* 1991;303:1019–1022

69. Rump P, Popp-Snidjers C, Heine RJ, Hornstra G. Components of the insulin resistance syndrome in seven-year-old children: relations with birth weight and the polyunsaturated fatty acid content of umbilical cord plasma phospholipids. *Diabetologia.* 2002;45:349–355

70. Schaefer-Graf U, Kojos S, Kilavuz O, et al. Determinants of fetal growth at different periods of pregnancies complicated by gestational diabetes mellitus or impaired glucose tolerance. *Diabetes Care.* 2003;26:193–198

71. Schaefer-Graf UM, Pawliczak J, Passow D, et al. Birth weight and parental BMI predict overweight in children from mothers with gestational diabetes. *Diabetes Care.* 2005;28:1734–1740

72. Vohr BR, McGarvey ST. Growth patterns of large-for-gestational-age and appropriate-for-gestational-age infants of gestational diabetic mothers and control mothers at age 1 year. *Diabetes Care.* 1997;20:1066–1072

73. Gillman MW, Rifas-Shiman R, Berkey CS, Field AE, Colditz GA. Maternal gestational diabetes, birth weight, and adolescent obesity. *Pediatrics.* 2003;111(3):e221–e226. Available at: http://pediatrics.aappublications.org/cgi/content/full/111/3/e221. Accessed September 25, 2007

74. Boney CM, Verma A, Tucker R, Bohr BR. Metabolic syndrome in childhood: association with birth weight, maternal obesity, and gestational diabetes mellitus. *Pediatrics*. 205;115(3):e290–e296

75. Pettitt DJ, Baird HR, Aleck KA, Knowler WC. Excessive obesity in offspring of Pima Indian women with diabetes during pregnancy. *N Engl J Med*. 1983;308:242–245

76. Pettitt DJ, Baird HR, Aleck KA, Bennett PH, Knowler WC. Excessive obesity in offspring of Pima Indian women with diabetes during pregnancy. *N Engl J Med*. 1983;308:242–245

77. Pettitt DJ, Knowler WC, Bennett PH, Aleck KA, Baird HR. Obesity in offspring of diabetic Pima Indian women despite normal birth weight. *Diabetes Care*. 1987;10:76–80

78. Pettitt DJ, Aleck KA, Baird HR, Carraher MJ, Bennett PH, Knowler WC. Congential susceptibility to NIDDM. Role of interauterine environment. *Diabetes*. 1988;37:622–628

79. Plagemann A. Perinatal programming and functional teratogenesis: impact on body weight regulation and obesity. *Physiol Behav*. 2005;86:661–668

80. Oken E, Huh SY, Taveras EM, Rich-Edwards JW, Gillman MW. Associations of maternal prenatal smoking with child adiposity and blood pressure. *Obes Res*. 2005;13:2021–2028

81. Kries Rv, Toschke A, Koletko B, Slikker W. Maternal smoking during pregnancy and childhood obesity. *Am J Epidemiol*. 2002;156:954–961

82. Gillman MW, Rifas-Shiman SL, Camargo CA Jr, et al. 2001 Risk of overweight among adolescents who were breastfed as infants. *JAMA*. 2002;285:2461–2467

83. von Kries R, Koletzko B, Sauerwald T, et al. Breast feeding and obesity: cross sectional study. *BMJ*. 1999;319:147–150

84. Nelson MC, Gordon-Larsen P, Adair LS. Are adolescents who were breast-fed less likely to be overweight? Analyses of sibling pairs to reduce confounding. *Epidemiology*. 2005;16:247–253

85. Hediger ML, Overpeck MD, Kuczmarski RJ, Ruan WJ. Association between infant breastfeeding and overweight in young children. *JAMA*. 2001;285:2453–2460

86. Agras WS, Kraemer HC, Berkowitz RI, Hammer LD. Influence of early feeding style on adiposity at 6 years of age. *J Pediatr*. 1990;116:805–809

87. Wolman P. Feeding practices in infancy and prevalence of obesity in preschool children. *J Am Diet Assoc*. 1984;84:436–438

88. Howard BV, Horn L, Hsia J, et al. Low-fat dietary pattern and risk of cardiovascular disease: the Women's Health Initiative Randomized Controlled Dietary Modification Trial. *JAMA*. 2006;295:655–666

89. Beresford SA, Johnson KC, Ritenbaugh C, et al. Low-fat dietary pattern and risk of colorectal cancer: the Women's Health Initiative Randomized Controlled Dietary Modification Trial. *JAMA*. 2006;295:643–654

90. Prentice RL, Caan B, Chlebowski RT. Low-fat dietary pattern and risk of invasive breast cancer: the Women's Health Initiative Randomized Controlled Dietary Modification Trial. *JAMA*. 2006;295:629–642

91. Kriska AM, Blair SN, Pereira MA. The potential role of physical activity in the prevention of non-insulin-dependent diabetes mellitus: the epidemiological evidence. *Exerc Sport Sci Rev*. 1994;22:121–143

92. Wei M, Schertner HA, Blair SN. The association between physical activity, physical fitness, and type 2 diabetes mellitus. *Compr Ther.* 2000;26:176–182

93. Manson JE, Nathan DM, Krowlewski AS, Stampfer MJ, Willett WC, Hennekens CH. A prospective study of exercise and incidence of diabetes among US male physicians. *JAMA.* 1992;268:63–67

94. Weinstein AR, Sesso HD, Lee IM, Manson J, Buring J, Gaziano J. Relationship of physical activity vs body mass index with type 2 diabetes in women. *JAMA.* 2004;292:1188–1194

95. Dietz WH Jr, Gortmaker SL. Do we fatten our children at the television set? Obesity and television viewing in children and adolescents. *Pediatrics.* 1985;75:807–812

96. Salbe AD, Nicolson M, Ravussin E. Total energy expenditure and physical activity correlate with plasma leptin concentrations in five-year-old children. *J Clin Invest.* 1997;99:592–595

97. Ku LC, Shapiro LR, Crayford PB, Huenemann RL. Body composition and physical activity in 8-year-old children. *Am J Clin Nutr.* 1981;34:2770–2775

98. Davies PS, Gregory J, White A. Physical activity and body fatness in pre-school children. *Int J Obes Relat Metab Disord.* 1995;19:6–10

99. Crespo CJ, Smit E, Troiano RP, Bartlett SJ, Macera CA, Andersen RE. Television watching, energy intake, and obesity in US children: results from the third National Health and Nutrition Examination Survey, 1988–1994. *Arch Pediatr Adolesc Med.* 2001;155:360–365

100. Borzekowski DL, Robinson TN. The 30-second effect: an experiment revealing the impact of television commercials on food preferences of preschoolers. *J Am Diet Assoc.* 2001;101: 42–46

101. Centers for Disease Control and Prevention. Prevalence of overweight among adolescents— United States, 1988–91. *MMWR Morb Mortal Wkly Rep.* 1994;43:818–821

102. Kuczmarski RJ. Trends in body composition for infants and children in the U.S. *Crit Rev Food Sci Nutr.* 1993;33:375–387

103. Flegal K, Ogden C, Wei R, Kuczmarski R, Johnson C. Prevalence of overweight in US children: comparison of US growth charts from the Centers for Disease Control and Prevention with other reference values for body mass index. *Am J Clin Nutr.* 2001;73:1086–1093

104. Wadden T. Treatment of obesity by moderate and severe caloric restriction. Results of clinical research trials. *Ann Intern Med.* 1993;229:688–693

105. Nuutinen O, Knip M. Long-term weight control in obese children: persistence of treatment outcome and metabolic changes. *Int J Obes Relat Metab Disord.* 1992;16:279–287

106. McGuire WT, Wing RR, Hill JO. The prevalence of weight loss maintenance among American adults. *Int J Obes Relat Metab Disord.* 1999;23:1314–1319

107. Klem ML, Wing RR, Lang W, McGuire MT, Hill JO. Does weight loss maintenance become easier over time? *Obes Res.* 2000;8:438–444

108. Klem M, Wing R, McGuire M, Seagle H, Hill J. A descriptive study of individuals successful at long term maintenance of substantial weight loss. *Am J Clin Nutr.* 1997;66:239–246

109. Wing RR, Hill JO. Successful weight loss maintenance. *Annu Rev Nutr.* 2001;21:323–341

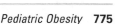

110. Belanger AJ, Cupples LA, D'Agostino RB. *The Framingham Study: The Epidemiological Investigation of Cardiovascular Disease. Section 36. Means at Each Examination and Interexamination Consistency of Specified Characteristics. Framingham Heart Study: 30-Year Follow-up*. Bethesda, MD: National Heart, Lung, and Blood Institute; 1988. Framingham Publication No. 88-2970

111. Johnston FE. Sex differences in fat patterning in children and youth. In: Bouchard C, Johnston F, eds. *Fat Distribution During Growth and Later Health Outcomes*. New York: Alan R. Liss Inc; 1988:85–102

112. Horlick M, Thornton J, Wang J, Fedun B, Levine L, Pierson R. The relationship of central adiposity to total body fatness in children and adolescents varies with sex, puberty, and black/white ethnicity (abstr). *Pediatr Res*. 2000;47:132A

113. Rosenbaum M, Leibel RL, Hirsch J. Obesity. *N Engl J Med*. 1997;337:396–407

114. Bouchard C, Bray GA, eds. 1995 *Regulation of Body Weight: Biological and Behavioral Mechanism*. Chichester, England: John Wiley & Sons Ltd; 1996

115. Sims EA, Goldman RF, Gluck CM, Horton ES, Kelleher PC, Rowe DW. Experimental obesity in man. *Trans Assoc Am Physicians*. 1968;81:153–170

116. Bouchard C, Tremblay A, Despres JP, et al. The response to long-term overfeeding in identical twins. *N Engl J Med*. 1990;322:1477–1482

117. Sims EA. Experimental obesity, dietary-induced thermogenesis, and their clinical implications. *Clin Endocrinol Metab*. 1976;5:377–395

118. Sims EA, Danforth E Jr, Horton ES, Bray GA, Glennon JA, Salans LB. Endocrine and metabolic effects of experimental obesity in man. *Rec Prog Horm Res*. 1973;29:457–496

119. Tremblay A, Despres JP, Theriault G, Fournier G, Bouchard C. Overfeeding and energy expenditure in humans. *Am J Clin Nutr*. 1992;56:857–862

120. Ravussin E, Lillioja S, Anderson TE, Christin L, Bogardus C. Determinants of 24-hour energy expenditure in man. Methods and results using a respiratory chamber. *J Clin Invest*. 1986;78:1568–1578

121. Geissler CA, Miller DS, Shah M. The daily metabolic rate of the post-obese and the lean. *Am J Clin Nutr*. 1987;45:914–920

122. Wadden TA, Foster GD, Letizia KA, Mullen JL. Long-term effects of dieting on resting metabolic rate in obese outpatients. *JAMA*. 1990;264:707–711

123. Elliot DL, Goldberg L, Kuehl KS, Bennett WM. Sustained depression of the resting metabolic rate after massive weight loss. *Am J Clin Nutr*. 1989;49:93–96

124. Dulloo A, Girardier L. 24 hour energy expenditure several months after weight loss in the underfed rat: evidence for a chronic decrease in whole-body metabolic efficiency. *Int J Obes Relat Metab Disord*. 1993;17:115–123

125. Schoeller DA. Balancing energy expenditure and body weight. *Am J Clin Nutr*. 1998;68:956S–961S

126. Raben A, Mygind E, Astrup A. Lower activity of oxidative key enzymes and smaller fiber areas in skeletal muscle of postobese women. *Am J Physiol*. 1998;275:e487–e494

127. Weigle DS, Brunzell JD. Assessment of energy expenditure in ambulatory reduced-obese subjects by techniques of weight stabilization and exogenous weight replacement. *Int J Obes*. 1990;14:69–77

128. Froidevaux F, Schutz Y, Christin L, Jequier E. Energy expenditure in obese women before and during weight loss, after refeeding, and in the weight-relapse period. *Am J Clin Nutr.* 1993;57:35–42

129. van Gemert WG, Westerterp KR, van Acker BA, et al. Energy, substrate and protein metabolism in morbid obesity before, during and after massive weight loss. *Int J Obes Relat Metab Disord.* 2000;24:711–718

130. deBoer JO, van Es AJ, van Raaij JM, Hautvast JG. Energy requirements and energy expenditure of lean and overweight women, measured by indirect calorimetry. *Am J Clin Nutr.* 1987;46:13–21

131. deBoer JO, van Es AJ, Roovers LC, van Raaij JM, Hautvast JG. Adaptation of energy metabolism of overweight women to low-energy intake, studied with whole-body calorimeters. *Am J Clin Nutr.* 1986;44:585–595

132. Leibel R, Rosenbaum M, Hirsch J. Changes in energy expenditure resulting from altered body weight. *N Engl J Med.* 1995;332:621–628

133. Rosenbaum M, Ravussin E, Matthews DE, et al. A comparative study of different means of assessing long-term energy expenditure in humans. *Am J Physiol.* 1996;270:R496–R504

134. Welle S, Forbes GB, Statt M, Bernard RR, Amatruda JM. Energy expenditure under free-living conditions in normal-weight and overweight women. *Am J Clin Nutr.* 1992;55:14–21

135. Weinsier RL, Hunter GR, Zuckerman PA, et al. Energy expenditure and free-living physical activity in black and white women: comparison before and after weight loss. *Am J Clin Nutr.* 2000;71:1138–1146

136. Astrup A, Buemann B, Christensen NJ, Madsen J. 24-hour energy expenditure and sympathetic activity in postobese women consuming a high carbohydrate diet. *Am J Physiol.* 1992;262:e282–e288

137. de Groot LC, van Es AJ, van Raaij JM, Vogt JE, Hautvast JG. Energy metabolism of overweight women 1 mo and 1 y after an 8-wk slimming period. *Am J Clin Nutr.* 1990;51:578–583

138. Mossberg H. 40-year follow-up of overweight children. *Lancet.* 1989;2:491–493

139. Maffeis C, Schutz Y, Pinnelli L. Effects of weight loss on resting energy expenditure in obese prepubertal children. *Int J Obes Relat Metab Disord.* 1992;16:41–47

140. Rosenbaum M, Leibel RL. The physiology of body weight regulation: relevance to the etiology of obesity in children. *Pediatrics.* 1998;101:525–539

141. Kiortsis DN, Durack I, Turpin G. Effects of a low-calorie diet on resting metabolic rate and serum tri-iodothyronine levels in obese children. *Eur J Pediatr.* 1999;158:446–450

142. Rosenbaum M, Hirsch J, Murphy E, Leibel RL. Effects of changes in body weight on carbohydrate metabolism, catecholamine excretion, and thyroid function. *Am J Clin Nutr.* 2000;71:1421–1432

143. Wardlaw SL. Clinical review 127: obesity as a neuroendocrine disease: lessons to be learned from proopiomelanocortin and melanocortin receptor mutations in mice and men. *J Clin Endocrinol Metab.* 2001;86:1442–1446

144. Rosenbaum M, Leibel R. Leptin: a molecule integrating somatic energy stores, energy expenditure, and fertility. *Trends Endocrinol Metab.* 1998;9:117–123

145. Ahima RS, Prabakaran D, Mantzoros C, et al. Role of leptin in the neuroendocrine response to fasting. *Nature*. 1996;382:250–252

146. Ahima RS, Kelly J, Elmquist JK, Flier JS. Distinct physiologic and neuronal responses to decreased leptin and mild hyperleptinemia. *Endocrinology*. 1999;140:4923–4931

147. Aronne L, Mackintosh R, Rosenbaum M, Leibel R, Hirsch J. Autonomic nervous system activity in weight gain and weight loss. *Am J Physiol*. 1995;38:R222–R225

148. Rosenbaum M, Nicolson M, Hirsch J, Murphy E, Chu F, Leibel RL. Effects of weight change on plasma leptin concentrations and energy expenditure. *J Clin Endocrinol Metab*. 1997;82:3647–3654

149. Roemmich JN, Sinning WE. Weight loss and wrestling training: effects on growth-related hormones. *J Appl Physiol*. 1997;82:1760–1764

150. Welt CK, Chan JL, Bullen J, et al. Recombinant human leptin in women with hypothalamic amenorrhea. *N Engl J Med*. 2004;351:987–997

151. Korner J, Aronne LJ. The emerging science of body weight regulation and its impact on obesity treatment. *J Clin Invest*. 2003;111:565–570

152. Schwartz MW, Morton GJ. Obesity: keeping hunger at bay. *Nature*. 2002;418:595–597

153. Leibel R, Chua S, Rosenbaum M. Obesity. In: Scriver CR, Beaudet AL, Sly WS, Valle D, eds. *The Metabolic and Molecular Bases of Inherited Disease*. Vol 3. 8th ed. New York, NY: McGraw-Hill; 2001:3965–4028

154. Vale W, Rivier C, Brown MR, et al. Chemical and biological characterization of corticotropin releasing factor. *Recent Prog Horm Res*. 1983;39:245–270

155. Farooqi IS, Keogh JM, Yeo GS, Lank EJ, Ceetham T, O'Rahilly S. Clinical spectrum of obesity and mutations in the melanocortin 4 receptor gene. *N Eng J Med*. 2003;348:1085–1095

156. Govaerts C, Srinivasan S, Shapiro A, et al. Obesity-associated mutations in the melanocortin 4 receptor provide novel insights into its function. *Peptides*. 2005;26:1909–1919

157. Leibel R. The molecular genetics of the melanocortin pathway and energy homeostasis. *Cell Metab*. 2006;3:79–81

158. Wellman P. Modulation of eating by central catecholamine systems. *Curr Drug Targets*. 2005;6:191–199

159. Saper C, Chou T, Elmquist J. The need to feed: homeostatic and hedonic control of eating. *Neuron*. 2002;36:199–211

160. Small CJ, Bloom SS. Gut hormones and the control of appetite. *Trends Endocrinol Metab*. 2004;15:259–263

161. Roth CL, Enriori PJ, Harz K, Woelfle J, Cowley MA, Reinehr T. Peptide YY is a regulator of energy homeostasis in obese children before and after weight loss. *J Clin Endocrinol Metab*. 2005;90:6386–6391

162. Korner J, Leibel RL. To eat or not to eat: how the gut talks to the brain. *N Engl J Med*. 2003;349:926–928

163. Chai BX, Neubig RR, Millhauser GL, et al. Inverse activity of agouti and agouti-related protein. *Peptides*. 2003;24:603–609

164. Farooqi IS, Jebb SA, Langmack G, et al. Effects of recombinant leptin therapy in a child with congenital leptin deficiency. *N Engl J Med*. 1999;16:879–884

165. Montague CT, Farooqi IS, Whitehead JP, et al. Congenital leptin deficiency is associated with severe early-onset obesity in humans. *Nature*. 1997;387:903–908

166. Clement K, Vaisse C, Lahlou N, et al. A mutation in the human leptin receptor gene causes obesity and pituitary dysfunction. *Nature*. 1998;392:398–401

167. Farooqi IS, Matarese G, Lord GM, et al. Beneficial effects of leptin on obesity, T cell hyporesponsiveness, and neuroendocrine/metabolic dysfunction of human congenital leptin deficiency. *J Clin Invest*. 2002;110:1093–1103

168. Ahima RS, Saper CB, Flier JS, Elmquist JK. Leptin regulation of neuroendocrine systems. *Front Neuroendocrinol*. 2000;21:263–307

169. Rosenbaum M, Goldsmith R, Bloomfield D, et al. Low dose leptin reverses skeletal muscle, autonomic, and neuroendocrine adaptations to maintenance of reduced weight. *J Clin Invest*. 2005;115:3579–3586

170. Heymsfield SB, Greenberg AS, Fujioka K, et al. Recombinant leptin for weight loss in obese and lean adults: a randomized, controlled, dose-escalation trial. *JAMA*. 1999;292:1568–1575

171. Munzberg H, Flier JS, Bjorbaek C. Region-specific leptin resistance within the hypothalamus of diet-induced obese mice. *Endocrinology*. 2004;145:4880–4889

172. Rahmouni K, Morgan DA, Morgan GM, Mark AL, Haynes WG. Role of selective leptin resistance in diet-induced obesity hypertension. *Diabetes*. 2005;54:2012–2018

173. Strader AD, Woods SC. Gastrointestinal hormones and food intake. *Gastroenterology*. 2005;128:175–191

174. Pagotto U, Marsicano G, Cota D, Lutz B, Pasquali R. The emerging role of the endocannabinoid system in endocrine regulation and energy balance. *Endocrinol Rev*. 2005;27:73–100

175. Klein TW, Newton C, Larsen K, et al. The cannabinoid system and immune modulation. *J Leuk Biol*. 2003;74:486–496

176. Ibrahim MM, Porreca F, Lai J, et al. CB2 cannabinoid receptor activation produces antinociception by stimulating peripheral release of endogenous opioids. *Proc Natl Acad Sci U S A*. 2005;102:3093–3098

177. Weyer C, Funahashi T, Tanaka S, et al. Hypoadiponectinemia in obesity and type 2 diabetes: close association with insulin resistance and hyperinsulinemia. *J Clin Endocrinol Metab*. 2001;86:1930–1935

178. Nemet D, Wang P, Funahashi T, et al. Adipocytokines, body composition, and fitness in children. *Pediatr Res*. 2003;53:148–152

179. Stern MP, Bartley M, Duggirala R, Bradshaw B. Birth weight and the metabolic syndrome: thrifty phenotype or thrifty genotype? *Diab Met Res Rev*. 2000;16:88–93

180. Stunkard AJ, Foch TT, Hrubec Z. A twin study of human obesity. *JAMA*. 1986;256:51–54

181. Sun M, Gower BA, Bartolucci AA, Hunter G, Figueroa-Colon R, Goran MI. A longitudinal study of resting energy expenditure relative to body composition during puberty in African American and white children. *Am J Clin Nutr*. 2001;73:308–315

182. Chung WK, Leibel RL. Molecular physiology of syndromic obesities in humans. *Trends Endocrinol Metab*. 2005;16:267–272

183. Must A, Jacques PF, Dallai GE, Bajema CJ, Dietz WH. Long-term morbidity and mortality of overweight adolescents. A follow-up of the Harvard Growth Study of 1922 to 1935. *N Engl J Med*. 1992;327:1350–1355

184. Webber LS, Srinivasan SR, Wattigneyy WA, Berenson GS. Tracking of serum lipids and lipoproteins from childhood to adulthood: The Bogalusa Heart Study. *Am J Epidemiol*. 1991;133:884–899

185. Field AE, Cook NR, Gillman MW. Weight status in childhood as a predictor of becoming overweight or hypertensive in early adulthood. *Obes Res*. 2005;13:163–169

186. Daniels S. Obesity in the pediatric patient: cardiovascular complications. *Prog Pediatr Cardiol*. 2001;12:161–167

187. Weiss R, Caprio S. The metabolic consequences of childhood obesity. *Best Pract Res Clin Endocrinol Metab*. 2005;19:405–419

188. Arslanian S, Suprasongsin C. Insulin sensitivity, lipids, and body composition in children: is "syndrome X" present? *J Clin Endocrinol Metab*. 1996;81:1058–1062

189. Dabelea D, Pettitt DJ, Jones KL, Arslanian SA. Type 2 diabetes mellitus in minority children and adolescents. An emerging problem. *Endocrinol Metab Clin North Am*. 1999;28:709–729, viii

190. Campaigne BN, Morrison JA, Schumann BC, et al. Indexes of obesity and comparisons with previous national survey data in 9- and 10-year-old black and white girls: the National Heart, Lung, and Blood Institute Growth and Health Study. *J Pediatr*. 1994;124:675–680

191. Morrison JA, Barton B, Biro FF, Sprecher DL, Falkner F, Obarzanek E. Sexual maturation and obesity in 9- and 10-year-old black and white girls: the National Heart, Lung, and Blood Institute Growth and Health Study. *J Pediatr*. 1994;124:889–895

192. Arslanian S, Suprasongsin C. Differences in the in vivo insulin sensitivity in healthy black vs white adolescents. *J Pediatr*. 1996;129:440–443

193. Gower BA, Nagy TR, Goran MI. Visceral fat, insulin sensitivity, and lipids in prepubertal children. *Diabetes*. 1999;48:1515–1521

194. Svec F, Nastasi K, Hilton C, Bao W, Srinivasan SR, Berenson GS. Black-white contrasts in insulin levels during pubertal development. The Bogalusa Heart Study. *Diabetes*. 1992;41:313–317

195. Yanovski JA, Yanovski SZ, Filmer KM, et al. Differences in body composition of black and white girls. *Am J Clin Nutr*. 1996;64:833–839

196. Caprio S, Tamborlane WV. The metabolic impact of obesity in childhood. *Endocrinol Metab Clin North Am*. 1999;28:731–747

197. Brambilla P, Manzoni P, Sironi S, et al. Peripheral and abdominal adiposity in childhood obesity. *Int J Obes Relat Metab Disord*. 1994;18:795–800

198. Ohlson LO, Larsson B, Bjorntorp P, et al. Risk factors for type 2 (non-insulin-dependent) diabetes mellitus. Thirteen and one-half years of follow-up of the participants in a study of Swedish men born in 1913. *Diabetologia*. 1998;31:798–805

199. Ashley MA, Buckley AJ, Criss AL, et al. Familial, anthropometric and metabolic associations of intramyocellular lipids levels in prepubertal males. *Pediatr Res*. 2002;51:81–86

200. Sinha R, Dufour S, Petersen KF, et al. Assessment of skeletal muscle triglyceride content by (1)H nuclear magnetic resonance spectroscopy in lean and obese adolescents: relationships to insulin sensitivity, total body fat, and central adiposity. *Diabetes*. 2002;51:1022–1027

201. Weiss R, Dufour S, Groszmann A, et al. Low adiponectin levels in adolescent obesity: a marker of increased intramyocellular lipid accumulation. *J Clin Endocrinol Metab.* 2003;88:2014–2018

202. Pugliese MT, Lifshitz F, Grad G, Fort P, Marks-Katz M. Fear of obesity. A cause of short stature and delayed puberty. *N Engl J Med.* 1983;309:513–518

203. Flegal KM. Epidemiological aspects of overweight and obesity in the United States. *Physiol Behav.* 2005;86:599–602

204. Keith S, Redden D, Katzmarzyk P, et al. Putative contributors to the secular increase in obesity: exploring the roads less traveled. *Int J Obes (Lond).* 2006;30:1585–1594

205. Barlow SE, Dietz WH. Obesity evaluation and treatment: Expert Committee recommendations. The Maternal and Child Health Bureau, Health Resources and Services Administration and the Department of Health and Human Services. *Pediatrics.* 1998;102(3):e29. Available at: http://pediatrics.aappublications.org/cgi/content/full/102/3/e29. Accessed September 25, 2007

206. Epstein LH. Family-based behavioural intervention for obese children. *Int J Obes Relat Metab Disord.* 1996;20:S14–S21

207. Blair SN. Evidence for success of exercise in weight loss and control. *Ann Int Med.* 1993;119:702–706

208. Gordon NF, Scott CB, Wilkinson WJ, Duncan JJ, Blair SN. Exercise and mild essential hypertension. Recommendations for adults. *Sports Med.* 1990;10:390–404

209. Wei M, Macera CA, Hornung CA, Blair SN. Changes in lipids associated with change in regular exercise in free-living men. *J Clin Epidemiol.* 1997;50:1137–1142

210. Epstein LH, Gordy CC, Raynor HA, Beddome M, Kilanowski CK, Paluch R. Increasing fruit and vegetable intake and decreasing fat and sugar intake in families at risk for childhood obesity. *Obes Res.* 2001;9:171–178

211. Roza AM, Shizgal HM. The Harris Benedict equation reevaluated: resting energy requirements and the body cell mass. *Am J Clin Nutr.* 1984;40:168–182

212. American Heart Association, Nutrition Committee. Diet and lifestyle recommendations revision 2006: a scientific statement from the American Heart Association Nutrition Committee. *Circulation.* 2006;114:82–96

213. Hernandez B, Gortmaker SL, Colditz GA, Peterson KE, Laird NM, Parra-Cabrera S. Association of obesity with physical activity, television programs and other forms of video viewing among children in Mexico city. *Int J Obes Relat Metab Disord.* 1999;23:845–854

214. Sugerman HJ, Sugerman EL, DeMaria EJ, Kennedy JKC, Mowery Y, Wolfe L. Bariatric surgery for severely obese adolescents. *J Gastrointest Surg.* 2003;7:102–107

215. Inge TH, Krebs NF, Garcia VF, et al. Bariatric surgery for severely overweight adolescents: concerns and recommendations. *Pediatrics.* 2004;114:217–223

216. Maggard M, Shugarman L, Suttorp M, et al. Meta-analysis: surgical treatment of obesity. *Ann Int Med.* 2005;142:547–559

217. Yanovski SZ. Pharmacotherapy for obesity—promise and uncertainty. *N Engl J Med.* 2005;353:2187–2189

218. Bray GA. A concise view of the therapeutics of obesity. *Nutrition.* 2000;16:953–960

219. Bray GA, Tartaglia LA. Medicinal strategies in the treatment of obesity. *Nature*. 2000;404:672–677

220. Lean ME. Sibutramine—a review of clinical efficacy. *Int J Obes Relat Metab Disord*. 1997;21:S30–S36

221. Stock M. Sibutramine: a review of the pharmacology of a novel anti-obesity agent. *Int J Obes Relat Metab Disord*. 1997;21:S25–S29

222. Finer N, James WP, Kopelman PG, Lean ME, Williams G. One-year treatment of obesity: a randomized, double-blind, placebo-controlled, multicentre study of orlistat, a gastrointestinal lipase inhibitor. *Int J Obes Relat Metab Disord*. 2000;24:306–313

223. Hill JO, Hauptman J, Anderson JW, et al. Orlistat, a lipase inhibitor, for weight maintenance after conventional dieting: a 1-y study. *Am J Clin Nutr*. 1999;69:1108–1116

224. Ozkan B, Bereket A, Turan S, Keskin S. Addition of orlistat to conventional treatment in adolescents with severe obesity. *Eur J Pediatr*. 2004;163:738–741

225. McDuffie JR, Calis KA, Booth SL, Uwaifo GI, Yanovski JA. Effects of orlistat on fat-soluble vitamins in obese adolescents. *Pharmacotherapy*. 2002;22:814–822

226. Lichtman A, Cravatt B. Food for thought: endocannabinoid modulation of lipogenesis. *J Clin Invest*. 2005;115:1130–1133

227. Jbilo O, Ravinet-Trillou C, Arnone M, et al. The CB1 receptor antagonist rimonabant reverses the diet-induced obesity phenotype through the regulation of lipolysis and energy balance. *FASEB J*. 2005;19:1567–1569

228. Ogden CL, Carroll MD, Flegal KM. Epidemiologic trends in overweight and obesity. *Endocrinol Metab Clin North Am*. 2003;32:741–760, vii

34 Food Sensitivity

Adverse reactions to foods have been implicated in causing many clinical problems ranging from life-threatening anaphylaxis to behavioral disorders.[1-5] However, in the past decade, the clinical spectrum and pathogenesis of many immunoglobulin (Ig)E- and non–IgE-mediated disorders have been well characterized, as described later in the chapter. Food allergic disorders are most common in early life and affect up to 8% of infants younger than 3 years.[3] Overall, approximately 2.5% of infants will experience allergic reactions to cow milk in the first 3 years of life, 1.5% will experience allergic reactions to egg, and 0.8% will experience allergic reactions to peanuts.[2] Fortunately, 60% to 80% of infants will "outgrow" their food allergies to egg and milk (ie, develop tolerance to them) within the first 5 to 7 years of life and 80% will outgrow them by 10 years of age. In contrast, approximately 20% of peanut-allergic infants will "outgrow" their peanut allergy during the first 5 years of life but rarely beyond this age.[6] Currently, food allergies represent the leading single cause of anaphylactic reactions treated in emergency departments in the United States, Europe, and Australia[7-9] and account for approximately 30 000 emergency department visits and 100 to 125 deaths per year in the United States.[10] Surveys suggest that peanut allergy is the leading cause of fatal and near-fatal food allergic reactions in the United States. At the present time, there is insufficient evidence to support the practice of delayed introduction of peanut products to prevent peanut allergy in infants identified as being at high risk of developing allergy as designated by a strong (biparental; parent and sibling) family history of allergy.[11] However, a complete allergy evaluation of any child suspected of having peanut allergy is suggested.[12]

Definitions

"Food allergy" is the term that has been used generically by physicians and patients to refer to many different types of clinical reactions and has resulted in confusion in terminology. To standardize nomenclature, the American Academy of Allergy and Immunology suggested that the following definitions be used for food-induced reactions[13]:

- *Adverse reaction to a food:* clinically abnormal response believed to be caused by an ingested food or food additive.

- *Food hypersensitivity (allergy):* clinically abnormal response believed to be caused by an immunologic reaction resulting from the ingestion of a food or food additive.

- *Food anaphylaxis:* classic allergic hypersensitivity reaction to food or food additives involving IgE antibody that occurs rapidly and may be life threatening.

- *Food intolerance:* general term describing an abnormal physiologic response to an ingested food or food additive (including metabolic, pharmacologic, or toxic reactions) or an idiosyncratic response to an ingested food or food additive. Note: in European literature, this term is used to mean an adverse reaction to food.

- *Food idiosyncrasy:* quantitatively abnormal response to a food or food additive; response differs from its physiologic or pharmacologic effect and resembles a hypersensitivity reaction but does not involve an immune mechanism.

- *Food toxicity (poisoning):* an adverse effect caused by direct action of a food or food additive on the host recipient without the involvement of immune mechanisms; nonimmune release of chemical mediators may occur; toxins may be from the food itself (eg, histamine in scombroid fish poisoning) or from micro-organisms within the food.

- *Pharmacologic food reaction:* adverse reactions to a food or food additive as a result of a naturally derived or added chemical that produces a drug-like or pharmacologic effect in the host (eg, caffeine in coffee).

- *Food aversions:* also may mimic adverse food reactions but are not reproducible when the patient ingests the food in a blinded fashion.

Clinical manifestations commonly ascribed to food hypersensitivity but not exclusively caused by food are as follows[1,2,14-17]:

1. *Systemic:* anaphylaxis, failure to thrive.
2. *Gastrointestinal:* vomiting, abdominal pain, diarrhea, malabsorption, enteropathies.[18,19]
3. *Respiratory:* rhinitis (nasal pruritus, rhinorrhea, and sneezing; ocular pruritus, tearing, and erythema), cough, throat tightness, hoarseness/dysphonia, wheezing, pulmonary infiltration.[20]
4. *Cutaneous:* pruritus, erythematous maculopapular rash, urticaria, angioedema, generalized flushing, atopic dermatitis.[1]

Hypersensitivity reactions to food may be categorized according to the interval between ingestion and the appearance of symptoms: immediate (minutes to 2 hours) or delayed (more than 2 hours, usually within 48 hours). These intervals may be associated with corresponding immunologic mechanisms involving IgE antibodies (immediate) or sensitized lymphocytes (delayed). Any of the manifestations may occur at any period during infancy or childhood. As depicted in Table 34.1, a number of food-allergic disorders have been clearly delineated.

Table 34.1
Food-Allergic Disorders

IgE-Mediated —————————— Mixed ——————————→ Non-IgE-Mediated		
Cutaneous: Urticaria Angioedema Erythematous macular rash Generalized flushing	Atopic dermatitis	Contact dermatitis Dermatitis herpetiformis
Gastrointestinal: Oral allergy syndrome Gastrointestinal anaphylaxis (immediate vomiting, colicky abdominal pain, and/or diarrhea)	Allergic eosinophilic esophagitis Allergic eosinophilic gastritis Allergic eosinophilic gastroenteritis	Food-induced enterocolitis Food-induced proctocolitis Food-induced enteropathy
Respiratory: Rhinoconjunctivitis Laryngeal edema Acute bronchospasm	Asthma	Food-induced pulmonary hemosiderosis (Heiner syndrome)

Diagnosis of Food Hypersensitivity

Symptoms associated with the ingestion of foods may stem from microbial, parasitic, or chemical contaminants; deficiencies of digestive enzymes; psychological aversion; hypersensitivity; and other causes.[1,2,14,21] Before making the diagnosis of food hypersensitivity, other possibilities that may account for adverse food reactions should be considered. A diagnosis of hypersensitivity to food requires: (1) verification that the food in question causes an adverse reaction; (2) exclusion of other causes of adverse reactions; and (3) identification of immunologic sensitization.

Complete delineation of the immunologic basis may be an elaborate undertaking that is not essential to the practical management of a food allergy but is necessary for full comprehension. Certain signs of an immunologic pathogenesis are discussed later.

Confirmation of Food as the Cause of Symptoms

Various symptoms are commonly ascribed to some foods recently eaten. A weak suspicion readily becomes a strong conviction, especially when no objective test is applied. Unwarranted enthusiasm can lead to erroneous incrimination of foods as the basis of many complaints.

The role of food as the cause of symptoms must be confirmed by some process that excludes the bias of the subject and observers. A double-blind placebo-controlled food challenge is the "gold standard" and may be necessary if errors in the diagnosis of adverse reactions to food and needless dietary restrictions are to be avoided. In some instances, the simpler open challenge-withdrawal test provides the same information.

Food Challenge

Recommended detailed procedures for performing a food challenge have been published.[1,14,22,23] Food challenges may be open, single-blind, or double-blind placebo-controlled. With infants and children up to 6 years of age, the suspected food may be successfully camouflaged by mixing it with some other food.* For older children, the suspected food or a placebo also may be camouflaged in a liquid or another food or, in some circumstances, administered in opaque capsules. These should be prepared by someone other than the subject or observer and designated by a code number. When capsules are used, early oral and laryngeal symptoms are not present, so progression to subsequent doses must be done cautiously to avoid excessive allergic symptoms, especially because capsule dissolution in the stomach may not be uniform. More often, the suspected food can be camouflaged in fruit shakes or other liquids (eg, Elecare [Abbott Nutrition, Columbus, OH] and Neocate One [Nutricia North America, Gaithersburg, MD]), applesauce, tapioca with fruit mix, etc, that mask the taste. The most common offending foods can be obtained in the dry state (eg, milk, eggs, peanut, soy, and cereal grain flours [wheat, barley, rye, oat, rice, corn]). Wet foods can be freeze-dried and powdered or blended in liquid vehicles.

Before the challenge, suspected foods are excluded from the diet for 2 weeks or longer for suspected delayed reactions (until symptoms subside). If the foods that may be provoking symptoms are unknown, a diet of foods unlikely to cause hypersensitivity may be given. Diets with decreasing levels

---

* Warning: Testing a food strongly implicated in the induction of an anaphylactic reaction is unnecessary and unsafe.

of food restriction have been helpful in formulating elimination diets for diagnostic and therapeutic reasons (Tables 34.2 through 34.4). The restricted diet is used in place of regular meals during the limited period of observation. Overly restrictive diets used for a prolonged period of time may result in nutritional deficiency, and in general, these should not be instituted without appropriate dietetic counseling.

Table 34.2
Allergy Diet No. 1*

Foods and Beverages Allowed[†]		Items to Be Avoided
Lamb	Poi	Milk, tea, coffee, cola, soft drinks
Rice, rice wafers, rice cereals	Pineapples, pears, loganberries, blueberries	Chewing gum
Lettuce,[†] spinach, artichokes, celery, beets, parsnips	Salt, sugar (cane or beet)	All medications except those prescribed by a physician
Water	Any vegetable oil, such as olive oil or Crisco,[‡] except oleomargarine[§]	All foods not listed under Foods and Beverages Allowed

* Modified from Golbert TM. Food allergy and immunologic diseases of the Gastrointestinal tract. In: Patterson R, ed. *Allergic Diseases: Diagnosis and Management*. 2nd ed. Philadelphia, PA: JB Lippincott Co; 1980:418

† All fruits and vegetables, except lettuce, must be cooked.

‡ The JM Smucker Co, Orville, OH.

§ Kosher pareve oleomargarines contain no milk and may be allowed.

During the challenge procedure, the suspected foods are administered under close supervision. The test dosing scheme is chosen according to the suspected severity of the reaction and typically ranges from 10 to 1000 mg as an initial dose, and doses are increased every 30 to 60 minutes. With immediate-type hypersensitivity, symptoms generally occur within several minutes to 4 hours. If 8 to 10 g of a dried food or 60 to 100 g of a wet food provokes no symptoms, usual portions of the food should be given openly to ensure that the food can be tolerated without reaction. A single unequivocal reaction in a double-blind challenge may be considered as definitive evidence of an adverse reaction to the food but is not unequivocal proof of an immunologic process without supporting laboratory evidence. Other mechanisms of adverse reactions, such as deficiency of digestive enzymes, may produce similar symptoms in some cases.

Table 34.3
Allergy Diet No. 2: Cereal-, Milk-, and Egg-Free Diet*

Foods and Beverages Allowed[†]		Items to Be Avoided
Lamb, chicken, turkey, beef, all-beef wieners, ham (boiled), bacon	Pineapples, apricots, cherries, blueberries, plums, prunes	Tea, coffee, cola, soft drinks
Arrowroot, potatoes, potato chips	Any vegetable shortening or oleomargarine that contains no milk solids[‡]	Chewing gum
Rice, yams, sweet potatoes, tapioca (whole or pearl, not minute)	Salt, sugar (cane or beet)	All medications except those prescribed by physician
Lettuce, artichokes, beets, spinach, celery, carrots, asparagus	Maple syrup or maple-flavored cane syrup	All foods not listed under Foods and Beverages Allowed
Lentils, navy beans, kidney beans	Water, ginger ale, white soda	
Soybeans, soy milk, soybean sprouts	Poi, olive oil, white vinegar, vanilla extract	

* Modified from Rowe's Cereal-Free 1-2-3 Diet. Adapted from Golbert TM. Food allergy and immunologic diseases of the gastrointestinal tract. In: Patterson R, ed. *Allergic Diseases: Diagnosis and Management.* Philadelphia, PA: JB Lippincott Co; 1972:363

† All fruits and vegetables, except lettuce, must be cooked.

‡ Kosher pareve oleomargarines, Mazola margarine (ACH Food Companies, Cordova, TN), and Crisco (The JM Smucker Co, Orville, OH) contain no milk.

With the use of blind food challenges in confirmation of delayed-type reactions, the interval between challenge doses should be as long as the time an adverse reaction is thought to have occurred after ingestion of the suspected food. Double-blind, placebo-controlled food challenges are particularly needed for confirmation of delayed adverse reactions to food, because the long interval between ingestion and the supposed reaction makes the association prone to error. The elimination diet, although not suitable for long-term use, can be used during the food-challenge period without concern.

Single-blind challenges, where the observer is not blinded as to the challenge content, are often sufficient in the clinical setting when outcome is based solely on objective symptoms. However, when more subjective symptoms are involved or the response seems unclear, the suspected foods must be evaluated with double-blind challenges. In many instances, adverse reactions to foods elicited by history will not be confirmed, and incriminated foods can be restored to the diet. Psychological and subjective complaints are especially susceptible to erroneous association with foods eaten; this can be verified through blind challenges.

Table 34.4
Allergy Diet No. 3*

Only Foods Allowed		
Rice	White potatoes	Lettuce
Lamb	Sweet potatoes, yams	Water
Beef	Squash	Ginger ale (dry)
Chicken, turkey	Carrots	Sugar (cane or beet)
Bacon	Soybeans	Salt
Apples	String beans	Maple or maple-flavored syrup
Peaches	Peas	White vinegar
Apricots	Spinach	Vanilla extract
Pears	Chard	Crisco†
Pineapples	Beets	Safflower oil margarine
Cranberries	Artichokes	Pearl tapioca
	Asparagus	
Possible milk substitutes: Alsoy‡ (corn-free), ProSobee,§ Isomil,‖ Coffee Rich¶		

Suggested Menu		
Breakfast	**Dinner**	**Supper**
Rice cereal	Lamb or beef patty	Chicken or turkey
Milk substitute	Baked potato	Mashed potatoes
Bacon	Lettuce and carrot salad	Peas
Tapioca and peaches	Baked pears	Lettuce and pineapple salad
Apple juice	Ginger ale	Frozen peaches
Water	Water	Water

* Adapted from Rowe AH. Elimination diets in the control of food allergy. In: Rowe AH Sr, Rowe AH Jr, eds. *Food Allergy, Its Manifestations and Control in the Elimination Diets.* Springfield, IL: Charles C Thomas Publisher; 1972:41–75

Eat and drink only the foods listed. Avoid coffee, tea, cola, and other soft drinks, and chewing gum.

† The JM Smucker Co, Orville, OH.

‡ Nestlé, Glendale, CA.

§ Mead Johnson, Evansville, IN.

‖ Abbott Nutrition, Columbus, OH.

¶ Coffee Rich, Cape Coral, FL.

Differential Diagnosis

When an adverse reaction to a food has been confirmed by blind challenge, customary procedures differentiate hypersensitivity disorders from various causes of disturbances of the gastrointestinal, respiratory, or cutaneous systems (ie, mucosal digestive enzyme deficiencies, cystic fibrosis, infections, and immunologic deficiencies). The diagnosis of hypersensitivity must be supported by detection of immunologic sensitization.[1,24]

Identification of an Immunologic Basis for an Adverse Reaction to Food

At present, a convenient technique for identification of a definitive component of the immunologic basis for a hypersensitivity reaction to food is available only for IgE-mediated food hypersensitivity reactions. The immunologic mechanisms responsible for delayed-type hypersensitivity reactions have not been elucidated sufficiently to permit selection of a definitive laboratory test for identification, although a number of investigators have been evaluating the utility of atopy patch tests in the diagnosis of such reactions.[25–27]

Symptoms of immediate food hypersensitivity are caused by release of mediators (eg, histamine) when food antigen combines with specific IgE antibody attached to mast cells and basophils. In children older than 6 months, the presence of IgE antibody to food generally may be identified by serologic tests (see "Diagnostic Approach to Food Hypersensitivity") or by a specific wheal-and-flare reaction on the skin induced by skin-prick testing. Certain precautions are necessary to make skin tests with food extracts reliable. Commercially prepared extracts must be subjected to verification.[28] The concentration and technique used must not cause reactions in the skin of persons not allergic but produce wheal-and-flare responses in hypersensitive individuals.

Food antigens used for skin testing should, in general, be obtained from reputable manufacturers as 1:20 weight-volume glycerinated extracts. After skin-prick testing with these materials, a mean wheal reaction at least 3 mm in diameter larger than the negative control (usually 0 mm in diameter) 15 minutes after application is considered a positive response. Because some food extracts (eg, fruits and vegetables) may lack appropriate antigens because of enzymatic degradation during preparation, direct skin-prick testing with the suspected food also should be performed; in these instances, a control individual should be tested simultaneously to exclude the possibility that a positive response is attributable to a local irritant effect.[29] The use of intradermal skin tests is not warranted, because they frequently evoke "nonspecific" irritant responses or wheal-and-flare reactions that indicate low-level sensitivity that is not associated with symptoms after ingestion of the food in a double-blind challenge. In addition, intradermal skin tests have been associated with systemic reactions, including fatal anaphylaxis.

Immediate skin test responses can be helpful in including or excluding possible culprit foods in equivocal cases.[1] Not all positive skin test results reflect clinical sensitivity to that food (ie, false-positive responses [clinically irrelevant]).[2] Standard radioallergosorbent tests (RASTs; see "Other Methods to Diagnose Hypersensitivity to Food") are no more diagnostic. Thus, it is potentially harmful to exclude foods from the diet on the basis of skin test results alone; careful comparisons between skin test results and clinical symptoms are necessary. Despite frequent false-positive skin test results, the incidence of false-negative results for IgE-mediated reactions is very low (<5%). Thus, a negative skin test response to a suspected food indicates a very low probability that an oral food challenge will result in immediate or early-onset hypersensitivity. In the last several years, it has been demonstrated that quantification of food-specific IgE antibodies are highly predictive of clinical reactivity and can be used to preclude the use of food challenges in some cases (see next section).[2,21]

Diagnostic Approach to Food Hypersensitivity

When a history is obtained that is suggestive of an adverse reaction to a specific food, the following is recommended:

1. For children older than 6 months, serologic tests or skin-prick skin tests with 1:20 food extract should be performed if an "immediate-type" (IgE-mediated) reaction is suspected. If the wheal response in the skin-prick test is less than 3 mm in diameter or the serologic test result is negative, significant clinical sensitivity to the food is unlikely (but rarely occurs). If the wheal response on the skin test is more than 3 mm in diameter, an oral food challenge should be performed to ascertain that the reaction is clinically significant. For serologic evaluation of egg, milk, peanut, and fish hypersensitivity, food-specific IgE concentrations may be obtained (eg, UniCAP or CAP System FEIA [Phadia, Portage, MI]). If the concentration exceeds the 95% predictive value (egg: 7 kU_A/L [2 kU_A/L for children <3 years]; milk: 15 kU_A/L [5 kU_A/L for children <2 years]; peanut: 14 kU_A/L; and fish: 20 kU_A/L), food challenges are not generally required to confirm the diagnosis of food hypersensitivity.[2]

2. For infants younger than 1 year, a double-blind food challenge should be performed if a response occurs to an open challenge. If positive, skin or serologic tests to determine that the reaction is based on immediate-type immunologic sensitization may be performed. Double-blind challenges are not always necessary, particularly if no response occurs with open challenge.

Radioallergosorbent Test

The RAST was developed for the estimation of allergen-specific IgE in serum. The concentration of specific IgE reflects the degree of sensitization but does not correlate with the severity of reaction that a patient may experience. As with skin tests, greater RAST concentrations are more likely to be correlated with clinical symptoms after exposure to the allergen. Except when the skin is unsuitable, as in patients with widespread atopic dermatitis, the standard RAST has no practical advantage over skin tests.[30] The same verification suggested for skin tests is required for RAST.

Serum Allergen-Specific IgE Quantification

The UniCAP or CAP System FEIA (fluorescein enzyme immunoassay) uses a cellulose matrix system that allows quantification of allergen-specific IgE antibodies. Studies comparing the outcome of double-blind placebo-controlled food challenges and the concentration of food-specific IgE antibodies have demonstrated a correlation between clinical reactions and the quantity of food-specific IgE (see Table 34.5).[2,31]

Table 34.5
Probability of Reactivity to Selected Foods

Food	>95% Probability of Reactivity*
Egg	7 kU_A/L (<1 y = 2 kU_A/L)
Milk	15 kU_A/L (<2 yr = 5 kU_A/L)
Peanut	14 kU_A/L
Fish	20 kU_A/L

* The probability of clinical reactivity decreases as the allergen-specific IgE decreases; <15% chance of reactivity when allergen-specific IgE <0.35 kU_A/L.

Food Hypersensitivity Not Involving IgE Antibody

In addition to immediate or anaphylactic-type food reactions that involve IgE antibody and mast-cell or basophil-mediator release, food antigens may induce a state of hypersensitivity through the formation of other classes of immunoglobulins (ie, IgG, IgM, or IgA) or sensitized lymphocytes. No clinically reliable tests exist to confirm an immune-mediated basis for non–IgE-mediated food hypersensitivity. Tests to determine serum concentrations of IgG antibodies to food antigens have not been shown to be clinically useful. With gastrointestinal manifestations, histopathologic examination of tissue may help determine the presence of immunoglobulins, complement, eosinophils, or lymphocytes. For example, ≥20 eosinophils per high-power field on esophageal biopsy tissue are indicative of allergic eosinophilic gastroenteritis.[32] Although these findings suggest an immunologic pathogenesis, they do not necessarily confirm a cause-and-effect relationship. However, until more precise diagnostic tools are available, these types of analyses have provided insight into potential immune mechanisms responsible for perplexing clinical symptomatology.

Milk Allergy

Cow milk hypersensitivity develops in 2.2% to 2.8% of infants, but approximately 80% of these children outgrow the reactivity (ie, develop tolerance) by 4 years of age.[2] Skin-prick tests at 1 year of age are valuable for predicting the outcome of the milk sensitivity and the likelihood of developing other food sensitivities.[33] Soy protein-based formulas are no less allergenic than are cow milk protein-based formulas.[34] The IgE-mediated symptoms may include diarrhea, vomiting, and failure to thrive.[33,35] Colitis with gastrointestinal bleeding and colic may occur, as may skin and respiratory symptoms.[1–3] Heiner syndrome, a rare syndrome alleviated by the elimination of milk, was described as recurrent otitis, bronchitis, sinusitis, and eosinophilia.[36] Pulmonary hemosiderosis with anemia and hemosiderin-laden cells in the saliva may be found.[37,38]

There is evidence that milk-induced enterocolitis, proctocolitis, eosinophilic esophagitis and gastroenterocolitis, and enteropathies (including celiac disease) induced by other foods are caused by immunologic mechanisms and fit the definition of food allergy.[3,15] Nevertheless, the diet of many infants who vomit, spit up, or have colicky symptoms is often altered without fulfilling the criteria as outlined.

If neither soy nor cow milk can be consumed, consideration should be given to consuming a greater amount of other foods with calcium (Appendix Q, Table Q-1) or a calcium supplement to meet the recommended dietary allowance.

Treatment

Rational treatment must be based on an accurate diagnosis. Clinically significant hypersensitivity to food occurs far less often than commonly perceived.[21] A relatively small number of foods are responsible for most confirmable hypersensitivity reactions to foods. Staple items, such as milk, eggs, and wheat, should be eliminated long-term only when clearly justified by proper diagnostic procedures. Infants with milk or soy hypersensitivity should be fed a substitute extensively hydrolyzed or elemental formula (Nutramigen [Mead Johnson, Evansville, IN], Alimentum [Abbott Nutrition, Columbus, OH], Neocate, or EleCare) until they are 1 year or older. A rechallenge with cow milk or soy should be undertaken after 1 year of age in a controlled setting in which intravenous fluids, intravenous medications (eg, corticosteroids), oxygen, and personnel familiar with resuscitation are available. For children, elimination diets should be designed with appropriate dietetic counseling.

Exclusion of a food for 2 to 4 weeks for IgE-mediated food allergy or 6 to 8 weeks for non–IgE-mediated food allergy (eg, allergic eosinophilic esophagitis) should serve to evaluate any contribution it may make to symptoms. Small amounts of a food may be tolerated, but larger quantities of it may cause symptoms. Because many antigens (eg, milk or soy proteins) are commonly found in many processed foods, dietetic consultation should take place to ensure complete elimination to avoid equivocal results and to establish a nutritionally adequate diet for various age groups. Drug therapy (eg, cromolyn sodium, leukotriene antagonists) has not been proven to be helpful, although the efficacy of anti-IgE therapy, which has not yet been approved for use in food allergy, has been shown to increase the amount of ingested peanut necessary to elicit an allergic reaction in patients at risk of peanut-induced anaphylaxis.[39] Patients who have had an anaphylactic reaction to food in the past, who have asthma and an IgE-mediated food allergy, or who are allergic to peanuts or tree nuts should carry an emergency plan and injectable form of epinephrine that can be used in case of inadvertent exposure to the offending food.

Prognosis

For IgE-mediated reactions, most children younger than 3 years will outgrow the clinical response in 1 to 7 years. Of infants with milk allergy, approximately 80% will tolerate milk by 4 years of age,[2] although a recent study suggested that milk allergy may be more persistent, with 80% of children with milk allergy tolerating milk by 16 years of age.[40] Overall, studies suggest that approximately 80% to 85% of young infants "outgrow" milk and egg allergies and that about 20% of infants who experience allergic reactions to peanuts will "outgrow" their sensitivity.[6,41] Children in whom food sensitivities develop after 3 years of age are less likely outgrow the problem. Although many children outgrow the clinical sensitivity, the immediate skin test response to the food allergen may remain positive for an extended period of time.

Prevention

For more than 50 years, investigators have debated as to whether early dietary intervention can prevent the development of food allergy and allergic disease. One randomized study comparing the effect of human milk compared with cow milk formula in preterm infants demonstrated a preventive effect of human milk against atopic disease in infants at risk of allergic disorders.[42] Similarly, meta-analyses of studies comparing the prophylactic effect of human milk and cow milk-based formula concluded that exclusive breastfeeding could prevent some atopic dermatitis and asthma.[43,44] There continues to be considerable debate as to whether the elimination of food allergens (eg, peanut, milk, and egg) from the diet of infants at high risk of atopic disease and their lactating mothers can further delay or prevent some food allergy and atopic disease. Although food allergens are clearly detectable in human milk,[45,46] a comprehensive review of a large number of studies evaluating dietary restriction during lactation concluded that there was no effect of an exclusionary diet on various allergy outcomes in most studies, especially if follow-up lasted beyond 4 years.[47] Furthermore, a recent study of dietary recall performed on a birth cohort failed to demonstrate any benefit of peanut exclusion in preventing peanut allergy.[48] The authors of virtually all studies concur that maternal dietary restrictions during pregnancy have not been shown to decrease the risk of food allergy or allergic diseases later in childhood.[49-51] Alternative infant formulas also have been evaluated for their beneficial effect in preventing food allergy and atopic disease. Recent meta-analyses concluded that there is no role for soy formula in the prevention of allergic disease[52] and that supplementing breastfeeding or exclusive infant feeding with extensively hydrolyzed casein-based formulas in place of cow milk formulas may prevent allergic disease and cow milk allergy.[53] On the basis of these studies, recommending the following guidelines for high-risk infants seems reasonable: (1) no maternal dietary avoidance during pregnancy is necessary; (2) exclusive breastfeeding is recommended for the first 4 to 6 months of life, or if breastfeeding is not possible or if supplementation is required, use of an extensively hydrolyzed or elemental formula (or possibly a partial hydrolysate formula, although the evidence to support this remains controversial) is recommended; and (3) introduction of solid foods should be delayed until 4 to 6 months of age.

| AAP | **In summary, the American Academy of Pediatrics states:** |

1. At the present time, there is lack of evidence that maternal dietary restrictions during pregnancy or lactation play a significant role in the prevention of atopic disease in the infant.
2. For infants at high risk of developing atopic disease, there is evidence that exclusive breastfeeding for at least 4 months, compared with feeding intact cow milk protein formula, decreases the cumulative incidence of atopic dermatitis and cow milk allergy in the first 2 years of life.
3. There is evidence that exclusive breastfeeding for at least 3 months protects against wheezing in early life. In infants at risk of developing atopic disease, the evidence that exclusive breastfeeding protects against allergic asthma occurring beyond 6 years of age is not convincing.
4. In studies of infants at high risk of developing atopic disease who are not breastfed exclusively for 4 to 6 months or who are formula fed, there is modest evidence that atopic dermatitis may be delayed or prevented by the use of extensively or partially hydrolyzed formulas in early childhood, compared with cow milk formula. For atopic disease in general, there is evidence that extensively hydrolyzed formulas may be more effective than partially hydrolyzed formulas compared with cow milk formula.
5. There is no convincing evidence for the use of soy-based infant formula for the purpose of allergy prevention.
6. Although solid foods should not be introduced before 4 to 6 months of age, there is no convincing evidence that delaying their introduction beyond this period has significant protective effect on the development of atopic disease.

Pediatrics. 2008;121:183–191

References

1. Sampson HA. Food allergy. Part 2: diagnosis and management. *J Allergy Clin Immunol.* 1999;103:981–999
2. Sampson HA. Update on food allergy. *J Allergy Clin Immunol.* 2004;113:805–819
3. Sicherer SH, Sampson HA. 9. Food allergy. *J Allergy Clin Immunol.* 2006;117(2 Suppl): S470–S475
4. Sampson HA. Food allergy. Part 1: immunopathogenesis and clinical disorders. *J Allergy Clin Immunol.* 1999;103:717–728
5. Sampson HA, Mendelson L, Rosen JP. Fatal and near-fatal anaphylactic reactions to food in children and adolescents. *N Engl J Med.* 1992;327:380–384
6. Skolnick HS, Conover-Walker MK, Koerner CB, Sampson HA, Burks W, Wood RA. The natural history of peanut allergy. *J Allergy Clin Immunol.* 2001;107:367–374
7. Yocum MW, Khan DA. Assessment of patients who have experienced anaphylaxis: a 3-year survey. *Mayo Clin Proc.* 1994;69:16–23

8. Novembre E, Cianferoni A, Bernardini R, et al. Anaphylaxis in children: clinical and allergologic features. *Pediatrics*. 1998;101(4):e8. Available at: http://pediatrics.aappublications.org/cgi/content/full/101/4/e8. Accessed September 25, 2007

9. Braganza SC, Acworth JP, McKinnon DR, Peake JE, Brown AF. Paediatric emergency department anaphylaxis: different patterns from adults. *Arch Dis Child*. 2006;91:159–163

10. Bock SA, Munoz-Furlong A, Sampson HA. Fatalities due to anaphylactic reactions to foods. *J Allergy Clin Immunol*. 2001;107:191–193

11. Greer FR, Sicherer SH, Burks AW, American Academy of Pediatrics, Committee on Nutrition and Section on Allergy and Immunology. The effects of early nutritional interventions on the development of atopic disease in infants and children: the role of maternal dietary restriction, breastfeeding, timing of introduction of complementary foods, and hydrolyzed formulas. *Pediatrics*. 2008;121: in press

12. Sampson HA. Clinical practice. Peanut allergy. *N Engl J Med*. 2002;346:1294–1299

13. Anderson JA. The establishment of common language concerning adverse reactions to foods and food additives. *J Allergy Clin Immunol*. 1986;78:140–144

14. Sicherer SH. Food allergy. *Lancet*. 2002;360:701–710

15. Bischoff SC, Crowe S. Gastrointestinal food allergy: new insights into pathophysiology and clinical perspectives. *Gastroenterology*. 2005;128:1089–1113

16. Sampson HA, Sicherer SH, Birnbaum AH. AGA technical review on the evaluation of food allergy in gastrointestinal disorders. American Gastroenterological Association. *Gastroenterology*. 2001;120:1026–1040

17. James JM, Bernhisel-Broadbent J, Sampson HA. Respiratory reactions provoked by double-blind food challenges in children. *Am J Respir Crit Care Med*. 1994;149:59–64

18. Wang LF, Lin JY, Hsieh K, Lin RH. Epicutaneous exposure of protein antigen induces a predominant Th2-like response with high IgE production in mice. *J Immunol*. 1996;156:4077–4082

19. Trier JS. Celiac sprue. In: Sleisenger MH, Fordtran JS, Scharschmidt BF, Feldman M, eds. *Gastrointestinal Disease: Pathophysiology/Diagnosis/Management*. 5th ed. Vol 2. Philadelphia, PA: WB Saunders Co; 1993:1078–1096

20. James JM, Eigenmann PA, Eggleston PA, Sampson HA. Airway reactivity changes in asthmatic children undergoing blinded food challenges. *Am J Respir Crit Care Med*. 1996;153:597–603

21. Sampson HA. Food allergy—accurately identifying clinical reactivity. *Allergy*. 2005;60(Suppl 79):19–24

22. Bock SA, Sampson HA, Atkins FM, et al. Double-blind, placebo-controlled food challenge (DBPCFC) as an office procedure: a manual. *J Allergy Clin Immunol*. 1988;82:986–997

23. Bahna SL. Diagnosis of food allergy. *Ann Allergy Asthma Immunol*. 2003;90(6 Suppl 3):77–80

24. Sampson HA. Differential diagnosis in adverse reactions to foods. *J Allergy Clin Immunol*. 1986;78:212–219

25. Niggemann B. Atopy Patch Test (APT)—its role in diagnosis of food allergy in atopic dermatitis. *Indian J Pediatr*. 2002;69:57–59

26. Spergel JM, Brown-Whitehorn T. The use of patch testing in the diagnosis of food allergy. *Curr Allergy Asthma Rep.* 2005;5:86–90

27. De Boissieu D, Waguet JC, Dupont C. The atopy patch tests for detection of cow's milk allergy with digestive symptoms. *J Pediatr.* 2003;142:203–205

28. Beyer K, Teuber SS. Food allergy diagnostics: scientific and unproven procedures. *Curr Opin Allergy Clin Immunol.* 2005;5:261–266

29. Rosen JP, Selcow JE, Mendelson LM, Grodofsky MP, Factor JM, Sampson HA. Skin testing with natural foods in patients suspected of having food allergies...is it necessary? *J Allergy Clin Immunol.* 1994;93:1068–1070

30. Sampson HA, Albergo R. Comparison of results of skin tests, RAST, and double-blind, placebo-controlled food challenges in children with atopic dermatitis. *J Allergy Clin Immunol.* 1984;74:26–33

31. Sampson HA. Utility of food-specific IgE concentrations in predicting symptomatic food allergy. *J Allergy Clin Immunol.* 2001;107:891–896

32. Liacouras CA, Spergel JM, Ruchelli E, et al. Eosinophilic esophagitis: a 10-year experience in 381 children. *Clin Gastroenterol Hepatol.* 2005;3:1198–1206

33. Host A. Cow's milk protein allergy and intolerance in infancy. Some clinical, epidemiological, and immunological aspects. *Pediatr Allergy Immunol.* 1994;5(Suppl):1–36

34. Zeiger RS, Heller S, Mellon M, Halsey J, Hamburger R, Sampson HA. Genetic and environmental factors effecting the development of atopy through age 4 in children of atopic parents: a prospective randomized study of food allergen avoidance. *Pediatr Allergy Immunol.* 1992;3:110–127

35. Baehler P, Chad Z, Gurbindo C, Bonin AP, Bouthillier L, Seidman EG. Distinct patterns of cow's milk allergy in infancy defined by prolonged, two-stage double-blind, placebo-controlled food challenges. *Clin Exp Allergy.* 1996;26:254–261

36. Lee SK, Kniker WT, Cook CD, Heiner DC. Cow's milk-induced pulmonary disease in children. *Adv Pediatr.* 1978;25:39–57

37. Boat TF, Polmar SH, Whitman V, Kleinerman JI, Stern RC, Doershuk CF. Hyperreactivity to cow milk in young children with pulmonary hemosiderosis and cor pulmonale secondary to nasopharyngeal obstruction. *J Pediatr.* 1975;87:23–29

38. Moissidis I, Chaidaroon D, Vichyanond P, Bahna SL. Milk-induced pulmonary disease in infants (Heiner syndrome). *Pediatr Allergy Immunol.* 2005;16:545–552

39. Leung DY, Sampson HA, Yunginger JW, et al. Effect of anti-IgE therapy in patients with peanut allergy. *N Engl J Med.* 2003;348:986–993

40. Skripak JM, Matsui EC, Mudd K, Wood RA. The natural history of IgE-mediated cow's milk allergy. *J Allergy Clin Immunol.* 2007;120:1172–1177

41. Perry TT, Matsui EC, Connover-Walker MK, Wood RA. The relationship of allergen-specific IgE levels and oral food challenge outcome. *J Allergy Clin Immunol.* 2004;114:144–149

42. Lucas A, Brooke OG, Morley R, Cole TJ, Bamford MF. Early diet of preterm infants and development of allergic or atopic disease: randomized prospective study. *BMJ.* 1990;300:837–840

43. Gdalevich M, Mimouni D, David M, Mimouni M. Breast-feeding and the onset of atopic dermatitis in childhood: a systematic review and meta-analysis of prospective studies. *J Am Acad Dermatol.* 2001;45:520–527

44. Gdalevich M, Mimouni D, Mimouni M. Breast-feeding and the risk of bronchial asthma in childhood: a systematic review with meta-analysis of prospective studies. *J Pediatr.* 2001;139:261–266

45. Kilshaw PJ, Cant AJ. The passage of maternal dietary proteins into human breast milk. *Int Arch Allergy Appl Immunol.* 1984;75:8–15

46. Vadas P, Wai Y, Burks W, Perelman B. Detection of peanut allergens in breast milk of lactating women. *JAMA.* 2001;285:1746–1748

47. Muraro A, Dreborg S, Halken S, et al. Dietary prevention of allergic diseases in infants and small children. Part III: critical review of published peer-reviewed observational and interventional studies and final recommendations. *Pediatr Allergy Immunol.* 2004;15: 291–307

48. Lack G, Fox D, Northstone K, Golding J. Factors associated with the development of peanut allergy in childhood. Avon Longitudinal Study of Parents and Children Study Team. *N Engl J Med.* 2003;348:977–985

49. Falth-Magnusson K, Kjellman NI. Allergy prevention by maternal elimination diet during late pregnancy—a 5-year follow-up of a randomized study. *J Allergy Clin Immunol.* 1992;89: 709–713

50. Lilja G, Dannaeus A, Foucard T, Graff-Lonnevig V, Johansson SG, Oman H. Effects of maternal diet during late pregnancy and lactation on the development of atopic diseases in infants up to 18 months of age—in-vivo results. *Clin Exp Allergy.* 1989;19:473–479

51. Hide DW, Matthews S, Matthews L, et al. Effect of allergen avoidance in infancy on allergic manifestations at age two years. *J Allergy Clin Immunol.* 1994;93:842–846

52. Osborn DA, Sinn J. Soy formula for prevention of allergy and food intolerance in infants. *Cochrane Database Syst Rev.* 2004;(3)CD003741

53. Osborn DA, Sinn J. Formulas containing hydrolysed protein for prevention of allergy and food intolerance in infants. *Cochrane Database Syst Rev.* 2006(4):CD003664

Introduction

Nutrients play integral roles in the development and function of the immune system. The keystones of an effective immune response are rapid cellular proliferation and early synthesis of regulatory and/or protective proteins, all of which require a ready supply of nutrients as substrates, cofactors, and structural components. Therefore, insufficiency of one or more essential nutrients is potentially rate limiting in the development and maintenance of immune responses. Similarly, inflammation and other immune responses alter a person's nutritional status through sequestration of minerals (eg, iron and zinc), impaired absorption, increased nutrient loss, or altered nutrient utilization. Although the effects of the immune system on nutritional status are important during inflammation and other acute disease states, this chapter focuses on the role of nutrition in immune system development and the effects of primary nutrient deficiencies on immune responses.

Nutrient-immune interactions are of special concern in infants and children because of the increased vulnerability of the developing immune system. Early in life, systemic humoral immunity is strongly dependent on maternal immunoglobulin (Ig) G acquired transplacentally, and specific mucosal immunity relies to a great extent on secretory IgA supplied via breastfeeding. This reliance on maternal factors is attributable to the paucity of production of those Ig isotypes during early infancy, the decreased repertoire of antibody-binding specificities during that period, and the slow development of antibody responses to polysaccharide antigens during the first 2 to 3 years of life.[1] Adult concentrations of serum IgM and IgG do not develop until 4 to 6 years of age.[2] The thymus and other immune tissues continue to grow and develop through puberty. Thus, definitions of "normal" immune status and responses depend on a child's age and stage of development. Factors such as preterm birth or low birth weight will further delay the development of the immune system.

To appreciate the importance to the child of nutrient-immune interactions, the ontogeny of the immune system must be considered in the context of the child's overall growth and development. Periods of rapid growth velocity increase the demands of muscle, organ, and other tissues on the available nutrient pool. If there is an insufficient supply of any nutrient, growth retardation and/or other functional deficits will occur. In some cases (eg, "catch-up" growth), nutrient repletion will promote nearly full recovery from a previous insult. In other cases (eg, cognitive development), moderate to severe nutritional insults early in life may overcome the system's plasticity and recovery may not be possible.

In the case of the immune system, the degree and reversibility of an immune defect depends on the timing, duration, severity, and type of nutritional insufficiency. Early and/or severe nutrient deficiencies appear to cause long-lasting effects on the immune system. Thymic involution and reduced immune responsiveness occur during moderate to severe general undernutrition and various single-nutrient deficiencies. Even after nutritional supplementation, immune responsiveness may not recover fully in previously malnourished children. Animal studies indicate that severe nutrient deficiencies during early development, especially in utero and in the preweaning period, may result in lifelong and even perhaps transgenerational immune deficiencies.[3] For example, in a mouse model of prenatal zinc deficiency, immune deficits appeared to carry over to the second and third generation.[4] Thus, in the growing child with nutrient deficiencies, the combination of increased nutrient demands and a rapidly developing immune system provide great potential for permanent adverse outcomes.

Nutritional status influences the immune system at different levels. Subclinical or frank deficiencies of some micronutrients (see "Micronutrients and Immunity") reduce the circulating amounts and functional capacities of key immune cells and proteins. Other micronutrient deficiencies, including essential fatty acids, folate, zinc, and vitamin A, cause mucosal lesions or reduce mucosal integrity, thus increasing susceptibility to infections. The most severe outcomes occur among children in developing nations where severe, combined nutrient deficiencies adversely affect many parts of the immune system. This chapter focuses on nutrient-immune interactions likely to be encountered among children in the United States or other industrialized countries.

Early Nutritional-Immunologic System Interactions

Current research amply documents the influence of early nutrition on (1) immunologic responses; (2) the immediate risks of acquiring infectious diseases; and (3) possibly, the risks of developing immune-related conditions expressed in later life stages. These influences have played major roles in the formulation of recommendations for the nutritional management of infants. Recognition of these influences comes principally from studies of infants fed human milk or synthetic formulas.[5,6]

Beyond the well-recognized nutritional roles of the major organic macronutrients (proteins, carbohydrates, and lipids), the macronutrients in human milk also play functional roles related to the infant's immune competence and ontogenic stage of development. These immunologic roles are expressed either actively (ie, by modulating the infant's ability to respond to an immunologic challenge) or passively (ie, by attenuating or preventing infection without altering the infant's immunologic development or ability to respond to a specific challenge).[7]

Several proteins in human milk have the potential to modulate specific and/or nonspecific immune responses before their degradation to amino acids and the subsequent fulfillment of the classical metabolic roles associated with dietary proteins. Among the 2 most frequently studied examples of proteins with this characteristic are secretory IgA and lactoferrin. Although the general protective roles of breastfeeding against infection are well documented, the only specific human milk component clinically proven to be protective is secretory IgA. Its efficacy against *Vibrio cholerae* O antigen and enterotoxin, *Campylobacter* species, and enterotoxin-producing *Escherichia coli* has been documented by various investigators.[8] Secretory IgA provides passive protection, presumably by neutralizing pathogens and their toxins and interfering with their adherence to the infant's gastrointestinal and upper respiratory tracts.

Human milk secretory IgA, however, also may provide a mechanism for active protection. The identification of anti-idiotypic antibodies in human milk suggests that breastfeeding may aid the infant's production of the corresponding idiotypic antibody.[8] Secretion of anti-idiotypic antibodies and excretion in human milk of potential pathogens such as cytomegalovirus concomitantly with the secretion of corresponding neutralizing antibodies may serve as important natural immunization strategies in early infancy.[9]

Other human milk proteins, such as cytokines, may influence the infant's immune system through alternative mechanisms. The identification in human milk of substantial amounts of immunomodulating cytokines, including those that are ordinarily proinflammatory (eg, tumor necrosis factor-alpha, interleukin [IL] 1-beta, IL-6),[10–13] anti-inflammatory (eg, transforming growth factor-beta and IL-10),[14,15] colony stimulating (eg, granulocyte colony-stimulating factor and macrophage colony-stimulating factor),[16,17] chemotactic (IL-8),[18] and others,[19] raises the possibility of roles for human milk cytokines in leukocyte development, mobilization, and activation; the regulation of cytokine production; the expression of class I and class II histocompatibility antigens; the up-regulation of secretory component production by epithelial cells; and the production of IgA dimers required for the assembly of secretory IgA in the recipient infant.

Earlier demonstrations of urinary excretion of intact and large fragments of lactoferrin by preterm infants fed human milk[20,21] and their maternal origin[22] raise the possibility of the postnatal uptake of other intact or biologically active fragments of immunoregulatory molecules of maternal origin by the infant at this and other developmental stages. The roles these and other immunoregulatory components and antigenic exposure play in determining disparate antibody responses to immunization and to differences in "baseline" serum immunoglobulin concentrations between breastfed and formula-fed infants remain unclear.[23]

The strong iron-binding capacity of lactoferrin is a well-described example of a "nonspecific" immune-modulating activity of a major human milk protein. This capacity presumably limits the availability to potentially pathogenic enteric flora of an essential mineral in the infant's gastrointestinal lumen by competing effectively with bacterial enterochelins for iron.[24] This competition limits the growth of iron-dependent pathogens in the infant's gastrointestinal lumen. Lactoferrin also appears to modulate inflammatory responses by influencing macrophage responses. Lactoferrin also is able to kill certain bacterial and fungal pathogens by the membrane-damaging effect of a peptide C (lactoferrin-H) located near the terminus of the lactoferrin molecule.

Anti-inflammatory capacity is not unique to lactoferrin. It is shared by several of the antimicrobial agents and other factors in human milk.[25] Beyond its actions as a single agent, lactoferrin also acts together with secretory IgA to mutually enhance each other's antibacterial efficacy.[23]

Although infants rely on carbohydrates as a key energy source, human milk carbohydrates also serve immune-related roles. Oligosaccharides and more complex glycoproteins and glycolipids serve as receptor analogs that interfere with the adherence of pathogens, such as pneumococci and *Haemophilus influenzae*, and enterotoxins, such as those of *V cholerae* and *E coli*, to epithelial cells.[26] These molecules may account partially for the protective effect of human milk against gastroenteritis, possibly otitis media, and respiratory infections.[8]

Similarly, lipids provide essential fatty acids for structuring membranes, serving as an important energy source and contributing to the infant's immunologic responses. The precursor role of essential fatty acids in the synthesis of functional components, such as prostaglandins, and the antiviral and antibacterial properties of the shorter-chain fatty acids, such as lauric acid, are examples of the immunologically related functions of dietary lipids.

Certain products from the hydrolysis of human lipids lyse enveloped viruses.[27] The human fat globule membrane and its mucin component's ability to bind s-fimbriated *E coli* suggest another potential protective property of the human milk's lipid fraction.[28]

Human milk also plays another important role. The normal development of the gastrointestinal tract is subdivided into 4 phases.[29] In the first phase, the infants' intestinal microflora resemble maternal flora and those of the surroundings encountered by infants during birth and the immediate postnatal period. Maternal intestinal flora is a source of colonization in the neonatal intestine. However, the vertical transmission of *E coli* strains from mother to infant during delivery is generally reported to be less than 50% in either industrialized or developing countries.[30,31] Transfer of enterobacteria other than *E coli* from mother to infant occurs infrequently, but horizontal transfer of enterobacteria, including *E coli*, occurs between neonates in the nursery.[32] The second phase is affected significantly by whether infants are breastfed or formula fed. Although there is some inconsistency among published studies, presumably because of methodologic differences, generally, initial similarities between the floras of breastfed and formula-fed infants on day 7 of postnatal life diminish substantially by day 30, especially in developing countries. Breastfed infants have less enterococci and clostridia in their flora than do formula-fed infants, and breastfed infants have more staphylococci and at younger ages.[33] Generally, breastfed infants have fewer *Klebsiella, Enterobacter*, and *Citrobacter* organisms in their flora, and the strains of *E coli* found in the flora differ between feeding groups. For example, P-fimbriated *E coli* are less common and type 1-fimbriated *E coli* are more common in the flora of breastfed infants than in the flora of formula-fed infants. P-fimbriae is the virulence factor most often associated with urinary tract infections.[33] Previous reports of highly marked differences between breastfed and formula-fed infants in the bifidobacteria content of their flora have not been confirmed for unexplained reasons by more recent investigations.[33] The third phase relates to the period after the initial introduction of solid foods. During this period, enterococci, bacteroides, clostridia, anaerobic streptococci, and other bacteria increase in the flora of breastfed infants. Less marked changes occur in the flora of formula-fed infants.[29] In the fourth phase (the time after the introduction of an adult diet), although the intestinal flora of infants remains distinct from that of adults, the flora increasingly resemble adult patterns.

The short-term benefits of these nutritional-immunologic interactions are clear.[5,34] The frequency of gastrointestinal tract infections in breastfed infants is lower in industrialized and industrially developing populations. Also, even when rates of infections are similar among breastfed and nonbreastfed infants, the duration and severity of infection often are less for breastfed infants. Attenuation of clinical responses has been reported for both gastrointestinal (eg, rotavirus infection) and respiratory tract infections (eg, respiratory syncytial virus infections). Such positive outcomes become progressively more significant as the frequency and severity of microbial challenges rise.

The possibility that the antimicrobial, anti-inflammatory, and immunoregulatory components in human milk have longer-lasting effects on the infant's immune system and the effects of breastfeeding on the development of allergic diseases remain controversial. If breastfeeding prevents certain allergic disorders, it is unclear whether those positive outcomes are attributable to delays in the introduction of potentially allergenic foods, to immunoregulatory components in the milk, or to the balance among specific nutrients. For example, Wright and Bolton[35] reported a significantly greater proportion of linoleic acid and a smaller proportion of dihomogamma-linolenic acid in the human milk lipid fraction of mothers of infants with atopic eczema compared with controls.

In addition, there is evidence that some breastfed infants become sensitized to certain maternally ingested foods by the passage of those food antigens into human milk.[36] However, the topic is controversial, because some of these same dietary proteins may be detected in human milk from mothers whose infants are asymptomatic, and one of the major suspected dietary allergens, bovine beta-lactoglobulin, immunologically cross-reacts with a fragment of human beta-casein.[37] Therefore, the diagnosis of allergic reactions in the breastfed infant attributable to food allergens passed via breastfeeding depends on tedious dietary elimination/oral provocation procedures in the lactating woman. The management of such problems requires either a cessation of breastfeeding or a long-term elimination of the food allergen from the maternal diet, and severely atopic infants may require support by a pediatric allergist. Recent studies suggest that prophylactic dietary elimination of suspected food allergens from the maternal diet, with the possible exception of peanuts (and subsequent development of peanut allergy) does not decrease the risk of the development of most atopic diseases in later childhood in breastfed infants (see also Chapter 34).[38]

Publications linking the length of breastfeeding to the risk of type 1 diabetes mellitus, childhood lymphoma, acute lymphocytic leukemia, and Crohn disease suggest that maturational changes may be brought about in early life by the provision of immunoactive components found in milk.[39–42]

These provocative, retrospective studies require the investigation of more specific mechanisms of action relating nutritional management in early life to immune system function in later development.

Preterm Birth and Infants With Low Birth Weight

Interactions between nutritional status and immune system function in infants of low birth weight attributable to preterm birth and/or intrauterine growth retardation have not been studied systematically. Therefore, these interactions are difficult to describe beyond the qualitative assessment of immune function deficiencies that are imposed by preterm birth[43] (eg, decreased placental transfer of maternal IgG to the fetus, developmental delays in many components of the immune system and/or intrauterine growth retardation) and are also linked inextricably to inadequate micronutrient status in infants with low birth weight. Preterm separation from the mother prevents the normal transfer of nutrients with key immunologic roles, because the transfer of nutrients, such as iron and zinc, mostly occurs in the third trimester. The vitamin status (eg, vitamin A) of such infants also is impaired. The inadequate nutrient transfer to the fetus that often accompanies growth retardation may be attributable to maternal nutrient deficiency states and/or secondary to impaired placental perfusion. In either case, the postnatal unavailability of adequate nutrient stores likely interferes with functions described in the nutrient-specific sections of this discussion. Schlesinger and Uauy[44] have reviewed potential nutrient-immune interactions in infants with low birth weight.

Micronutrients and Immunity

Primary nutrient deficiencies are seen rarely in children in the United States, with the exception of iron deficiency. On the other hand, aberrant diets lacking key nutrients (eg, ascorbic acid[45]), certain medical conditions (eg, fat malabsorption, acrodermatitis enteropathica) and lifestyle choices (eg, vegan or macrobiotic diets) can induce moderate or severe nutrient deficiencies that may influence immune competence. Even in mild cases of nutrient deficiency, concern has been raised that immunologic effects of nutrient deficiency may precede the appearance of classic nutritional deficiency sequelae. Unfortunately, the bulk of scientific literature on nutritional deficiency and immune competence is based largely on data from severely malnourished individuals, cell culture experiments, animal models, and clinical trials with adult or elderly subjects. The greatest caution must be taken in extrapolating suggestive data from animals or adults into recommendations for children.

V

Conversely, a number of vitamins, minerals, and other dietary ingredients are marketed and sold in the United States for their putative immune system-enhancing properties. Given the high rates of common infectious diseases (eg, cold, influenza) among young children, parents may choose to use such supplements. A recent population survey found that half of all mothers gave vitamin supplements to their preadolescents.[46] Thus, pediatricians often are challenged by the need to be familiar with the scientific evidence about individual nutrients and other dietary supplement ingredients.

Iron

Iron deficiency is the most prevalent micronutrient deficiency among children in the United States, affecting 2% to 3% of children 3 to 11 years of age and 9% to 11% of girls 12 to 19 years of age.[47] The prevalence is higher among certain at-risk groups, such as Hispanic individuals.[48] Studies in France[49] and the United States[50] showed that iron supplementation of children of low socioeconomic status who are iron deficient can normalize blood T-lymphocyte counts, delayed-type hypersensitivity skin responses, or in vitro IL-2 production, but the clinical consequences are unknown. A small placebo-controlled trial among 6- to 36-month-old children in Togo, West Africa (n = 163), found no change in infectious disease incidence after 6 months of iron supplementation.[51] Apparently, B-lymphocyte and antibody formation are not affected by iron deficiency. Iron supplementation of iron-replete children is not known to improve immune function further, and increased availability of elemental iron in the gut has the potential to promote the growth and survival of pathogenic organisms.[52] High-dose supplementation with iron alone can also interfere with zinc absorption and, therefore, exacerbate zinc deficiency.[53]

Zinc

Moderate or severe zinc deficiency can impair both lymphocyte and phagocyte cell function in humans,[54] but this degree of zinc deficiency is encountered rarely in the United States. In developing countries, zinc supplementation reduces infectious disease morbidity, especially respiratory and diarrheal diseases, among infants and preschool children.[55-57] In a randomized, placebo-controlled trial of more than 1700 cases of acute diarrhea in Nepalese children, zinc supplementation reduced the duration of diarrhea and was not enhanced or dependent on concomitant vitamin A supplementation.[58] Zinc supplements have been used to modify the immune status of elderly patients in institutions[59] or as high-dose oral lozenges to treat the common cold in adults,[60] but there is no direct evidence that zinc supplementation may benefit zinc-replete children. Furthermore, there is a risk of zinc supplements impairing copper absorption at daily intakes >7 mg for children younger than 3 years, >12 mg for children 4 to 8 years of age, or >23 mg for children 9 to 13 years of age.[61]

Vitamin A

In developing countries, vitamin A supplementation of deficient children reduces overall mortality[62,63] and morbidity from diarrhea,[64] measles,[65] and possibly other diseases.[66] Vitamin A-deficient animals in experimental models have impaired T-lymphocyte responses to mitogens and antigens, reduced natural killer cell activity, and decreased production of interferon.[67] However, there is no direct evidence that vitamin A supplementation benefits the immune system of vitamin A-replete children. Daily intakes of retinol >600 µg for children younger than 3 years, >900 µg for children 4 to 8 years of age, or >1700 µg for children 9 to 13 years of age[61] should be avoided to reduce the risk of vitamin A toxicity. This form of toxicity is not seen when vitamin A is supplied by provitamin A carotenoids (eg, beta-carotene, alpha-carotene).

Vitamin E

Although high-dose vitamin E supplements can improve immune function in healthy elderly subjects,[68] it is unclear whether this occurs in children. Vitamin E supplements did not affect tetanus antibody titers in 2-month-old infants[69] or neutrophil function in preterm infants.[70] On the other hand, smaller increases in vitamin E intake may serve the child's overall nutritional adequacy, because few children in the United States consume the recommended amounts of vitamin E.[71]

Vitamin C

Vitamin C commonly has been believed to benefit the immune system since Nobel laureate Linus Pauling advocated high-dose vitamin C supplementation to prevent the common cold.[72] A recent, comprehensive meta-analysis indicates that high-dose vitamin C (1 g or more daily) does not reduce the incidence of the common cold but may slightly reduce the duration of the infection.[73] Five of the 11 studies evaluated in this meta-analysis were conducted in children, and the results in this subset were consistent with the overall finding. Few studies have addressed the role of vitamin C more generally in the immune system, although neutrophils are known to maintain high concentrations of the vitamin in vivo,[74] and vitamin C may inactivate histamine chemically.[75] Overall, it is unclear whether high-dose vitamin C supplements have any general immunologic benefit for pediatric populations.

B Vitamins

Moderate to severe deficiencies of vitamin B$_6$,[76,77] vitamin B$_{12}$,[78,79] pantothenic acid,[80,81] folate,[82] or biotin[83,84] suppress immune responses in adult humans and/or animal models. Biotin and pantothenic acid are nearly ubiquitous in the US diet,[85] and deficiency only occurs in unusual circumstances. Vitamin B$_{12}$ deficiency may occur in breastfed infants of vegan mothers[86] or, theoretically, in vegan children who do not consume a supplemental source of vitamin B$_{12}$. Much less information is available on the effects of B-vitamin supplements on immune responses, although a few preliminary studies indicate that pharmacologic intakes of riboflavin[87] or vitamin B$_6$[88–90] can affect immunologic parameters. B-vitamin deficiency or supplementation studies have not been conducted in children, and the clinical relevance of these findings for the pediatric population is unknown.

Nucleotides

Nucleotides (components of RNA and DNA) normally are found in human milk at concentrations of approximately 189 ± 70 μmol/L.[91] Currently, nucleotides are added to several infant formulas in the United States. The mechanism by which dietary nucleotides may modify immune function is unknown,[92] although recent mouse-model studies indicate they may augment T helper 1-biased immune responses.[93,94] Studies in human infants have reported that adding nucleotides to infant formula increases natural killer cell activity, IL-2 production by monocytes, serum IgM and IgA concentrations, and serum antibody titers to food antigens.[95–97] The clinical relevance of these changes is unknown. Two studies have reported more clinically specific endpoints. One study showed higher antibody titers to *H influenzae* type b vaccine in treated infants,[98] and another study reported a reduced duration and frequency of diarrheal disease in a group of children of low socioeconomic status.[99] Such data are promising, but additional studies are needed to understand the mechanism of action, confirm clinical endpoints, and monitor the long-term effects of adding nucleotides to infant formula.

Long-Chain Polyunsaturated Fatty Acids

Human milk fat contains 0.10% to 0.35% docosahexaenoic acid (DHA) and 0.30% to 0.65% arachidonic acid (ARA), depending on the mother's polyunsaturated fatty acid intake.[100] Some term infant formulas now also contain DHA and ARA.[101] Both DHA and ARA may contribute to visual acuity and cognitive development,[102,103] but their effects on infant immune function are not well understood. Arachidonic acid is the precursor for prostaglandins and leukotrienes that regulate normal inflammatory processes.[104,105] In vivo, DHA feeding can inhibit both inflammation responses and T-lymphocyte signaling in animal models and adult humans.[106,107] Infant data related to these responses are limited and difficult to interpret. Observational studies indicate that mothers of infants with atopy have lower concentrations of DHA and ARA in their milk compared with mothers of infants without atopy.[108,109] On the other hand, Field et al[110] found that preterm infants fed formula with DHA and ARA had more mature CD4+ T-lymphocytes with higher ex vivo IL-10 production (indicating a potential bias toward antibody and atopic responses) than did infants fed formula without DHA and ARA. Additional studies are needed to determine whether DHA and ARA can have clinically significant effects on in vivo inflammation, immune responses, mucosal immune system development, or long-term immunocompetence.

Probiotics

Yogurt, certain other milk-based products, and some dietary supplements contain live, nonpathogenic bacteria of *Lactobacillus* or *Bifidobacterium* species, collectively termed "probiotics." Certain human milk carbohydrates naturally enhance the growth of probiotic bacteria in the infant's gut[111] that may benefit the child by competitively reducing colonization of the gastrointestinal tract with pathogenic organisms. A number of studies have used probiotic-containing foods or infant formula to successfully prevent or treat chronic,[112,113] acute,[114-118] or antibiotic-induced diarrhea[119] in children, although not all studies showed an effect.[120] Some infants with atopic dermatitis have benefited from probiotic supplements,[121] and pre- and postnatal probiotic consumption by mothers with at least 1 first-degree atopic relative may reduce the frequency of atopic dermatitis in their infants.[122] A wide range of other health effects have been ascribed to probiotic organisms, but considerably fewer data are available to substantiate other claims.[123]

Herbal Products

An emergent issue in children's nutrition is the use of dietary supplements or fortified foods for purposes other than achieving nutritional adequacy. Herbal supplements—a subcategory of dietary supplements—often are promoted and claimed to be safe on the basis of history of use in folk remedies or among aboriginal cultures. Health care professionals should be aware that there are currently no premarket federal standards of quality, safety, or efficacy testing for herbal treatments. The Food and Drug Administration can exercise enforcement power only if (1) the manufacturer claims the herb works like a drug; (2) the herb contains illegal substances or substances not declared on the label; or (3) the herb causes unambiguous, serious harm to people who have purchased and used the supplement. With these cautions in mind, the health care professional must discern judiciously between benign actions that may have special significance for the family (religion, tradition, self-empowerment) and potentially hazardous misuse of potent bioactive compounds. Additional information on common dietary supplements is available from the American Dietetic Association's *The Health Professional's Guide to Popular Dietary Supplements*[124] and the *Physician's Desk Reference (PDR) for Herbal Medicines*.[125] The Natural Medicines Comprehensive Database provides evidence-based, clinical information on natural medicines and is available online (www.naturaldatabase.com).

Summary

Adequate nutrition is necessary for proper development and function of a child's immune system. Both human milk and synthetic formula can provide adequate nutrition, but human milk is clearly best for infants, because it provides unique components proven to protect and stimulate the developing immune system and contributes positively to growth and development in other ways. In older children, immune function appears to be preserved except in the most severe micronutrient deficiencies. The use of high-dose nutrient supplements and other dietary components to stimulate immune function in otherwise well-nourished children is controversial. Overall, considerably more research is needed to better understand how the maturation and function of the immune system interacts with the changing nutrient requirements of growth.

References

1. Adderson EE, Johnston JM, Shackerford PG, Carroll WL. Development of the human antibody repertoire. *Pediatr Res.* 1992;32:257–263
2. Burgio GR, Ugazio AG, Notarangelo LD. Immunology of the neonate. *Curr Opin Immunol.* 1989–1990;2:770–777
3. Gershwin ME, Beach RS, Hurley LS. Nutritional factors and immune ontogeny. In: *Nutrition and Immunity.* Orlando, FL: Academic Press, Inc; 1985:99–127
4. Beach RS, Gershwin ME, Hurley LS. Gestational zinc deprivation in mice: persistence of immunodeficiency for three generations. *Science.* 1982; 218:469–471

5. Institute of Medicine. *Nutrition During Lactation.* Washington, DC: National Academy Press; 1991

6. Stevens S. Maturation of the immune system in breast-fed and bottle-fed infants. In: Cunningham-Rundles S, ed. *Nutrient Modulation of the Immune Response.* New York, NY: Marcel-Dekker, Inc; 1993:301–318

7. Garza C, Schanler RJ, Butte NF, Motil KJ. Special properties of human milk. *Clin Perinatol.* 1987;14:11–32

8. Hanson LA, Adlerberth I, Carlsson BUM, et al. Human milk antibodies and their importance for the infant. In: Cunningham-Ruddles S, ed. *Nutrient Modulation of the Immune Response.* New York, NY: Marcel Dekker, Inc; 1993:525–532

9. Peckham CS, Johnson C, Ades A, Pearl K, Chin KS. Early acquisition of cytomegalovirus infection. *Arch Dis Child.* 1987;62:780–785

10. Rudloff HE, Schmalstieg FC Jr, Mushtaha AA, Palkowetz KH, Liu SK, Goldman AS. Tumor necrosis factor-alpha in human milk. *Pediatr Res.* 1992;31:29–33

11. Munoz C, Endres S, van der Meer J, Schlesinger L, Arevalo M, Dinarello C. Interleukin-1 beta in human colostrum. *Res Immunol.* 1990;141:505–513

12. Saito S, Maruyama M, Kato Y, Moriyama I, Ichijo M. Detection of IL-6 in human milk and its involvement in IgA production. *J Reprod Immunol.* 1991;20:267–276

13. Rudloff HE, Schmalstieg FC Jr, Palkowetz KH, Paszkiewicz EJ, Goldman AS. Interleukin-6 in human milk. *J Reprod Immunol.* 1993;23:13–20

14. Okada M, Ohmura E, Kamiya Y, et al. Transforming growth factor (TGF)-alpha in human milk. *Life Sci.* 1991;48:1151–1156

15. Garofalo R, Chheda S, Mei F, et al. Interleukin-10 in human milk. *Pediatr Res.* 1995;37: 444–449

16. Gilmore WS, McKelvey-Martin VJ, Rutherford S, et al. Human milk contains granulocyte colony stimulating factor. *Eur J Clin Nutr.* 1994;48:222–224

17. Hara T, Irie K, Saito S, et al. Identification of macrophage colony-stimulating factor in human milk and mammary gland epithelial cells. *Pediatr Res.* 1995;37: 437–443

18. Palkowetz KH, Royer CL, Garofalo R, Rudloff HE, Schmalstieg FC Jr, Goldman AS. Production of interleukin-6 and interleukin-8 by human mammary gland epithelial cells. *J Reprod Immunol.* 1994;26:57–64

19. Garofalo RP, Goldman AS. Cytokines, chemokines, and colony-stimulating factors in human milk: the 1997 update. *Biol Neonate.* 1998;74:134–142

20. Goldblum RM, Schanler RJ, Garza C, Goldman AS. Human milk feeding enhances the urinary excretion of immunologic factors in low birth weight infants. *Pediatr Res.* 1989;25:184–188

21. Goldman AS, Garza C, Schanler RJ, Goldblum RM. Molecular forms of lactoferrin in stool and urine from infants fed human milk. *Pediatr Res.* 1990;27:252–255

22. Hutchens TW, Henry JF, Yip TT, et al. Origin of intact lactoferrin and its DNA-binding fragments found in the urine of human milk-fed preterm infants. Evaluation by stable isotopic enrichment. *Pediatr Res.* 1991;29:243–250

23. Stephens S, Dolby JM, Montreuil J, Spik G. Differences in inhibition of the growth of commensal and enteropathogenic strains of *Escherichia coli* by lactotransferrin and secretory immunoglobulin A isolated from human milk. *Immunology*. 1980; 41:597–603

24. Griffiths E, Humphreys J. Bacteriostatic effect of human milk and bovine colostrum on *Escherichia coli*: importance of bicarbonate. *Infect Immun*. 1977;15:396–401

25. Goldman AS, Thorpe LW, Goldblum RM, Hanson LA. Anti-inflammatory properties of human milk. *Acta Paediatr Scand*. 1986;75:689–695

26. Newburg DS. Oligosaccharides and glycoconjugates in human milk: their role in host defense. *J Mammary Gland Biol Neoplasia*. 1996;1:271–283

27. Isaacs CE, Thormar H. The role of milk-derived antimicrobial lipids as antiviral and antibacterial agents. *Adv Exp Med Biol*. 1991;310:159–165

28. Schroten H, Hanisch FG, Plogmann R, et al. Inhibition of adhesion of S-fimbriated Escherichia coli to buccal epithelial cells by human milk fat globule membrane components: a novel aspect of the protective function of mucins in the nonimmunoglobulin fraction. *Infect Immun*. 1992;60:2893–2899

29. Orrhage K, Nord CE. Factors controlling the bacterial colonization of the intestine in breastfed infants. *Acta Paediatr Suppl*. 1999;88:47–57

30. Gothefors L, Carlsson B, Ahlstedt S, Hanson LA, Winberg J. Influence of maternal gut flora and colostral and cord serum antibodies on presence of *Escherichia coli* in faeces of the newborn infant. *Acta Paediatr Scand*. 1976;65:225–232.

31. Adlerberth I. Bacterial adherence and intestinal colonization in newborn infants [dissertation]. Göteborg, Sweden: Göteborg University, 1996

32. Fryklund B. Epidemiology of enterobacteria and risk factors for invasive Gram-negative bacterial infection in neonatal special-care units [dissertation]. Stokholm: Stockholm University, 1994

33. Wold AE, Adlerberth I. Breast feeding and the intestinal microflora of the infant— implications for protection against infectious diseases. *Adv Exp Med Biol*. 2000;478:77–93

34. Kramer MS, Chalmers B, Hodnett ED, et al. Promotion of Breastfeeding Intervention Trial (PROBIT): a randomized trial in the Republic of Belarus. *JAMA*. 2001;285:413–420

35. Wright S, Bolton C. Breast milk fatty acids in mothers of children with atopic eczema. *Br J Nutr*. 1989;62:693–697

36. Goldman AS. Association of atopic diseases with breast-feeding: food allergens, fatty acids, and evolution. *J Pediatr*. 1999;134:5–7

37. Conti A, Giuffrida MG, Napolitano L, et al. Identification of the human beta-casein C-terminal fragments that specifically bind to purified antibodies to bovine beta-lactoglobulin. *J Nutr Biochem*. 2000;11:332–337

38. Herrmann ME, Dannemann A, Gruters A, et al. Prospective study of the atopy preventive effect of maternal avoidance of milk and eggs during pregnancy and lactation. *Eur J Pediatr*. 1996;155:770–774

39. Davis MK, Savitz DA, Graubard BI. Infant feeding and childhood cancer. *Lancet*. 1988; 2:365–368

40. Koletzko S, Sherman P, Corey M, Griffiths A, Smith C. Role of infant feeding practices in development of Crohn's disease in childhood. *BMJ*. 1989;298:1617–1618

41. Mayer EJ, Hamman RF, Gay EC, Lezotte DC, Savitz DA, Klingensmith GJ. Reduced risk of IDDM among breast fed children. The Colorado IDDM Registry. *Diabetes.* 1988;37:1625–1632

42. Shu XO, Linet MS, Steinbuch M, et al. Breast-feeding and risk of childhood acute leukemia. *J Natl Cancer Inst.* 1999;91:1765–1772

43. Goldman AS. Back to basics: host responses to infection. *Pediatr Rev.* 2000;21:342–349

44. Schlesinger L, Uauy R. Nutrition and neonatal immune function. *Semin Perinatol.* 1991; 15:469–477

45. Tamura Y, Welch DC, Zic JA, Cooper WO, Stein SM, Hummell DS. Scurvy presenting as painful gait with bruising in a young boy. *Arch Pediatr Adolesc Med.* 2000; 154:732–735

46. Roche Vitamins. *Vitamin Consumption in the US.* Parsippany, NJ: Roche Vitamins Inc; 2000

47. Centers for Disease Control and Prevention. Recommendations to prevent and control iron deficiency in the United States. *MMWR Recomm Rep.* 1998;47(RR-3):1–29

48. Frith-Terhune AL, Cogswell ME, Khan LK, Will JC, Ramakrishnan U. Iron deficiency anemia: higher prevalence in Mexican American than in non-Hispanic white females in the third National Health and Nutrition Examination Survey, 1988–1994. *Am J Clin Nutr.* 2000;72:963–968

49. Thibault H, Galan P, Selz F, et al. The immune response in iron-deficient young children: effect of iron supplementation on cell-mediated immunity. *Eur J Pediatr.* 1993;152:120–124

50. Krantman HJ, Young SR, Ank BJ, O'Donnell CM, Rachelefsky GS, Stiehm ER. Immune function in pure iron deficiency. *Am J Dis Child.* 1982;136:840–844

51. Berger J, Dyck JL, Galan P, et al. Effect of daily iron supplementation on iron status, cell-mediated immunity, and incidence of infections in 6–36 month old Togolese children. *Eur J Clin Nutr.* 2000;54:29–35

52. Kent S, Weinberg ED, Stuart-Macadam P. The etiology of the anemia of chronic disease and infection. *J Clin Epidemiol.* 1994;47:23–33

53. Couzy F, Keen C, Gershwin ME, Mareschi JP. Nutritional implications of the interactions between minerals. *Prog Food Nutr Sci.* 1993;17:65–87

54. Shankar AH, Prasad AS. Zinc and immune function: the biological basis of altered resistance to infection. *Am J Clin Nutr.* 1998;68(2 Suppl):447S–463S

55. Sazawal S, Black RE, Bhan MK, Bhandari N, Sinha A, Jalla S. Zinc supplementation in young children with acute diarrhea in India. *N Engl J Med.* 1995;333:839–844

56. Rosado JL, Lopez P, Munoz E, Martinez H, Allen LH. Zinc supplementation reduced morbidity, but neither zinc nor iron supplementation affected growth or body composition of Mexican preschoolers. *Am J Clin Nutr.* 1997;65:13–19

57. Sazawal S, Black RE, Jalla S, Mazumdar S, Sinha A, Bhan MK. Zinc supplementation reduces the incidence of acute lower respiratory infections in infants and preschool children: a double-blind, controlled trial. *Pediatrics.* 1998;102:1–5

58. Strand TA, Chandyo RK, Bahl R, et al. Effectiveness and efficacy of zinc for the treatment of acute diarrhea in young children. *Pediatrics.* 2002;109:898–903

59. Girodon F, Galan P, Monget AL, et al. Impact of trace elements and vitamin supplementation on immunity and infections in institutionalized elderly patients: a randomized controlled trial. MIN. VIT. AOX. Geriatric Network. *Arch Intern Med.* 1999;159:748–754

60. Mossad SB, Macknin ML, Medendorp SV, Mason P. Zinc gluconate lozenges for treating the common cold. A randomized, double-blind, placebo-controlled study. *Ann Intern Med.* 1996;125:81–88

61. Institute of Medicine. *Dietary Reference Intakes for Vitamin A, Vitamin K, Arsenic, Boron, Chromium, Copper, Iodine, Iron, Manganese, Molybdenum, Nickel, Silicon, Vanadium, and Zinc.* Washington, DC: National Academies Press; 2000

62. West KP Jr, Pokhrel RP, Katz J, et al. Efficacy of vitamin A in reducing preschool child mortality in Nepal. *Lancet.* 1991;338:67–71

63. Rahmathullah L, Underwood BA, Thulasiraj RD, et al. Reduced mortality among children in southern India receiving a small weekly dose of vitamin A. *N Engl J Med.* 1990;323:929–935

64. Glasziou PP, Mackerras DE. Vitamin A supplementation in infectious diseases: a meta-analysis. *BMJ.* 1993;306:366–370

65. Hussey GD, Klein M. A randomized, controlled trial of vitamin A in children with severe measles. *N Engl J Med.* 1990;323:160–164

66. Shankar AH, Genton B, Semba RD, et al. Effect of vitamin A supplementation on morbidity due to *Plasmodium falciparum* in young children in Papua New Guinea: a randomised trial. *Lancet.* 1999;354:203–209

67. Scrimshaw NS, SanGiovanni JP. Synergism of nutrition, infection, and immunity: an overview. *Am J Clin Nutr.* 1997; 66:464S–477S

68. Meydani SN, Meydani M, Blumberg JB, et al. Vitamin E supplementation and in vivo immune response in healthy elderly subjects. A randomized controlled trial. *JAMA.* 1997;277:1380–1386

69. Kutukculer N, Akil T, Egemen A, et al. Adequate immune response to tetanus toxoid and failure of vitamin A and E supplementation to enhance antibody response in healthy children. *Vaccine.* 2000;18:2979–2984

70. Mino M. Clinical uses and abuses of vitamin E in children. *Proc Soc Exp Biol Med.* 1992;200:266–270

71. US Department of Agriculture-Agricultural Research Service. *Food and Nutrient Intakes by Children 1994–96, 1998.* Table Set 17. Available at: http://www.ars.usda.gov/SPSUserFiles/Place/12355000/pdf/scs_all.pdf. Accessed November 2, 2007

72. Pauling L. The significance of the evidence about ascorbic acid and the common cold. *Proc Natl Acad Sci U S A.* 1971;68:2678–2681

73. Douglas RM, Chalker EB, Treacy B. Vitamin C for preventing and treating the common cold. *Cochrane Database Syst Rev.* 2000;(2):CD000980

74. Muggli R. Vitamin C and phagocytes. In: Cunningham-Rundles S, ed. *Nutrient Modulation of the Immune Response.* New York, NY: Marcel-Dekker; 1993:75–90

75. Johnston CS. The antihistamine action of ascorbic acid. *Subcell Biochem.* 1996; 25:189–213

76. Frydas S, Reale M, Vacalis D, et al. IgG, IgG1 and IgM response in *Trichinella spiralis*-infected mice treated with 4-deoxypirydoxine or fed a vitamin B_6-deficient diet. *Mol Cell Biochem.* 1999;194:47–52

77. Rall LC, Meydani SN. Vitamin B_6 and immune competence. *Nutr Rev.* 1993; 51:217–225

78. Tamura J, Kubota K, Murakami H, et al. Immunomodulation by vitamin B$_{12}$: augmentation of CD8+ T lymphocytes and natural killer (NK) cell activity in vitamin B$_{12}$-deficient patients by methyl-B$_{12}$ treatment. *Clin Exp Immunol*. 1999;116: 28–32

79. Fata FT, Herzlich BC, Schiffman G, Ast AL. Impaired antibody responses to pneumococcal polysaccharide in elderly patients with low serum vitamin B$_{12}$ levels. *Ann Intern Med*. 1996;124:299–304

80. Hodges RE, Bean WB, Ohlson MA, Bleiler RE. Factors affecting human antibody response. IV. Pyridoxine deficiency. *Am J Clin Nutr*. 1962;11:180–186

81. Hodges RE, Bean WB, Ohlson MA, Bleiler RE. Factors affecting human antibody response. V. Combined deficiencies of pantothenic acid and pyridoxine. *Am J Clin Nutr*. 1962;11:187–199

82. Dhur A, Galan P, Hercberg S. Folate status and the immune system. *Prog Food Nutr Sci*. 1991;15:43–60

83. Baez-Saldana A, Diaz G, Espinoza B, Ortega E. Biotin deficiency induces changes in subpopulations of spleen lymphocytes in mice. *Am J Clin Nutr*. 1998;67: 431–437

84. Rabin BS. Inhibition of experimentally induced autoimmunity in rats by biotin deficiency. *J Nutrition*. 1983;113:2316–2322

85. Institute of Medicine. *Dietary Reference Intakes for Thiamin, Riboflavin, Niacin, Vitamin B$_6$, Folate, Vitamin B$_{12}$, Pantothenic Acid, Biotin, and Choline*. Washington, DC: National Academies Press; 1998

86. Specker BL, Black A, Allen L, Morrow F. Vitamin B$_{12}$: low milk concentrations are related to low serum concentrations in vegetarian women and to methylmalonic aciduria in their infants. *Am J Clin Nutr*. 1990;52:1073–1076

87. Araki S, Suzuki M, Fujimoto M, Kimura M. Enhancement of resistance to bacterial infection in mice by vitamin B$_2$. *J Vet Med Sci*. 1995;57:599–602

88. Gebhard KJ, Gridley DS, Stickney DR, Shulz TD. Enhancement of immune status by high levels of dietary vitamin B$_6$ without growth inhibition of human malignant melanoma in athymic nude mice. *Nutr Cancer*. 1990; 14:15–26

89. Talbott MC, Miller LT, Kerkvliet NI. Pyridoxine supplementation: effect on lymphocyte responses in elderly persons. *Am J Clin Nutr*. 1987;46:659–664

90. Debes SA, Kirksey A. Influence of dietary pyridoxine on selected immune capacities of rat dams and pups. *J Nutr*. 1979;109:744–759

91. Motil KJ. Infant feeding: a critical look at infant formulas. *Curr Opin Pediatr*. 2000;12: 469–476

92. Grimble GK, Westwood OM. Nucleotides as immunomodulators in clinical nutrition. *Curr Opin Clin Nutr Metab Care*. 2001;4:57–64

93. Jyonouchi H, Sun S, Abiru T, Winship T, Kuchan MJ. Dietary nucleotides modulate antigen-specific type 1 and type 2 T-cell responses in young c57bl/6 mice. *Nutrition*. 2000; 16:442–446

94. Nagafuchi S, Hachimura S, Totsuka M, et al. Dietary nucleotides can up-regulate antigen-specific Th1 immune responses and suppress antigen-specific IgE responses in mice. *Int Arch Allergy Immunol*. 2000;122:33–41

95. Carver JD, Pimentel B, Cox WI, Barness LA. Dietary nucleotide effects upon immune function in infants. *Pediatrics*. 1991;88:359–363

96. Martinez-Augustin O, Boza JJ, Del Pino JI, Lucena J, Martinez-Valverde A, Gil A. Dietary nucleotides might influence the humoral immune response against cow's milk proteins in preterm neonates. *Biol Neonate*. 1997;71:215–223

97. Navarro J, Maldonado J, Narbona E, et al. Influence of dietary nucleotides on plasma immunoglobulin levels and lymphocyte subsets of preterm infants. *Biofactors*. 1999; 10:67–76

98. Pickering LK, Granoff DM, Erickson JR, et al. Modulation of the immune system by human milk and infant formula containing nucleotides. *Pediatrics*. 1998; 101:242–249

99. Brunser O, Espinoza J, Araya M, Cruchet S, Gil A. Effect of dietary nucleotide supplementation on diarrhoeal disease in infants. *Acta Paediatr*. 1994;83:188–191

100. Jensen RG, Bitman J, Carlson SE, Couch SC, Hamosh M, Newburg DS. Milk lipids: A. Human milk lipids. In: Jensen RG, ed. *Handbook of Milk Composition*. San Diego, CA: Academic Press; 1995:495–575

101. Rulis AM, Lewis CJ. FDA agency response letter to Martek Biosciences Corp. regarding GRAS notice GRN 000041. FDA Office of Premarket Approval. Available at: http://www.cfsan.fda.gov/~rdb/opa-g041.html. Accessed April 8, 2003

102. SanGiovanni JP, Berkey CS, Dwyer JT, Colditz GA. Dietary essential fatty acids, long-chain polyunsaturated fatty acids, and visual resolution acuity in healthy fullterm infants: a systematic review. *Early Hum Dev*. 2000;57:165–188

103. Gibson RA, Makrides M. The role of long chain polyunsaturated fatty acids (LCPUFA) in neonatal nutrition. *Acta Paediatr*. 1998;87:1017–1022

104. Griffiths RJ. Prostaglandins and inflammation. In: Gallin JI, Snyderman R, eds. *Inflammation: Basic Principles and Clinical Correlates*. 3rd ed. Philadelphia, PA: Lippincott Williams and Wilkins; 1999:349–360

105. Penrose JF, Austen KF, Lam BK. Leukotrienes: biosynthetic pathways, release, and receptor-mediated actions with relevance to disease states. In: Gallin JI, Snyderman R, eds. *Inflammation: Basic Principles and Clinical Correlates*. 3rd ed. Philadelphia, PA: Lippincott Williams and Wilkins; 1999:361–372

106. Calder PC. N-3 polyunsaturated fatty acids, inflammation and immunity: pouring oil on troubled waters or another fishy tale? *Nutr Res*. 2001;21:309–341

107. McMurray DN, Jolly CA, Chapkin RS. Effects of dietary n-3 fatty acids on T cell activation and T cell receptor-mediated signaling in a murine model. *J Infect Dis*. 2000;182(suppl):S103–S107

108. Duchen K, Casas R, Fageras-Bottcher M, Yu G, Björkstén B. Human milk polyunsaturated long-chain fatty acids and secretory immunoglobulin A antibodies and early childhood allergy. *Pediatr Allergy Immunol*. 2000;11:29–39

109. Businco L, Ioppi M, Morse NL, Nisini R, Wright S. Breast milk from mothers of children with newly developed atopic eczema has low levels of long chain polyunsaturated fatty acids. *J Allergy Clin Immunol*. 1993;91:1134–1139

110. Field CJ, Thomson CA, Van Aerde JE, et al. Lower proportion of CD45RO+ cells and deficient interleukin-10 production by formula-fed infants, compared with human-fed, is corrected with supplementation of long-chain polyunsaturated fatty acids. *J Pediatr Gastroenterol Nutr*. 2000;31:291–299

111. Kunz C, Rudloff S, Baier W, Klein N, Strobel S. Oligosaccharides in human milk: structural, functional, and metabolic aspects. *Annu Rev Nutr*. 2000;20:699–722

112. Boudraa G, Touhami M, Pochart P, Soltana R, Mary JY, Desjeux JF. Effect of feeding yogurt versus milk in children with persistent diarrhea. *J Pediatr Gastroenterol Nutr*. 1990;11: 509–512

113. Touhami M, Boudraa G, Mary JY, Soltana R, Desjeux JF. [Clinical consequences of replacing milk with yogurt in persistent infantile diarrhea.] [Article in French]. *Ann Pediatr (Paris)*. 1992;39:79–86

114. Oberhelman RA, Gilman RH, Sheen P, et al. A placebo-controlled trial of Lactobacillus GG to prevent diarrhea in undernourished Peruvian children. *J Pediatr*. 1999;134:15–20

115. Pant AR, Graham SM, Allen SJ, et al. Lactobacillus GG and acute diarrhoea in young children in the tropics. *J Trop Pediatr*. 1996;42:162–165

116. Raza S, Graham SM, Allen SJ, Sultana S, Cuevas L, Hart CA. Lactobacillus GG promotes recovery from acute nonbloody diarrhea in Pakistan. *Pediatr Infect Dis J*. 1995;14:107–111

117. Majamaa H, Isolauri E, Saxelin M, Vesikari T. Lactic acid bacteria in the treatment of acute rotavirus gastroenteritis. *J Pediatr Gastroenterol Nutr*. 1995;20:333–338

118. Saavedra JM, Bauman NA, Oung I, Perman JA, Yolken RH. Feeding of Bifidobacterium bifidum and Streptococcus thermophilus to infants in hospital for prevention of diarrhoea and shedding of rotavirus. *Lancet*. 1994;344: 1046–1049

119. Contardi I. [Oral bacterial therapy in prevention of antibiotic-induced diarrhea in childhood.] [Article in Italian]. *Clin Ter*. 1991;136:409–413

120. Millar MR, Bacon C, Smith SL, Walker V, Hall MA. Enteral feeding of premature infants with Lactobacillus GG. *Arch Dis Child*. 1993;69:483–487

121. Isolauri E, Arvola T, Sutas Y, Moilanen E, Salminen S. Probiotics in the management of atopic eczema. *Clin Exp Allergy*. 2000;30:1604–1610

122. Kalliomaki M, Salminen S, Arvilommi H, Kero P, Koskinen P, Isolauri E. Probiotics in primary prevention of atopic disease: a randomized placebo-controlled trial. *Lancet*. 2001;357: 1076–1079

123. Naidu AS, Bidlack WR, Clemens RA. Probiotic spectra of lactic acid bacteria (LAB). *Crit Rev Food Sci Nutr*. 1999;39:13–126

124. Sarubin A. *The Health Professional's Guide to Popular Dietary Supplements*. Chicago, IL: American Dietetic Association; 2000

125. Medical Economics Co. *PDR for Herbal Medicines*. 2nd ed. Montvale, NJ: Medical Economics Co; 2000

36 Nutritional Support For Children With Developmental Disabilities

Introduction

Feeding difficulties and poor growth are well-recognized problems in children with neurologic impairments. Despite the well-documented growth abnormalities in this population, the exact cause remains unclear. Both nutritional and nonnutritional factors may contribute to linear growth failure. In patients with moderate to severe cerebral palsy, poor nutritional status is associated with increased health care utilization and limitation in social activities for both the child and the parents.[1] Improvement of nutritional status improves growth, enhances quality of life and well-being, decreases irritability and spasticity, and leads to better resistance to infections and better healing of decubitus ulcers.[2-4] Nutritional repletion can also improve lower esophageal sphincter tone and gastroesophageal reflux.[5]

Monitoring of nutritional status and provision of adequate nutrition are essential in the care of the patient with neurologic impairment. Promotion of growth and well-being must be an integral part of medical management. Because of the numerous factors that need to be considered, nutritional intervention is best accomplished by a multidisciplinary team involving dietitians, speech-language and occupational therapists, psychologists, physicians, and nurses.[6]

Growth Abnormalities in Children With Neurologic Impairments

Prevalence

Children with developmental disabilities are at high risk of malnutrition. They are often in a poor nutritional state, exhibiting marked linear growth failure, poor weight gain, and decreased lean body mass and fat stores.[7-11] The true prevalence of malnutrition in this population is not known, but a significant proportion are shorter and lighter than the reference standard, and this worsens as the child grows older.[12] The growth and nutritional status of children with spastic quadriplegia is generally more severely affected, but 30% of children with diplegia or hemiplegia also exhibit signs of malnutrition with decreased weight and triceps skin fold thickness, and 23% are stunted.[8] A small proportion of patients with cerebral palsy (8%–14%) are overweight. Growth charts for patients with quadriplegic cerebral palsy have been developed (www.kennedykrieger.org).[12] These growth charts reflect the malnutrition still affecting these patients and should not be considered a standard. In recent years, progress has been made in the nutritional care of patients with neurologic impairments, but there is still room for improvement.

Pathophysiology

Nutritional factors play a major role in the growth of children with neurologic impairements.[3,7] Nutrition-related factors, such as inappropriate intake, oral motor dysfunction, increased losses, and abnormal energy expenditure, clearly affect the growth of patients with neurologic disability.[13-22] Their condition may increase the risk of developing specific nutrient deficiencies. However, nonnutritional factors may also contribute to growth abnormalities in this population.[11,23]

Nonnutritional Factors Affecting Growth

In patients with cerebral palsy, height and weight z-score are highly correlated, indicating that nutritional factors indeed play a role in linear growth failure. However, height z-score declines with advancing age independently of weight z-score, suggesting that nonnutritional factors also contribute to linear growth failure.[11] The severity of the neurologic disease correlates with an increased risk of growth failure. Height z-score is significantly lower in children with seizures, those who are nonambulatory, and those with spastic quadriplegia.[11] Linear growth of children with diplegia or hemiplegia is less affected than linear growth of those with spastic quadriplegia.[8] In children with spastic hemiplegia, significantly smaller measures of breadth and length on the affected side suggest the influence of the neurologic disease on growth.[23] Endocrine factors, immobility, and lack of weight-bearing activity may also have an effect on growth.

Inappropriate Intake

Children with cerebral palsy spontaneously consume less calories than age-matched controls.[19,21,22] The major nutritional deficit seems to be quantitative rather than qualitative.[19] Inadequate caloric intake is a major factor contributing to malnutrition, because aggressive nutritional supplementation using nasogastric or gastrostomy tube feedings improves growth.[2-4,10,24] The first year of life and the adolescent growth spurt are the 2 periods in which the child with neurologic impairment is most vulnerable, because caloric intake cannot adapt to support increased needs associated with rapid growth.

Because of their poor oral and fine motor skills, more than half of children with neurologic impairments are totally dependent on a caregiver for feedings.[25] Because they are often unable to communicate hunger and satiety, the caregiver regulates their intake. It has been shown that the caregiver often overestimates caloric intake and time spent feeding the child.[22,25] The task of feeding such a child is difficult and time consuming, and inadequate intake may ensue.[21] On the other hand, it is possible to overfeed a child with cerebral palsy; therefore, careful monitoring of growth is important, especially after initiating tube feedings, to avoid deleterious effects of obesity.

Oral-Motor Dysfunction
Feeding difficulties are common in the pediatric population with neurologic impairments.[25,26] Problems such as poor suck, vomiting, gagging, and choking are often reported as the first indication that something is wrong with the child.[21] In fact, in 60% of patients, severe feeding problems preceded the diagnosis of cerebral palsy.[25] In a study of children with cerebral palsy, more than 90% had oral-motor dysfunction, 57% had sucking problems, 38% had swallowing problems, and 80% had been fed nonorally on at least 1 occasion in the first year of life.[25] Sucking and swallowing problems, inadequate lip closure, drooling, and persistent extrusion reflex make oral feedings difficult. Feeding efficiency in patients with severe cerebral palsy is far below normal, as it may take them 2 to 12 times longer than children without cerebral palsy to swallow pureed food and up to 15 times longer to chew and swallow solid food.[27] Mealtime becomes very frustrating and time consuming for the caregiver and for the child. Prolonged feeding time (more than 3 hours/day) was reported by 28% of parents of children with neurologic impairments.[18] On average, mothers of children with disabilities spend 3.3 hours/day feeding their children, whereas parents of typical children spend 0.8 hours.[28] Even longer mealtime does not compensate for the child's feeding impairment, and as a consequence, caloric intake is often insufficient.[27] In addition, some children may have significant episodes of hypoxemia during feeding resulting from aspiration.[29]

Oral-motor dysfunction is a major factor in the pathogenesis of malnutrition in patients with cerebral palsy. Oral intake, weight, height, and weight-for-height z-scores are significantly lower in patients with oral-motor dysfunction than in patients without dysfunction.[13–20] Persistent, severe feeding difficulties are associated with poor growth and can help to identify children who will benefit from gastrostomy feeding.[16,17]

Increased Losses

In addition to decreased intake, excessive losses may occur from spillage because of poor hand-to-mouth coordination or inadequate swallowing. Abnormal gastric motility and gastroesophageal reflux (GER) are frequently encountered in patients with neurologic impairment. Gastroesophageal reflux may contribute to increased loss of nutrients as a result of frequent emesis.[30–32] Esophagitis, which may occur with GER, often causes discomfort and may lead to food aversion.

Abnormal Energy Requirements

Nutrient requirements and expected growth pattern are difficult to determine in this heterogeneous population. Defining energy needs is very important because of the patient's inability to communicate hunger and satiety and because of abnormal physical activity and body composition. Patients with spastic quadriplegic cerebral palsy fed exclusively by gastrostomy tube can grow normally with 60% ± 15% of Recommended Dietary Allowances (RDAs) for gender and age or 103% ± 32% of RDAs for weight.[33] Some patients may become obese despite relatively low caloric intake. This can be explained by the fact that resting energy expenditure (REE) is reduced in children with neurologic impairments.[22,34,35] When measured by indirect calorimetry in patients with spastic quadriplegic cerebral palsy, REE was significantly less than typical age-matched controls without cerebral palsy or from those calculated from World Health Organization equations based on weight, age, and gender.[34] Calculation of total energy needs based on World Health Organization standards for healthy children (1.5–1.6 × calculated REE) overestimates energy requirements in children with cerebral palsy (1.1 × measured REE).

Muscle tone (hypotonicity, spasticity, and athetosis) and activity level (bedridden, moderately active, ambulatory) will influence energy needs. Patients who are ambulatory or who have athetosis have higher energy needs.[36,37] Additional calories must be given to achieve normal growth and catch-up growth. Energy needs also may be increased during periods of infection, such as aspiration pneumonia.

Osteopenia

Osteoporosis is very common in children with neurologic impairments, and pathologic bone fractures may affect as many as 26% of children with cerebral palsy.[38,39] Fractures often heal poorly, increasing the need for medical care and diminishing the child's quality of life. Inadequate intake of calcium, phosphorus, and vitamin D; malnutrition; use of anticonvulsants;

lack of weight-bearing activity; and lack of sun exposure contribute to poor bone mineralization in children with cerebral palsy.[33,40–45] Calcium, phosphorus, and vitamin D intake are often insufficient in patients with cerebral palsy.[33,40,46] In addition, anticonvulsants are known to interfere with vitamin D metabolism by increasing its conversion to inactive metabolites and have been shown to be associated with osteomalacia in patients after prolonged treatment.[43,44] Ambulatory status is also important in the pathogenesis of osteopenia.[46,47] A low weight-for-age z-score is a strong predictor of low bone mineral density.[45] Measuring bone mineral density using bone densitometry may be difficult in some patients with skeletal deformities or involuntary movements or in patients with poor collaboration ability. Bone quantitative ultrasonography may be an alternative method in such situations.[48] Supplemental vitamin D should be given to patients with neurologic impairments, especially if they are taking anticonvulsants, have lack of exposure to sunlight, or are nonambulatory.[44] In a small controlled trial, bisphosphonates increased bone mineral density in children with cerebral palsy by 89% over 18 months.[49]

Assessment

Assessment of the child with neurologic impairment should include medical, nutritional, and growth history as well as a family and social history. A physical examination, including anthropometric measurements, should be performed. Meal observations and appropriate investigation will complete the evaluation.

Medical History

Assessment of health status must include knowledge of the underlying disease to better understand its natural history. Some patients have a static condition with little or no potential for improvement, others have a degenerative disease, and some have a reversible temporary neurologic impairment. The duration, severity, and prognosis of the neurologic impairment will influence the type of nutritional intervention required by the patient.

The review of systems will focus on respiratory and gastrointestinal symptoms, because they influence the type of nutritional intervention required by the child. Chronic respiratory problems and recurrent pneumonias may be caused by aspiration from GER or swallowing dysfunction. Frequent emesis and food refusal are suggestive of GER and esophagitis. Constipation is frequently seen in children with neurologic impairments and may be exacerbated by insufficient fluid and fiber intake.

It is important to review the medications used by the patient. Among the medications commonly used by children with neurologic impairments are anticonvulsants that may affect consciousness level, appetite, and vitamin D metabolism. The use of laxatives, prokinetics, and H-2 blockers or proton-pump inhibitors reflects the presence of gastrointestinal problems.

Nutritional and Growth History

The nutritional history must review all aspects of the feeding process, including the child's appetite and ability to self feed, the efficiency of the feeding process with different textures, and the time required to feed the child.

A good evaluation of oral-motor skills and swallowing function, including adequacy of lip closure, drooling, spilling, extrusion reflex, incoordination, gagging, and delayed swallowing, must be performed, because oral-motor impairment is a major factor leading to malnutrition.[13–19] Choking and coughing during meals are suggestive of aspiration, and fatigue progressing during meals may result from aspiration-induced hypoxia.[29] The amount of time spent feeding the child should be estimated. Sixty percent of patients with cerebral palsy are totally dependent on a caregiver for their intake.[25] For the caregiver, often the parent, too much time spent around meals may impair the parent-child relationship and take time away from other activities. It is also important to assess the parental perception of mealtime, as it is often perceived as a stressful and not enjoyable experience.[18,21] Parents are under constant pressure to adequately feed their child to ensure sufficient weight gain.[50]

Keeping in mind that parental report often overestimates intake, a review of a typical day's food intake or a full 3-day food record will help assessing caloric intake but also adequacy of fiber, vitamin, and mineral intake. Food refusal or a recent change in feeding pattern may be indicative of an underlying problem.

A careful review of previous growth pattern is very important. Birth weight and length and subsequent available height, weight, and head circumference measurements should be plotted on growth charts to evaluate growth and to detect changes in growth patterns, such as weight loss, abnormal weight gain, or growth faltering. Infants with cerebral palsy who had a low birth weight are at greater nutritional risk.

Family History

The height of the biologic parents should be recorded to estimate the patient's genetic potential for linear growth.

Social History

The social situation, including the child's school and therapy schedule; the family situation, including the presence of siblings and the parents' work schedule; and medical insurance and available home care must be considered. The amount of care required by a child with neurologic impairment has a great effect on the family's social life and financial situation, the parents' work, and the patient's siblings. Nutritional intervention should be well planned and integrated into the family's routine and environment as efficiently as possible.

Growth Assessment

Weight and length or height must be obtained at every visit and should be as accurate as possible, always using the same technique and equipment. Weight should be measured on the same scale every time with the child wearing little or no clothing. Length should be obtained in the supine position for children younger than 2 years or for older children who are unable to stand. Standing height is obtained when possible. Head circumference must also be measured for children younger than 3 years but may be of limited use in children with brain damage.

Reliable length measurements may be difficult to obtain in children with severe contractures or scoliosis. For these patients, alternative techniques, such as knee height,[51] upper arm length (UAL), or lower leg length (LLL) may be used to assess body length.[52] The right side is measured unless the patient is hemiplegic, in which case the less-affected side is used. In children younger than 2 years, the UAL represents the distance between the top of the shoulder and the bottom of the elbow with joints at a right angle, and the LLL is the distance between the top of the knee to the sole of the heel, again with both joints at a right angle. In children older than 2 years, the UAL is obtained using an anthropometer to measure the distance between the acromion and the head of the radius, and the LLL is obtained using a tape to measure the distance between the superomedial border of the tibia and the inferior border of the medial malleolus with the child sitting, one leg crossed horizontally across the other. UAL is usually less compromised than LLL in patients with cerebral palsy.[9] References standards are available for children older than 2 years.[52]

Mid-arm circumference and triceps skinfold thickness are useful to estimate upper-arm muscle and fat area. Measurements should be obtained by the same observer every time to improve reliability. Subscapular skinfold measurement may also be obtained but may be less affected than triceps skinfold in malnourished patients with neurologic impairment (85% vs 60% of typical controls).[7] This pattern of retention of truncal fat is often seen in malnutrition. Triceps skinfold thickness is an excellent indicator of nutrition and is more sensitive than weight-for-height z-score to identify malnourished patients. A triceps skinfold value less than the 10th percentile identified 96% of malnourished children; weight-for-height z-score less than the 10th percentile failed to identify 45% of children with depleted fat stores.[53] Normal values for mid-arm circumference and triceps skinfold thickness are available in Appendix W.

Physical Examination

Physical examination will reveal signs of malnutrition or specific nutrient deficiencies. The skin examination may reveal pallor, edema, petechiae, decubitus ulcers, or rashes. Cheilitis, smooth tongue, or gingival bleeding can be seen. The chest should be examined to detect abnormal breath sounds suggesting lung disease attributable to chronic aspiration, and abdominal examination may reveal signs of constipation. Assessment of muscle tone and activity level will help determine energy needs. Skeletal deformities, such as scoliosis and contractures, should be noted, because they may interfere with adequate positioning during meals or with the installation of a percutaneous gastrostomy tube.

Meal Observation

Observation of a meal, preferably in the home environment, provides important information with regard to positioning, food intake and spillage, aspiration, and parent-child interaction during meals. Poor positioning is often observed even when an adequately adapted seat has been provided.[21] Mealtime can be a stressful time for the caregiver, and the parent-child interaction during the meal may be poor.[21] Monitoring of oxygen saturation during the meal may help detect hypoxemia.

Laboratory Evaluation

In general, laboratory evaluation adds very little to the clinical evaluation of nutritional status. Selected blood tests may be useful to assess specific conditions when clinically suspected. Serum albumin and prealbumin concentrations reflect nutritional adequacy in the previous month and week, respectively. However, in a study involving patients with cerebral palsy, albumin and prealbumin concentrations were rarely below normal and showed little correlation with nutritional status.[54] Therefore, normal values may lead to a false sense of security when assessing these children.

A complete blood cell count and iron studies will detect iron-deficiency anemia that may occur with inadequate iron intake or chronic blood loss from reflux esophagitis. Serum electrolyte and blood urea nitrogen (BUN) concentrations may help assess hydration status, but BUN concentration may not be reliable because of significantly decreased muscle mass. Vitamin D and serum calcium, phosphorus, and alkaline phosphatase concentrations should be verified, especially in patients taking anticonvulsants. Parathyroid hormone concentration may be determined and bone densitometry may be performed if necessary.

Specific Investigation

Additional specific investigation is often warranted, according to the medical history, the physical findings, and the intervention plan.

Videofluoroscopy evaluates the efficiency of the swallowing process using liquids and different food textures. It provides a better assessment of the risk of aspiration, especially in patients who aspirate without the typical history of coughing and choking. The study should be performed in a setting that mimics the conditions in which the child is fed at home, because positioning and length of the meal affect the risk of aspiration. The results of the videofluoroscopy may help in adapting the patient's diet to decrease the risk of aspiration.

An upper gastrointestinal tract series is useful to detect anatomic abnormalities, such as peptic stricture, hiatal hernia, malrotation, or superior mesenteric artery syndrome, but should not be used for diagnosing GER. In a patient with severe scoliosis, the stomach is often abnormally located in the thorax, and an upper gastrointestinal tract series should be obtained before a percutaneous gastrostomy tube is placed to determine the position of the stomach.

Although GER can be diagnosed clinically in most instances, a 24-hour esophageal pH monitoring may help uncover subclinical reflux in patients with food refusal or chronic respiratory symptoms. It is especially important if a gastrostomy tube is considered to evaluate the need for an antireflux procedure. Gastric emptying scans can help determine the presence of delayed gastric emptying and possible aspiration from reflux.

Nutritional Intervention

After careful evaluation of nutritional status, feeding abilities, medical condition, and social situation, an intervention plan taking into account the patient's unique needs is determined by a multidisciplinary team. The team initiates nutritional therapy and should also provide continuous support and periodic reevaluation of the patient's condition and nutritional status.

Early intervention is important, because the best response to nutritional repletion is seen in children with the shortest duration between the neurologic insult and institution of nutritional therapy. When enteral nutrition was initiated within a year of the insult, weight, length, and weight-for-length improved. Between 1 and 8 years after the insult, nutritional therapy improved both linear growth and weight-for-length but led to a lesser weight gain. After 8 years, nutritional intervention led to minimal weight gain and did not improve linear growth.[4] Children with neurologic impairments who had a gastrostomy tube placed in the first year of life were more likely to exceed the fifth percentile for weight and height.[10]

Nutritional Requirements

Energy needs are difficult to determine in this heterogeneous population. Dietary Reference Intakes (DRIs) for age are based on healthy individuals and overestimate the needs of children with neurologic impairments. Caloric needs should be individualized according to the patient's condition. Because measuring REE in each individual is impossible in most clinical settings, alternative methods to determine energy needs were developed.

Height has been used to estimate caloric needs. Children without motor dysfunction required 14.7 kcal/cm, ambulatory patients with motor dysfunction required 13.9 kcal/cm, and nonambulatory patients with motor dysfunction needed 11.1 kcal/cm.[55]

The following formula using basal metabolic rate (BMR) and taking into consideration muscle tone, activity level, and growth factors has been developed to calculate energy needs in children with severe cerebral palsy[56]:

$$\text{Calories (kcal/day)} = (\text{BMR} \times \text{muscle tone factor} \times \text{activity factor}) + \text{growth factor}$$

Where:

- BMR (kcal/day) = body surface area (m^2) × standard metabolic rate (kcal/m^2/hour) × 24 hours;

- muscle tone factor: 0.9 if decreased, 1.0 if normal, 1.1 if increased;

- activity factor: 1.15 if bedridden, 1.2 if dependant, 1.25 if crawling, 1.3 if ambulatory; and

- growth factor: 5 kcal/g of desired weight gain.

Formulas based on weight, height, and age to determine REE in healthy individuals are not adequate to estimate the energy needs of children with neurologic impairments.[34,57-59] If REE can be measured, the caloric requirements of children with spastic quadriplegic cerebral palsy are usually 1.1 × measured REE.[34]

However, the best way to evaluate the adequacy of nutritional therapy is to monitor the response in terms of weight gain. Caloric intake should be readjusted accordingly. This is particularly important after initiation of tube feedings, because excessive weight gain may occur.[10]

Goal of Nutritional Intervention

Forcing the weight-for-height z-score to or above 0 in children with quadriplegic cerebral palsy may lead to excessive body fat accumulation.[24] Ideally, body weight for children whose activity level is typical should be on the 50th percentile on the weight-for-height chart. For patients who are wheelchair bound but able to accomplish independent transfers, weight-for-height z-score should approximately that of the 25th percentile, and for patients who are bedridden, the 10th percentile is sufficient for adequate nutrition but low enough to facilitate the care and mobilization of the child. An exception should be made for patients younger than 3 years (chronologic or height age), for which weight-for-height z-score should be between the 25th and the 50th percentile independent of activity level.[56]

Source of Nutrients

The choice of formula depends on the age of the patient, the presence of any specific nutrient deficiencies or medical problems, and caloric requirements. Before 1 year of age, infant formula is preferred. The formula may be concentrated (see Table 36.1) to increase calories in patients with high caloric needs and to reduce the volume in those with feeding intolerance (see also Chapter 23: Enteral Nutrition).

Table 36.1
Concentration of Formula

kcal/oz	Liquid Concentrate Formula	Water
24	13 oz	8 oz
28	13 oz	5.5 oz
30	13 oz	4 oz

Nutrient modules, such as carbohydrates or lipids, may be used to increase caloric density or to change the composition of the diet (see Table 36.2). Carbohydrates may be added in the form of glucose polymers. Lipids can be supplied as long- or medium-chain triglycerides; they are calorically dense and have little influence on osmolality but may aggravate delayed gastric emptying. Medium-chain triglyceride oil is absorbed without the need for chylomicron formation but does not contain essential fatty acids.

Table 36.2
Modular Nutrients

Product	Description	Caloric Content
Carbohydrate		
Polycose powder (Abbott Nutrition, Columbus, OH)	Glucose polymer	23 kcal/tbsp
Moducal (Nestlé, Glendale, CA)	Maltodextrin	30 kcal/tbsp
Fat		
Microlipid (Nestlé, Glendale, CA)	Safflower oil emulsion	4.5 kcal/mL
MCT oil	Coconut oil	7.7 kcal/mL

Precautions should be taken to avoid preparation errors. By concentrating the formula, the renal solute load (RSL) increases and the amount of free water decreases. RSL should not exceed 250 mOsm/L and can be estimated as follows:

$$RSL \ (mOsm) = (protein \ [g] \times 4) + (Na \ [mEq] + K \ [mEq] + Cl \ [mEq])$$

When nutrient modules are used to modify the caloric content, the final composition of the diet must be determined to ensure that the final diet provides 35% to 65% of the calories as carbohydrates, 7% to 16% as protein, and 30% to 55% as fat. Ketosis may develop if more than 55% of calories are fat, excess carbohydrate may overwhelm absorption capacity and cause diarrhea, and protein intakes exceeding 5 g/kg per day may cause azotemia.

After 1 year of age, a pediatric 1-kcal/mL formula is generally used. Adult formulas should be avoided in the pediatric population with neurologic impairments. The calorie-to-nutrient ratio in an adult solution may be inadequate in children with low calorie needs and may lead to micronutrient deficiencies. Pediatric solutions have a higher vitamin and mineral content and should be used to avoid vitamin D, phosphorus, calcium, and iron deficiencies.[33] The use of high-energy formulas (1.5 or 2 kcal/mL) requires careful monitoring of hydration status and micronutrient intake. A fiber-containing formula may improve constipation. In children with neurologic impairments who have GER, the use of whey-based formula compared with casein-based formula is associated with better tolerance and faster gastric emptying.[60,61] Amino-acid based formulas may be useful in patients with refractory esophagitis.[62]

Fluid intake must be carefully monitored in patients with neurologic impairments. Because their caloric needs are low, they are often given a relatively small volume of formula that may not provide an adequate amount of fluid. In addition, formula may be concentrated to avoid emesis in patients who do not tolerate large volumes, further decreasing free water intake. Daily free water intake should be sufficient to ensure adequate urine output and to avoid constipation.

Route of Enteral Feedings
In patients with adequate oral motor skill and low risk of aspiration, oral intake may be maintained. It is often necessary to increase the caloric density of the food and to add oral supplements to provide sufficient caloric intake. Food consistency should be adjusted according to the swallowing function study. Thickening agents may be added to liquids and purees. An occupational therapist can provide adapted utensils and adequate positioning during meals. Oral feeding therapy may improve oral feeding skills but have lead to limited results in promoting feeding efficiency or weight gain.[63,64] Assistive feeding devices may provide more consistent food presentation but did not improve feeding efficiency.[65]

In view of the daily commitment and effort required to feed the child orally, everyday reality must be considered. Some caregivers spend a considerable amount of time feeding the child with disappointing results in terms of weight gain. In patients who require an excessive amount of time to ingest sufficient calories and/or who are unable to maintain adequate weight gain, oral intake may be supplemented with tube feedings. The decision to initiate tube feedings is often difficult for parents. Tube feedings may be perceived by them as a failure, and they may feel guilty about not being able to feed their child.[50] Parents are often reluctant to agree to tube feedings, because they think that their child will lose the ability to eat by mouth.[66] Therefore, unless there is a medical contraindication to feed the child orally, parents should be involved in the decision-making process. The decision to initiate tube feedings should be made with the parents with the goal of improving their quality of life as well as the child's. In children with severe neurologic impairment, most parents (90%) considered that tube feedings, despite frequent minor complications, improved their quality of life.[67] Enteral nutrition often improves the patients' nutritional status dramatically.[2,4,10] Tube-fed children with cerebral palsy have significantly higher weight-for-height z-scores than do orally fed children with cerebral palsy.[24]

The decision to initiate tube feedings does not preclude maintaining oral intake. Without the stress of having to provide sufficient calories orally, eating may become an enjoyable activity. However, patients with significant oral-motor dysfunction and high risk of aspiration should be tube fed exclusively.

Nasogastric Feedings

Nasogastric feedings are minimally invasive. They may be attempted initially in some patients but should not be used for long-term nutrition support. The nasogastric tube is unaesthetic and uncomfortable and is easily dislodged. A short trial of nasogastric feedings is often helpful to determine the patient's tolerance to gastric feedings or to improve nutritional status before a more permanent solution is determined.

Nasojejunal Feedings

Nasojejunal feedings are preferred in patients with significant gastroesophageal reflux who do not tolerate nasogastric feedings. Nasojejunal tubes can be inserted in the stomach and allowed to migrate into the small intestine with or without the help of prokinetics.[68,69] Other techniques include pH probe-assisted placement[70,71] and fluoroscopic or endoscopic placement. Nasojejunal feedings should not be used on a long-term basis.

Gastrostomy

If long-term enteral nutrition is required (>3 months), a gastrostomy tube is preferred. Evidence-based literature examining risk versus benefits associated with gastrostomy tube feedings is lacking.[72–74] However, it seems that the use of a gastrostomy tube relieves the stress associated with feedings,[18,50] promotes weight gain,[75] and improves quality of life for the caregivers.[76]

The gastrostomy tube can be placed surgically or percutaneously using radiologic or endoscopic techniques. The choice between a surgical and a percutaneous gastrostomy tube will depend on the presence or absence of GER requiring antireflux procedures and on the existence of contraindication(s) to percutaneous placement.

Placement of the percutaneous endoscopic gastrostomy (PEG) tube is a simple technique that requires short anesthesia or conscious sedation and involves minimal postoperative discomfort, and the tube can be used within 6 hours of placement. In some patients with severe scoliosis, the stomach may not be accessible percutaneously, which precludes placement of a PEG tube. Other contraindications to PEG tube placement include the presence of ascites, hepatomegaly or splenomegaly, portal hypertension, and in some cases, previous abdominal surgery. Bowel perforation, pneumoperitoneum, peritonitis, gastrocolic fistulas, bleeding, exacerbation of GER, and local infections may occur with PEG tube placement. The rate of major complications (requiring surgery) after PEG tube placement is 2% to 17.5% in the pediatric population.[77–79] Minor complications (infection, granulation tissue formation, leakage from the stoma, or tube dysfunction) occur in 4% to 22%.[78,79] Gastroesophageal reflux occurred after PEG tube placement in 25% to 27% of patients without previous clinical symptoms of GER, and 17% of patients required an antireflux procedure (ARP).[80,81] Among those with pre-existing GER, 18.5% subsequently required an ARP or a gastrojejunal tube.[81] Preoperative esophageal pH monitoring for evaluation of GER should be considered, because 5% patients with neurologic impairment with a normal pH probe study result before PEG tube placement eventually required an ARP, compared with 29% if the pH probe study result was abnormal.[77] In patients with mild to moderate GER, a PEG tube is a good option. If GER develops after the procedure, medical treatment should be attempted before considering an ARP.

In patients with severe GER, placement of a surgical gastrostomy tube with an ARP should be considered. The patient must be evaluated carefully, because ARP failures, postoperative complications, and need for reintervention are more common in patients with neurologic impairments than in those without impairments. In the population with neurologic impairments, the failure rate of ARPs is between 19% and 28%, and the incidence of major complications is between 10% and 33%.[82–84] Surgical complications of ARPs include prolonged ileus, intussusception, bleeding, bowel perforation, wound infection or dehiscence, wrap herniation, tight wrap, and pneumonia. Furthermore, the Nissen procedure may induce myoelectrical disturbances and inappropriate activation of the emetic reflex, inducing postoperative retching.[85] Patients with neurologic impairments are particularly at risk of developing dumping and gas bloat syndrome after an ARP. A careful evaluation of gastric emptying is necessary to identify patients who require a pyloroplasty in conjunction with an ARP. There is no role for a prophylactic ARP in patients with no previous GER.

Surgical gastrostomy tube placement alone should be reserved for patients with contraindications to PEG tube placement or in patients whose stomach cannot be accessed percutaneously. Postgastrostomy GER occurs more frequently with surgical gastrostomy tubes than with PEG tubes. Sixty-six percent of patients with normal pH probe study results before surgical gastrostomy tube placement had a positive study result after the procedure.[86] In patients with neurologic impairment without GER undergoing a surgical gastrostomy tube placement, between 14% and 44% developed GER and 14% to 33% subsequently required an ARP.[87,88]

Gastrojejunostomy

Percutaneously placed gastrojejunal feeding tubes may be a reasonable alternative to a gastrostomy tube and an ARP for some patients.[89–91] They can be used for patients with GER who are not good candidates for prolonged anesthesia or patients with recurrence of GER after an ARP. The gastrojejunal tube does not treat GER, and the patient will continue to require medication. A percutaneous gastrojejunal tube carries less risk of major complications in patients with neurologic impairment than does a Nissen procedure with a surgical gastrostomy tube placement (11.8% vs 33.3%) but a higher risk of minor complications (44.1% vs 6.6%). Most of the minor complications associated with the gastrojejunal tube relate to tube malfunction.[91]

Method of Administration

The preferred mode of administration is bolus feeding. Bolus feedings physiologically mimic meals and are more convenient in ambulatory patients. Initially, continuous infusions at night may be required in combination with daytime boluses for patients with poor nutritional status and high caloric needs. Subsequent change to daytime boluses may be attempted if tolerated. Some patients with reflux or delayed gastric emptying may not tolerate boluses and may require long-term continuous feeds. When the child requires transpyloric feeds, a continuous infusion is necessary.

Approach to Feeding Intolerance

Vomiting and feeding intolerance occurs commonly after tube feedings are initiated. Although the nasogastric or gastrostomy tube is frequently blamed, feeding intolerance may be the results of the major changes in the diet occurring with the initiation of tube feedings in terms of texture (mostly purees to liquid) and in terms of volume. A conservative approach should be favored. In the absence of intercurrent infections and anatomic problems, the feeding regimen should be reevaluated. Changing the feeding schedule from boluses to continuous feeds, decreasing the rate of infusion, or concentrating the formula to decrease the volume may improve tolerance. Medical treatment of GER with acid-suppressing therapy and/or prokinetics should be considered. If feeding intolerance persists, an ARP may be needed.

Ethical Considerations

With advances in medicine, children with developmental disabilities are surviving longer and are often cared for at home by their parents. There is increasing awareness that improving nutritional status improves their health and quality of life. Nutritional intervention should be carefully planned and discussed with the family. The decision to initiate tube feedings and, most of all, to have a gastrostomy tube installed is often difficult. Medical and parental opinions may be different, and parental concerns should not be overlooked. Parents may think of tube feedings as a failure on their part to adequately feed their child and to care for their child altogether. They may see this as burden or as additional evidence of their child's disease.[92] Nutritional intervention is more than improving nutritional status; it should be viewed as a tool to improve the patient's and the parents' quality of life.

Conclusion

Children with neurologic disabilities cannot be nutritionally evaluated against conventional standards because of growth retardation, abnormal energy requirements, and abnormal body composition, but they should not be expected to be malnourished. One of the most basic components of care is provision of adequate nutrition. Therefore, medical management of these patients must include careful monitoring of their nutritional status, and early, multidisciplinary nutritional intervention is essential to promote growth and well-being. It is extremely important to provide continuous support to the families of children with developmental disabilities and feeding problems to ensure the success of nutritional therapy.

References

1. Samson-Fang LJ, Fung E, Stallings VA, et al. Relationship of nutritional status to health and societal participation in children with cerebral palsy. *J Pediatr.* 2002;141:637–643
2. Patrick J, Boland M, Stoski D, Murray GE. Rapid correction of wasting in children with cerebral palsy. *Dev Med Child Neurol.* 1986;28:734–739
3. Shapiro BK, Green P, Krick J, Allen D, Capute AJ. Growth of severely impaired children: neurological versus nutritional factors. *Dev Med Child Neurol.* 1986;28:729–733

V

4. Sanders KD, Cox K, Cannon R, et al. Growth response to enteral feeding by children with cerebral palsy. *JPEN J Parenter Enteral Nutr.* 1990;14:23–26

5. Lewis D, Khoshoo V, Pencharz PB, Golladay ES. Impact of nutritional rehabilitation on gastroesophageal reflux in neurologically impaired children. *J Pediatr Surg.* 1994;29:167–169

6. Wodarski LA. An interdisciplinary nutrition assessment and intervention protocol for children with disabilities. *J Am Diet Assoc.* 1990;90:1563–1568

7. Stallings VA, Charney EB, Davies JC, Cronk CE. Nutrition-related growth failure of children with quadriplegic cerebral palsy. *Dev Med Child Neurol.* 1993;35:126–138

8. Stallings VA, Charney EB, Davies JC, Cronk CE. Nutritional status and growth of children with diplegic or hemiplegic cerebral palsy. *Dev Med Child Neurol.* 1993;35:997–1006

9. Stallings VA, Cronk CE, Zemel BS, Charney EB. Body composition in children with spastic quadriplegic cerebral palsy. *J Pediatr.* 1995;126:833–839

10. Rempel GR, Colwell SO, Nelson RP. Growth in children with cerebral palsy fed via gastrostomy. *Pediatrics.* 1988;82:857–862

11. Stevenson RD, Hayes RP, Cater LV, Blackman JA. Clinical correlates of linear growth in children with cerebral palsy. *Dev Med Child Neurol.* 1994;36:135–142

12. Krick J, Murphy-Miller P, Zeger S, Wright E. Pattern of growth in children with cerebral palsy. *J Am Diet Assoc.* 1996;96:680–685

13. Krick J, Van Duyn MA. The relationship between oral-motor involvement and growth: a pilot study in a pediatric population with cerebral palsy. *J Am Diet Assoc.* 1984;84:555–559

14. Thommessen M, Riis G, Kase BF, Larsen S, Heiberg A. Energy and nutrient intakes of disabled children: do feeding problems make a difference? *J Am Diet Assoc.* 1991;91:1522–1525

15. Thommessen M, Heiberg A, Kase BF, Larsen S, Riis G. Feeding problems, height and weight in different groups of disabled children. *Acta Paediatr Scand.* 1991;80:527–533

16. Motion S, Northstone K, Emond A, Stucke S, Golding J. Early feeding problems in children with cerebral palsy: weight and neurodevelopmental outcomes. *Dev Med Child Neurol.* 2002;44:40–43

17. Troughton KE, Hill AE. Relation between objectively measured feeding competence and nutrition in children with cerebral palsy. *Dev Med Child Neurol.* 2001;43:187–190

18. Sullivan PB, Lambert B, Rose M, Ford-Adams M, Johnson A, Griffiths P. Prevalence and severity of feeding and nutritional problems in children with neurological impairment: Oxford Feeding Study. *Dev Med Child Neurol.* 2000;42:674–680

19. Sullivan PB, Juszczak E, Lambert BR, Rose M, Ford-Adams ME, Johnson A. Impact of feeding problems on nutritional intake and growth: Oxford Feeding Study II. *Dev Med Child Neurol.* 2002;44:461–467

20. Fung EB, Samson-Fang L, Stallings VA, et al. Feeding dysfunction is associated with poor growth and health status in children with cerebral palsy. *J Am Diet Assoc.* 2002;102:361–373

21. Reilly S, Skuse D. Characteristics and management of feeding problems of young children with cerebral palsy. *Dev Med Child Neurol.* 1992;34:379–388

22. Stallings VA, Zemel BS, Davies JC, Cronk CE, Charney EB. Energy expenditure of children and adolescents with severe disabilities: a cerebral palsy model. *Am J Clin Nutr.* 1996;64:627–634

23. Stevenson RD, Roberts CD, Vogtle L. The effect of non-nutritional factors on growth in cerebral palsy. *Dev Med Child Neurol*. 1995;37:124–130

24. Kong CK, Wong HS. Weight-for-height values and limb anthropometric composition of tube-fed children with quadriplegic cerebral palsy. *Pediatrics*. 2005;116(6):e839–e845. Available at: http://pediatrics.aappublications.org/cgi/content/full/116/6/e839. Accessed September 27, 2007

25. Reilly S, Skuse D, Poblete X. Prevalence of feeding problems and oral motor dysfunction in children with cerebral palsy: a community survey. *J Pediatr*. 1996;129:877–882

26. Dahl M, Thommessen M, Rasmussen M, Selberg T. Feeding and nutritional characteristics in children with moderate or severe cerebral palsy. *Acta Paediatr*. 1996;85:697–701

27. Gisel EG, Patrick J. Identification of children with cerebral palsy unable to maintain a normal nutritional state. *Lancet*. 1988;1:283–286

28. Johnson CB, Deitz JC. Time use of mothers with preschool children: a pilot study. *Am J Occup Ther*. 1985;39:578–583

29. Rogers BT, Arvedson J, Msall M, Demerath RR. Hypoxemia during oral feeding of children with severe cerebral palsy. *Dev Med Child Neurol*. 1993;35:3–10

30. Sondheimer JM, Morris BA. Gastroesophageal reflux among severely retarded children. *J Pediatr*. 1979;94:710–714

31. Ravelli AM, Milla PJ. Vomiting and gastroesophageal motor activity in children with disorders of the central nervous system. *J Pediatr Gastroenterol Nutr*. 1998;26:56–63

32. Zangen T, Ciarla C, Zangen S, et al. Gastrointestinal motility and sensory abnormalities may contribute to food refusal in medically fragile toddlers. *J Pediatr Gastroenterol Nutr*. 2003;37:287–293

33. Fried MD, Pencharz PB. Energy and nutrient intakes of children with spastic quadriplegia. *J Pediatr*. 1991;119:947–949

34. Azcue MP, Zello GA, Levy LD, Pencharz PB. Energy expenditure and body composition in children with spastic quadriplegic cerebral palsy. *J Pediatr*. 1996;129:870–876

35. Bandini LG, Schoeller DA, Fukagawa NK, Wykes LJ, Dietz WH. Body composition and energy expenditure in adolescents with cerebral palsy or myelodysplasia. *Pediatr Res*. 1991;29:70–77

36. Rose J, Gamble JG, Burgos A, Medeiros J, Haskell WL. Energy expenditure index of walking for normal children and for children with cerebral palsy. *Dev Med Child Neurol*. 1990;32:333–340

37. Rose J, Medeiros JM, Parker R. Energy cost index as an estimate of energy expenditure of cerebral-palsied children during assisted ambulation. *Dev Med Child Neurol*. 1985;27:485–490

38. Brunner R, Doderlein L. Pathological fractures in patients with cerebral palsy. *J Pediatr Orthop B*. 1996;5:232–238

39. Henderson RC, Lark RK, Gurka MJ, et al. Bone density and metabolism in children and adolescents with moderate to severe cerebral palsy. *Pediatrics*. 2002;110(1):e5. Available at: http://pediatrics.aappublications.org/cgi/content/full/110/1/e5. Accessed September 27, 2007

40. Duncan B, Barton LL, Lloyd J, Marks–Katz M. Dietary considerations in osteopenia in tube-fed nonambulatory children with cerebral palsy. *Clin Pediatr (Phila)*. 1999;38:133–137

41. Henderson RC, Lin PP, Greene WB. Bone-mineral density in children and adolescents who have spastic cerebral palsy. *J Bone Joint Surg Am.* 1995;77:1671–1681

42. Morijiri Y, Sato T. Factors causing rickets in institutionalised handicapped children on anticonvulsant therapy. *Arch Dis Child.* 1981;56:446–449

43. Tolman KG, Jubiz W, Sannella JJ, et al. Osteomalacia associated with anticonvulsant drug therapy in mentally retarded children. *Pediatrics.* 1975;56:45–50

44. Bischof F, Basu D, Pettifor JM. Pathological long-bone fractures in residents with cerebral palsy in a long-term care facility in South Africa. *Dev Med Child Neurol.* 2002;44:119–122

45. Henderson RC, Kairalla J, Abbas A, Stevenson RD. Predicting low bone density in children and young adults with quadriplegic cerebral palsy. *Dev Med Child Neurol.* 2004;46:416–419

46. Baer MT, Kozlowski BW, Blyler EM, Trahms CM, Taylor ML, Hogan MP. Vitamin D, calcium, and bone status in children with developmental delay in relation to anticonvulsant use and ambulatory status. *Am J Clin Nutr.* 1997;65:1042–1051

47. Chad KE, McKay HA, Zello GA, Bailey DA, Faulkner RA, Snyder RE. Body composition in nutritionally adequate ambulatory and non-ambulatory children with cerebral palsy and a healthy reference group. *Dev Med Child Neurol.* 2000;42:334–339

48. Hartman C, Brik R, Tamir A, Merrick J, Shamir R. Bone quantitative ultrasound and nutritional status in severely handicapped institutionalized children and adolescents. *Clin Nutr.* 2004;23:89–98

49. Henderson RC, Lark RK, Kecskemethy HH, Miller F, Harcke HT, Bachrach SJ. Biphosphonates to treat osteopenia in children with quadriplegic cerebral palsy: a randomized, placebo-controlled clinical trial. *J Pediatr.* 2002;141:644–651

50. Sleigh G. Mothers' voice: a qualitative study on feeding children with cerebral palsy. *Child Care Health Dev.* 2005;31:373–383

51. Hogan SE. Knee height as a predictor of recumbent length for individuals with mobility-impaired cerebral palsy. *J Am Coll Nutr.* 2005;18:201–205

52. Spender QW, Cronk CE, Charney EB, Stallings VA. Assessment of linear growth of children with cerebral palsy: use of alternative measures to height or length. *Dev Med Child Neurol.* 1989;31:206–214

53. Samson-Fang LJ, Stevenson RD. Identification of malnutrition in children with cerebral palsy: poor performance of weight for height centiles. *Dev Med Child Neurol.* 2000;42:162–168

54. Lark RK, Williams CL, Stadler D, et al. Serum prealbumin and albumin concentrations do not reflect nutritional state in children with cerebral palsy. *J Pediatr.* 2005;147:695–697

55. Culley WJ, Middleton TO. Caloric requirements of mentally retarded children with and without motor dysfunction. *J Pediatr.* 1969;75:380–384

56. Krick J, Murphy PE, Markham JF, Shapiro BK. A proposed formula for calculating energy needs of children with cerebral palsy. *Dev Med Child Neurol.* 1992;34:481–487

57. Dickerson RN, Brown RO, Gervasio JG, Hak EB, Hak LJ, Williams JE. Measured energy expenditure of tube-fed patients with severe neurodevelopmental disabilities. *J Am Coll Nutr.* 1999;18:61–68

58. Dickerson RN, Brown RO, Hanna DL, Williams JE. Validation of a new method for estimating resting energy expenditure of non-ambulatory tube-fed patients with severe neurodevelopmental disabilities. *Nutrition.* 2002;18:578–582

59. Bandini LG, Puelzl-Quinn H, Morelli JA, Fukagawa NK. Estimation of energy requirements in persons with severe central nervous system impairment. *J Pediatr.* 1995;126:828–832

60. Fried MD, Khoshoo V, Secker DJ, Gilday DL, Ash JM, Pencharz PB. Decrease in gastric emptying time and episodes of regurgitation in children with spastic quadriplegia fed a whey-based formula. *J Pediatr.* 1992;120:569–572

61. Khoshoo V, Zembo M, King A, Dhar M, Reifen R, Pencharz P. Incidence of gastroesophageal reflux with whey- and casein-based formulas in infants and children with severe neurological impairment. *J Pediatr Gastroenterol Nutr.* 1996;22:48–55

62. Miele E, Staiano A, Tozzi A, Auricchio R, Paparo F, Troncone R. Clinical response to amino acid-based formula in neurologically impaired children with refractory esophagitis. *J Pediatr Gastroenterol Nutr.* 2002;35:314–319

63. Gisel EG, Applegate-Ferrante T, Benson JE, Bosma JF. Effect of oral sensorimotor treatment on measures of growth, eating efficiency and aspiration in the dysphagic child with cerebral palsy. *Dev Med Child Neurol.* 1995;37:528–543

64. Gisel EG. Effect of oral sensorimotor treatment on measures of growth and efficiency of eating in the moderately eating-impaired child with cerebral palsy. *Dysphagia.* 1996;11:48–58

65. Pinnington L, Hegarty J. Effects of consistent food presentation on efficiency of eating and nutritive value of food consumed by children with severe neurological impairment. *Dysphagia.* 1999;14:17–26

66. Corwin DS, Isaacs JS, Georgeson KE, Bartolucci AA, Cloud HH, Craig CB. Weight and length increases in children after gastrostomy placement. *J Am Diet Assoc.* 1996;96:874–879

67. Smith SW, Camfield C, Camfield P. Living with cerebral palsy and tube feeding: a population-based follow-up study. *J Pediatr.* 1999;135:307–310

68. Taylor B, Schallom L. Bedside small bowel feeding tube placement in critically ill patients utilizing a dietician/nurse approach. *Nutr Clin Pract.* 2001;16:258–262

69. Kalliafas S, Choban PS, Ziegler D, Drago S, Flancbaum L. Erythromycin facilitates postpyloric placement of nasoduodenal feeding tubes in intensive care unit patients: randomized, double-blinded, placebo-controlled trial. *JPEN J Parenter Enteral Nutr.* 1996;20:385–388

70. Dimand RJ, Veereman-Waters G, Braner DA. Bedside placement of pH-guided transpyloric small bowel feeding tubes in critically ill infants and small children. *JPEN J Parenter Enteral Nutr.* 1997;21:112–114

71. Krafte-Jacobs B, Persinger M, Carver J, Moore L, Brilli R. Rapid placement of transpyloric feeding tubes: a comparison of pH-assisted and standard insertion techniques in children. *Pediatrics.* 1996;98:242–248

72. Sleigh G, Brocklehurst P. Gastrostomy feeding in cerebral palsy: a systematic review. *Arch Dis Child.* 2004;89:534–539

73. Samson-Fang L, Butler C, O'Donnell M. Effects of gastrostomy feeding in children with cerebral palsy: an AACPDM evidence report. *Dev Med Child Neurol.* 2003;45:415–426

74. Sleigh G, Sullivan PB, Thomas AG. Gastrostomy feeding versus oral feeding alone for children with cerebral palsy. *Cochrane Database Syst Rev.* 2004;(2):CD003943

75. Sullivan PB, Juszczak E, Bachlet AM, et al. Gastrostomy tube feeding in children with cerebral palsy: a prospective, longitudinal study. *Dev Med Child Neurol.* 2005;47:77–85

76. Sullivan PB, Juszczak E, Bachlet AM, et al. Impact of gastrostomy tube feeding on the quality of life of carers of children with cerebral palsy. *Dev Med Child Neurol.* 2004;46:796–800

77. Sulaeman E, Udall JN Jr, Brown RF, et al. Gastroesophageal reflux and Nissen fundoplication following percutaneous endoscopic gastrostomy in children. *J Pediatr Gastroenterol Nutr.* 1998;26:269–273

78. Khattak IU, Kimber C, Kiely EM, Spitz L. Percutaneous endoscopic gastrostomy in paediatric practice: complications and outcome. *J Pediatr Surg.* 1998;33:67–72

79. Behrens R, Lang T, Muschweck H, Richter T, Hofbeck M. Percutaneous endoscopic gastrostomy in children and adolescents. *J Pediatr Gastroenterol Nutr.* 1997;25:487–491

80. Heine RG, Reddihough DS, Catto-Smith AG. Gastro-oesophageal reflux and feeding problems after gastrostomy in children with severe neurological impairment. *Dev Med Child Neurol.* 1995;37:320–329

81. Isch JA, Rescorla FJ, Scherer LR III, West KW, Grosfeld JL. The development of gastroesophageal reflux after percutaneous endoscopic gastrostomy. *J Pediatr Surg.* 1997; 32:321–322

82. Pearl RH, Robie DK, Ein SH, et al. Complications of gastroesophageal antireflux surgery in neurologically impaired versus neurologically normal children. *J Pediatr Surg.* 1990; 25:1169–1173

83. Smith CD, Othersen HB Jr, Gogan NJ, Walker JD. Nissen fundoplication in children with profound neurologic disability. High risks and unmet goals. *Ann Surg.* 1992;215:654–658

84. Spitz L, Roth K, Kiely EM, Brereton RJ, Drake DP, Milla PJ. Operation for gastrooesophageal reflux associated with severe mental retardation. *Arch Dis Child.* 1993;68:347–351

85. Richards CA, Andrews PL, Spitz L, Milla PJ. Nissen fundoplication may induce gastric myoelectrical disturbance in children. *J Pediatr Surg.* 1998;33:1801–1805

86. Jolley SG, Smith EI, Tunell WP. Protective antireflux operation with feeding gastrostomy. Experience with children. *Ann Surg.* 1985;201:736–740

87. Langer JC, Wesson DE, Ein SH, et al. Feeding gastrostomy in neurologically impaired children: is an antireflux procedure necessary? *J Pediatr Gastroenterol Nutr.* 1988;7:837–841

88. Wheatley MJ, Wesley JR, Tkach DM, Coran AG. Long-term follow-up of brain-damaged children requiring feeding gastrostomy: should an antireflux procedure always be performed? *J Pediatr Surg.* 1991;26:301–304

89. Wales PW, Diamond IR, Dutta S, et al. Fundoplication and gastrostomy versus image-guided gastrojejunal tube for enteral feedings in neurologically impaired children with gastroesophageal reflux. *J Pediatr Surg.* 2002;37:407–412

90. Peters JM, Simpson P, Tolia V. Experience with gastrojejunal feeding tubes in children. *Am J Gastroenterol.* 1997;92:476–480

91. Albanese CT, Towbin RB, Ulman I, Lewis J, Smith SD. Percutaneous gastrojejunostomy versus Nissen fundoplication for enteral feeding of the neurologically impaired child with gastroesophageal reflux. *J Pediatr.* 1993;123:371–375

92. Craig GM, Scambler G, Spitz L. Why parents of children with neurodevelopmental disabilities requiring gastrostomy feeding need more support. *Dev Med Child Neurol.* 2003;45:183–188

37 Nutrition of Infants and Children Who Are Critically Ill

Critical illness is often accompanied by a profound and predictable constellation of metabolic aberrations. More than 60 years ago, Cuthbertson described the fundamental aspects of this metabolic response in adults.[1] The metabolic sequelae of illness and surgery seen in neonates and children qualitatively resemble those of adults, although marked quantitative differences exist. To design optimal nutritional therapy for the critically ill child, an understanding of these metabolic changes and their effects on nutrient requirements is necessary.

Metabolic Reserves and Baseline Requirements

The most striking difference in body composition between the healthy adult and child is the quantity of protein available in times of injury. As a percentage of body weight, the protein stores of adults are twice those of neonates (Table 37.1). Lipid stores are also decreased in children as compared with adults, whereas carbohydrate reserves are constant across age groups. Neonates and children not only have reduced stores but also have much higher baseline requirements. The resting energy expenditure for neonates with low birth weight is 3 times that for adults. Protein requirements for the preterm neonate to maintain growth rates approximating those in utero are 3.5 times the requirement for protein balance in the adult.[2] Thus, critically ill children are potentially much more susceptible to the deleterious effects of protracted catabolic stress. Compounding this, most critically ill children do not receive even the recommended dietary intake of protein or energy for healthy children until after a full week in the intensive care unit.[3–5]

Table 37.1

The Body Composition of Neonates, Children, and Nonobese Adults as a Percent of Total Body Weight

Age	Percent Protein	Percent Fat	Percent Carbohydrates
Neonates	11	14	0.4
Children (10 y)	15	17	0.4
Adults	18	19	0.4

Based on the data of Forbes and Bruining,[6] Fomon et al,[7] and Munro.[8]

Protein Metabolism

Amino acids are the key building blocks required for growth and tissue repair. Most amino acids reside in proteins, and the remaining amino acids circulate in the free amino acid pool. These pools are dynamic, with continuous protein degradation and synthesis resulting in a process termed "protein turnover." This process allows reutilization of amino acids from protein breakdown and contributes more than 2 times the amino acids derived from protein intake. In critically ill children, such as those with severe burn injury or respiratory failure requiring extracorporeal membrane oxygenation (ECMO), protein turnover is doubled when compared with normal subjects.[9] Generally in critical illness, amino acids are redistributed away from skeletal muscle for repair of injured tissues, the activity of cells involved in the inflammatory response, and the synthesis of acutely needed enzymes, serum proteins, and glucose (by way of gluconeogenesis) in the liver. There is also a marked increase in the circulation of hepatically derived acute-phase proteins (eg, C-reactive protein, fibrinogen, haptoglobin, alpha$_1$-antitrypsin, and alpha$_1$-acid glycoprotein) and a concomitant decrease in hepatically derived nutrient transport proteins (eg, albumin and retinol-binding protein). A salient advantage of high protein turnover is that it allows for the immediate synthesis of proteins needed for the inflammatory response and tissue repair. The process does require energy, derived from either an increase in resting energy expenditure or a redistribution of energy normally used for growth. Although critically ill children demonstrate both an increase in whole-body protein degradation and whole-body synthesis, it is the former that predominates. Thus, these patients manifest net negative protein balance, which clinically may be noted by weight loss, negative nitrogen balance, and skeletal muscle wasting.

The catabolism of skeletal muscle for gluconeogenesis is necessary, because glucose is the preferred substrate for the brain, red blood cells, and the renal medulla and provides an energy source for repair of injured tissues. Gluconeogenesis is enhanced by illness in adults and children. On a per-kg-of-body-weight basis, gluconeogenesis seems to be particularly high in ill neonates with low birth weight (presumably because of their relatively large ratio of brain to body weight).[10] Interestingly, the provision of dietary glucose is relatively ineffective in quelling endogenous glucose production in stressed states and often results in significant hyperglycemia.[11]

Skeletal muscle catabolism to generate glucose is an excellent short-term adaptation in the ill child; however, it is limited in duration because of the reduced stores available. Without elimination of the inciting stress for catabolism, the progressive loss of diaphragmatic and intercostal muscle as well as cardiac muscle can precipitate cardiopulmonary failure. Fortunately, nutritional supplementation of amino acids improves protein balance. The mechanism for this change in ill and preterm neonates appears to be an increase in protein synthesis with relatively unaffected protein degradation rates.[12,13]

The amount of protein required to optimally enhance protein accretion is higher in sick than in healthy children. Infants demonstrate 25% higher protein degradation after surgery, 100% increase in urinary nitrogen excretion with bacterial sepsis, and 100% increase in protein breakdown if they are ill enough to require ECMO.[9] Children treated for cancer also show increased net protein breakdown.[14] The single most important nutritional intervention in ill children is the provision of dietary protein sufficient to optimize protein synthesis, facilitate wound healing and the inflammatory response, and preserve skeletal muscle protein mass. The quantity of protein (or amino acid solution) administered in critical illness should be 3 to 4 g/kg per day for infants with low birth weight, 2 to 3 g/kg per day for full-term neonates, and 1.5 g/kg per day for older children.[15] Certain severely stressed states may require additional protein supplementation with careful monitoring of growth rates in chronically ill patients. Excessive protein administration should be avoided, because toxicity is possible, particularly in patients with marginal renal function. Neonates with low birth weight fed protein allotments of 6 g/kg per day have demonstrated azotemia, pyrexia, a higher incidence of strabismus, and somewhat lower IQ.[16,17]

Two important issues regarding the protein metabolism of critically ill children remain to be elucidated. At present, there is no specific recommendation regarding a special amino acid composition that may be of specific benefit to critically ill children. One study of prophylactic arginine supplementation in preterm neonates demonstrated a decrease in morbidity in treated patients; however, a larger trial is needed before specific clinical recommendations can be made.[18,19] The use of glutamine supplementation remains investigational and, in contrast with adult studies, does not result in appreciable benefit over standard amino acid formulations postoperatively or in preterm critically ill infants.[20,21] Similarly, quelling the extreme protein catabolism found in sick children using hormonal modulation also remains experimental. Specifically, studies of growth hormone have not demonstrated a significant benefit in pediatric critically ill patients, and the utility of insulin as an anabolic hormone continues to be under investigation.[22,23]

Energy Metabolism

A careful appraisal of energy requirements in critically ill children is required, because both underestimates and overestimates are associated with potentially deleterious consequences. Inadequate caloric allotment will result in poor protein retention, particularly if protein administration is marginal. Excessive caloric provision, in the form of surplus glucose, in neonates receiving ECMO results in increased carbon dioxide production rates (hence, exacerbating ventilatory failure) and an apparent paradoxic increase in net protein degradation.[24]

The energy needs of critically ill patients are governed by the severity and persistence of the illness. The resting energy expenditure in the flow phase of injury is increased by 50% in children with severe burns and returns to normal during convalescence.[25] Preterm neonates with bronchopulmonary dysplasia similarly have a 25% increase in energy needs over basal requirements.[26] Conversely, stable extubated neonates, including those with shunts from large ventricular septal defects, have resting energy expenditures that resemble those of healthy infants.[27,28] Neonates undergoing major surgery have only a transient 20% increase in energy expenditure that returns to baseline levels within 12 hours, unless complications develop.[29] Neonates with very low birth weight undergoing patent ductus arteriosus ligation do not manifest any discernable increase in resting energy expenditure the first day after surgery.[30]

Total energy requirements encompass resting energy expenditure, energy needed for physical activity, and diet-induced thermogenesis. Resting energy expenditure itself includes the caloric requirement for growth. Although critically ill children have increased energy requirements as a result of increased protein turnover, their growth is often halted during extreme physiologic stress. As a result of intrinsic illness and sedation, the levels of physical activity are low in critical illness. Using a stable isotopic technique, the mean energy expenditures of critically ill neonates receiving ECMO and an age- and diet-matched nonstressed control were found to be nearly identical.[31] The critically ill cohort did, however, have a greater variability in energy expenditure. Further, as previously noted, a surfeit of calories in critically ill neonates does not necessarily result in improved protein accretion. Thus, for practical purposes, the recommended dietary caloric intake for healthy children is a reasonable starting point in critically ill patients. Postoperative parenterally fed neonates provided with an adequate amino acid intake require a total of 85 to 90 kcal/kg per day of energy to achieve adequate protein accretion rates during the first 3 days after surgery.[12]

Ventilated neonates with extremely low birth weight receiving 3.0 g/kg per day of protein and 105 kcal/kg per day remain in positive protein balance before and after patent ductus arteriosus ligation.[30] Enterally fed critically ill children, as a rule, require an additional 10% increment in calories because of obligate malabsorption.

Once protein needs have been met, both carbohydrate and lipid energy sources have similar beneficial effects on net protein synthesis in ill patients.[32] A rational partitioning of these energy-yielding substrates is predicated on the knowledge of carbohydrate and lipid utilization in illness.

Carbohydrate Metabolism

Glucose production and availability is a priority in ill children to supply glucose-dependent organs and cells adequate energy. Adults with injuries and sepsis have a threefold increase in glucose turnover and oxidation and an elevation in gluconeogenesis.[33,34] An important feature of the metabolic stress response is that the provision of dietary glucose does not halt gluconeogenesis; consequently, the catabolism of muscle proteins continues.[11] It is clear, however, that a combination of glucose and amino acids effectively improves protein balance in illness, even in preterm neonates with respiratory distress during the first week of life. This combination therapy improves protein balance primarily by augmenting protein synthesis.[35] In early nutritional support regimens for surgical patients, glucose and amino acid formulations with minimal lipids (only enough to obviate fatty acid deficiency) were often used. Another common practice provided energy allotments well over requirements. As may be predicted, the excess glucose was synthesized to fat, resulting in a net generation of carbon dioxide. The synthesis of fat from glucose has a respiratory quotient (RQ), defined as the ratio of carbon dioxide produced to oxygen consumed, of approximately 8.7. In clinical situations, this high RQ is not attained, because glucose is never purely used for fatty acid synthesis. Nonetheless, the provision of excess glucose results in an elevated RQ and, thus, increases the ventilatory burden placed on the child. The mean RQ in neonates fed a high-glucose diet after surgery is approximately 1.0, whereas comparable neonates fed with less glucose and lipids at 4.0 g/kg per day have an RQ of 0.83.[32] In contrast with glucose metabolism, excess lipids are merely stored as triglycerides and do not result in an augmentation of carbon dioxide production. Hypermetabolic adult patients fed excess caloric allotments with high-glucose total parenteral nutrition have a 30% increase in oxygen consumption, a 57% increase in carbon dioxide production, and a 71% increase in minute ventilation.[36] Thus, avoidance of overfeeding and the use of a mixed-fuel system of nutrition using both glucose and lipids to yield energy are of theoretic and practical utility in stressed patients, many of whom also have respiratory failure. Such an approach also often obviates the increase in morbidity and mortality associated with significant or prolonged hyperglycemia in the relatively insulin-resistant ill child.[37,38]

Lipid Metabolism

Lipid metabolism, analogous to protein and carbohydrate metabolism, is generally accelerated by illness and trauma.[39] During the initial, brief ebb phase, a period of relative hypometabolism after trauma or in early septic shock, lipid utilization is compromised, and triglyceride concentrations increase with an attendant decrease in the metabolism of intravenously administered lipids. However, in the predominant flow phase of injury, a prolonged period of increased metabolic activity after the ebb phase, adult patients demonstrate lipid turnover rates two- to fourfold higher than comparable controls in proportion to the degree of injury.[40,41] Conceptually similar to the increased protein turnover noted in illness, this process involves the recycling of free fatty acids and glycerol into, and hydrolysis from, triglycerides. Both metabolic processes result in a continual stream of substrates through the plasma pool, with an energy cost reflected by an increase in the resting metabolic rate. Approximately 30% to 40% of the released fatty acids are oxidized for energy, and the RQ values post injury are in the vicinity of 0.8. This suggests that free fatty acids are, in fact, the prime source of energy in stressed patients. When subjected to uncomplicated abdominal surgery, infants and children have a decrease in RQ and in plasma triglyceride concentration, implying an increased oxidation of free fatty acids.[42] The glycerol, released along with free fatty acids from triglycerides, may be converted to pyruvate, which, in turn, is used as a gluconeogenic precursor. Importantly, as with other catabolic processes in illness and trauma, the provision of dietary glucose does not decrease glycerol clearance or diminish lipid recycling.

Normal ketone body metabolism is markedly altered by severe illness. The product of incomplete fatty acid and pyruvate oxidation is acetyl-coenzyme A, which, through a condensation reaction within the hepatocyte, forms the ketone bodies acetoacetate and beta-hydroxybutyric acid. In starved healthy subjects, a major adaptation to help preserve skeletal muscle mass is the use of ketone bodies generated by the liver as an energy source for the brain (which cannot directly oxidize free fatty acids). However, in the 3-day period after trauma, there is a negligible increase in serum ketone body concentrations when compared with healthy fasting subjects.[43] This observation may be understood in light of serum insulin concentrations. Ketogenesis is inhibited by even low concentrations of the hormone, a phenomenon evident to physicians by the absence of ketotic problems in type 2 diabetes mellitus. Hence, the high insulin concentrations seen in severe injury and after major surgery ablate the ketotic adaptation of starvation.

The energy needs of the injured patient are met largely by the mobilization and oxidation of free fatty acids. In conjunction with increased demands, ill neonates have limited lipid stores. Thus, they may suffer biochemical essential fatty acid deficiency within 1 week if administered a fat-free diet.[44,45] In infants, linoleic and linolenic acid are considered essential, and both arachidonic acid and docosahexaenoic acid are considered conditionally essential. When there is a lack of dietary linoleic acid, the formation of arachidonic acid (a tetraene) by desaturation and chain elongation cannot occur, and the same pathway entrains available oleic acid to form 5,8,11-eicosatrienoic acid (a triene). Empirically, a triene-to-tetraene ratio of greater than 0.4 is characteristic of essential fatty acid deficiency. The clinical syndrome consists of dermatitis, alopecia, thrombocytopenia, susceptibility to bacterial infection, and failure to thrive.[44,45] To obviate essential fatty acid deficiency in injured infants, the prompt administration of linoleic acid and linolenic acid is recommended.

The provision of commercially available lipid solutions to parenterally fed critically ill neonates obviates the risk of essential fatty acid deficiency, results in improved protein utilization, and does not significantly increase carbon dioxide production or metabolic rate.[46] These advantages, however, are balanced by some potential risks of excess administration, including hypertriglyceridemia, increased infections, and decreased alveolar oxygen diffusion capacity.[47–49] Although the evidence does not demonstrate any difference in growth, chronic lung disease, or death in preterm infants with early lipid introduction (≤5 days), the possible adverse effects of lipid administration have resulted in most centers starting lipid supplementation in ill neonates and children at 0.5 to 1 g/kg per day and advancing over a period of days to 2 to 4 g/kg per day while closely monitoring triglyceride concentrations.[50] Lipid administration is usually restricted to a maximum of 30% to 40% of total calories, although this practice has not been validated by clinical trials.

Vitamin and Trace Mineral Metabolism

Vitamin and trace mineral metabolism in ill and postoperative pediatric patients has not been well studied. For the neonate and child, the fat-soluble vitamins A, D, E, and K, as well as the water-soluble vitamins ascorbic acid, thiamine, riboflavin, pyridoxine, niacin, pantothenate, biotin, folate, and vitamin B_{12}, are all required and are routinely administered. Because vitamins are not stoichiometrically consumed in biochemical reactions but rather act as catalysts, the administration of large supplements of vitamins in stressed states is not logical from a nutritional standpoint. The trace minerals that are required for normal development are zinc, iron, copper, selenium, manganese, iodide, molybdenum, and chromium. Trace minerals are usually used in the synthesis of the active sites of a ubiquitous and extraordinarily important class of enzymes called metalloenzymes. As with vitamins, the role of metalloenzymes is to act as catalysts. Hence, unless there are excessive losses, such as enhanced zinc loss with severe diarrhea, large nutritional requirements would not be anticipated in illness. The vitamin and trace mineral needs of healthy children and neonates are outlined in Appendix J. These levels have been used in critically ill patients, and little evidence exists that they are nutritionally inadequate. In children with severe hepatic failure, such as those with severe parenteral nutrition-related cholestasis, copper and manganese accumulation occurs and, thus, parenteral trace mineral supplementation should be limited to once per week with monitoring of serum mineral concentrations.

The pharmacologic use of vitamins and trace minerals in pediatric illness is controversial. Although deficiency has obvious implications for growth, immune competence, and other vital physiologic functions, reviews of both vitamin and trace mineral toxicity demonstrate that excessive dosage is clearly a health risk.[51,52] Again, vitamin and trace element supplementation in critically ill neonates and children according to current guidelines and with appropriate monitoring is prudent.

Routes of Nutrient Provision

In the critically ill child, the enteral route of nutrient provision is preferable to parenteral nutrition whenever the gastrointestinal tract is functional. Enteral nutrition is physiologic, safer, and more cost-effective. The use of nasojejunal feeding tubes placed at bedside or through interventional radiologic techniques is a very useful adjunct to the nutritional management of the critically ill child, with significant improvements in the amount of nutrition successfully delivered when compared with gastric feeding.[53]

Continuous feedings using standard formulas can adequately nourish most patients. At the time of extubation, feeds are held for a period of 6 to 12 hours. If parenteral nutrition is necessary, central venous access is sought. Peripheral percutaneously placed intravenous lines that are threaded centrally and central lines are the preferred routes of administration. Central access may be garnered at bedside in most intensive care unit patients. Groin lines are not a favored access route for nutritional therapy because of their propensity for infection.

Conclusion

Neonates and children are particularly susceptible to the loss of lean body mass and its attendant increased morbidity and mortality. Critical illness results in increased protein, carbohydrate, and lipid utilization and net negative protein balance. The judicious administration of carbohydrates, lipids, vitamins, trace minerals, and particularly, protein can optimize wound healing and reduce or even eliminate the consequences of this catabolic response.

Bibliography

1. Cuthbertson DP. Further observations on the disturbance of metabolism caused by injury, with particular reference to the dietary requirements of fracture cases. *Br J Surg.* 1936;23:505–520

2. Kashyap S, Schulze KF, Forsyth M, et al. Growth, nutrient retention, and metabolic response in low birth weight infants fed varying intakes of protein and energy. *J Pediatr.* 1988;113:713–721

3. Taylor RM, Preedy VR, Baker AJ, Grimble G. Nutritional support in critically ill children. *Clin Nutr.* 2003;22:365–369

4. Rogers EJ, Gilbertson HR, Heine RG, Henning R. Barriers to adequate nutrition in critically ill children. *Nutrition.* 2003;19:865–868

5. Hulst JM, van Goudoever JB, Zimmermann LJ, et al. The effect of cumulative energy and protein deficiency on anthropometric parameters in a pediatric ICU population. *Clin Nutr.* 2004;23:1381–1389

6. Forbes GB, Bruining GJ. Urinary creatinine excretion and lean body mass. *Am J Clin Nutr.* 1976;29:1359–1366

7. Fomon SJ, Haschke F, Ziegler EE, Nelson SE. Body composition of reference children from birth to age 10 years. *Am J Clin Nutr.* 1982;35(5 Suppl):1169–1175

8. Munro HN. Nutrition and muscle protein metabolism: introduction. *Fed Proc.* 1978;37: 2281–2282

9. Keshen TH, Miller RG, Jahoor F, Jaksic T. Stable isotopic quantitation of protein metabolism and energy expenditure in neonates on- and post-extracorporeal life support. *J Pediatr Surg.* 1997;32:958–962

10. Keshen T, Miller R, Jahoor F, Jaksic T, Reeds PJ. Glucose production and gluconeogenesis are negatively related to body weight in mechanically ventilated, very low birth weight neonates. *Pediatr Res.* 1997;41:132–138

11. Long CL, Kinney JM, Geiger JW. Nonsuppressability of gluconeogenesis by glucose in septic patients. *Metabolism.* 1976;25:193–201

12. Duffy B, Pencharz P. The effects of surgery on the nitrogen metabolism of parenterally fed human neonates. *Pediatr Res.* 1986;20:32–35

13. Denne SC, Karn CA, Ahlrichs JA, Dorotheo AR, Wang J, Liechty EA. Proteolysis and phenylalanine hydroxylation in response to parenteral nutrition in extremely premature and normal newborns. *J Clin Invest.* 1996;97:746–754

14. Daley SE, Pearson AD, Craft AW, et al. Whole body protein metabolism in children with cancer. *Arch Dis Child.* 1996;75:273–281

15. Premji SS, Fenton TR, Sauve RS. Higher versus lower protein intake in formula-fed low birth weight infants. *Cochrane Database Syst Rev.* 2006;(1):CD003959

16. Goldman HI, Freudenthal R, Holland B, Karelitz S. Clinical effects of two different levels of protein intake on low-birth-weight infants. *J Pediatr.* 1969;74:881–889

17. Goldman HI, Liebman OB, Freudenthal R, Reuben R. Effects of early dietary protein intake on low-birth-weight infants: evaluation at 3 years of age. *J Pediatr.* 1971;78:126–129

18. Amin HJ, Zamora SA, McMillan DD, et al. Arginine supplementation prevents necrotizing enterocolitis in the premature infant. *J Pediatr.* 2002;140:425–431

19. Shah P, Shah V. Arginine supplementation for prevention of necrotising enterocolitis in preterm infants. *Cochrane Database Syst Rev.* 2004;(4):CD004339

20. Albers MJ, Steyerberg EW, Hazebroek FW, et al. Glutamine supplementation of parenteral nutrition does not improve intestinal permeability, nitrogen balance, or outcome in newborns and infants undergoing digestive-tract surgery: results from a double-blind, randomized, controlled trial. *Ann Surg.* 2005;241:599–606

21. Tubman TR, Thompson SW, McGuire W. Glutamine supplementation to prevent morbidity and mortality in preterm infants. *Cochrane Database Syst Rev.* 2005;(1):CD001457

22. Scolapio JS. Short bowel syndrome: recent clinical outcomes with growth hormone. *Gastroenterology.* 2006;130(2 Suppl):S122–S126

23. Agus MS, Javid PJ, Ryan DP, Jaksic T. Intravenous insulin decreases protein breakdown in infants on extracorporeal membrane oxygenation. *J Pediatr Surg.* 2004;39:839–844

24. Shew SB, Keshen TH, Jahoor F, Jaksic T. The determinants of protein catabolism in neonates on extracorporeal membrane oxygenation. *J Pediatr Surg.* 1999;34:1086–1090

25. Jahoor F, Desai M, Herndon DN, Wolfe RR. Dynamics of the protein metabolic response to burn injury. *Metabolism.* 1988;37:330–337

26. Weinstein MR, Oh W. Oxygen consumption in infants with bronchopulmonary dysplasia. *J Pediatr.* 1981;99:958–961

27. Shew SB, Beckett PR, Keshen TH, Jahoor F, Jaksic T. Validation of a [13C]bicarbonate tracer technique to measure neonatal energy expenditure. *Pediatr Res.* 2000;47:787–791

28. Ackerman IL, Karn CA, Denne SC, Ensing GJ, Leitch CA. Total but not resting energy expenditure is increased in infants with ventricular septal defects. *Pediatrics.* 1998;102:1172–1177

29. Jones MO, Pierro A, Hammond P, Lloyd DA. The metabolic response to operative stress in infants. *J Pediatr Surg.* 1993;28:1258–1262

30. Shew SB, Keshen TH, Glass NL, Jahoor F, Jaksic T. Ligation of a patent ductus arteriosus under fentanyl anesthesia improves protein metabolism in premature neonates. *J Pediatr Surg.* 2000;35:1277–1281

31. Jaksic T, Shew SB, Keshen TH, Dzakovic A, Jahoor F. Do critically ill surgical neonates have increased energy expenditure? *J Pediatr Surg.* 2001;36:63–67

32. Jones MO, Pierro A, Garlick PJ, McNurlan MA, Donnell SC, Lloyd DA. Protein metabolism kinetics in neonates: effect of intravenous carbohydrate and fat. *J Pediatr Surg.* 1995; 30:458–462

33. Long CL, Spencer JL, Kinney JM, Geiger JW. Carbohydrate metabolism in normal man and effect of glucose infusion. *J Appl Physiol.* 1971;31:102–109

34. Long CL, Spencer JL, Kinney JM, Geiger JW. Carbohydrate metabolism in man: effect of elective operations and major injury. *J Appl Physiol.* 1971;31:110–116

35. Rivera A, Jr., Bell EF, Bier DM. Effect of intravenous amino acids on protein metabolism of preterm infants during the first three days of life. *Pediatr Res.* 1993;33:106–111

36. Askanazi J, Rosenbaum SH, Hyman AI, Silverberg PA, Milic-Emili J, Kinney JM. Respiratory changes induced by the large glucose loads of total parenteral nutrition. *JAMA.* 1980; 243:1444–1447

37. Faustino EV, Apkon M. Persistent hyperglycemia in critically ill children. *J Pediatr.* 2005; 146:30–34

38. Alaedeen DI, Walsh MC, Chwals WJ. Total parenteral nutrition-associated hyperglycemia correlates with prolonged mechanical ventilation and hospital stay in septic infants. *J Pediatr Surg.* 2006;41:239–244

39. Jeevanandam M, Young DH, Schiller WR. Nutritional impact on the energy cost of fat fuel mobilization in polytrauma victims. *J Trauma.* 1990;30:147–154

40. Wiener M, Rothkopf MM, Rothkopf G, Askanazi J. Fat metabolism in injury and stress. *Crit Care Clin.* 1987;3:25–56

41. Nordenstrom J, Carpentier YA, Askanazi J, et al. Metabolic utilization of intravenous fat emulsion during total parenteral nutrition. *Ann Surg.* 1982;196:221–231

42. Powis MR, Smith K, Rennie M, Halliday D, Pierro A. Effect of major abdominal operations on energy and protein metabolism in infants and children. *J Pediatr Surg.* 1998;33:49–53

43. Birkhahn RH, Long CL, Fitkin DL, Busnardo AC, Geiger JW, Blakemore WS. A comparison of the effects of skeletal trauma and surgery on the ketosis of starvation in man. *J Trauma.* 1981;21:513–519

44. Paulsrud JR, Pensler L, Whitten CF, Stewart S, Holman RT. Essential fatty acid deficiency in infants induced by fat-free intravenous feeding. *Am J Clin Nutr.* 1972;25:897–904

45. Friedman Z, Danon A, Stahlman MT, Oates JA. Rapid onset of essential fatty acid deficiency in the newborn. *Pediatrics*. 1976;58:640–649

46. Van Aerde JE, Sauer PJ, Pencharz PB, Smith JM, Heim T, Swyer PR. Metabolic consequences of increasing energy intake by adding lipid to parenteral nutrition in full-term infants. *Am J Clin Nutr*. 1994;59:659–662

47. Cleary TG, Pickering LK. Mechanisms of intralipid effect on polymorphonuclear leukocytes. *J Clin Lab Immunol*. 1983;11:21–26

48. Periera GR, Fox WW, Stanley CA, Baker L, Schwartz JG. Decreased oxygenation and hyperlipemia during intravenous fat infusions in premature infants. *Pediatrics*. 1980;66: 26–30

49. Freeman J, Goldmann DA, Smith NE, Sidebottom DG, Epstein MF, Platt R. Association of intravenous lipid emulsion and coagulase-negative staphylococcal bacteremia in neonatal intensive care units. *N Engl J Med*. 1990;323:301–308

50. Simmer K, Rao SC. Early introduction of lipids to parenterally-fed preterm infants. *Cochrane Database Syst Rev*. 2005;(2):CD005256

51. Marks J. The safety of the vitamins: an overview. *Int J Vitam Nutr Res Suppl*. 1989;30:12–20

52. Flodin NW. Micronutrient supplements: toxicity and drug interactions. *Prog Food Nutr Sci*. 1990;14:277–331

53. Meert KL, Daphtary KM, Metheny NA. Gastric vs small-bowel feeding in critically ill children receiving mechanical ventilation: a randomized controlled trial. *Chest*. 2004;126:872–878

38 Anorexia Nervosa and Bulimia Nervosa

Anorexia nervosa and bulimia nervosa are associated with significant health problems resulting from nutritional and weight control practices used by patients either to lose weight or to minimize weight gain.[1] Therefore, medical and nutritional consultation is of particular importance in the management of these conditions, which are generally classified as disorders of mental health. Affected individuals are typically intellectually bright and strong willed, making them receptive to professional input but also resistant to suggestions for change, making them challenging clinically. Health care professionals working with young people with an eating disorder require: (1) general knowledge about the disorder and specific understanding of the individual (and her or his family) affected by the disorder; and (2) practical information regarding the management of common problems related to health, food, nutrition, and weight-control. This chapter focuses on these elements as they relate to pediatric practice and nutrition consultation.[2]

Clinical Features

Weight and Food-Related Characteristics

Common features of eating disorders include dysfunctional eating habits (frequently related to underlying psychosocial issues involving developing autonomy and identity, low self-esteem, family dynamics, or environmental problems), body image disturbance (generally focused on the abdomen, hips, and thighs) and change in weight (ranging from extreme loss of weight in anorexia nervosa to fluctuation around a normal to moderately high weight in bulimia nervosa). The *Diagnostic and Statistical Manual for Primary Care (DSM-PC), Child and Adolescent Version*, published by the American Academy of Pediatrics, classifies conditions on a continuum of severity from variations (minor deviations from normal that might still be of concern), to problems (more serious manifestations representing subthreshold eating disorders), to full eating disorders (meeting full criteria of the *Diagnostic and Statistical Manual of Mental Disorders, Fourth Edition* [DSM-IV]), as shown in Tables 38.1 and 38.2.

Anorexia nervosa is an eating disorder characterized by an insufficient and voluntarily restricted caloric intake resulting in weight loss (or failure to gain weight during puberty) that is accompanied by an obsession to be thinner and a delusion of being fat. Weight loss can be extreme, but there is no specific amount of weight loss required in diagnostic criteria. The DSM-IV suggests, as an example, 85% of ideal body weight. However, patients with less severe eating patterns in the DSM-PC categories of "variations" or "problems" (Tables 38.1 and 38.2) may not experience this degree of emaciation but still deserve medical and nutritional attention. More than 75% of people with anorexia nervosa exercise compulsively to accelerate weight loss. Fewer than 10% attempt to rid themselves of calories by vomiting or taking laxatives; such purging is more commonly associated with bulimia nervosa.

Table 38.1
Combined DSM-PC/DSM-IV Criteria for Eating Disorders: Dieting-Anorexia Nervosa Spectrum

V65.49 Dieting/Body Image Variation
<ul><li>A significantly overweight child changes eating habits in a realistic, healthy way.</li><li>The child does not completely eliminate any food group but generally decreases intake of food, especially of sweets and fats, or is eating an appropriate diet.</li><li>The child favors a thin appearance but has a realistic image.</li><li>The individual can stop dieting voluntarily.</li></ul>
V69.1 Dieting/Body Image Problem
<ul><li>Dieting and voluntary food restrictions are more restrictive and result in weight loss or failure to gain weight as expected during growth, but these behaviors are not sufficiently intense to qualify for the diagnosis of anorexia nervosa or eating disorder, not otherwise specified.</li><li>The individual begins to become obsessed with the pursuit of thinness and develops systematic fears of gaining weight.</li><li>The individual also begins to develop a consistent disturbance in body perception and starts to deny that weight loss or dieting is a problem.</li></ul>
307.1 Anorexia Nervosa (from DSM-IV)
<ul><li>Refusal to maintain body weight at or above a minimally normal weight for age and height (eg, weight loss leading to maintenance of body weight less than 85% of that expected; or failure to make expected weight gain during period of growth, leading to body weight less than 85% of that expected).</li><li>Body mass index (BMI) is <17.5 for older adolescents.</li><li>Intense fear of gaining weight or becoming fat, even though underweight.</li><li>Disturbance in the way in which one's body weight, shape, or size is experienced; undue influence of body weight or shape on self-evaluation; or denial of the seriousness of the current low body weight.</li><li>In postmenarchal females, amenorrhea (ie, the absence of at least 3 consecutive menstrual cycles. A female is considered to have amenorrhea if her periods occur only following hormone [eg, estrogen] administration.)</li></ul>

Sources: American Academy of Pediatrics. *The Classification of Child and Adolescent Mental Diagnoses in Primary Care: Diagnostic and Statistical Manual for Primary Care (DSM-PC), Child and Adolescent Version.* Wolraich ML, Felice ME, Drotar D, eds. Elk Grove Village, IL: American Academy of Pediatrics: 1996; and American Psychiatric Association. *Diagnostic and Statistical Manual of Mental Disorders, Fourth Edition (DSM-IV).* Washington, DC: American Psychiatric Association; 1994.

Table 38.2

Combined DSM-PC/DSM-IV Criteria for Eating Disorders: Purging/Binge Eating-Bulimia Nervosa Spectrum

V65.49 Purging/Binge-Eating Variation

- Occasional overeating or perception of overeating or either objective or subjective binges occurs.
- Intermittent concern about body image or getting fat is present in specific situations during which too much food was eaten. Concerns are not pervasive or cross-situational and do not change eating behaviors.
- Normal weight gain is typically present.

V69.19 Purging/Binge-Eating Problem

- Experimentation with vomiting, laxatives, fasting, or exercises to prevent weight gain.
- Isolated episodes are far apart in time.
- Individual has increased episodes of uncontrolled eating, and perceptions of body shape or size become more systematically distorted. Negative self-evaluation is often influenced by weight and body shape.
- The behaviors are not sufficiently intense to qualify for a diagnosis of bulimia nervosa or eating disorder, not otherwise specified.

307.51 Bulimia Nervosa (from DSM-IV)

- Recurrent episodes of binge eating, characterized by both of the following:
  - Eating, in a discrete period of time (eg, within any 2-hour period), an amount of food that is definitely larger than most people would eat during a similar period of time and under similar circumstances.
  - A sense of lack of control over eating during the episode (eg, a feeling that one cannot stop eating or control what or how much one is eating).
- Recurrent inappropriate compensatory behavior in order to prevent weight gain, such as self-induced vomiting; misuse of laxatives, diuretics, enemas, or other medications; fasting; or excessive exercise.
- The binge eating and inappropriate compensatory behaviors both occur, on average, at least twice a week for 3 months.
- Body shape and weight unduly influence self-evaluation.
- The disturbance does not occur exclusively during episodes of anorexia nervosa.

Sources: American Academy of Pediatrics. *The Classification of Child and Adolescent Mental Diagnoses in Primary Care: Diagnostic and Statistical Manual for Primary Care (DSM-PC), Child and Adolescent Version.* Wolraich ML, Felice ME, Drotar D, eds. Elk Grove Village, IL: American Academy of Pediatrics: 1996; and American Psychiatric Association. *Diagnostic and Statistical Manual of Mental Disorders, Fourth Edition (DSM-IV).* Washington, DC: American Psychiatric Association; 1994.

   Bulimia nervosa has the key feature of repeated episodes of consuming large amounts of food in a brief period (binge eating). Binges are followed by compensatory behavior intended to rid the body of the effects of food: fasting; "purging" through vomiting, laxatives, or diuretics; or exercise. Depending on the balance between intake and output, patients range from moderately thin to moderately overweight. An individual's weight can fluctuate depending on the pattern of weight control over time. Episodic binges make binge-eating disorder similar to bulimia nervosa, but binge-eating disorder does not include compensatory behaviors to rid the body of the effects of excessive calories. In fact, for patients with binge-eating disorder, self-deprecating thoughts after a binge may best be relieved by another binge. Thus, individuals with binge-eating disorder may become massively overweight.

Typically, patients with bulimia nervosa have strong feelings of guilt, shame, and embarrassment about both the binge eating and the compensatory behaviors, such as vomiting. However, the relief of anxiety that patients experience after "getting rid of the food" temporarily helps them feel better. This relief is short-lived, because the cycle of behaviors tends to repeat itself in an addictive fashion. A personal and/or family history of depression and/or addictions is commonly found in patients with bulimia nervosa.

Meals

Meals are typically restricted to small amounts of a monotonously narrow range of low-calorie, low-fat foods and low-calorie beverages.[3] Breakfast is generally avoided, with excuses such as, "I can't eat that early in the morning," or "I have to do my workout," or "I'll eat at school." If not entirely vegetarian, the intake of meat is typically severely restricted and eaten primarily at dinner—under duress from parents—and confined to small amounts of grilled skinless poultry or broiled fish. Snacks and desserts are assiduously avoided in anorexia nervosa. When they occur, binges typically consist of "forbidden foods" considered to be "fattening" and occur in the late afternoon or evening. Immediately after a binge, patients may go to the bathroom to vomit, take laxatives, or exercise.

Clinical Approach

Comerci[4] has noted 4 main elements of successful treatment of eating disorders: (1) early recognition and restoration of physiologic stability; (2) establishment of a trusting, therapeutic partnership with the patient; (3) involvement of the family in treatment; and (4) a team approach. Levenkron[5] has emphasized the "nurturant-authoritative" approach, in contrast to an unsupportive, authoritarian one. With respect to medical and nutritional management, eating disorders are a final common pathway allowing affected individuals to cope with unresolved adolescent developmental conflicts. Parents often search for a specific cause, emotional flaw, set of family traits, or precipitating event, but this is rarely helpful in the short-term. Mental health services may focus on these issues over a period of months to years, but emerging evidence regarding the effectiveness of the "Maudsley" approach points out the importance of ensuring adequate caloric intake and weight stabilization as an essential first step in the treatment of adolescents with eating disorders. This approach, described by Lock and LeGrange,[6] emphasizes the important role that parents have in helping their daughter or son begin to normalize eating. At one level, the conflict about eating and weight gain is metaphoric and has nothing to do with food, eating, or weight. The struggle for control over these concrete issues is symbolic of the intangible, confusing, and often illusory internal struggles that accompany adolescent development. However, this conflict also can result in serious health consequences that perpetuate dysfunctional patterns. It is essential that both levels be addressed in treatment. Nutritional, medical, and psychological interventions should occur simultaneously and with active parental involvement.[7]

Epidemiology, Prevalence, and Genetics

Eating disorders most commonly affect white, adolescent females. There is an increasing awareness of these conditions, especially bulimia nervosa, among females in minority groups and among males, however. Prevalence is estimated at between 0.5% and 5% of adolescent females.[7] Certain groups, such as athletes or dancers, may have a substantially higher risk of developing anorexia nervosa. However, the prevalence of unrecognized, atypical, or subclinical anorexia nervosa is undoubtedly several-fold greater, and these individuals may be at greater risk of health consequences, because they are less likely to come to clinical attention and more likely to persist in unhealthy nutritional and weight-control habits.

There is clearly a genetic predisposition to eating disorders, with chromosomes 1, 2, and 13 revealing regions of interest[8] for restrictive anorexia nervosa. Relatives of patients with eating disorders have approximately a 10-fold greater lifetime risk of developing an eating disorder compared with relatives of unaffected individuals,[8] with the highest risk occurring for a monozygotic twin of a person with anorexia nervosa. However, emerging data indicate that the strongest association is with mood or anxiety disorders. That is, eating disorders are not inherited directly. Rather, "inheritance" is best considered as a "vulnerability" to developing an eating disorder on the basis of being depressed and/or anxious, both of which are recognized familial genetic traits.

Assessment

General Issues

The initial assessment of the adolescent with an eating disorder should focus on weight loss and health, per se, and should not to attempt to determine underlying psychological or emotional factors.[7,9] The denial and resistance to change that patients frequently display when threatened with direct confrontation about their eating disorder is less likely to be exhibited when they are questioned about their nutritional habits, physical symptoms, and health. The first step in the assessment is to determine whether weight loss is intentional and/or desired and ensure that the symptoms are not related to a medical disease, such as inflammatory bowel disease, endocrinopathy, cancer, or an occult infection. However, some patients recover from a medical condition, such as infectious mononucleosis, only to continue to lose weight because they then diet intentionally. This occurs because of positive reinforcement that they receive for the weight loss that accompanied the initial illness. Pubertal adolescents, on the other hand, may fail to increase caloric intake during their growth spurt or may increase their caloric expenditure playing sports and lose weight unintentionally. Finally, many healthy adolescents lose weight while attempting to "get in shape" or "look better."

The second step in the assessment of a person with a suspected eating disorder is to determine whether weight control habits are excessive or unhealthy. Young people with eating disorder variations or problems in the DSM-PC classification may have health problems associated with weight control. Questionnaires assessing symptoms related to malnutrition, such as those in Table 38.3, can be used to identify individuals who may be experiencing health problems associated with weight control.

Table 38.3
Questionnaire for Adolescents With Weight Loss

I. Symptoms: Do you have any of the following symptoms?	NO	YES
Cold or blue hands or feet	☐	☐
Constipation	☐	☐
Dizziness or fainting	☐	☐
Headaches	☐	☐
Tiredness or weakness	☐	☐
Loss of appetite	☐	☐
Difficulty concentrating or making decisions	☐	☐
Feeling irritable	☐	☐
Being sad or bored	☐	☐
Not wanting to be around friends or family	☐	☐
Thinking about food	☐	☐
Worrying about gaining weight	☐	☐
Loss or irregularity of menstrual periods (females)	☐	☐

Table 38.3 *(Continued)*
Questionnaire for Adolescents With Weight Loss

II. Weight and Activity History

1. What is the *most* you have ever weighed?............................. _____
2. What is the *least* you have weighed in the last year?................ _____
3. What do you weigh *now*? .... _____
4. What would you *like* to weigh? .... _____

	NO	YES
5. Are you trying to lose weight?	☐	☐
6. Do you exercise at least once a week?..............................	☐	☐

If yes, check all that apply:

	No	Yes	Hours/Week
Running/jogging	☐	☐	_____
Aerobics/calisthenics.............................	☐	☐	_____
Dancing/ballet..	☐	☐	_____
Gymnastics	☐	☐	_____
Swimming...	☐	☐	_____
Team sport(s)	☐	☐	_____
Other: _____			_____

	NO	YES
7. Do you exercise to lose weight?	☐	☐

8. Check all the methods that you have used to try to control your weight in the past 2 months.

Dieting	Exercising	Diet Pills	Vomiting	Laxatives
☐	☐	☐	☐	☐

III. Eating History

1. Rate on a scale of 0 to 5 how much you eat at each of the following times during a typical day. (Nothing = 0; Snack = 1; Small meal = 2; Meal = 3; Large meal = 4; Binge = 5)

At...	Between...	After...
Breakfast _____	Breakfast and lunch _____	Going to bed _____
Lunch _____	Lunch and dinner _____	Something upsetting _____
Dinner _____	Dinner and bedtime _____	

2. Please describe your typical breakfast, lunch, and dinner.

	Food/Beverage	Amount
Breakfast	_____	_____
	_____	_____
Lunch	_____	_____
	_____	_____
Dinner	_____	_____
	_____	_____
	_____	_____

V

The third step in conducting the nutritional assessment is to determine the degree to which the pursuit of thinness is an overriding concern and a driving force in the individual's daily activities. Typically, adolescents with anorexia nervosa restrict intake to <1000 kcal/day, are unwilling to accept a body weight >85% of average weight for height, and have a self-concept that is directly linked to their weight or how they feel about their weight. It is useful to have the patient identify a desired goal weight, especially if body weight is still within a normal weight range for age, height, and gender. Adolescents with anorexia nervosa either have an unrealistically low goal weight or cannot identify a specific weight with which they would be satisfied. Although a distorted body image is included in diagnostic criteria for anorexia nervosa, many adolescent females without eating disorders are also dissatisfied with their bodies, especially their hips, buttocks, and thighs, limiting the specificity of this finding. Instruments such as the Eating Disorder Inventory can also be used to measure features, including body dissatisfaction or drive for thinness.

If the evidence indicates that the adolescent has anorexia nervosa, the fourth step is to determine an immediate plan of action. The biopsychosocial approach recognizes that patients require attention to their biological, psychological, and social needs. For patients who have lost a significant amount of weight and are exhibiting signs of starvation and hypometabolism or who have intractable vomiting and electrolyte imbalance, hospitalization should be considered. However, with early recognition, hospitalization can usually be avoided—even if the child or adolescent is an unwilling participant in treatment—as long as appropriate outpatient treatment is available and the parents are actively engaged in all aspects of it.

Physical Health Issues

No organ system is spared the effects of the malnutrition that occurs in anorexia nervosa.[1,7] Keys and colleagues studied young adult males who were "voluntarily" starved to determine the effects of starvation and the best means of refeeding extremely malnourished individuals.[10] These subjects exhibited findings remarkably similar to those found in anorexia nervosa; much of the clinical syndrome can be traced to the physiologic adaptation to low caloric intake. Among patients with eating disorders, the most concerning health problems are amenorrhea, hypothermia, bradycardia, and orthostatic cardiovascular instability; low weight, amenorrhea, and poor nutrition predispose females to osteoporosis. Hypothermia can be extremely uncomfortable and profound, so temperature measurement is essential.

Cardiovascular instability can lead to weakness, fatigue, dizziness, loss of energy, fainting, and death. Orthostatic pulse change of more than 30 beats/minute indicates significant compromise.

Cardiovascular instability can also occur in bulimia nervosa, but it is generally attributable to volume depletion and electrolyte imbalance (hypokalemic, hypochloremic metabolic alkalosis). Erosion of the dental enamel (caused by stomach acid), abrasion of the knuckles of metacarpophalangeal joints (rubbing against the maxillary central incisors), and enlargement of the salivary glands indicate significant binge eating and vomiting.

Anthropometry

The most important anthropometric measurements in the assessment of an adolescent with an eating disorder are accurate height and weight. The latter should be determined with the patient in a gown, immediately after voiding. The body mass index (BMI) is a calculated anthropometric variable that standardizes weight for height (see Appendix D). The BMI is of more value in screening for excessive weight gain than in identifying the presence of an eating disorder, because it tends to increase in children and adolescents until adult stature is attained. Although a BMI of <17.5 translates to less than the 85th percentile weight for height for adults and is considered a lower weight threshold for the diagnosis of anorexia nervosa, a BMI of 17.5 represents the 50th percentile for an 11-year-old female.

Skinfold thickness, either as triceps or multiple-site determination, can be used to assess subcutaneous fat, but the standards apply only for older adolescents, and skilled personnel using research-quality instruments must obtain the measurements. Thus, plastic calipers are unreliable and should not be used. The 4-site (triceps, biceps, subscapular, iliac) method of body fat determination is probably the most accurate. Also, the measurement may not be accurate in states of dehydration, and there have been few studies in which skinfold thickness in adolescents with anorexia nervosa has been compared with reference methods of body composition determination. The primary use of this tool is in following the progress of a patient during treatment rather than to define a level of body fat at any one time. Electronic scales that provide a digital read-out of body weight and of "body fat" using bioelectrical impedance analysis, actually indirectly measure body water,[11] so disturbances in fluid or electrolyte concentrations impair their validity in measuring body composition.

Early in recovery from anorexia nervosa, more than two thirds of the weight gained is lean body mass.[12,13] As the body approaches a more normal distribution of lean and fat mass, an increasing amount of tissue is fat. The composition does not appear to be influenced by dietary content but can be influenced by activity. That is, if patients increase their energy intake in a well-balanced diet and also engage in a combination of aerobic exercise and resistance training, the majority of tissue that is added will be lean. This point deserves emphasis, because most patients believe that all of their weight gain is, or will be, as fat. In addition, it is worthwhile to emphasize to patients that lean body mass has a higher metabolic rate than fat, which is relatively inert. Thus, an increase in temperature can be interpreted as an increase in lean body tissue, not fat. Likewise, cold, acrocyanotic hands and feet with poor peripheral circulation and slow capillary refill can be interpreted to mean a low lean body (muscle) mass, whereas warm hands and feet with good circulation and rapid capillary refill indicate an improved metabolic rate and lean, not fat, body mass.

Laboratory Studies

The laboratory evaluation of patients with anorexia nervosa is primarily directed at detecting unsuspected underlying medical conditions.[7] Nutrition-related tests include concentrations of hepatic secretory proteins, measures of immune function, and measurement of vitamin or mineral concentrations.[14] Serum prealbumin (transthyretin), with a half-life of 2 days, can be used to assess energy balance and protein synthesis in the liver. Concentrations of these proteins are typically normal as a result of adequate protein intake in the context of extreme restriction of carbohydrates and fat or as a result of dehydration. Transferrin, with a half-life of 8 days, tends to be nonspecifically increased in anorexia nervosa. Visceral protein concentrations can be assessed with the calculation of creatinine height index (CHI) and then compared with reference standards.[15] A 20% to 40% reduction of CHI is evidence of moderate visceral protein depletion, and severe depletion is indicated by a reduction of more than 40%. Measurement of immune function by various methods have not produced consistent results in the literature but can sometimes be useful in assessing the physiologic response to nutritional status. Vitamin and mineral concentrations in circulating compartments, such as the serum, may not be related to actual deficiencies at the tissue level. In vitro assay of dependent enzymes with and without the vitamin cofactor may be a more useful measure but is not routinely available.

Routine laboratory tests obtained during medical evaluation usually include a complete blood cell count and erythrocyte sedimentation rate (ESR), chemistry panel, and urinalysis. The results of these tests may be normal, a reflection of the remarkable ability of the body to maintain homeostatic balance. Patients who have lost weight most commonly show a low white blood cell count but a normal ESR. Patients who vomit several times a day may show hypochloremic, hypokalemic metabolic alkalosis and have concentrated alkaline urine. Thyroid screening is often performed but rarely useful, because the clinical picture in anorexia nervosa combines symptoms of hyper- and hypothyroidism. An unusual finding is elevated serum cholesterol concentration, with both high and normal low-density lipoprotein fractions being reported, despite an extremely low intake of both fat and cholesterol. Electrocardiography may be indicated if there is significant bradycardia or rhythm disturbance. Before performing any tests, one should explicitly state whether normal results are expected and that the tests represent baseline measures. Otherwise, "normal" findings may be interpreted as "nothing is wrong."

Diet and Activity Records

Recording food and drink intake by an adolescent is helpful both in assessment and in treatment. It helps the health care professional to identify dietary patterns, deficiencies, excesses, and strengths, and it helps the patient become more aware of her or his nutritional habits.[16] Seven-day food diaries are superior to 24-hour recall. However, because adolescents with anorexia nervosa overestimate their serving size (often by as much as 50%), it is important to verify their reports. In this respect, food models are helpful tools that simultaneously inform the professional about the patient's intake and teach the patient how to estimate serving size. The weekly journals used to evaluate nutrition can also be used to determine dysfunctional habits (such as eating a rice cake for breakfast), associated mood disturbances (such as not eating dinner because of an argument with a parent), and episodes in which the patient makes a breakthrough toward recovery (such as eating a "forbidden food" like peanut butter). In the Maudsley approach, parents have much more active and prescriptive involvement in determining dietary intake.[17]

To understand the balance between energy intake and output, it is also important to record the type, intensity, frequency, and duration of exercise. In addition, one should determine whether there are other ways in which energy is expended without qualifying as "exercise." For example, walking to and from school while carrying a heavy book bag, bounding repeatedly up and down stairs at home to "get something," or "stretching" twice a day all add to the daily expenditure of calories, but generally go unmeasured. Again, parents may need to be actively involved in this aspect of monitoring as well, because patients tend to underestimate either the intensity or duration of their activity.[17]

Energy Intake and Needs

The measurement of metabolic rate by indirect calorimetry can be helpful in determining the metabolic needs of the patient. This allows the expected decrease in resting energy expenditure (REE) that occurs with starvation as well as the increase in REE that occurs with refeeding to be monitored. Measurement of REE is not widely available, so an estimate of energy needs is usually required, generally between 2000 and 3000 kcal/day, sometimes more.[18] When patients ask how many calories they need to eat, it may be helpful to remind them that a calorie is a unit of energy required to raise the temperature of 1 cm^3 of water by 1°C. By emphasizing to patients that food provides their body with energy and heat, it may become easier to increase their energy intake. Patients who have a high level of anxiety or who engage in "fidgeting" (formally known as "nonexercise activity thermogenesis") appear to need a much higher energy intake than calculated by REE or mathematic formula. Thus, the answer to the question of "how many calories are needed to gain weight" is "enough to cover the amount that are expended each day, plus an additional amount for new tissue."

Vitamins and Minerals

Elevated plasma concentrations of retinol (the primary form of vitamin A in plasma) and retinyl esters (a transient form of vitamin A associated with chylomicrons) in anorexia nervosa have been reported by some investigators. These changes are not typical of protein-energy malnutrition and may be attributable to altered metabolism (closely related to low triiodothyronine concentrations) or delayed clearance of chylomicrons. It is not clear why adolescents with anorexia nervosa have a tendency to become hypercarotenemic. The intake of beta-carotene can be quite high in patients whose diet consists largely of yellow vegetables. However, Rock and Curran-Celentano[15] pointed out that elevated plasma carotenoid concentrations in anorexia nervosa may also indicate a diminished ability to clear or metabolize these compounds. There is little evidence for these increased concentrations posing a risk of hypervitaminosis A, however.

Investigators have reported increased, decreased, and normal plasma concentrations of tocopherol in anorexia nervosa. Because vitamin E is known to be associated with lipoproteins, concentrations may reflect the effects of binding to blood lipids rather than tissue concentrations. Vitamin E deficiency has been related to cognitive and neuropsychological problems, even though there is no consistent pattern of deficiency yet recognized. Further investigation is required to elucidate the circumstances in which alteration of vitamin E status might be expected. Deficiencies of thiamin, riboflavin, and vitamin B_6 may also contribute to cognitive problems and physiological features associated with semistarvation in many patients with anorexia nervosa. The dietary requirements for these vitamins are determined by substrate utilization, the severity of malnutrition, the refeeding process, and the stage of recovery. Measurements of blood concentrations are of little clinical use unless the history and physical examination suggest the presence of a specific deficiency.

The primary minerals that are of concern in anorexia nervosa are calcium and zinc.[14] Although calcium intake is typically much less than the Recommended Dietary Allowance, serum concentrations are usually normal and urinary excretion is often increased. This may be attributable to the resorption of bone that commonly occurs in association with the low estrogen and high cortisol concentrations typically found in patients with anorexia nervosa. There is little evidence that variation in calcium intake has measurable effects on bone density over the short term, possibly because the high resorptive state makes skeletal calcium available, even if dietary calcium is reduced. On the other hand, adequate calcium and vitamin D need to be included in the daily intake, because it is impossible to predict how long the patient will engage in the dysfunctional eating habits. Ideally, this should be in the form of high nutritional-value foods and beverages, including dairy products. The American Academy of Pediatrics recommends that if a patient relies on calcium-fortified foods or nondairy foods that are low in vitamin D, then another source of vitamin D is needed to provide the adequate intake of 200 IU/day (5 µg/day).[15] For example, orange juice can also be fortified with both calcium and vitamin D. Calcium intake is of concern for all female adolescents, because only 10% of them achieve the recommended adequate dietary intake of calcium of 1300 mg/day. The most commonly available calcium supplements contain 300 to 600 mg of elemental calcium per tablet but should also contain vitamin D to optimize absorption of calcium.[15,19]

Zinc is known to be lost in catabolic states such as occurs in anorexia nervosa, but serum concentrations are difficult to measure and interpret; balance studies are probably more useful clinically than are serum concentrations. There is also theoretic evidence to consider zinc deficiency as possibly related to some of the symptoms of anorexia nervosa but little evidence to suggest that it is clinically relevant. A double-blind, placebo-controlled clinical trial of zinc supplementation demonstrated improvement in some psychological functioning but no effect on weight gain. Furthermore, it is important to note that excessive zinc supplementation can cause copper deficiency.

Daily Structure

The daily structure should include eating 3 meals a day.[9] Eating an adequate breakfast (not merely a rice cake) maximizes the likelihood of adequate daily caloric intake and deserves repeated emphasis. If approximately half of the daily energy requirement is not consumed by the end of lunch, patients tend to put off eating until late in the day and find themselves unable to consume adequate nutrition without binge eating. The consequence of eating an insufficient amount of food at meals will be failure to gain weight, which will elicit responses by the treatment team, which should include the parents, who can ensure that healthy food is available and that mealtimes are planned into the day. Although parents should avoid becoming the "food police," the importance of their role in ensuring adequate caloric intake cannot be overestimated. Parents need to avoid battles that cannot be won. Likewise, if the adolescent acquiesces and eats merely to please parents, there is the possibility that purging will develop as a means of avoiding weight gain after being "forced" to eat. Specific guides are now available to assist parents in developing a daily structure.[17]

Nutrition Prescription

"Food is medicine" needs to be a central theme in the treatment of eating disorders. The initial caloric prescription is generally between 1000 and 1400 kcal/day, although the use of 130% of REE as determined by indirect calorimetry or adjusted Harris-Benedict equation are more precise methods of determining actual resting energy requirements. These values need to be adjusted for estimated energy expenditure in daily activity, especially for adolescents involved in sports or vigorous physical exercise. The nutrition prescription should work toward gradually increasing weight at the rate of about 0.5 to 1 lb/week, by increasing energy intake at 100- to 200-kcal increments every few days. In addition, the gradual inclusion of "forbidden foods" should be part of the nutrition prescription once the adolescent has shown evidence of being able to eat adequately to gain weight. A standard nutritional balance of 15% to 20% protein, 55% to 60% carbohydrate, and 20% to 25% fat is appropriate. However, the fat content may need to be lowered to 15% to 20% early in treatment because of continued fat phobia.

Rock and Curran-Celentano note that if refeeding is accomplished with an increasing energy-containing diet consisting of a variety of regular foods, sufficient amounts of vitamins and minerals will be provided, so correction of deficiencies without supplementation is anticipated.[16] Treating the nutritional problems with nutrient-dense foods will also help to correct the multitude of metabolic and physiological abnormalities associated with semistarvation in addition to reversing specific micronutrient deficiencies. Low-dose multiple vitamins with minerals at Recommended Dietary Allowances may be appropriate for chronically ill adolescents who are unable to maintain adequate nutrition. On the other hand, the use of high-dose supplements can have unfavorable effects either through excessive concentrations of the micronutrient itself or through adverse interactions with other elements (such as occurs between zinc and copper).

Nutrition-Specific Issues

It is useful to remind the patient of the physical evidence that nutrition is inadequate (low body temperature, pulse, and blood pressure; orthostatic cardiovascular changes and dizziness; and cold, blue hands and feet) when discussing meal planning. Emphasizing food as fuel for the body, the source of energy in our daily lives grounds the goal of increasing a patient's energy level, endurance, and strength in the need for food. It is also important to recognize cognitive distortions of adolescents with anorexia nervosa. Examples include dichotomous, all-or-none thinking; overgeneralization; jumping to conclusions; catastrophizing; emotional reasoning; personalization; and the use of "should" statements. These generate behaviors such as classifying down into "good" or "bad" categories, having a day "ruined" because of one unexpected event, or choosing foods based on rigid restrictions rather than personal desires or wishes. In combination with the perfectionism that characterizes adolescents with anorexia nervosa, cognitive patterns can lead to extreme levels of fat restriction (<5 g/day) or strict vegetarianism or a totally vegan diet. These dietary patterns are almost always related to limitation or elimination of fat, although their "health" benefits are most commonly touted by patients.

Finally, delayed gastric emptying occurs with malnutrition, leading to early satiety and fullness with small meals. Although this generally abates with a few weeks of healthy eating, it can preclude adequate nutrition, especially if low-calorie foods and drinks continue to be ingested. Therefore, frequent, small meals that are high in carbohydrates, starting early in the day can be helpful. Some patients find liquid nutritional supplements helpful, because they occupy a small volume and have more rapid transit time than solid food. Prokinetic agents, such as metoclopramide, can be used if these symptoms are debilitating but may be associated with limiting adverse effects.

Hospitalization

Some health care professionals include falling below a predetermined minimum weight as an indication for hospitalization for an adolescent with moderate anorexia nervosa. Low weight is only one index of malnutrition.[1,7] Weight should not be used as the sole criterion for admission to the hospital. Most adolescents with moderate anorexia nervosa realize the wisdom in the adage "a pint is a pound the world around." They may drink fluids or hide heavy objects in their underwear before a "weigh-in" if weight, alone, determines hospital admission. This may result in acute hyponatremia or dangerous degrees of unrecognized weight loss. A focus on health that includes a physical examination and consideration of body temperature, pulse, blood pressure, and orthostatic cardiovascular changes generally is more physiologically defensible than an arbitrary minimum. However, some patients need to know a concrete minimum threshold to avoid hospitalization. Increasing emphasis on, and availability of, more intensive outpatient service models, such as partial hospitalization programs, can help patients and parents avoid inpatient hospitalization. Partial hospitalization programs typically (1) operate 6 to 8 hours a day, 4 to 5 days a week; (2) ensure that patients take in adequate calories; (3) preclude dysfunctional habits, such as vomiting or compulsive exercise; (4) provide the patient with new knowledge, skills, and positive experiences with eating; and (5) engage patients in developing alternative coping skills based on group processes.

Energy Needs and Dietary Prescription for Hospitalized Patients

Most adolescents with severe anorexia nervosa who are hospitalized require at least 1500 kcal/day to maintain weight. Their reduced basal metabolic rate may be as low as 800 to 1000 kcal/day, and maintenance requirements are 130% to 150% of basal metabolic rate. Approximately 1 g of weight is gained for every 5 kcal of intake in excess of output; to accrue 100 additional g of weight requires an excess of 500 kcal. At low weight, few calories are expended in exercise than at higher weights; even with 1 hour of vigorous exercise, the patient expends ≤400 kcal. If an adolescent appears to eat >3500 kcal daily and still does not gain weight, it is likely that food is being vomited or discarded or that unrecognized exercise is occurring. Younger patients require slightly more energy to gain weight than do older patients, because some of their intake is allocated to growth.

In prescribing an initial caloric intake, the health care professional must recognize that gaining weight is frightening and that patients who demonstrate decreased metabolic rate (hypothermia, bradycardia, hypotension, and lethargy) may gain weight more readily than physiologically stable individuals. Initial weight gain can be rapid for 3 reasons. First, many malnourished adolescents are hypovolemic and gain weight in the form of extracellular fluid. Second, their basal metabolic rate can be half of normal. This reduction in energy expenditure enables calories ingested to exceed calories expended even at low levels of intake, resulting in weight gain in the form of body tissues. Third, these newly formed tissues are two thirds lean, not entirely fat as presumed by most patients, regardless of the protein content of the diet. It requires much less energy to produce protein-rich lean tissue than it does to produce fat-rich storage tissue (that is formed in quantity only after restoration of the lean body mass). Thus, more weight is gained initially for each excess calorie over expenditure than will be gained later as the patient approaches normal weight and body composition.

Therefore, although the daily requirement may eventually exceed 2500 kcal, one should not attempt to prescribe an increase of more than 50% over current average daily intakes of energy. Not only is the patient unlikely to respond favorably to a "normal" diet, but also it is unnecessary and can be physically and psychologically dangerous if the patient gains weight too quickly. Parents, especially, need to recognize that "more" is not necessarily "better" with respect to eating and weight gain. By focusing on a gradual, monitored increased intake, the health care professional can often lessen the adolescent's resistance to changing her eating habits.

The minimal daily caloric intake can begin at approximately 1000 to 1200 kcal but may need to be lower if the patient was ingesting only a few hundred kcal/day before admission. Intake is increased, as necessary, at 250- to 500-kcal increments every 2 days. In severely malnourished patients, fluid retention, congestive heart failure,[20] hypophosphatemia[21] and other manifestations of the "refeeding syndrome" can occur with too rapid replacement. Rarely is it advisable to decrease the daily caloric minimum once it is established at a higher level. Only if the patient has demonstrated consistent weight gain not attributable to fluid should lowering energy intake be considered.

Food Choices

Adolescents with anorexia nervosa typically agonize obsessively over decisions relating to choosing and consuming food, because eating means they will disappoint themselves by "giving in," but not eating means they will disappoint those they want to please. Therefore, they should be allowed ≤10 minutes to make menu selections and ≤30 minutes to complete a meal.

If the patient is unable to choose sufficient food within the 10-minute allotment, additional foods are chosen by the dietitian. If the patient does not clear a food tray within the 30-minute allotment, the tray can be removed, and the uneaten portions can be returned at the next meal time or replaced with fresh food. Alternatively, the balance of energy needs for the meal can be taken as a liquid supplement. In extremely resistant cases in which the medical stability of the patient is tenuous, that nutrition may need to be supplied via nasogastric tube or by parenteral nutrition.[22] Attempts to increase appetite with medications, such as with cyproheptadine or olanzapine, are generally not supported by data.[23,24] Likewise, selective serotonin reuptake inhibitors have not been found to be effective in low-weight anorexia nervosa,[25] and pharmacotherapy is not recommended unless also combined with adequate nutrition.[26] Selective serotonin reuptake inhibitors are approved for use in bulimia nervosa but often need to be taken at higher doses (≥60 mg) than generally prescribed in routine pediatric practice,[27] and their prescription should be overseen by a physician experienced in the treatment of eating disorders.

References

1. Rome ES, Ammerman S, Rosen DS, et al. Children and adolescents with eating disorders: the state of the art. *Pediatrics*. 2003;111(1):e98–e108. Available at: http://pediatrics.aappublications.org/cgi/content/full/111/1/e98. Accessed October 1, 2007

2. American Dietetic Association. Position of the American Dietetic Association: nutrition intervention in the treatment of anorexia nervosa, bulimia nervosa, and eating disorders not otherwise specified (EDNOS). *J Am Diet Assoc*. 2001;101:810–819

3. van der Ster Wallin G, Norring C, Lennemas MA, Holmgren S. Food selection in anorectics and bulimics: food items, nutrient content and nutrient density. *J Am Coll Nutr*. 1995;14:271–277

4. Comerci GD. Eating disorders in adolescents. *Pediatr Rev*. 1988;10:37–47

5. Levenkron S. *Anatomy of Anorexia*. New York, NY: W. W. Norton & Co; 2000

6. Lock J, le Grange D. Family-based treatment of eating disorders. *Int J Eating Disord*. 2005;37(Suppl):S64–S67

7. American Academy of Pediatrics, Committee on Adolescence. Identifying and treating eating disorders. *Pediatrics*. 2003;111:204–211

8. Bulik CM. Exploring the gene-environment nexus in eating disorders. *J Psychiatry Neurosci*. 2005;30:335–339

9. Kreipe RE, Dukarm CP. Eating disorders in adolescents and older children. *Pediatr Rev*. 1999;20:410–420

10. Keys A, Brozek J, Henschel A. *The Biology of Human Starvation*. Minneapolis, MN: University of Minnesota Press; 1950

11. Powell LA, Nieman DC, Melby C, et al. Assessment of body composition change in a community-based weight management program. *J Am Coll Nutr.* 2001;20:26–31

12. Forbes GB, Kreipe RE, Lipinski BA, Hodgman CH. Body composition changes during recovery from anorexia nervosa: comparison of two dietary regimes. *Am J Clin Nutr.* 1984;40:1137–1145

13. Scalfi L, Marra M, Caldara A, Silvestri E, Contaldo F. Changes in bioimpedance analysis after stable refeeding of undernourished anorexic patients. *Int J Obes Relat Metab Disord.* 1999;23:133–137

14. Hadigan CM, Anderson EJ, Miller KK, et al. Assessment of macronutrient and micronutrient intake in women with anorexia nervosa. *Int J Eat Disord.* 2000;28:284–292

15. Greer FR, Krebs NF, American Academy of Pediatrics, Committee on Nutrition. Optimizing bone health and calcium intakes of infants, children, and adolescents. *Pediatrics.* 2006;117:578–585

16. Rock CL. Curran-Celentano J. Nutritional management of eating disorders. *Psychiatr Clinic North Am.* 1996;19:701–713

17. Lock J, LeGrange D. *Help Your Teenager Beat an Eating Disorder.* New York, NY: Guilford Press; 2005

18. Melchior JC. From malnutrition to refeeding during anorexia nervosa. *Curr Opin Clin Nutr Metab Care.* 1998;1:481–485

19. Marcason W. Nutrition therapy and eating disorders: what is the correct calorie level for clients with anorexia? *J Am Diet Assoc.* 2002;102:644

20. Kohn MR, Golden NH, Shenker IR. Cardiac arrest and delirium: presentations of the refeeding syndrome in severely malnourished adolescents with anorexia nervosa. *J Adolesc Health.* 1998;22:239–243

21. Fisher M, Simpser E. Schneider M. Hypophosphaternia secondary to oral refeeding in anorexia nervosa. *Int J Eat Disord.* 2000;28:181–187

22. Mehler PS, Weiner KA. Treatment of anorexia nervosa with total parenteral nutrition. *Nutr Clin Pract.* 1995;10:183–187

23. Halmi KA, Eckert E, LaDu TH, Cohen J. Anorexia nervosa: treatment efficacy of cyproheptadine and amitriptyline. *Arch General Psychiatry.* 1986;43:177–181

24. Malina A, Gaskill J, McConaha C, et al. Olanzapine treatment of anorexia nervosa: a retrospective study. *Int J Eat Disord.* 2003;33:234–237

25. Ferguson CP, La Via MC, Crossan PJ. Kaye WH. Are serotonin selective reuptake inhibitors effective in underweight anorexia nervosa? *Int J Eat Disord.* 1999;25:11–17

26. Casper RC. How useful are pharmacological treatments in eating disorders? *Psychopharmacol Bull.* 2002;36:88–104

27. Pederson KJ, Roerig JL, Mitchell JE. Towards the pharmacotherapy of eating disorders. *Expert Opin Pharmacother.* 2003;4:1659–1678

Nutrition of Children With HIV-1 Infection

Infection with human immunodeficiency virus (HIV) is a worldwide problem of increasing magnitude. The World Health Organization estimates that 34.6 to 42.3 million adults and children were living with HIV infection in 2005, the majority of whom were in developing countries.[1] In 2005, the cause of death worldwide in up to 670 000 children 0 through 14 years of age was attributed to HIV or acquired immunodeficiency syndrome (AIDS).[1] Although the number of individuals infected with HIV has increased, the number of children dying of AIDS has remained essentially unchanged in the last 5 years because of expanded use of antiretroviral therapy and improved prophylactic regimens worldwide. In industrialized nations, HIV infection has become a chronic illness as highly active antiretroviral therapy (HAART) has become the mainstay of treatment. With the increasing number of children surviving with HIV infection and AIDS, the need for appropriate supportive care is paramount. Health care professionals who care for children with HIV or AIDS should be aware of potential nutritional problems and their consequences. In the past, wasting syndrome was the primary nutritional concern for HIV-infected individuals. Now, nearly 10 years since the advent of HAART, we are facing new and different nutritional issues. Knowledge and implementation of effective nutritional therapies are important to improve medical outcomes and quality of life. With appropriate combination of antiretroviral therapy and nutritional support, many HIV-infected children are now able to lead relatively normal lives.

Wasting Syndrome

During the early 1980s, AIDS was first recognized in Africa as an epidemic and was initially termed "slim disease," because people in Uganda were dying of severe malnutrition for otherwise unknown reasons.[2] Eventually, HIV, the virus causing AIDS, was discovered. Wasting is included as one of the principle criteria for the diagnosis of severely symptomatic AIDS (category C, Table 39.1).[3]

Although the prevalence of AIDS and AIDS-associated wasting have declined in the industrialized world as a result of advances in antiretroviral therapy, wasting is still of significant concern for children in both industrialized and developing nations. The Centers for Disease Control and Prevention (CDC)[3] defines wasting in children younger than 13 years as: (1) persistent weight loss of more than 10% of baseline; (2) downward crossing of at least 2 percentile lines on the weight-for-age chart in a child 1 year or older; or (3) being at less than the 5th percentile on weight-for-height or body mass index (BMI) charts on 2 consecutive measurements at least 30 days apart, plus chronic diarrhea or documented fever for at least 30 days, whether intermittent or constant.

Table 39.1
Pediatric Criteria for Diagnosis of AIDS*

Immunologic Category, by Evidence of Suppression	Clinical Category, by Symptom Severity			
	N, None	A, Mild	B, Moderate	C, Severe
1. None	N1	A1	B1	C1
2. Moderate	N2	A2	B2	C2
3. Severe	N3	A3	B3	C3

* Centers for Disease Control and Prevention classification system of human HIV infection in children younger than 13 years (revised 1994). Children born to HIV-infected women and whose status is not confirmed are classified by using the above grid with a letter E (for perinatally exposed) placed before the appropriate classification code (eg, EN2). From Centers for Disease Control and Prevention.[3]

The relationship between protein-energy malnutrition (PEM) and adverse effects on the immune system, resulting in immune deficiency states, has been recognized for many years.[4] Table 39.2 lists the differences and similarities between the effects of PEM and HIV infection on the immune system. On a basic level, PEM may exacerbate the immunologic effects of HIV infection. Epidemiologic studies of both adult and pediatric patients with HIV infection suggest that nutritional status can independently affect quality of life and survival, in part because of the deleterious effect of malnutrition on immune function. Wasting is related to length of survival.[5,6] Weight loss has been associated with increased infectious complications in patients with AIDS. Conversely, HIV infection and its complications have been associated with nutritional disorders. Higher HIV viral load has been associated with a greater risk of growth failure.[7,8] In addition, other factors, such as lower CD4 T-lymphocyte counts; infectious complications, such as pneumonia; maternal drug use during pregnancy; lower infant CD4+ T-lymphocyte count; and exposure to antiretroviral therapy (nonprotease inhibitor), have been associated with growth problems.[9,10]

A variety of disturbed growth patterns, most noted in the pre-HAART era, have been described for HIV-infected children,[9–14] ranging from symmetric delays in weight and height to severe wasting with normal height. The differences in growth patterns are likely attributable to the variable manifestations of the disease in HIV-infected children, associated with factors such as viral load and infections, as mentioned previously. In industrialized countries in the pre-HAART era, HIV-infected children showed declines in both weight and length as early as the first 1 to 3 months of life. Sequential follow-up showed that growth of HIV-infected children remained below that in age- and gender-matched uninfected children. However, fetuses are now treated prenatally with antiretroviral medications[15] given to the mother during the second or third trimester of pregnancy to decrease the risk of transmission of HIV from mother to infant. This intervention has caused transmission rates to decrease to less than 2%.[16,17]

Table 39.2

Comparison of Body Composition, Energy Expenditure, and Immunologic Function in Protein-Energy Malnutrition (PEM), Sepsis, and HIV Infection

Condition	Body Composition	Energy Expenditure	Immune Function
PEM (starvation)	Decreased fat leading to decreased lean body mass	Decreased	Decreased white blood cell count, cell-mediated immunity, and T-lymphocyte function; decreased immunoglobulin (Ig) A and E; increased or decreased IgG
Sepsis	Decreased lean body mass leading to decreased fat	Increased	Activated (effective)
HIV	Decreased lean body mass leading to decreased fat	Unchanged to increased according to severity of infection	Increased IgG; decreased CD4 T-lymphocyte count and function

Several pediatric studies in the pre-HAART era have shown progressive decreases in lean body mass over time in children with HIV or AIDS, and measures of fat stores remained constant, yet low.[11,12] There is conflicting literature on whether there is more of a pattern of cachexia (preferential wasting of muscle over fat) or normal weight loss with initial loss of fat over lean body mass[18,19] in adults with HIV or AIDS. Cytokines may be responsible for some of the growth and metabolic and immunologic effects associated with HIV infection,[20] and there are positive changes in cytokine patterns after HAART therapy.[21]

Causes of Malnutrition in HIV and AIDS

In general, malnutrition and its consequences are more common in the child in whom AIDS is diagnosed. Malnutrition in children with HIV or AIDS may be attributable to several mechanisms working independently or synergistically. These causes are summarized in Table 39.3. Insufficient consumption of nutrients is a factor that may lead to undernutrition. A variety of potential factors may lead to abnormal intake, as outlined in Table 39.3. For example, inflammation and ulcers of the upper gastrointestinal tract can lead to anorexia as a result of odynophagia, dysphagia, or abdominal pain that is associated with eating. In a series in the pre-HAART era, 70% of upper gastrointestinal tract endoscopies in HIV-infected children revealed histologic abnormalities.[22] These lesions can be attributable to peptic injury or infectious pathogens, such as *Candida albicans*, cytomegalovirus, or herpes simplex virus, all of which may cause inflammation and pain with swallowing or after eating. Furthermore, oral ulcers that are attributable to viral pathogens or "idiopathic" oral ulcers[23] are common and may cause pain with eating and reduce oral intake. These opportunistic upper intestinal conditions are unusual in children who have a CD4 T-lymphocyte frequency of greater than 15%.[24]

Pancreatic and biliary tract disease can also cause vomiting and abdominal pain in HIV-infected children leading to poor oral intake. Pancreatic disease has been linked to medications (eg, pentamidine, 2', 3'-dideoxyinosine [ddI], sulfa medications, some protease inhibitors [Table 39.4]) and opportunistic infections (eg, cytomegalovirus, *Cryptosporidium* species, and mycobacterial disease).[25,26] Biliary tract disease with sclerosing cholangitis and papillary stenosis has been linked to *Cryptosporidium* species, cytomegalovirus, and *Microsporidia* species.[27,28] Primary anorexia, described in patients with cancer and other chronic conditions, may also contribute to inadequate oral intake. It is postulated that increased cytokine production (eg, tumor necrosis factor, interferon-gamma, and interleukins 1 and 6) may be associated with anorexia.[29] In animal models, administration of exogenous tumor-necrosis factor has produced anorexia and cachexia.[30] Tumor necrosis factor also causes delayed gastric emptying, which can increase anorexia as well.[31] The scientific data that implicate these cytokines as mediators of anorexia are controversial.[32]

Human immunodeficiency virus encephalopathy, which could be present in up to 16% of children with HIV infection in the pre-HAART era[33] yet has lower prevalence rates with successful viral suppression,[34] may result in the physical inability to consume enough calories to sustain growth. Oral administration of feedings under this condition may also be dangerous because of the high risk of aspiration in neurologically compromised children. Finally, many medications that HIV-infected children are required to take may result in gastric irritation, vomiting, nausea, and diarrhea. These medications are listed in Table 39.4.

Table 39.3
Causes of Nutritional Deficiencies and Wasting in HIV and AIDS*

1. Decreased nutrient intake
Primary anorexia
Peptic disease
Opportunistic infections of upper gastrointestinal tract (*Candida* species, cytomegalovirus, herpes simplex virus)*
Idiopathic aphthous ulcers
Dysgeusia (zinc deficiency)
Pancreatic/hepatobiliary disease
Encephalopathy
2. Malabsorption
Mucosal disease
Infectious*
Inflammatory
Disaccharidase deficiency
Protein-losing enteropathy
Fat malabsorption
Hepatobiliary
Sclerosing cholangitis
Chronic pancreatitis
Coinfection with hepatitis B or hepatitis C virus
3. Increased nutritional requirements or tissue catabolism
Protein wasting
Hypermetabolism/related to degree of immune suppression
Futile metabolic cycling
Secondary to:
Fever, infections, sepsis*
Neoplasms (Kaposi sarcoma, lymphoma)*
Medications
Release of catabolic factors (cytokines)
4. Psychosocial factors
Poverty
Illness in biologic family members
Limited access to health care
Substance abuse

*These causes are more common in children with CD4 T-lymphocyte frequencies of <15%.

V

Differences have been demonstrated in total energy intake between HIV-infected and -uninfected children, suggesting that substandard intakes may relate to growth differences.[8] However, a large prospective study has shown that stable, HIV-infected children in an ambulatory setting whose growth was below that of a control group received well over the Recommended Dietary Allowance (RDA) in total calories and protein, similar to the uninfected control children.[35] In this study, however, even in this group of infected children, a higher intake of nutrients was associated with improvement in weight and fat mass, a finding confirmed in at least one other study.[36] Intake of critical immune-modulating micronutrients, such as iron, vitamin C, and vitamin A, have been shown to be low in the earlier stages of HIV infection in adolescents.[37]

Malabsorption may also contribute to malnutrition. The etiology of malabsorption is multifactorial but includes gastrointestinal mucosal abnormalities leading to macro- and micronutrient malabsorption. These mucosal changes can be attributable to local HIV infection of the gut or secondary enteric infections. There is evidence that certain gastrointestinal epithelial cells bind and selectively transfer HIV from the cells' apical to basolateral surface, where viral translocation across the epithelium encounters lamina propria macrophages and T-lymphocytes.[38,39] As a result of either local HIV infection (that induces proinflammatory changes in the gastrointestinal mucosa) or of the damage caused by a secondary infection, mucosal function is compromised, with resulting malabsorption. Because of the difficulty in treating many of these infections, the diarrhea may be unremitting and predispose to the severe malnutrition that may lead to eventual mortality, especially in developing nations.

The evaluation of diarrhea in patients with AIDS yields a specific cause in 50% to 85% of patients, with most being effectively treated.[40] The nonspecific AIDS enteropathy[41] may be attributable, in part, to undiagnosed infections or to HIV infection itself (secondary to inflammatory changes induced by HIV in mucosal lymphocytes).[42] Several investigators have reported impaired carbohydrate, fat, and protein absorption in children with HIV or AIDS[43,44]; the extent of malabsorption is not always correlated with the degree of malnutrition.[43]

In addition to nutrient losses as a result of diarrhea, gastrointestinal bleeding attributable to mucosal ulcerations leads to loss of nutrients with the loss of blood. Opportunistic infections affect the hepatobiliary system and pancreas in addition to the gastrointestinal tract and may lead to malabsorption. The site and severity of infection vary according to the infecting organism (Table 39.5).

Table 39.4
Medications and Common Gastrointestinal Adverse Effects

Class/Medication	Adverse Effects
Nucleoside/nucleotide analogue reverse transcriptase inhibitors (NRTIs/NtRTIs) Abacavir (ABC, Ziagen*) Didanosine (ddl, Videx†) Emtricitabine (FTC, Emtriva‡) Lamivudine (3TC, Epivir*) Stavudine (d4T, Zerit†) Tenofovir (TDF, Viread‡) Zalcitabine (ddC, Hivid§) Zidovudine (ZDV, AZT, Retrovir*)	**Class:** nausea, vomiting, abdominal pain, diarrhea, pancreatitis, abnormal liver function tests; rare severe hepatomegaly acidosis with hepatic steatosis
Nonnucleoside analogue reverse transcriptase inhibitors (NNRTIs) Delavirdine (DLV, Rescriptor‖) Efavirenz (EFV, Sustiva†) Nevirapine (NVP, Viramune¶)	**Class:** nausea, vomiting, abnormal liver enzymes
Protease inhibitors (PIs) Amprenavir (APV, Agenerase*) Atazanavir (ATV, Reyataz†) Fosamprenavir (f-APV, Lexiva*) Indinavir (IDV, Crixivan#) Lopinavir/Ritonavir (LPV/RTV, Kaletra**) Nelfinavir (NFV, Viracept‖) Ritonavir (RTV, Norvir**) Saquinavir (SQV, Invirase§, Fortovase§) Tipranavir (TPV, Aptivus¶)	**Class:** nausea, vomiting, diarrhea, fatigue, stomatitis, abnormal liver enzymes, interactions with other drugs metabolized by liver, hypertriglyceridemia, hyperlipidemia (except Atazanavir) **Specific:** Atazanavir: increased unconjugated bilirubin concentrations, jaundice; Indinavir: hyperbilirubinemia; Ritonavir: pancreatitis; Saquinavir: dyspepsia; Tipranavir: elevated amylase
Fusion inhibitors Enfuvirtide (T-20, Fuzeon§)	Nausea, vomiting, elevated liver enzymes, all as part of rare hypersensitivity reaction

* GlaxoSmithKline, Research Triangle Park, NC.
‖ Pfizer, New York, NY.
† Bristol-Myers Squibb, New York, NY.
¶ Boehringer Ingelheim, Ridgefield, CT.
‡ Gilead Sciences, Foster City, CA.
# Merck & Co, Whitehouse Station, NJ.
§ Hoffman-La Roche, Nutley, NJ.
** Abbott Laboratories, Abbott Park, IL.

Table 39.5
Infectious Gastrointestinal Manifestations of HIV and AIDS*

Site	Manifestations or Infecting Organisms	
Oral	Candidiasis	Oral hairy leukoplakia
	HSV	Kaposi sarcoma
	Human papillomavirus	Lymphoma
Esophagus	Candidiasis	Cryptosporidiosis
	CMV	Kaposi sarcoma
	HSV	Lymphoma
Stomach	CMV	Kaposi sarcoma
	Cryptosporidiosis	Helicobacter pylori
Small intestine	Giardiasis	*Salmonella* species
	Cryptosporidiosis	Enteroaggregative *Escherichia coli*
		Blastocystis hominis
	CMV	*Isospora belli*
	Shigella species	Rotavirus, calicivirus, astrovirus, coronavirus, picornavirus
	Mycobacterium species	Adenovirus
	Lymphoma	
Colon	CMV	*Entamoeba* species
	Salmonella species	Lymphoma
	Shigella species	*Clostridium difficile*
	Campylobacter species	Adenovirus
Anus/rectum	Kaposi sarcoma	Squamous cell carcinoma
	Lymphoma	Papovavirus
Hepatobiliary	*Mycobacterium* species	Cryptosporidiosis
	CMV	Kaposi sarcoma
	Cryptococcus, histoplasmosis	Microsporida
	Hepatitis B, C, or D	
Pancreas	CMV	Cryptosporidiosis
	Mycobacterium species	

HSV indicates herpes simplex virus; CMV, cytomegalovirus.

Other nutrient deficiencies often seen in patients with AIDS-related gastrointestinal disease include vitamin B_{12}, folic acid, thiamine, zinc, selenium, calcium, and magnesium deficiencies. Fat-soluble vitamins, particularly vitamins A and D, may be malabsorbed, and deficiencies of these vitamins have been described. Fat malabsorption and protein-losing enteropathy are likely a result of severe enteritis usually caused by secondary infections. Small-bowel bacterial overgrowth, a result of gastrointestinal dysmotility or hypochlorhydria, may also predispose the individual to malabsorption. Pancreatic insufficiency is more rare, although it has been described in some HIV-infected patients.[45] Diarrhea may also be caused by antiretroviral therapy (Table 39.4), other medications (especially antibiotic agents), malignancies, and rarely, inflammatory bowel disease.

Asymptomatic chronic viral infections may have some effect on energy utilization and can predispose children to secondary infections, which can alter energy utilization patterns. These infections can increase or shunt effective use of energy substrates from normal, healthy growth patterns to abnormal ones, as in many children with chronic illness, including cystic fibrosis, inflammatory bowel disease, congenital heart disease, and cancer.[44-46] The chronic viral activity of HIV is likely no different. In small studies of energy expenditure, there are, in general, no differences in resting energy expenditure[8,36,46] or total energy expenditure[7,8] between HIV-infected children with growth failure and those with normal rates of growth. However, adults with HIV-1 infection show increasing resting energy expenditure with increasing severity of illness,[47] especially with secondary infection and more advanced HIV disease.[48,49] As HIV-infected children are treated with HAART, previously noted increases in protein catabolism decrease to more normal rates, suggesting that chronic viral activity leads to increased protein catabolism and can be brought to more normal levels with successful viral suppression.[50]

Psychosocial factors are also important contributors to suboptimal growth of HIV-infected children. An unstable home environment and inadequate emotional and social support may obviously affect growth in both HIV-infected[51] and -uninfected children.[52,53] Children with HIV infection are more likely than uninfected children to live with parents who are ill, who have limited access to social services and support, and who may have ongoing problems with substance abuse.[54] Investigators have found maternal crack and cocaine use during pregnancy to be a predictor of growth and nutritional problems for the child.[9,10] This finding is not unique for HIV infection; it has been reported in other uninfected cohorts.[55] Children born to drug-using women are often small, suggesting that drugs have a prenatal effect, but the postnatal home environment is likely to influence growth as well. Recent studies have also found that caregivers can positively or negatively influence functional status of HIV-infected children.[51]

The Nutritional Effects of HAART

Protease inhibitors are highly potent antiretroviral agents that act by selectively blocking HIV protease, an enzyme necessary for HIV replication in the later stages of virus production.[56] Studies in children suggest that protease inhibitor therapy is associated with a reduction in viral load and an increase in CD4 T-lymphocyte count,[57,58] and longitudinal studies suggest that this immune response may be sustained over time.[59] Current pediatric treatment guidelines include a protease inhibitor in the recommended combination therapy regimen for any HIV-infected child with clinical symptoms (CDC class A, B, C), immune suppression (CDC class 2, 3), or HIV RNA levels ≥100 000 copies/mL or any child younger than 1 year in whom HIV infection is diagnosed because of the high viral load during this period.[24] Thus, most children with HIV infection in industrialized countries are given these medications. The term HAART refers to a combination of antiretroviral agents, generally including a protease inhibitor, which is highly effective against HIV replication.

Over the past several years, coincident with the introduction of HAART therapy, a clinical syndrome of body fat redistribution and metabolic changes has been described initially in adults,[60] yet with increasing reports in children.[61–64] Patients infected with HIV who are receiving HAART regimens have developed a syndrome of peripheral insulin resistance, hyperlipidemia, and lipodystrophy (truncal obesity, dorsocervical fat pad, and extremity and facial wasting).[60] Clinical and biochemical abnormalities associated with the lipodystrophy syndrome are shown in Table 39.6. Risk factors associated with developing fat redistribution syndrome in adults include female gender, increasing age, and higher pretherapy body weight.[65] Complications associated with fat redistribution syndrome include higher rates of diabetes mellitus and premature cardiovascular disease.[66] Medical compliance with drug therapy may be poorer because of the cosmetic adverse effects of therapy.

Lipodystrophy has now increasingly been described in children as well.[61–64] One of the earlier studies in children with HIV infection showed that protease inhibitor therapy improves weight, weight-for-height, and mid-arm muscle circumference of HIV-infected children, independent of the concurrent decrease in HIV viral load, and improved CD4 T-lymphocyte counts.[67] Immediate treatment effects were most apparent with an improvement in weight and mid-arm muscle circumference, and there was a trend toward increased height and lean body mass. In addition to the positive improvement in growth and lean body mass, however, HAART is also associated with abnormalities in fat distribution in children. In another study, there were decreased limb-trunk fat ratios in HIV-infected children receiving HAART when compared with healthy controls.[62] These findings suggest that both peripheral lipoatrophy and central obesity occur in these children. Additional studies have shown that most children have evidence of these abnormalities in fat distribution within 3 years of initiating a protease inhibitor-containing regimen and that these changes progress over time.[63] Other studies have identified metabolic abnormalities induced by specific classes of drugs.[68] In particular, protease inhibitor therapy seems to cause more abnormalities in lipid profiles, and nonnucleoside transcriptase inhibitors may be more protective.[68,69] It is of interest that serum hyper-cholesterolemia and subsequent fat redistribution seem to be particularly pronounced during puberty, suggesting that there is an interaction with HAART and physiologic changes occurring during this time.[70]

Table 39.6
Clinical and Biochemical Abnormalities Associated With Lipodystrophy Syndrome

Clinical Features	Laboratory Features
Increased abdominal (visceral) fat	Hyperlipidemia
Increased waist-to-hip ratio (more reliable in adults)	Increased triglycerides
	Increased total cholesterol
Buffalo hump	Increased low-density lipoprotein
Fat atrophy	Decreased high-density lipoprotein
Wasting of extremities	Insulin resistance
Wasting of buttocks	Normal to increased serum glucose
Loss or thinning of facial fat, prominence of nasolabial fold	Increased insulin
	Increased C peptide
No change to increased weight	Decreased glucose tolerance/insulin resistance
Fatigue and weakness	

New evidence suggests that HIV infection also affects bone mineral density in children receiving HAART.[71,72] In a recent study, HIV-infected children had lower bone mineral density compared with age- and gender-matched controls, despite the fact that they had normal nutritional status and were not growth stunted.[73] In this group, multivitamin use positively affected bone mineral density and would be an important nutritional consideration in all HIV-infected children.

The long-term concerns of the metabolic changes that occur with HAART are the potential cardiac implications of hyperlipidemia, insulin resistance, and obesity. In adults with HAART-related fat maldistribution, several studies have suggested an increase in the risk of myocardial infarction related to duration of protease inhibitor therapy.[69,74,75] Such long-term evaluation in children is still needed, but children could be exposed to protease inhibitors for significantly longer periods over their lifetime, compared with adults, and cardiac risk factors may prove to be more pronounced at an earlier age.

There are currently no guidelines for therapeutic intervention in children with lipid abnormalities and insulin resistance. Therapeutic strategies to diminish the clinical and biochemical features of the fat redistribution syndrome in adults include oral hypoglycemic agents such as metformin[76] and troglitazone (although liver toxicity limits its use).[77] These agents have not been used extensively in children, and large-scale studies evaluating their use are not yet available. Medications to lower serum cholesterol concentration also need to be studied in children; however, caution should be exercised in prescribing lipid-lowering medications, because there may be potential interactions between these medications and antiretroviral medications.[78] It is clear, however, that interventions such as exercise and diet control can be useful,[79,80] and these should be the primary focus in children with metabolic changes at this time.

Recommendations for Nutritional Support

Wasting contributes significantly to the morbidity and mortality of patients infected with HIV. With the advent of HAART and its attendant nutritional consequences, increasing metabolic complications are likely to ensue over the years as children with HIV infection become older. The most effective role the pediatrician can play in the nutritional care of the HIV-infected child is close surveillance of nutritional and metabolic complications over time and with evolving medical therapy. Specifically, vigilant screening for lipid and metabolic abnormalities, including vascular thrombotic events, should become standard of care for all children with HIV infection. The efficacy of nutritional support in children with HIV infection and AIDS is an important ancillary treatment. A gross assessment of nutritional status can be achieved by careful monitoring of weight status (ie, weight-for-age, weight-for-height [younger than 2 years], and BMI [older than 2 years]. The very early detection of failure to gain weight allows the opportunity for prevention of malnutrition, clearly a more effective intervention approach than repletion once malnutrition or failure to thrive has occurred. In addition, changes in body composition become a very important sign of disease progression and can be determined through serial measurements of mid-arm circumference, triceps skinfold measurements, and bioelectric impedance analysis.

Enteral tube feeding can be administered in the hospital and at home to children with HIV infection and failure to thrive. Children supported with enteral nutrition show an increase in weight-for-age, weight-for-height, or BMI scores and adipose stores but no improvement in height-for-age or lean body mass over the short-term.[6,81] There is evidence that nutritional status independently predicts morbidity and mortality; children whose weight improved with gastrostomy tube feedings survived longer than those whose weight did not improve.[6] Nutrition also improves functional status.[51] The influence of socioeconomic factors on the development of wasting syndrome, HIV infection itself, and nutritional status needs to be considered and targeted, because patients from families of lower socioeconomic status who are at higher risk of nutritional and other health problems predominate among populations with HIV infection and AIDS. The influence of the socioeconomic environment on the provision of adequate nutrition may be particularly critical. Limiting factors that may be present include poor health of the caregiver because of HIV infection or AIDS, inadequate cooking facilities, poverty and limited food availability, emotional deprivation, and inexperienced parenting.

Complete data on which to base nutrition interventions for HIV-infected children are lacking. Optimal treatment to decrease viral load is important, because high viral loads are directly linked with poorer nutritional state. However, successful viral suppression is also linked to higher prevalence of metabolic abnormalities. The following are guidelines to provide optimal nutritional care of HIV-infected children.

1. *Nutrition assessment* should be performed on all patients, regardless of symptoms. This assessment should include a review of the medical and dietary history, a dietary diary with calorie count, anthropometric measurements (ie, weight, height, BMI, head circumference [younger than 3 years], mid-arm muscle circumference, and skinfold measurements [4 sites]), and measurement of baseline laboratory values (eg, complete blood cell count, albumin, prealbumin, iron, zinc, lipid profile, and absorptive tests as indicated). When inadequate weight gain or weight loss is identified, aggressive diagnostic evaluation should be pursued to detect opportunistic infections or other inflammatory lesions of the gastrointestinal tract. With clinical symptoms, an evaluation of gastroin-

testinal absorption is indicated. Treatment of underlying infections will likely improve the response to nutritional and medical management. Determining the degree and extent of gastrointestinal malabsorption will help guide dietary recommendations. With clinically evident fat redistribution syndrome, fasting serum glucose and insulin concentrations should be obtained and a homeostatic model assessment-insulin resistance score (as a marker of insulin resistance) can be calculated as fasting insulin (U/mL) × fasting glucose (mmol/L)/22.5.[82] If abnormal, an oral glucose tolerance test, hemoglobin A_1C, and C-peptide concentrations should be ascertained. If these results are abnormal, dietary and exercise advice and an oral hypoglycemic agent should be considered.

2. *Nutritional counseling* should provide guidance for patients to maintain a diet that provides the RDAs or dietary reference intakes of nutrients. The intake and dietary composition should be adjusted according to the degree of gastrointestinal dysfunction and insulin resistance and may include a low-fat, lactose-free, low-fiber, caffeine-free diet. Infants may benefit from formulas for which the caloric density has been increased by adding cereal or modular nutrient supplements (eg, glucose polymers, protein powders, medium-chain triglycerides if needed [this is an expensive supplement], and vegetable oils) or by preparing the formula at a different concentration. Patients with diarrhea may benefit from an elemental formula. Fad diet techniques, including megavitamins and amino acid supplementation, should be discouraged. Frequent nutritional assessment is necessary to determine the response to the nutritional intervention. Further recommendations should be made if the child fails to respond to a specific intervention.

3. *Specialized nutrition support* is indicated before the onset of malnutrition, because undernutrition will complicate the disease course for patients with HIV infection and AIDS. Oral nutrition supplementation is preferable. However, enteral tube feedings (eg, nasogastric or gastrostomy tube) may be necessary to provide supplemental or total nutritional support for patients with inadequate oral intake. Appropriate diagnostic studies to treat an underlying gastrointestinal tract disorder that results in inadequate intake should be performed before initiating supplemental enteral feedings. If inadequate intake is attributable to delayed feeding skills, support by a team including a speech or occupational therapist, a behavioral therapist, and a registered dietitian may be effective.

Parenteral nutrition is reserved for children in whom the enteral route is not feasible and includes those with severe malabsorption, gastrointestinal dysfunction attributable to infection or dysmotility, and pancreatitis. Parenteral nutrition should not be instituted with an ongoing disseminated infection.

4. *Vitamin and mineral supplementation* should be provided so the dietary intake of vitamins and minerals is 1 to 5 times the RDA. Megadoses (10 times the RDA) are discouraged. Routine monitoring and supplementation of selected micronutrients (calcium, vitamin A, vitamin E, folate, vitamin B_{12}, iron, zinc) are recommended.

5. *Nutritional appetite stimulants and growth hormone* may be useful in selected patients. Megestrol acetate should not be used in children who have documented insulin resistance, because this therapy may exacerbate it. Growth hormone may be useful in the preadolescent whose growth is significantly stunted, although it is unclear whether overall adult height ultimately will be improved.

6. *Drug-nutrient interactions* should be considered. In addition, many of the antiretroviral drugs and medications used to treat illness or symptoms related to HIV infection may cause nausea, anorexia, abdominal pain, diarrhea, dry mouth, and alterations in taste. The adverse effects of medications and their administration schedules on intake should be considered.

7. *A nutrition support team* should be involved to ensure optimal nutrition monitoring and care. A core team of a physician, a nurse-specialist, a nutritionist, and a social worker collaborating with other health care professionals offers the best opportunity to achieve optimal nutritional health for individual patients.

8. *Metabolic complications of HAART* should be carefully evaluated and monitored. As HAART has been in use for nearly 10 years, lipodystrophy, insulin resistance, hyperlipidemia, abnormalities in bone mineral density, metabolic syndrome, and frank obesity will become more evident. Children receiving HAART will be overall healthier and will also be affected by the epidemic obesity seen in general today. Routine evaluation of lipid profiles, insulin concentrations, and dual energy x-ray absorptiometry measurements should be performed. Exercise regimens and appropriate nutritional counseling targeting metabolic problems should be implemented early on.

Conclusion

The cause of nutritional problems in children with HIV infection is complex and likely multifactorial. Although the incidence of malnutrition in industrialized countries has decreased with the advent of HAART therapy, a significant number of children continue to have problems with malnutrition and gastrointestinal dysfunction. However, greater numbers of children with HIV infection, who now have better viral suppression because of effective HIV therapies, are suffering from increasing rates of obesity, lipodystrophy, hyperlipidemia, and prediabetes and diabetic conditions and are at risk of developing sequelae associated with these problems. Optimal nutritional support includes complete nutritional assessment and follow-up of every child and adolescent with HIV infection or AIDS. The long-term metabolic and cardiac complications of HAART will shape nutritional issues in HIV-infected children in industrialized nations in the future.

References

1. Joint United Nations Programme on HIV/AIDS. Report on the global HIV/AIDS epidemic 2006. Geneva, Switzerland: UNAIDS; 2006. Available at: www.unaids.org. Accessed October 2, 2007

2. Serwadda D, Mugerwa RD, Sewankambo NK, et al. Slim disease: a new disease in Uganda and its association with HTLV-III infection. *Lancet.* 1985;2:849–852

3. Centers for Disease Control and Prevention. 1994 revised classification system for human immunodeficiency virus infection in children less than 13 years of age. *MMWR Morb Mortal Wkly Rep.* 1994;43(RR–12):1–10

4. Chandra RK, Kumari S. Nutrition and immunity: an overview. *J Nutr.* 1994;124(Suppl 8): 1433S–1435S

5. Carey VJ, Yong FH, Frenkel LM, McKinney RE Jr. Pediatric AIDS prognosis using somatic growth velocity. *AIDS.* 1998;12:1361–1369

6. Miller TL, Awnetwant EL, Evans S, Morris VM, Vazquez IM, McIntosh K. Gastrostomy tube supplementation for HIV-infected children. *Pediatrics.* 1995;96:696–702

7. Johann-Liang R, O'Neill L, Cervia J, et al. Energy balance, viral burden, insulin-like growth factor-1, interleukin-6 and growth impairment in children infected with human immunodeficiency virus. *AIDS.* 2000;14:683–690

8. Arpadi SM, Cuff PA, Kotler DP, et al. Growth velocity, fat-free mass and energy intake are inversely related to viral load in HIV-infected children. *J Nutr.* 2000;130:2498–2502

9. Moye J, RichK C, Kalish LA, et al. Natural history of somatic growth in infants born to women infected by human immunodeficiency virus. Women and Infants Transmission Study Group. *J Pediatr.* 1996;128:58–69

10. Miller TL, Easley KA, Zhang W, et al. Maternal and infant factors associated with failure to thrive in children with vertically transmitted human immunodeficiency virus-1 infection: the prospective P2C2 human immunodeficiency virus multicenter study. *Pediatrics.* 2001;108:1287–1296

11. Miller TL, Evans SJ, Orav EJ, McIntosh K, Winter HS. Growth and body composition in children infected with the human immunodeficiency virus-1. *Am J Clin Nutr.* 1993;57:588–592

12. Arpadi SM, Horlick MN, Wang J, Cuff P, Bamji M, Kotler DP. Body composition in prepubertal children with human immunodeficiency virus type 1 infection. *Arch Pediatr Adolesc Med.* 1998;152:688–693

13. Saavedra JM, Henderson RA, Perman JA, Hutton N, Livingston RA, Yolken RH. Longitudinal assessment of growth in children born to mothers with human immunodeficiency virus infection. *Arch Pediatr Adolesc Med.* 1995;149:497–502

14. McKinney RE, Robertson RW. Effect of human immunodeficiency virus infection on the growth of young children. Duke Pediatric AIDS Clinical Trials Unit. *J Pediatr.* 1993;123:579–582

15. Connor EM, Sperling RS, Gelber R, et al. Reduction of maternal-infant transmission of human immunodeficiency virus type 1 with zidovudine treatment. Pediatric AIDS Clinical Trials Group Protocol 076 Study Group. *N Engl J Med.* 1994;331:1173–1180

16. Dorenbaum A, PACTG 316 Study Team. Report of results of PACTG 316: an international phase III trial of standard antiretroviral (ARV) prophylaxis plus nevirapine (NVP) for prevention of perinatal HIV transmission [abstr LB7]. Paper presented at the 8th Conference on Retroviruses and Opportunistic Infections; February 4–8, 2001; Chicago, IL. Available at: http://www.retroconference.org/2001/Abstracts/Abstracts/Abstracts/LB7.htm. Accessed November 2, 2007

17. The European Mode of Delivery Collaboration. Elective caesarean-section versus vaginal delivery in prevention of vertical HIV-1 transmission: a randomised clinical trial. *Lancet.* 1999;353:1035–1039

18. Kotler DP, Wang J, Pierson RN. Body composition studies in patients with acquired immunodeficiency syndrome. *Am J Clin Nutr.* 1985;42:1255–1265

19. Mulligan K, Tai VW, Schambelan M. Cross-sectional and longitudinal evaluation of body composition in men with HIV infection. *J Acquir Immune Defic Syndr Hum Retrovirol.* 1997;15:43–48

20. de Martino M, Galli L, Chiarelli F, et al. Interleukin-6 release by cultured peripheral blood mononuclear cells inversely correlates with height velocity, bone age, insulin-like growth factor-I, and insulin-like growth factor binding protein-3 serum levels in children with perinatal HIV-1 infection. *Clin Immunol.* 2000;94:212–218

21. Resino S, Galan I, Perez A, et al. HIV-infected children with moderate/severe immune-suppression: changes in the immune system after highly active antiretroviral therapy. *Clin Exp Immunol.* 2004;137:570–577

22. Miller TL, McQuinn L, Orav EJ. Endoscopy of the upper gastrointestinal tract as a diagnostic tool for children with human immunodeficiency virus infection. *J Pediatr.* 1997;130:766–773

23. Kotler DP, Reka S, Orenstein JM, Fox CH. Chronic idiopathic esophageal ulceration in the acquired immunodeficiency syndrome: characterization and treatment with corticosteroids. *J Clin Gastroenterol.* 1992;15:284–290

24. Oeske J, Scott GB, Havens P, Working Group on Antiretroviral Therapy and Medical Management of HIV-Infected Children. *Guidelines for the Use of Antiretroviral Agents in Pediatric HIV Infection.* Bethesda, MD: National Institutes of Health; 2005. Available at: http://aidsinfo.nih.gov/ContentFiles/PediatricGuidelines11032005052.pdf. Accessed November 2, 2007

V

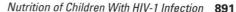

25. Miller TL, Winter HS, Luginbuhl LM, Orav EJ, McIntosh KS. Pancreatitis in pediatric human immunodeficiency virus infection. *J Pediatr*. 1992;120:223–227

26. Butler KM, Venson D, Henry N, et al. Pancreatitis in human immunodeficiency virus-infected children receiving dideoxyinosine. *Pediatrics*. 1993;91:747–751

27. Bouche H, Housset JL, Dumont JL, et al. AIDS-related cholangitis: diagnostic features and course in 15 patients. *Hepatology*. 1993;17:34–39

28. Pol S, Romana CA, Richard S, et al. Microsporidia infection in patients with human immunodeficiency virus and unexplained cholangitis. *N Engl J Med*. 1993;328:95–99

29. Morley JE, Thomas DR, Wilson MM. Cachexia: pathophysiology and clinical relevance. *Am J Clin Nutr*. 2006;83:735–743

30. Beutler, B, Milsark IW, Cerami AC. Passive immunization against cachectin/tumor necrosis factor protects mice from lethal effect of endotoxin. *Science*. 1985; 229:869–871

31. Langhans W. Bacterial products and the control of ingestive behavior: clinical implications. *Nutrition*. 1996;12:303–315

32. Rimaniol AC, Zylberberg H, Zavala F, Viard JP. Inflammatory cytokines and inhibitors in HIV infection: correlation between interleukin-1 receptor antagonist and weight loss. *AIDS*. 1996;10:1349–1356

33. Tardieu M, Le Chenadec J, Persoz A, Meyer L, Blanche S, Mayaux MJ. HIV-1-related encephalopathy in infants compared with children and adults. French Pediatric HIV Infection Study and the SEROCO Group. *Neurology*. 2000;54:1089–1095

34. Chiriboga CA, Fleishman S, Champion S, Gaye-Robinson L, Abrams EJ. Incidence and prevalence of HIV encephalopathy in children with HIV infection receiving highly active antiretroviral therapy (HAART). *J Pediatr*. 2005;146:402–407

35. Henderson RA, Talusan K, Hutton N, Yolken RH, Caballero B. Resting energy expenditure and body composition in children with HIV infection. *J Acquir Immune Defic Syndr Hum Retrovirol*. 1998;19:150–157

36. Miller TL, Evans SE, Vasquez I, Orav EJ. Dietary intake is an important predictor of nutritional status in HIV-infected children [abstr]. *Pediatr Res*. 1997;41:85A

37. Kruzich LA, Marquis GS, Carriquiry AL, Wilson CM, Stephensen CB. US youths in the early stages of HIV disease have low intake of some micronutrients important for optimal immune function. *J Am Diet Assoc*. 2004;104:1095–1101

38. Meng G, Sellers MT, Mosteller-Barnum M, Rogers TS, Shaw GM, Smith PD. Lamina propria lymphocytes, not macrophages, express CCR5 and CXCR4 and are the likely target cell for human immunodeficiency virus type 1 in the intestinal mucosa. *J Infect Dis*. 2000;182: 785–791

39. McDonald D, Wu L, Bohks SM, KewalRamani VN, Unutmaz D, Hope TJ. Recruitment of HIV and its receptors to dendritic cell-T cell junctions. *Science*. 2003;300:1295–1297

40. Weber R, Ledergerber B, Zbinden R, et al. Enteric infections and diarrhea in human immunodeficiency virus-infected persons: prospective community-based cohort study. *Arch Int Med*. 1999;159:1473–1480

41. Ullrich R, Zeitz M, Heise W, L'age M, Hoffken G, Riecken EO. Small intestinal structure and function in patients infected with human immunodeficiency virus (HIV): evidence for HIV-induced enteropathy. *Ann Intern Med*. 1989;111:15–21

42. Kotler DP. HIV infection and the gastrointestinal tract. *AIDS*. 2005;19:107–117
43. Miller TL, Orav EJ, Martin SR, Cooper ER, McIntosh K, Winter HS. Malnutrition and carbohydrate malabsorption in children with vertically transmitted human immunodeficiency virus 1 infection. *Gastroenterology*. 1991;100:1296–1302
44. Yolken RH, Hart W, Oung I, Shiff C, Greenson J, Perman JA. Gastrointestinal dysfunction and disaccharide intolerance in children infected with human immunodeficiency virus. *J Pediatr*. 1991;118:359–363
45. Carroccio A, Fontana M, Spagnuolo MI, et al. Pancreatic dysfunction and its association with fat malabsorption in HIV infected children. *Gut*. 1998;43:558–563
46. Alfaro MP, Siegel RM, Baker RC, Heubi JE. Resting energy expenditure and body composition in pediatric HIV infection. *Pediatr AIDS HIV Infect*. 1995;6:276–280
47. Melchior JC, Raguin G, Boulier A, et al. Resting energy expenditure in human immunodeficiency virus-infected patients: comparison between patients with and without secondary infections. *Am J Clin Nutr*. 1993;57:614–619
48. Grunfeld C, Pang M, Shimizu L, Shigenaga JK, Jensen P, Feingold KR. Resting energy expenditure, caloric intake, and short-term weight change in human immunodeficiency virus infection and the acquired immunodeficiency syndrome. *Am J Clin Nutr*. 1992;55:455–460
49. Hommes MJ, Romijn JA, Godfried MH, et al. Increased resting energy expenditure in human immunodeficiency virus-infected men. *Metabolism*. 1990;39:1186–1190
50. Hardin DS, Ellis KJ, Rice J, Doyle ME. Protease inhibitor therapy improves protein catabolism in prepubertal children with HIV infection. *J Pediatr Endocrinol Metab*. 2004;17:321–325
51. Missmer S, Speigelman D, Gorbach SL, Miller TL. Predictors of change in the functional status of children with human immunodeficiency virus infection. *Pediatrics*. 2000;106(2):e24. Available at: http://pediatrics.aappublications.org/cgi/content/full/106/2/e24. Accessed October 3, 2007
52. Money J. The syndrome of abuse dwarfism (psychosocial dwarfism or reversible hyposomatotropism). *Am J Dis Child*. 1977;131:508–513
53. Boulton TJ, Smith R, Single T. Psychosocial growth failure: a positive response to growth hormone and placebo. *Acta Paediatr*. 1992; 81:322–325
54. Health Protection Agency. Children whose mothers are infected with HIV. *Commun Dis Rep CDR Wkly*. 1995;5:111
55. Lifschitz MH, Wilson GS, Smith EO, Desmond MM. Fetal and postnatal growth of children born to narcotic-dependent women. *Pediatrics*. 1983;102:686–690
56. Kakuda TN, Struble KA, Piscitelli SC. Protease inhibitors for the treatment of human immunodeficiency virus infection. *Am J Health Syst Pharm*. 1998;55:233–254
57. Mueller BU, Sleaseman J, Nelson RP Jr, et al. A phase I/II study of the protease inhibitor indinavir in children with HIV infection. *Pediatrics*. 1998;102:101–109
58. Rutstein RM, Feingold A, Meislich D, Word B, Rudy B. Protease inhibitor therapy in children with perinatally acquired infection. *AIDS*. 1997;11:F107–F111
59. Soh CH, Oleske JM, Brady MT, et al. for the Pediatric AIDS Clinical Trials Group. Long-term effects of protease-inhibitor-based combination therapy on CD4 T-cell recovery in HIV-1-infected children and adolescents. *Lancet*. 2003;362:2045–2051

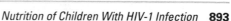

60. Carr A, Samaras K, Chisholm DJ, Cooper DA. Pathogenesis of HIV-1 protease inhibitor-associated peripheral lipodystrophy, hyperlipidemia, and insulin resistance. *Lancet*. 1998;351:1881–1883

61. Arpadi SM, Cuff PA, Horlick M, Kotler DP. Visceral obesity, hypertriglyceridemia and hypercortisolism in a boy with perinatally acquired HIV infection receiving protease inhibitor-containing antiviral treatment [lett]. *AIDS*. 1999;13:2312–2313

62. Brambilla P, Bricalli D, Sala N, et al. Highly active antiretroviral-treated HIV-infected children show fat distribution changes even in absence of lipodystrophy. *AIDS*. 2001;15:2415–2422

63. Vigano A, Mora S, Testolin C, et al. Increased lipodystrophy is associated with increased exposure to highly active antiretroviral therapy in HIV-infected children. *J Acquir Immune Defic Syndr Hum Retrovirol*. 2003;32:482–489

64. Miller T. Nutritional aspects of HIV-infected children receiving highly active antiretroviral therapy. *AIDS*. 2003;17:S130–S140

65. Bartnof HS. New anti-HIV drug interactions, toxicities, and dosing options. *BETA*. 1999;12:60–63

66. Friis-Moller N, Sabin CA, Weber R, et al. Data Collection on Adverse Events of Anti-HIV Drugs (DAD) Study Group. Combination antiretroviral therapy and the risk of myocardial infarction. *N Engl J Med*. 2003;349:1993–2003

67. Miller TL, Mawn BE, Orav EJ, et al. The effect of protease inhibitors on growth and body composition in HIV-infected children. *Pediatrics*. 2001;107(5):e77. Available at: http://pediatrics.aappublications.org/cgi/content/full/107/5/e77. Accessed October 3, 2007

68. Sharma T, Orav EJ, Duggan C, et al. Visceral adiposity and cardiac risk profiles in human immunodeficiency virus-1 infected children. Paper presented at the Pediatric Academic Societies Meeting; April 29–May 2, 2006; San Francisco, CA

69. McComsey GA, Leonard E. Metabolic complications of HIV therapy in children. *AIDS*. 2004;18:1753–1768

70. Taylor P, Worrell C, Steinberg SM, et al. Natural history of lipid abnormalities and fat redistribution among human immunodeficiency virus-infected children receiving long-term, protease inhibitor-containing, highly active antiretroviral therapy regimens. *Pediatrics*. 2004;114(2):e235–e242. Available at: http://pediatrics.aappublications.org/cgi/content/full/114/2/e235. Accessed October 3, 2007

71. Arpadi SM, Horlick M, Thornton J, Cuff PA, Wang J, Kotler DP. Bone mineral content is lower in prepubertal HIV-infected children. *J Acquir Immune Defic Syndr Hum Retrovirol*. 2002;29:450–454

72. Mora S, Zamproni I, Beccio S, Bianchi R, Giacomet V, Vigano A. Longitudinal changes of bone mineral density and metabolism in antiretroviral-treated human immunodeficiency virus-infected children. *J Clin Endocrinol Metab*. 2004;89:24–28

73. Jacobson DL, Spiegelman D, Duggan C, et al. Predictors of bone mineral density in human immunodeficiency virus-1 infected children. *J Pediatr Gastroenterol Nutr*. 2005;41:339–346

74. Friis-Moller N, Weber R, Reiss P, et al. Cardiovascular disease risk factors in HIV patients—association with antiretroviral therapy. Results from the DAD Study. *AIDS*. 2003;17:1179–1193

75. Mary-Krause M, Cotte L, Simon A, Partisani M, Costagliola D. Increased risk of myocardial infarction with duration of protease inhibitor therapy in HIV-infected men. Clinical Epidemiology Group from the French Hospital Database. *AIDS*. 2003;17:2479–2486

76. Hadigan C, Corcoran C, Basgoz N, Davis B, Sax P, Grinspoon S. Metformin in the treatment of HIV-1 lipodystrophy syndrome: a randomized controlled trial. *JAMA*. 2000;284:472–477

77. Walli RK, Michl GM, Muhlbayer D, Brinkmann L, Geobel FD. Effects of troglitazone on insulin sensitivity in HIV-1-infected patients with protease inhibitor-associated diabetes mellitus. *Res Exp Med (Berl)*. 2000;199:253–262

78. Ratz Bravo AE, Tchambaz L, Krahenbuhl-MelcherA, Hess L, Schlienger RG, Krahenbuhl S. Prevalence of potentially severe drug-drug interactions in ambulatory patients with dyslipidemia receiving HMG-CoA reductase inhibitor therapy. *Drug Saf*. 2005;28:263–275

79. Malita FM, Karelis AD, Toma E, Rabasa-Lhoret R. Effects of different types of exercise on body composition and fat distribution in HIV-infected patients: a brief review. *Can J Appl Physiol*. 2005;30:233–245

80. Smit E. Balancing the health benefits and the risks of obesity among HIV-infected youth. *J Amer Diet Assoc*. 2004;104:1549–1553

81. Henderson RA, Saavedra JM, Perman JA, Hutton N, Livingston RA, Yolken RH. Effect of enteral tube feeding on growth of children with symptomatic human immunodeficiency virus infection. *J Pediatr Gastroenterol Nutr*. 1994;18:429–434

82. Matthews DR, Hosker JP, Rudenski AS, Naylor BA, Treacher DF, Turner RC. Homeostasis model assessment: insulin resistance and beta-cell function from fasting plasma glucose and insulin concentrations in man. *Diabetologia*. 1985;28:412–419

Nutrition For Children With Sickle Cell Disease

Sickle cell disease (SCD) is a general term for the genetic disorder related to the production of hemoglobin S, anemia, and a collection of acute and chronic clinical events caused by the blockage of blood flow by the abnormal sickle-shaped red blood cells. The hallmark is a chronic hemolytic anemia with acute and chronic tissue injury.

Sickle cell anemia, the homozygous hemoglobin S state, is the most common variant type of sickle cell disease and affects more than 50 000 black people. The prevalence of hemoglobin SS in black newborn infants is estimated to be approximately 1 in 375. There are 2 less common types of sickle cell disease in the United States. In the black population, hemoglobin SC disease occurs in approximately 1 in 835 live births, and sickle beta-thalassemia occurs in approximately 1 in 1700 live births. Thus, sickle cell disease, with an autosomal-recessive inheritance pattern, is the most common, medically significant genetic condition in black children but also occurs in people with Mediterranean, East Indian, Middle Eastern, Caribbean, and South and Central American ancestry. The discussion that follows uses hemoglobin SS disease (SCD) as the example, because it is the most common and presents the greatest nutritional care challenges.

Sickle cell disease is frequently associated with growth failure, delayed pubertal development, and poor nutritional status.[1-6] The exact etiology of this pattern of poor growth and abnormal body composition has not been completely established. Yet, it is generally recognized that nutritional factors are implicated and are likely a major cause. Various nutrition factors have been identified, including increased energy requirements as the result of increased resting energy expenditure, poor dietary intake, and increased caloric and micronutrient requirements as a result of the chronic hemolysis and increased erythropoiesis and increased protein turnover,[7-17] although a recent study suggests that the bone marrow turnover does not account for the energy requirements.[18]

Several studies have documented increased resting energy expenditure in children and adults with SCD in the United States and other counties. Generally, the increase is in the range of 10% to 20% above predicted or above the measured energy expenditure of healthy control children. Children with SCD do not necessarily show the desired, adaptive increase in dietary intake, although dietary intake is always difficult to accurately document in free-living children. In one study, children with SCD showed approximately a 15% increase in resting energy expenditure compared with control children. These same children with SCD did not increase their dietary intake and showed a trend toward decreasing energy used for normal childhood physical activity.[1] These findings were supported by an additional study in which total energy expenditure was similar, resting energy expenditure was higher, and physical activity-associated energy expenditure was lower in children with SCD compared with healthy age- and gender-matched adolescents.[16] The common SCD acute illness event does not appear to increase the resting energy expenditure[17]; however, illness events were associated with decreased energy intakes.[19] Some of the new treatments, such as oral glutamine supplementation and hydroxyurea therapy, may decrease the elevated resting energy expenditure.[20,21]

When comparing children and adolescents with SCD with healthy control children and national reference data, those with SCD have many indications of growth faltering and abnormal body composition.[22] This is shown by a variety of anthropometric measures, including lower body weight, height, mid-arm circumference, arm fat stores, and arm muscle stores. In addition, bone ages are often delayed, indicating delayed sexual maturation. More direct measures of body composition by several research methods showed lower total body mass, total fat stores, and total body fat-free mass stores.[23] Acute illness episodes in infants and younger children may be accompanied by decreased fat stores but not muscle mass.[19] This is a pattern of impaired growth, delayed puberty, and poor nutritional status with low energy stores and muscle wasting in a group of children with a common chronic disease.

Bone health is another important nutritional consideration for children with sickle cell anemia. Dactylitis during childhood is a consequence of necrosis of the epiphysis and bone marrow within the fingers, resulting in permanent shortening of the carpels and metacarpals. People with sickle cell disease are also at increased risk of developing necrosis of the femoral head. Bone area and bone mineral content deficits are also present in children with SCD, even when adjusting for age, height, pubertal status, and lean body mass.[24] Studies suggest that this is more common in boys, and the decreased bone mineral content is associated with delayed growth and maturation. The cortical bone compartment is thought to be most affected in studies using dual energy x-ray absorptiometry and peripheral quantitative computed tomography. Multiple factors most likely contribute to this poor bone health, including decreased vitamin D and calcium intake.[24,25] Bone marrow hyperplasia in response to increased red blood cell turnover expands the marrow medullary space in long bones, thinning the cortical bone compartment. This likely results in increased bone fragility and increased lifelong risk of fracture. Increases in protein and energy metabolism are also associated with increased bone turnover in SCD.[26] Increased protein turnover and decreased lean body mass may be significant when considering the concept of the bone-muscle unit. Forces produced by muscle contractions influence the restructuring of bone, and changes in muscle mass affect bone mass, size, and strength and may be relevant to SCD.

In addition, there is evidence that some micronutrients are at risk, in addition to the growth failure-related macronutrient risk (calories and possibly protein intake). Folate, vitamin B_6, vitamin B_{12}, and zinc status have all been shown to be suboptimal in some children and adolescents with SCD.[27–30] Low folate status was documented in a group of patients who were prescribed a daily folate supplement (1 mg/day). This study was conducted before the recent changes in food folate fortification in the United States. Folate supplementation is a common but not universal practice in SCD care centers in the United States. Iron status in patients with SCD is unclear, although a recent study suggested that iron depletion and deficiency are uncommon in children and adolescents with SCD.[31] Vitamin B_6 status was found to be suboptimal in these children with SCD, as indicated by low serum concentrations.[30,32] In the study in which nutritional and growth status were assessed, the vitamin B_6 status correlated with weight and body mass index[30] and was negatively associated with the reticulocyte count. Vitamin B_6, vitamin B_{12}, folic acid, and homocysteine are linked along the 1-methyl metabolism pathway. Homocysteine, in addition to serving as a functional biomarker of folate status, when increased, is linked to endothelial dysfunction and is a prospective indicator of risk for atherosclerotic disease. Children with SCD have had homocysteine concentrations documented to be slightly higher than in age-matched healthy control children; in this study, these children also had lower vitamin B_6 concentrations and an inverse correlation of homocysteine to vitamin B_{12} concentration.[32] Supplementation of folic acid and vitamins B_6 and B_{12} in children with SCD resulted in decreased plasma homocysteine concentrations,[33] suggesting a potential role for supplementation with these vitamins in this population. Vitamin A status may be suboptimal and is associated with poor growth and hematologic status, increased pain, and more frequent hospitalizations in children.[34] Zinc supplementation has been shown to be of benefit in linear growth and weight gain in prepubertal children with SCA, even in those with normal plasma zinc concentrations before supplementation.[29] Additional studies suggested that vitamin D[24] and antioxidant concentrations, in addition to vitamin A (ie, vitamin E and selenium) concentrations, are low in children and adolescents with SCD.[35-37] Vitamin C supplementation in children with SCA has been demonstrated to increase hemoglobin, packed cell volume, and percentage of fetal hemoglobin.[38] Vitamin C serves as an important antioxidant system associated with the cell membrane and may act to decrease osmotic fragility in this disorder.

Children with sickle cell anemia are not iron deficient. Some of these children are at increased risk of more frequent sickling episodes, anemia, and stroke. Chronic transfusion therapy in this higher-risk group results in higher hemoglobin, fewer strokes, reduced pain and acute chest syndrome, and better growth as measured by weight for age and height for age than children with sickle cell anemia not receiving chronic transfusion therapy.[39] Chronic transfusion therapy, however, increases the risk of iron overload syndromes and should be monitored for closely by health care professionals.

Given these general findings in children with SCD, careful nutrition and growth assessment should be a routine component of care. However, there are neither nutrition intervention trials nor nutrition consensus statements to suggest a standard of care. In usual practice, there is rarely a pediatric nutritionist or dietitian in the hematology outpatient care area on a routine basis. Therefore, the nutrition assessment (see Chapter 24) and nutrition support care is based on good practice patterns for infants, children, and adolescents with chronic disease.

The nutritional concern that is routinely addressed and stressed by most clinical care teams is the importance of maintaining adequate hydration and encouraging fluid intake, particularly during warm weather.[40] Children with SCD have increased fluid needs as a result of hyposthenuria.[40] Dehydration can precipitate an acute pain event. Some care must be taken to avoid use of fluids that contain only water and carbohydrates and few other nutrients. This may lead to inadequate dietary nutrient density as a result of consuming excess fluids from "empty calories." Anorexia and/or nausea secondary to fever, pain, or analgesic or other medications may contribute to poor overall caloric intake. The suboptimal intake during periods of illness at home and when hospitalized may contribute to the pattern of poor growth.[17]

The major concern for nutritional support is to ensure that children with SCD routinely consume adequate calories to maintain a normal pattern of growth (weight, height, and pubertal) and a normal pattern of fat stores (assessment of subcutaneous fat stores at the triceps site). Protein needs are somewhat increased, but for most patients living in the United States, this is not a clinical problem, because the typical diet contains 1.5 to 2 times the recommended protein intake. Routine longitudinal growth and nutritional status assessment is essential to care. These data should be the basis of diagnosis of growth failure or malnutrition and should provide the basis for planning the nutrition intervention strategy. Given the common occurrence of linear growth failure, the biologic parental heights should be obtained, recorded on the patient's growth chart, and used to assess the pattern of linear growth. Short stature is not a part of the genetic expression of this hemoglobinopathy. With optimal nutritional intake, most children will be able to grow to their genetic potential for height. The care team should take this into account and not accept poor height growth as an unavoidable part of SCD. An accurate record of longitudinal growth (length, height, weight, head circumference) and body composition (measurement of fat stores) is essential to monitoring nutritional status and evaluating the results of nutrition intervention efforts. At least every 6 months, the progression through pubertal development should be documented in the physical examination and nutrition assessment sections of the health record for children 10 years and older.

Given the recent data on micronutrient status, there appears to be a dietary or metabolic risk, but specific recommendations cannot be made for vitamin or mineral supplementation above a usual age- and gender-based Recommended Dietary Allowance. Current commercially available children's vitamin and mineral compounds routinely contain iron, and because of concerns regarding iron overload syndrome, generally are not recommended for children with SCD. There are no data to demonstrate safety or efficacy of higher than Recommended Dietary Allowances of vitamin and mineral intake.

Many black children have a low intake of dairy products because of either lactose intolerance or family dietary or cultural practices that limit dietary intake. This information should be noted, and an effort should be made to maintain adequate calcium and vitamin D intake. Families and patients should also be asked about other important nutrition information, such as the use of a vegetarian diet or other restrictive food practices.

In summary, the goal for infants, children, and adolescents with SCD is to grow and develop within the typical pattern and not be limited by the nutritional effects of SCD. The increased energy requirements can be met most often by nutrition and behavioral education (patient, family) for a diet that is dense in calories and nutrients. When necessary, specific caloric supplements and feeding tubes are important components of care. Less is known about increased micronutrient requirements, and appropriate tests for monitoring, usually blood concentrations, should be obtained before and after implementation of additional supplementation in any individual patient.

References

1. Barden EM, Zemel BS, Kawchak DA, Goran MI, Ohene-Frempong K, Stallings VA. Total and resting energy expenditure in children with sickle cell disease. *J Pediatr.* 2000;136:73–79

2. Platt OS, Rosenstock W, Espeland MA. Influence of sickle hemoglobinopathies on growth and development. *N Engl J Med.* 1984;311:7–12

3. Phebus CK, Gloninger MF, Maciak BJ. Growth patterns by age and sex in children with sickle cell disease. *J Pediatr.* 1984;105:28–33

4. Heyman MB, Vichinsky E, Katz R, et al. Growth retardation in sickle cell disease treated by nutritional support. *Lancet.* 1985;1:903–906

5. Stevens MC, Maude GH, Cupidore L, Jackson H, Hayes RJ, Serjeant GR. Prepubertal growth and skeletal maturation in children with sickle cell disease. *Pediatrics.* 1986;78:124–132

6. Finan AC, Elmer MA, Sasanow SR, McKinney S, Russel MO, Gill FM. Nutritional factors and growth in children with sickle cell disease. *Am J Dis Child.* 1988;142:237–240

7 Kopp-Hoolihan, LE, van Loan MD, Mentzer WC, Heyman MB. Elevated resting energy expenditure in adolescents with sickle cell anemia. *J Am Diet Assoc.* 1999;99:195–199

8. Borel MJ, Buchowski MS, Turner EA, Peeler BB, Goldstein RE, Flakoll PJ. Alterations in basal nutrient metabolism increase resting energy expenditure in sickle cell disease. *Am J Physiol.* 1998;274:e357–e364

9. Modebe O, Ifenu SA. Growth retardation in homozygous sickle cell disease: role of calorie intake and possible gender-related differences. *Am J Hematol.* 1993;44:149–154

10. Gray NT, Barlett JM, Kolasa KM, Marcuard SP, Holbrook CT, Horner RD. Nutritional status and dietary intake of children with sickle cell anemia. *Am J Pediatr Hematol Oncol.* 1992;14:57–61

11. Badaloo A, Jackson AA, Jahoor F. Whole body protein turnover and resting metabolic rate in homozygous sickle cell disease. *Clin Sci (Lond).* 1989;77:93–97

12. Salman EK, Haymond MW, Bayne E, et al. Protein and energy metabolism in prepubertal children with sickle cell anemia. *Pediatr Res.* 1996;40:34–40

13. Singhal A, Davies P, Sahota A, Thomas PW, Serjeant GR. Resting metabolic rate in homozygous sickle cell disease. *Am J Clin Nutr.* 1993;57:32–34

14. Singhal A, Thomas P, Cook R, Wierenga K, Serjeant G. Delayed adolescent growth in homozygous sickle cell disease. *Arch Dis Child.* 1994;71:404–408

15. Singhal A, Davies P, Wierenga KJ, Thomas P, Serjeant G. Is there an energy deficiency in homozygous sickle cell disease? *Am J Clin Nutr.* 1997;66:386–390

16. Buchowski MS, Townsend KM, Williams R, Chen KY. Patterns and energy expenditure of free-living physical activity in adolescents with sickle cell anemia. *J Pediatr.* 2002;140:86–92

17. Fung EB, Malinauskis BM, Kawchak DA, et al. Energy expenditure and intake in children with sickle cell disease during acute illness. *Clin Nutr.* 2001; 20:131–138

18. Harmatz P, Heyman MB, Cunningham J, et al. Effects of red blood cell transfusion on resting energy expenditure in adolescents with sickle cell anemia. *J Pediatr Gastroenterol Nutr.* 1999;29:127–31

19. Malinauskas BM, Gropper SS, Kawchak DA, Zemel BS, Ohene-Frempong K, Stallings VA. Impact of acute illness on nutritional status of infants and young children with sickle cell disease. *J Am Diet Assoc.* 2000;100:330–334

20. Williams R, Olivi S, Li CS, et al. Oral glutamine supplementation decreases resting energy expenditure in children and adolescents with sickle cell anemia. *J Pediatr Hematol Oncol.* 2004;26:619–625

21. Fung EB, Barden EM, Kawchak DA, Zemel BS, Ohene-Frempong K, Stallings VA. Effect of hydroxyurea therapy on resting energy expenditure in children with sickle cell disease. *J Pediatr Hematol Oncol.* 2001;23:604–608

22. Barden EM, Kawchak DA, Ohene-Frempong K, Stallings VA, Zemel BS. Body composition in children with sickle cell disease. *Am J Clin Nutr.* 2002;76:218–225

23. VanderJagt DJ, Harmatz P, Scott-Emuakpor AB, Vichinsky E, Glew RH. Bioelectrical impedance analysis of the body composition of children and adolescents with sickle cell disease. *J Pediatr.* 2002;140:681–687

24. Buison AM, Kawchak DA, Schall JI, et al. Bone area and bone mineral content deficits in children with sickle cell disease. *Pediatrics.* 2005;116:943–949

25. Lal A, Fung EB, Pakbaz Z, Hackney-Stephens E, Vichinsky EP. Bone mineral density in children with sickle cell anemia. *Pediatr Blood Cancer.* 2006;47:901–906

26. Buchowski MS. De la Fuente A, Flakoll PJ, Chen KY, Turner EA. Increased bone turnover is associated with protein and energy metabolism in adolescents with sickle cell anemia. *Am J Physiol Endocrinol Metab.* 2001;280:e518–e527

27. Kennedy TS, Fung EB, Kawchak DA, Zemel BS, Ohene-Frempong K, Stallings VA. Red blood cell folate and serum vitamin B_{12} status in children with sickle cell disease. *J Pediatr Hematol Oncol.* 2001;23:165–169

28. Leonard MB, Zemel BS, Kawchak DA, Ohene-Frempong K, Stallings VA. Plasma zinc status, growth and development in children with sickle cell disease. *J Pediatr.* 1998;132:467–471

29. Zemel BS, Kawchak D, Fung E, Ohene-Frempong K, Stallings VA. Effect of zinc supplementation on growth and body composition in children with sickle cell disease. *Am J Clin Nutr.* 2002;75:300–307

30. Nelson MC, Zemel BS, Kawchak DA, et al. Vitamin B_6 status of children with sickle cell disease. *J Pediatr Hematol Oncol.* 2002;24:463–469

31. Stettler N, Zemel BS, Kawchak DA, Ohene-Frempong K, Stallings VA. Iron status of children with sickle cell disease. *JPEN J Parenter Enteral Nutr.* 2001;25:36–38

32. Segal JB, Miller ER III, Brereton NH, Resar LM. Concentrations of B vitamins and homocysteine in children with sickle cell anemia. *So Med J.* 2004;97:149–155

33. van der Dijs FPL, Fokkema MR, Dijck-Brouwer J, et al. Optimization of folic acid, vitamin B_{12} and vitamin B_6 supplements in pediatric patients with sickle cell disease. *Am J Hematol.* 2002;69:239–246

34. Schall JI, Zemel BS, Kawchak D, Ohene-Frempong K, Stallings VA. Vitamin A status and outcomes in young children with sickle cell disease. *J Pediatr.* 2004;145:99–106

V

35. Chiu D, Vichinsky E, Yee M, Kleman K, Lubin B. Peroxidation, vitamin E and sickle cell anemia. *Ann N Y Acad Sci.* 1982;393:323–335

36. Marwah SS, Wheelwright D, Blann AD, et al. Vitamin E correlates inversely with non-transferrin-bound iron in sickle cell disease. *Br J Haematol.* 2001;114:917–919

37. Natta CL, Chen LC, Chow CK. Selenium and gluthione peroxidase levels in sickle cell anemia. *Acta Haematol.* 1990;83:130–132

38. Jaja SI, Ikotun AR, Gbenebitse S, Temiye EO. Blood pressure, hematologic and erythrocyte fragility changes in children suffering from sickle cell anemia following ascorbic acid supplementation. *J Trop Pediatr.* 2002;48:366–370

39. Wang W, Morales KH, Scher CD, et al. Effect of long-term transfusion on growth in children with sickle cell anemia: results of the STOP Trial. *J Pediatr.* 2005;147:244–247

40. Smith JA, Wethers DL. Health care maintenance. In: Embury SH, Hebbel RP, Mohandas N, Steinberg MH, eds. *Sickle Cell Disease: Basic Principles and Clinical Practice.* New York, NY: Raven Press; 1994:739–744

Nutritional Management of Children With Renal Disease

Introduction

Individuals with normal renal function have great latitude in the quantity (and quality) of the nutrients they can ingest. Unfortunately, individuals with kidney disease have less latitude in their nutritional choices, either because of decreased renal waste excretion and/or increased renal tubular losses. In addition, these infants and children may have decreased appetites and insufficient energy intakes, which can further limit nutrition and growth.[1] Nutritional prescriptions can be complex, and it is often necessary to restrict the intake of some nutrients (see Table 41.1) while at the same time supplementing other nutrients necessary to maintain homeostasis and support growth. Reasonable starting points for diet prescriptions are noted in Table 41.2.

This chapter will discuss nutritional considerations in a variety of renal conditions that affect infants, children, or adolescents. Whenever possible, evidence-based recommendations for nutritional support of children with specific kidney disorders will be given and controlled studies will be cited, but unfortunately, critical studies in children are often lacking, and studies performed in adults may be cited. The Food and Nutrition Board of the National Research Council has presented standards in the form of Dietary Reference Intakes (DRIs). Previously, this information was presented as Recommended Dietary Allowances (RDA). For the nutrients to be discussed, there is often little difference between the 2 values. Within this paper, the term RDA is used when describing experimental results performed using the RDAs as standards, and the term DRI is used when noting current standards.

Urinary Tract Infections, Vesicoureteral Reflux, and Urinary Incontinence

Urinary tract infections (UTIs [often associated with vesicoureteral reflux]) are among the most common pediatric renal problems. There are no data that demonstrate a clear role for special nutritional management of children with recurrent UTIs whether there is associated reflux or not. However, recurrent UTIs have been associated with constipation, which certainly may respond to dietary manipulation. There are some preliminary data suggesting that cranberry juice may be helpful in minimizing the risk of infection, but no compelling data are available from studies in children.[2,3]

Table 41.1
Food Sources of Selected Nutrients

Sodium	Fast food, microwavable products, and snack foods, such as chips, contribute significant sodium to the diet. Appealing to parents to make lifestyle changes for the entire family may be effective and necessary.
	Foods that should be limited when sodium restriction is recommended include the following: • Convenience products (frozen, packaged, or canned), including pizza, macaroni and cheese, meat stew, spaghetti, and burritos. **Use** frozen entrees with the lowest sodium content. • Cured, salted, canned, or smoked meats, including ham, corned beef, jerky, salt pork, luncheon meats, bacon, sausage, hot dogs/frankfurters, sausage, canned tuna or salmon, and sardines. **Use** fresh meats or those frozen without added sauces. • Processed cheese, cheese spreads, or buttermilk. **Use** low-sodium cheese, ricotta/mozzarella cheese, and cream cheese. • Regular canned or frozen soups and bouillon cubes and instant soup or dried noodle cups. **Use** low-sodium soups or homemade soups without salt or bouillon cubes and fresh-cooked pasta and grains. • Salted crackers and snack foods, such as potato chips. **Use** unsalted chips, pretzels, and unsalted popcorn or crackers. • Regular canned vegetables, vegetable juices, or those frozen with salt. **Use** fresh or frozen vegetables without added salt; if canned, use "no salt added" vegetables and sauces.
Potassium	Juices, fruits, vegetables, and nuts contribute the most significant sources of potassium to the diet. If restricted, a multivitamin supplement may be necessary to provide micronutrient needs. Herbal products may provide significant potassium and should be avoided in children.
	Examples of high-potassium foods: orange juice, carrot juice; avocados, bananas, cantaloupe, dried fruits (raisins, apricots, bananas, etc), oranges; potatoes, sweet potatoes, tomatoes; chocolate; lentils, dried beans (cooked); and nuts. **Examples of low-potassium foods:** cranberry juice and apple juice; apples, grapes, peaches, pears, pineapple, strawberries, watermelon; green beans, lettuce, zucchini; bread; dried pasta (cooked); and tortillas.
Phosphorus	Milk and milk products, plus meat, chicken, fish, eggs, and nuts provide the most significant sources of phosphorus in the diet. Ironically, dairy products generally are the most popular protein source for children. Limiting dairy products and utilizing phosphate binders with meals is the treatment goal. Calcium supplementation may be required, because limiting phosphorus in the diet automatically limits calcium as well.

Table 41.2

Reasonable Starting Points for Diet Prescription in Kidney Disease

Overview	Evaluating patient and family lifestyle eating patterns may reveal areas that can be improved without limiting all sources of the nutrient in question. Ongoing nutritional follow-up is important to monitor nutrient intake and assess adequacy.
	Obtain a detailed diet history to determine current food and beverage intake. All diet changes are based on evaluation of this current intake. Focus on decreasing the amount of frequently consumed high sources of elevated nutrients.
	Resist the temptation to restrict nutrients until there is a need demonstrated.
	The word "low" in front of a nutrient ("low sodium," "low potassium") is not a diet order. Be specific (suggestions below). "Renal" is not a diet order.
	Selective micronutrient restrictions may result in the patient refusing to consume adequate amounts of macronutrients (calories, protein, and fat). Follow-up is important to ensure adequacy of intake to meet growth needs.
	Limit as few nutrients as possible to optimize intake.

Nutrient	Possible Diet Order	Description	Recommended Starting Points	Comments
Sodium	3–4 g sodium (formerly No Added Salt)	Food is cooked with some salt; high sources such as pizza, hot dogs, chips are limited or avoided	<20 kg Outpatient: begin with 2 g/day Inpatient with severe edema: 1 g/day	A sodium restriction will automatically decrease fat intake in most children.
	2 g sodium	Food is prepared with no salt; high sources are eliminated	>20 kg Outpatient: begin with 3 g/day Inpatient with severe edema: 2 g/day	
	1 g sodium	Food is prepared with no salt; low-sodium products are used exclusively		
Potassium	Limit food sources with high potassium content	Frequently consumed high-potassium foods (see Table 41.1) are decreased or eliminated	Limit only high sources of potassium child is currently eating/drinking	Often, initially limiting frequently consumed foods like potatoes, bananas, and orange juice is sufficient to control serum potassium concentrations. Correct acidosis, bleeding, and other potential causes of elevated potassium.

V

Table 41.2 *(Continued)*
Reasonable Starting Points for Diet Prescription in Kidney Disease

Nutrient	Possible Diet Order	Description	Recommended Starting Points	Comments
Phosphorus	800 mg/day	High sources are limited to 8 oz of milk/day or the phosphorus equivalent of cheese, yogurt, ice cream, beans, nuts.	Start with 800 mg/day, smaller children will consume less because of smaller portion sizes	Infants require higher serum phosphorus concentrations for adequate bone mineralization. Start phosphorus binders with meals as necessary. Phosphorus limitation will automatically limit protein and potassium intake. Calcium intake may be insufficient (unless calcium binders are given).
	600 mg/day	Milk, milk products, beans, nuts, chocolate are eliminated.		
Protein	Regular diet	Highest sources include meat, poultry, fish, egg, dairy products.	Start with a diet history to determine need, if any, to restrict protein.	Children with rising blood urea nitrogen (BUN) concentrations rarely consume more than the DRI because of poor appetite and phosphorus restriction. Ensure adequate calorie intake for protein sparing; otherwise, BUN may be elevated as a result of protein catabolism. Protein needs are increased in dialysis; see Table 41.5.

Primary nocturnal enuresis is a common pediatric condition. A recent systematic review has documented only 2 controlled studies assessing nutritional therapy.[4] The overall results are insufficient to recommend this form of treatment. Although it has been suggested that the introduction of a low-allergen diet can successfully cure enuresis, only 2 controlled studies are available; the number of treated patients is low, making the results less reliable; and the studies have not been replicated.[4] It is generally agreed that limiting fluid intakes in the evening or after dinner is ineffective and unwarranted. There are also no nutritional issues associated with urinary incontinence, although there is anecdotal evidence that elimination diets have been of benefit for children with nocturnal enuresis.[5]

Hypertension

There is good epidemiologic data on the association between childhood obesity and high blood pressure.[6] Body weights track from childhood through adulthood and there is strong evidence that obesity or increased body mass index (BMI) is related to hypertension.[7-9] Dietary modification aimed at weight stabilization (or slow weight loss in the older adolescent) to normalize BMI (see also Chapter 33: Obesity) is appropriate.[10] The reported increase in the incidence of childhood obesity, the development of the metabolic syndrome, and implications for the development of hypertension have been noted.[6,11-13] It is clear that for individuals of any age, weight loss is difficult both to achieve and to maintain. In the past, attention was focused on having the individual lose most or all of their excess weight, but it has become evident that moderate weight reduction (weight loss in the range of 5%–10% of initial body weight) is also effective in lowering blood pressure.[14] The DASH (Dietary Approach to Stop Hypertension) eating plan, a diet high in fruits and vegetables, has been associated with modest weight loss and a significant decease in blood pressure in adults.[15-17]

Sodium restriction is often recommended, although the safety and efficacy of long-term sodium restriction in children and adolescents has not been established.[4,18-21] In adults, lowering sodium intakes has an additive effect on the decrease in blood pressure seen with the DASH diet.[22] In addition, high-sodium foods are often calorically dense and should, therefore, be limited in the diet of the obese hypertensive child. The National Health and Nutrition Examination Survey III noted that average sodium intakes for children between 3 and 18 years of age range between 2.8 and 4.6 g/day. The Institute of Medicine has suggested that a much lower quantity of sodium is adequate for otherwise healthy infants and children (Table 41.3).[23] Unfortunately, it is often difficult to achieve these levels of sodium intake, but they are certainly a safe and an appropriate goal. Depending on the child's usual sodium intake, restricting sodium intake to 2 to 3 g/day may be a reasonable starting point.

Table 41.3
Dietary Reference Intakes (DRIs): Recommended Intakes for Individuals, Macronutrients

Age Group	Protein (g/day)	Protein g/kg per day	Sodium g/day	Phosphorous mg/day	Calcium mg/day	Potassium g/day
Infants						
0–6 mo	9.1	1.5	0.12	100	210	0.4
7–12 mo	11	**1.5**	0.37	275	270	0.7
Children						
1–3 y	13	1.1	1	**460**	500	3
4–8 y	19	0.95	1.2	**500**	800	3.8
Males						
9–13 y	34	0.95	1.5	**1250**	1300	4.5
14–18 y	52	0.85	1.5	**1250**	1300	4.7
Females						
9–13 y	34	0.95	1.5	1250	1300	4.5
14–18 y	46	0.85	1.5	1250	1300	4.7

* Unbolded values are adequate intakes (AIs)—the recommended average daily intake level based on observed or experimentally determined approximations or estimates of nutrient intake by a group (or groups) of apparently healthy people that are assumed to be adequate—used when an DRI cannot be determined.

† Values in **bold** typeface are listed as the DRIs—adequate for 97.5% of the population.

Source: Food and Nutrition Board, Institute of Medicine.[23]

Epidemiologic and some clinical data are accumulating that suggest that increased dietary calcium and potassium may be effective in helping to lower blood pressures,[24–29] but there are few data that either potassium or calcium supplements are effective. By virtue of its fruit and vegetable content, the DASH diet is an example of such a diet. Manipulations of dietary magnesium or fiber may prove to be beneficial, but data in children are lacking.[30,31] Studies in adults and infants suggest that diets or infant formulas supplementing long-chain polyunsaturated fatty acids are associated with lower blood pressures,[32] but data in children are lacking.

Kidney Stone Disorders

The main constituents of the renal stones that occur in childhood are calcium and oxalate. Less commonly, cystine or uric acid stones are found. Although there are a variety of conditions that predispose children to renal stones, there are certain common therapeutic interventions. In all cases, a high fluid intake is the primary recommendation. Children should be encouraged to drink at least 1.5 to 2 times their calculated maintenance fluid requirements (opinion-based recommendation). If necessary, children should be encouraged to get up in the middle of the night to urinate and then drink additional fluid before going back to bed. The fluids the child chooses to drink may have an effect on the child's total caloric intake, and the family should be instructed to provide at least 50% of the intake as water. A simple method to assess the adequacy of fluid intake is to tell the child and family that the urine should be clear and not yellow in color (opinion-based recommendation).

Renal sodium reabsorption is linked to the reabsorption of a variety of other chemicals, including calcium and the amino acid cystine (the source of kidney stones in the inherited condition cystinuria). High sodium intakes lead to increased sodium excretion and, hence, increased calcium and cystine excretion. Conversely, low-sodium diets lead to decreased calcium and cystine excretion[33-36] so that salt restriction should be advised. When a low-salt diet is insufficient to lower calcium or cystine excretion, a distal tubule diuretic is often added.

In adults, protein restriction has been associated with decreased renal stone formation. Because of the importance of protein intake to growth, low-protein diets cannot be recommended, but there is little harm in limiting protein intake to the DRI for age (Table 41.2).

There is no role for dietary calcium restriction, and calcium should be provided at the level of the DRI (Table 41.3). Epidemiologic data in adults suggest that high-calcium diets may be effective in decreasing the risk of recurrent calcium stones.[36-39]

Hyperoxaluria can be divided into primary (hereditary) and secondary forms. There is no evidence that limiting dietary oxalate is of value in patients with the metabolic defects associated with primary hyperoxaluria. For children with secondary hyperoxaluria or with hypercalciuria and mild hyperoxaluria, avoidance of high-oxalate foods (see Table 41.4) may be prudent.[40,41] Vitamin C should be limited to 100 mg/day or less, because ascorbate is converted to oxalate in alkaline urine.

A small proportion of children with recurrent renal stones pass stones composed predominantly of uric acid. There is no evidence that restricting the intake of foods with a high purine content alters the rate of stone formation.[42,43] The goal is to achieve but not exceed the DRI for protein (Table 41.3).

Table 41.4
Foods With High Oxalate Content[41]

Spinach
Rhubarb
Beets
Nuts
Chocolate
Tea
Wheat bran
Strawberries

Renal Tubular Defects

The tubules serve to reabsorb water and chemicals lost to the body as a consequence of glomerular filtration. Within the proximal tubule, these defects may be isolated to a single compound (eg proximal renal tubular acidosis, hypophosphatemia) or present as multiple proximal renal tubular defects, a condition known as Fanconi syndrome. Disorders within the loop of Henle or the distal convoluted tubule are associated with the loss of electrolytes and water and/or inability to acidify urine. Each of these abnormalities results in the development of abnormal serum electrolyte concentrations and necessitates the administration of supplements.

Infants and children with proximal renal tubular acidosis present with short stature, failure to thrive, and hypokalemic, hypochloremic metabolic acidosis. Appropriate treatment includes oral administration of large amounts of bicarbonate (often 10–20 mEq/kg per day) as well has supplemental potassium.

The proximal tubule is the main site for renal reabsorption of phosphorus. A proximal tubular defect in phosphorus reabsorption leads to hypophosphatemic rickets, a condition characterized by short stature and a variety of other associated findings.[44,45] Treatment consists of phosphorus supplementation, and doses of 30 to 90 mg/kg per day administered 3 or 4 times during the day may be necessary. Unfortunately, this dose of phosphorus may cause diarrhea, and supplementation must begin with lower doses, slowly increasing the daily intake as needed and tolerated. Although serum calcium concentrations are often normal before therapy, the administration of phosphorus leads to hypocalcemia and secondary hyperparathyroidism, necessitating the concurrent administration of one of the activated forms of vitamin D. When the proximal tubule is affected, replenishment must be frequent, because the renal loss is continuous. Nasogastric and gastrostomy supplements overnight have been used.

Children with distal tubular defects may have distal renal tubular acidosis (dRTA), a condition characterized by an inability to excrete acid urine. Children with dRTA require alkali in the range of 1 to 5 mEq/kg per day, a significantly lower dose than that required by children with proximal renal tubular acidosis. Individuals with dRTA are also at risk of developing renal calculi and nephrocalcinosis as a result of hypercalciuria and inability to excrete acid urine. Other disorders of the loop of Henle or distal tubule (most commonly Bartter or Gitelman syndromes) are associated with renal potassium or magnesium wasting. In these conditions, oral supplementation of potassium and/or magnesium replacement is indicated in doses dependent on measured serum concentrations.

Nephrotic Syndrome

Nephrotic syndrome is defined clinically by the presence of proteinuria, hypoalbuminemia, edema, and hypercholesterolemia. The development of edema is attributable to the abnormal salt (and water) retention seen in this condition. The mainstay of dietary therapy for children with nephrotic syndrome is sodium restriction. Although no studies define the optimal level to which sodium should be restricted in these children, reasonable estimates are noted in Table 41.2. This level of sodium restriction requires that the entire family adjust their eating habits, at the least taking the salt shaker off the table, limiting processed foods, and eliminating salted snack foods. Most pediatric patients respond to corticosteroids and can be weaned off of steroids within 3 to 6 months. Unfortunately, most will relapse and require the reinstitution of steroid therapy. Some children will require the use of additional medications to limit proteinuria and keep them free of edema. Because most forms of nephrotic syndrome recur, it should be explained to the family that it would be best for them to adopt healthy dietary habits and limit their salt intake indefinitely. Given the associations among steroid use, weight gain, and hypertension, all patients would benefit from nutritional counseling as well as increased physical activity.

At times, children with severe edema may have to be hospitalized for aggressive fluid removal. One common error is the provision of intravenous "maintenance" or "partial maintenance" fluids. In the absence of intravascular volume depletion, there is no need to provide intravenous fluids, and unnecessary salt and water administration can be avoided. Although it is possible to aggressively limit oral sodium intake in hospitalized patients, very low-sodium diets are generally unpalatable and will be successful only for a limited time during the inpatient period and will generally not be followed outside the hospital.

Serum albumin concentrations cannot be restored to normal by nutritional supplementation, and there are both animal and adult human data that demonstrate that serum albumin concentrations actually improve using low-protein diets.[46] However, there are no data that address this in pediatric patients, and again, low protein intakes must be weighed against the concern for the development of malnutrition and poor growth in pediatric patients. Suggested protein intakes are, therefore, set no lower than the DRI for age (Table 41.3).

Infants with congenital nephrotic syndrome typically have very high degrees of proteinuria and do develop clinical evidence of protein depletion. Nutritional care in this group of infants is complex, often requiring both enteral feeding and repeated albumin infusions to prevent severe hypoproteinemia and edema formation.[47]

Hypercholesterolemia is common in these patients both as component of the nephrotic syndrome and steroids administration. Although prolonged hyperlipidemia is a recognized cardiovascular risk factor, it does not appear that the transient hypercholesterolemia seen in children who recovered from the nephrotic syndrome has any negative effect on cardiovascular mortality later in life.[48] Unfortunately, there are few data supporting the use of low-fat diets to decrease cholesterol concentrations[49] and only minimal pediatric data on the use of cholesterol-lowering agents in this condition.[50] However, because in a given patient, the outcome of the nephrotic syndrome may be unknown and steroid usage as well as high-fat diets encourage weight gain, attention to dietary lipid content is prudent. Fortunately, limiting dietary sodium also limits the consumption of high-fat foods popular with children (hot dogs, pizza, and cheese). The ubiquitous presence of high-sodium, high-fat foods makes dietary recommendations complex, and families often benefit from dietary counseling by a registered dietitian.

Glomerulonephritis

Clinically, glomerulonephritis is characterized by the presence of both hematuria and proteinuria. Renal function may be reduced, and patients often
develop hypervolemia and/or hypertension. If the nephrotic syndrome is
also present, hyperlipidemia is likely. The nutritional management of these
patients depends on how well renal function is maintained. In the setting of
hypervolemia and hypertension, sodium restriction is often required. There
are significant differences between acute and chronic renal insufficiency,
because in the former, there is little time for the development of the renal
compensatory adjustments that are often seen in the chronic state. The care
of children with glomerulonephritis is, therefore, dependent on whether the
condition is acute or chronic as well as on the presence of associated finings,
such as hypertension or the nephrotic syndrome.

Acute Renal Failure

Acute renal failure (ARF) is defined as an abrupt decline in the glomerular filtration rate and is most often caused either by underperfusion of the kidneys
(eg, during hypovolemic shock) or as the result of intrinsic renal disease.
Intrinsic renal diseases are usually forms of acute glomerulonephritis or the
hemolytic-uremic syndrome. Acute renal failure may be associated either
with low levels of urinary water output (oliguria/anuria) or with normal or
even increased urine volumes (nonoliguric renal failure). In general, patients with acute renal failure cannot adjust urine output effectively, and the
physician will be called on to manage fluid intakes to prevent either volume
overload or volume depletion. Irrespective of the volume of urine output,
individuals with acute renal failure are unable to control the excretion of
metabolic wastes such as urea, sodium, potassium, phosphorus, and acid.
Specific dietary requirements will depend on the clinical circumstances, but
general recommendations are possible. When hypertension and volume
overload are a concern, sodium (and often fluid volume) should be limited.
Individuals with oligoanuria who are not clinically volume overloaded
should receive daily fluid intakes equivalent to their urine output plus
estimated insensible water loss. Potassium and phosphate intakes are often
restricted, with allowable intakes based on the clinical setting.

There is no evidence to suggest that ARF, per se, leads to an increase in
energy requirements. Even when ARF is associated with other conditions
(eg, sepsis, multiple organ failure), recent studies using indirect calorimetry
have shown that standard formulas used to compute energy requirements

are inaccurate and overestimate actual energy requirements.[51,52] In the absences of direct measurements, caloric requirements should be provided at the level of the DRI for chronologic age (Table 41.5).

Table 41.5
Recommended Energy and Protein Intakes in Children by Age

Age Group	Predialysis		Hemodialysis		Peritoneal Dialysis	
	Energy*	Protein[†]	Energy*	Protein[‡]	Energy[§]	Protein[‖]
0–6 mo	100–110	2.2	100–110	2.6	100–110	3
6–12 mo	95–105	1.5	95–105	2	95–105	2.4
1–3 y	90	1.1	90	1.6	90	2.0
4–10 y	70	0.95	70	1.6	70	1.8–2.0
11–14 y (boys)	55	0.95	55	1.4	55	1.8
11–14 y (girls)	47	0.95	47	1.4	47	1.8
15–18 y (boys)	45	0.85	45	1.3	45	1.5
15–18 y (girls)	40	0.85	40	1.2	40	1.5

* kcal/kg per day.

[†] g/kg per day.

[‡] Protein intakes increased by approximately 0.4 g/kg per day to account for hemodialysis losses.

[§] Note: up to 10% of the total caloric intake (10 kcal/kg per day) can be absorbed as dextrose via the dialysate. Obesity may become a concern for some children and adolescents on peritoneal dialysis.

[‖] Protein requirements on peritoneal dialysis reflect the significant loss of proteins through the dialysis fluid.

Adapted from the National Research Council,[23] the National Kidney Foundation,[64] and Wassner and Baum.[65]

Although there are good reasons to limit excess protein intake in ARF, a minimum protein intake of 1 g/kg per day is important to minimize protein catabolism. Amino acids that are not used for protein anabolism are degraded, with their nitrogen contributing to excess urea production. In addition, for enteral feeding, phosphorus and acid intakes are linearly related to protein intake. The best method available to maximize the efficiency of protein utilization is to provide adequate nonprotein calories. In the absence of dialysis therapy, a reasonable goal is for the serum urea nitrogen concentration to increase at a rate of between 10 and 20 mg/dL per day.

Whenever possible, enteral nutrition should be used, but depending on the child's age and ability to tolerate enteral nutrition or to ingest solid foods, parenteral nutrition may be necessary.

Nutritional goals in these individuals include assessing and reversing negative nitrogen balance, meeting energy needs, maintaining appropriate hydration, establishing and maintaining electrolyte and bone-mineral balance, and providing appropriate vitamin and mineral supplementation.[53] With the widespread availability of pediatric dialysis, including forms of continual renal replacement therapy, it is now possible to provide adequate nutritional intake for most infants and children with ARF. Currently, dialysis therapies are instituted at an early stage to allow the provision of adequate nutrition.

Chronic Renal Failure

Current terminology divides chronic kidney disease (CKD) into 5 categories (Table 41.6). When renal function declines to a glomerular filtration rate of <60 mL/min/1.73 m² (stage 3), changes in blood chemistries become apparent and growth failure becomes more likely. Spontaneous food (energy) intake is low in children with CKD.[1,54,55] Energy intake should be provided at approximately 100% to 120% of the DRI for age.[55]

Table 41.6
Classification of the Stages of Chronic Kidney Disease[75]

Stage	GFR (mL/min per 1.73 m²)	Description	Action Plan
1	≥90	Kidney damage with normal or increased GFR	Treat primary and comorbid conditions. Slow CKD progression, CVD risk reduction
2	60–89	Kidney damage with mild reduction of GFR	Estimate rate of progression of CKD.
3	30–59	Moderate reduction of GFR	Evaluate and treat complications.
4	15–29	Severe reduction of GFR	Prepare for kidney replacement therapy.
5	<15	Kidney failure	Kidney replacement therapy

GFR indicates glomerular filtration rate; CVD, cardiovascular disease.

There is no evidence that restricting protein intake to less than the DRI is effective in delaying progression of renal insufficiency[56,57] and some evidence that, at least in infants, low protein intakes may actually inhibit growth.[56] Because high protein intakes should also be avoided in CKD, the most appropriate recommendations are for protein intakes to be set at the DRI for age.[57-59] This is a modest restriction, because when allowed unrestricted diets, children with CKD eat an average 120% to 150% of the DRI.[1,60,61]

The kidney has a remarkable ability to excrete potassium, but as renal function declines, it is reasonable to limit intake of foods with high potassium content. Hyperkalemia presenting in individuals with moderate CKD generally indicates an acute potassium overload (eg, dietary indiscretion, intravenous administration), a significant catabolic event, or dehydration. Analogous to the setting of acute renal failure, children with significant chronic renal disease may need more stringent potassium restriction.

The control of serum calcium and phosphorus is complex. Calcium absorption is decreased as a result of decreased oral intake and decreased vitamin D hydroxylation. Phosphorus excretion is dependent on renal function, and urinary excretion decreases with progressive CKD. In children older than 1 year, phosphorus intakes should be restricted when the serum phosphate concentration is >5.5. For children younger than 7 to 8 years, a limit of 600 to 800 mg/day is a reasonable starting point. Older children and adolescents should be limited to 800 to 1000 mg/day. In practice, these patients often receive oral calcium compounds that serve as phosphate binders as well as activated vitamin D analogues to increase enteral calcium absorption. Poor control of serum calcium and phosphorus concentrations is associated with hyperparathyroidism and renal osteodystrophy and increased risk of cardiac calcification.[62] A National Kidney Foundation Kidney Disease Outcomes and Quality Initiative guideline for the management of renal osteodystrophy was recently published,[63] as was a more general guideline for the management of children and adults with CKD.[64]

In the absence of hypertension or volume overload, it is reasonable to limit sodium intake to 3 to 4 g. When volume overload is present, sodium intake should be limited, and diuretics may have to be administered. Because individuals drink to isotonicity, there is rarely a reason to specifically limit water intake.

One subset of children with CRF requires special mention—infants and toddlers with nonoliguric CRF, usually as a result of congenital hydronephrosis or renal dysplasia. These children may not be able to conserve sodium and bicarbonate despite advanced degrees of renal failure and often require sodium chloride and alkali supplementation. Signs of sodium depletion are often subtle and include listlessness, failure to gain weight despite adequate caloric intake, hyperkalemia, and hypercalcemia. It is reasonable to initiate supplementation with approximately 2 to 3 mEq/kg per day of sodium chloride. Substantially greater amounts of sodium may be necessary to ensure optimal growth. Sodium bicarbonate cannot substitute for sodium chloride to restore intravascular volume, and severe acidosis may not be apparent until the infants receive sufficient sodium chloride. Supplementation should be continued until the serum sodium concentration is greater than 140 mEq/L or the infant develops either hypertension or volume overload.[65]

Vitamins and Trace Minerals

With the exception of vitamin D, there is no evidence to indicate that the metabolism of fat-soluble vitamins is abnormal in CKD, and supplementation is not necessary. Vitamin A supplements should be specifically avoided, because vitamin A can accumulate in children with CKD, resulting in vitamin A toxicity.[66] Vitamin E supplements are not necessary as a standard nutritional supplement.

Current recommendations state that children receiving well-balanced diets may not require vitamin supplementation.[64] Appropriate nutritional follow-up is required to be certain that limitations in dietary intake do not excessively restrict micronutrient intakes. Because of these concerns, supplements of the water-soluble vitamins are often provided to patients with CKD and end-stage renal disease. Excessive amounts of vitamin C can lead to increased serum oxalate concentrations. Particular attention should be paid to folate, because folate depletion can limit the effectiveness of administered erythropoietin. Hyperhomocysteinemia has been shown to be an independent predictor of heart disease. Although supplementation with vitamin B_6, folate, and vitamin B_{12} improves homocysteine concentrations in patients with normal renal function and those after transplantation, there is no consensus on their efficacy in other individuals with CKD.[67]

Carnitine, a transporter of fatty acids, may be deficient in CKD, and carnitine supplementation has been suggested as a treatment for both hyperlipidemia and anemia.[68,69] Studies involving carnitine supplementation are difficult to interpret, at least in part because of the variety of dosages, time courses, and delivery methods used. There is little pediatric evidence available to support carnitine supplementation in pediatric patients, and consequently, routine supplementation is not recommended.[70,71]

V

There is little information available on the need for trace mineral supplementation for infants and children with CKD, but it would appear that for most individuals, supplements are not required. In individual clinical situations, it may be prudent to assess serum concentrations as an approximation of body stores and supplement as necessary.

Children on Dialysis

The National Kidney Foundation recently addressed dietary and nutritional issues related to children on dialysis.[64] The following summarizes the recommendations. There are 2 common forms of maintenance dialysis for children with end-stage renal disease—peritoneal dialysis and hemodialysis. The National Kidney Foundation separated its recommendations for these 2 dialysis types when there were data to justify that separation. Protein and energy requirements were based on the Recommended Dietary Allowance (DRIs were not yet established) for the child's chronologic age and gender as a starting point for the diet prescription with additional protein intake to account for protein and amino acid losses during dialysis (Table 41.5). Supplemental vitamins were not routinely recommended for children whose diet achieved the recommended amounts for the individual vitamins. Supplemental nutritional support (oral and/or enteral) is suggested for those children who cannot consistently consume DRIs of protein and energy or who are not growing despite good biochemical control and seemingly adequate intake.[64]

Renal Transplantation

Current immunosuppressive regimens for children after a renal transplant most often include the use of corticosteroids and calcineurin inhibitors. In part as a result of this therapy, a high proportion of children are hypertensive after transplantation. In the initial post-transplant period, the focus of medical nutrition therapy should be on limitation of sodium (3–4 g/day), weight control, and adequate fluid intake, especially for smaller children who receive adult-size kidneys. Long-term goals include achieving or maintaining age- and gender-appropriate BMI, regular physical activity, and eating a variety of foods, including fruits and vegetables, with moderate consumption of high-fat and high-sodium foods. Adequate fluid intake remains a long-term goal. Children should have their lipid concentrations monitored after transplantation.[72-74]

References

1. Foreman JW, Abitbol CL, Trachtman H, et al. Nutritional intake in children with renal insufficiency: a report of the growth failure in children with renal diseases study. *J Am Coll Nutr*. 1996;15:579–585

2. Jepson RG, Mihaljevic L, Craig J. Cranberries for preventing urinary tract infections. *Cochrane Database Syst Rev*. 2004;(1):CD001321

3. Henig YS, Leahy MM. Cranberry juice and urinary-tract health: science supports folklore. *Nutrition*. 2000;16:684–687

4. Glazener CM, Evans JH, Cheuk DK. Complementary and miscellaneous interventions for nocturnal enuresis in children. *Cochrane Database Syst Rev*. 2005;(2):CD005230

5. Hjalmas K, Arnold T, Bower W, et al. Nocturnal enuresis: international evidence based management strategy. *J Urol*. 2004;171:2545–2561

6. Sorof J, Daniels S. Obesity hypertension in children: a problem of epidemic proportions. *Hypertension*. 2002;40:441–447

7. Freedman DS, Dietz WH, Srinivasan SR, Berenson GS. The relation of overweight to cardiovascular risk factors among children and adolescents: the Bogalusa Heart Study. *Pediatrics*. 1999;103:1175–1182

8. Rosner B, Prineas R, Daniels SR, Loggie J. Blood pressure differences between blacks and whites in relation to body size among US children and adolescents. *Am J Epidemiol*. 2000;151:1007–1019

9. Dyer AR, Elliott P. The INTERSALT study: relations of body mass index to blood pressure. INTERSALT Co-operative Research Group. *J Hum Hypertens*. 1989;3:299–308

10. Rocchini AP, Katch V, Anderson J, et al. Blood pressure in obese adolescents: effect of weight loss. *Pediatrics*. 1988;82:16–23

11. Daniels SR, Arnett DK, Eckel RH, et al. Overweight in children and adolescents: pathophysiology, consequences, prevention, and treatment. *Circulation*. 2005;111: 1999–2012

12. Rosenberg B, Moran A, Sinaiko AR. Insulin resistance (metabolic) syndrome in children. *Panminerva Med*. 2005;47:229–244

13. Vivian EM. Type 2 diabetes in children and adolescents—the next epidemic? *Curr Med Res Opin*. 2006;22:297–306

14. Mertens H, Van Gaal L. Overweight, obesity, and blood pressure: the effects of modest weight reduction. *Obes Res*. 2000;8:270–278

15. The DASH Eating Plan. Available at: http://www.nhlbi.nih.gov/health/public/heart/hbp/dash/. Accessed October 3, 2007

16. Appel LJ, Moore TJ, Obarzanek E, et al. A clinical trial of the effects of dietary patterns on blood pressure. *N Engl J Med*. 1997;336:1117–1124

17. Harsha DW Lin PH, Obarzanek E, Karanja NM, Moore TJ, Calballero B. Dietary approaches to stop hypertension: a summary of study results. *J Am Diet Assoc*. 1999;(8 Suppl):S35–S39

18. Falkner B, Michel S. Blood pressure response to sodium in children and adolescents. *Am J Clin Nutr*. 1997;65(Suppl 2):618S–621S

19. Geleijnse J, Grobbee D, Hofman A. Sodium and potassium intake and blood pressure change in childhood. *Br Med J.* 1990;300:899–902

20. Mo R, Omvik P, Lund-Johansen P, Myking O. The Bergen blood pressure study: sodium intake and ambulatory blood pressure in offspring of hypertensive and normotensive families. *Blood Press.* 1993;2:278–283

21. Staessen JA, Lijnen P, Thijs L, Fagard R. Salt and blood pressure in community-based intervention trials. *Am J Clin Nutr.* 1997;65(Suppl 2):661S–670S

22. Vollmer WM, Sacks FM, Ard J, et al. Effects of diet and sodium intake on blood pressure: subgroup analysis of the DASH-Sodium Trial. *Ann Intern Med.* 2001;135:1019–1028

23. Institute of Medicine. *Dietary Reference Intakes for Energy, Carbohydrate, Fiber, Fat, Fatty Acids, Cholesterol, Protein and Amino Acids (Macronutrients).* Washington, DC: National Academies Press; 2005

24. Allender PS, Cutler JA, Follmann D, Cappuccio FP, Pryer J, Elliott P. Dietary calcium and blood pressure: a meta-analysis of randomized clinical trials. *Ann Intern Med.* 1996;124:825–831

25. Falkner B, Sherif K, Michel S, Kushner H. Dietary nutrients and blood pressure in urban minority adolescents at risk for hypertension. *Arch Pediatr Adolesc Med.* 2000;154:918–922

26. Karanja N, Morris CD, Rufolo P, Snyder G, Illingworth DR, McCarron DA. Impact of increasing calcium in the diet on nutrient consumption, plasma lipids, and lipoproteins in humans. *Am J Clin Nutr.* 1994;59:900–907

27. Kristal-Boneh E, Green MS. Dietary calcium and blood pressure—a critical review of the literature. *Public Health Rev.* 1990;18:267–300

28. Resnick LM. The role of dietary calcium in hypertension: a hierarchical overview. *Am J Hypertens.* 1999;12:99–112

29. Sorof JM, Forman A, Cole N, Jemerin JM, Morris RC. Potassium intake and cardiovascular reactivity in children with risk factors for essential hypertension. *J Pediatr.* 1997;131:87–94

30. Mizushima S, Cappuccio FP, Nichols R, Elliott P. Dietary magnesium intake and blood pressure: a qualitative overview of the observational studies. *J Hum Hypertens.* 1998;12:447–453

31. Whelton SP, Hyre AD, Pedersen B, Yi Y, Whelton PK, He J. Effect of dietary fiber intake on blood pressure: a meta-analysis of randomized, controlled clinical trials. *J Hypertens.* 2005;23:475–481

32. Ulbak J, Lauritzen L, Hansen HS, Michaelsen KF. Diet and blood pressure in 2.5-y-old Danish children. *Am J Clin Nutr.* 2004;79:1095–1102

33. Norman RW, Manette WA. Dietary restriction of sodium as a means of reducing urinary cystine. *J Urol.* 1990;143:1193–1195

34. Rodriguez LM, Santos F, Malaga S, Martinez V. Effect of a low sodium diet on urinary elimination of cystine in cystinuric children. *Nephron.* 1995;71:416–418

35. Borghi L, Schianchi T, Meschi T, et al. Comparison of two diets for the prevention of recurrent stones in idiopathic hypercalciuria. *N Engl J Med.* 2002;346:77–84

36. Cirillo M, Ciacci C, Laurenzi M, Mellone M, Mazzacca G, De Santo NG. Salt intake, urinary sodium and hypercalciuria. *Miner Electrolyte Metab.* 1997;23:265–268

37. Burtis WJ, Gay L, Insogna KL, Ellison A, Broadus AE. Dietary hypercalciuria in patients with calcium oxalate kidney stones. *Am J Clin Nutr.* 1994;60:424–429

38. Hess B, Jost C, Zipperle L, Takkinen R, Jaeger P. High-calcium intake abolishes hyperoxaluria and reduces urinary crystallization during a 20-fold normal oxalate load in humans. *Nephrol Dial Transplant.* 1998;13:2241–2247

39. Osorio AV, Alon US. The relationship between urinary calcium, sodium, and potassium excretion and the role of potassium in treating idiopathic hypercalciuria. *Pediatrics.* 1997;100:675–681

40. Laminski NA, Meyers AM, Kruger M, Sonnekus MI, Margolius LP. Hyperoxaluria in patients with recurrent calcium oxalate calculi: dietary and other risk factors. *Br J Urol.* 1991;68: 454–458

41. Massey LK, Sutton RA. Modification of dietary oxalate and calcium reduces urinary oxalate in hyperoxaluric patients with kidney stones. *J Am Diet Assoc.* 1993;93:1305–1307

42. Cattini Perrone H, Bruder Stapleton F, Toporovski J, Schor N. Hematuria due to hyperuricosuria in children: 36-month follow-up. *Clin Nephrol.* 1997;48:288–291

43. La Manna A, Polito C, Marte A, Iovene A, Di Toro R. Hyperuricosuria in Children: Clinical Presentation and Natural History. *Pediatrics.* 2001;107:86–90

44. Reid IR, Hardy DC, Murphy WA, Teitelbaum SL, Bergfeld MA, Whyte MP. X-linked hypophosphatemia: a clinical, biochemical, and histopathologic assessment of morbidity in adults. *Medicine (Baltimore).* 1989;68:336–352

45. Tieder M, Modai D, Samuel R, et al. Hereditary hypophosphatemic rickets with hypercalciuria. *N Engl J Med.* 1985;312:611–617

46. Kaysen GA, Gambertoglio J, Jiminez I, Jones H, Hutchison F. Effect of dietary protein intake on albumin homeostasis in nephrotic patients. *Kidney Int.* 1986;29:572–577

47. Papez KE, Smoyer WE. Recent advances in congenital nephrotic syndrome. *Curr Opin Pediatr.* 2004;16:165–170

48. Lechner BL, Bockenhauer D, Iragorri S, Kennedy TL, Siegel NJ. The risk of cardiovascular disease in adults who have had childhood nephrotic syndrome. *Pediatr Nephrol.* 2004; 19:744–748

49. D'Amico G, Gentile MG, Manna G, et al. Effect of vegetarian soy diet on hyperlipidaemia in nephrotic syndrome. *Lancet.* 1992;339:1131–1134

50. Coleman JE, Watson AR. Hyperlipidaemia, diet and simvastatin therapy in steroid-resistant nephrotic syndrome of childhood. *Pediatr Nephrol.* 1996;10:171–174

51. Briassoulis G, Venkataraman S, Thompson AE. Energy expenditure in critically ill children. *Crit Care Med.* 2000;28:1166–1172

52. Vazquez Martinez JL, Martinez-Romillo PD, Diez Sebastian J, Ruza Tarrio F. Predicted versus measured energy expenditure by continuous, online indirect calorimetry in ventilated, critically ill children during the early postinjury period. *Pediatr Crit Care Med.* 2004;5:19–27

53. Abitbol CL, Rossique M, Rios M. Nutrition support for pediatric patients with acute renal failure. In: Merritt R, ed. A.S.P.E.N. Nutrition Support Practice Manual. 2nd ed. Silver Springs, MD: American Society for Parenteral and Enteral Nutrition; 2005:287–295

54. Abitbol CL, Warady BA, Massie MD, et al. Linear growth and anthropometric and nutritional measurements in children with mild to moderate renal insufficiency: a report of the Growth Failure in Children with Renal Diseases Study. *J Pediatr.* 1990;116:S46–S54

55. Wingen A, Mehls O. Nutrition in children with preterminal chronic renal failure. Myth or important therapeutic aid. *Pediatr Nephrol.* 2002;17:111–120

56. Uuay RD, Hogg RJ, Brewer ED, Reisch JS, Cunningham C, Holliday MA. Dietary protein and growth in infants with chronic renal insufficiency: a report from the Southwest Pediatric Nephrology Study Group and the University of California, San Francisco. *Pediatr Nephrol.* 1994;8:45–50

57. Wingen AM, Fabian-Bach C, Schaefer F, Mehls O. Randomized, multicentre study of a low-protein diet on the progression of renal failure in children. *Lancet.* 1997;349:1117–1123

58. Hellerstein S, Holliday MA, Grupe WE, al. Nutritional management of children with chronic renal failure. Summary of the Task Force on Nutritional Management of Children with Chronic Renal Failure. *Pediatr Nephrol.* 1987;1:195–211

59. Sedman A, Friedman A, Boineau F, Strife CF, Fine R. Nutritional management of the child with mild to moderate chronic renal failure. *J Pediatr.* 1996;129:S13–S18

60. Ratsch IM, Catassi C, Verrina E, et al. Energy and nutrient intake of patients with mild to moderate chronic renal failure compared with healthy children: an Italian multicentre study. *Eur J Pediatr.* 1992;151:701–705

61. Wingen AM, Fabian-Bach C, Mehls O. Evaluation of protein intake by dietary diaries and urea-N excretion in children with chronic renal failure. European Study Group for Nutritional Treatment of Chronic Renal Failure in Childhood. *Clin Nephrol.* 1993;40:208–215

62. Oh J, Wunsch R, Turzer M, et al. Advanced coronary and carotid arteriopathy in young adults with childhood-onset chronic renal failure. *Circulation.* 2002;106:100–105

63. National Kidney Foundation. Clinical practice guidelines for bone metabolism and disease in children with chronic kidney disease. *Am J Kidney Dis.* 2003;42:S1–S201

64. National Kidney Foundation. Clinical practice guidelines for nutrition in chronic renal failure. *Am J Kidney Dis.* 2000;35(6 Suppl 2):S1–S140

65. Wassner SJ, Baum M. Chronic renal failure: physiology and management. In: Barratt TM, Avner ED, Harmen WE, eds. *Pediatric Nephrology.* 4th ed. Baltimore, MD: Lippincott, Williams &Wilkins; 1999:1155–1182

66. Yatzidis H, Digenis P, Fountas P. Hypervitaminosis A accompanying advanced chronic renal failure. *Br Med J.* 1975;110:352–353

67. Shemin D, Bostom AG, Selhub J. Treatment of hyperhomocysteinemia in end-stage renal disease. *Am J Kidney Dis.* 2001;38(4 Suppl 1):S91–S94

68. Calvani M, Benatti P, Mancinelli A, et al. Carnitine replacement in end-stage renal disease and hemodialysis. *Ann N Y Acad Sci.* 2004;1033:52–66

69. Hurot J, Cucherat M, Haugh M, Fouque D. Effects of L-carnitine supplementation in maintenance hemodialysis patients: a systemic review. *J Am Soc Nephrol.* 2002;13:708–714

70. Lilien MR, Duran M, Quak JM, Frankhuisen JJ, Schroder CH. Oral L-carnitine does not decrease erythropoietin requirement in pediatric dialysis. *Pediatr Nephrol.* 2000;15(1–2): 17–20

71. Schroder CH, European Pediatric Peritoneal Dialysis Working Group. The management of anemia in pediatric peritoneal dialysis patients. Guidelines by an ad hoc European committee. *Pediatr Nephrol.* 2003;18:805–809

72. Baker S, Barlow S, Cochran W, et al. Overweight children and adolescents: a clinical report of the North American Society for Pediatric Gastroenterology, Hepatology and Nutrition. *J Pediatr Gastroenterol Nutr.* 2005;40:533–543

73. Broyer M, Tete M, Laudat MH, Goldstein S. Plasma lipids in kidney transplanted children and adolescents: influence of pubertal development, dietary intake and steroid therapy. *Eur J Clin Invest.* 1981;11:397–402

74. Locsey L AL, Kincses Z, Berczi C, Paragh G. The importance of obesity and hyperlipidaemia in patients with renal transplants. *Int Urol Nephrol.* 1998;30:767–775

75. Hogg R, Furth S, Lemley K, et al. National Kidney Foundation's Kidney Disease Outcomes Quality Initiative clinical practice guidelines for chronic kidney disease in children and adolescents: evaluation, classification and stratification. *Pediatrics.* 2003;111:1416–1421

Nutritional Management of Children With Cancer

Malnutrition in pediatric oncology patients is often related to the location and extent of disease and the complications of therapy.[1-4] Malnutrition may be associated with poor growth and development, decreased immune function (including anergy to intradermal antigens), decreased tolerance for chemotherapy, and increased rates of infection. Studies suggest that children with cancer who are malnourished have a higher risk of developing chemotherapy toxicity, have a higher incidence of infectious complications, and tolerate chemotherapy more poorly when compared with children with normal nutritional status.[5-9]

Whether malnutrition leads to less favorable outcomes in children with cancer is currently not clear.[10-16] Nevertheless, the effects of poor nutrition on a child's physical and emotional well-being and quality of life is well established.[15,16] The goals for nutrition support in children with cancer are to promote normal growth and development, minimize morbidity and mortality, and maximize quality of life. The pathogenesis of malnutrition in children with cancer is multifactorial and includes the effects of the tumor(s), the host response to the malignancy, the effects of therapy, and psychological factors.

Nutritional Status at Diagnosis

Childhood cancer often presents with an acute onset (eg, acute leukemia) and a relatively stable state of nutrition at the time of diagnosis. However, children with solid tumors, especially those causing intestinal obstruction or demonstrating widespread metastatic disease, may have a higher incidence of malnutrition.[8] Malnutrition in pediatric oncology patients is commonly seen in children with advanced disease and those who relapse or do not respond to treatment and often is related to a certain type of intensive therapy.[2,5] The incidence of malnutrition has been reported to range from 6% in children with newly diagnosed leukemia to as high as 50% in patients with stage IV neuroblastoma.[6,8] At the other end of the spectrum, the incidence of overweight or obesity among children at the time of the diagnosis of cancer is increasing.[17]

Host-Related Effects on Nutritional Status

Metabolic effects of cancer, known as cancer cachexia, have been demonstrated both in animal models and humans.[18] Cachexia is a complicated process that varies by the site of tumor and is marked by early satiety, weight loss, and abnormal utilization of substrates, such as protein, fat, and carbohydrate.[18–20] Changes in substrate metabolism include an increase in protein turnover and loss of the normal compensatory mechanisms seen in starvation, which may result in skeletal muscle depletion.[19–23] Additionally, accelerated lipolysis results in depletion of fat stores and increased free fatty acid turnover with the net effect of wasting of body fat and hyperlipidemia.[18,19] Changes in carbohydrate metabolism result in an energy-losing cycle. Studies of adult patients with large tumor burdens have shown that tumors consume glucose by anaerobic glycolysis, producing lactic acid. Lactic acidosis, during infusions of glucose, has also been reported in children with cancer.[2,5,19] The data regarding changes in a patient's metabolic rate attributable to a malignancy tend to be inconsistent; mixed results have been reported in adult and pilot pediatric trials.[5,19]

The most common characteristic of cancer-associated malnutrition is anorexia. Anorexia occurs as a result of both the malignancy and the cancer therapy.[20,23] Adverse effects of chemotherapy, such as nausea, vomiting, diarrhea, mucositis, food aversion, and an altered sense of taste and smell, are major causes of anorexia in children undergoing cancer treatment. Furthermore, infection, chemotherapy-induced ulcers, delayed gastric emptying, pain, and psychological factors can play a significant role in the development of anorexia. There appears to be a clear relationship between treatments for cancer and anorexia, malnutrition, and growth retardation.[8,24,25]

Therapy-Related Effects on Nutritional Status

Multimodal treatments (chemotherapy, radiation, surgery, and biologic and immunologic therapies) may contribute either directly or indirectly to an altered nutritional status in children with cancer. Most chemotherapeutic agents adversely affect dietary intake. In a study of 100 pediatric oncology patients with a recent diagnosis of cancer, 44 were found to be consuming less than 80% of their estimated caloric requirements, compared with none of the controls.[2,26] Oral mucositis is one of the common adverse effects of intensive cancer treatment.[8,27] Many chemotherapy agents cause nausea and vomiting, altered food intake, impaired digestion and absorption, and increased nutrient losses. Antineoplastic drugs can cause diarrhea, constipation, ileus, and morphologic changes in the intestine resulting in an alteration of digestive enzyme.[8,28] Factors such as constipation, related to use of vincristine or narcotics, and lactose malabsorption with diarrhea can result in significant abdominal discomfort and loss of appetite.

Toxicity of chemotherapy treatment is related to the type of agent, the dose, and combination of chemotherapeutic medications. The child receiving chemotherapy may experience significant dysphagia and an alteration in nutritional status. Although new approaches in supportive care established by the Children's Oncology Group have decreased the nausea, vomiting, and mucositis associated with some of the treatment protocols, these adverse effects continue to present challenges in care of children with cancer.[29]

Radiation therapy alone or in combination with chemotherapy can severely affect one's nutritional status. The adverse effect may be influenced by dose, fractionation, location, and field size.[8,30] Radiotherapy to the head and neck can result in anorexia, altered taste sensation, and mucositis. Radiation to the chest can cause dysphagia or swallowing difficulties. Therapy to the abdomen or pelvis can result in gastrointestinal adverse effects (nausea, vomiting with poor food intake) or late effects on intestinal mucosa leading to radiation enteritis.[8,30]

Infection is a common occurrence in children with cancer. Among the factors that contribute to an increased risk of infection are myelosuppression and changes in humoral and cellular immunity, which may in part be a result of poor nutrition.[31] A child with an infection who is myelosuppressed may experience a poor appetite with suboptimal nutritional intake. Antibiotics as well as antifungal agents can cause gastrointestinal and urinary losses of nutrients, malabsorption, and anorexia with associated weight loss.

Psychological Factors

The adverse effects of anti-cancer therapy often create many psychosocial challenges.[32] Loss of appetite, eating discomfort associated with nausea or vomiting, separation from home environment at meal time, disruption of normal life, alteration in body image, and frequent medical procedures may all have significant effects on children's and adolescents' oral intake. Using a team approach, including the involvement of psychosocial, medical, nursing, and nutrition staff, may reduce some of the anxiety related to eating and may improve nutritional intake. Knowledge of treatment protocols and expected adverse effects of therapy will permit early intervention to prevent significant nutrition deterioration.

Nutritional Screening

The nutritional status of all children with cancer should be evaluated at the time of diagnosis and throughout therapy. The purpose of a nutrition evaluation is to identify the child at risk of malnutrition and to establish baseline nutrition information for future follow-up examinations.

The following criteria are used to identify children at risk[33,34]:

- Total weight loss of >5% of the preillness body weight over the past month
- Weight <10th or >90th percentile for age
- Height <10th percentile for age
- Weight for height <10th or >90th percentile
- Weight <90% of ideal body weight for height
- Triceps skinfold thickness <10th percentile and mid-arm circumference <5th percentile (arm anthropometry appears to be a more sensitive measure of malnutrition than weight for height in children with large solid tumors[33])
- BMI <5th or >85th percentile for age
- Oral intake <80% of estimated needs

Children receiving high-dose chemotherapy or combination therapy for aggressive cancers are at high risk of developing malnutrition and may need early nutrition intervention on the basis of their oral intake and the treatment protocol.

Nutritional Assessment

The goals of nutrition assessment are to identify and define nutrition problems, to establish individual nutrition needs and care plans, and to assess the appropriate route of nutrition. Follow-up is essential in monitoring the effectiveness of nutrition support therapy. The nutritional assessment of a child diagnosed with cancer should include:

- Medical and surgical history, including history of gastrointestinal symptoms, such as diarrhea, vomiting, and constipation
- Medication history, to include review of chemotherapy, antibiotics, and antifungal agents and their potential effects on nutritional status

- Anthropometric assessment (see below)

- Biochemical assessment (see below)

- Diet history to include:
  - Type and amount of foods or formula consumed
  - Feeding and eating patterns
  - Feeding problems and skills
  - Food aversions or intolerance
  - Food preferences
  - Food intake in relation to treatment schedule
  - Supplements, herbs, and/or complementary therapies

Anthropometric Assessment

Appropriate growth in children is the best indicator of adequate nutrition during the growth period. The National Center for Health Statistics (NCHS) growth charts are used to determine the percentile of height (length) for age, weight for age, weight for length (height), and head circumference for age (<3 years). These measurements are the most sensitive indicators of growth and should be a routine aspect of nutritional evaluation of the child with cancer at the time of diagnosis and throughout therapy.[7,8,33,34] The percent weight loss from the child's usual body weight and percent of ideal body weight for height can be used to determine nutritional status in children with cancer.[8,34] A significant deviation from the 50th percentile of weight for height is indicative of under- or overnutrition. Longitudinal data on each child's growth pattern is most helpful for detecting deviations from a child's normal growth pattern. Flattening of the weight/growth curve may be an early indicator of decreased energy and protein intake.

Rapid weight gain throughout therapy should also be recognized, and early intervention should be implemented to prevent excessive weight gain during and after treatment. Body mass index (BMI [weight/height^2]) is an indirect measure of lean body mass and fat stores.[34] In adolescents, BMI for age correlates with total body fatness and can be used as a screening tool to determine over- and undernutrition.[33]

Biochemical Assessment

Biochemical determinations in combination with anthropometric data are helpful in the evaluation of the patient's nutritional status. Serum albumin and prealbumin concentrations are obtained to determine visceral protein status. These values are altered by poor protein intake, impaired absorption, inadequate synthesis, chronic losses, hydration status, and abnormal liver and renal function.[7,8,34] Their specificity is limited, because they are also acute phase reactant proteins. An abnormal serum albumin concentration may more often reflect the acute metabolic response to fever and infection or chronic catabolic stress from infection rather than the depletion of lean body mass.

The concentration of transthyretin (prealbumin), with its shorter half-life of 2 to 3 days versus 21 days for serum albumin, is often used to determine the effectiveness of nutrition interventions. Other serum biochemical indices, such as concentrations of sodium, potassium, chloride, bicarbonate, glucose, creatine, urea nitrogen, calcium, phosphorous, magnesium, triglycerides, and transaminases, should be monitored closely, because dietary intake as well as chemotherapy and antibiotic medications can alter their values.

Clinical Evaluation

The clinical evaluation of the child with cancer should include monitoring for signs of muscle or fat depletion, wasting, edema, or mouth sores and must be a routine part of the comprehensive nutritional assessment.

Estimating Nutrient Requirements

Actual nutrient requirements of children with cancer may vary with individual needs, disease activity, and treatment modalities. It is necessary to establish intake goals for calories, protein, vitamins, minerals, and fluids, especially for children receiving parenteral and enteral nutrition support. Different tables and equations are used to determine calorie and other nutrient requirements in children with cancer. The Dietary Reference Intakes (DRIs) for age and sex and World Health Organization equations for basal metabolic rate are often used.[8,33,34] The DRIs may not be the most appropriate method for estimating the calorie requirements of children with cancer.[8] Children receiving intensive therapy are generally less active and require less energy than their healthy counterparts. However, they may need additional calories during infections or other stresses. World Health Organization equations for basal metabolic rate, with a broad range of additional calories for growth and stress, is commonly used. Protein requirements for children with cancer are not known. Children with significant metabolic stress (eg, major surgery, infection) or increased losses may have a higher protein requirement. During stress-related illness, the usual estimate of the protein requirement in children is 1.5 to 2.5g/kg per day, which is approximately 50% higher than normal.[35]

There is little information regarding vitamin and mineral requirements of children with cancer. Recommendations for vitamins and minerals are based on the DRIs for age and gender. If the oral intake is suboptimal, or if there are increased losses of certain nutrients through vomiting, diarrhea, or malabsorption, individual or multivitamin-mineral supplement is recommended. Additional iron supplementation is not recommended for children receiving blood products frequently. It is generally accepted that children receiving methotrexate should not receive additional folic acid as a supplement.

Mineral wasting and deficiencies associated with the adverse effects of chemotherapy are commonly seen in children. The nutrients most frequently affected include magnesium, calcium, phosphorus, potassium, and zinc.[7] Intravenous or oral electrolyte supplementation is often needed. In these cases, monitoring of serum electrolyte concentrations is essential. The provision of adequate fluid is important throughout therapy.

Fluid requirements are highly individualized; however, the following guidelines may be used as estimates of maintenance fluid requirements[34]:

- <10 kg: 100 mL/kg per day
- >10 kg–20 kg: 1000 mL plus 50 mL/kg for each kg >10 kg per day
- >20 kg–30 kg: 1500 mL plus 20 mL/kg for each kg >20 kg per day
- >30 kg: 1500 mL/m² per day or 35 mL/kg per day

Nutrition Therapy

Nutrition therapy involves oral feeding, enteral tube feeding, and parenteral nutrition. Although the oral route is the preferred method of providing nutrition, the challenges for children on intensive treatment protocols are their inability to eat an adequate amount of food in the face of nausea, vomiting, aversion to smells and tastes, mucositis, and stomatitis. Children should be encouraged to try calorically dense foods. They should not be forced, threatened, or punished for not being able to eat enough food.

Initial nutritional counseling regarding the effects of cancer and its treatment on nutrition is an important part of the comprehensive care of children with cancer. Information regarding appropriate food choices to meet daily nutrient requirements with or without supplements may be adequate for some children on maintenance therapy. Guidelines for management of nutritional complications resulting from therapy should be provided during initial or ongoing counseling. Food safety and appropriate food handling should be a part of overall nutrition education for the caregiver.

Special diets, such as the neutropenic or low-bacteria diet, are used in some oncology centers to minimize the introduction of pathogenic organisms into the gastrointestinal tract; however, recent studies do not support the effectiveness of such restrictions.[36,37] Appetite stimulants, such as megestrol acetate and dronabinol, are used to treat weight loss in some patients experiencing cachexia, anorexia, and nausea. The potential adverse effects of these drugs should be considered.

Tube Feeding

When oral intake remains inadequate, tube feedings may provide an effective and safe method for nutrition support. Although nasogastric tube feeding has been accepted for nutrition support of children with other illnesses,[38] it is generally accepted that this is not the preferred approach for children with cancer because of the discomfort of nasogastric tube placement, the psychological effects of alterations in body image, and poor compliance. An additional concern with nasogastric tube feeding is possible trauma to the fragile mucosal surfaces of a patient with a low platelet and white blood cell count, resulting in bacterial translocation into the bloodstream. Yet, there are pilot data that have demonstrated the safety and feasibility of nasogastric tube feedings for the nutritional support of children with cancer when other routes of feeding are inappropriate.[39]

Gastrostomy tube feedings have been used for nutritional support in pediatric oncology patients with some concern for site infections, leakage of gastric contents onto the skin, and poor healing at the site.[40–42] In general, enteral tube feedings have a number of distinct advantages over parenteral nutrition.[43,44] These advantages include:

- Decreased risk of infection;
- Maintenance of structural and functional gastrointestinal integrity;
- Decreased potential for bacterial translocation;
- Greater ease and safety of administration;
- Decreased hepatobiliary complications; and
- Lower cost.

Tube feeding should be the first choice for nutritional support of children with an inadequate oral intake. The following criteria should be considered when tube feeding is recommended:

- The patient and family consent;

- A functional gastrointestinal tract;

- The inability of the child to maintain normal nutrition by the oral route;

- The patient's status regarding nausea, vomiting, and diarrhea;

- An adequate platelet count (>20 000); and

- A normal mucosal surface in the upper gastrointestinal tract.

A team approach including a dietitian, child life specialist, social workers, psychiatrist, oncologists, and nurses helps facilitate the successful initiation and continuation of nasogastric tube feedings on a child with cancer.[39] It is necessary to follow institutional guidelines for use of anti-emetic and prokinetic medications for successful enteral feeding.

The optimal access route for enteral nutrition is determined on the basis of anticipated duration of the tube feeding, the neurologic status of the patient, and the risk of aspiration. In general, nasoenteric tubes are considered for short-term use (<6 weeks), although successful long-term use of nasogastric tube feeding has been reported.[39] Other routes of enteral tube feeding include nasoduodenal, nasojejunal, gastrostomy, and jejunostomy tubes. The use of a silicone or polyurethane tube with the smallest diameter (6–8 French) is recommended for nasoenteric tubes.

Enteral formulas are selected on the basis of age and gastrointestinal function. Infant formulas with 20 to 30 kcal/oz are appropriate choices for oral or enteral tube feedings of infants. Lactose-free infant formulas may be required because of chemotherapy-induced lactose intolerance. The need for nutrient-dense formulas (>20 kcal/oz) is based on fluid tolerance. Increasing the formula concentration may increase renal solute load or cause gastrointestinal intolerance with abdominal distention, vomiting, or diarrhea. Thus, the concentration of a formula should be increased slowly with close monitoring of potential adverse effects. A concentrated formula may be achieved by adding "modular" supplements to standard infant formulas. Age-appropriate standard formulas may be used for patients with normal gut function. Unflavored formulas with lower osmolality are better tolerated than flavored ones and are recommended for tube feedings. Children with

V

abnormal gastrointestinal tract function may benefit from protein hydro-lysate or elemental formulas (see Appendix U).

Tube feeding may be administered by continuous drip using a feeding pump for a reliable, constant infusion rate. Continuous feeding may be better tolerated with delayed gastric emptying. Tube feedings may also be delivered by intermittent bolus feeding, which is more physiologic and mimics normal feeding. Nocturnal continuous feedings with daytime oral and/or bolus feedings work well to meet nutritional goals. Small bowel feedings should be considered for children with neurologic impairment who have a higher risk of aspiration and those with frequent vomiting. Continuous tube feedings may be initiated with full-strength isotonic formula at 1 to 2 mL/kg per hour per day. They may be advanced by 1 to 2 mL/kg per hour per day as tolerated until the volume goal is achieved.[34,35]

Parenteral Nutrition

Parenteral nutrition is indicated when the child's nutrition status cannot be maintained by enteral route. This may occur with tumors producing gastrointestinal tract obstruction, severe mucositis, uncontrolled nausea and vomiting, or inability to absorb nutrients. Children receiving hematopoietic stem cell transplants with severe mucositis and enteritis, those with a diagnosis of typhlitis, and postsurgical patients with ascites may also be candidates for parenteral nutrition. The parenteral route may also be required to supplement enteral tube feedings. The use and risk of parenteral nutrition in children with cancer has been extensively reviewed.[45–49] The risk of catheter-related infections and gastrointestinal and metabolic complications should be considered when parenteral nutrition is selected for nutritional support of a child with normal gastrointestinal tract function. An aggressive approach with enteral tube feedings has greatly reduced the need for total parenteral nutrition, thereby reducing potential adverse effects and cost.[39]

The Relationship Between Diet and Cancer

Although the roles of diet and lifestyle in cancer prevention have received considerable attention in adults,[50] to date there is no evidence to suggest a link between childhood cancer and any specific dietary choices or nutrient imbalances. Healthy habits, including eating a healthy diet, staying physically active, maintaining a normal weight during the maintenance phase of treatment and after treatment, may help keep a child with cancer healthy and reduce the late effects of therapy. It would be prudent to emphasize a diet consisting of a wide variety of foods including plant food sources, whole grains, fruits, and vegetables as illustrated in the US Department of Agriculture's "MyPyramid" (see Chapter 6).

There has been an increased focus on supportive care of children with cancer. This includes efforts to develop uniform guidelines for nutritional management of children with cancer through the Children's Oncology Group[51] as well as clinical trials to investigate the role of certain nutrients, such as glutamine, arginine, omega-3 fatty acids, antioxidants, and herbal products in childhood cancer.

References

1. Novy MA, Saavedra JM. Nutrition therapy for pediatric cancer patient. *Top Clin Nutr.* 1997;12:16–25

2. Bechard LJ, Adiv OE, Jaksic T, Duggan C. Nutritional supportive care. In: Pizzo P, Poplack DG, eds. *Principles and Practice of Pediatric Oncology.* 4th ed. Philadelphia, PA: Lippincott Williams & Wilkins; 2002:1285–1300

3. Reilly JJ, Weir J, McColl JH, Gibson BE. Prevalence of protein-energy malnutrition at diagnosis in children with lymphoblastic leukemia. *J Pediatr Gastroenterol Nutr.* 1999;194–197

4. Elhasid R, Laor A, Lischinskys S, Postovsky S, Weyl Ben Arush M. Nutritional status of children with solid tumors. *Cancer.* 1999;86:119–125

5. Mauer A, Burgess J, Donaldson SS, et al. Special nutritional needs of children with malignancies: a review. *JPEN J Parenter Enteral Nutr.* 1990;14:315–324

6. Sala A, Pencharz P, Barr RD. Children, cancer and nutrition—a dynamic triangle in review. *Cancer.* 2004;100:677–687

7. Ladas EJ, Sacks N, Meacham L, et al. A multidisciplinary review of nutrition considerations in the pediatric oncology population: a perspective from children's oncology group. *Nutr Clin Pract.* 2005;20:377–393

8. Barale KV, Charuhas PM. Oncology and hematopoietic cell transplantation. In: Samour PQ, King K, eds. *Handbook of Pediatric Nutrition.* 3rd ed. Sudbury, MA: Jones & Bartlett Publishers; 2005:459–481

9. Lobato-Mendizabal E, Lopez-Martinez B, Ruiz-Arguelles GJ. A critical review of the prognostic value of the nutritional status at diagnosis in the outcome of therapy of children with acute lymphoblastic leukemia. *Rev Invest Clin.* 2003;55:31–35

10. Lange BJ, Gerbing RB, Feusner J, et al. Mortality in overweight and underweight children with acute myeloid leukemia. *JAMA.* 2005;293:203–211

11. Murry DJ, Riva L, Poplack DG. Impact of nutrition on pharmacokinetics of anti-neoplastic agents. *Int J Cancer Suppl.* 1998;11:48–51

12. Viana MB, Murao M, Ramos G, et al. Malnutrition as a prognostic factor in lymphoblastic leukemia: a multivariate analysis. *Arch Dis Child.* 1994;71:304–310

13. Taj MM, Pearson AD, Mumford DB, Price L. Effect of nutritional status on the incidence of infection in childhood cancer. *J Pediatric Hematol Oncol.* 1993;10:283–287

V

14. Barr RD, Gibson BE. Nutritional status and cancer in childhood. *J Pediatr Hematol Oncol.* 2000;22:491–494

15. Pedrosa F, Bonilla M, Liu A, et al. Effect of malnutrition at the time of diagnosis on the survival of children treated for cancer in El Salvador and Northern Brazil. *J Pediatr Hematol Oncol.* 2000;22:502–505

16. Van Eys J. Benefits of nutritional intervention on nutritional status, quality of life and survival. *Int J Cancer Suppl.* 1998;11:66–88

17. Rogers PC, Meacham LR, Oeffinger KC, Henry DW, Lange BJ. Obesity in pediatric oncology. *Pediatr Blood Cancer.* 2005;45:881–891

18. Picton S. Aspects of altered metabolism in children with cancer. *Int J Cancer Suppl.* 1998;11:62–64

19. Langer CJ, Hoffman JP, Ottery FD. Clinical significance of weight loss in cancer patients: rationale for use of anabolic agents in the treatment of cancer-related cachexia. *Nutrition.* 2001;17(1 Suppl):S1–S20

20. Strasser F, Bruera ED. Update on anorexia and cachaexia. *Hematol Oncol Clin North Am.* 2002;160:589–617

21. Kurzer M, Meguid MM. Cancer and protein metabolism. *Surg Clin North Am.* 1986;66:969–1001

22. Pencharz P. Aggressive oral, enteral or parenteral nutrition: prescriptive decisions in children with cancer. *Int J Cancer Suppl.* 1998;11:73–75

23. Kern KA, Norton JA. Cancer cachexia. *JPEN J Parenter Enteral Nutr.* 1988;12:286–298

24. Katz JA, Chambers B, Everhart C, Marks JF, Buchanan GR. Linear growth in children with acute lymphoblastic leukemia treated without cranial irradiation. *J Pediatr.* 1991;118:575–578

25. Katz JA, Pollock BH, Jacaruso D, Morad A. Final attained height in patients successfully treated for childhood acute lymphoblastic leukemia. *J Pediatr.* 1993;123:546–552

26. Smith DE, Stevens MC, Booth IW. Malnutrition at diagnosis of malignancy in childhood: common but mostly missed. *Eur J Pediatr.* 1991;150:318–322

27. Bryant R. Managing side effects of childhood cancer treatment. *J Pediatr Nurs.* 2003; 18:113–125

28. Wohlschlaeger A. Prevention and treatment of mucositis: a guide for nurses. *J Pediatr Oncol Nurs.* 2004;21:281–287

29. Betcher DL, Bond D, Graner K, Lorenzen A. Chemotherapy induced nausea and vomiting. In: Altman AJ, ed. *Supportive Care of Children with Cancer.* 3rd ed. Baltimore, MD: Johns Hopkins University Press; 2004:181–199

30. Pieters RS, Marcus K, Marcus RB. Side effects of radiation therapy. In: Altman AJ, ed. *Supportive Care of Children with Cancer.* 3rd ed. Baltimore, MD: Johns Hopkins University Press; 2004:156–180

31. Altman AJ, Wolff LJ. The prevention of infection. In: Altman AJ, ed. *Supportive Care of Children with Cancer.* 3rd ed. Baltimore, MD: Johns Hopkins University Press; 2004:1–12

32. Lesko LM. Psychosocial issues in the diagnosis and management of cancer cachexia and anorexia. *Nutrition.* 1989;5:114–116

33. Hendricks KM, Duggan C, eds. *Manual of Pediatric Nutrition.* Hamilton, Ontario: B.C. Decker; 2005

34. Sacks N, Ringwald-Smith K, Hale G. Nutrition support. In: Altman AJ, ed. *Supportive Care of Children with Cancer.* 3rd ed. Baltimore, MD: Johns Hopkins University Press; 2004:243–261

35. Sheard NF, Clark N. Nutritional management of pediatric oncology patients. In: Baker SS, Baker RD, Davis A, eds. *Pediatric Enteral Nutrition.* New York, NY: Chapman Hall; 1994:387–398

36. Ladas E. The neutropenic diet: an examination of evidence. *Oncology Nutrition Dietetic Practice Group.* 2002;10(2). Available at: www.oncologynutrition.org. Accessed October 8, 2007

37. Moody K, Charlson ME, Finlay J. The neutropenic diet: what is the evidence? *J Pediatr Hematol Oncol.* 2002;24:717–721

38. Heyland DK, Cook DJ, Guyatt GH. Enteral nutrition in the critically ill patient: a critical review of evidence. *Intensive Care Med.* 1993;19:435–442

39. Deswarte-Wallace J, Firouzbakhsh S, Finklestein JZ. Using research to change practice: enteral feedings for pediatric oncology patients. *J Pediatr Oncol Nurs.* 2001;18:217–223

40. Mathew P, Bowman L, Williams R, et al. Complications and effectiveness of gastrostomy feedings pediatric cancer patients. *J Pediatr Hematol Oncol.* 1996;18:81–85

41. Szeluga DJ, Stuart BK, Brookmeyer R, Utermohlen V, Santos GW. Nutritional support of bone marrow transplant recipients: a prospective, randomized clinical trial comparing total parenteral nutrition to an enteral feeding program. *Cancer Res.* 1987;47:3309–3316

42. Skolin I, Hernell O, Larsson MV, Wahlgren C, Wahlin YB. Percutaneous endoscopic gastrostomy in children with malignant disease. *J Pediatr Oncol Nurs.* 2002;19:154–163

43. Ford C, Whitlock JA, Pietsch JB. Glutamine-supplemented tube feedings versus total parenteral nutrition in children receiving intensive chemotherapy. *J Pediatr Oncol Nurs.* 1997;14:68–72

44. Han-Markey T. Nutrition consideration in pediatric oncology. *Semin Oncol Nurs.* 2000; 16:146–151

45. Deitch E, Winterton J, Li M, Berg R. The gut as a portal of entry for bacteremia. Role of protein malnutrition. *Ann Surg.* 1987;205:681–692

46. Pietsch JB, Ford C, Whitlock JA. Nasogastric tube feedings in children with high-risk cancer: a pilot study. *J Pediatr Hematol/Oncol.* 1999;2:111–114

47. Charuhas PM, Gautier ST. Parenteral nutrition in pediatric oncology. In: Baker SS, Baker RD, Davis A, eds. *Pediatric Parenteral Nutrition.* New York, NY: Chapman & Hall; 1997:331–353

48. ASPEN Board of Directors and Clinical Guidelines Task Force. Guidelines for the use of parenteral and enteral nutrition in adult and pediatric patients. *JPEN J Parenter Enteral Nutr.* 2002:26(Suppl):1SA–138SA

49. Mirtallo J, Canada T, Johnson D, et al. Safe practices for parental nutrition. *JPEN J Parenter Enteral Nutr.* 2004;28:S39–S70

50. Chan JM, Gann PH, Giovannucci EL. Role of diet in prostate cancer development and progression. *J Clin Oncol.* 2005;23:8152–8160

51. Lads EJ, Sacks N, Brophy P, Rogers P. Standards of nutritional care in pediatric oncology: result from a nationwide survey on the standards of practice in pediatric oncology. A Children's Oncology Group Study. *Pediatr Blood Cancer.* 2006;46:339–344

Growth Failure

Prevalence

Height velocity is the most sensitive parameter by which impaired linear growth can be recognized. The percentage of children with Crohn disease whose growth is affected varies with the definition of growth impairment and with the nature of the population under study (eg, tertiary referral center versus total population). Weight loss or a failure to gain weight appropriately for age may precede the decrease in height velocity.

Impairment of linear growth is common in children before the recognition of Crohn disease and during the subsequent years. As a result, height at maturity is often compromised. In contrast, linear growth is less often impaired at the time of diagnosis of ulcerative colitis and, in follow-up, growth impairment is much less frequently observed.

Pathophysiology

Several interrelated factors may contribute to growth impairment in children with Crohn disease. Chronic undernutrition has long been implicated as a remediable cause of growth retardation. However, a simple nutritional hypothesis fails to explain all the observations related to growth patterns among children with inflammatory bowel disease (IBD). More recently, the direct growth-inhibiting effects of proinflammatory cytokines released from the inflamed intestine have been increasingly recognized. Enhancement of linear growth is best achieved through control of intestinal inflammation and ensuring adequate nutritional intakes.

Role of Cytokines and Endocrine Mediators

Insulin growth factor-1 (IGF-1), produced by the liver in response to growth hormone (GH) stimulation, normally mediates GH effects on the growth plate of bones. The association between impaired growth in Crohn disease and low IGF-1 concentrations is well recognized. Several interrelated factors may influence IGF-1 concentrations, including malnutrition, direct cytokine effects, and suppression by chronic daily corticosteroid therapy.

Elevated concentrations of cytokines, such as tumor necrosis factor (TNF)-alpha, previously referred to as "cachectin," explain, in part, the anorexia that often accompanies Crohn disease, even in the absence of symptoms. Although anti-TNF-alpha antibodies reduce disease activity, a direct association between TNF-alpha and growth failure remains elusive. Animal studies also support a role for interleukin (IL)-6 in growth inhibition in chronic inflammatory states. Transgenic mice that overexpress IL-6 have reduced growth rates because of reduced IGF-1 production.

Aside from providing additional calories, nutritional interventions can potentially improve the inflammation in IBD via modulation of pro- and anti-inflammatory cytokine profiles. For instance, short-chain fatty acids can regulate cytokine and chemokine gene expression by intestinal epithelial cells. Transforming growth factor (TGF)-beta, a polypeptide that modulates intestinal epithelial cell growth and development and has anti-inflammatory effects, is biologically active in human and cow milk. An open, uncontrolled trial[1] using a polymeric formula containing TGF-beta-2 as the sole source of nutrition in children with Crohn disease reported remission in 79% of cases, associated with down-regulation of intestinal mRNA expression of IL-1, interferon (IFN)-gamma, and IL-8, whereas TGF-beta-1 concentrations increased. It remains to be seen whether the addition of anti-inflammatory cytokines to treatment protocols will prove beneficial in controlled, blinded trials.

Monitoring of Nutritional Status

Screening and assessing children with IBD for under- or overnutrition is an essential component of medical care. Screening includes, at a minimum, obtaining data on body weight for age and height for age, including calculation of the body mass index (BMI [kg/m^2]). These data should be plotted and followed longitudinally on appropriate growth charts (see Appendix D).

Assessment of nutritional status includes history, physical examination, and laboratory testing. Essential in the history is a review of recent weight changes (especially weight loss that has been correlated with increasing morbidity and mortality). It is important to obtain preillness heights so the effects of chronic intestinal inflammation can be fully appreciated. It is essential to note appetite changes and obtain a dietary history (often with the assistance of a clinical nutritionist or a registered dietitian who can perform a 24-hour dietary intake history). Documentation of the use of medications, including corticosteroids and other immunosuppressive medications, and nutritional supplements, including vitamins and minerals, is also important. It is vital to review the symptoms of the underlying illness that might affect nutrient requirements, such as difficulty swallowing, nausea, vomiting, or diarrhea. A review of social factors is valuable, including the home environment, economic factors, and access to appropriate foods.

Physical examination includes anthropometric assessment of body habitus, including weight, height, BMI, head circumference in children younger than 3 years, and triceps skinfold thickness and mid-arm circumference to estimate body fat and muscle mass. It is important to plot all measurements on appropriate standardized charts, record sexual maturation by Tanner staging, and document physical signs of generalized undernutrition (eg, marasmus and kwashiorkor) or specific nutrient deficiencies, including skin rash, hair changes, oral lesions, hepatomegaly, clubbing of the nail beds, and edema.

Laboratory tests of nutritional status, including serum albumin concentration, may be helpful, but interpretation is complicated by gastrointestinal losses and concurrent medication use (particularly that of corticosteroids). Serum albumin concentration is better correlated with inflammation of the intestinal tract than with nutritional state in patients with IBD. Serum prealbumin (transthyretin) has a much shorter half-life (2 days) than does albumin (18–20 days), and its concentration has been used to assess the efficacy of nutrition support. Other serum protein concentrations proposed for assessing nutritional status include serum transferrin and retinol-binding protein, but these have little advantage over albumin and prealbumin. Anergy also has been used as a marker of undernutrition, but this test is also compromised by immunosuppressive medications. Other laboratory tests that are available but not typically used in the clinical setting include the ratio of urinary creatinine to height and 3-methylhistidine determinations, both measures of somatic (muscle) protein status, and a 24-hour urine urea nitrogen concentration, reflecting protein catabolism. Because of the difficulty obtaining accurate specimens and assumptions that have to be made to interpret these tests, they are not used in most clinical settings.

Research techniques that assess nutritional status have not yet been widely applied to patients with IBD. Such techniques include bioelectric impedance analysis and total body electrical conductance to determine total body water and fat mass and isotopic labeling of various molecules to determine energy expenditure and metabolic turnover rates. Recent application of dual-energy x-ray absorptiometry scanning for patients with IBD has yielded important information regarding bone mineral deficiencies among children and adolescents with IBD.[2–4]

Specific nutrient deficiencies are found in children with IBD, more commonly in Crohn disease than in ulcerative colitis. However, micronutrient deficiencies are likely reflective of disease activity rather than specific nutritional deficiencies.

Selected Nutrient Requirements

Daily nutrient requirements may be higher than the Dietary Reference Intakes because of malabsorption, enteric losses associated with diarrhea, and the obligatory metabolic cost of growth and inflammation. During disease exacerbation, energy consumption in children with Crohn disease may decrease by approximately 20% of the Recommended Dietary Allowance. Energy deficits have been estimated to be 400 kcal/day. Children with Crohn disease generally have greater nutrient needs on the basis of age, gender, and weight than do children with ulcerative colitis. Current consensus is that the diet of pediatric patients with IBD be well balanced, based on MyPyramid from the US Department of Agriculture (www.mypyramid. gov), and follow the Dietary Reference Intakes recommended by the Institute of Medicine. Dietary restrictions are avoided unless intestinal obstruction or specific abnormalities of digestion exist. Dietary supplementation of selected nutrients may be warranted on the basis of inferences from newer information accumulated in the last 15 years.

Energy

Resting energy expenditure (REE [kcal/day]) in well-nourished children with Crohn disease is not different from values obtained in healthy children; the apparent increase in REE in children with Crohn disease is a result of their lower fat-free mass. In well-nourished children who underwent ileocolectomy for Crohn disease, REE decreased approximately 5% after accounting for the energy expended by the resected gut. Although REE was reported to be lower in undernourished children with Crohn disease than in healthy children, when expressed in terms of lean body mass, REE was not different between the 2 groups.[5] In a subset of these undernourished children with Crohn disease, REE was 35% higher compared with malnourished female patients with anorexia nervosa, implying that adaptation of REE in children with active Crohn disease in response to weight loss is offset by the metabolic consequences of mucosal inflammation. These changes in REE are reversible and sustainable with aggressive enteral refeeding. High-fat diets may be used more efficiently for body fat deposition in adults with Crohn disease. However, low-fat diets are equally as effective as high-fat diets in restoring body fat mass in undernourished children with Crohn disease. Approximately 90% of dietary fat is absorbed, regardless of the quality or quantity consumed. Short-term refeeding studies in undernourished children with Crohn disease demonstrate rapid weight gain (average 8.7 kg/6 weeks) with dietary energy intakes that approximated 170% of REE. Long-term refeeding studies in undernourished children with Crohn disease show catch-up growth, with average height and weight gains of 7 to 9 cm/year and 7 kg/year, respectively, with daily dietary energy intakes approximating 133% of recommended values for ideal body weight or 60 to 75 kcal/kg actual body weight. Taken together, these studies suggest that energy needs may be increased above recommended dietary intakes by as little as 5% and as much as 35% in children with Crohn disease, depending on their nutritional status and the degree of inflammatory disease activity.

Protein

Whole body protein turnover is increased in children with increased disease activity, which can be reduced with either corticosteroid therapy or an elemental diet. Although the efficiency of dietary nitrogen absorption is high with peptide-based formulas, refeeding studies using elemental formulas suggest that the efficiency of nitrogen utilization in children with Crohn disease depends on dietary proteins rich in aromatic and sulfur amino acids, particularly tyrosine and cystine. A glutamine-enriched diet offers no advantage over a low-glutamine diet in children with Crohn disease. However, if glutamine supplementation of the diet occurs at the expense of a reduction in other potentially conditionally essential amino acids (glycine and proline), thereby lowering the protein quality of the diet, no benefit may be seen. Short-term refeeding studies in undernourished children with Crohn disease demonstrate that lean body mass constitutes 80% of body weight gain when daily dietary protein intakes approximate 3 g/kg and the protein-energy ratio of the peptide-based formulas averages 1:6.25. Dietary protein is not a limiting nutrient in Western diets; nevertheless, the metabolic costs of inflammation and growth on protein nutriture in children with Crohn disease have not yet been fully elucidated. As such, no specific recommendations for quantitative and qualitative protein and/or amino acid needs can be made at this time.

Vitamins, Trace Minerals, and Antioxidants

Deficiencies for virtually every vitamin, mineral, and trace element have been reported in children with Crohn disease. During disease exacerbation, dietary intakes of iron, zinc, copper, folic acid, and vitamin C, but not vitamins A or E, may decrease, on average, 20% to 50% below their Recommended Dietary Allowance. Altered serum or plasma concentrations often are used to define the deficiency state; however, these values may correlate with markers of inflammation and not reflect body tissue stores or functional deficits. With severe, extensive inflammation or after extensive resection of the terminal ileum, parenteral vitamin B_{12} supplementation may be necessary.

Vitamcin D

Bone mineralization is an important consideration in the care of the growing child with IBD. The World Health Organization defines osteopenia as the loss of bone mineral and matrix z-scores >1 standard deviation (SD) and osteoporosis as matrix z-scores >2 standard deviations below the mean for male and female populations. High rates of osteopenia and osteoporosis are reported in pediatric patients with IBD.[2,6-8] Vertebral compression fracture has been reported as a presenting manifestation of the disease, and there is a higher rate of bone fracture in children after corticosteroid treatment.

Gender and pubertal staging are important considerations in understanding reported rates of osteopenia and osteoporosis. In most studies, a greater proportion of adolescent boys exhibited osteoporosis. However, when osteoporosis occurs in girls with Crohn disease, it tends to persist. Because bone density is heavily influenced by growth and puberty, correction for height age, bone age, or BMI reduces the apparent prevalence of osteoporosis. An independent risk factor may be genetic predisposition. Patient groupings can be further subdivided by disease classification (Crohn disease vs ulcerative colitis), treatment with corticosteroids, or previous surgery. Patients with Crohn disease have far greater impairment of bone density than do patients with ulcerative colitis. Bone mineral density has consistently been reported to be low at diagnosis in pediatric patients with Crohn disease, after 2 years of treatment, and in adults with longstanding disease.

Corticosteroids reduce calcium absorption, down-regulate calcitriol synthesis, decrease gene expression of calcium-binding protein, inhibit osteoblast proliferation, and stimulate osteoclastic bone resorption. Corticosteroid use at >7.5 mg/day, 5 g lifetime cumulative dose, or >12 months of lifetime exposure are risk factors for a low bone mineral density z-score.

Patients with newly diagnosed Crohn disease exhibit hypercalciuria, indicating negative calcium balance, because of the effects of systemic inflammation. Serum from pediatric patients with Crohn disease inhibits osteoblastic activity in bone cell culture that is attributed to the effects of IL-6, TNF-alpha, and other cytokines. There also is a genetic component in the response of bone in patients with Crohn disease to proinflammatory cytokines (ie, noncarriage of the 240-base pair allele of the IL-1ra gene).

Treatment of Bone Disease

Effective therapy of the underlying disease is the most powerful treatment for osteoporosis. Provision of adequate calcium and vitamin D is also essential. New guidelines have increased recommended intakes of calcium in growing adolescents to 1300 mg/day and maintained the vitamin D recommendation at 400 IU/day. Ensuring adequate calcium intake is important in patients with lactose intolerance, dietary restriction, decreased intake, and malabsorption. Patients may be monitored by bone density assessment correlated to height age, bone age, or BMI. Results of serum osteocalcin, a measure of bone turnover, are highly variable in adolescents. Monitoring patients for low alkaline phosphatase concentrations may be a useful screening technique.

Patients with IBD are at greater risk of physical inactivity, an independent risk factor for osteoporosis. Immobilization and bed rest compound other risk factors in patients with acute illness. Maintaining activity, encouraging full participation in sports, and minimizing bed rest are important factors. Smoking exacerbates Crohn disease and should be particularly discouraged in adolescents.

The use of calcitonin has not been widely studied in children. Newer calcitonin preparations are not recommended for children because of an increased risk of osteosarcoma. The bisphosphonate drugs inhibit osteolysis and have been used to prevent osteoporosis and prevent the risk of fracture in adults. A Cochrane meta-analysis of 13 trials involving 842 patients showed that the use of bisphosphonate is effective in preventing and treating bone loss treated with corticosteroids.[9] Bisphosphonate use has been studied in children with osteogenesis imperfecta and other diseases.[10,11] Increasing bone strength is a separate consideration from bone density. There are no published data supporting use of bisphosphonates in children with IBD. The early implementation of nutritional or immunosuppressive therapies as an alternative to chronic corticosteroid treatment may reduce the prevalence of osteoporosis in children with IBD.

Zinc

Zinc is a critical trace metal in humans, because it functions as a cofactor in more than 300 metalloenzymes, with critical function in RNA and DNA synthesis, lymphocyte proliferation, cytokine production, free radical activity, and wound healing. Zinc deficiency contributes to growth retardation, anorexia, impaired cell-mediated immunity, hypogonadism, and acrodermatitis, all of which have been documented in patients with IBD. Serum zinc concentrations do not accurately reflect total body zinc depletion, because more than 95% of the zinc is intracellular, and serum concentrations depend on albumin-binding availability.

Reduced serum zinc concentrations are reported in patients with Crohn disease and ulcerative colitis, and reduced zinc content is demonstrated in mucosal biopsy specimens from patients with IBD. Reduced serum zinc concentrations in Crohn disease correlate with disease activity but not with disease location or nutritional status. Patients with Crohn disease complicated by acrodermatitis experience response to zinc supplementation.

In vitro epithelial cell line restitution is enhanced by supraphysiologic supplementation of zinc. Twelve patients with Crohn disease in remission received pharmacologic doses of zinc (25 mg of elemental zinc 3 times/day for 8 weeks), which reversed increased small bowel permeability in 10 of 12 patients. Supplemental zinc, as an antioxidant, in combination with selenium and vitamin E, is increasingly used in patients with IBD, with no controlled studies to confirm their value.

Folate

Folate may protect against colonic cancer in IBD because of its essential role in the synthesis, methylation, and repair of DNA. Epidemiologic evidence in support of an association between folate status and colon cancer was first observed in patients with ulcerative colitis.[12] Folate deficiency is well described in children with IBD; however, the folic acid requirement of children with Crohn disease has not been determined. The minimum daily folic acid requirement for healthy adults is approximately 50 µg, but it may increase sixfold to eightfold in IBD. Adult patients with Crohn disease who receive total parenteral nutrition (TPN) with folic acid have low concentrations of red blood cell folate when receiving 400 µg of folic acid per day, whereas red blood cell folate concentrations increased with a daily infusion of 800 µg of folic acid. Such studies lend some credence to the clinical practice of folate supplementation in subjects with Crohn disease; however, the recommended dose of folic acid (1 mg/day, orally) is empiric. Folate supplementation is also common practice for those receiving medications that may interfere with folate metabolism, such as sulfasalazine and methotrexate. However, evidence to substantiate this practice is lacking.

The prevalence of thromboembolic complications is increased in patients with Crohn disease because of the procoagulant effects associated with inflammation. Hyperhomocysteinemia, a risk factor for venous and arterial thrombosis, is common in IBD. Hyperhomocysteinemia results from genetic or environmental factors, the latter including dietary deficiencies of folate, cobalamin, and pyridoxine. Despite these relationships, hyperhomocysteinemia appears not to contribute to the development of venous or arterial thrombosis in adults with IBD, regardless of nutritional vitamin status.

Antioxidants

Oxidant stress is considered important in the pathogenesis of IBD. Nutritional antioxidants, such as alpha-tocopherol, ascorbic acid, and selenium, as well as other biologic antioxidants, such as glutathione peroxidase and glutathione, are presumed to protect cells from free radical injury. Antioxidant vitamin and mineral supplements may be of potential therapeutic value in IBD. Low serum retinol and alpha-tocopherol concentrations are found in 6% of children with IBD, although the mean values were not different among children with Crohn disease or ulcerative colitis or healthy control subjects. However, alpha-tocopherol concentrations are not affected by the nutritional status of these children or by the use of multivitamin supplements. Alpha-tocopherol, beta-carotene, and gamma-tocopherol concentrations are comparable in children with Crohn disease and healthy children. Others report that whole blood concentrations of alpha-tocopherol, glutathione, and glutathione peroxidase are higher in children with Crohn disease. Firm recommendations for vitamin and mineral supplementation in children with IBD await future studies that provide information on the qualitative and quantitative aspects by which nutrients regulate immune function in relation to inflammation.

Nutritional Therapy for IBD

Elemental Versus Polymeric Diets

Three meta-analyses have concluded that enteral nutrition, as primary therapy for Crohn disease, is statistically inferior to corticosteroid use in inducing clinical remission. Treatment failures are attributable to intolerance of the defined formula diets or the tube feeding, leading to high dropout rates. In another analysis that was limited to randomized clinical trials involving only pediatric patients (5 trials comprising 127 patients), exclusive enteral nutrition was as effective as corticosteroid use in inducing clinical remission.[13] No subanalysis by type of defined formula was performed. The authors concluded that improved growth and development, without the adverse effects of steroids, made enteral nutrition a better first choice for first-line therapy in children with active Crohn disease.

However, from a practical point of view, issues of compliance, as well as a less favorable response rate in patients with extensive colitis (whether Crohn disease or ulcerative colitis), render nutritional therapy less attractive for these subgroups. Enteral nutrition is most commonly used to induce remission in children with active Crohn disease involving the small bowel (with or without proximal colonic disease) who have either growth failure or intolerable steroid-induced adverse effects.

Both elemental and polymeric diets are associated with improved disease activity scores, histologic healing, and down-regulation of proinflammatory cytokines.[1,14] A recent meta-analysis considered results from 9 trials comprising fewer than 300 patients treated with elemental and nonelemental diets. No differences existed between the diet formulations. However, several types of defined formula diets were included in the nonelemental group. A recent double-blind, randomized trial compared the effect of a polymeric and an elemental diet in patients with active Crohn disease. The 2 preparations were identical except for the nitrogen source (ie, amino acid vs intact protein). Remission rates were better for elemental versus polymeric formula (80% vs 55%, respectively [$P = .01$]), although the total number of patients studied was small (n = 21).

Elemental diets may support mucosal healing because of their high content of glutamine. However, a recent double-blind randomized controlled trial of a glutamine-enriched polymeric diet failed to substantiate this hypothesis.

An alternate explanation for the potential advantage of specific formulas for patients with Crohn disease may be the fat, rather than protein, content. To address this issue, a recent randomized, controlled double-blind trial compared 2 single whole protein formulas with long-chain triglycerides supplying either 5% or 30% of total energy.[15] Remission rates were comparably low, reaching only 26% and 33% for the low- and higher-triglyceride formulas, respectively. Once again, a high proportion of the patients in this adult patient trial (21 of 54) were unable to tolerate the diet, accounting for the high failure rates. Finally, 2 recent studies examined the type, rather than the amount, of fat in the defined formula diet. The use of medium-chain triglycerides did not affect the ability of an elemental diet to induce remission, achieved in approximately two thirds of patients.[16] In the second study,[17] a polymeric diet containing lipids at a concentration of 35 g/1000 kcal high in oleic acid (79%) and low in linoleic acid (6.5%) was compared with an identical diet except for the lower oleic acid (45%) and higher linoleic acid (28%) content. Overall, the high-oleic acid formula induced remission in 20%, compared with 52% for a high-linoleic acid diet ($P = .05$). Both formulas were inferior to the use of corticosteroids (79% [$P = .001$]). With all of these results taken together, there is no firm evidence supporting the use of amino acid-, peptide-, or whole protein-based formulas for the primary treatment of active Crohn disease. However, the type of fat may be of more importance with regard to the therapeutic efficacy of nutritional findings for active Crohn disease. Recently, formulas with anti-inflammatory cytokines, prebiotics, and probiotics have become available for the treatment of IBD. There is insufficient evidence at this time to support the routine use of these formulas in the treatment of children with IBD.

Total Parenteral Nutrition as Primary Therapy

When considering studies of TPN in patients with IBD, 2 points are significant. First, there are few studies reported in children. Second, enteral nutrition is the preferred method of nutritional support for patients with IBD because of reduced complications and lower cost. Nevertheless, the use of TPN in IBD can be considered as primary or adjunct therapy when the enteral route cannot be used or the enteral route is ineffective in maintaining nutritional support. TPN also is indicated in selected patients before and after surgery, including individuals who are severely undernourished or those whose disease is complicated by fistula(s), short bowel syndrome, toxic megacolon, intestinal obstruction, or perforation.

Preoperative parenteral nutrition has been shown to be efficacious in reducing postoperative complications in 1 study when therapy was administered for at least 5 days. Total parenteral nutrition given before surgery particularly benefited only those patients with IBD who are severely undernourished.[18,19] A more recent analysis of the literature on perioperative TPN reported that preoperative TPN decreased complications by approximately 10%. In contrast, when TPN is initiated only during the postoperative period, complications are approximately 10% higher than those observed in untreated control subjects.

Bowel rest and TPN reduce intestinal inflammation and decrease disease activity in selected patients with Crohn disease. Several retrospective analyses performed since 1990 have examined the effectiveness of TPN as primary medical therapy. Most patients with severe, but uncomplicated, Crohn colitis experience response to TPN and aggressive medical therapy. However, TPN induced no additional benefits over corticosteroids in patients with ulcerative colitis. Although most studies have failed to demonstrate a therapeutic effect of TPN in ulcerative colitis, some confirm nutritional benefits to such patients.

Total parenteral nutrition may be as effective as enteral nutrition when severe malnutrition is present or luminal feedings are not tolerated because of gut failure.

Several studies have examined the effects of TPN on the closure of intestinal fistula(s) in patients with Crohn disease. When the data are pooled, there was only a 44% initial closure rate of fistula(s), and of these, only 37% remain closed for an extended period of time. Recent studies also have reported that short-bowel syndrome may occur in patients with Crohn disease and repeated operations. These patients often require home TPN.

Home TPN and home enteral nutritional therapy use across the United States was recently evaluated. Patients with Crohn disease made up the third-largest group (after neoplasms and miscellaneous conditions), constituting 11% to 12% of patients receiving home TPN. The prevalence of home TPN and home enteral nutritional therapy in the United States is as much as 10 times higher than that in other industrialized countries. Both therapies are relatively safe. The primary disease requiring the home nutrition therapy strongly influenced patient survival.

Fish Oil

Attention has recently been directed at the immunomodulatory role of polyunsaturated fatty acids. Increased amounts of the omega-6 fatty acid, linoleic acid, increases arachidonic acid concentrations in the serum and cell membrane. The resulting increase in the synthesis of leukotriene B_4 and thromboxane A_2 stimulates the proinflammatory response. In Japan, the incidence of Crohn disease is reported to correlate with omega-6 fatty acid intake.[20]

In contrast, the omega-3 fatty acid eicosapentaenoic acid (EPA) competes with arachidonic acid. This shifts synthesis to leukotriene B_5, a far less potent proinflammatory product, while inhibiting the synthesis of inflammatory cytokines, such as TNF-alpha, and increasing the scavenging of free radicals. Fish oil, a rich source of omega-3 fatty acids, has been investigated as therapy in patients with IBD. In adults with mild to moderate ulcerative colitis, 4 studies using doses of 2.7 g to 4.2 g daily of omega-3 fatty acids demonstrated a modest clinical improvement and reduction of concurrent steroid requirements. Other studies showed no benefit from fish oil treatment for maintaining ulcerative colitis in remission. In adults with Crohn disease in clinical remission but with markers of active inflammation, enteric-coated fish oil preparation in daily doses of 2.7 g for 1 year led to a reduction in relapse rates from 74% in patients treated with placebo to 41% in those receiving fish oil. However, a randomized, controlled study of a regimen of 5 g of fish oil daily for 2 years did not confirm a reduction in relapse rates.

Glutamine

Glutamine supplementation maintains mucosal thickness and villus height in animal models of colitis, reduces endotoxemia, and enhances mucosal barrier function. Supplemental glutamine prevents increased intestinal permeability to lactulose and mannitol in patients with active IBD receiving postoperative TPN. However, there appears to be no advantage of a glutamine-enriched polymeric diet compared to a standard diet in active Crohn disease. Other factors, such as epidermal growth factor and recombinant GH, also could be added to enteral formulas to potentially provide advantage to the enterocyte by enhancing uptake of glutamine.

Short-Chain Fatty Acids

Colonic bacteria metabolize unabsorbed carbohydrate, protein, and fiber to form short-chain fatty acids, hydrogen, and carbon dioxide. The short-chain fatty acids, primarily acetate, propionate, and butyrate (ratio of 60:20:20, respectively), are weak electrolytes but constitute the predominant luminal anions in colonic fluid. Recognition that luminal short-chain fatty acid concentrations are decreased in severe ulcerative colitis led to an interest in the potential role of these substances as therapy in IBD. Butyrate is a preferred metabolic substrate for colonocytes and is a trophic factor in the colon.

Initial observations with either mixtures of short-chain fatty acids or butyrate alone given as enemas produced apparent clinical benefit. However, 2 prospective, randomized, placebo-controlled studies did not show a therapeutic effect of short-chain fatty acids on colitis. Thus, the role of short-chain fatty acids in maintaining mucosal integrity requires additional investigation.

Psychosocial Effects of Nutritional Interventions in the Care of Children With IBD

Inflammatory bowel disease represents a major, lifelong health threat that challenges the psychological resources of both the affected child and his or her family. Acute, active disease may necessitate hospital admittance, causing major disruptions in children's academic, social, and family life. Most children with IBD experience considerable worry, distress, and concern about their disease and its effects on school absences, academic achievement, and participation in family and social activities away from home. As a chronic condition, IBD poses continual demands on patients and their families to cope with fluctuating degrees of illness, prolonged use of medications, uncomfortable treatments, and dietary limitations.

The complications of growth failure and delayed puberty in some children add to the psychological stress associated with IBD. Indeed, a recent meta-analysis indicates that children with IBD have more psychological disturbances than do age-matched groups with other chronic illnesses. Empirical studies indicate that psychological problems of an internalizing nature, including depression, anxiety, low self-esteem, separation anxiety, fearfulness, social withdrawal, relationship difficulties, and body image problems, are common in children and adolescents with IBD. Depression is particularly common, especially in patients with newly diagnosed disease.[21] However, an effective multidisciplinary team approach enables aggressive immune suppression and nutritional therapy and favorable psychosocial outcomes. There is also evidence that psychosocial dysfunction is more common among families of children with IBD than in those with healthy children or children with diabetes. These findings indicate that stress associated with IBD can have a strong adverse effect on the family system at large.

There are few published reports regarding the effects of nutrition support on psychosocial functioning in patients with IBD. In one study, adults receiving TPN experienced transient depressive states, body image changes, and alexithymia (ie, difficulty in describing or recognizing one's own emotions) but did not show serious psychopathologic characteristics. This finding contradicts the results of an earlier study reporting serious psychopathologic problems during the early stages of TPN. However, because neither study included a comparison group, it is not known whether patients were reacting to the disease or to the TPN. Navarro et al[22] examined the psychological outcome of constant-rate enteral nutrition in 17 children and adolescents with moderate to severe Crohn disease. The authors reported that subjects showed excellent psychological tolerance, expressed feelings of well-being, and reported improved daily functioning. However, the study did not include a control group, did not report objective measurements, and failed to describe the statistical analyses employed.

Treatment interventions can have both direct and indirect effects on psychosocial functioning. Although enteral nutrition does not entail the adverse effects of steroid treatment, it does have drawbacks. Enteral nutrition requires high patient motivation and necessitates tube feeding. Social factors, including support from family and friends, as well as peer pressure at school, are recognized as important influences on tolerance of enteral nutrition.

It is not difficult to imagine how enteral nutrition can affect psychosocial functioning. During treatment, patients endure prolonged periods of oral food deprivation and can experience frustration because of disruption of social and family activities during meals. Enteral nutrition can be difficult for children who eat their meals at school, particularly if they are already embarrassed about the disease. Enteral nutrition can also exacerbate feelings of being different and, thus, further contribute to a sense of alienation. There is the additional consideration that the feeding tube and pump apparatus make the disease more visible, both to patients and to those around them. This can accentuate feelings of self-consciousness and heighten embarrassment in social situations. In addition, patients initially experience the insertion of a nasal gastric tube as intrusive. The psychologic meanings that patients attribute to treatment procedures, as well as emotional reactions such as anxiety, fear, and depression, may well be more influential than physical status in determining adherence to treatment and the success of nutritional therapies.

Summary

Impairment of linear growth is common in children with Crohn disease, both before recognizing the presence of the disease and thereafter. Growth impairment is much less prevalent in pediatric patients with ulcerative colitis. Chronic undernutrition, nutrient losses, medications, and proinflammatory mediators are increasingly recognized as contributing to the observed growth failure in Crohn disease and ulcerative colitis. Children with Crohn disease generally have greater nutrient needs on the basis of gender, age, and weight than do those with ulcerative colitis. Important clinical practices can enhance the growth and nutritional status of children and adolescents with IBD (see Table 43.1).

Table 43.1
Clinical Approach to Nutritional Support of Pediatric Patients With IBD

1.	Screening and assessing pediatric patients with IBD for malnutrition and growth failure is an essential component of medical care. At a minimum, this includes height, weight, and BMI followed serially and plotted on standardized reference growth charts. Biochemical tests of nutrient and micronutrient status and, in patients at high risk of developing bone disease, imaging of selected bones for mineral content and density also may yield useful information and are considered an integral part of the medical regimen.
2.	A diet well balanced in all nutrients on the basis of MyPyramid and following the reference dietary intakes for gender and age is advisable for all pediatric patients with IBD. Dietary supplementation of selected nutrients, such as energy, protein, zinc, vitamins, and calcium, may be warranted based on the basis of a nutritional assessment of the individual patient.

Table 43.1 *(Continued)*
Clinical Approach to Nutritional Support of Pediatric Patients With IBD

3.	Ensuring adequate calcium (1300 mg/day for adolescents) and vitamin D (400 IU/day for all ages) is essential in children with IBD. Patients at greatest risk of developing osteopenia and osteoporosis may be monitored by bone mineral density assessment. Maintaining full physical activity and minimizing bed rest are important to reduce the risk of bone disease. Data on the efficacy and safety of bisphosphonates in children with bone disease and IBD is insufficient to permit definitive recommendations at this time.
4.	Elemental and polymeric enteral diets may be equally effective in inducing remission for active Crohn disease; definitive evidence to recommend one over the other is lacking. Enteral nutrition is considered before parenteral nutrition, because it is safer and less costly.
5.	Total parenteral nutrition is considered for nutrition support in children with IBD when the enteral route cannot be used or is ineffective in nutrition support. Total parenteral nutrition is effective as primary therapy in pediatric patients with Crohn disease whose nutrient needs cannot be supported enterally or who are resistant to corticosteroid therapy. Preoperative TPN may reduce postoperative complications in malnourished patients who are not candidates for enteral nutrition support.
6.	Data at this time are too limited to allow definitive recommendations regarding the use of glutamine, fish oil, or short-chain fatty acids as primary therapy to control inflammation in children with IBD.
7.	Psychosocial dysfunction is common in children with active IBD. Total enteral and parenteral nutrition may also have negative effects on social and psychologic functioning. For such children, ongoing support by a mental health professional who is experienced in helping children develop coping strategies to deal with the effects of chronic illness and the treatments used for IBD is a critical component of the child's therapy.

Adapted with permission.[23]

References

1. Fell JM, Paintin M, Arnaud-Battandier F, et al. Mucosal healing and a fall in mucosal pro-inflammatory cytokine mRNA induced by a specific oral polymeric diet in paediatric Crohn's disease. *Aliment Pharmacol Ther.* 2000;14:281–289

2. Boot AM, Bouquet J, Krenning EP, de Muinck Keizer-Schrama SM. Bone mineral density and nutritional status in children with chronic inflammatory bowel disease. *Gut.* 1998;42:188–194

3. Sentongo TA, Semaeo EJ, Stettler N, Piccoli DA, Stallings VA, Zemel BS. Vitamin D status in children, adolescents, and young adults with Crohn disease. *Am J Clin Nutr.* 2002;76:1077–1081

4. Semeao EJ, Jawad AF, Zemel BS, Neiswender KM, Piccoli DA, Stallings VA. Bone mineral density in children and young adults with Crohn's disease. *Inflamm Bowel Dis.* 1999;5:161–166

5. Azcue M, Rashid M, Griffiths A, Pencharz PB. Energy expenditure and body composition in children with Crohn's disease: effect of enteral nutrition and treatment with prednisolone. *Gut.* 1997;41:203–208

6. Abitbol V, Roux C, Chaussade S, et al. Metabolic bone assessment in patients with inflammatory bowel disease. *Gastroenterology.* 1995;108:417–422

7. Gokhale R, Favus MJ, Karrison T, Sutton MM, Rich B, Kirschner BS. Bone mineral density assessment in children with inflammatory bowel disease. *Gastroenterology.* 1998;114:902–911

8. Issenman RM, Atkinson SA, Radoja C, Fraher L. Longitudinal assessment of growth, mineral metabolism, and bone mass in pediatric Crohn's disease. *J Pediatr Gastroenterol Nutr.* 1993;17:401–406

9. Homik J, Cranney A, Shea B, et al. Bisphosphonates for steroid induced osteoporosis. *Cochrane Database Syst Rev.* 2000;(2):CD001347

10. Glorieux FH, Bishop NJ, Plotkin H, Chabot G, Lanoue G, Travers R. Cyclic administration of pamidronate in children with severe osteogenesis imperfecta. *N Engl J Med.* 1998;339:947–952

11. Bianchi ML, Cimaz R, Bardare M, et al. Efficacy and safety of alendronate for the treatment of osteoporosis in diffuse connective tissue diseases in children: a prospective multicenter study. *Arthritis Rheum.* 2000;43:1960–1966

12. Lashner BA, Provencher KS, Seidner DL, Knesebeck A, Brzezinski A. The effect of folic acid supplementation on the risk for cancer or dysplasia in ulcerative colitis. *Gastroenterology.* 1997;112:29–32

13. Heuschkel RB, Menache CC, Megerian JT, Baird AE. Enteral nutrition and corticosteroids in the treatment of acute Crohn's disease in children. *J Pediatr Gastroenterol Nutr.* 2000;31:8–15

14. Teahon K, Smethurst P, MacPherson A, et al. Intestinal permeability in Crohn's disease and its relation to disease activity and relapse following treatment with elemental diet. *Eur J Gastroenterol Hepatol.* 1993;5:79–84

15. Leiper K, Woolner J, Mullan MM, et al. A randomized controlled trial of high versus low long chain triglyceride whole protein feed in active Crohn's disease. *Gut.* 2001;49:790–794

16. Sakurai T, Matsui T, Yao T, et al. Short-term efficacy of enteral nutrition in the treatment of active Crohn's disease: a randomized, controlled trial comparing nutrient formulas. *JPEN J Parenter Enteral Nutr.* 2002;26:98–103

17. Gassull MA, Fernandez-Banares F, Cabre E, et al. Fat composition may be a clue to explain the primary therapeutic effect of enteral nutrition in Crohn's disease: results of a double blind randomized multicentre European trial. *Gut.* 2002;51:164–168

18. Han PD, Burke A, Baldassano RN, Rombeau JL, Lichtenstein GR. Nutrition and inflammatory bowel disease. *Gastroenterol Clin North Am.* 1999;28:423–443, ix.

19. Gouma DJ, von Meyenfeldt MF, Rouflart M, Soeters PB. Preoperative total parenteral nutrition (TPN) in severe Crohn's disease. *Surgery.* 1988;103:648–652

20. Shoda R, Matsueda K, Yamato S, Umeda N. Epidemiologic analysis of Crohn disease in Japan: increased dietary intake of n-6 polyunsaturated fatty acids and animal protein relates to the increased incidence of Crohn disease in Japan. *Am J Clin Nutr.* 1996;63:741–745

21. Burke P, Meyer V, Kocoshis S, et al. Depression and anxiety in pediatric inflammatory bowel disease and cystic fibrosis. *J Am Acad Child Adolesc Psychiatry.* 1989;28:948–951

22. Navarro J, Vargas J, Cezard JP, Charritat JL, Polonovski C. Prolonged constant rate elemental enteral nutrition in Crohn's disease. *J Pediatr Gastroenterol Nutr.* 1982;1:541–546

23. Kleinman RE, Baldassano RN, Caplan A, et al. Nutrition support for pediatric patients with inflammatory bowel disease: a clinical report of the North American Society for Pediatric Gastroenterology, Hepatology and Nutrition. *J Pediatr Gastroenterol Nutr.* 2004;39:15–27

44 Liver Disease

The liver is the "powerhouse" for metabolic activity in the body. It is the major site for (1) the synthesis of serum proteins, such as albumin and coagulation factors; (2) urea synthesis for normal nitrogen metabolism and ammonia clearance; (3) glucose production for maintaining normoglycemia; and (4) lipid metabolism by producing lipoproteins and converting fatty acids to ketone bodies. These metabolic functions require a considerable amount of energy. The liver consumes approximately 20% of resting energy requirements while constituting only 2% of body weight.[1] Patients who have significant liver disease demonstrate impaired hepatic metabolic function as well as extrahepatic alterations in glucose (insulin resistance and impaired glucose tolerance), lipid (increased lipolytic rates), and protein (decreased protein synthesis and increased amino acid oxidation rates) metabolism.

Nutritional support of an infant or child with liver disease is dependent on the type of liver disease. Acute liver disease, as seen with viral hepatitis, may require no special nutritional therapy unless encephalopathy ensues. With acute liver disease, anorexia, vomiting, and diarrhea may result in acute weight loss. Malnutrition, however, is uncommon.

Nutritional support of the child with chronic liver disease is altered depending on whether cholestasis is present or not. With cholestasis, fat-soluble vitamins and medium-chain triglycerides (MCTs) are usually required to optimize growth. Children who are anicteric but who have cirrhosis present a different challenge, because hypermetabolism, enteropathy, and increased protein oxidation may occur. Various inborn errors of metabolism that cause liver disease (ie, galactosemia, tyrosinemia, hereditary fructose intolerance, Wilson disease) have specific nutritional requirements and dietary restrictions. The success of pediatric liver transplantation has made the recognition of the importance of nutritional support in the pretransplant period imperative to optimize the success of the transplant.

Protein-energy malnutrition occurs commonly in patients with advanced liver disease and may be caused by several factors. Decreased nutrient intake occurs because of anorexia and nausea. The presence of tense ascites, especially in an infant, makes food intake much more difficult as a result of the intra-abdominal pressure on the stomach. Diminished food intake may result from depression caused by hospitalization or the unpalatable nature of many restricted diets. Malabsorption of fat and fat-soluble vitamins frequently complicates childhood chronic cholestatic liver disease. Fat and fat-soluble vitamins require a critical concentration of intraluminal bile acids for micellar solubilization. Cholestasis, with diminished bile flow, results in reduced biliary secretion of bile acids and consequent fat and fat-soluble vitamin malabsorption. Supplementation with the fat-soluble vitamins A, D, E, and K is required to avoid potential deficiencies of these vitamins (see Table 44.1). Cirrhosis and portal hypertension may lead to enteropathy and malabsorption secondary to increased mesenteric venous system pressure and villous atrophy from malnutrition. Some liver diseases (Alagille syndrome, progressive familial intrahepatic cholestasis type 1, primary sclerosing cholangitis, hepatic fibrosis) may be associated with extrahepatic organ dysfunction such as pancreatic insufficiency (eg, cystic fibrosis), inflammatory bowel disease, or other syndromes (eg, Joubert, Johanson-Blizzard) that will aggravate the malabsorption.

Table 44.1
Vitamin Supplementation in Children With Cholestasis

Vitamin	Recommended Dose	Preparation	Dose Provided
Vitamin A	Oral supplementation of vitamin A ranges from 5000 to 25 000 IU/day of water-miscible vitamin A	Vitamin A capsules, generic	10 000 U/capsule or 25 000 U/capsule
		ADEK drops (Axcan Pharma, Birmingham, AL)	3170 IU/mL of vitamin A as palmitate and 50% as beta-carotene
		ADEK tablets	9000 IU of vitamin A as palmitate and 60% as beta-carotene
		Vitamin A parenteral (Aquasol A Parenteral [Hospira, Lake Forest, IL)	50 000 U/mL (15 mg retinol)
Vitamin D	600–2000 IU/day	Oral vitamin D supplementation (Drisdol, sanofi-aventis, Bridgewater, NJ)	Ergocalciferol, 50 000 IU/capsule, 8000 U/mL
	0.02 µg/kg	1,25-OH vitamin D (Calcijex calcitriol injection [Abbott Laboratories, Abbott Park, IL])	1 µg/mL
Vitamin E	In infants, 50–100 IU/day	α-tocopherol, Aqua-E (Yasoo Health, Johnson City, TN)	20 IU/mL
	In older children with vitamin E deficiency, 15–25 IU/kg per day	Liqui-E (TPGS-D-alpha tocopheryl polyethylene glycol 1000 succinate [Twinlab/Ideasphere, American Fork, UT])	400 IU/15 mL

Table 44.1 *(Continued)*
Vitamin Supplementation in Children With Cholestasis

Vitamin	Recommended Dose	Preparation	Dose Provided
Vitamin K	Daily or twice-weekly dose of 2.5–10 mg depending on response to therapy	Mephyton (Merck and Co, Whitehouse Station, NJ [vitamin K_1])	5-mg tablets
	Subcutaneous or intravenous vitamin K administration (1–5 mg dependent on size)	AquaMephyton (Merck and Co, Whitehouse Station, NJ [vitamin K_1])	2 mg/mL or 10 mg/mL

Nutritional Assessment of the Child With Liver Disease

It is imperative that any child with chronic liver disease undergo a thorough nutritional assessment to determine the degree of malnutrition, if present, and to tailor the nutritional intervention (see also Chapter 24: Assessment of Nutritional Status). The severity of malnutrition may not correlate with the degree of vitamin or trace mineral deficiency or the degree of hepatic dysfunction. A number of obstacles complicate the ability to accurately assess the nutritional status of a child with liver disease.

Body weight may be deceptive, because organomegaly from an enlarged liver or spleen, edema, or ascites can mask weight loss and actually increase the weight. Height (or length in infants and young children) is a better indicator of malnutrition in these children and can be a reliable tool to determine chronic malnutrition. A decrease in height or length for age percentile may be indicative of prolonged malnutrition.

In addition to weight and height or length measurements, triceps skin-fold thickness and mid-arm circumference measurements provide sensitive indicators of nutritional status in children with chronic liver disease. Lower extremities are more prone to peripheral edema and fluid retention than upper extremities; thus measurements of upper extremities are a better indicator of body fat stores and muscle mass. Reduced fat-fold thickness and mid-arm circumference have been observed in children before measured effects in weight or height or length. In children, early reduction in fat and muscle stores reflects the preferential utilization of fat stores to conserve protein stores for energy in the malnourished state. To optimize the accuracy of anthropometric measurements, it is best to use a single observer using a standard technique with serial measurements.

Measurement of the concentrations of plasma proteins that are synthesized by the liver, including albumin, transferrin, prealbumin, and retinol-binding protein, has been used to determine visceral protein nutriture. However, diminished serum concentrations of these proteins may not accurately reflect the body's visceral protein status. The serum concentrations of these proteins more closely correlate with the severity of liver injury rather than the degree of malnutrition as assessed by anthropometric measurements. Hypoalbuminemia in chronic liver disease patients often results from third spacing of fluid and protein in ascites or the extravascular compartment. Further, increased catabolism of albumin without a compensatory increase in albumin synthesis because of inadequate reserves and malabsorption of amino acids and peptides often makes albumin an inaccurate measure of nutritional status. Poor oral intake may further contribute to hypoalbuminemia.

Nitrogen balance studies are difficult to evaluate in children with chronic liver disease. Impairment of hepatic urea synthesis leads to underestimation of urinary nitrogen losses. Further, ammonia accumulates in the intra- and extracellular compartments instead of being excreted by the kidneys. The creatinine-height index is a good indicator of lean body mass if renal function is unimpaired. When utilizing the creatinine-height index, dietary protein intake, trauma, and infection must be considered, because they all can alter creatinine excretion.

Immune status is sometimes used as an indirect measure of nutritional status. However, because liver disease and, in particular, hypersplenism can result in lymphopenia, abnormal skin test results for delayed hypersensitivity, or decreased concentrations of complement irrespective of nutritional status, these immunologic markers are of limited usefulness in children with liver disease.

Another problem with using biochemical measurements to determine nutritional status in children with liver disease is that many of the drugs used to treat children with liver disease may alter the blood concentrations of vitamins. For example, cholestyramine and colestipol, bile acid-binding resins, may deplete enteral bile acids and interfere with fat-soluble vitamin absorption from the intestines. Diphenylhydantoin and phenobarbital increase the hepatic metabolism of vitamin D and, thus, decrease 25-OH-cholecalciferol concentrations in plasma.

A well-prepared 24-hour diet diary can be invaluable in assessing the usual caloric intake and should always account for use of dietary supplements or any dietary restrictions that have been imposed. Problems such as nausea, vomiting, diarrhea, or anorexia should be recorded, because these may contribute to poor intake. A careful and thorough physical examination can determine the degree of muscle wasting, depletion of subcutaneous fat and any evidence of vitamin or mineral deficiencies.

Malabsorption in Chronic Liver Disease

Fat

Steatorrhea (fat malabsorption) is frequently observed in patients with cirrhosis and/or chronic cholestasis, although the degree of biliary obstruction correlates poorly with the amount of fat excreted in the stools. Even in the absence of biliary obstruction, intraluminal bile salt concentrations are thought to be below the critical micellar concentration such that intraluminal products of lipolysis cannot form micellar solutions.[2] Typically, the prothrombin time is prolonged. A trial of parenteral vitamin K administration daily will often correct the prothrombin time and points to poor fat-soluble vitamin absorption. Anorexia, failure to thrive, ascites, prolongation of the prothrombin time (unresponsive to vitamin K supplementation), and steatorrhea progress in conjunction with worsening of the underlying liver disease and cirrhosis.

Treatment with a low-fat diet supplemented with formulas containing MCT (C8-C12 fatty acids [Pregestimil {Mead Johnson, Evansville, IN}, approx 60% MCT; Alimentum {Abbott Nutrition, Columbus, OH}, approx 50% MCT; or Portagen {Mead Johnson, Evansville, IN}, approx 87% MCT]) or MCT oil helps to decrease the degree of steatorrhea and may help to improve the nutritional status of the infant. Elemental formulas are not necessary in these infants. Diets enhanced with MCTs can also improve energy intake in older children with cholestasis. MCT does not require intraluminal bile salts for micellar formation to be absorbed in the intestinal lumen. MCTs are relatively water soluble and directly absorbed into the portal circulation. However, when decompensation ensues, although steatorrhea may be diminished with MCT dietary supplementation, failure to thrive may progress.

Essential Fatty Acids

The malabsorption of fat, especially long-chain triglycerides, and inadequate intake can lead to essential fatty acid (EFA) deficiency. EFAs are fatty acids that cannot be synthesized by desaturation or elongation of shorter fatty acids. Linoleic acid and linolenic acid are EFAs. Deficiency of EFAs may result in growth impairment; a dry, scaly rash; thrombocytopenia, and impaired immune function.[3] Long-chain triglycerides are poorly absorbed if cholestasis is present. Infants have a small linoleic acid store.[4] Cholestasis in infants places them at an increased EFA deficiency risk. Pregestimil and Alimentum provide only 7% to 14% of calories as linoleic acid. To prevent EFA deficiency, in a healthy individual, at least 3% to 4% of calories should be linoleic acid. If cholestasis is severe enough to allow 30% to 40% of dietary fat to be malabsorbed, then EFA deficiency may ensue.[5] Portagen, containing 87% MCTs and <3% EFAs, is not recommended for long-term use in children with cholestatic liver disease, because EFA deficiency may occur if supplementation is not provided.[6] Corn oil or safflower oil containing linoleic acid can be added to foods or a lipid emulsion (Microlipid [Nestlé, Glendale, CA]) can be added to formula to provide additional linoleic acid.

Fat-Soluble Vitamins

Bile acids in the intestinal lumen are important not only for fat absorption from the lumen but also for fat-soluble vitamin absorption. Vitamins A, D, E, and K are all dependent on intraluminal bile acid concentration. When the intraluminal bile acid concentration falls below a critical micellar concentration (1.5–2.0 mM), malabsorption of fat-soluble vitamins ensues. Cholestyramine and colestipol, bile acid-binding resins, may deplete enteral bile acids and interfere with fat-soluble vitamin absorption from the intestines. Vitamins A and E require hydrolysis by an intestinal esterase that is bile acid dependent before intestinal absorption. In infants, cholestasis leads to rapid depletion of body stores of fat-soluble vitamins with both biochemical and clinical features of deficiency evident unless adequate supplementation is used. Evaluation of fat-soluble vitamin deficiency, supplementation, and follow-up monitoring are all necessary for infants and children with cholestasis.

To alleviate the malabsorption of fat-soluble vitamins in chronic liver disease, a daily dose of an aqueous preparation of vitamins A, D, E, and K may be prescribed at twice the Recommended Dietary Allowance as a starting dose. Periodic determination of serum concentrations of vitamins A, 25 OH-D, and E may be necessary to optimize nutritional support and may result in supplementation of individual fat-soluble vitamins. As a surrogate for vitamin K, prothrombin time and/or international normalized ratio may be serially followed.

Hypocalcemia resulting from dietary calcium deficiency or malabsorption can lead to rickets and osteopenia on bone radiographs. Large doses of vitamin D supplements (5000–20 000 IU/day) may be required to correct this condition. Each fat-soluble vitamin will be discussed individually, because evaluation, supplementation, and monitoring differ.

Vitamin A

Vitamin A (see Table 44.2) refers to retinol and its derivatives having similar biologic activities. The principle vitamin A compounds include retinol, retinal (retinaldehyde), retinoic acid, and retinyl esters that differ in the terminal group at the end of the side chain. Dietary vitamin A predominantly is derived from animal sources (liver, fish liver oils, dairy products, kidney, eggs) and carotenoids (provitamin A, beta carotene) in darkly colored vegetables, oily fruits, and red palm oil. The adequate intake for vitamin A for infants is 400 to 500 µg/day. The Recommended Dietary Allowance of vitamin A is 300 µg/day for children 1 to 3 years of age, 400 µg/day for children 4 to 8 years of age, and 600–1000 µg/day for older children and adults (see Appendix J).

Table 44.2
Indices of Vitamin A Status

Index	Normal Range
Fasting serum retinol concentration	>20 µg/dL (>0.693 µmol/L)
Fasting serum retinol binding protein	>1 mg/dL
Retinol/retinol binding protein ratio	>0.8 mol/mol
Modified relative dose response (+TPGS)	<10% at 10 hours

As a fat-soluble vitamin, vitamin A absorption can be adversely affected by cholestasis. Vitamin A nutritional status can be determined by assessing vitamin A concentration in liver tissue, corneal examination, conjunctival impression cytology, and dark-field adaptation tests.[7] Conjunctival impression cytology uses cellulose acetate filter paper that is applied to the eye, and specimens are examined under a microscope and then graded on the basis of goblet cells and epithelial cells. From a practical standpoint, determinations of serum retinol and/or retinol-binding protein concentrations are routinely used to screen for vitamin A nutritional status in children with chronic liver disease. Vitamin A deficiency is reported in 35% to 69% of children with cholestatic liver disease. However, serum concentrations of retinol and/or retinol-binding protein may not accurately reflect vitamin A sufficiency or deficiency states, particularly in cholestatic liver disease because vitamin A is stored in the liver. The best noninvasive test of vitamin A status is the relative dose response. The relative dose response is based on the observation that if hepatic vitamin A stores are normal, plasma retinol concentration does not change significantly after a small oral loading dose of exogenous vitamin A (1500 IU; 450 μg). However, when hepatic vitamin A stores are low, the plasma retinol concentration markedly increases in response to a relatively small oral loading dose of exogenous vitamin A, reaching a peak several hours after administration. The standard relative dose response assesses plasma retinol concentration 5 hours after an oral loading dose of vitamin A. However, in children with chronic cholestasis, poor absorption of the oral vitamin A may interfere with interpretation of vitamin A stores. To bypass the possibility of poor absorption, intravenous or intramuscular doses of vitamin A have been used to better assess vitamin A hepatic stores. Also, oral vitamin A in combination with oral D-alpha-tocopheryl polyethylene glycol-1000 succinate (TPGS [25 IU/kg]), a water-soluble form of vitamin E, which aids in absorption of lipid-soluble compounds, may also be used in a modified relative dose response to improve vitamin A oral absorption in cholestasis. A modified relative dose response of >20% increase at 10 hours is considered a positive test result indicative of low hepatic vitamin A stores.

Detecting vitamin A deficiency is important, because vitamin A deficiency may lead to xerophthalmia, keratomalacia, irreversible damage to the cornea of the eye, night blindness, and pigmentary retinopathy. Although these ocular findings are rare in cholestatic children, the potential for eye damage and visual disturbance is real.

Oral supplementation of vitamin A in children with liver disease ranges from 5000 to 25 000 IU/day of water-miscible vitamin A. Oral water-miscible vitamin A is not readily available for use in infants. Vitamin A capsules (10 000 U/capsule or 25 000 U/capsule, generic) are available. ADEK drops (Axcan Pharma, Birmingham, AL) contain 3170 IU/mL of vitamin A as palmitate and 50% as beta-carotene; ADEK tablets contain 9000 IU of vitamin A as palmitate and 60% as beta-carotene. Vitamin A parenteral (Aquasol A Parenteral [Mayne Pharma, Lake Forest, IL], 50 000 U/mL-15 mg retinol) may be used for vitamin A replacement therapy intramuscularly.

Vitamin A toxicity has been well recognized and can cause hepatotoxicity. Monitoring during vitamin A supplementation is obligatory. Vitamin A toxicity may cause fatigue; malaise; anorexia; vomiting; increased intracranial pressure; painful bone lesions, including osteopenia, and higher risk of fractures; hypercalcemia; and a massive desquamation dermatitis.[8] Vitamin A hepatotoxicity is associated with elevated retinyl esters and can be assayed.[9] Recent studies suggest that relatively little excess vitamin A can lead to toxicity, so close monitoring of vitamin A status and of any supplementation is warranted.[10]

Vitamin D

Vitamin D (calciferol) includes vitamin D_2 (ergocalciferol) and vitamin D_3 (cholecalciferol). Vitamin D_2 is found in very few foods naturally but is found in plants and fungi and added to supplement cow milk. Vitamin D may also be photosynthesized in the skin of vertebrates by the action of ultraviolet B radiation. Vitamin D is biologically inert and requires hydroxylation to form its biologically active hormone 1,25-dihydroxyvitamin D. Hydroxylation at the 1 position occurs in the kidney, and 25-hydroxylation occurs in the liver. Vitamin D's major biologic function in humans is to maintain serum calcium and phosphorus concentrations within the normal range by enhancing the efficiency of the small intestine to absorb these minerals from the diet. The adequate intake for vitamin D (calciferol) is 5 µg/day (200 IU) for infants, children, and adults (see Appendix J).

Vitamin D deficiency is demonstrated by its effect on calcium metabolism, resulting in hypocalcemia, hypophosphatemia, tetany, osteomalacia, and rickets. Children with chronic liver disease may develop hepatic osteodystrophy manifested by rickets, bone demineralization (osteopenia), or pathologic fractures.[11] These findings have been presumed attributable to fat malabsorption, the result of diminished bile outflow leading to steatorrhea and associated calcium and vitamin D malabsorption. Hypocalcemia and vitamin D insufficiency results in secondary hyperparathyroidism and increased bone resorption. Despite vitamin D repletion by supplementation to normal values, some patients continue to have poor bone mass, implying that vitamin D status alone does not account for hepatic osteodystrophy.[12] Magnesium deficiency has been proposed as playing a role in the development of this bone disease.[13] Liver transplantation has demonstrated remarkable improvement in bone mineral density of these children.[14]

Clinically, bone mineral content is often assessed by dual-energy x-ray absorptiometry. Biochemical tests for vitamin D include serum vitamin D (vitamin D_2 and D_3), 25-OH vitamin D_2 and D_3, 1,25-OH_2 vitamin D, and vitamin-D binding protein. Serum concentrations of calcium, phosphorous, magnesium, alkaline phosphatase, and parathyroid hormone can be useful in assessing for osteomalacia, osteopenia, and rickets. Dietary calcium and phosphorus content must also be assessed. The most common indicator of vitamin D status in children with chronic cholestasis is the plasma concentration of 25-hydroxycholecalciferol (25-OH-D). A serum 25-OH-D concentration below 14 to 15 ng/mL is suggestive of vitamin D deficiency. Periodic assessment of serum 25-OH-D concentrations, adequate sunlight exposure, and adequate dietary intake of calcium and phosphorous is recommended for children with cholestasis. Vitamin D deficiency can be treated with oral vitamin D supplementation (ergocalciferol [Drisdol, sanofi-aventis, Bridgewater, NJ], 50 000 IU/capsule [8000 U/mL]), usually at a dose range of 600 to 2000 IU/day. It is often possible to normalize plasma 25-OH-D concentrations in children with chronic cholestasis by providing 2 to 4 µg/kg per day. Serum 25-OH-D concentrations must be closely monitored along with calcium and phosphorus concentrations during supplementation.

Because of increased costs and risks of toxicity, use of parenteral vitamin D preparations should be used only if patients fail to respond to oral therapy and will comply with parenteral therapy. Availability of various vitamin D preparations has been problematic. 1,25-OH vitamin D (Calcijex [Abbott Laboratories, Abbott Park, IL], calcitriol injection, 1 µg/mL) at a dose of 0.02 µg/kg may be judiciously used with monitoring for vitamin D intoxication by determining urine calcium-to-creatinine ratio and serum calcium, phosphorus, and 25-OH-D concentrations. Vitamin D toxicity may include hypercalcemia, causing central nervous system depression; ectopic calcifications; hypercalciuria, causing nephrocalcinosis; and nephrolithiasis. Bisphosphonate use for children with chronic liver disease has been limited to its use in treating hypercalcemia in children awaiting liver transplantation.[15]

Vitamin E

Vitamin E refers to a group of 8 compounds, including the tocopherols and the tocotrienols. The 4 major forms of vitamin E (α, β, δ, γ) differ by the position and number of methyl group substitutions and their bioactivity. α-Tocopherol is the predominant form found in food and has the highest biologic activity. γ-Tocopherol is found in high concentrations in soy oil. Foods high in vitamin E include grain, plant, and vegetable oils. The recommended dietary intake for adequate vitamin E is 4 mg/day in infants 0 to 6 months of age, 5 mg/day in infants 7 to 12 months of age, 6 mg/day in children 1 to 3 years of age, 7 mg/day in children 4 to 8 years of age, 11 mg/day in children 9 to 13 years of age, and 15 mg/day in older adolescents and adults (see Appendix J). Oral vitamin E requires solubilization by bile acids to mixed micelles and esterase hydrolysis by pancreatic or intestinal esterases that are bile acid dependent before absorption by the intestinal enterocyte. In blood, vitamin E is transported in low-density and high-density lipoprotein.

In infants and children with cholestasis, impaired secretion of bile acids results in malabsorption of vitamin E.[16] Vitamin E is the most hydrophobic of the fat-soluble vitamins and has the greatest need for bile acids intraluminally for absorption. Vitamin E absorption, as determined by an oral vitamin E tolerance test, is profoundly diminished in children with cholestasis who are vitamin E deficient and can be improved by coadministration of bile acids.[15] Vitamin E is necessary to maintain the structure and function of the nervous system. Peripheral neuropathy, ataxia, ophthalmoplegia, and muscle weakness characterize vitamin E deficiency in children with cholestasis.[17] Reversal of these findings may be accomplished before permanent injury occurs if supplementation and normalization of serum vitamin E concentrations is accomplished before 3 years of age.[18] The best predictor of vitamin E status in children with cholestasis is the ratio of serum vitamin E to total serum lipids (the sum of the serum cholesterol, triglycerides, and phospholipids), because vitamin E partitions into the plasma lipoproteins that may be increased in cholestasis.[19] The serum vitamin E concentration may be increased into the normal range as a result of its partitioning into the plasma lipoproteins. The ratio of serum vitamin E to lipid compensates for this phenomenon. Biochemical vitamin E deficiency in older children and adults is <0.8 mg of total tocopherol/g of total lipid and in infants younger than 1 year is <0.6 mg/g. The target vitamin E-to-lipid ratio for correction of vitamin E deficiency is 0.8 to 1.0 mg/g. Although measurement of vitamin E in adipose tissue assesses vitamin E stores, it is impractical, because it requires adipose biopsies and is not readily available. Other functional assays of vitamin E status include red blood cell (RBC) hydrogen peroxide hemolysis and the RBC malondialdehyde release test.[20,21] Vitamin E deficiency is suggested if >10% of RBCs hemolyze on hydrogen peroxide exposure. Unfortunately, hydrogen peroxide hemolysis of RBCs or measurement of malondialdehyde (a lipid peroxidation product) may be affected by selenium or polyunsaturated fatty acids, so these tests are not specific for vitamin E deficiency. Breath ethane and pentane measurements have been used to assess antioxidant deficiency as a measure of vitamin E sufficiency.[22] Ethane and pentane are volatile gasses released during peroxidation of fatty acids. Although noninvasive, the cost, special equipment necessary for collection and detection of the gasses, and low specificity for vitamin E deficiency, because selenium deficiency also interferes, make this test impractical.

To prevent vitamin E deficiency in infants and children with cholestasis, vitamin E supplementation is indicated. In infants, 50 to 100 IU/day of vitamin E (alpha-tocopherol [Aqua-E {Yasoo Health}, 20 IU/mL]; TPGS [Liqui-E

{Twinlabs}, 400 IU/15 mL]) may be prescribed. In older children with vitamin E deficiency, 15 to 25 IU/kg per day of vitamin E therapy is begun. Vitamin E dosing should be careful to not interfere with medications that might hamper its intestinal absorption (ie, cholestyramine) and may benefit from morning dosing when bile flow may be maximal after an overnight fast. Monitoring the ratio of vitamin E to lipid and performing a neurologic examination will help determine the need to increase vitamin E dosing if normalization does not occur within several weeks of therapy. Vitamin E toxicity is rare and may present as bleeding in children taking anticoagulants or sepsis in neonates.

Vitamin K

Vitamin K is a member of the naphthoquinone family and has 3 forms.[23] Phylloquinone (vitamin K_1) is found in leafy vegetables, soybean oil, fruits, seeds, and cow milk. Menaquinone (vitamin K_2) is produced by intestinal bacteria. Menadione (vitamin K_3) is a synthesized form of vitamin K and has better water solubility. Because of the lack of data to estimate an average requirement, a recommended adequate intake is based on representative dietary intake data from healthy individuals. The adequate intake for vitamin K is 2.0 µg/day for infants 0 to 6 months of age, 2.5 µg/day for infants 7 to 12 months of age, 30 µg/day for children 1 to 3 years of age, 55 µg/day for children 4 to 8 years of age, 60 µg/day for children 9 to 13 years of age, and 75 µg/day for adolescents 14 to 18 years of age. The adequate intake for men and women is 120 and 90 µg/day, respectively (see Appendix J). No adverse effect has been reported for individuals consuming higher amounts of vitamin K.

Absorption of vitamin K_1 requires bile and pancreatic secretions that are impaired by cholestasis. Intestinal absorption of vitamin K_1 is an active process, whereas vitamin K_2 absorption is by passive diffusion. Absorbed vitamin K is incorporated into chylomicrons and is transported to the blood via the lymph. Little vitamin K is stored in the liver.

Vitamin K functions as a coenzyme during the synthesis of the biologically active form of a number of proteins involved in blood coagulation and bone metabolism. The vitamin K-dependent coagulation proteins include factors II, VII, IX, and X; protein C; and protein S.[24] Another family of vitamin K-dependent proteins includes the gla proteins. Osteocalcin is one of these proteins involved in bone mineralization.[25] Vitamin K deficiency in infancy can cause coagulopathy resulting in intracranial bleeding.[26] In children with cholestasis, malabsorption of vitamin K accompanied by antibiotic suppression of intestinal flora vitamin K production predisposes to vitamin K deficiency.[27]

Vitamin K status is frequently measured by using the prothrombin time, which is dependent on vitamin K-dependent clotting factors. If the prothrombin time is prolonged in comparison with the partial thromboplastin time, then vitamin K deficiency is likely. Liver disease may prolong the prothrombin time because of impaired synthesis of clotting factors active in the intrinsic coagulation pathway. Although impractical for routine use, vitamin K concentrations may also be directly measured by high-performance liquid chromatography. Vitamin K status can be more sensitively ascertained by the plasma protein induced in vitamin K absence II (PIVKA-II) assay (enzyme-linked immunosorbent assay). Plasma PIVKA-II values greater than 3 ng/mL are indicative of vitamin K deficiency, although this test also has not proved to be clinically useful, because abnormal concentrations may also be found in normal patients. Plasma conjugated bilirubin, total bile acids, and severity of liver disease all have positively correlated with plasma PIVKA-II concentrations. Measurement of vitamin K-dependent clotting factors are costly, are not easily obtainable, and offer no advantage over monitoring prothrombin time for assessing vitamin K deficiency.

Vitamin K deficiency in children with cholestasis should be avoided. Supplementation with oral vitamin K should be provided (Mephyton [Merck and Co, Whitehouse Station, NJ], vitamin K_1, 5-mg tablets) in a daily or twice-weekly dose of 2.5 to 10 mg, dependent on response to therapy. Failure to respond to oral vitamin K supplementation may require subcutaneous or intravenous vitamin K administration (AquaMephyton [Merck and Co], vitamin K_1, 2 mg/mL or 10 mg/mL). If given intravenously, the dose should be given slowly (not to exceed 1 mg/minute) to avoid anaphylaxis. To attempt correction of coagulopathy, vitamin K may be given subcutaneously or intravenously for 3 days consecutively. Failure to respond to this regimen suggests significant hepatic dysfunction.

Water-Soluble Vitamins

Although, theoretically, decreased intake and malabsorption secondary to enteropathy are risk factors for deficiencies of water-soluble vitamins in children with chronic liver diseases, the incidence of deficiencies of these vitamins in these conditions has not been reported. Deficiencies of water-soluble vitamins in children with chronic liver disease are likely to be uncommon, because infant and enteral formulas used to feed children with chronic liver disease are supplemented with these vitamins.

Trace Elements

Zinc

Although children with chronic liver disease are often considered at risk of trace element deficiencies, no systematic studies of these deficiencies have been reported. Zinc is an important trace metal that is essential for normal cellular growth and differentiation, immune function, wound healing, and protein synthesis. Zinc deficiency is associated with acrodermatitis, diarrhea, and poor growth. Zinc metabolism is altered in children and adults with chronic liver disease. Infants and children with biliary atresia have been observed to have lower plasma zinc concentrations compared with controls.[28] Plasma zinc concentrations do not correlate with age, episodes of cholangitis, or repeated surgical procedures. Inappropriate urinary zinc excretion has been documented in children with chronic liver disease and hypozincemia and may be the pathogenesis for the observed deficiency in chronic liver disease.[29] Other potential causes for zinc deficiency in patients with chronic liver disease include decreased intestinal absorption, decreased dietary intake, and reduced portal-venous extraction secondary to portosystemic shunting. After liver transplantation, the abnormal zinc homeostasis observed is rapidly improved and biochemical zinc deficiency reversed.[30] Serum zinc concentrations may not reflect total body zinc status. Identification of zinc deficiency may be difficult, although occasionally, a low-alkaline phosphatase, a zinc-dependent enzyme, can indicate zinc deficiency state. If clinical signs of zinc deficiency are suspected (acrodermatitis, diarrhea, and poor growth), an empiric trial of zinc supplementation is warranted. The standard dose of zinc for supplementation is 1 to 2 mg/kg per day of elemental zinc.

Copper

Copper is an essential trace element and functions as a cofactor for several important enzymes, such as lysyl oxidase, elastase, monoamine oxidase, cytochrome oxidase, ceruloplasmin, and superoxide dismutase. Deficiency of copper may be expressed by impaired activity of these enzymes. Signs of copper deficiency include neutropenia, microcytic anemia nonresponsive to iron supplementation, bone abnormalities, skin disorders, and depigmentation of hair and skin. The immune system is affected, resulting in diminished phagocytic activity of neutrophils and impaired cellular immunity. The anemia is the result of low concentrations of ceruloplasmin or ferroxidase, an enzyme that is required for the incorporation of iron into hemoglobin.

Wilson disease is an autosomal-recessive disorder of copper metabolism that results in toxic effects of copper. In patients with Wilson disease, excess copper is stored in the body, especially in the liver and brain. Clinically, patients develop cirrhosis, eye lesions (Kayser-Fleisher rings), kidney abnormalities, and neurologic disease. Despite high amounts of copper in the liver, serum concentrations of copper and ceruloplasmin are often low. Treatment includes chelation therapy with D-penicillamine or triethylenetetramine (trietine) and oral zinc therapy to reduce intestinal copper absorption. For advanced cases, liver transplantation can be life saving.

Copper is excreted into the intestinal tract via the biliary route. Thus, copper deficiency is unlikely to occur in children with cholestasis. However, in contrast, when children with cholestasis receive parenteral nutrition, copper is often excluded from trace mineral supplementation to avoid excessive accumulation of systemic copper.

Chromium

Chromium functions as a cofactor for insulin. Chromium deficiency is associated with poor growth and impaired glucose, lipid, and protein metabolism. Although peripheral insulin resistance and glucose intolerance occur in liver disease and chromium deficiency occurs in adults, studies of the utility of chromium supplementation in adults or children with chronic liver disease are nonexistent. Chromium deficiency in infants is probably rare and only associated with protein-calorie malnutrition or prolonged parenteral nutrition without supplementation. Other than occasional development of glucose intolerance and hyperglycemia, the only indicator of chromium deficiency is the demonstration of a beneficial effect to chromium supplementation.

Manganese

Manganese is a cofactor for enzymes such as arginase, glutamate-ammonia ligase, manganese superoxide dismutase, and pyruvate carboxylase. Deficiency of manganese has not been reported in infants and children. Toxic effects of manganese accumulation in the basal ganglia are reported in adults with cirrhosis and liver disease may cause lack of coordination and balance, mental confusion, and muscle cramps and may contribute to hepatic encephalopathy. Extrapyramidal effects may resemble Parkinson's disease. Because manganese is excreted in bile, children with cholestatic liver disease may develop elevated plasma concentrations.[31] Further, children with liver disease who receive parenteral nutrition, as with copper, should have manganese eliminated or reduced in trace mineral supplementation in parenteral nutrition solutions.

Selenium

Selenium deficiency has been demonstrated in children receiving long-term parenteral nutrition without supplementation. Selenium deficiency results in macrocytosis and loss of hair and skin pigmentation.[32] Selenium is a required part of several proteins, such as selenium-dependent glutathione peroxidase, selenoprotein P, and deiodinase. Serum selenium concentration may be decreased in adults with liver disease. No studies have addressed the distribution of selenium into bioactive forms, such as glutathione peroxidase and selenoprotein P, in patients with liver disease.

Ascites Management

Ascites development usually signifies advanced liver disease with portal hypertension. Significant hypoalbuminemia results from protein leakage into the peritoneal space and diminished albumin synthesis as a result of the liver disease. Most children with ascites have developed the condition slowly over time and are well compensated. Respiratory distress from the fluid compressing the diaphragms or concern for infected ascitic fluid (usually accompanied by fever) should prompt a paracentesis for both diagnostic and therapeutic indications. The fluid may be cultured for organisms and a cell count and differential can be obtained. Large fluid withdrawal should be avoided to prevent rapid fluid shifts from the intravascular space to the peritoneal cavity that could result in shock, preventable with careful observation and intravascular volume replacement (preferably albumin).

Treatment of ascites begins with strict observance of sodium and fluid restriction. All sources of sodium, whether dietary, in intravenous fluids, from medications, or otherwise, must be counted. Unfortunately, food palatability is related to sodium content. A diet that is sodium free or severely sodium restricted may be highly unpalatable for a child. Urinary sodium excretion is frequently assessed to determine the adequacy of sodium restriction. Approximately 140 mEq of sodium will translate into approximately 1 L of water loss. Adequate calories, carbohydrates, proteins, and vitamins remain an important goal of therapy.

Fluid restriction is also an important part of the dietary treatment of ascites. A stepwise, gentle approach to fluid restriction is warranted.[33,34] If, in response to therapy, the child is losing weight, maintaining serum sodium concentrations, and showing evidence of appropriate urinary sodium excretion, then allowing the child to regulate his or her fluid intake may be acceptable. However, inappropriate fluid retention (weight gain, increasing abdominal girth), hyponatremia, or poor urinary sodium excretion should lead to fluid restriction to two thirds to three quarters of maintenance fluid therapy. If there is no improvement, diuretics are added. Spironolactone (3–6 mg/kg per day, divided twice daily) is often used as first-line diuretic therapy for ascites in children and will take approximately 5 days to begin demonstrating a noticeable effect. If additional diuretic therapy is required, addition of furosemide (1–2 mg/kg per day, divided twice daily) may be used. Diuretic dosages should be tailored to the individual child with the goal of using the smallest effective dose. The goal of sodium and fluid restriction and diuretics should not be complete elimination of the ascites. Further, close monitoring of serum electrolyte concentrations, intake and output balance, and vital signs is mandatory and may require consequent nutrient supplementation or adjustments. Attention to avoiding renal compromise resulting from the restrictions is paramount.[35]

Liver Failure

Children with fulminant liver failure may develop hepatic encephalopathy (hepatic coma). Ammonia, the result of protein metabolism, is considered to be a contributing factor in the development and progression of encephalopathy. Thus, protein restriction is recommended for children with hepatic encephalopathy, and for children in deep coma, a completely protein-free diet may be warranted. However, to regenerate new liver tissue, some protein is advisable (1 mg/kg per day) in children who can tolerate even small amounts so that anabolism, and not catabolism, of protein stores occurs.

Branched-chain amino acid (BCAA)-enriched formulas for enteral and parenteral use have been postulated to aid in the therapy of patients in acute or chronic liver failure in adults.[36] These formulas are expensive, and their role for children with liver failure has not been defined.

Altering the type of dietary protein may benefit certain patients with chronic hepatic encephalopathy. Most, but not all, studies that compared vegetable with animal dietary protein found that vegetable protein diets were better tolerated than were animal protein diets. Vegetable diets reduce urea production rate by increasing dietary fiber intake and increasing incorporation and elimination of nitrogen in fecal bacteria. Most patients with cirrhosis can tolerate an increasing amount of standard protein without worsening encephalopathy. Formulas with high concentrations of BCAAs

V

(leucine, isoleucine, valine) and small amounts of aromatic amino acids (phenylalanine, tyrosine) have been proposed for use in patients with hepatic encephalopathy on the basis of the observation that the ratio of plasma BCAAs to aromatic amino acids is reduced in patients who have cirrhosis. Liquid formulas enriched with BCAAs, which contain approximately 35% of total amino acids as BCAAs, may be useful in a small percentage of patients with cirrhosis who are truly intolerant of increasing dietary protein. As much as 80 g of protein given as BCAA-enriched solutions has been tolerated in patients who could not tolerate 40 g of standard dietary protein. The large expense of BCAA-enriched solutions discourages their use in most settings.

The clinical efficacy of parenteral BCAA-enriched conventional parenteral nutrition solutions in patients with acute hepatic encephalopathy has been evaluated in clinical trials.[37] Patients who received BCAA-enriched solutions demonstrated a statistically significant improvement in mental recovery from high-grade encephalopathy during short-term (7–14 days) nutritional therapy. Considerable heterogeneity in mortality rates among studies precluded meaningful aggregation of mortality data. Although the pooled analysis of trials suggests a beneficial effect of BCAA-enriched formulas as a primary therapy in patients with acute hepatic encephalopathy, the studies have several shortcomings that limit enthusiasm for this relatively expensive therapy. The control groups usually received suboptimal, and possibly harmful, nutritional support, consisting of high-dextrose solutions without amino acids. Only one study compared BCAA-enriched parenteral nutrition with a standard amino acid parenteral nutrition solution. None of the studies reported on complications associated with nutritional therapy, and none evaluated whether short-term benefits of nutritional therapy led to a long-term reduction in complications.

Protein-energy malnutrition is prevalent in children with chronic cholestasis and liver disease. Significant increases in growth and nitrogen balance are observed in children with cholestatic liver disease supplemented with BCAA, suggesting that BCAA requirements are increased in chronic cholestasis.[38] Measurements using indicator amino acid oxidation demonstrate that the mean requirement of total BCAA in children with mild to moderate liver disease is greater than the mean requirement for the total BCAA established in healthy children.[39]

The clinical features of hepatic encephalopathy, although well defined in adults, are not as evident in children. The Pediatric Acute Liver Failure Study Group classified hepatic encephalopathy in stages from 0 to IV. In stage 0, clinical signs or symptoms are absent, and reflexes and electroencephalographic and neurologic signs are normal. In stages I and II, children are often inconsolable, crying, and inattentive to task and have normal or hyperreflexic reflexes. In stage III, the child may become somnolent, stuporous, and combative with hyperreflexic reactions. In stage IV, the child is comatose, arouses with painful stimuli (stage IVa) or no response (stage IVb), and has absent reflexes. The child may have decerebrate or decorticate posturing and abnormal, very slow delta activity on electroencephalography. False neurotransmitters, fatty acids, mercaptans, and other toxins likely play a role in the development of encephalopathy.[40] Potential precipitating factors (sepsis, hemorrhage, medications) must be identified and managed proactively. Protein restriction may be necessary, and absorption and production of ammonia within the intestines should be prevented using lactulose or nonabsorbable antibiotic agents.

Lactulose, a nonabsorbable carbohydrate composed of galactose and fructose, can be metabolized by intraluminal bacteria to form organic acids.[41] The result is the acidification of the colonic pH allowing for the conversion of ammonia to ammonium ion that can be trapped in the colon and then evacuated via stool. Lactulose also causes increased numbers of stools, which aids in ammonia elimination via the intestine. Patients in deep coma can have lactulose instilled directly into the colon via an enema to avoid the possibility of aspiration.

Antibiotics have also been used to diminish ammonia production intraluminally in the intestines. Neomycin and gentamicin have frequently been used in this capacity. Unfortunately, both of these antibiotic agents are not completely nonabsorbable. If absorbed in sufficient quantities with chronic use, ototoxicity and nephrotoxicity have been reported.

Parenteral Nutrition-Associated Liver Disease

Parenteral nutrition-associated liver disease results from prolonged use of total parenteral nutrition and is especially prevalent among neonates with recurrent sepsis, those having undergone surgical procedures, or those born preterm and leads to total parenteral nutrition-associated cholestasis (see Chapter 22: Parenteral Nutrition). The incidence of this problem appears to be decreasing as more aggressive use of enteral nutrition has been used. Prevention has involved early initiation and steady progression of enteral feedings and prevention of sepsis. Specific nutrient regimens have been attempted to diminish the risk of total parenteral nutrition-associated cholestasis, including using amino acid preparations that promote a plasma amino acid pattern resembling those in breastfed infants; limiting potentially toxic amino acids, such as methionine; adding antioxidant nutrients (eg, glutathione, vitamin E); and limiting fat and/or carbohydrate loads in at-risk infants. Further investigations are ongoing to determine efficacy of all of these treatments. Infants and older children sustaining severe liver toxicity that leads to cirrhosis and irreversible liver injury may require liver transplantation, with or without small intestinal transplantation, as a life-saving measure.

References

1. Powell DW. Approach to the patient with liver disease. In: Goldman L, Ausiello D, eds. *Cecil Textbook of Medicine.* 22nd ed. Philadelphia, PA: Saunders; 2004:894–896

2. Bradley BW, Murphy GM, Bouchier IA, Sherlock S. Diminished micellar phase lipid in patients with chronic nonalcoholic liver disease and steatorrhea. *Gastroenterology.* 1970;58:781–789

3. Wene JD, Connor WE, Den Besten L. The development of EFA deficiency in healthy men fed fat free diets intravenously and orally. *J Clin Invest.* 1975;56:127–134

4. Clandinin MT, Chappell JE, Heim T, Swyer PR, Chance GW. Fatty acid utilization in perinatal de novo synthesis of tissues. *Early Hum Dev.* 1981;5:355–366

5. Pettei MJ, Daftary S, Levine JJ. Essential fatty acid deficiency associated with the use of a medium-chain-triglyceride infant formula in pediatric hepatobiliary disease. *Am J Clin Nutr.* 1991;53:1217–1221

6. Kaufman SS, Scrivner DJ, Murray ND, Vanderhoof JA, Hart MH, Antonson DL. Influence of Portagen and Pregestimil on essential fatty acid status in infantile liver disease. *Pediatrics.* 1992;89:151–154

7. Feranchak AP, Gralla J, King R, et al. Comparison of indices of vitamin A status in children with chronic liver disease. *Hepatology.* 2005;42:782–792

8. Lippe B, Hensen L, Mendoza G, Finerman A, Welch M. Chronic vitamin A intoxication. A multisystem disease that could reach epidemic proportions. *Am J Dis Child.* 1981;135:634–636

9. Smith FR, Goodman DS. Vitamin A transport in human vitamin A toxicity. *New Engl J Med.* 1976;294:805–808

10. Penniston KL, Tanumihardjo SA. The acute and chronic toxic effects of vitamin A. *Am J Clin Nutr.* 2006;83:191–201

11. Heubi JE, Hollis BW, Specker B, Tsang RC. Bone disease in chronic childhood cholestasis. 1. Vitamin D absorption and metabolism. *Hepatology.* 1989;9:258–264

12. Bucuvalas JC, Heubi JE, Specker BL, Gregg DT, Yergey AL, Vieira NE. Calcium absorption in bone disease associated with liver cholestasis during childhood. *Hepatology.* 1990; 12:1200–1205

13. Heubi JE, Higgins JV, Argao EA, Sierra RI, Specker BL. The role of magnesium in the pathogenesis of bone disease in childhood cholestatic liver disease: a preliminary report. *J Pediatr Gastroenterol Nutr.* 1997;25:301–306

14. Argao EA, Balistreri WF, Hollis BW, Ryckman FC, Heubi JE. Effect of orthotopic liver transplantation on bone mineral content and serum vitamin D metabolites in infants and children with chronic cholestasis. *Hepatology.* 1994;20:598–603

15. Attard TM, Dhawan A, Kaufman SS, Collier DS, Langnas AN. Use of disodium pamidronate in children with hypercalcemia awaiting liver transplantation. *Pediatr Transplant.* 1998;2:157–159

16. Sokol RJ, Heubi JE, Iannaccone S, Bove KE, Balisteri WF. Mechanism causing vitamin E deficiency during chronic childhood cholestasis. *Gastroenterology.* 1983;85:1172–1182

17. Guggenheim MA, Jackson V, Lilly J, Silverman A. Vitamin E deficiency and neurologic disease in children with cholestasis: a prospective study. *J Pediatr.* 1983;102:577–579

18. Sokol RJ, Guggenheim MA, Iannaccone ST, et al. Improved neurologic function after long-term correction of vitamin E deficiency in children with chronic cholestasis. *N Engl J Med.* 1985;313:1580–1586

19. Sokol RJ, Heubi JE, Iannaccone ST, Bove KE, Balisteri WF. Vitamin E deficiency with normal serum vitamin E concentration in children with chronic cholestasis. *N Engl J Med.* 1984;310:1209–1212

20. Gordon HH, Nitowsky HM, Cornblath M. Studies of tocopherol deficiency in infants and children. 1. Hemolysis of erythrocytes in hydrogen peroxide. *AMA Am J Dis Child.* 1955;90:669–681

21. Cynamon HA, Isenberg JN, Nguyen CH. Erythrocyte malondialdehyde release in vitro: a functional measure of vitamin E status. *Clin Chim Acta.* 1985;151:169–176

22. Refat M, Moore TJ, Kazui M, Risby TH, Perman JA, Schwarz KB. Utility of breathe ethane as a noninvasive biomarker of vitamin E status in children. *Pediatr Res.* 1991;30:396–403

23. Olson RE. The function and metabolism of vitamin K. *Annu Rev Nutr.* 1984;4:281–337

24. Shah DV, Suttie JW. The vitamin K dependent, in vitro production of prothrombin. *Biochem Biophys Res Commun.* 1974;60:1397–1402

25. Price PA, Parthemore JG, Deftos LJ. New biochemical marker for bone metabolism. Measurement by radioimmunoassay of bone GLA protein in the plasma of normal subjects and patients with bone disease. *J Clin Invest.* 1980;66:878–883

26. Bancroft J, Cohen MB. Intracranial hemorrhage due to vitamin K deficiency in breast-fed infants with cholestasis. *J Pediatr Gastroenterol Nutr.* 1993;16:78–80

27. Yanofsky RA, Jackson VG, Lilly JR, Stellin G, Klingensmith WC III, Hathaway WE. The multiple coagulopathies of biliary atresia. *Am J Hematol.* 1984;16:171–180

28. Goksu N, Ozsoylu S. Hepatic and serum levels of zinc, copper and magnesium in childhood cirrhosis. *J Pediatr Gastroenterol Nutr.* 1986;5:459–462

29. Hambidge KM, Krebs NF, Lilly JR, Zerbe GO. Plasma and urine zinc in infants and children with extrahepatic biliary atresia. *J Pediatr Gastroenterol Nutr.* 1987;6:872–877

30. Narkewicz MR, Krebs N, Karrer F, Orban-Eller K, Sokol RJ. Correction of hypozincemia following liver transplantation in children is associated with reduced urinary zinc loss. *Hepatology.* 1999;29:830–833

31. Bayliss EA, Hambidge KM, Lilly JR, Sokol RJ, Stewart B. Hepatic concentrations of zinc, copper and manganese in infants with extrahepatic biliary atresia. *J Trace Elem Med Biol.* 1995;9:40–43

32. Vinton NE, Dahlstrom KA, Strobel CT, Ament ME. Macrocytosis and pseudoalbinism: manifestations of selenium deficiency. *J Pediatr.* 1987;111:711–717

33. Runyon BA. Treatment of patients with cirrhosis and ascites. *Semin Liver Dis.* 1997;17: 249–260

34. Garcia-Tsao G. Current management of the complications of cirrhosis and portal hypertension: variceal hemorrhage, ascites, and spontaneous bacterial peritonitis. *Gastroenterology.* 2001;120:726–748

35. Sort P, Navasa M, Arroyo V, et al. Effect of intravenous albumin on renal impairment and mortality in patients with cirrhosis and spontaneous bacterial peritonitis. *N Engl J Med.* 1999;341:403–409

36. Cerra FB, Cheung NK, Fischer JE, et al. Disease-specific amino acid infusion (F080) in hepatic encephalopathy: a prospective, randomized, double-blind, controlled trial. *JPEN J Parenter Enteral Nutr.* 1985;9:288–295

37. Marchesini G, Marzocchi R, Noia M, Bianchi G. Branched-chain amino acid supplementation in patients with liver diseases. *J Nutr.* 2005;135:1596S–1601S

38. Chin SE, Shepherd RW, Thomas BJ, et al. Nutritional support in children with end-stage liver disease: a randomized crossover trial of a branched-chain amino acid supplement. *Am J Clin Nutr.* 1992;56:158–163

39. Mager DR, Wykes LJ, Roberts EA, Ball RO, Pencharz PB. Branched-chain amino acid needs in children with mild-to-moderate chronic cholestatic liver disease. *J Nutr.* 2006;136:133–139

40. Jalan R, Hayes PC. Hepatic encephalopathy and ascites. *Lancet.* 1997;350:1309–1315

41. Debray D, Yousef N, Durand P. New management options for end-stage chronic liver disease and acute liver failure: potential for pediatric patients. *Paediatr Drugs.* 2006;8:1–13

45 Cardiac Disease

Growth retardation is prevalent in children with congenital heart disease (CHD). Growth failure in heart disease, once termed cardiac cachexia, has a multifactorial etiology and follows a pattern identical to acute and chronic protein-calorie undernutrition, with wasting of body mass and stunting of linear growth. Cyanosis, congestive heart failure (CHF), and pulmonary hypertension (pulmonary-to-systemic pressure ratio >0.4) are the sentinel features of CHD implicated in growth failure. Growth failure attributable to congenital heart malformation may begin before birth in a neonate with intrauterine growth retardation. Infants with most forms of cardiac malformations (transposition of the great arteries [TGA] being a notable exception) have a lower-than-normal birth weight.[1] Approximately 6% of infants with symptomatic heart disease may present with intrauterine growth retardation.[2] In addition, extracardiac malformations or recognizable syndromes (eg, trisomy 21, trisomy 18, Turner syndrome, VACTERL [vertebral, anal, cardiac, tracheoesophageal, renal, limb] syndrome, CHARGE [coloboma of the eye, heart defects, atresia of the choanae, retardation of growth and/or development, genital and/or urinary abnormalities, and ear abnormalities and deafness] syndrome) with noncardiac reasons for impaired growth are also more common in children with heart disease.[3]

Acute undernutrition, defined as reduced weight relative to the median weight predicted by length (wasting), and chronic undernutrition, based on reduced length relative to the median length predicted for age (stunting), are more prevalent among hospitalized patients with CHD. Acute undernutrition or wasting may affect up to one third of patients and chronic undernutrition or stunting may be found in approximately two thirds of patients. As many as 60% of patients with left-to-right shunts and up to 70% of patients with either cyanosis or CHF meet criteria for undernutrition.[4] The most severe undernutrition may occur in severe CHF associated with ventricular septal defect (VSD), patent ductus arteriosus, TGA, or coarctation of the aorta. Infants with these defects may present as appropriate for gestational age at birth but incur early weight deficits or wasting, followed by linear growth deficits or stunting. In cyanotic lesions, such as tetralogy of Fallot or TGA, symmetric failure to thrive is observed with weight and length gain depressed concurrently. In acyanotic lesions such as atrial septal defect (ASD), VSD, or patent ductus arteriosus, slow weight gain or wasting predominates over linear growth retardation or stunting, especially with CHF and/or large left-to-right shunts. The incidence of growth failure is highest in patients with VSD, perhaps because of the greater prevalence of pulmonary hypertension and CHF in children with large left-to-right shunts.[5] A recent retrospective study of 123 children with CHD showed the worst growth retardation in patients with a large VSD (CHF) and tetralogy of Fallot (cyanotic heart disease). Delay in skeletal maturation as assessed by bone age is related to severity of hypoxemia in cyanotic heart disease but also is seen in CHF.[5] Conversely, asymptomatic acyanotic lesions (aortic stenosis, coarctation, pulmonary stenosis) without congestive heart failure or pulmonary hypertension may not be associated with undernutrition. Surgical repair or correction allows normalization of most height deficits.[6]

The following text describes the components of undernutrition in CHD, the nutritional effects of the hemodynamic features of CHD, and the effects of nutrients on cardiac function, providing a basis for optimal nutritional management and monitoring.

Undernutrition in CHD

Undernutrition occurs when metabolic demands for protein or energy (expenditure), combined with nutrient losses (regurgitation or malabsorption), exceed energy and protein nutrient intake. Investigators have attempted to study each of these components of nutrient balance. In addition to deficits in these macronutrients affecting growth and body composition, clinically important deficiency in certain micronutrients may also occur.

Energy Expenditure

A number of studies have confirmed that total daily energy expenditure (TDEE), including components of physical activity such as cardiorespiratory work associated with movement and dietary thermogenesis, is increased significantly in children with CHD, with relatively insignificant increases in resting energy expenditure (REE) relative to lean body mass. Total daily energy expenditure comprises REE, physical activity, and dietary-induced thermogenesis. Metabolizable, or absorbed, energy intake must exceed TDEE to permit normal growth. Although REE in children with CHD seems to be similar to age-matched reference children, infants with CHD from 3 to 5 months of age have approximately 40% increased TDEE (94.2 + 6.9 kcal/ kg per day vs 67.1 + 7.3 kcal/kg for healthy infants).[7-11] Surgery does not seem to alter REE.[5]

Nutrient Losses

Some patients with CHD have abnormalities of gastrointestinal function or renal losses that may affect nutrition. Urinary losses of energy as glucosuria and proteinuria may be significant in certain patients with renal disease or glucose intolerance. Approximately 8% of infants with CHD have associated major gastrointestinal tract malformations, such as tracheoesophageal fistula and esophageal atresia, malrotation, or diaphragmatic hernia, which generally will limit intake and cause losses of nutrients.[12] Fecal losses of energy in subclinical steatorrhea or of protein in protein-losing enteropathy may be more significant and prevalent than expected, affecting up to 50 % of patients with a variety of congenital heart lesions. In one study, protein-losing enteropathy was found in 8 of 21 infants with severe CHD[13] and is a major complication common to patients who undergo the Fontan procedure or have severe right-sided CHF. Steatorrhea, indicative of disturbed digestion or absorption, was found in 5 of 21 infants with CHD (1 of 8 patients with CHF and 4 of 12 patients with cyanotic heart disease).[13] In these patients, mucosal small-bowel biopsies were normal. Mean resting oxygen consumption was higher in infants with CHF than in those with cyanotic heart disease.[13]

No significant malabsorption of energy or fat in stools was observed in the study of children receiving diuretics by Vaisman et al.[14] Total body water and extracellular water excess were measured and correlated directly with fat losses and inversely with energy intake suggesting a relationship to the degree of CHF and diuretic efficacy. Therefore, infants with increased total body water (ie, not effectively diuresed) had more malabsorption than euvolemic diuresed patients.

Yahav et al[15] studied malabsorption relative to energy requirements in 14 infants with CHD from 2 to 36 months of age (mean, 10.4 months). Ten infants with CHF and 4 with cyanosis were studied in 3 periods of 3 to 7 days each, comparing baseline oral intake, supplemented oral intake, and nasogastric tube feedings of a formula with high caloric density. Nasogastric tube feedings of a formula with high caloric density (1.5 kcal/mL or 45 kcal/oz) were administered to 11 patients. Consistent weight gain averaging 13 g/day was observed only in patients receiving >170 kcal/kg per day, with only 50% of the children gaining weight on 149 kcal/kg per day. Increased cardiac and respiratory rates were observed in patients after feeding and were attributed to dietary thermogenesis but did not appear to be clinically significant. Minor intestinal losses of fat were observed in 3 patients and protein-losing enteropathy was not observed in any patients, and these were not considered significant limiting factors.[15]

Nutrient Intake

Several studies have examined energy and nutrient intake requirements of infants and young children with CHD (Table 45.1). Approximately 140 to 150 kcal/kg per day is required for linear growth and to increase subcutaneous fat and muscle in infants with CHD and CHF. In one study of 19 infants randomly assigned to 3 groups, only the group receiving continuous 24-hour nasogastric tube feedings over a 5-month study period were able to achieve intake >140 kcal/day (mean, 147 kcal/day).[16] Only this group of patients was able to demonstrate improved nutritional status manifested as increased weight, length, and anthropometric measures of fat and muscle stores. The groups who received either 12-hour supplemental nocturnal infusions or oral feedings failed to achieve such intakes and growth responses, perhaps because of increased REE. The group receiving 12-hour oral feedings plus infusions received only 122 kcal/kg, well below the threshold for growth. Fatigue during oral feedings was considered a limiting factor in both of these groups. In addition, in the 12-hour infusion group, daytime oral intake (52 kcal/kg) actually dropped to approximately 50% of the prestudy mean caloric intake (98 kcal/kg). The investigators concluded that only 24-hour continuous enteral feeding by nasogastric tube of a 1-kcal/mL formula was able to provide >140 kcal/kg per day and result in improved nutritional status.[16]

Table 45.1
Energy Requirements for Normal Growth in Infants With CHD

Study	Age Range	Mode	% IBW	kcal/kg per Day	kcal/kg IBW
Bougle[40]	2 wk–6 mo	NG	—	137	—
Vanderhoof[41]	1 wk–9 mo	NG	—	120–150	—
Schwarz[16]	1–10 mo	NG	82	147	120
Yahav[15]	2–36 mo	NG/PO	76	149–169	113–128
Barton[7]	0–3 mo	NG/PO	80	143	114
Summary	0–36 mo	NG	80	145	115

IBW indicates ideal body weight or weight for height; NG, nasogastric; PO, oral.

Two studies have concluded that children with CHD who are not growing appear to consume insufficient calories, because they respond to supplementation, supporting the fact that failure to gain weight can be simply a matter of inadequate intake, not intrinsic genetic or cardiac factors. The type of cardiac defect does not necessarily predict or limit the response to dietary counseling and oral supplementation.[17,18]

Delayed gastric emptying[19] and gastroesophageal reflux[20] in children with CHD as well as oral aversion may be significant features that reduce voluntary intake and compromise nutrition. There may be early satiety induced by gastroparesis and gut hypomotility related to edema or hypoxia as well as by distention from hepatomegaly associated with CHF.

Congestive Heart Failure

Growth failure in children with CHF is common. The pathogenesis of this growth failure in CHF is not always clear and is likely to be multifactorial. Congestive heart failure may impair growth as a consequence of increased energy requirements caused by increased myocardial and respiratory work, increased catecholamines, and intestinal malabsorption, anorexia, or fatigability during feedings. In adults with CHF, total energy expenditure appears to be lower than that in controls. High protein-calorie feeds do not reverse growth impairment, suggesting that the wasting has a metabolic basis rather than one of negative protein and energy balance.[21] In addition, malnutrition in adults with CHF is associated with increased right atrial pressure and tricuspid regurgitation.[22] Elevated right atrial pressures may cause intestinal protein losses and fat malabsorption and/or anorexia because of splanchnic and mesenteric venous congestion. In adults, REE is increased and may be caused by the increased work of breathing or elevated sympathetic innervation.[23] Cytokines, such as tumor necrosis factor, are increased in adults with heart failure and may contribute to the cachexia seen in this condition.[24]

Both oxygen consumption and basal metabolic rate are increased in infants with CHF when compared with normal children or children with cyanotic CHD.[13,25,26] Traditionally, growth failure has been most common in infants with CHF as a result of pulmonary overcirculation from large left-to-right shunts, such as a VSD or atrioventricular septal defect. This has been most evident in children with a VSD and large left-to-right shunt and pulmonary hypertension.[18] Fortunately, the increasing success of complete repairs of such defects in infancy has greatly lessened this problem.

There are many possible reasons for growth failure in children with CHF. There may be insufficient caloric intake because of inability to consume adequate calories for growth, intestinal malabsorption attributable to passive congestion and/or low cardiac output, or increased metabolic demands primarily attributable to increased work of breathing. Insufficient caloric intake could be caused by a variety of factors, including excessive fatigue with oral feeding, excessive vomiting, or iatrogenic fluid restriction and diuresis because of the severity of heart failure.[16,27] Decreased gastric capacity caused by pressure on the stomach from an enlarged, congested liver, or from ascites may also interfere with the amount of nutrients a patient can ingest.[28] Children with CHF also may have abnormal intestinal function. They can demonstrate excessive intestinal protein losses, possibly secondary to elevated venous and lymphatic pressure.[13] Because of the obvious negative consequences of chronic fluid (and, thus, caloric) restriction in children, fluid restriction is now only temporarily used in patients who are either awaiting some type of intervention (eg, surgery or heart transplantation) or recovering from some type of acute process (eg, surgery, acute decompensation, pleural effusions, etc).

Cyanotic Heart Disease

The role of hypoxemia as a primary cause of growth retardation in children is unclear. Cyanotic CHD (eg, tetralogy of Fallot, tricuspid atresia) with chronic hypoxemia is frequently associated with undernutrition and linear growth retardation, especially if prolonged and if complicated by CHF (TGA or single ventricle). Isolated hypoxemia or desaturation does not necessarily result in tissue hypoxia, because tissue aerobic metabolism may not be impaired until arterial partial pressure of oxygen falls below 30 mm Hg, a threshold also affected by such factors as oxygen-carrying capacity determined by erythroid mass or hemoglobin and tissue perfusion. Therefore, the added complication of CHF probably contributes to chronic tissue hypoxia, which limits growth.

Some studies have demonstrated significant differences in growth between cyanotic and acyanotic children, whereas others have failed to do so.[5] Cyanotic children without pulmonary hypertension can demonstrate a normal nutritional state, with stunting of growth being more common than poor weight gain.[29] Children with cyanotic CHD have also been shown to have excessive stool protein loss.[13] Cyanotic patients with pulmonary hypertension had the worst growth, with hypoxemia or cyanosis (right-to-left shunting) and pulmonary hypertension having additive effects.[29] However, after surgical repair of cyanotic CHD, these children had REE and TDEE that were no different than those of controls.[30]

Circulatory Shunts

Cardiac lesions with nutritional implications may also be categorized by shunt direction and magnitude: left-to-right shunts associated with CHF and right-to-left shunts associated with hypoxemia or cyanosis. As previously described, cyanotic patients with pulmonary hypertension appear to have the worst growth, with hypoxemia or cyanosis (right-to-left shunting) and pulmonary hypertension having additive effects.[18,29] Infants with a clinically significant VSD have significantly higher TDEE than healthy control infants, suggesting that they are unable to meet additional energy demands from activity of dietary thermogenesis, resulting in growth retardation.[31]

Pulmonary Hypertension

Increased resting oxygen consumption in CHD has been demonstrated, especially in patients with CHF or pulmonary hypertension, and attributed to the oxygen demands of increased catecholamine secretion and other factors. Pulmonary hypertension is a complication frequently implicated in growth failure, correlated with stunting in VSD, an acyanotic lesion.[32] Children with both cyanotic heart disease and pulmonary hypertension demonstrated both moderate to severe wasting and linear growth retardation.[29]

Surgery

Significant protein calorie undernutrititon may delay surgical correction and impair postoperative recovery and growth. Growth failure has been added to the heart transplant criteria for the United Network for Organ Sharing, such that children with growth failure complicating CHD are listed at a higher status than children without growth failure.[33] Children demonstrate improvement in growth after corrective or palliative repair of a congenital heart lesion, and available data support the use of early surgical correction of major cardiac malformations to optimize growth.[9,30]

Within 1 week of surgery in infants with heart disease, energy expenditures fall sharply to reach levels significantly below preoperative levels. By approximately 2.5 years after surgery, weight, body composition, REE, TDEE, and energy expended during physical activity are similar to those in healthy children without CHD.[30] Studies have demonstrated a reversal of decreased growth velocity in infants who have undergone repair of VSD, tetralogy of Fallot, and TGA in the first year of life.[34] There are conflicting data regarding somatic growth in patients who have undergone the Fontan procedure. Some studies have demonstrated improvement in growth parameters,[35] whereas others have shown persistent growth failure.[36] These differences may relate to many factors, including different malformations or timing of surgery. Catch-up linear growth is more likely with corrective than

V

palliative surgery and with early repair. Residual, although reduced, CHF or shunt may still prevent normal nutritional recovery.[34,37]

Nutritional Assessment

A complete nutritional history includes feeding pattern and schedule, including frequency, duration, and volume of feedings. The volume of each feeding may actually be inversely related to the duration of feeding as the child fatigues. Diaphoresis with feedings reflects autonomic stimulation effects. Gastrointestinal function should be assessed to identify reflux and vomiting losses, irritability attributable to esophagitis or cramping, diarrhea or constipation, and early satiety, which may respond to acid control and motility medications or may be signs of associated anomalies. The physical examination must include accurate nude weight, length or height, and head circumference plotted on a growth curve. Consider changes in rate of growth or growth velocity as well as the relation of actual body weight to the ideal body weight predicted by height or length age. Use appropriate charts for children who were born preterm and for those with Down syndrome (see Appendix D), Turner syndrome (see www.kidsgrowth.com/resources/articledetail.cfm?id =521), or trisomy 18 (see http://members.optushome.com.au/karens/growth.htm). Assessment of subcutaneous fat and muscle mass may be helpful, if measured by a skilled dietitian with calipers, although dehydration or edema may affect validity. Signs of CHF, pulmonary hypertension, clubbing, cyanosis, and hepatomegaly connote increased risk of nutritional failure.

Laboratory evaluation initially should include hemoglobin, oxygen saturation, and albumin and prealbumin concentrations. Protein-losing enteropathy as a cause of hypoalbuminemia can be confirmed by fecal $alpha_1$-antitrypsin assay and is encountered in conditions of systemic venous hypertension, which occur with right-sided CHF, constrictive pericardial disease, restrictive cardiac disease, or post-Fontan operation. A low alkaline phosphatase or cholesterol concentration may signify zinc deficiency, which may affect taste and linear growth.

Nutritional Support

The goals of nutritional intervention are to (1) achieve nutritional balance by providing sufficient energy to stop catabolism of lean body mass and sufficient protein to match nitrogen losses; (2) provide additional nutrients to restore deficits and allow growth, thus normalizing weight for height and promoting linear growth; (3) provide enteral feedings to replace parenteral nutrition as tolerated by the gastrointestinal system; (4) develop and maintain oral feeding competence to enable voluntary independent feeding.

Nutrient Prescription

Optimal nutritional support should provide sufficient energy and protein not only to prevent breakdown or catabolism of protein and maintain body composition and weight but also to restore deficits and permit growth toward genetic potential. Electrolyte losses with diuretics and deficiencies in micronutrients, such as the trace minerals iron and zinc or vitamins, may be limiting factors. As a general principle, for any given level of nitrogen (or protein) provided in the diet, increasing the energy (calories) will improve nitrogen balance and protein synthesis or accretion. Similarly, for a given level of energy intake, increasing the protein intake will improve the nitrogen balance or protein accretion. If energy provided by carbohydrate and fat in the diet is below the patient's requirements, protein will be catabolized as an energy source and not used in synthesis of lean body mass. Even if sufficient calories are provided to stop gluconeogenesis and restore body glycogen and fat stores, enough protein must be provided as a nitrogen source to allow accretion of lean body protein mass and effective growth. A marginal or negative electrolyte balance, such as low net sodium or potassium intake in the setting of fluid restriction and diuretic use, required for some patients in CHF, may impair growth independent of energy and protein sufficiency. Iron and zinc deficiencies have been implicated in cases of failure to thrive, with improved growth demonstrated after supplementation.

Energy Requirement

Additional energy above the Recommended Dietary Allowance for age is required to permit normal growth rates, with even greater amounts required to restore nutritional deficits in "catch-up" or accelerated growth. A portion of this incremental energy requirement may be explained by simply calculating needs on the basis of the patient's ideal or median body weight predicted from body length or even head circumference. This calculation assumes that metabolic needs for energy and protein are determined by the relatively preserved brain, visceral, and lean body mass with a minimal contribution from the adipose or fat mass that is depleted with undernutrition. In this reasoning, a lean but longer infant's energy requirement would exceed that of a robust infant of the same weight, whose lean mass is less and reflected in a shorter length. In undernutrition, the ratio of metabolically active lean body mass to total weight is increased. For example, 150 kcal/kg of actual body weight in the typical lean child with CHD, who may be 80% of the expected or "ideal" weight for length, corresponds to 120 kcal/kg for a healthy, robust infant of the same length but at ideal body weight because of increased fat mass. Therefore, energy requirements may be more reliably based on the child's "ideal" body weight for length or height (Table 45.1).

Increased cardiac and respiratory work in the child with CHF, shunt, or cyanosis undoubtedly adds to the energy requirement. Increased catecholamines in CHF will increase energy expenditure, as will the demands of increased respiratory rate and hematopoiesis in cyanotic heart disease. The myocardium itself is a significant consumer of energy, with demands increased with pulmonary hypertension, hypertrophy, shunting, and CHF. Barton et al[7] estimated the energy requirement of an infant with CHD; the energy cost of normal tissue deposition is 21 kJ/g (5 kcal/g).[38] This energy cost is 30% less than the 31 kJ/g (7.4 kcal/g) estimated in infants with CHD on high-energy feeds.[39] This difference is consistent with a greater fat content (more energy per weight) of the tissue replenished in infants with CHD and is supported by measuring increased skinfold thickness during high-energy feeding.[39] Assuming 75% of energy cost of growth is stored in this new tissue and the remainder is used during synthesis (part of TDEE), an intake of 600 kJ/kg per day (143 kcal/kg per day) is required to allow average weight gain during the first 3 months of life.[7] Table 45.1 summarizes a number of studies of energy required to achieve growth in patients with CHD, comparing requirements calculated for actual body weight and ideal body weight for height or age. The parenteral requirements for energy will be approximately 70% to 80% of these enteral estimates.

One must also consider the metabolic load imposed by feeding. Cardiac output is determined by tissue metabolic demand. As additional nutrients are provided, cardiac output must increase to oxygenate these tissues, and ventilatory demands on the lungs increase to eliminate the carbon dioxide generated by metabolic activity. This phenomenon of increased energy demands of nutrition support known as dietary thermogenesis, the thermic effect of food or specific dynamic action, varies for different nutrients, being minimal for fat metabolism and quite significant—up to 5% of calories—for carbohydrate. Carbohydrates are used for fat synthesis when carbohydrates or equivalent glucose amounts are administered at a rate exceeding 8 mg/kg per minute. This endothermic process requires energy and oxygen and liberates carbon dioxide, which must be expired. For this reason, the energy provided should be distributed between fat and carbohydrate, with fat providing at least 30% of the total caloric intake. At least 6% of the fat should be long-chain triglycerides (linoleic acid as in corn, soy, safflower oils) and some linolenic acid to provide essential fatty acids. The value and safety of additional omega-3 fatty acids beyond essential fatty acid requirements are the subject of research.

Overfeeding or overly rapid increments in nutrition support can precipitate or worsen CHF. A refeeding syndrome has been described in which over-zealous nutritional support has caused complications, not only with cardiac failure, but also with conduction disturbances and dysrhythmias related to electrolyte and mineral shifts with anabolism. Provision of glucose leads to an insulin-mediated influx of potassium and intermediary metabolism demands for phosphorus (phosphorylated intermediate metabolites and production of adenosine triphosphate) lead to an intracellular shift, causing profound hypokalemia, hypophosphatemia, hypomagnesemia, and hypocalcemia. Prolongation of QT_c interval may be observed. Sudden death suspected to be related to lethal arrhythmias, such as torsade de pointes, has been attributed to the rapid refeeding of patients accommodated to the undernourished state.

In preterm and term neonates with CHD, there is a higher incidence of necrotizing enterocolitis. This fact dictates gradual advancement of feeding in the newborn period and monitoring tolerance in terms of abdominal distention, accumulating gastric residual, and hematochezia. For those on parenteral nutrition, trophic feedings of approximately 10 mL/kg of formula, preferably expressed human milk, for enteral and enterohepatic stimulation is beneficial.

Protein Intake

There is little discussion in the literature about nitrogen balance or protein intake in children with CHD. In general, if sufficient nonprotein energy is provided to prevent gluconeogenesis from catabolism of dietary amino acids, provision of more protein (up to specific limits) leads to greater incorporation of protein and its nitrogen in lean body mass. Protein generally constitutes 5% to 12% of total calories, reflected in the composition of human milk and infant formulas modeling human milk. Fomon and Ziegler suggested a formula caloric composition of 9% protein, 60% carbohydrate, and 31% fat provided in a density of 1 kcal/mL for infants with CHD.[42] The ratio of energy to protein in infant formulas is 30 to 50 kcal/g of protein (corresponding to nonprotein calorie-to-nitrogen ratios of 287:140). Thus, a child receiving 140 kcal/kg per day of energy would receive 2.9 to 4.25 g/kg of protein, if derived from standard or concentrated formula, with protein constituting 8% to 12% of total calories. To avoid excessive hepatic protein metabolic and renal solute load, assuming a limit of 3.5 g/kg per day of protein, the additional energy required above 120 kcal/kg on the basis of ideal body weight for length should be provided by either glucose polymers (polycose or starch) or by fat (microlipid or oils) added to the formula, unless using a standard infant formula or human milk (see Table 45.2). These formulas are low enough in protein content that their high calorie-to-protein ratio allows concentration of the formula to achieve a higher calorie intake without exceeding the threshold for protein tolerance. Once the child is older than 1 year, an intact protein-based 1 kcal/mL formula (Pediasure [Abbott Laboratories, Abbott Park, IL], Kindercal [Mead Johnson, Evansville, IN]), a protein-hydrolysate formula (Peptamen Jr [Nestlé, Glendale, CA]), or an amino acid-based formula (Neocate 1+ [Nutricia North America, Gaithersburg, MD], Elecare [Abbott Laboratories], Vivonex Pediatric [Nestlé]) should be substituted for standard infant formula.

Table 45.2
Protein Load in Relation to Energy Provided in Selected Formulas

Formula	Protein g/dL (% kcal)	kcal/mL	kcal/g of Protein	kcal/kg at 3.5 g of Protein/kg	Protein g/kg at: 140 kcal/kg per Day	150 kcal/kg per Day
Human milk	0.9 (5)	0.69	77	268	1.83	1.96
Enfamil*/Similac†	1.4 (8)	0.67	48	167	2.9	3.1
PediaSure†	3 (12)	1	33	116	4.25	4.5
Portagen*	2.4 (14)	0.67	28	98	5	5.36
Nutramigen*	1.9 (11)	0.67	35	123	4	4.25
Pregestimil*	1.9 (11)	0.67	35	123	4	4.25
Neocate‡	2 (12)	0.69	35	121	4	4.3
Vivonex Pediatric§	2.4 (12)	0.8	33	117	4.2	4.3

* Mead Johnson, Evansville, IN.

† Abbott Laboratories, Abbott Park, IL.

‡ Nutricia North America, Gaithersburg, MD.

§ Nestlé, Glendale, CA.

Protein-losing enteropathy is diagnosed by hypoalbuminemia, lack of proteinuria, and positive fecal alpha$_1$-antitrypsin assay. Typically, protein-losing enteropathy is encountered in patients with Fontan anatomy or constrictive pericarditis. Additional protein is probably necessary, and the fat provided may be limited to predominantly medium-chain triglycerides (MCTs), transported via portal circulation, to reduce mesenteric lymphatic flow and pressures contributing to the protein loss. A similar rationale leads to the use of MCTs in patients with chylothorax or chylous ascites. Formulas with a predominant fat source of MCTs are Portagen (Mead Johnson), a lactose-free protein hydrolysate formula with 85% of its fat as MCT oil, Vivonex Pediatric (68% of fat as MCT oil), Peptamen Jr (60% of fat as MCT oil), Pregestimil (Mead Johnson [55% of fat as MCT oil]), and Alimentum (Abbott Laboratories [50% of fat as MCT oil]). The older child may be given Lipo-Sorb (Symmetry Corp, Milpitas, CA [85% of fat as MCT oil]), similar in content to Portagen. Human milk will be unable to supply these protein needs without supplementation and is very high in long-chain triglycerides, which require assimilation via the lymphatic system.

Electrolytes, Minerals, and Micronutrients

Disturbances in electrolyte and mineral homeostasis accompany diuretic therapy or refeeding. Hypokalemia or hypocalcemia may cause changes in myocardial conduction and contractility. Diuretic therapy is irrational if sodium intake is not controlled. Potassium and chloride depletion commonly occur and may require supplementation. Calcium, magnesium, and zinc may also be depleted. Calciuria may be diminished by using chlorothiazide instead of furosemide. Calcium absorption from the gut is limited in magnesium deficiency (magnesium-dependent adenosine triphosphatase). Potassium may be spared by addition of spironolactone in selected cases.

Zinc depletion may manifest as a low alkaline phosphatase activity and cholesterol concentration (zinc-dependent enzymatic products). Iron needs are increased in cyanotic heart disease to maintain the increased erythroid mass demanded by hypoxemia. Anemia contributes to tissue hypoxia in patients with ventricular pressure overload, volume overload, CHF, or hypoxemia/cyanosis. In aortic valve stenosis, anemia may contribute to subendocardial ischemia, causing angina or arrhythmia. In patients with a large VSD, anemia causes decreased blood viscosity and pulmonary vascular resistance that allows increased left-to-right shunting and increased CHF and pulmonary blood flow.[43] Selenium and carnitine deficiency may occur in unsupplemented parenteral nutrition and may manifest as cardiomyopathy.

Thiamine (vitamin B_1) deficiency may present as the syndrome of wet beriberi with varying severity of CHF as a result of impaired myocardial function and impaired autonomic regulation of circulation. Clinical manifestations include edema, fatigue, dyspnea, and tachycardia with signs of CHF.

Shoshin is a severe form of beriberi that may affect infants with pulmonary edema and CHF. Thiamine depletion may occur in settings of high carbohydrate intake without thiamine, as in a nursing mother on an inadequate diet or consuming alcohol, and settings of prolonged parenteral nutrition or glucose administration without a multivitamin supplement. Thiamine requirements are increased with the stress of surgery and critical illness, and losses of thiamine increase with loop diuretics such as furosemide, putting patients with CHD at risk of deficiency. Shamir et al[44] identified thiamine deficiency in 4 of 22 children with CHD before surgery, 3 of whom had adequate thiamine intakes, and 6 of 22 after surgery. However, no relationship to the level of undernutrition, thiamine intake, or furosemide use could be proven. Vitamin K-containing foods, such as green, leafy vegetables, may interfere with the effectiveness of warfarin sodium.

Fluids

Many patients, especially those with CHF, are restricted in fluid intake with or without diuretic treatment. Providing adequate calories while restricting fluids is challenging and requires a concentrated formula, often requiring continuous administration via nasogastric or transpyloric tube.

Feeding Strategies

Oral or enteral feedings are preferred. There need be no restriction in volume of formula in infants with CHF or cyanosis if they feed voluntarily. Many patients with CHD have limited oral voluntary intake insufficient to supply nutrient requirements to maintain growth. The increased cardiopulmonary demands of eating or associated problems such as gastrointestinal dysmotility, preterm birth, and airway or pulmonary disease may prevent adequate intake. Volume may also be restricted, especially in patients with lesions associated with CHF or pulmonary hypertension requiring diuretic therapy and fluid and sodium restriction. Reparative or palliative surgery may be safer if performed after achieving a target weight. Formula concentration is frequently increased to provide more energy and protein in a restricted volume. If volume is the limiting factor, a more concentrated formula will be necessary to provide up to 3.5 g/kg per day of protein, above which additional calories may be added with carbohydrates (polycose powder or liquid) or fats (microlipid). Medium-chain triglycerides may contribute to diarrhea and cramping but are valuable as the principal fat source in patients with chylothorax. Concentrating a formula leads to increased protein and solute load, osmolarity, or tonicity and decreased free water. A recent study of postoperative infants showed that advancement to a high concentration formula within 2 days rather than 5 days to a lower concentration safely improved energy intake and weight gain and decreased length of stay.[45]

Supplemental enteral nutrition is frequently instituted to achieve nutritional goals via nasogastric or gastrostomy tube. Some studies have concluded that only 24-hour continuous enteral feeding by nasogastric tube of a concentrated or augmented formula is able to provide the minimum of 140 kcal/kg per day necessary to improve nutritional status.[16] Consequences of coercive oral feeding efforts or nasopharyngeal tube placement and feeding include a high incidence of oral aversion, which may prove quite refractory long after the cardiac issues have improved. Patients who are considered likely to require chronic nasogastric tube feedings for longer than 6 months should be considered early for gastrostomy tube placement. Given the possibility that gastrostomy tube placement may alter motility and increase gastroesophageal reflux, evidence of airway penetration; impaired airway protective reflexes, such as absent gag or cough; or lower respiratory tract disease may mandate protective antireflux surgery (Nissen fundoplication or variants). If airway protective reflexes are intact (eg, no vocal cord recurrent laryngeal nerve palsy) and there is no evidence of respiratory compromise, such as reactive airway disease, laryngospasm/stridor, or aspiration pneumonia, then percutaneous gastrostomy tube placement without antireflux surgery is a safe and effective option.[46] The anatomy of the upper gastrointestinal tract should be evaluated by contrast studies to exclude associated anomalies of tracheoesophageal fistula; vascular ring; gross airway penetration, directly or with reflux; and intestinal rotational anomalies. For patients with aspiration risks who are not considered safe candidates for antireflux fundoplication surgery, transpyloric feeding with a nasojejunal or percutaneous gastrojejunal tube is an alternative. Although transpyloric duodenal or jejunal tube feeding may prevent formula entry into the stomach, gastroduodenal motility may be inhibited and duodenogastric reflux of bile or gastroesophageal reflux of acid and/or bile may still occur.

The breastfed infant may require manual or pump expression of the milk if there are fatigue or problems suckling because of inability to latch on, excessive respiratory effort, and/or tachypnea competing with sucking and swallowing. Tube feeding either fortified human milk or a formula with high caloric density continuously to augment a marginal nursing intake will be required for sufficient calories.

Parenteral nutrition is reserved for patients who cannot be fed effectively or safely by the enteral routes described previously. Examples would be patients with associated gastrointestinal tract disease, such as necrotizing enterocolitis, or those at risk of aspiration because of tachypnea and gastroesophageal reflux. Because cardiac output is determined by the demands of peripheral tissue metabolism, advancement of feedings, whether parenteral or enteral, in the patient accommodated to chronic malnutrition should be gradual and monitored for refeeding complications. Peripheral capillary vasodilation in response to tissue anabolism can lead to high-output cardiac failure; excessive volume administration can provoke CHF and anasarca. Glucose uptake and metabolism will cause intracellular influx of potassium, magnesium, calcium, and most dramatically, phosphate. Dysrhythmias, particularly atrial arrhythmias related to changes in venous return, and ventricular arrhythmias related to conduction disturbances may be associated with electrolyte fluxes (hypokalemia, hypocalcemia, hypophosphatemia) and can manifest in changes in the corrected QT interval on electrocardiography. Other cardiac complications of nutritional support include volume overload, increased viscosity and pulmonary artery pressures with high lipid infusions (exceeding 0.15 g/kg per hour or 3.5 g/kg per day), increased tissue metabolic demand for cardiac output, arrhythmias, and endocarditis/sepsis related to the central venous catheter.

Monitoring Outcome

Precise weights and lengths (or standing heights for patients older than 3 years) should be obtained at each encounter and plotted on the appropriate growth curve (eg, specific curve for children with Down syndrome, infants 0–36 months of age [length], or children 2–18 years of age [heights]). The same dietitian should obtain measurements of mid-arm circumference and triceps skinfold thickness to help assess muscle and fat stores, understanding that fluid status and edema may affect the measures. Review of the diet is important. The current formula and methods for mixing and adding supplements should be reviewed to eliminate errors in formulation. The family should be instructed to bring a 3- or 5-day diet record to the clinic visit for evaluation by the dietitian for nutrient analysis. Attention should be paid to total caloric intake, proportion of fat and carbohydrate intake, protein intake, and adequacy of micronutrients, including iron, zinc, and vitamins. Fluid volume intake, urinary frequency, and hydration status in the context of diuretic therapy should be assessed. More sophisticated measures of body composition, including bone mineral status, may be obtained in certain groups or research settings, if technology such as dual-energy x-ray absorptiometry or bioelectrical impedance analysis is available. Indirect calorimetry can assess REE and respiratory quotient to assess energy requirements and avoid overfeeding in patients in the intensive care unit. In the absence of direct measures of lean body mass or energy requirements, the surrogate parameter of weight expected for length or age or ideal body weight for length can be helpful in estimating energy and protein requirements for the very lean or obese child (see Table 45.1). However, serial measurement of changes in weight, length, and anthropometry are the best indicators of nutrient adequacy.

References

1. Levy RJ, Rosenthal A, Castaneda AR, Nadas AS. Growth after surgical repair of simple D-transposition of the great arteries. *Ann Thorac Surg.* 1978;25:225–230
2. Levy RJ, Rosenthal A, Fyler DC, Nadas AS. Birthweight of infants with congenital heart disease. *Am J Dis Child.* 1978;132:249–254
3. Rosenthal GL, Wilson PD, Permutt T, Boughman JA, Ferencz C. Birth weight and cardiovascular malformations: a population-based study. The Baltimore-Washington Infant Study. *Am J Epidemiol.* 1991;133:1273–1281
4. Cameron JW, Rosenthal A, Olson AD. Malnutrition in hospitalized children with congenital heart disease. *Arch Pediatr Adolesc Med.* 1995;149:1098–1102
5. Leitch CA. Growth, nutrition and energy expenditure in pediatric heart failure. *Progr Pediatr Cardiol.* 2000;11:195–202
6. Schuurmans FM, Pulles-Heintzberger CF, Gerver WJ, Kester AD, Forget PP. Long-term growth of children with congenital heart disease: a retrospective study. *Acta Paediatr.* 1998;87:1250–1255
7. Barton JS, Hindmarsh PC, Scrimgeour CM, Rennie MJ, Preece MA. Energy expenditure in congenital heart disease. *Arch Dis Child.* 1994;70:5–9
8. Leitch CA, Karn CA, Peppard RJ, et al. Increased energy expenditure in infants with cyanotic congenital heart disease. *J Pediatr.* 1998;133:755–760
9. Mitchell IM, Davies PS, Day JM, Pollock JC, Jamieson MP. Energy expenditure in children with congenital heart disease, before and after cardiac surgery. *J Thorac Cardiovasc Surg.* 1994;107:374–380
10. Huse DM, Feldt RH, Nelson RA, Novak LP. Infants with congenital heart disease. Food intake, body weight, and energy metabolism. *Am J Dis Child.* 1975;129:65–69
11. Menon G, Poskitt EM. Why does congenital heart disease cause failure to thrive? *Arch Dis Child.* 1985;60:1134–1139
12. Rosenthal A. Congenital cardiac anomalies and gastrointestinal malformations. In: Pierpont MEM, Moller JH, eds. *Genetics of Cardiovascular Disease.* Boston, MA: Martinus Nijhoff; 1987:113–126
13. Sondheimer JM, Hamilton JR. Intestinal function in infants with severe congenital heart disease. *J Pediatr.* 1978;92:572–578

14. Vaisman N, Leigh T, Voet H, Westerterp K, Abraham M, Duchan R. Malabsorption in infants with congenital heart disease under diuretic treatment. *Pediatr Res.* 1994;36:545–549

15. Yahav J, Avigad S, Frand M, et al. Assessment of intestinal and cardiorespiratory function in children with congenital heart disease on high-caloric formulas. *J Pediatr Gastroenterol Nutr.* 1985;4:778–785

16. Schwarz SM, Gewitz MH, See CC, et al. Enteral nutrition in infants with congenital heart disease and growth failure. *Pediatrics.* 1990;86:368–373

17. Unger R, DeKleermaeker M, Gidding SS, Christoffel KK. Calories count. Improved weight gain with dietary intervention in congenital heart disease. *Am J Dis Child.* 1992;146:1078–1084

18. Salzer HR, Haschke F, Wimmer M, Heil M, Schilling R. Growth and nutritional intake of infants with congenital heart disease. *Pediatr Cardiol.* 1989;10:17–23

19. Cavell B. Gastric emptying in infants with congenital heart disease. *Acta Paediatr Scand.* 1981;70:517–520

20. Forchielli ML, McColl R, Walker WA, Lo C. Children with congenital heart disease: a nutrition challenge. *Nutr Rev.* 1994;52:348–353

21. Sole MJ, Jeejeebhoy KN. Conditioned nutritional requirements and the pathogenesis and treatment of myocardial failure. *Curr Opin Clin Nutr Metab Care.* 2000;3:417–424

22. Carr JG, Stevenson LW, Walden JA, Heber D. Prevalence and hemodynamic correlates of malnutrition in severe congestive heart failure secondary to ischemic or idiopathic dilated cardiomyopathy. *Am J Cardiol.* 1989;63:709–713

23. Freeman LM, Roubenoff R. The nutrition implications of cardiac cachexia. *Nutr Rev.* 1994;52:340–347

24. Feldman AM, Combes A, Wagner D, et al. The role of tumor necrosis factor in the pathophysiology of heart failure. *J Am Coll Cardiol.* 2000;35:537–544

25. Krauss AN, Auld PA. Metabolic rate of neonates with congenital heart disease. *Arch Dis Child.* 1975;50:539–541

26. Stocker FP, Wilkoff W, Miettinen OS, Nadas AS. Oxygen consumption in infants with heart disease. Relationship to severity of congestive failure, relative weight, and caloric intake. *J Pediatr.* 1972;80:43–51

27. Weintraub RG, Menahem S. Growth and congenital heart disease. *J Paediatr Child Health.* 1993;29:95–98

28. Gervasio MR, Buchanan CN. Malnutrition in the pediatric cardiology patient. *CCQ.* 1985;8:49–56

29. Varan B, Tokel K, Yilmaz G. Malnutrition and growth failure in cyanotic and acyanotic congenital heart disease with and without pulmonary hypertension. *Arch Dis Child.* 1999;81:49–52

30. Leitch CA, Karn CA, Ensing GJ, Denne SC. Energy expenditure after surgical repair in children with cyanotic congenital heart disease. *J Pediatr.* 2000;137:381–385

31. Ackerman IL, Karn CA, Denne SC, Ensing GJ, Leitch CA. Total but not resting energy expenditure is increased in infants with ventricular septal defects. *Pediatrics.* 1998;102:1172–1177

32. Levy RJ, Rosenthal A, Miettinen OS, Nadas AS. Determinants of growth in patients with ventricular septal defect. *Circulation.* 1978;57:793–797

33. Renlund DG, Taylor DO, Kfoury AG, Shaddy RS. New UNOS rules: historical background and implications for transplantation management. United Network for Organ Sharing. *J Heart Lung Transplant.* 1999;18:1065–1070

34. Sholler GF, Celermajer JM. Cardiac surgery in the first year of life: the effect on weight gains of infants with congenital heart disease. *Aust Paediatr J.* 1986;22:305–308

35. Stenbog EV, Hjortdal VE, Ravn HB, Skjaerbaek C, Sorensen KE, Hansen OK. Improvement in growth, and levels of insulin-like growth factor-I in the serum, after cavopulmonary connections. *Cardiol Young.* 2000;10:440–446

36. Cohen MI, Bush DM, Ferry RJ Jr, et al. Somatic growth failure after the Fontan operation. *Cardiol Young.* 2000;10:447–457

37. Baum D, Beck RQ, Haskell WL. Growth and tissue abnormalities in young people with cyanotic congenital heart disease receiving systemic-pulmonary artery shunts. *Am J Cardiol.* 1983;52:349–352

38. Payne PR, Waterlow JC. Relative energy requirements for maintenance, growth, and physical activity. *Lancet.* 1971;2:210–211

39. Jackson M, Poskitt EM. The effects of high-energy feeding on energy balance and growth in infants with congenital heart disease and failure to thrive. *Br J Nutr.* 1991;65:131–143

40. Bougle D, Iselin M, Kahyat A, Duhamel JF. Nutritional treatment of congenital heart disease. *Arch Dis Child.* 1986;61:799–801

41. Vanderhoof JA, Hofschire PJ, Baluff MA, et al. Continuous enteral feedings. An important adjunct to the management of complex congenital heart disease. *Am J Dis Child.* 1982;136:825–7

42. Fomon SJ, Ziegler EE. Nutritional management of infants with congenital heart disease. *Am Heart J.* 1972;83:581–588

43. Lister G, Hellenbrand WE, Kleinman CS, Talner NS. Physiologic effects of increasing hemoglobin concentration in left-to- right shunting in infants with ventricular septal defects. *N Engl J Med.* 1982;306:502–506

44. Shamir R, Dagan O, Abramovitch D, Abramovitch T, Vidne BA, Dinari G. Thiamine deficiency in children with congenital heart disease before and after corrective surgery. *JPEN J Parenter Enteral Nutr.* 2000;24:154–158

45. Pillo-Blocka F, Adatia I, Sharieff W, McCrindle BW, Zlotkin S. Rapid advancement to more concentrated formula in infants after surgery for congenital heart disease reduces duration of hospital stay: a randomized clinical trial. *J Pediatr.* 2004;145:761–766

46. Ciotti G, Holzer R, Pozzi M, Dalzell M. Nutritional support via percutaneous endoscopic gastrostomy in children with cardiac disease experiencing difficulties with feeding. *Cardiol Young.* 2002;12:537–541

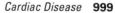

Nutrition in Cystic Fibrosis

Cystic fibrosis (CF) is an autosomal-recessive disease affecting multiple organ systems, including the airways, exocrine pancreas, intestine, and hepatobiliary system, as well as the genital tract in males. There is considerable heterogeneity of disease phenotype. It is caused by mutations in the CF conductance regulator gene (CFTR), which encodes a cyclic adenosine monophosphate-activated chloride channel localized on the apical surface of epithelial cells. Since the CF gene was cloned in 1989, more than 1300 different CFTR gene mutations have been identified. At least some of the variability of the CF phenotype can be explained by genotype, but it is now recognized that there are other genetic modifiers of disease affecting several organs, including the lungs, intestinal tract, and liver.[1] The strongest relation between the genotype and the phenotype is observed in the exocrine pancreas.[2,3] Most patients with CF conventionally diagnosed have evidence of pancreatic insufficiency (PI). Most patients with the PI phenotype present with signs and symptoms of maldigestion and/or failure to thrive at an early age. A subset of patients have evidence of pancreatic dysfunction but retain sufficient residual pancreatic function to permit normal digestion without the need for exogenous pancreatic enzyme supplements with meals.[4] The term pancreatic sufficiency (PS) is used to describe patients with this phenotype, who tend to have a milder form of CF disease. Analysis of large patient cohorts have revealed that different mutations in the CFTR gene confer either the PI or the PS phenotypes.[3] Specifically, the PI phenotype is associated with 2 mutations that are classified as "severe," whereas a single "mild" mutation, which appears to be dominant over the "severe" allele, confers the PS phenotype. From a nutritional perspective, patients with the PI phenotype are at greatest risk of developing malnutrition and/or growth failure.

V

Diagnosis

In some states and in certain countries throughout the world, the diagnosis of CF is established by newborn screening using measurement of the immunoreactive trypsinogen concentration with or without complementary CF genotyping in dried blood spots. Many patients are asymptomatic at diagnosis and may remain pancreatic sufficient for a period of time.[5] However, a surprisingly large number of patients with pancreatic insufficiency have evidence of malnutrition at approximately 7 weeks of age, when the diagnosis is usually confirmed after screening.[6] If newborn screening is not performed, the diagnosis of CF is established by characteristic signs and symptoms or, in some cases, on the basis of the knowledge of an affected first-degree relative. Common presenting signs and symptoms of CF, which can occur alone or in combination, include:

- Meconium ileus at birth (can be diagnosed in utero)
- Failure to thrive
- Severe malnutrition with anemia, hypoalbuminemia, and edema
- Greasy, foul smelling, and bulky stools
- Pulmonary disease (recurrent pneumonia, persistent cough, or wheezing)
- Excessive appetite with increased energy intake
- Poor appetite with decreased energy intake
- Hyponatremia attributable to excessive salt loss from sweating (especially hot climates)
- Salty taste (parents often describe a salty taste when kissing their infants)

In most cases, the diagnosis of CF is confirmed by characteristic clinical features of the disease plus an elevated sweat chloride concentration (>60 mmol/L), which should be performed on 2 occasions in a medical center with significant experience in the diagnosis of CF. In the United States, these centers should be certified by the Cystic Fibrosis Foundation. Other clinical evaluations of the patient are helpful in establishing the diagnosis and/or to perform a baseline assessment. These include:

- Analysis of CF genotypes
- Chest radiography
- Pulmonary function tests and sputum analysis (if older than 5–7 years)
- Liver function tests
- Serum albumin and protein concentrations
- Complete blood cell count, prothrombin time
- Serum vitamin A, vitamin E, and 25-hydroxyvitamin D (25-OH-D) concentrations

- 72-hour fecal fat balance study or alternative tests of pancreatic function, such as fecal chymotrypsin, fecal elastase-1, and serum trypsinogen

- Height, weight, weight as a percentage of ideal body weight (IBW) for height for children younger than 2 years, body mass index (BMI) percentile for children and adolescents 2 to 18 years of age and BMI for adults older than 18 years, skinfold measurements

Assessment of Pancreatic Function Status

Exocrine pancreatic function should be assessed in the following situations: (1) at diagnosis (before enzyme therapy is initiated) to provide objective evaluation of pancreatic status and to determine the severity of nutrient maldigestion; (2) to monitor patients with PS for evidence of developing fat maldigestion attributable to PI, particularly when frequent bulky bowel movements or unexplained weight loss occur; and (3) before and after changes in enzyme therapy and/or initiation of adjunctive treatment to provide objective evidence of a response to treatment. At diagnosis, a 72-hour fecal fat balance study provides the most information about nutrient absorption.[7] It can be completed at home or in hospital. If stools are to be collected at home, the family should be given a dietary scale and equipment for collecting the bowel movements, including a stool collection can. Details of the test should be carefully explained to the patient and/or family and clear written instructions should be provided. Food should be weighed and recorded so that fat intake can be accurately calculated. If food or the formula contains medium-chain triglycerides, the stool must be analyzed by a specialized method.[8] For infants younger than 6 months, fat losses exceeding 15% of fat intake are indicative of PI. In patients older than 6 months, fat losses exceeding 7% of intake are considered to be abnormal.[9]

Seventy-two hour fecal fat studies cannot be performed accurately in the infant who is being breastfed, because the nutrient content and volume of human milk cannot be determined accurately. The fat content of human milk, in particular, varies considerably. In these circumstances, health care professionals should encourage the mother to breastfeed and rely on other clinical and laboratory evidence of PI before initiating enzyme therapy. The vast majority of patients who present with meconium ileus will have PI. In addition, young infants with severe failure to thrive, with or without hypoalbuminemia and edema, are likely to have PI. The presence of hypovitaminosis A and/or E,[10,11] microscopic evidence of fat droplets in stool, and

V

low fecal elastase-1 concentrations[12,13] are strongly suggestive of PI. In these circumstances, a 72-hour fecal fat balance study may still be recommended but should be deferred until breastfeeding has been discontinued.

Fecal elastase-1 is a specific test of pancreatic function. A small sample of formed stool (approx 20 g) is required. Fecal elastase-1 is measured by an enzyme-linked immunosorbent assay.[14] Because the test measures only human pancreatic elastase, oral pancreatic enzymes of other origin will not affect the test results. Values <100 μg/g of stool are highly suggestive of PI.[13] It should be noted that a watery stool, as in cases of watery diarrhea or stool from an ileostomy, may give a false-negative result because of dilution of the fecal effluent. In such circumstances, it would be advised to wait until the diarrhea resolves or calculate 72-hour losses of fecal elastase-1 adjusted for fecal output.[13]

Nutritional Care

Goals

The goal of nutritional care in patients with CF is to achieve normal growth and nutritional status.[15] In addition, for those with PI, the aim of enzyme therapy is to optimize macronutrient absorption (see "Enzyme Therapy")[16] and to maintain normal micronutrient concentrations, such as serum fat-soluble vitamin concentrations (see "Vitamin Therapy"). A high-energy, nutritionally balanced diet is encouraged with liberal use of fat to provide additional calories. In patients with impaired glucose tolerance, careful monitoring by the CF and endocrine teams is recommended.[17] In patients with type 1 diabetes mellitus, careful control of blood sugars with appropriate insulin therapy must be balanced with the need to maintain energy balance through regular meals and snacks.[17–19]

Assessment and Monitoring

A complete nutritional assessment includes a diet history and relevant laboratory and clinical data. Height and weight measurements, appropriate mid-arm circumference parameters, and assessment of pubertal development in the adolescent are used to assist in the determination of nutritional status.

Nutritional monitoring is considered to be a routine part of every clinic visit, which in most CF centers, occurs every 3 to 4 months. Routine assessment should include measurement of height and weight and mid-arm circumference. Written dietary records may be obtained along with documentation of enzyme intake if growth or weight gain is a concern. Attention should be given to determine compliance with enzyme therapy.

Seventy-two hour fecal fat collections should be arranged if indicated, particularly if there is poor growth or weight gain. If the patient exhibits evidence of severe steatorrhea, adjustments should be made to enzymes, or adjuvants may be used (see "Enzyme Therapy"). Recent studies reveal that subjective abdominal symptoms or frequency of bowel movements are not correlated with the severity of fat absorption, so objective evaluation is encouraged to evaluate the response to enzyme therapy.[20,21] Laboratory indices of nutritional status should be obtained at least once each year or more frequently if there is a concern. This should include concentrations of vitamin A, vitamin E, and 25-OH-D; albumin concentration; liver function tests; complete blood cell count; and prothrombin time.

Nutritional Requirements

For most patients with CF, energy requirements only moderately exceed the Recommended Dietary Allowance (RDA).[22] If a patient is healthy and has minimal pulmonary disease, energy requirements hardly ever exceed 5% to 10% of the RDA. In patients with severe lung disease (ie, 1-second forced expiratory volume <40%) or in those who have severe maldigestion or malabsorption, energy requirements may be significantly increased, ranging from 20% to 50% or more of the RDA.[23] However, some patients, particularly those with advanced lung disease, may reduce energy expenditure by decreasing physical activity. To calculate energy needs, the following formulae are used (modified from CF consensus report[24]).

Younger than 1 year:

$$\frac{\text{RDA} \times 1.25^* \times \text{IBW (kg)}}{\text{Actual weight (kg)}} = \text{kcal/kg per day}$$

Older than 1 year:

$$\text{Basal metabolic rate [using actual weight]} \times (1.5\text{--}1.7 \text{ [activity factor]}) \times \frac{0.93}{0.85} = \text{kcal/day}$$

- Add 200–400 kcal/day to achieve weight gain if <90%–95% IBW or if BMI is <19

- Use actual fraction of absorption if available from 72-hour fat balance studies (ie, replace 0.85 with known value)

___

* After diagnosis, infants may require 125% of the RDA to achieve catch-up weight gain

Vitamins

Supplemental fat-soluble vitamins (A, D, E, and K) are usually required to counter malabsorption of these micronutrients in patients with PI.[10] In most patients, daily requirements for vitamins A and D are approximately 1 to 2 times the Dietary Reference Intakes (DRIs), and for vitamin E are estimated to be approximately 5 to 20 times the DRI.[25,26] Recent evidence suggests that vitamin D requirements may be higher than the current recommendation. In fact, some patients show a poor serum 25-OH-D response to very high oral doses of vitamin D.[27] The precise requirement for vitamin K has not been established, and patients with CF exhibit abnormal biochemical concentrations of protein in vitamin K absence-2 when no supplements are given,[28] and small supplemental doses of vitamin K fail to correct values in most patients. Because vitamin K is also associated osteocalcin function, its potential in maintaining bone mineral density should be considered.[29] For patients with clinically significant liver disease with evidence of portal hypertension attributable to multilobular cirrhosis, additional fat-soluble vitamins may be required. In particular, supplemental vitamin K (5 mg/day) is recommended, particularly in a patient with laboratory evidence of vitamin K deficiency (see also Chapter 19).

Salt

Patients with CF, particularly young infants, are at risk of developing hyponatremia if sweat losses are excessive. The risk is greatest in patients exposed to hot environments or to those who are overdressed or in overheated rooms in cooler temperatures (ie, infants). To prevent hyponatremia, a liquid mineral mix (1 mL = 1.6 mmol of sodium, 1.6 mmol of potassium, 2 mmol of chloride, and 0.84 mmol of phosphate) can be offered to infants receiving only human milk or formula. A mineral mix solution weight can be added to the patient's food or formula (1 mL/100 mL of formula [based on 150–180 mL of formula/kg of body weight] or 1.5 mL/kg per day for breastfed infant, divided into 6–8 doses/day) to provide approximately 3.5 to 4.5 mmol of sodium/kg of body weight. The dose may require adjustment depending on individual salt losses. Electrolyte status in infants should be monitored or assessed if there is any suspicion of electrolyte imbalance, for example in an infant with excessive sweating. This can be done noninvasively by testing urine or serum electrolyte concentrations. Signs of electrolyte depletion include unexplained lethargy and poor feeding. In children younger than 1 year, addition of 1/8 tsp (12 mmol of sodium) of table salt twice a day or a saline solution containing the equivalent amount of salt in 5 mL of water (made by a pharmacist) may be advised. Salt tablets are usually unnecessary for older children. Sports drinks that contain significant quantities of electrolytes are recommended for older individuals who are undertaking strenuous exercise or individuals who are living in or visiting hot climates.

Patient and Parent Education

Education of patients and their caregivers is a vital and routine component of the multidisciplinary care of patients with CF. A solid grounding in the special nutritional needs of a patient with CF should be established at diagnosis. This should include an explanation of the role of the pancreas and how enzyme replacement therapy helps to correct maldigestion. Parents should be given specific instructions on how to provide an appetizing, high-energy, nutritionally balanced diet, particularly with a liberal use of fat to provide extra calories. It is important to communicate the expectation that most children with CF are able to grow and gain weight normally. Patients and their parents require education about the importance of fat-soluble vitamins. Details on when to administer enzymes and vitamins must be reviewed on several occasions. In older children, concerns about compliance should be emphasized at diagnosis and assessed at each follow-up visit.

Specific Guidelines

Infants

Breastfeeding is encouraged, although some patients may require fortification with formula or a concentrated formula as a supplement. Milk-based formulas are recommended as an alternative to breastfeeding. There is no evidence that hydrolyzed or medium-chain triglyceride-containing formulas offer any nutritional advantage to the patient with CF.[30] If a young infant with CF is not thriving or is failing to exhibit catch-up growth, strategies should include supplementing breastfeeding with formula (by bottle or with the use of a lactation aid) or increasing the strength of formula to at least 3300 kJ/L (24 kcal/oz) to ensure adequate energy intake.

When solids are introduced into the diet, extra energy can be provided by adding 2.5 to 5 mL (1/2–1 tsp) of butter, margarine, or oil to each 128-mL (4-oz) jar of meat or vegetables. Commercially prepared infant foods contain very little salt, and additional table salt (1/8 tsp or approx 12 mmol of sodium) should be added twice daily to solids.

Children Older Than 1 Year

Most children with CF take in similar amounts of energy and nutrients as do children without CF.[31] Therefore, strategies to provide a high-energy diet are required for children with CF who are undernourished. In addition to 3 regular meals, 3 daily snacks are recommended. Adding butter or margarine to food will increase total energy intake. Milkshake supplements may be offered if required. Homemade milkshakes are less expensive than commercially prepared ones. Commercial dietary supplements are not proven to be of benefit to the nutritional status of patients with CF.[32] Nevertheless, these expensive sources of energy are often used in CF centers, despite lack of evidence to support their use. Nutritional supplements may actually substitute for normal dietary energy intake rather than as a supplement to increase total energy intake. Strategies to improve nutritional intake through enriching the energy content of regular meals and snacks should be entertained before costly supplements are introduced.

Aggressive Nutritional Support

Provided lung function is not severely compromised or impaired, most patients will grow normally in childhood and remain well nourished during adulthood. Pulmonary exacerbations may cause acute weight loss, but following appropriate therapy, healthy patients will regain weight quite rapidly. Unfortunately, a subset of individuals, especially those with advanced lung disease, will be unable to maintain energy balance.[33] In such cases, more aggressive approaches to nutritional therapy may be indicated, because patients are incapable of increasing energy intake voluntarily.

Supplemental nutritional support via gastrostomy or jejunostomy tube is indicated in patients who exhibit poor weight gain over a period of 6 months to 1 year or show persistent malnutrition (weight as a percentage of IBW for height of <85% or BMI <18).[34,35] Patients with end-stage lung disease who are listed for lung transplantation frequently experience reduced energy intake and decline in weight. In these circumstances, early and careful use of supplemental tube feedings may help to maintain energy balance.

Feeds are usually run overnight by continuous pump infusion. The energy needs and rate of infusion are determined on an individual basis. Patients are encouraged to eat normal meals during the day. However, voluntary intake, particularly at breakfast time, may be decreased. The choice of feed depends on individual tolerance and cost. Most patients can tolerate a complete formula (1.0–2.0 kcal/mL),[36] provided adequate enzyme therapy is prescribed (1000–2000 U of lipase/g of fat) and adjusted according to individual needs. Enzymes should be taken at intervals—at the beginning of the infusion, at bedtime, and at the end of the tube feeding. In patients who experience cramping or diarrhea, lowering the concentration of the formula may help to alleviate symptoms. Predigested feeds are more expensive than regular complete formulas, but those with a low fat content can be given without the use of supplemental enzymes and may be better tolerated by some patients. Lower carbohydrate-containing formulas may be chosen for individuals with CF-related diabetes mellitus. Occasionally, initiation of tube feedings will expose clinical or biochemical manifestations of CF-related diabetes mellitus, especially in older patients with PI. To anticipate this problem, an oral glucose tolerance test should be considered before placing the gastrostomy tube. To determine supplemental energy requirements from tube feeding, total energy requirements, normal dietary intake, nutritional status, and the degree of malabsorption must be considered. Initially higher supplemental energy requirements may be required to achieve catch-up growth and/or nutritional rehabilitation. Once patients achieve catch-up-growth, maintenance needs may be lower. In most patients, delivery of approximately one third of total energy needs by tube feeding will achieve improvement of nutritional status. However, the amount will vary considerably according to various factors, including individual energy needs, severity of malnutrition, degree of malabsorption, and the patient's ability to ingest calories voluntarily. In our experience, very few patients are able to discontinue enteral tube feeding completely. However, once nutritional status is improved, it may be possible to decrease the amount of energy provided by enteral tube feeding, either by decreasing the total volume of feeds per night or by decreasing the number of nights per week that the feeds are given.

Total parenteral nutrition is rarely indicated in patients with CF. Total parenteral nutrition may be important to nourish neonates immediately after surgery for meconium ileus. In addition, short-term total parenteral nutrition may be required if oral intake is inadequate because of vomiting or severe respiratory distress, especially if symptoms are accompanied by acute weight loss.

Commonly Encountered Nutritional Problems

Feeding Difficulties or Poor Growth in Infancy

When the diagnosis of CF is established in infancy, the patient may be severely malnourished. In these circumstances, it may take more than a year to achieve full catch-up growth. Young infants have high energy requirements and frequently have severe malabsorption, which may require several adjustments to enzyme therapy in the first year after diagnosis. If poor weight gain is observed or the patient is failing to exhibit catch-up growth, careful assessment of energy intake and/or malabsorption may be needed. Breastfed infants may require formula supplements, and those receiving formula may require additional energy by increasing the concentration of the formula. Gastroesophageal reflux is quite common in the infant with CF,[37] particularly in those with respiratory disease. Drugs to suppress gastric acid may be indicated if reflux is severe. A hydrolyzed formula offers no advantage and should be only considered in individuals who have had significant bowel resection after complicated meconium ileus.[30]

Malabsorption

A large number of patients with CF continue to have maldigestion despite adequate dosing with potent pancreatic enzymes.[38,39] Subjective symptoms, such as abdominal bloating or cramps or bulky stools, cannot reliably assess the severity of maldigestion.[21,40] Instead, objective assessment is advocated by a 72-hour fat collection (while eating a regular diet) and the prescribed dose of enzymes. If severe fat maldigestion is identified (fecal fat losses exceeding 20% of intake) and is clearly contributing to abdominal symptoms or malnutrition, the dose of enzymes could be increased up to the maximum recommended amount. Alternatively, inhibition of gastric acid secretion with a histamine antagonist or a proton-pump inhibitor may raise intestinal pH and improve the efficacy of enzyme therapy (see "Enzyme Therapy"). Several weeks after the adjustment to therapy has been made, the individual patient should be reassessed by a repeat 72-hour fecal fat collection.

Distal Intestinal Obstruction Syndrome and Constipation

Distal intestinal obstruction syndrome (DIOS) is unique to CF and is characterized by cramping abdominal pain, which may be periumbilical or in the right lower quadrant. A mass is usually palpable in the ileocecal area. Unlike simple constipation, the frequency and consistency of bowel motions are usually normal. It should be emphasized that simple constipation is a common problem in individuals with CF. Consequently, a careful history, abdominal examination, and abdominal radiography are indicated when abdominal pain attributable to DIOS is suspected to distinguish it from constipation and other CF-associated complications, such as intussusception and appendiceal abscess. Distal intestinal obstruction syndrome is treated by several different approaches. If DIOS is severe, a balanced electrolyte solution (used for cleansing the bowel before colonoscopy) is very effective in relieving the subacute obstruction. Complete bowel obstruction is an absolute contraindication to the use of these solutions. Volumes of 4 to 8 L, delivered at 1 L/hour, are usually required for a complete cleanout in children older than 10 years. In younger children, the electrolyte solution should be administered at a rate of 20 mL/kg per hour for 4 to 6 hours. In children older than 2 years, mineral oil given in doses of 2 to 4 tbsp by mouth before bedtime is often successful in preventing recurring episodes of DIOS. N-Acetylcysteine and, in severe cases, large-volume enemas with hyperosmolar contrast agents are also used. More recently, a polyethylene-glycol solution without electrolytes has been used by some health care professionals to help with the management of DIOS and/or constipation in CF. Anecdotal reports suggest that this solution, a powder mixed with any choice of beverage, at volumes of approximately 2 to 4 cups per day, depending on the patient's weight, is effective in children with CF. Its use, however, has only been confirmed in children without CF who have constipation and for those who require a bowel cleanout when preparing for colonoscopy.[41]

Insulin Dependent Diabetes

Adolescents and adults with CF and pancreatic insufficiency are at increased risk of developing CF-associated diabetes mellitus.[17,18] The prevalence of CF-related diabetes mellitus is reported to be between 5% and 15% in children younger than 18 years and up to 50% in adults with CF.[19,42] In many instances, patients exhibit no clear-cut signs and symptoms of diabetes mellitus. Furthermore, determination of hemoglobin A1C is not a reliable test for the diagnosis of CF-related diabetes mellitus. The diagnosis should be considered in any patient who is exhibiting weight loss or poor weight gain. Some CF centers are recommending annual screening for diabetes mellitus by a modified oral glucose tolerance test after the age of 10 years. In the patient who has CF-related diabetes mellitus, high-energy meals and snacks are encouraged, but energy needs and insulin requirements must be carefully balanced. Foods high in simple sugars may be limited according to insulin needs. Multidisciplinary care and the support of an endocrinologist is essential. In individuals who have impaired glucose tolerance, close monitoring by both the CF and endocrine teams are required, because these patients are at increased risk of developing CF-related diabetes mellitus.

Bone Health

Bone mineral density may be reduced in patients with CF.[43] Nutrition plays an important role in bone health. Well-nourished prepubertal children with CF can have normal bone mineral density.[44] However, poor bone mass gains during childhood and adolescence can contribute to poor bone mineral-ization in adults.[45] Ensuring good nutritional status along with adequate intake of calcium and vitamin D as well as physical activity are factors that may be related to bone health in CF.[44] It should be noted that an increase in childhood fractures has been reported in children without CF.[46] Causes may include a decrease in overall activity and decline in intake of calcium and vitamin D-containing foods, such as milk.[47,48] Other factors, such as increased fecal calcium loss, possibly attributable to increased intestinal permeability,[49] could potentially place patients with CF at a greater risk of decreased bone mineral density. Attention to serum vitamin D concentrations, bone mineral density, level of dietary calcium intake, and physical activity level in child-hood and adolescence may help protect patients from osteoporosis later in life. Use of steroids may also increase risk of reduced bone mineral density. Additional vitamin D and or calcium supplements may be required in patients receiving long-term steroid treatment.

Enzyme Therapy

Patients with CF who have PI are treated with pancreatic enzyme extracts of porcine origin. A large variety of enzyme products are available, including enteric-coated microspheres, enteric-coated tablets, and conventional powder enzymes.[38,39] All products contain the various enzymes synthesized by the pancreas, including amylase, proteases, and lipase. The actual activity of these enzymes and the ratio to one another varies considerably according to specific batches and the commercial manufacturer. Enzyme potency is based on the content of amylase, protease, and lipase in each capsule. However, many health care professionals use lipase content to determine enzyme dosing to treat fat maldigestion. Commercial products are sold in capsules with varying lipase activity, ranging from 4000 to 25 000 U of lipase/capsule. The stated activity in each product is the minimum amount of activity during its shelf-life, as dictated by national regulatory agencies. The actual activity may be considerably higher than stated (sometimes by as much as 200%), but during the shelf-life of the product, there could be considerable loss of activity.[50]

The enteric-coated forms vary considerably in their biochemical coating, biophysical dissolution properties, and size of microspheres or microtab-lets.[38,51] There are few carefully performed clinical studies comparing the different formulations and few in vivo data are available that demonstrate the superiority of a single product. In fact, all currently available enzyme products fail to completely correct nutrient maldigestion in all patients with CF.[20,38,40] The reasons are multiple, are likely to vary from patient to patient, and in some cases may be attributable to factors unrelated to failed pancreatic digestion.[52] The enteric coating of enzyme microsphere or microtablets requires a pH >5.2 to 6.0 for dissolution to occur in the proximal intestine, which may be acidic in the CF patient. Unprotected powder enzymes are subject to destruction by the harsh acid-peptic gastric environment.[53] Patients with CF and PI have gastric acid hypersecretion and a relative deficiency of bicarbonate secretion from the pancreatico-biliary tree. This may result in a more acidic proximal intestinal environment, which may be below the ideal optimal pH for maximal pancreatic enzyme activity and may hasten the inactivation of enzymes, especially lipase within the small intestine. Histamine (H_2)-antagonists or proton-pump inhibitors may be used to improve the intestinal milieu, but studies have revealed mixed results.[54,55] Even if nutrient digestion is achieved, malabsorption of nutrients may occur because of thick intestinal mucus, which may affect the unstirred water layer, reducing absorption of fatty acids in the small intestinal epithelium.[52,56] Nevertheless, enzymes do improve nutrient digestion and absorption in CF patients, but the caregiver must be aware of the less-than-ideal efficacy of these products in individual patients.

Enzyme Administration

Dosing guidelines (see Table 46.1) have been established by the Cystic Fibrosis Foundation and the US Food and Drug Administration.[57] These guidelines were established when it was recognized that many CF centers were giving excessive doses of enzymes. Excessive dosing was, in turn, strongly associated with a newly recognized and severe intestinal complication termed "fibrosing colonopathy."[58] Response to treatment by individual patients will vary considerably, as will their required dosing schedule. Although dosing is best calculated using U of lipase/g of fat ingested, it is perhaps more practical to use a dosing schedule with age-adjusted guidelines.[57] This takes into account the fact that fat intake varies at different ages, with infants taking much larger amounts per body weight than adults. Age-adjusted guidelines, with a limit of 4000 U of lipase/g of fat or 2500 U of lipase/kg per meal beyond 1 year of age, would avoid overdosing (see Table 46.1).

Table 46.1
Dosing Guidelines for Administration of Enzymes

Age	Conventional Products	Enteric-Coated Products*
Infants	8–16 000 U of lipase/120 mL (4 oz) of formula 8000 U of lipase/60 mL (4 tbsp) of solids 8–16 000 U of lipase/breastfeeding session	8000 U of lipase/240 mL (8 oz) of formula 8000 U of lipase/120 mL (8 tbsp) of solids 4–8000 U of lipase/breastfeeding session
1–4 y	—	16–24 000 U of lipase/meal[†] 8–1600 U of lipase/snack[‡]
5–12 y	—	24–40 000 U of lipase/meal[†] 8–24 000 /snack[‡]
>12 y	—	40–64 000 U of lipase/meal[†] 16–24 000 U of lipase/snack[‡]

*The majority of patients with CF require approximately 1800–2000 U of lipase/g of fat per day (range, 500–4000).

[†] Infants and children <4 y: 1000 U of lipase/kg per meal; children and adults >4 y: 500 U of lipase/kg per meal, to a maximum of 2500 U of lipase/kg per meal.

[‡] The dose should vary according to the size of each snack. This should be assessed for each patient individually.

There are no convincing data concerning timing of enzyme dosing with meals, but for practical reasons, it is recommended that enzymes be taken in 2 to 3 divided doses before and during meals.[59] Theoretically, this will result in more even mixing and gastric emptying of enzymes, although this has not been clinically proven. Enzymes are not required with simple carbohydrates (ie, hard candy, popsicles, pop, gelatin dessert) but are needed for foods containing fat, protein, and starch (rice, potatoes, etc). Suggested guidelines for administration of enzymes in infants and older children are outlined below.

Infants
Conventional unprotected powder enzymes or enteric-coated products should be offered before feeding. Enzymes can be mixed with 2 to 3 mL (1/2 tsp) applesauce and given by spoon. Unprotected powder enzymes should be offered in applesauce immediately after mixing, because the acidity of the applesauce will destroy the enzymes. Other strained fruit can be tried if applesauce is not taken, but parents should be encouraged to use only one type of food to avoid problems with overall food refusal if many different types of food are used as the vehicle for enzyme delivery.

Mouth care is important for infants before administration of enzymes. Petroleum jelly should be applied around the outside of the mouth for skin protection. After administration, the inside of the mouth should be cleaned with an oral sponge or cotton swab soaked in water to avoid irritation of the mouth by residual enzymes. Once an infant is taking solids, mouth cleaning is not necessary, because the action of saliva and food mixing in the mouth cleans the mouth. A zinc-based cream is recommended for buttocks care at the start of enzyme therapy and for a few weeks or months afterward. A "home-made" cream consisting of approximately one-third nystatin, two thirds zinc-containing cream, and a small amount of 1% hydrocortisone is often useful, which should be applied generously to buttocks with each diaper change.

Children Older Than 1 Year

At 1 year of age, children can be offered enteric-coated products, mixed with 1 food. Patients should be discouraged from chewing the capsules, as this will destroy the protective coating. Swallowing of capsules is encouraged as soon as parents consider the child is ready. This varies considerably from patient to patient but occurs usually around 4 to 5 years of age. Some older patients continue to experience difficulties swallowing capsules. In this case, they should open the capsule and sprinkle the beads in the mouth and then drink a liquid.

Adjunctive Therapy

H_2-antagonists and proton-pump inhibitors inhibit gastric acid and, in some cases, may improve enzyme activity either by: (1) decreasing gastric acidity, resulting in less destruction of unprotected conventional powder enzymes in the stomach; or (2) increasing pH in the upper intestine, allowing for more rapid dissolution of the enteric coating and optimal conditions for enzymes to catalyze nutrients. As mentioned, efficacy of this treatment is not clear, because results in 1 study proved proton-pump inhibitors to be helpful,[54] and another found no benefit.[55] The health care professional providing care for the patient with CF should be cautioned that there are no safety data on the long-term use of these medications in children.

For patients who continue to have symptoms of maldigestion and malabsorption with maximum prescribed enzyme dose for age, a combination of enteric-coated and conventional enzymes should be tried. Although the efficacy of the combination approach was not proven to be more effective in reducing fat malabsorption compared with enteric-coated enzymes alone in a recent study,[20] some patients in the study did respond to this treatment. It is recommended to substitute approximately 25% of the enteric-coated product with conventional products. For example, if a patient is receiving six 8000-U enteric-coated products per meal, then offer 4 enteric-coated products and 2 conventional enzymes of the same strength.

Vitamin Therapy

The fat-soluble vitamins (A, D, E, and K) are absorbed with dietary fat and, therefore, need to be supplemented in the CF diet (see Table 46.2). Multivitamins containing the fat-soluble vitamins A, D, E, and K have been formulated for patients with CF. Products available include ADEKs (drops or chewables [Axcan Pharma, Birmingham, AL]), SourceCF (softgels [SourceCF, Huntsville, AL]), and Vitamax (chewables [Cystic Fibrosis Services Pharmacy, Bethesda, MD]). Compliance with vitamin therapy is important and should be assessed on a regular basis. Deficiency of the fat-soluble vitamins (especially vitamins A, E, and D) are not uncommon.[10] Therefore, yearly monitoring of vitamin concentrations is recommended.

Table 46.2
Vitamin Therapy

Vitamins*	<2 y		2–8 y		8 y–adult
A	1500 IU		5000 IU		5000–10 000 IU
D	400 IU		400 IU		400–800 IU
	0–6 y	6–12 y	1–4 y	4–10 y	>10 y
E	25 IU	50 IU	100 IU	100–200 IU	200–400 IU
K	Unknown: see text				

* Vitamins should be taken with meals, because enzymes will help assimilation.

   Adverse effects of severe vitamin deficiencies have been reported, including severe xerophthalmia (vitamin A), hematologic and neurologic complications (vitamin E), clotting abnormalities (vitamin K), and loss of bone density (vitamin D).[60]

   Because overdosing of fat-soluble vitamins (especially vitamins A and D) can be harmful and high concentrations of vitamins A and E have been reported in patients with CF after lung transplantation,[61] it is important to instruct patients to take only the amount prescribed and to ensure that they are not taking other over-the-counter vitamin products in addition to the prescribed vitamins. Again, yearly monitoring of serum vitamin concentrations is recommended.

References

1. Drumm ML, Konstan MW, Schluchter MD, et al. Genetic modifiers of lung disease in cystic fibrosis. *N Engl J Med*. 2005;353:1443–1453

2. Kerem E, Corey M, Kerem BS, et al. The relation between genotype and phenotype in cystic fibrosis—analysis of the most common mutation (delta F508). *N Engl J Med*. 1990;323:1517–1522

3. Kristidis P, Bozon D, Corey M, et al. Genetic determination of exocrine pancreatic function in cystic fibrosis. *Am J Hum Genet*. 1992;50:1178–1184

4. Gaskin K, Gurwitz D, Durie P, Corey M, Levison H, Forstner G. Improved respiratory prognosis in patients with cystic fibrosis with normal fat absorption. *J Pediatr*. 1982;100:857–862

5. Waters DL, Dorney SF, Gaskin KJ, Gruca MA, O'Halloran M, Wilcken B. Pancreatic function in infants identified as having cystic fibrosis in a neonatal screening program. *N Engl J Med*. 1990;322:303–308

6. Reardon MC, Hammond KB, Accurso FJ, et al. Nutritional deficits exist before 2 months of age in some infants with cystic fibrosis identified by screening test. *J Pediatr*. 1984;105:271–274

7. van de Kamer JH, ten Bokkel Huinink H, Weyers HA. Rapid method for the determination of fat in feces. *J Biol Chem*. 1949;177:347–355

8. Jeejeebhoy KN, Ahmad S, Kozak G. Determination of fecal fats containing both medium and long chain triglycerides and fatty acids. *Clin Biochem*. 1970;3:157–163

9. Fomon SJ, Ziegler EE, Thomas LN, Jensen RL, Filer LJ Jr. Excretion of fat by normal full-term infants fed various milks and formulas. *Am J Clin Nutr*. 1970;23:1299–1313

10. Feranchak AP, Sontag MK, Wagener JS, Hammond KB, Accurso FJ, Sokol RJ. Prospective, long-term study of fat-soluble vitamin status in children with cystic fibrosis identified by newborn screen. *J Pediatr*. 1999;135:601–610

11. Kalnins D, Corey M, Durie P, Ellis L, Ellis G. Do serum vitamin E levels correlate with 72-hour fecal fat at time of CF diagnosis? [abstr]. *Pediatr Pulmonol*. 1995;12(Suppl):266

12. Loser C, Mollgaard A, Folsch UR. Faecal elastase 1: a novel, highly sensitive, and specific tubeless pancreatic function test. *Gut*. 1996;39:580–586

13. Beharry S, Ellis L, Corey M, Marcon M, Durie P. How useful is fecal pancreatic elastase 1 as a marker of exocrine pancreatic disease? *J Pediatr*. 2002;141:84–90

14. Scheefers-Borchel U, Schefferrs H, Arnold R, Fischer P, Sziegoliet A. Pankreatische Elastase-1: parameter Fur die chronische und akute Pankreatitis. *Lab Med*. 1992;16:427–474

15. Borowitz D, Baker RD, Stallings V. Consensus report on nutrition for pediatric patients with cystic fibrosis. *J Pediatr Gastroenterol Nutr*. 2002;35:246–259

16. Pencharz PB, Durie PR. Nutritional management of cystic fibrosis. *Annu Rev Nutr*. 1993;13:111–136

17. Moran A, Hardin D, Rodman D, et al. Diagnosis, screening and management of cystic fibrosis related diabetes mellitus: a consensus conference report. *Diabetes Res Clin Pract*. 1999;45:61–73

18. Lanng S, Thorsteinsson B, Lund-Andersen C, Nerup J, Schiotz PO, Koch C. Diabetes mellitus in Danish cystic fibrosis patients: prevalence and late diabetic complications. *Acta Paediatr*. 1994;83:72–77

19. Solomon MP, Wilson DC, Corey M, et al. Glucose intolerance in children with cystic fibrosis. *J Pediatr*. 2003;142:128–132

20. Kalnins D, Corey M, Ellis L, Durie PR, Pencharz PB. Combining unprotected pancreatic enzymes with pH-sensitive enteric-coated microspheres does not improve nutrient digestion in patients with cystic fibrosis. *J Pediatr*. 2005;146:489–493

21. Baker SS, Borowitz D, Baker RD. Pancreatic exocrine function in patients with cystic fibrosis. *Curr Gastroenterol Rep*. 2005;7:227–233

22. National Research Council. *Recommended Dietary Allowances*. 10th ed. Washington, DC: National Academies Press; 1989

23. Fried MD, Durie PR, Tsui LC, Corey M, Levison H, Pencharz PB. The cystic fibrosis gene and resting energy expenditure. *J Pediatr*. 1991;119:913–916

24. Ramsey BW, Farrell PM, Pencharz P. Nutritional assessment and management in cystic fibrosis: a consensus report. The Consensus Committee. *Am J Clin Nutr*. 1992;55:108–116

25. Institute of Medicine. *Dietary Reference Intakes for Vitamin A, Vitamin K, Arsenic, Boron, Chromium, Copper, Iodine, Iron, Manganese, Molybdenum, Nickel, Silicon, Vanadium, and Zinc*. Washington, DC: National Academies Press; 2000

26. Institute of Medicine. *Dietary Reference Intakes for Vitamin C, Vitamin E, Selenium, and Carotenoids*. Washington, DC: National Academies Press; 2000

27. Boyle MP, Noschese ML, Watts SL, Davis ME, Stenner SE, Lechtzin N. Failure of high-dose ergocalciferol to correct vitamin D deficiency in adults with cystic fibrosis. *Am J Respir Crit Care Med*. 2005;172:212–217

28. Rashid M, Durie P, Andrew M, et al. Prevalence of vitamin K deficiency in cystic fibrosis. *Am J Clin Nutr*. 1999;70:378–382

29. Conway SP, Wolfe SP, Brownlee KG, White H, Oldroyd B, Truscott JG, et al. Vitamin K status among children with cystic fibrosis and its relationship to bone mineral density and bone turnover. *Pediatrics*. 2005;115:1325–1331

30. Ellis L, Kalnins D, Corey M, Brennan J, Pencharz P, Durie P. Do infants with cystic fibrosis need a protein hydrolysate formula? A prospective, randomized, comparative study. *J Pediatr*. 1998;132:270–276

31. Powers SW, Patton SR, Rajan S. A comparison of food group variety between toddlers with and without cystic fibrosis. *J Hum Nutr Diet*. 2004;17:523–527

32. Kalnins D, Corey M, Ellis L, Pencharz PB, Tullis E, Durie PR. Failure of conventional strategies to improve nutritional status in malnourished adolescents and adults with cystic fibrosis. *J Pediatr*. 2005;147:399–401

33. Pencharz PB, Durie PR. Pathogenesis of malnutrition in cystic fibrosis, and its treatment. *Clin Nutr*. 2000;19:387–394

34. Levy LD, Durie PR, Pencharz PB, Corey ML. Effects of long-term nutritional rehabilitation on body composition and clinical status in malnourished children and adolescents with cystic fibrosis. *J Pediatr*. 1985;107:225–230

35. Efrati O, Mei-Zahav M, Rivlin J, et al. Long term nutritional rehabilitation by gastrostomy in Israeli patients with cystic fibrosis: clinical outcome in advanced pulmonary disease. *J Pediatr Gastroenterol Nutr*. 2006;42:222–228

36. Erskine JM, Lingard CD, Sontag MK, Accurso FJ. Enteral nutrition for patients with cystic fibrosis: comparison of a semi-elemental and nonelemental formula. *J Pediatr.* 1998;132:265–269

37. Heine RG, Button BM, Olinsky A, Phelan PD, Catto-Smith AG. Gastro-oesophageal reflux in infants under 6 months with cystic fibrosis. *Arch Dis Child.* 1998;78:44–48

38. Durie P, Kalnins D, Ellis L. Uses and abuses of enzyme therapy in cystic fibrosis. *J R Soc Med.* 1998;91(Suppl 34):2–13

39. Lebenthal E, Rolston DD, Holsclaw DS Jr. Enzyme therapy for pancreatic insufficiency: present status and future needs. *Pancreas.* 1994;9:1–12

40. Kalnins D, Stewart C, Corey M, Tullis E, Pencharz P, Durie P. Does the addition of bicarbonate to an enzyme microsphere preparation improve efficacy? [abstr]. *Pediatr Pulmonol.* 1998;(Suppl 15):355

41. Pashankar DS, Uc A, Bishop WP. Polyethylene glycol 3350 without electrolytes: a new safe, effective, and palatable bowel preparation for colonoscopy in children. *J Pediatr.* 2004;144:358–362

42. Moran A, Doherty L, Wang X, Thomas W. Abnormal glucose metabolism in cystic fibrosis. *J Pediatr.* 1998;133:10–17

43. Aris RM, Merkel PA, Bachrach LK, et al. Guide to bone health and disease in cystic fibrosis. *J Clin Endocrinol Metab.* 2005;90:1888–1896

44. Buntain HM, Greer RM, Schluter PJ, et al. Bone mineral density in Australian children, adolescents and adults with cystic fibrosis: a controlled cross sectional study. *Thorax.* 2004;59:149–155

45. Buntain HM, Schluter PJ, Bell SC, et al. Controlled longitudinal study of bone mass accrual in children and adolescents with cystic fibrosis. *Thorax.* 2006;61:146–154

46. Khosla S, Melton LJ III, Dekutoski MB, Achenbach SJ, Oberg AL, Riggs BL. Incidence of childhood distal forearm fractures over 30 years: a population-based study. *JAMA.* 2003;290:1479–1485

47. Greer FR, Krebs NF, American Academy of Pediatrics, Committee on Nutrition. Optimizing bone health and calcium intakes of infants, children, and adolescents. *Pediatrics.* 2006;117:578–585

48. Striegel-Moore RH, Thompson D, Affenito SG, et al. Correlates of beverage intake in adolescent girls: the National Heart, Lung, and Blood Institute Growth and Health Study. *J Pediatr.* 2006;148:183–187

49. Schulze KJ, O'Brien KO, Germain-Lee EL, Baer DJ, Leonard AL, Rosenstein BJ. Endogenous fecal losses of calcium compromise calcium balance in pancreatic-insufficient girls with cystic fibrosis. *J Pediatr.* 2003;143:765–771

50. Kraisinger M, Hochhaus G, Stecenko A, Bowser E, Hendeles L. Clinical pharmacology of pancreatic enzymes in patients with cystic fibrosis and in vitro performance of microencapsulated formulations. *J Clin Pharmacol.* 1994;34:158–166

51. Carroccio A, Pardo F, Montalto G, et al. Effectiveness of enteric-coated preparations on nutritional parameters in cystic fibrosis. A long-term study. *Digestion.* 1988;41:201–206

52. Borowitz D, Durie PR, Clarke LL, et al. Gastrointestinal outcomes and confounders in cystic fibrosis. *J Pediatr Gastroenterol Nutr.* 2005;41:273–285

53. Barraclough M, Taylor CJ. Twenty-four hour ambulatory gastric and duodenal pH profiles in cystic fibrosis: effect of duodenal hyperacidity on pancreatic enzyme function and fat absorption. *J Pediatr Gastroenterol Nutr.* 1996;23:45–50

54. Heijerman HG, Lamers CB, Bakker W. Omeprazole enhances the efficacy of pancreatin (pancrease) in cystic fibrosis. *Ann Intern Med.* 1991;114:200–201

55. Francisco MP, Wagner MH, Sherman JM, Theriaque D, Bowser E, Novak DA. Ranitidine and omeprazole as adjuvant therapy to pancrelipase to improve fat absorption in patients with cystic fibrosis. *J Pediatr Gastroenterol Nutr.* 2002;35:79–83

56. Laiho KM, Gavin J, Murphy JL, Connett GJ, Wootton SA. Maldigestion and malabsorption of 13C labelled tripalmitin in gastrostomy-fed patients with cystic fibrosis. *Clin Nutr.* 2004;23:347–353

57. Borowitz DS, Grand RJ, Durie PR. Use of pancreatic enzyme supplements for patients with cystic fibrosis in the context of fibrosing colonopathy. Consensus Committee. *J Pediatr.* 1995;127:681–684

58. FitzSimmons SC, Burkhart GA, Borowitz D, et al. High-dose pancreatic-enzyme supplements and fibrosing colonopathy in children with cystic fibrosis. *N Engl J Med.* 1997;336: 1283–1289

59. Brady MS, Rickard K, Yu PL, Eigen H. Effectiveness of enteric coated pancreatic enzymes given before meals in reducing steatorrhea in children with cystic fibrosis. *J Am Diet Assoc.* 1992;92:813–817

60. Bhudhikanok GS, Wang MC, Marcus R, Harkins A, Moss RB, Bachrach LK. Bone acquisition and loss in children and adults with cystic fibrosis: a longitudinal study. *J Pediatr.* 1998;133:18–27

61. Stephenson A, Brotherwood M, Robert R, et al. Increased vitamin A and E levels in adult cystic fibrosis patients after lung transplantation. *Transplantation.* 2005;79:613–615

47　The Ketogenic Diet

The ketogenic diet is a high-fat, low-carbohydrate, and minimal-protein diet designed to mimic the fasting state. It is used most commonly to treat intractable epilepsy but is also a primary therapy for some metabolic defects involving glucose transport and metabolism. The diet increases the body's reliance on fatty acids rather than on glucose for energy. This chapter briefly reviews the history, physiology, efficacy, indications, contraindications, and mechanisms of action of the ketogenic diet. The emphasis is on implementing and maintaining the classic ketogenic diet while preventing and managing its complications. Alternative dietary therapies for epilepsy, including the modified Atkins diet and the low-glycemic index treatment, are also mentioned.

History

The benefits of fasting for seizure control have been known for ages.[1] Although the first scientific report did not appear until 1911 in France, fasting for seizure therapy was used by Hippocrates and was also recommended in the Bible (Mark 9:14-29). In the United States, the first report of fasting as a treatment for epilepsy was presented to the American Medical Association in 1921 by endocrinologist Geyelin (New York Presbyterian Hospital, New York, NY) on the basis of his observation of patients treated by the osteopath Conklin (Battle Creek, MI), who believed that epilepsy could be caused by toxic secretions from intestinal Peyer patches.[2] Because fasting is not a practical long-term treatment, Wilder (Mayo Clinic, Rochester, MN) described a high-fat, low-carbohydrate, "ketogenic" diet to mimic fasting; the first efficacy studies of this ketogenic diet in 1925 and 1926 showed remarkable efficacy, with 50% to 60% of patients becoming seizure free.[2] Interest in the diet waned after the introduction of phenytoin in 1938, but a resurgence of interest in the diet occurred in the 1990s, in part as a result of the advocacy of the Charlie Foundation (http://www.charliefoundation.org) and the media attention surrounding the 1997 movie *First Do No Harm*.[1] The diet is currently administered at major medical centers around the United States as well as at least 70 medical centers in 41 other countries.[3]

Physiologic Basis

The basis of the ketogenic diet is apparently the brain's ability to obtain 30% to 60% or more of its energy during fasting from serum ketone bodies derived from beta-oxidation of fatty acids.[4-8] Some of the most relevant aspects are briefly reviewed here (Fig 47.1).

Fig 47.1

Summary of ketogenesis.

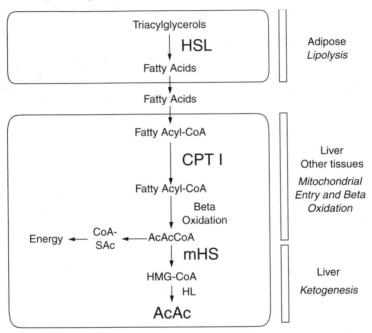

SL indicates hormone-sensitive lipase; CPT I, carnitine palmitoyltransferase I; AcAcCoA, acetoacetyl-CoA; CoA, coenzyme A; mHS, mitochondrial HMG-CoA synthetase; HMG, 3-hydroxy-3-methyl glutaric acid; HL, HMG-CoA lyase; AcAc, acetoacetate.

Adapted from Mitchell and Fukao.[6]

Fasting lowers serum glucose concentration, resulting in a low ratio of insulin to glucagon. The decrease in this ratio and changes in other hormones, such as epinephrine, stimulate lipolysis in adipocytes. The free fatty acids released into the blood cannot cross the blood-brain barrier and, therefore, cannot be used directly to sustain brain metabolism. Instead, fatty acids are converted by the liver to ketone bodies that cross the blood-brain barrier and serve as a major energy source for the brain.

Fatty acids from lipolysis undergo beta-oxidation to acetyl-coenzyme A (acetyl-CoA) in the mitochondria of liver, cardiac muscle, and skeletal muscle cells. Acetyl-CoA ordinarily condenses with oxaloacetate to enter the tricarboxylic acid (TCA) cycle (or Krebs cycle). However, liver oxaloacetate concentration is low during fasting, because it is used to synthesize glucose. The liver, therefore, converts excess acetyl-CoA to acetoacetate and then to beta-hydroxybutyrate, 2 ketone bodies, which are then released into the bloodstream and cross the blood-brain barrier.

In the brain as in other tissues, beta-hydroxybutyrate and acetoacetate are converted back to acetyl-CoA and enter the TCA cycle (Fig 47.2), yielding biosynthetic carbon compounds and energy (in the form of reduced nicotinamide adenine dinucleotide and reduced flavin adenine dinucleotide). The mitochondrial electron transport chain then oxidizes nicotinamide adenine dinucleotide and flavin adenine dinucleotide to yield adenosine triphosphate.

Fig 47.2
Pathways of ketone utilization.

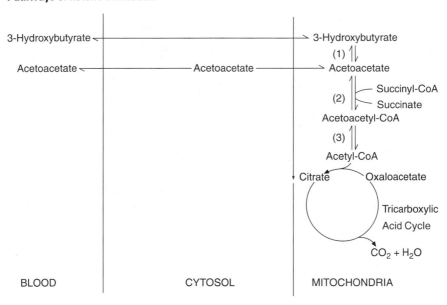

1 = hydroxybutyrate dehydrogenase; 2 = 3-oxoacid-coenzyme A (CoA) transferase; 3 = acetoacetyl-CoA thiolase.
Adapted from Williamson.[8]

Beta-oxidation of fatty acids in the liver occurs in the mitochondrial matrix; therefore, free fatty acids must cross the outer and inner mitochondrial membranes. The carnitine cycle is required for this transmembrane transport of long-chain fatty acids but not for short- or medium-chain fatty acids.[9]

Mechanisms of Action

The mechanisms by which the ketogenic diet acts as an anticonvulsant remain unknown, although many hypotheses have been proposed.[5,10,11] Some hypotheses involve a direct or indirect anticonvulsant effect of ketone bodies. For example, there is evidence that acetone has a direct anticonvulsant effect on neurons, but it is unclear what the mechanism of this effect might be or whether the anticonvulsant effect of the ketogenic diet is related to acetone.[12] Acetoacetate and beta-hydroxybutyrate do not appear to act on synapses or directly alter neurotransmitter function.[13] However, metabolism of ketone bodies by the TCA cycle may result in increased levels of glutamate and, therefore, increased gamma-aminobutyric acid, a major inhibitory neurotransmitter.[10,14]

It is also possible that anticonvulsant effects may not result directly from ketone bodies but instead from other physiologic consequences of the ketogenic diet. Changes in cerebral pH have been suggested but appear unlikely.[15] The amount of polyunsaturated fatty acids is elevated in the ketogenic diet, which has been shown to modulate voltage-gated sodium channels and L-type calcium channels, which may affect neuronal excitability.[10] Fatty acids may also have a neuroprotective effect by inducing mitochondrial uncoupling proteins and, therefore, reducing reactive oxygen species formation.[10] Because glucose uptake is greater during seizures than during any other brain activity, the decreased availability of glucose as a rapidly mobilized energy source may provide an anticonvulsant effect.[11] The changes in energy homeostasis associated with the diet may also affect the activity of adenosine triphosphate-sensitive potassium channels, or other physiologic changes may affect 2-pore domain potassium channels.[10,16] Given the complex nature of the metabolic changes involved, it is likely that no single mechanism will explain the anticonvulsant effect of the ketogenic diet.

Indications

Intractable Epilepsy

The ketogenic diet is indicated in the treatment of intractable epilepsy. It effectively treats multiple seizure types (including generalized seizures, partial-onset seizures, and infantile spasms[17–19]) and seizure syndromes (including Lennox-Gastaut syndrome,[20] Dravet syndrome [severe myoclonic epilepsy of infancy],[21] and Doose syndrome [myoclonic-astatic epilepsy of early childhood][22]). It is also effective for seizures caused by tuberous sclerosis complex[23,24] and other inherited disorders. The ketogenic diet is usually considered too difficult for use as a first-line agent. Furthermore, like other treatments, the ketogenic diet is associated with a risk of adverse events (see "Adverse Effects"). Although it has occasionally been used as first- or second-line therapy,[25] most neurologists would recommend fair trials of 2 or 3 antiepileptic drugs, appropriate for seizure type and at therapeutic doses, before attempting the ketogenic diet.

The ketogenic diet is indicated for patients of all ages. Good efficacy has been demonstrated in infants, who may receive the diet in the form of a ketogenic formula (see "Calculation of the Ketogenic Diet").[18,26] In most studies, efficacy in adolescents and adults is similar to that in children,[27–29] although some studies suggest slightly lower tolerability in older patients.[19]

Inborn Metabolic Disorders

The ketogenic diet may also be indicated for certain congenital disorders affecting glucose metabolism and transport, including pyruvate dehydrogenase complex deficiency[30] and glucose transporter type 1 deficiency. [31,32] Pyruvate dehydrogenase normally converts pyruvate (from glycolysis) to acetyl-CoA, which normally enters the TCA cycle. Glucose transporter type 1 is responsible for facilitated tran sport of glucose across the blood-brain barrier. In both disorders, mutations result in an inability of the brain to use glucose as its primary energy substrate. The ketogenic diet should be considered soon after diagnosis of these metabolic disorders.

Experimental Uses

Ketogenic diets have recently been tried as alternative therapy for a range of diseases, including type 2 diabetes mellitus,[33] polycystic ovary syndrome,[34] autism spectrum disorder,[35] bipolar disorder,[36] and even malignant astrocytoma.[37,38] Efficacy and safety have not been demonstrated for any of these indications; therefore, the use of the diet for each of these conditions is strictly experimental.

Efficacy

Since the early 1920s, multiple case series and open-label studies, mostly retrospective, have been published describing the efficacy of the ketogenic diet for intractable epilepsy. A 2003 meta-analysis of 720 patients in 9 studies published by 1998 showed 37% of patients achieving >90% reduction in seizure frequency compared with baseline, 30% achieving 50% to 90% reduction, and 33% achieving <50% reduction.[39] Several efficacy series have been published since that time: of those, 5 large studies (>40 patients) published between 1998 and 2005 that presented efficacy data at 6 and 12 months[40-44] were reviewed. A total of 425 patients were included in this meta-analysis. At 6 months, 146 (34.4%) had discontinued the diet, 109 (25.6%) had >90% reduction in seizure frequency compared with baseline, 98 (23.1%) had 50% to 90% reduction in seizures, 55 (12.9%) had <50% reduction in seizures, and 17 (4.0%) were lost to follow-up. At 12 months, 229 (53.9%) had discontinued the diet, 80 (18.9%) had >90% reduction in seizure frequency compared with baseline, 60 (14.1%) had 50% to 90% reduction in seizures, 29 (6.8%) had <50% reduction in seizures, and 27 (6.4%) were lost to follow-up. Described another way, at 12 months, 169 patients remained on the diet, of which 35.5% had >90% reduction in seizure frequency compared with baseline, 47.3% had 50% to 90% reduction in seizures, and 17.2% had <50% reduction in seizures.

Of note, no randomized, controlled trials of the ketogenic diet have been published to date.[45] Nevertheless, the evidence from class II and III studies overwhelmingly supports the conclusion that the ketogenic diet is an effective treatment for many patients with intractable epilepsy. This conclusion is further supported by the observation that patients who have failed trials of 2 antiepileptic drugs have a limited chance of achieving seizure control with a third drug. On the ketogenic diet, such patients with intractable epilepsy have approximately a one-third chance of achieving seizure control and another one-third chance of attaining a meaningful but incomplete reduction in seizures.

Most studies have not found significant differences in outcome with respect to age, sex, seizure type, or etiology, although some suggest that the diet may be slightly more effective in younger children and in primary generalized epilepsies.[19,46] Even patients who do not experience decreased seizure frequency may still benefit from the diet: many patients on the ketogenic diet have reduced seizure intensity, improved alertness, improved behavior, and reduced number or dosage of antiepileptic drugs. In a prospective study, significant improvements in developmental quotient, attention, and social functioning were observed in 34 children who continued on the ketogenic diet for 1 year.[47]

Contraindications

The ketogenic diet is contraindicated for patients with fatty acid oxidation defects, including defects involving fatty acid transportation, enzymes of beta-oxidation, and ketone body production.[48] It is contraindicated in patients with primary carnitine deficiency or other carnitine cycle defects.[7] It is contraindicated in pyruvate carboxylase deficiency.[49] Candidates for the ketogenic diet should be screened for metabolic disorders, including a comprehensive metabolic blood panel, before diet initiation. Although high-fat diets can exacerbate ketotic hypoglycemia, the ketogenic diet is not absolutely contraindicated in this condition but requires careful monitoring.[50]

No drugs are absolutely contraindicated with the ketogenic diet, but cotherapy with some drugs may increase the risk of certain adverse events. Because cotherapy may provide optimal seizure control for some patients, the risks and benefits must be weighed. Furthermore, all medications must be reviewed for carbohydrate content (see "Concurrent Medications and Occult Carbohydrates").

Carbonic anhydrase inhibitors (including acetazolamide, topiramate, and zonisamide), like the ketogenic diet, are associated with increased risk of metabolic acidosis and should be used with caution. Careful monitoring of serum bicarbonate concentrations is appropriate with these drugs.[51,52] Prophylaxis with potassium citrate or other buffering agents may be appropriate in patients at increased risk of metabolic acidosis. Carbonic anhydrase inhibitors are also associated with an increased risk of renal stones.[53] Nevertheless, patients cotreated with topiramate and the ketogenic diet do not appear to have higher risk of nephrolithiasis than other patients treated with the ketogenic diet.[51,54] Adequate hydration and buffering agents, such as potassium citrate, are especially important to prevent calculi in patients cotreated with carbonic anhydrase inhibitors. With appropriate prophylaxis, carbonic anhydrase inhibitors and the ketogenic diet can usually be safely coadministered.

Cotherapy with valproate is also somewhat controversial. Rare adverse events associated with valproate include acute pancreatitis and hepatic failure. Long-term use of valproate can also induce carnitine deficiency. It has been suggested, therefore, that cotherapy with valproate and the ketogenic diet may induce hepatotoxicity by a carnitine-related mechanism in some patients or may unacceptably increase the risk of other adverse effects, such as pancreatitis.[9,55] However, recent studies have not found that valproate increases the risk of adverse events on the ketogenic diet.[40,56] Liver function, pancreatic amylase concentration, and carnitine concentration should be monitored carefully in patients cotreated with valproate and the ketogenic diet, but valproate is not an absolute contraindication to the ketogenic diet.

Adverse Effects

Common short-term adverse effects of the ketogenic diet include dehydration, hypoglycemia, acidosis, vomiting, diarrhea, constipation, and loss of appetite.[55] These complications are generally treated symptomatically. The first 3 symptoms may be prevented with a diet protocol that includes no fasting, no fluid restriction, and prophylactic administration of potassium citrate (see "Calculation of the Ketogenic Diet"). Constipation is very common and can usually be managed with polyethylene glycol.

Common longer-term adverse effects include growth retardation (see "Growth Retardation"), hypertriglyceridemia (see "Lipid Profiles"), renal stones (see "Renal Stones"), increased bruising, irritability, and lethargy. Some patients on the ketogenic diet may be more susceptible to infection, but it is unclear whether impaired immune function is attributable to the diet or whether patients on the diet have impaired immune function for other reasons.[57] Rare but serious adverse events have been reported with the ketogenic diet, including acute (possibly hypertriglyceridemia-induced) pancreatitis,[58] cardiomyopathy associated with prolonged QT_c interval,[59] and acute hemolytic anemia.[55] Hepatotoxicity and Fanconi renal tubular acidosis have been reported in a few patients cotreated with the ketogenic diet and valproate,[55] but this combination has been used in many other patients without adverse effects.[40]

Growth Retardation

Since 1999, 5 studies have addressed growth in children on the ketogenic diet.[60–64] Studies assessing growth after 4 or 6 months of treatment have had inconsistent results, but studies assessing children after 12 months of treatment consistently show decreased height-for-age and weight-for-age z-scores. Changes in weight-for-age appear to be greatest within the first several months on the diet, while the greatest changes in height-for-age occur only after 6 months on the diet. Younger children may be at greater risk of growth retardation. There is anecdotal evidence that some children may experience catch-up growth after completing ketogenic diet treatment. The risk of growth retardation, especially with long-term treatment, should be considered when weighing the risks and benefits of the ketogenic diet. Height and weight should be monitored closely (at least every 3 months). Protein and total kilocalories should be adjusted in patients with suboptimal growth.

Renal Stones

The ketogenic diet is associated with an increased risk of nephrolithiasis.[53,65] Renal calculi occur in approximately 3% to 10% of children treated with the diet.[65] Certain medications (eg, zonisamide) may increase the risk of calculi (see "Contraindications"). Calculi may be composed of uric acid, calcium oxalate, or calcium phosphate. Patients with hematuria (gross or microscopic), crystalluria, abdominal pain, or flank pain should be evaluated for possible nephrolithiasis. Analgesia and hydration are appropriate for acute episodes, and lithotripsy and/or medical expulsive therapy may be indicated in some cases. Further incidence may be prevented by liberalization of fluids and alkalinization of urine with potassium citrate or other buffering agents.

Lipid Profiles

The ketogenic diet increases triglyceride, total cholesterol, and low-density lipoprotein concentrations and decreases high-density lipoprotein concentration.[61,66] The long-term consequences of these alterations in lipid profile are unknown, especially because they may normalize after the patient is weaned from the diet.

The Keto Team

The ketogenic diet requires a multidisciplinary team approach. At the heart of the "keto team" are the patient and his or her family, the neurologist, the dietitian, the pediatrician, and nurse(s). The inpatient pediatric house staff, a gastroenterologist, the hospital foodservice staff, a social worker, a pharmacist, and other specialists are typically involved as well. Close coordination and excellent communication are mandatory. Implementing the ketogenic diet is very time intensive for families and for clinicians.

Calculation of the Ketogenic Diet

The ketogenic diet is traditionally calculated at a 4:1 ketogenic ratio (4 g of fat/1 g of protein and carbohydrate), although this ratio may be modified to suit different needs of some patients. Lower ratios may be necessary to meet some patients' protein requirements or to improve tolerability. During follow-up, the diet may be recalculated with an increased ketogenic ratio if necessary for improved seizure control or with increased calories and/or protein if necessary for growth.

The caloric requirements of children with intractable epilepsy, especially those with impaired mobility, often differ substantially from other children. In preinitiation consultation, the dietitian collects and analyzes a 3-day food record, measures height and weight, and assesses activity level. After considering all of these variables, a caloric recommendation for the ketogenic diet can be formulated. Because weight gain may compromise ketosis, some clinicians calculate caloric intake at 75% of the Recommended Dietary Allowance; however, the 3-day food record may provide a more reliable estimate of an individual's caloric requirement.

The calculation of macronutrient requirements for the ketogenic diet is outlined in Table 47.1. Menus should be calculated by, or in consultation with, a registered dietitian with experience in the ketogenic diet. These calculations can be performed by hand, but the process is greatly facilitated by ketogenic diet software (eg, KetoCalculator [Nutricia North America, Gaithersburg, MD]). Many families rely exclusively on menus calculated by the dietitian; some parents learn to calculate menus for their own children. Menus are calculated to the nearest g, and foods should be weighed to the nearest tenth of a g.

Table 47.1
Ketogenic Diet Macronutrient Calculations

1. Calculate kcal needed per day
Example: 15-kg child × 68 kcal/kg per day = 1000 kcal/day
2. Calculate number of dietary units needed per day*
For example, on a 4:1 diet, each dietary unit (4 g fat + 1 g protein or carbohydrate) = 40 kcal (1000 kcal/day)/(40 kcal/unit) = 25 units/day
3. Calculate the number of g of fat required per day
Fat: 25 units/day × 4 g/unit = 100 g per day
4. Calculate the remainder of units/kcal, allotted to protein and carbohydrate
Protein and carbohydrate: 25 units/day × 1 g/unit = 25 g/day
5. Maintain at least the minimum protein requirement (1 g/kg per day)
Protein: 1 g/kg per day × 15 kg = 15 g/day of protein
6. Calculate remainder, allotted to carbohydrate
Carbohydrate: 25 g/day − 15 g/day protein = 10 g/day carbohydrate
7. Divide the allotments into 3 meals per day

* The kcal per dietary unit vary with the ratio of the ketogenic diet as follows: for a 2:1 diet, 22 kcal per dietary unit; for a 3:1 diet, 31 kcal per dietary unit; for a 4:1 diet, 40 kcal per dietary unit; and for a 5:1 diet, 49 kcal per dietary unit.

In constructing menus to satisfy the daily allotment of macronutrients, fat (from heavy cream, butter or margarine, oils, mayonnaise, and other sources) is a critical part of the equation. Heavy cream (36% fat) may be drunk, whipped, or flavored and frozen as ice cream. Consistent use of the same brand of heavy cream and careful calculations using nutritional tables[67] or standard software are mandatory. Once fat is allotted, protein sources (eg, meat, fish, poultry, egg, and cheese) are added, taking into account the protein already present in cream. Carbohydrate-containing foods (eg, fruits and vegetables) are added last, taking into account the carbohydrates already present in cream, protein sources, and medications. Small quantities of certain "free foods" (eg, a lettuce leaf, 2 macadamia nuts, or 2 olives) may be added to increase dietary flexibility and palatability.

A powdered formula with a 4:1 ketogenic ratio is available (KetoCal, Nutricia North America, Gaithersburg, MD) and can be used as a meal substitute. For children who are fed via tube, KetoCal can be used, or Ross Carbohydrate Free soy-based formula (Abbott Nutrition, Columbus, OH) can be combined with a glucose polymer (Polycose, Abbott Nutrition, Columbus, OH) and emulsified safflower oil (Microlipid, Nestlé, Glendale, CA) to yield the desired ketogenic ratio.

Micronutrient Supplementation

The ketogenic diet is deficient in several vitamins (including vitamins D and B) and minerals (including magnesium, potassium, and calcium). Children on the ketogenic diet must receive supplements of these vitamins and minerals. Parents must understand that these supplements are not elective. Before the requirements of these vitamins became understood in the 1920s and 1930s, patients developed serious complications of vitamin and mineral deficiencies. Patients should receive an age-appropriate low-carbohydrate multivitamin (such as One-a-Day Bugs Bunny Sugar-Free [Bayer Consumer Care Products, Morristown, NJ] or Centrum [Wyeth Consumer Healthcare, Madison, NJ]) per day as well as a carbohydrate-free calcium supplement. Some health care professionals also recommend vitamin D supplementation in addition to the multivitamin.[67] Because carnitine is important for fatty acid transport, carnitine concentrations should be monitored; patients who develop carnitine deficiency should receive carnitine supplementation.[9]

Initiation Protocol

Before scheduling diet initiation, parents should meet with a dietitian familiar with the ketogenic diet. In addition to assessing the patient's anthropometric and nutritional status, the dietitian educates the family about the ketogenic diet and the initiation protocol. Baseline laboratory studies (complete blood cell count; complete metabolic panel; lipid profile; determination of electrolyte, serum carnitine, and serum beta-hydroxybutyrate concentrations; and urinalysis) are performed to detect any possible contraindications. The family should commit to maintain the diet under close supervision for at least 2 months to determine whether the diet will be effective.

Traditionally, the ketogenic diet is initiated with a 24- to 48-hour fast, followed by the introduction of ketogenic meals once the patient is in documented ketosis (large ketones on urine dipstick). In recent years, this approach has been called into question; some medical centers have introduced modified initiation protocols that do not involve fasting.[68–70] There is some evidence that fasting may not accelerate ketosis or improve outcomes; there is also evidence that nonfasting protocols may be more easily tolerated and may reduce the likelihood of some complications (including symptomatic acidosis, hypoglycemia, and electrolyte imbalances). This topic remains controversial.

Whether fasting or not, standard practice is to initiate the ketogenic diet on an inpatient basis, although at least one medical center has offered the ketogenic diet on an outpatient basis.[71] Hospital admission has many benefits: it allows monitoring for adverse events, treatment of complications, and adjustment of medications. Furthermore, it provides an ideal opportunity for the keto team to meet with the patient and family to provide education and support.

If a classic fasting protocol is used (eg, Johns Hopkins Children's Center, Baltimore, MD), the patient is asked to fast after dinner the night before the admission.[44] After 48 hours of fasting, ketogenic meals are introduced, first at one third of calculated calories for 24 hours, then at two thirds of calculated calories for 24 hours, then at full strength. Alternatively, using 1 nonfasting protocol (Massachusetts General Hospital, Boston, MA), full-strength ketogenic meals are given from day 1. Under another protocol (Children's Hospital of Pennsylvania, Philadelphia, PA), full-calorie meals are given from day 1 at a 1:1 ketogenic ratio. The ratio is then increased daily to 2:1, to 3:1, and finally, to 4:1.[68]

During the course of the hospital admission, blood glucose concentration is generally monitored every 6 hours, or more often if hypoglycemia is detected, until the child is in ketosis and tolerating the full-ketogenic diet. Once eating the diet and in ketosis, the child is monitored clinically and blood glucose concentration measurements are performed only if there are symptoms of hypoglycemia. Unless the child is symptomatic, blood glucose concentrations as low as 25 mg/dL are not treated. Urine ketone dipsticks are typically checked every void. Serum bicarbonate concentration is checked every 24 hours; concentrations as low as 15 mmol are considered normal, but symptoms of acidosis (lethargy, vomiting) or serum bicarbonate concentration <15 mmol should be treated. Potassium citrate may be given prophylactically.

The traditional ketogenic diet involves restricted fluid intake on the basis of the observation that urine ketone concentrations may decrease with increased hydration. However, fluid intake generally does not affect serum beta-hydroxybutyrate, which is a more reliable indicator of ketosis than urine ketone concentration.[72] To reduce the risk of dehydration and nephrolithiasis, many health care professionals now recommend a ketogenic diet without fluid restriction.[65,69] Preliminary data suggest that fluid liberalization does not decrease efficacy.

Maintenance and Follow-Up

A child on the ketogenic diet requires close supervision by his or her pediatric neurologist/epileptologist, dietitian, and pediatrician. Ketogenic diet clinic follow-up visits are typically at 1 month, 3 months, and every 3 months thereafter. At these visits, the child's parents or caregivers should provide records of seizure frequency, records of urine dipsticks for ketones, and food diaries to the neurologist and the dietitian. Height and weight are measured, and routine laboratory studies are performed, as during the preinitiation consult. Clinicians should ask about common adverse effects. The diet may be adjusted at these visits to optimize growth and seizure control.

Minor viral illnesses and more serious infections typically make it difficult to maintain ketosis and may increase metabolic acidosis. During intercurrent illnesses, breakthrough seizures can often be managed with a benzodiazepine pulse (eg, lorazepam or diazepam).

Concurrent Medications and Occult Carbohydrates

Most oral drug formulations and almost all syrups contain carbohydrates in the form of sugars, starches, or reduced carbohydrates, such as glycerin. Parents or caregivers should be instructed to check with the dietitian before giving any new prescription or over-the-counter medications to children on the ketogenic diet. Other occult carbohydrates include sugar in toothpaste and sorbitol in lotions (including sunscreen) and shampoos, which may be absorbed transdermally. Only sugar-free toothpastes (such as Tom's of Maine [Kennebunk, ME]) should be used. Hidden sources of carbohydrate should be considered if seizure exacerbations occur.

Likewise, physicians who care for children on the ketogenic diet should consult with the dietitian and with appropriate references regarding choice of medications.[73,74] A compounding pharmacy should be identified that can prepare carbohydrate-free drug formulations, and the hospital pharmacist may be contacted for inpatient hospital stays, including diet initiations. During inpatient hospital stays, physicians, pharmacists, and nursing staff should be reminded to avoid intravenous solutions containing dextrose, glucose, or other sugars. Any added carbohydrates in medication formulations must be included in diet calculations.

Adjusting the Diet for Optimal Seizure Control

The experienced pediatric neurologist and dietitian will learn to adjust the ketogenic diet like an antiepileptic drug. Breakthrough seizures may occur at times of day when ketosis is suboptimal; in these cases, the diet may be adjusted to optimize seizure control. For example, breakthrough seizures on waking in the morning might be treated with a small, high-fat snack at bedtime (eg, olives) to help sustain ketosis overnight.

Discontinuation of the Ketogenic Diet

Children who have experienced 1 or 2 years of seizure freedom may be weaned from the ketogenic diet by reducing the ketogenic ratio gradually over several months. If seizures recur during the weaning process, the diet can be immediately reincreased to the original ratio without necessitating hospital admission. Of 150 patients in a prospective study, 11 were seizure free after 1 year on the diet and subsequently discontinued the diet. At 3- to 6-year follow-up, 8 remained seizure free and 2 maintained a 90% to 99% reduction from baseline, suggesting an excellent long-term prognosis for those who achieve seizure freedom on the ketogenic diet.[75]

Most children who try the diet without significant improvement discontinue within months. Occasionally, children experience significant improvement on the ketogenic diet and stay on the ketogenic diet for many years. Such patients should be monitored at a major pediatric epilepsy center.

Alternative Dietary Therapy

Although the ketogenic diet has been used for more than 80 years with good efficacy, it remains difficult for patients to tolerate. More than half of patients typically discontinue within 1 year (see "Efficacy"); of those who discontinue, roughly half are unable to tolerate its restrictions or find it unpalatable. Therefore, several variations on the classic ketogenic diet have been introduced. In the 1970s, Huttenlocher et al[76] introduced the medium-chain triglyceride (MCT) oil version of the ketogenic diet. Because MCT oil is, gram-for-gram, more ketogenic than other fats, the MCT oil diet allowed liberalized quantities of protein and carbohydrate. Although efficacy was similar to the classic ketogenic diet, it was considered equally unpalatable with increased adverse effects of bloating, nausea, and vomiting.

More recently, a modified Atkins diet has been used in 20 children with 6-month efficacy similar to that observed in the ketogenic diet; approximately one third of patients experienced >90% reduction in seizure frequency, one third experienced 50% to 90% reduction in seizures, and one third experienced <50% reduction in seizures.[77]

A low-glycemic index treatment may also provide a more liberal dietary therapy for intractable epilepsy.[78] This approach permits greater total intake of carbohydrate than the traditional ketogenic diet but uses foods with a relatively low glycemic index (ie, foods that produce a relatively low increase in blood glucose per gram of carbohydrate). Among 20 children on a low-glycemic index treatment at 1- or 3-month follow-up, 52% had >90% reduction, 16% had 50% to 90% reduction, 21% had <50% reduction, and 11% had no reduction in seizure frequency compared with baseline.[78] Reductions in seizure frequency on the modified Atkins diet and low-glycemic index treatment suggest that successful dietary therapy for epilepsy may not require ketosis at the level once thought necessary. These observations have interesting implications for the possible mechanisms of action of the ketogenic diet.

Conclusions

The ketogenic diet is the most effective available treatment for intractable epilepsy, although it carries with it a significant risk of adverse effects. An expert ketogenic team is required to ameliorate this risk and to guide patients and families through diet initiation and maintenance. Parents should attempt the ketogenic diet only with the guidance of an experienced dietitian, neurologist, and support staff.

References

1. Bailey EE, Pfeifer HH, Thiele EA. The use of diet in the treatment of epilepsy. *Epilepsy Behav.* 2005;6:4–8

2. Wheless JW. History and origin of the ketogenic diet. In: Stafstrom CE, Rho JM, eds. *Epilepsy and the Ketogenic Diet.* Totowa, NJ: Humana Press; 2004:31–50

3. Kossoff EH, McGrogan JR. Worldwide use of the ketogenic diet. *Epilepsia.* 2005;46:280–289

4. Cullingford TE. Molecular regulation of ketogenesis. In: Stafstrom CE, Rho JM, eds. *Epilepsy and the Ketogenic Diet.* Totowa, NJ: Humana Press; 2004:201–215

5. Nordli DR, DeVivo DC. Effects of the ketogenic diet on cerebral energy metabolism. In: Stafstrom CE, Rho JM, eds. *Epilepsy and the Ketogenic Diet.* Totowa, NJ: Humana Press; 2004:179–184

6. Mitchell GA, Fukao T. Inborn errors of ketone body metabolism. In: Scriver CR, Beaudet AL, Sly WS, Valle D, eds. *The Metabolic and Molecular Bases of Inherited Disease.* Vol 2. 8th ed. New York, NY: The McGraw-Hill Companies; 2001:2327–2356

7. Sankar R, Sotero de Menezes. Metabolic and endocrine aspects of the ketogenic diet. *Epilepsy Res.* 1999;37:191–201

8. Williamson DH. Ketone body metabolism during development. *Fed Proc.* 1985;44:2342–2346

9. De Vivo DC, Bohin TP, Coulter DL, et al. L-carnitine supplementation in childhood epilepsy: current perspectives. *Epilepsia.* 1998;39:1216–1225

10. Freeman J, Veggiotti P, Lanzi G, Tagliabue A, Perucca E. The ketogenic diet: from molecular mechanisms to clinical effects. Institute of Neurology IRCSS C. Mondino Foundation. *Epilepsy Res.* 2006;68:145–180

11. Greene AE, Todorova MT, Seyfried TN. Perspectives on the metabolic management of epilepsy through dietary reduction of glucose and elevation of ketone bodies. *J Neurochem.* 2003;86:529–537

12. Likhodii SS, Burnham WM. The effects of ketone bodies on neuronal excitability. In: Stafstrom CE, Rho JM, eds. *Epilepsy and the Ketogenic Diet.* Totowa, NJ: Humana Press; 2004:217–228

13. Thio LL, Wong M, Yamada KA. Ketone bodies do not directly alter excitatory or inhibitory hippocampal synaptic transmission. *Neurology.* 2000;54:325–331

14. Yudkoff M, Daikhin Y, Nissim I, Nissim I. The ketogenic diet: interactions with brain amino acid handling. In: Stafstrom CE, Rho JM, eds. *Epilepsy and the Ketogenic Diet.* Totowa, NJ: Humana Press; 2004:185–199

15. Al-Mudallal AS, LaManna JC, Lust WD, Harik SI. Diet-induced ketosis does not cause cerebral acidosis. *Epilepsia.* 1996;37:258–261

16. Vamecq J, Vallee L, Lesage F, Gressens P, Stables JP. Antiepileptic popular ketogenic diet: emerging twists in an ancient story [review]. *Prog Neurobiol.* 2005;75:1–28

17. Eun SH, Kang HC, Kim DW, Kim HD. Ketogenic diet for treatment of infantile spasms. *Brain Dev.* 2006;28:566–571

18. Kossoff EH, Pyzik PL, McGrogan JR, Vining EP, Freeman JM. Efficacy of the ketogenic diet for infantile spasms. *Pediatrics.* 2002;109:780–783

19. Maydell BV, Wyllie E, Akhtar N, et al. Efficacy of the ketogenic diet in focal versus generalized seizures. *Pediatr Neurol.* 2001;25:208–212

20. Trevathan E. Infantile spasms and Lennox-Gastaut syndrome. *J Child Neurol.* 2002;17 (Suppl 2):2S9–2S22

21. Caraballo RH, Cersosimo RO, Sakr D, Cresta A, Escobal N, Fejerman N. Ketogenic diet in patients with Dravet syndrome. *Epilepsia.* 2005;46:1539–1544

22. Caraballo RH, Cerosimo RO, Sakr D, Cresta A, Escobal N, Fejerman N. Ketogenic diet in patients with myoclonic-astatic epilepsy. *Epileptic Disord.* 2006;8:151–155

23. Coppola G, Klepper J, Ammendola E, et al. The effects of the ketogenic diet in refractory partial seizures with reference to tuberous sclerosis. *Eur J Pediatr Neurol.* 2006;10:148–151

24. Kossoff EG, Thiele EA, Pfeifer HH, McGrogan JR, Freeman JM. Tuberous sclerosis complex and the ketogenic diet. *Epilepsia.* 2005;46:1684–1686

25. Rubenstein JE, Kossoff EH, Pyzik PL, Vining EP, McGrogan JR, Freeman JM. Experience in the use of the ketogenic diet as early therapy. *J Child Neurol.* 2005;20:31–34

26. Nordli DR Jr, Kuroda MM, Carroll J, et al. Experience with the ketogenic diet in infants. *Pediatrics.* 2001;108:129–133

27. Sperling MR, Nei M. The ketogenic diet in adults. In: Stafstrom CE, Rho JM, eds. *Epilepsy and the Ketogenic Diet.* Totowa, NJ: Humana Press; 2004:103–109

28. Mady MA, Kossoff EH, McGregor AL, Wheless JW, Pyzik PL, Freeman JM. The ketogenic diet: adolescents can do it, too. *Epilepsia.* 2003;44:847–851

29. Sirven J, Whedon B, Caplan D, et al. The ketogenic diet for intractable epilepsy in adults: preliminary results. *Epilepsia.* 1999;40:1721–1726

30. Wexler ID, Hemalatha SG, McConnell J, et al. Outcome of pyruvate dehydrogenase deficiency treated with ketogenic diets. Studies in patients with identical mutations. *Neurology.* 1997;49:1655–1661

31. Wang D, Pascual JM, Yang H, et al. Glut-1 deficiency syndrome: clinical, genetic, and therapeutic aspects. *Ann Neurol.* 2005;57:111–118

32. Klepper J, Scheffer H, Leiendecker B, et al. Seizure control and acceptance of the ketogenic diet in GLUT1 deficiency syndrome: a 2- to 5-year follow-up of 15 children enrolled prospectively. *Neuropediatrics.* 2005;36:302–308

33. Yancy WS Jr, Foy M, Chalecki AM, Vernon MC, Westman EC. A low-carbohydrate, ketogenic diet to treat type 2 diabetes. *Nutr Metab (Lond).* 2005;2:34

34. Mavropoulos JC, Yancy WS, Hepburn J, Westman EC. The effects of a low-carbohydrate, ketogenic diet on the polycystic ovary syndrome: a pilot study. *Nutr Metab (Lond).* 2005;2:35

35. Evangeliou A, Vlachonikolis I, Mihailidou H, et al. Application of a ketogenic diet in children with autistic behavior: pilot study. *J Child Neurol.* 2003;18:113–118

36. Yaroslavsky Y, Stahl Z, Belmaker RH. Ketogenic diet in bipolar illness. *Bipolar Disord.* 2002;4:75

37. Seyfried TN, Sanderson TM, El-Abbadi MM, McGowan R, Mukherjee P. Role of glucose and ketone bodies in the metabolic control of experimental brain cancer. *Br J Cancer.* 2003;89:1375–1382

38. Nebeling LC, Miraldi F, Shurin SB, Lerner E. Effects of a ketogenic diet on tumor metabolism and nutritional status in pediatric oncology patients: two case reports. *J Am Coll Nutr.* 1995;14:202–208

39. Thiele EA. Assessing the efficacy of antiepileptic treatments: the ketogenic diet. *Epilepsia.* 2003;44(Suppl 7):26–29

40. Lyczkowski DA, Pfeifer HH, Ghosh S, Thiele EA. Safety and tolerability of the ketogenic diet in pediatric epilepsy: effects of valproate combination therapy. *Epilepsia.* 2005;46:1533–1538

41. Kang HC, Kim JY, Kim DW, Kim HD. Efficacy and safety of the ketogenic diet for intractable childhood epilepsy: Korean multicentric experience. *Epilepsia.* 2005;46:272–279

42. DiMario FJ, Holland J. The ketogenic diet: a review of the experience at Connecticut Children's Medical Center. *Pediatr Neurol.* 2002;26:288–292

43. Coppola G, Veggiotti P, Cusmai R, et al. The ketogenic diet in children, adolescents and young adults with refractory epilepsy: an Italian multicentric experience. *Epilepsy Res.* 2002;48:221–227

44. Vining EP, Freeman JM, Ballaban-Gil K, et al. A multicenter study of the efficacy of the ketogenic diet. *Arch Neurol.* 1998;55:1433–1437

45. Levy R, Cooper P. Ketogenic diet for epilepsy [review]. *Cochrane Database Syst Rev.* 2003;(3):CD001903

46. Freeman JM, Vining EP, Pillas DJ, Pyzik PL, Casey JC, Kelly LM. The efficacy of the ketogenic diet-1998: a prospective evaluation of intervention in 150 children. *Pediatrics.* 1998;102:1358–1363

47. Pulsifer MB, Gordon JM, Brandt J, Vining EP, Freeman JM. Effects of ketogenic diet on development and behavior: preliminary report of a prospective study. *Dev Med Child Neurol.* 2001;43:301–306

48. Bergqvist AGC. Indications and contraindications of the ketogenic diet. In: Stafstrom CE, Rho JM, eds. *Epilepsy and the Ketogenic Diet.* Totowa, NJ: Humana Press; 2004:111–121

49. DeVivo DC, Haymond MW, Leckie MP, Bussman YL, McDougal DB Jr, Pagliara AS. The clinical and biochemical implications of pyruvate carboxylase deficiency. *J Clin Endocrinol Metab.* 1977;45:1281–1296

50. DeVivo DC, Pagliara AS, Prensky AL. Ketotic hypoglycemia and the ketogenic diet. *Neurology.* 1973;23:640–649

51. Takeoka M, Riviello JJ Jr, Pfeifer H, Thiele EA. Concomitant treatment with topiramate and ketogenic diet in pediatric epilepsy. *Epilepsy.* 2002;43:1072–1075

52. Taillan KB, Nahata MC, Tsao CY. Role of the ketogenic diet in children with intractable seizures. *Ann Pharmacother.* 1998;32:349–361

53. Furth SL, Casey JC, Pyzik PL, et al. Risk factors for urolithiasis in children on the ketogenic diet. *Pediatr Nephrol.* 2000;15:125–128

54. Kossoff EH, Pyzik PL, Furth SL, Hladky HD, Freeman JM, Vining EP. Kidney stones, carbonic anhydrase inhibitors, and the ketogenic diet. *Epilepsia.* 2002;43:1168–1171

55. Ballaban-Gil K, Callahan C, O'Dell C, Pappo M, Moshé S, Shinnar S. Complications of the ketogenic diet. *Epilepsia.* 1998;39:744–748

56. Kang HC, Cheung DE, Kim DW, Kim HD. Early- and late-onset complications of the ketogenic diet for intractable epilepsy. *Epilepsia.* 2004;45:1116–1123

57. Woody RC, Steele RW, Knapple WL, Pilkington NS Jr. Impaired neutrophil function in children with seizures treated with the ketogenic diet. *J Pediatr.* 1989;115:427–430

58. Stewart WA, Gordon K, Camfield P. Acute pancreatitis causing death in a child on the ketogenic diet. *J Child Neurol.* 2001;16:682

59. Best TH, Franz DN, Gilbert DL, Nelson DP, Epstein MR. Cardiac complications in patients on the ketogenic diet. *Neurology.* 2000;54:2328–2330

60. Peterson SJ, Tangney CC, Pimentel-Zablah EM, Hjelmgren B, Booth G, Berry-Kravis E. Changes in growth and seizure reduction in children on the ketogenic diet as a treatment for intractable epilepsy. *J Am Diet Assoc.* 2005;105:718–725

61. Liu YM, Williams S, Basualdo-Hammond C, Stephens D, Curtis R. A prospective study: growth and nutritional status of children treated with the ketogenic diet. *J Am Diet Assoc.* 2003;103:707–712

62. Vining EP, Pyzik P, McGrogan J, et al. Growth of children on the ketogenic diet. *Dev Med Child Neurol.* 2002;44:796–802

63. Williams S, Basualdo-Hammond C, Curtis R, Schuller R. Growth retardation in children with epilepsy on the ketogenic diet: a retrospective chart review. *J Am Diet Assoc.* 2002;102:405–407

64. Couch SC, Schwarzman F, Carroll J, et al. Growth and nutritional outcomes of children treated with the ketogenic diet. *J Am Diet Assoc.* 1999;99:1573–1575

65. Kielb S, Koo HP, Bloom DA, Faerber GJ. Nephrolithiasis associated with the ketogenic diet. *J Urol.* 2000;164:464–466

66. Kwiterovich PO Jr, Vining EP, Pyzik P, Skolasky R Jr, Freeman JM. Effect of a high-fat ketogenic diet on plasma levels of lipids, lipoproteins, and apolipoproteins in children. *JAMA.* 2003;290:912–920

67. Freeman JM, Freeman JB, Kelly MT. *The Ketogenic Diet: A Treatment for Epilepsy.* 3rd ed. New York, NY: Demos Medical Publishing; 2000

68. Bergqvist AGC, Schall JI, Gallagher PR, Cnaan A, Stallings VA. Fasting versus gradual initiation of the ketogenic diet: a prospective, randomized clinical trial of efficacy. *Epilepsia.* 2005;46:1810–1819

69. Kim DW, Kang HC, Park JC, Kim HD. Benefits of the nonfasting ketogenic diet compared with the initial fasting ketogenic diet. *Pediatrics.* 2004;114:1627–1630

70. Wirrell EC, Darwish HZ, Williams-Dyjur C, Blackman M, Lange V. Is a fast necessary when initiating the ketogenic diet? *J Child Neurol.* 2002;17:179–182

71. Vaisleib II, Buchhalter JR, Zupanc ML. Ketogenic diet: outpatient initiation, without fluid, or caloric restrictions. *Pediatr Neurol.* 2004;31:198–202

72. Gilbert DL, Pyzik PL, Freeman JM. The ketogenic diet: seizure control correlates better with serum beta-hydroxybutyrate than with urine ketones. *J Child Neurol.* 2000;15:787–790

73. Karvelas G, Lebel D, Carmant L. The carbohydrate and caloric content of drugs [Appendix A]. In: Stafstrom CE, Rho JM, eds. *Epilepsy and the Ketogenic Diet.* Totowa, NJ: Humana Press; 2004:311–344

74. McGhee B, Katyal N. Avoid unnecessary drug-related carbohydrates for patients consuming the ketogenic diet. *J Am Diet Assoc.* 2001;101:87–101

75. Hemingway C, Freeman JM, Pillas DJ, Pyzik PL. The ketogenic diet: a 3- to 6-year follow-up of 150 children enrolled prospectively. *Pediatrics.* 2001;108:898–905

76. Huttenlocher PR, Wilbourn AJ, Signore JM. Medium-chain triglycerides as a therapy for intractable childhood epilepsy. *Neurology.* 1971;21:1097–1103

77. Kossoff EH, McGrogan JR, Bluml RM, Pillas DJ, Rubenstein JE, Vining EP. A modified Atkins diet is effective for the treatment of pediatric epilepsy. *Epilepsia.* 2006;47:421–424

78. Pfeifer HH, Thiele EA. Low-glycemic-index treatment: a liberalized ketogenic diet for treatment of intractable epilepsy. *Neurology.* 2005;65:1810–1812

Introduction

The oral health of children living in industrialized countries has improved over the last 2 decades in a remarkable way, but there are many children who continue to suffer the effects of dental decay.[1] By kindergarten age, 40% of children have experienced early childhood caries (ECC).[2] It has been reported that ECC is 5 times more common than asthma.[3] Segments of the population continue to experience a disproportionate amount of caries and have a difficult time obtaining care. Children who experience ECC tend to remain at high risk of caries in the primary as well as the permanent dentition. Children have a 32 times greater chance of having caries by 3 years of age if they come from a low socioeconomic background, eat sugary foods, and have a mother with a low education level.[4]

Dental Caries—An Infectious Disease

The group of cariogenic bacteria that is well established to have the highest association with caries is *Streptococcus mutans*. These bacteria are not detectable in children's mouths until the teeth have begun eruption. The predominant source of this infection seems to be associated with the mother's saliva. Studies have shown that mothers with high concentrations of salivary *S mutans* tended to have children with high concentrations. This places the child at a high risk of developing caries. Dental caries is an infectious disease. These findings give support for the need to address oral issues and preventive measures in mothers during their pregnancy in hopes of reducing the mother's overall concentrations of *S mutans*.

As the carbohydrate intake increases, *S mutans* colonizes in plaque and metabolizes carbohydrates, creating an acidic environment. This provides for a drop in the plaque pH, and demineralization of the enamel can occur. Saliva serves an important role as a buffering agent by remineralizing the demineralized enamel. Saliva provides calcium and phosphate minerals, which increases remineralization. In addition, the presence of fluoride helps in the formation of fluoridated hydroxyapatite and fluorapatite. Both of these are less soluble than hydroxyapatite when placed in an acidic environment. If demineralization exceeds remineralization over time, cavitation of the enamel surface will occur, leading to frank caries. As the carious lesion continues to grow in size, eventually the pulp/nerve of the tooth will become involved, leading to pain, infection, early tooth loss, and potential crowding problems. Severe dental infections can lead to hospitalizations and emergency surgeries for removal of infected teeth.

Dietary Influences

Early childhood caries, in many cases, is thought to be the result of the inappropriate use of a bottle or sippy cup while sleeping or its unsupervised use during the day with a liquid other than water. Early childhood caries usually affects the maxillary anterior teeth first, followed by the primary molars. The lower anterior teeth are usually not involved because of the protective nature of the tongue. A study by Kaste and Gift[5] demonstrated that approximately 95% of children 6 months to 5 years of age have used a bottle at some time, with nearly 20% of these children using a bottle in bed with contents other than water. More than 8% of children 2 to 5 years of age still used a bottle. Most infant formulas have been shown to be acidogenic and promote the development of caries.[6]

There have also been reports of ECC associated with at-will breastfeeding. The role at-will breastfeeding plays in contributing to ECC has been controversial. Although there have been some studies that have implicated this practice with caries, this may be misleading if the remainder of the child's diet is overlooked. On the basis of a study by Erickson et al[7] (Table 48.1), breastfeeding alone did not cause any significant decrease in the pH of plaque and was found not to be cariogenic in an in vitro study. Human milk was demonstrated to be a poor buffering agent when acid from other carbohydrate sources were added. With the addition of sucrose to human milk, the rate of in vitro caries formation was faster than for sucrose alone. It was concluded from this study that human milk alone was not cariogenic. However, if a child is given a sugar-rich food in combination with on-demand breastfeeding, the combination is highly cariogenic. Once the first tooth erupts, the American Academy of Pediatric Dentistry (AAPD) recommends that breastfeeding should be limited to normal meal times and not at will while sleeping.[8] Because of the decrease in salivary flow during sleep, there is a decrease in the clearance of sugars from formula, human milk, juices, etc by saliva in the mouth. This, in-turn, allows these substrates to have an increased cariogenic effect.

In the United States by the 1 year of age, almost 90% of infants have been introduced to fruit juice. Some juice products have been shown to

Table 48.1
Relative Decay Potential of Beverages[4,6,7]

Source Relative Decay Potential	
Standards	
Water	0.00
10% sucrose solution	1.00
Human milk	
Human milk alone	0.01
Human milk with 10% sucrose	1.30
Formula*	
Enfamil ProSobee LIPIL[†]	1.11
Isomil Advance[‡]	0.79
Enfamil LactoFree LIPIL[†]	0.68
Nestlé Good Start 2 Supreme[§]	0.62
Enfamil LIPIL[†]	0.57
Enfamil Next Step LIPIL[†]	0.51
Similac Advance[‡]	0.51
Nestlé Good Start Supreme[§]	0.01
Nutramigen LIPIL[†]	0.01
Other beverages	
Yo-J[∥] (yogurt-based drink)	0.32
Apple juice	0.80
Orange juice	0.85
Grape juice	0.74
Fruit drinks (10% juices)	0.93
Soft drinks ("soda" or "pop")	1.05

* The Committee on Nutrition recommends the use of iron-supplemented (not low-iron supplemented) formulas for infants being fed formula.

[†] Mead Johnson, Evansville, IN.

[‡] Abbott Nutrition, Columbus, OH.

[§] Nestlé, Glendale, CA.

[∥] Kemps LLC, St Paul, MN.

contain more sugar than some soft drinks.[9] Juice should be limited to 4 to 6 oz per day in children younger than 5 years.[10,11] Sucrose, glucose, and fructose found in fruit juices are probably the main sugars associated with

ECC. A study by Neff[12] suggests that fructose and glucose are as cariogenic as sucrose in their abilities to cause a decrease in the oral pH. In addition, starchy foods, such as breads or biscuits, have been shown to cause a variable pH decrease. As the levels of starch increased, the acid production found in plaque also increased.[13]

The frequency of eating and drinking also plays a role in the decay process for children. Children who are constantly snacking and drinking sugar-containing substances are at higher risk of developing caries than are children who eat 3 meals and few snacks per day. The more frequent the dietary intake, the greater the risk of caries. The amount of calories that can be attributed to sugars has increased by 16% between 1982 and 1996. Today, 155 pounds of sugar are eaten by the average person annually, which is equivalent to 39 teaspoonfuls per day.[9] Consumption of soft drinks has been on the rise, with 56% to 85% of children in school consuming at least 1 serving of soda each day and some children consuming even greater amounts.[14] Between 1989 and 1995, the consumption of carbonated beverages has increased by 41% in children 12 to 17 years of age. These increased amounts of soda, which have no nutritional value, can cause intake of needed nutrients, such as vitamin A, calcium, magnesium, and B vitamins, not to be adequate because of less consumption of whole milk.[9] Between 1965 and 1996, the intake of dairy products has decreased by as much as 30% with the amount of soft drinks doubling.[15]

With the high sugar content that oral bacteria are able to metabolize to acid and the highly acidic nature of soft drinks (even diet drinks), demineralization of the teeth occurs, eventually leading to tooth decay.[14] Studies by Erickson et al (Table 48.1)[6,7] have demonstrated the decay potential of several beverages, including formulas. Parents must be reminded that their child should not use a bottle or sippy cup containing these sweetened drinks during leisure activities around the house. These drinks should be limited to meal and snack times only.

The teeth are most susceptible to caries the first few years after their eruption because of their immaturity. In addition to the lack of maturation of the teeth, there could be a possibility that the teeth may have actual structural defects or hypoplastic areas. This could be the result of hereditary diseases, birth trauma, preterm birth and low birthweight, infections, malnutrition, metabolic disorders, and chemical toxicity.[16] Enamel defects can be common in newborn infants, ranging from 12.8% in children weighing >2500 g to more than 62% in those born preterm with very low birth weight (<1500 g).[17] In children intubated at birth, left-sided defects of the maxillary anterior teeth occurred twice as frequently as right-sided defects. Defects were noted to have occurred in

85% of the 40 intubated children in this study, compared with approximately 22% of nonintubated children.[18] Chronically ill children are also at high risk of developing ECC. These children can have increased enamel hypoplastic areas as well. In addition, many of these children may be comforted with bottles containing sweetened liquids or frequently ingest medications that have high sugar content. This allows the teeth to be surrounded by a constant source of sugar, leading to rapid demineralization of the enamel. Enamel erosions have also been reported in children with gastroesophageal reflux disease.

Poor nutritional intake has resulted not only in ECC but also an increase in childhood obesity. The American Academy of Pediatrics (AAP) has stated that the prevalence of overweight children has been on the increase.[19] Data collected from the National Health and Nutrition Examination Survey from 1999–2000 demonstrated that 13% of children 6 to 11 years of age were overweight, which more than tripled the numbers noted in a similar survey from 1971–1974. This increase in weight can partially be attributed to foods that are packaged for convenience, making them easy targets for snacking. Many of them contain sucrose and other refined carbohydrates that are highly cariogenic, leading not only to weight gain but also caries.[20]

In counseling these patients, it is important that bad habits be dealt with as early as possible to limit the possible lifetime implications. It is important to attempt to achieve goals one step at a time rather than trying to change everything at once. Reinforcement of the risks of poor dietary habits may help to change poor behavior. Finally, showing families alternatives and how to accomplish good dietary habits may provide better long-term success than just telling them what not to do.[11]

The Costs Are Enormous

The prevalence of caries in 3- to 5-year-olds in the US Head Start program has been reported as high as 90% in some groups.[21] Untreated dental decay leads to pain, poor eating, infection, speech problems, crowding of the permanent teeth, and self-esteem issues. In a study by Acs,[22] 8.7% of children with ECC weighed less than 80% of their ideal weight, compared with only 1.7% of the control group. In addition, 19.1% of children with ECC were in the 10th percentile or less for weight, compared with only 7% of the control group. ECC has also been implicated in contributing to other health problems, such as otitis media.

Many times, treatment for ECC has to be completed in the operating room under general anesthesia because of the amount of treatment required and the situational anxiety of the child. The costs of dental treatment in a hospital setting can be very expensive. Not only can treatment of ECC be expensive to society, but also, the child's overall health and well-being can be compromised.

Nutritional Effects

The teeth may reflect nutritional disturbances that occur during their formation. Tooth development begins during the second month of embryonic life, and by 8 years of age, the crowns of all permanent teeth except the third molars are formed. Enamel and dentin have no powers of biologic regeneration, and any defect in their structure is permanent.

A published longitudinal study[23] of Peruvian children confirmed previous studies in animals and indirect epidemiologic evidence in humans that suggested a cause-and-effect relationship between early malnutrition and increased dental caries. The study also reported the eruption of primary teeth was significantly delayed.

Vitamin A deficiency during tooth formation is reported to interfere with calcification and result in hypoplasia of the enamel. The effect of vitamin C deficiency in humans occurs chiefly in the gingival and periodontal tissues. The gingiva is bright red with a swollen, smooth, shiny surface that may become boggy, ulcerate, and bleed.

When vitamin D deficiency occurs during childhood, eruption of the deciduous and permanent teeth is delayed, and the sequence of eruption is disturbed. Histologically, widening of the predentin layer, the presence of interglobular dentin, and interference with enamel formation has been reported. Some authors report hypoplasia of the enamel with a symmetrical distribution of thinning and pitting enamel defects.

In riboflavin deficiency, glossitis begins with soreness of the tip and lateral margins of the tongue. The tongue surface appears reddened and coarsely granular. The lips are pale, and cheilosis develops at the oral commissures.

Niacin deficiency leads to pellagra. In the acute stages, the oral mucosa becomes fiery red and painful, accompanied by profuse salivation. As pellagra progresses, the epithelium of the tongue sloughs.[24]

Fluoride Background

Water fluoridation was named as one of the top 10 public health achievements in the 20th century by the Centers for Disease Control and Prevention. Since the introduction of fluoride through water fluoridation and topical fluorides, there has been a significant reduction in caries. Studies have shown that caries in the primary teeth of children have decreased by as much as 60%. Fluoride has been shown to reduce dental decay by 3 specific mechanisms: (1) it reduces the solubility of enamel; (2) it reduces the bacteria's ability to produce acid; and (3) it promotes remineralization. At one time, fluoride was thought to exert a pre-eruptive effect on teeth through the use of prenatal fluoride, but now it is generally accepted that its main benefit is topical in nature. Systemically, fluoride exerts its topical effects through secretion from the salivary glands.

Fluoridation protects more than 170 million individuals throughout the United States. By 2010, it is hoped that 75% of the United States water supply will be fluoridated. The benefits of fluoridation extend across all ethnic groups and income and education levels. The cost of water fluoridation is $0.50/person annually in larger communities and $3.00/person annually in smaller ones.[25]

Fluoride Supplements

For children living in a fluoride-deficient area, fluoride supplements may be of some benefit. Table 48.2 shows the most recent guidelines on fluoride supplementation that have been accepted by the American Dental Association, AAPD, and AAP.[26]

Table 48.2
Fluoride Supplementation Schedule*[26]

Age	Fluoride Concentration in Local Water Supply, ppm		
	<0.3	0.3–0.6	>0.6
Birth–6 mo	0.00	0.00	0.00
6 mo–3 y	0.25	0.00	0.00
3–6 y	0.50	0.25	0.00
6 y–at least 16 y	1.00	0.50	0.00

* Must know fluoride values of drinking water prior to making a prescription. All values are mg of fluoride supplement/day.

When considering whether a fluoride supplement is needed, more time should be spent considering all sources of fluoride that a child may have access to on a given day. Allowing the sole fact of no fluoride in the community water to dictate the need for a fluoride prescription may be premature and lead to an overall underestimation of the child's total fluoride intake on a daily basis. For example, a child may be living in a nonfluoridated community but attend school in an area where fluoride is at optimal levels. If the fluoride content of a child's water source is unknown, then it is important to have the water tested at a local laboratory for the fluoride content before prescribing a fluoride supplement. Foods and beverages that are processed in communities with optimally fluoridated water are consumed not only in the area where they are processed but also can be shipped to a neighboring community that is nonfluoridated. This added benefit of fluoride is termed the "halo" or "diffusion" effect and can benefit people in nonfluoridated communities. A child's overall risk of decay should also be considered before prescribing a fluoride supplement.

As a result of the widespread availability of fluoride, the difference in the decay rate in communities with fluoridated water compared with those that are not fluoridated has lessened. According to Burt, the question was raised as to the need for fluoride supplements in the United States, given the fact that fluoride can be found in so many various sources, such as drinking water, toothpaste, gels, rinses, professionally applied fluorides, and processed foods and beverages. The argument was made that the evidence for the benefit of fluoride supplements when used from birth or soon after was weak and that supplements were a risk factor for fluorosis.[27] It is essential, as ways to reduce caries are devised, that the risks of fluorosis are minimized. Given that as a guideline, it could be concluded that the risk of using fluoride supplements outweigh the benefits, because the risk of fluorosis has been proven.

Some may argue that fluoride supplements should not be eliminated. Moss states that dietary supplements alone are unlikely to be the cause of the reported increase in fluorosis because compliance continues to be extremely poor.[28] Other authors have also noted the lack of compliance of patients with prescriptions.[29,30] In addition, few children use supplements for more than a year and a half at best.[28] Horowitz states[29] that it would be wrong in his opinion to eliminate the availability of dietary fluoride supplementation as a caries-preventive regimen. Many children are still at high risk of dental caries, and for a variety of reasons, may not have access to fluoridated drinking water or professionally administered fluoride regimens. He goes on to say that postponing the use of fluoride supplements until 2 or 3 years of age, as some propose, will reduce the supplements' potential effectiveness in caries prevention. Some studies have shown the greatest benefit for the primary and permanent teeth is when fluoride supplements are given before 2 years of age.[31] In addition, Horowitz feels that a downward revision in dosage is very different than the recommendation for the elimination of fluoride supplements altogether.[29]

Prescriptions for supplemental fluoride should be specific about when and how the supplement is to be given. Fluoride ingested on an empty stomach is 100% bioavailable, whereas fluoride administered with milk or a meal will not be completely absorbed. The best time to administer the supplement is at bedtime or at least 1 hour before eating.[32]

Another factor that may need to be considered in assessing a child's total fluoride exposure is the increasing popularity of bottled water and home water-filtration systems. The question that arises is what effect these may have on the total fluoride content. The majority of bottled water sold on the market today does not contain adequate amounts of fluoride (0.7–1.2 ppm). In a 1991 study of 39 different bottled water brands, 34 of them had fluoride levels less than 0.3 ppm.[33] Home water-treatment systems also have the ability to reduce fluoride levels. It has been well established that reverse osmosis and distillation units remove significant amounts of fluoride. Therefore, it is conceivable that a preschool child could live in an optimally fluoridated area but not receive adequate amounts of fluoride. A common type of home water-filtration is the carbon or charcoal filter systems. Generally, they do not remove significant levels of fluoride. Studies have also shown that water softeners caused no significant changes in fluoride levels.[34,35] The optimum concentration of fluoride in the drinking water ranges from 0.7 to 1.2 ppm. These ranges effectively reduce dental decay while minimizing the risk of dental fluorosis.

Fluorosis

How much fluoride a child should receive on a daily basis varies with both age and body weight. Table 48.3[36] demonstrates the adequate intake of fluoride from all sources on a daily basis to be 0.05 mg/kg per day. This is the amount of fluoride needed for optimal health without the risk of fluorosis. It has been calculated by gender and age group. The maximum level has been set at 0.10 mg/kg per day for infants, toddlers, and children up to 8 years of age. For older children who are not at risk of fluorosis, the upper limit has been set at 10 mg/day.

Over the past several years, an increase in enamel fluorosis has been noted in both optimally fluoridated and nonfluoridated areas. Fluorosis is the result of too much fluoride and affects approximately 22% of children. Of these children, 94% have only a very mild to mild form of fluorosis.[25]

This condition results in a change in the appearance of the teeth when higher-than-optimal levels of fluoride are ingested before 7 years of age during the calcification stage of tooth development. Dental fluorosis is a cosmetic effect with few known health problems. The risk of fluorosis can be greatly reduced by proper supervision of children around the use of fluoride-containing products. Clinically, fluorosis can range from minor white lines running across the teeth to a more severe form that exhibits a very chalky appearance with possible pitting and brown staining.

Table 48.3
Dietary Reference Intake for Fluoride

Age Group	Adequate Intake (mg/day)	Tolerable Upper Intake (mg/day)
Infants 0–6 mo	0.01	0.7
Infants 7–12 mo	0.5	0.9
Children 1–3 y	0.7	1.3
Children 4–8 y	1.0	2.2
Children 9–13 y	2.0	10
Boys 14–18 y	2.0	10
Girls 14–18 y	3.0	10
Males 19 y and older	4.0	10
Females 19 y and older	3.0	10

Institute of Medicine. *Dietary Reference Intakes for Calcium, Phosphorous, Magnesium, Vitamin D, and Fluoride.* Washington, DC: National Academies Press; 1997 (see also Appendix J).

One factor that has contributed to the overall increase in fluorosis has been the inappropriate prescribing of fluoride supplements for children already in optimally fluoridated communities. Pendrys[37] found that inappropriate supplementation accounted for 25% of the fluorosis cases of children living in an optimally fluoridated area.

In Europe and Canada, fluoride supplement schedules are used as guidelines for only children considered to be at high risk of caries, and fluoride supplementation does not start until the child reaches 3 years of age.[27] One reason for this may be the fact that there are many alternative forms of fluoride to choose from today.

Many studies over the past few years have shown strong evidence of an association between dental fluorosis and the use of fluoride toothpaste in early childhood. A study conducted in Asheville, North Carolina found that using a fluoride toothpaste before 2 years of age increased a child's chances of developing fluorosis by 3 times.[38] Another study conducted in Canada showed that 72% of the fluorosis cases could be attributed to early fluoride toothpaste use during the first 2 years of life.[39] It is recommended that children should not use fluoridated toothpaste until after reaching the age of 2, and then, only a small pea-sized amount. Over the past several years, many companies have marketed toothpaste with special colors and flavors to increase use by children. There is concern this type of marketing may encourage children to use more toothpaste and potentially ingest significant amounts of fluoride, thereby contributing to dental fluorosis. A study by Adair[40] demonstrated that children used significantly more children's toothpaste than the adult brands and that they brushed their teeth for a longer period of time. His study demonstrated that only approximately 50% of the children expectorated and only approximately 25% rinsed after brushing. The number of children who rinsed and expectorated were even smaller. Parents should be reminded of the need to supervise their preschool children during toothbrushing to ensure that the proper amount of toothpaste is used regardless of whether their water is optimally fluoridated or not. Parents should encourage their children to expectorate and rinse with water as soon as possible to lessen the amount swallowed. Horowitz stated that because nearly all children use fluoride toothpaste and relatively few take fluoride supplements, fluoride toothpaste undoubtedly has had a greater overall effect on the rate of fluorosis in the United States than have fluoride supplements.[29]

Having considered the risks and benefits of fluoride, the idea of assessing the child's overall risk of developing caries becomes important. One can look at the child's previous dental history, the family history, medical complications, diet, hygiene, fluoride status, and use of chronic medications in determining a child's risk of developing caries and the need for a fluoride supplement. The AAPD has also established a Caries-risk Assessment Tool[41] (available at http://aapd.org/media/Policies_Guidelines/P_CariesRiskAssess. pdf) that will help in determining what a child's risk of developing future decay could be and help in forming an overall treatment plan for a child.

Fluoride Toxicity

Although fluoride has been shown to be beneficial, it can be toxic to children if taken in high doses. The acute toxic dose of fluoride has been determined to be 5 mg/kg, for which medical intervention will be necessary. Because most toothpaste products on the market in the United States contain fluoride, it is theoretically possible for a child to ingest enough toothpaste to lead to toxicity. The probable toxic dose for a 1-year-old (10-kg) child is contained in 50 mL of a 1000-ppm fluoride toothpaste. For a 5-year-old (19-kg) child, it is found in 95 mL. For these reasons, parents are to be reminded that close supervision of all fluoride products is essential for their children. Children should be encouraged not to swallow or eat toothpaste. All fluoride products should be stored out of reach of young children. Symptoms include nausea, vomiting, electrolyte imbalance, arrhythmias, central nervous system excitation, and coma followed by death within a few hours.[42]

Role of the Pediatrician

Tooth decay is the most common chronic disease of childhood. Despite the clear importance of health insurance, an estimated 1.3 million children with special health care needs were uninsured during the period of 1994–1995. These children were disproportionately represented among low-income families. It was also pointed out that there are access problems for some children with special health care needs, despite having insurance.[43] Children with dental problems lose more than 51 million school hours annually,[44] and substantial numbers of children with untreated caries are seen in emergency departments around the United States. According to 1 study, 27% of the children that were seen had never been to the dentist. For those that were 3.5 years and younger, this was the first visit for 52% of the children.[45] Only 1 in 5 children covered by Medicaid received preventive oral care for which they were eligible.[46]

The infectious nature of dental caries, its early onset, and the potential of early interventions require an emphasis on preventive oral care in the primary pediatric setting.[46] Most caries in children today occur in approximately 25% of children. These children could greatly benefit from early referral for appropriate care. Pediatric primary health care professionals see many more children than do dentists and can be sure to provide early intervention. An early examination of children may identify children at greatest risk of dental disease. The presence of plaque on the upper front teeth of infants is predictive of future caries. In a study of children 19 months of age, the prevalence of plaque was the best predictor of future caries risk in 91% of the children.[47] Undetected caries can present dramatically if left untreated.

When the decay spreads to the nerve of the tooth, infection can result, leading to a cellulitis.

The AAPD and AAP recommend that all infants obtain an oral health risk assessment by their primary health care professional or other qualified professional by 6 months of age. This risk assessment should be obtained using the Caries-risk Assessment Tool[41] (available at http://aapd.org/media/Policies_Guidelines/P_CariesRiskAssess.pdf). A child should see a dentist by 12 months of age.[8,48]

The number of dentists available to treat young children with significant dental disease is insufficient and eroding, and it is essential for primary health care professionals to help ensure timely oral screenings. Fewer than 3% of dentists are trained as pediatric specialists, and roughly, only 1 pediatric dentist exists for every 15 pediatricians in the United States.[49] There are approximately 4500 practicing pediatric dentists. Over the last 10 years, the AAPD has increased the number of residency training program slots by 100, bringing the total to 280. The goal of reducing children's oral health disparities also supports increased integration of dentistry with medicine and other health disciplines. Children with special health care needs have the potential for significant oral-systemic interactions, which necessitates integrated approaches. Although hospitalized children typically receive complete pediatric examinations, it is rare that their oral health and its effects on the systemic health are fully evaluated.[46] These children require additional oral health promotion efforts by pediatricians if poor oral health and significant oral health problems are to be eliminated. These children face such complex and demanding health care needs, oral health issues tend to be of secondary concern. As a result, these children often suffer avoidable dental problems that further affect the quality of their life. The more demanding a child's medical issues, the more necessary it is to ensure early and timely referral for dental care.[49]

The US Surgeon General David Satcher has called for a national oral health plan to eliminate disparities in oral health for all Americans. Surgeon General Satcher stated, "Everyone has a role in improving and promoting oral health. Together we can work to broaden public understanding of the importance of oral health and its relevance to general heath and well-being, and to ensure that existing and future preventive, diagnostic and treatment measures for oral diseases and disorders are made available to all Americans."[3]

References

1. Nowak AJ. Rationale for the timing of the first oral evaluation. *Pediatr Dent.* 1997;19:8–11

2. Pierce KM, Rozier RG, Vann WF Jr. Accuracy of pediatric primary care providers' screening and referral for early childhood caries. *Pediatrics.* 2002;109(5):e82. Available at: http://pediatrics.aappublications.org/cgi/content/full/109/5/e82. Accessed October 22, 2007

3. Oral health in America: a report of the Surgeon General. *J Calif Dent Assoc.* 2000;28: 685–695

4. Nowak AJ, Warren JJ. Infant oral health and oral habits. *Pediatr Clin North Am.* 2000; 47:1043–1066, vi

5. Kaste LM, Gift HC. Inappropriate infant bottle feeding. Status of the Healthy People 2000 objective. *Arch Pediatr Adolesc Med.* 1995;149:786–791

6. Sheikh C, Erickson PR. Evaluation of plaque pH changes following oral rinse with eight infant formulas. *Pediatr Dent.* May–Jun 1996;18:200–204

7. Erickson PR, Mazhari E. Investigation of the role of human breast milk in caries development. *Pediatr Dent.* Mar–Apr 1999;21:86–90

8. American Academy of Pediatric Dentistry, Clinical Affairs Committee, Infant Oral Health Subcommittee, Council on Clinical Affairs. Guideline on Infant Oral Health Care, Pediatric Dentistry Reference Manual. *Pediatric Dentistry.* 2005–2006;27(7 Reference Manual):68–71

9. Falco MA. The lifetime impact of sugar excess and nutrient depletion on oral health. *Gen Dent.* Nov-Dec 2001;49:591–595

10. American Academy of Pediatrics, Committee on Nutrition. The use and misuse of fruit juice in pediatrics. *Pediatrics.* 2001;107:1210–1213

11. Marshall TA. Diet and nutrition in pediatric dentistry. *Dent Clin North Am.* 2003;47:279–303

12. Neff D. Acid production from different carbohydrate sources in human plaque in situ. *Caries Res.* 1967;1:78–87

13. Mormann JE, Muhlemann HR. Oral starch degradation and its influence on acid production in human dental plaque. *Caries Res.* 1981;15:166–175

14. Kaplowitz G. *The Dangers of Soda Pop.* Academy of Dental Therapeutics and Stomatology; 2004. Available at: http://www.ineedce.com/pdf_files/adts_the_dangers_of_soda_pop.pdf. Accessed November 2, 2007

15. Cavadini C, Siega-Riz AM, Popkin BM. US adolescent food intake trends from 1965 to 1996. *Arch Dis Child.* 2000;83:18–24

16. Seow WK. Enamel hypoplasia in the primary dentition: a review. *ASDC J Dent Child.* 1991; 58:441–452

17. Seow WK, Humphrys C, Tudehope DI. Increased prevalence of developmental dental defects in low birth-weight, prematurely born children: a controlled study. *Pediatr Dent.* 1987;9: 221–225

18. Seow WK, Brown JP, Tudehope DI, O'Callaghan M. Developmental defects in the primary dentition of low birth-weight infants: adverse effects of laryngoscopy and prolonged endotracheal intubation. *Pediatr Dent.* 1984;6:28–31

19. Krebs NF, Jacobson MS, American Academy of Pediatrics, Committee on Nutrition. Prevention of pediatric overweight and obesity. *Pediatrics.* 2003;112:424–430

20. Adair SM. Dietary counseling—time for a nutritionist in the office? *Pediatr Dent*. 2004; 26:389

21. Tinanoff N, O'Sullivan DM. Early childhood caries: overview and recent findings. *Pediatr Dent*. 1997;19:12–16

22. Acs G, Lodolini G, Kaminsky S, Cisneros GJ. Effect of nursing caries on body weight in a pediatric population. *Pediatr Dent*. 1992;14:302–305

23. Alvarez JO, Caceda J, Woolley TW, et al. A longitudinal study of dental caries in the primary teeth of children who suffered from infant malnutrition. *J Dent Res*. 1993;72:1573–1576

24. Shafer WG, Hine MK, Levy BM. *A Textbook of Oral Pathology*. 4th ed. Philadelphia, PA: Saunders; 1983

25. American Dental Association. Fluoridation Facts. Available at: www.ada.org/public/topics/fluoride/facts/index.asp. Accessed October 22, 2007

26. American Academy of Pediatric Dentistry, Council on Clinical Affairs. Guideline on fluoride therapy. *Pediatr Dent*. 2005–2006;27(7 Reference Manual):90–91

27. Burt BA. The case for eliminating the use of dietary fluoride supplements for young children. *J Public Health Dent*. 1999;59:269–274

28. Moss SJ. The case for retaining the current supplementation schedule. *J Public Health Dent*. 1999;59:259–262

29. Horowitz HS. The role of dietary fluoride supplements in caries prevention. *J Public Health Dent*. 1999;59:205–210

30. Adair SM. Overview of the history and current status of fluoride supplementation schedules. *J Public Health Dent*. 1999;59:252–258

31. Mellberg JR, Ripa LW. *Fluoride in Preventive Dentistry: Theory and Clinical Applications*. Chicago, IL: Quintessence Publishing Co; 1983

32. Shulman ER, Vallejo M. Effect of gastric contents on the bioavailability of fluoride in humans. *Pediatr Dent*. 1990;12:237–240

33. Tate WH, Chan JT. Fluoride concentrations in bottled and filtered waters. *Gen Dent*. 1994; 42:362–366

34. Robinson SN, Davies EH, Williams B. Domestic water treatment appliances and the fluoride ion. *Br Dent J*. 1991;171:91–93

35. Warren JJ, Levy SM. Current and future role of fluoride in nutrition. *Dent Clin North Am*. 2003;47:225–243

36. Institute of Medicine. *Dietary Reference Intakes for Calcium, Phosphorus, Magnesium, Vitamin D, and Fluoride*. Washington, DC: National Academies Press; 1997

37. Pendrys DG. Risk of fluorosis in a fluoridated population. Implications for the dentist and hygienist. *J Am Dent Assoc*. 1995;126:1617–1624

38. Lalumandier JA, Rozier RG. The prevalence and risk factors of fluorosis among patients in a pediatric dental practice. *Pediatr Dent*. 1995;17:19–25

39. Osuji OO, Leake JL, Chipman ML, Nikiforuk G, Locker D, Levine N. Risk factors for dental fluorosis in a fluoridated community. *J Dent Res*. 1988;67:1488–1492

40. Adair SM, Piscitelli WP, McKnight-Hanes C. Comparison of the use of a child and an adult dentifrice by a sample of preschool children. *Pediatr Dent*. 1997;19:99–103

41. American Academy of Pediatric Dentistry, Council on Clinical Affairs. Use of a Caries-risk Assessment Tool (CAT) for infants, children, and adolescents. *Pediatric Dentistry Reference Manual*. 2005–2006;27(7 Reference Manual):25–27

42. Whitford GM. Fluoride in dental products: safety considerations. *J Dent Res*. 1987;66: 1056–1060

43. Newacheck PW, McManus M, Fox HB, Hung YY, Halfon N. Access to health care for children with special health care needs. *Pediatrics*. 2000;105:760–766

44. Gift HC, Reisine ST, Larach DC. The social impact of dental problems and visits. *Am J Public Health*. 1992;82:1663–1668

45. Sheller B, Williams BJ, Lombardi SM. Diagnosis and treatment of dental caries-related emergencies in a children's hospital. *Pediatr Dent*. 1997;19:470–475

46. Mouradian WE, Wehr E, Crall JJ. Disparities in children's oral health and access to dental care. *JAMA*. 2000;284:2625–2631

47. Alaluusua S, Malmivirta R. Early plaque accumulation—a sign for caries risk in young children. *Community Dent Oral Epidemiol*. 1994;22:273–276

48. Hale KJ, American Academy of Pediatrics, Section on Pediatric Dentistry. Oral health risk assessment timing and establishment of the dental home. *Pediatrics*. 2003;111:1113–1116

49. Edelstein BL. Public and clinical policy considerations in maximizing children's oral health. *Pediatr Clin North Am*. 2000;47:1177–1189, vii

49 Community Nutrition Services

Promoting the nutritional health of children and their families is a common goal of the nutrition services offered by a wide variety of public and private agencies, organizations, and individuals in communities across the nation. These include federal government agencies; state health and education departments; local health agencies, such as city and county health departments; community health centers; health maintenance and preferred provider organizations; hospital and ambulatory outpatient clinics; nutritionists and dietitians in public and private practice; voluntary health agencies, such as the American Diabetes Association and the American Heart Association; social service agencies; elementary and secondary schools; colleges and universities; and business and industry.

Nutrition Services Provided Through Federal, State, and Local Health and Nutrition Agencies

Each year, Congress appropriates funds for a variety of nutrition and health programs, many of which are targeted to low-income mothers and children. Such programs are administered at the national level by the US Department of Agriculture (USDA) and the US Department of Health and Human Services (DHHS). The USDA services include Child Nutrition Programs (National School Lunch Program, School Breakfast Program, Summer Food Service Program, and Child and Adult Care Food Program), the Special Supplemental Nutrition Program for Women, Infants, and Children (WIC), the Food Stamp Program, and the Commodity Supplemental Food Program. Services of the DHHS include maternal and child health services block grant programs; preventive health services block grant programs; Early and Periodic Screening, Diagnostic, and Treatment (EPSDT) program under Medicaid; Indian Health Services; and programs from the Centers for Disease Control and Prevention (CDC). There are also programs such as community health centers and migrant health projects that serve at-risk populations.[1]

In addition to federal support, considerable state and local funds also support child health programs. An example of a local resource is community-based food programs that are nonprofit, nongovernmental, grass-roots, self-help community developmental programs. One such resource is America's Second Harvest: The Nation's Food Bank Network, which coordinates a vast network of local food pantries and meal programs across the country.

Many of these food programs are tied to other services that low-income mothers and children may need.

Physicians and other primary health care professionals should be knowledgeable about the local food and nutrition programs so they can assist families to become informed consumers and appropriate referrals can be made to food and nutrition programs. An informed health care professional can also serve as an advocate to strengthen policy and budget decisions that guide the provision of quality cost-effective nutrition programs focused on improving the health of the nation.

Although nutrition services were introduced into public health programs as early as the late 1920s, Title V of the Social Security Act of 1935 (Pub L No. 74-721) initiated the federal-state partnership for maternal and child health that served as the major impetus for the development of nutrition services for mothers and children.[2] A census of public health nutrition personnel in 1999–2000 showed that approximately 10 904 public health nutritionists are employed in federal, state, and local public health agencies.[3] Public health nutritionists provide a wide range of services on the basis of core public health functions, which include assessment, assurance, and policy development. These include provision of direct clinical services (eg, screening, assessment, nutrition counseling, monitoring); population-based research; development and implementation of nutrition services and policies that focus on disease prevention and health promotion; provision of technical assistance to a range of providers and consumers; collection and analysis of health-related data, including nutrition surveillance and monitoring; investigation and control of disease, injuries, and responses to natural disasters; protection of the environment, housing, food, water, and workplaces; public information, education, and community mobilization; quality assurance; training and education; leadership, planning, policy development, and administration; targeted outreach and linkage to personal services; and other direct clinical services.[4]

Many community nutrition services include screening, education, counseling, and treatment to improve the nutritional status of an individual or a population. These services are designed to meet the preventive, therapeutic, and rehabilitative health care needs of all segments of the population. The focus of nutrition services in an agency is based on several factors, including the mission of the agency, funding, analysis of data from a community-needs assessment, resources, and politics.[5] Nutrition services are provided in a variety of inpatient and outpatient settings. Public agencies provide nutrition services for individuals throughout the life cycle. The broadest range of nutrition services may be most evident in community-based nutrition programs, in which services are based on the core public health functions. The physician and other primary health care professionals must know where services are provided in their community. Professional and federal resources for nutrition services are listed in Table 49.1. The Maternal and Child Health (MCH) Library at Georgetown University maintains the MCH Organizations Database (www.mchlibrary.info/databases/aboutorg.html), listing more than 2000 government, professional, and voluntary organizations involved in MCH activities primarily at a national level—this is a useful resource for pediatricians and other primary care providers. Qualified providers of nutrition services include physicians, registered dietitians (RDs) and/or licensed dietitians, licensed nutritionists, nurses, and other qualified professionals. The American Dietetic Association (ADA), the largest organization of professional dietitians and nutritionists, has identified qualified providers as the RD and other qualified professionals who meet licensing and other standards prescribed at the state level.[6]

Health and Nutrition Agencies: A Nutrition Resource to Provide Services and Identify Qualified Providers

Federal, state, and local health and nutrition agencies, particularly those employing public health nutritionists, can be helpful resources for physicians and other primary health care professionals. Nutritionists provide extensive technical assistance to clients and their families and physicians, especially for children with special health care needs. One example is services for children with an inborn error of metabolism. The diet prescription includes special medical formulas and foods that are modified to meet medical and socioeconomic needs. The formulas and foods are expensive, and the costs are generally not reimbursed by insurance companies. Many states have provisions for coverage for special formulas and foods.[7] Physicians should contact the special needs program of their state health department for information about patient eligibility for coverage for these formulas and foods and procedures for obtaining them. Another example in which a nutritionist and nutrition services are instrumental in supporting feeding and growth is an early intervention program. In an early intervention program, nutritionists work with the child's family, other team members, and the child's primary health care professional to optimize development from birth to 3 years of age.[8]

Table 49.1
Selected Professional and Federal Resources for Nutrition Services

Selected Professional Nutrition Organizations
American Dietetic Association (ADA) 120 S. Riverside Plaza, Suite 2000 Chicago, IL 60606-6995 Phone: 800-877-1600; Consumer Nutrition Hot Line: 800-366-1655 www.eatright.org
School Nutrition Association (SNA) 700 S. Washington Street, Suite 300 Alexandria, VA 22314 Phone: 703-739-3900; Fax 703-739-3915 www.schoolnutrition.org
Association of State and Territorial Public Health Nutrition Directors PO Box 1001 Johnstown, PA 15907-1001 Phone: 814-255-2829 www.astphnd.org/
National WIC Association 2001 S Street, NW, Suite 580 Washington, DC 20009–3405 Phone: 202-232-5492; fax: 202-387-5281 www.nwica.org/
American Public Human Services Association (APHSA) 810 First Street, NE Suite 500 Washington, DC 20002 Phone: 202-682-0100 Fax: 202-289-6555 www.aphsa.org/Home/home_news.asp
America's Second Harvest 35 E. Wacker Drive, Suite 2000 Chicago, IL 60601 Phone: 800-771-2303 www.secondharvest.org (Web site has a search function to locate local services)
Selected Federal Resources
US Department of Agriculture Resources
US Department of Agriculture Food and Nutrition Service (FNS) 3101 Park Center Drive Alexandria, VA 22302 Phone: 703-305-2062 Information on USDA nutition assistance programs including associated research, nutrition educaion initiatives, such as WIC Loving Support Breastfeeding Campaign, Team Nutrition, Eat Smart Play Hard, State Nutrition Action Plans (SNAP), and Food Stamp Nutrition Education, are found at: http://fns.usda.gov/fns/ Fact sheets on the USDA nutrition assistance programs are available at: http://fns.usda.gov/cga/FactSheets/ProgramFactSheets.htm

Table 49.1 *(Continued)*
Selected Professional and Federal Resources for Nutrition Services

US Department of Agriculture Center for Nutrition Policy and Promotion (CNPP) 3101 Park Center Drive Alexandria, VA 22302 Phone: 703-305-7600 The CNPP develops and promotes dietary guidance that links scientific research to the nutrition needs of consumers. For information on CNPP resources, the Dietary Guidelines for Americans, and MyPyramid, see www.cnpp.usda.gov/.
US Department of Agriculture Cooperative State Research, Education, and Extension Service (CSREES) 1400 Independence Avenue, SW, Stop 2201 Washington, DC 20250-2201 Phone: 202-720-7441 The CSREES provides linkages between federal and state components of a broad-based national agricultural higher education, research, and extension system designed to address national problems and needs related to agriculture, the environment, human health and well-being, and communities; see www.csrees.usda.gov
National Agricultural Library (NAL) US Department of Agriculture Abraham Lincoln Building 10301 Baltimore Avenue Beltsvile, MD 20705-2351 Phone: 301-504-5414 (for FNIC); Fax: 301-504-6409 (for FNIC) The NAL sponsors the Food and Nutrition Information Center (FNIC), the Healthy Meals Resource System for schools and child care programs, the WIC Works Resource System, the Food Stamp Nutrition Connection Resource System, and the USDA/FDA Foodborne Illness Education Information Center. The FNIC/NAL also sponsors the "Nutrition.gov" Web site, which provides easy access to the best food and nutrition information from across the federal government.
US Department of Health and Human Services Resources
Centers for Disease Control and Prevention Division of Nutrition and Physical Activity 4770 Buford Highway, Mailstop K25 Atlanta, GA 30341 Phone: 770-488-6042 Information and resources on infant and child nutrition, physical activity, and the obesity epidemic are available from the CDC Web site at www.cdc.gov/nccdphp/dnpa.
Food and Drug Administration 5600 Fishers Lane Rockville, MD 20857 For general inquiries: 1-888-INFO-FDA (1-888-463-6332) For Office of Public Affairs: 301-827-6250 This Web site is a central source of information about FDA activities and resources and includes a section on consumer advice and publications on food safety and nutrition: www.fda.gov.

V

Table 49.1 *(Continued)*
Selected Professional and Federal Resources for Nutrition Services

The National Center for Education in Maternal and Child Health (NCEMCH) Georgetown University Box 571272 Washington, DC 20057-1272 Phone: 202-784-9770; fax 202-784-9777 Funded by the Maternal and Child Health Bureau, Health Resources and Services Administration, Department of Health and Human Services, the NCEMCH Web site (www.ncemch.org) provides online access to NCEMCH initiatives, educational resources, and publications; a virtual MCH library and MCH databases; bibliographies; and knowledge paths.
US Department of Health and Human Services 200 Independence Avenue, SW Washington, DC 20201 For more information by mail, write: National Health Information Center PO Box 1133 Washington, DC 20013-1133 Phone: 301-565-4167 Toll Free: 1-800-336-4797 The HealthierUS initiative is a national effort, sponsored by the Department of Health and Human Services and the Executive Office of the President, to improve people's lives, prevent and reduce the costs of disease, and promote community health and wellness. See the Web site, which includes information on nutrition, physical activity, and healthy choices: www.Healthier US.gov.
National Heart, Lung, and Blood Institute PO Box 30105 Bethesda, MD 20824-0105 Phone: 301-592-8573 or toll-free 866-35-WECAN *We Can!* or "Ways to Enhance Children's Activity and Nutrition" is a national education program from the National Institutes of Health designed for families and caregivers to help children 8 to 13 years of age achieve a healthy weight. This program offers communities and families resources including materials for healthcare providers, physicians, and parents. See the Web site: http://wecan.nhlbi.nih.gov.
Indian Health Service The Reyes Building 801 Thompson Avenue, Ste. 400 Rockville, MD 20852-1627 Phone: 301-443-1083 For information on how the Indian Health Service works to improve the health of patients with nutrition related diseases, and prevent these illnesses in future generations through interventions in schools, community health programs, and hospital and clinic based services, see the Web site: www.ihs.gov.

The national program for Infants and Toddlers with Disabilities and their Families, created by Congress in 1986 under the Education for All Handicapped Children Act (Pub L No. 99-457), is administered by state agencies. The Education for All Handicapped Children Act was renamed the Individuals with Disabilities Education Act (IDEA) and was amended several times. The most recent amendment to IDEA (Pub L No. 108-446) occurred in December 2004.

To be eligible for services, children must be younger than 3 years and have a confirmed disability or established developmental delay, as defined by the state, in 1 or more of the following areas of development: physical, cognitive, communication, social-emotional, and/or adaptive. A complete evaluation of the child and family must be conducted, at no cost to the family, to determine whether a child is eligible for this early intervention program. The evaluation would include an assessment of the child's nutritional history and dietary intake; anthropometric, biochemical, and clinical variables; feeding skills and feeding problems; and food habits and food preferences. If a child and family are found eligible for services, the parents and a team will develop a written plan (individualized family service plan [IFSP]) for providing early intervention services to the child and, as necessary, to the family. The child's and family's IFSP can include nutrition, or nutrition may be listed as another service that the child receives but is not provided or paid for by the early intervention system. Depending on the child's assessed nutritional needs, a qualified nutritionist, as a member of the IFSP team, would develop and monitor appropriate goals and objectives to address any nutritional needs and also make referrals to appropriate community resources to carry out nutrition goals, if needed. For more information on disabilities in infants, toddlers, children, and youth and the Individuals with Disabilities Education Act, which is the law authorizing special education and the early intervention program, see the Web site of the National Dissemination Center for Children with Disabilities (www.nichcy.org).

Other types of nutrition services provided by many state and local health agencies include nutrition counseling, classes on specific aspects of nutrition (eg, infant feeding, breastfeeding, diet and prevention of heart disease, and weight management), radio and cable television programs on nutrition topics, publications and educational materials on a wide range of topics for the lay public, and nutrition seminars and workshops. Local nutrition education resources are available from the USDA-funded Cooperative Extension Service. This service provides up-to-date information about the science of nutrition and its practical application in planning low-cost, nutritious meals. Many nutrition publications provided by the Cooperative Extension Service and other public health agencies are available in various foreign languages and for clients with low literacy skills.[5,9]

The USDA's Cooperative State Research, Education, and Extension Service operates the Expanded Food and Nutrition Education Program (EFNEP) in all 50 states and in American Samoa, Guam, Micronesia, Northern Marianas, Puerto Rico, and the Virgin Islands. The Expanded Food and Nutrition Education Program is designed to assist limited-resource audiences in acquiring the knowledge, skills, attitudes, and behavior changes necessary to follow nutritionally sound diets and to contribute to their personal development and improvement of the total family diet and nutritional well-being (for more information, see http://www.csrees.usda.gov/nea/food/efnep/efnep.html).

The director of the nutrition department at the state health department is another excellent resource for identifying specific state, regional, or national resources and services. Similar information can be obtained from the Association of State and Territorial Public Health Nutrition Directors (Table 49.1). The state affiliate of the ADA or the ADA consultant directory can help identify an RD with specific clinical expertise (Table 49.1). Consumers may also call the ADA consumer hotline number and speak directly to an RD who can assist them with answers to general questions ranging from food labeling to food sanitation and other topics.

In addition to federal, state, and local health agencies, agencies such as visiting nurse associations, the American Diabetes Association, the American Heart Association, health maintenance organizations, and hospital inpatient and outpatient departments frequently employ personnel with nutrition expertise. They usually provide technical consultation in nutrition to physicians and nurses and nutrition counseling to patients and other agencies in the community. An increasing number of RDs have also established private or independent practices.

Nutrition-Assistance Programs

National policy has long provided for publicly supported nutrition-assistance programs to safeguard the health of individuals whose nutrition status is compromised because of poverty or complex physiologic, social, or other stressors. The National School Lunch Act of 1946 (Pub L No. 79-396) provided for a major federal role in food service for school children. Two major types of nutrition-assistance programs are operated nationally by the USDA: the Food Stamp Program and the special nutrition programs that include the Child Nutrition Programs and WIC. The USDA Food and Nutrition Service

(FNS) provides updated fact sheets on each of its nutrition-assistance programs (Table 49.1).

Food Stamp Program

The Food Stamp Program (FSP) is a nutrition-assistance program that enables people with low income and few resources to buy nutritious food and make healthy food choices within a limited budget.[10] It is the largest of the federal nutrition-assistance programs. States have the option to include nutrition education activities to food stamp participants and eligible individuals as part of their administrative services. Every state now conducts nutrition education activities for current and potential food stamp clients. The average monthly household benefit level in fiscal year 2007 was $215. Food stamp benefits are provided on an electronic card that is used by participants at authorized retail stores to buy food. Food stamp benefits redeemed at local stores not only provide nutrition benefits for the participants but also provide an economic boost to the local community. Every $5 in new food stamp benefits generates $9.20 in total community spending.

The Food Stamp Program is a federal program but it is administered by state and local agencies. As an entitlement program, it is available to all who meet the eligibility standards. However, only 56% of those who are eligible actually participate in the Food Stamp Program. Half of the participants are children and another 8% are older than 60 years. The FNS, which oversees the Food Stamp Program, offers numerous resources and tools to help community and faith-based organizations, state and local offices, food retailers, and other health and social service providers teach their clients with low income about the nutrition benefits of food stamps and help them enroll. These materials are available free online (http://www.fns.usda.gov/fsp/outreach/default.htm).

To qualify for food stamp benefits, a person must apply through a local food stamp office and have income and resources under certain limits. The FNS Web site offers the "step 1" online prescreening tool (www.foodstamps-step1.usda.gov) in English and Spanish, which privately tells users whether they may be eligible for benefits and how much they could receive. The FNS Web site also provides Food Stamp application and local office locators (http://www.fns.usda.gov/fsp/outreach/map.htm) and state Food Stamp information/hotline numbers (http://www.fns.usda.gov/fsp/contact_info/hotlines.htm).

V

School Nutrition Programs

The National School Lunch Program (NSLP), the School Breakfast Program (SBP), and the Special Milk Program are administered in most states by the state education agency, which enters into agreements with officials of local schools or school districts to operate nonprofit food services. Most public and private schools in the United States participate in the National School Lunch Program. Participating schools receive cash subsidies and donated USDA commodities. Any public or nonprofit private school of high school grade or less is eligible. Public and licensed, nonprofit, private residential child care institutions, such as orphanages, community homes for disabled children, juvenile detention centers, and temporary shelters for runaway children, are also eligible. For more information on USDA school meals programs, visit http://www.fns.usda.gov/cnd.

Schools participating in the federal school meals programs agree to serve nutritious meals at a reduced price or free to children who are determined to be eligible on the basis of uniform national poverty guidelines, determined annually by the USDA. A child's eligibility to receive reduced-price or free meals is based on their household size and income. Additionally, a child from a household currently certified to receive food stamps or benefits under the Food Distribution Program on Indian Reservations or Temporary Assistance to Needy Families (TANF) is categorically eligible for free benefits. The school meals program provides federal subsidies for program meals served to children from all income levels; however, free and reduced-price meals served to children determined to be eligible by income criteria are subsidized at a higher rate.

Federal nutrition requirements are specified in program regulations to ensure that the nutrition goals of the school meal programs are met. The nutrient standards, averaged over a week's menu cycle, are one-third and one-quarter of the Recommended Dietary Allowances for protein, vitamin A, vitamin C, iron, calcium, and calories for various age/grade groupings for school lunch and school breakfast, respectively.

Through the 1994 Healthy Meals for Healthy Children Act (Pub L No. 104-149), the USDA, in 1995, undertook the first major reform in the nutritional quality of school meals since the program began, with the School Meals Initiative for Healthy Children. In addition to the Recommended Dietary Allowances for key nutrients, starting in 1996, school were also required to comply with the Dietary Guidelines for Americans (DGAs), which call for less fat, saturated fat, cholesterol, and sodium and more fruits, vegetables, and grains. The Dietary Guidelines for Americans are the cornerstone of federal nutrition policy and nutrition education activities. They are jointly issued and updated every 5 years by the USDA and DHHS. The MyPyramid food guidance system provides food-based guidance to help implement the recommendations of the DGAs. The DGAs provide authoritative advice for people 2 years and older about how good dietary habits can promote health and reduce risks of major chronic diseases. For more information the DGAs, see http://www.health.gov/dietaryguidelines and for more information on MyPyramid, see http://www.mypyramid.gov.

To help schools implement the updated nutritional standards, the USDA launched the Team Nutrition initiative in June 1995. In addition to expanding training and technical assistance resources for schools, Team Nutrition brings together public and private networks to promote food choices for a healthy diet through 6 channels: the classroom, food service providers, the media, the entire school, families, and the community. Team Nutrition funds a limited number of competitive grants to states each year for Team Nutrition initiatives at the state and local levels. The Nutrition, Education and Training Program, authorized in 1978, provided the state and local infrastructure for the delivery of the Team Nutrition materials and resources to the local schools; however, although the Nutrition, Education, and Training (NET) Program is still authorized under current legislation, no funding has occurred since 1998. More information on Team Nutrition can be found at http://teamnutrition.usda.gov.

The Special Milk Program reduces the cost of each half-pint of milk served to children by providing cash reimbursement at an annually adjusted rate. A school district can choose to provide milk free to children who meet the eligibility guidelines. This program is available only to schools, child care institutions, and summer camps that do not participate in other federal meal service programs.

School Wellness Policies

Under the Child Nutrition and WIC Reauthorization Act of 2004 (Pub L No. 108-265), each local educational agency participating in a program authorized by the National School Lunch Act or the Child Nutrition Act of 1966 (Pub L No. 89-642) was required to establish a local school wellness policy by school year 2006. The purpose of implementing local wellness policies is to create healthy school nutrition environments that promote healthy eating and physical activity for students.

The legislation placed the responsibility of developing and implementing a wellness policy at the local level so that the individual needs of each local educational agency can be addressed. Preventing childhood obesity is a collective responsibility requiring the family, school, community, corporate, and governmental commitments. The key is to implement changes through coordinated and collaborative efforts from all sectors. For more information, visit the USDA Web site at http://teamnutrition.usda.gov/Healthy/wellnesspolicy.html.

The American Academy of Pediatrics (AAP) has encouraged its membership to become involved in assisting their local school districts in developing and implementing school wellness policies. The AAP and the ADA are cooperating with the Action for Healthy Kids, a national nonprofit organization, to address the epidemic of overweight, undernourished, and sedentary youth through tangible changes in the school environment. Useful information for how pediatricians can become involved in school wellness policies is available (www.actionforhealthykids.org).

Child and Adult Care Food Program

The Child and Adult Care Food Program (CACFP) provides cash reimbursement and commodities for the provision of meals and snacks to facilities providing nonresidential child care for children. Institutions eligible to participate include nonprofit child care centers, Head Start centers, and family or group child care homes. Some for-profit child care centers serving children from families with low income may also be eligible to participate in the program.

Although federal subsidies continue to be provided for meals served to children from all income levels, program benefits are primarily directed to needy children. Children 12 years and younger are eligible to receive up to 2 meals and 1 snack each day at a child care home or center. Children who reside in homeless shelters may receive up to 3 meals each day. Migrant children 15 years and younger and persons with disabilities, regardless of their age, are eligible to receive reimbursable meals. After-school care snacks are available to children through 18 years of age. For more information on the Child and Adult Care Food Program, visit the Web site (http://www.fns.usda.gov/cnd/care).

Summer Food Service Program

The Summer Food Service Program (SFSP) provides nutritious meals for children 18 years and younger during school vacations at centrally located sites, such as schools or community centers in neighborhoods with low incomes, or at summer camps. Meals are served free to all eligible children and must meet the nutritional standards established by the USDA. Sponsors of the program must be public or private nonprofit schools, public agencies, or private nonprofit organizations. For more information on the Summer Food Service Program, visit the Web site (http://www.fns.usda.gov/cnd/summer).

Supplemental Food Programs

WIC Program

The WIC program is the premier public health nutrition program serving low-income, nutritionally at-risk pregnant, breastfeeding, and nonbreast-feeding postpartum women, infants, and children up to 5 years of age. The WIC program is administered at the federal level by the FNS of the USDA and was created by Congress to serve as an adjunct to health care during critical times of growth and development. The benefits of the WIC program include nutritious supplemental foods, nutrition education, and referrals for health and social services, which are all provided to participants at no cost. Many studies show that the WIC program has made many contributions toward improving maternal and child health and saving children's lives.[11–14]

The WIC program is available in all 50 states, 34 Indian Tribal Organizations, American Samoa, the District of Columbia, Guam, Puerto Rico, the Virgin Islands, and the Commonwealth of the Northern Marianas Islands. As of 2006, these state agencies administered the WIC program through 1835 local agencies and 9000 clinic sites. Of the 8.0 million people who received WIC benefits each month in fiscal year 2006, approximately 3.99 million were children, 2.07 million were infants, and 2.02 million were women. Approximately one half of the infants born in the United States today receive WIC benefits. Services under WIC are provided in county health departments, hospitals, mobile clinics (vans), community centers, schools, public housing sites, Indian reservations, migrant health centers and camps, and Indian Health Service facilities.

Since the piloting of the WIC program in 1972, funding has grown to approximately $5.086 billion yearly. Program funds are allocated to state agencies according to a formula that considers both administrative and food costs. The food packages provided for the different categories of WIC participants are designed to provide nutrients frequently lacking in the diets of the target population. The food items currently authorized are milk, eggs, cheese, iron-fortified infant formula, iron-fortified infant and adult cereal, fruit and vegetable juice, and dried beans/peas or peanut butter. Participants generally receive food instruments that can be redeemed at approved grocery stores for specified foods. In some instances, participants receive food through home delivery or a warehouse distribution system. Women who exclusively breastfeed can receive an enhanced food package that includes tuna and carrots. The average monthly food package cost for fiscal year 2006 was $37.14.

The Institute of Medicine (IOM) recently reviewed the WIC food packages in a 22-month study. The final report from the IOM, *WIC Food Packages: Time for a Change,*[15] was released on April 27, 2005. On August 7, 2006, the FNS published in the *Federal Register* a proposal that would implement the first comprehensive revisions to the WIC food packages since 1980. The proposed changes largely follow recommendations made by the IOM as well as the latest nutrition science and the DGAs. On December 6, 2007, an interim final rule revising the WIC food packages was published in the *Federal Register*. The new food packages align with the 2005 Dietary Guidelines for Americans and infant feeding practice guidelines of the American Academy of Pediatrics.

Interim Final Rule Provisions—Major Food Package Changes

The revised food packages retain the same current food categories and add new food categories as well as optional substitutions for some current food categories to better meet the needs of WIC's diverse population, including:

- Addition of fruits and vegetables for women and children—participants may choose fruits and vegetables (fresh and processed) that provide ethnic variety and appeal.

- Addition of soy-based beverage and tofu as milk alternatives for women and children—medical documentation is required for children to ensure that the child's health care professional is aware that milk is being replaced with soy-based beverage or tofu.

- Addition of whole-grain foods for women and children—participants may choose whole-grain cereals and in addition receive whole-wheat bread or brown rice, bulgur, oatmeal, whole-grain barley, or soft corn or whole-wheat tortillas, at state option.

- Reductions in some food allowances, including milk, cheese, eggs, and juice for women and children—the new food packages are consistent with dietary recommendations from the DGAs, and the reductions in some food allowances allow a more balanced food package to be provided. Fully breastfeeding women receive the most variety and largest quantity of food.

- Provision of only fat-reduced milk to women and children 2 years and older and provide only whole milk to children 1 year of age. Whole milk would be available for women and children older than 2 years only with medical documentation.

- Revision of infant food packages—infants will receive food packages designed for the categories of fully breastfeeding, partially breastfeeding, or fully formula feeding. Compared with previous food packages, partially breastfed infants receive less infant formula to allow mothers to feed more human milk to their infants. Partially breastfeeding mothers are offered counseling and support to help them establish their milk supply and are provided an individualized amount of infant formula based on an assessment of need. Jarred infant foods (fruits and vegetables) have been added for all infants 6 months and older, and the quantity of infant formula is reduced. Jarred infant food meat has been added for fully breastfed infants 6 months and older, and juice has been eliminated from the infant food packages. Low-iron infant formula is no longer authorized.

- For the complete provisions and requirements for foods in the new WIC food packages, refer to the full regulation at www.fns.usda.gov/wic. Although federal regulations specify the minimum nutritional requirements for the WIC foods, state agencies determine which foods, under the new regulation, to include on state-authorized food lists.

The food packages better promote and support the establishment of successful, long-term breastfeeding, provide WIC participants with a wider variety of foods including fruits and vegetables and whole grains, provide less saturated fat and cholesterol and more fiber to women and children, reinforce the nutrition messages provided to participants, and provide WIC state agencies greater flexibility in prescribing food packages to accommodate the cultural food preferences of WIC participants. WIC state agencies must implement the provisions no later than August 5, 2009. An interim final rule allows FNS to obtain feedback on the major changes to the food packages as recommended by IOM while allowing implementation to move forward. The comment period for the interim final rule ends on February 1, 2010. The USDA will issue a final rule after review and analysis of public comments.

Nutrition education is an important benefit of the WIC program. Efforts are made to provide client-centered nutrition education that focuses on the individual participant's nutritional needs, cultural preferences, and education level. Breastfeeding promotion and support activities are an important component of WIC nutrition education.

The WIC Farmers' Market Nutrition Program provides additional coupons to WIC recipients that can be used to buy fresh fruits and vegetables from authorized farmers, farmers markets, or roadside stands.

For more information on the WIC program, see the WIC Web site at http://www.fns.usda.gov/wic.

> ### AAP
> **The American Academy of Pediatrics policy statement on the WIC program**
>
> Highlights the important collaboration between pediatricians and local WIC programs to ensure that infants and children receive high-quality, cost-effective health care and nutrition services.
> *Pediatrics.* 2001;108:1216–1217

Food Distribution Programs

These programs include the Commodity Supplemental Food Program, the Emergency Food Assistance Program, the Food Distribution Program on Indian Reservations, Nutrition Services Incentive Program (NSIP [formerly the Nutrition Program for the Elderly]); and Schools/Child Nutrition Commodity Programs, which includes the National School Lunch Program; Summer Food Service Program; and the Child and Adult Care Food Program.

Commodity Supplemental Food Program

The Commodity Supplemental Food Program (CSFP) operates in 32 states (of which the District of Columbia is included) and on 2 Indian reservations. The program provides food packages to low-income pregnant, lactating, and postpartum women up to 1 year, to infants and children up to 6 years of age, and to elderly people 60 years or older.

Like the WIC program, the Commodity Supplemental Food Program provides food packages to supplement the diets of participants. The foods offered include infant formula and cereal, nonfat dry and evaporated milk, juice, farina, oats, ready-to-eat cereal, rice, pasta, egg mix, dehydrated potatoes, peanut butter, dried beans or peas, canned meat or poultry or tuna, and canned fruits and vegetables. Food packages through the Commodity Supplemental Food Program do not provide a complete diet but, rather, are good sources of the nutrients typically lacking in the diets of the target population.

Unlike the WIC program, the Commodity Supplemental Food Program distributes food rather than vouchers for redemption at grocery stores. Eligible people cannot participate concurrently in both programs. In fiscal year 2006, an average of more than 462 000 people each month participated in the Commodity Supplemental Food Program, including more than 422 000 elderly people and more than 40 000 women, infants, and children.

State agencies set eligibility standards, store the food, and select local public and nonprofit private agencies to which they distribute the food. Local agencies determine the eligibility of applicants, distribute the foods, and may provide nutrition education and referrals for health care and social services. In addition to donated food, the USDA provides funds to cover some of the administrative costs of outreach, warehousing, and client transportation. For more information on the Commodity Supplemental Food Program, see the Web site (http://www.fns.usda.gov/fdd/programs/csfp).

The Emergency Food Assistance Program

The Emergency Food Assistance Program (TEFAP) is a federal program, administered by the USDA, that helps supplement the diets of low-income Americans, including elderly people, by providing them with emergency food and nutrition assistance at no cost. Under the Emergency Food Assistance Program, the USDA makes commodity foods available to state distributing agencies. States provide the food to local agencies that they have selected, usually food banks, which in turn distribute the food to soup kitchens and food pantries that directly serve the public. These organizations distribute the commodities for household consumption or use them to prepare and serve meals in a congregate setting. Recipients of food for home use must meet income eligibility criteria set by the states. States also provide the food to other types of local organizations, such as community action agencies, which distribute the foods directly to needy households. State agencies receive the food and supervise overall distribution. For more information on the Emergency Food Assistance Program, see the Web site (http://www.fns.usda.gov/fdd/programs/tefap).

Food Distribution Program on Indian Reservations

The Food Distribution Program on Indian Reservations (FDPIR) provides commodity foods to low-income households on Indian reservations and to American Indian households residing in approved areas near reservations or in Oklahoma. Many households participate in the Food Distribution Program on Indian Reservations, as an alternative to the Food Stamp Program, because they do not have easy access to food stamp offices or authorized food stores. The program is administered at the federal level by the FNS. The Food Distribution Program on Indian Reservations is administered locally by either Indian Tribal Organizations or an agency of a state government. As of 2006, there are approximately 257 tribes receiving benefits under the through 98 Indian Tribal Organizations and 5 state agencies. Average monthly participation for fiscal year 2006 was 89 867 individuals.

Each month, participating households receive a food package to help them maintain a nutritionally balanced diet. Participants may select from more than 70 products, including: frozen ground beef and chicken, canned meats, poultry, and fish; canned fruits and vegetables, canned soups, and spaghetti sauce; macaroni and cheese, pastas, cereals, rice, and other grains; cheese, egg mix, and nonfat dry and evaporated milk; flour, cornmeal, bakery mix, and reduced sodium crackers; low-fat refried beans, dried beans, and dehydrated potatoes; canned juices and dried fruit; peanuts and peanut butter; and corn syrup, vegetable oil, and shortening. Participants on most reservations can choose fresh produce instead of canned fruits and vegetables. For more information on the Food Distribution Program on Indian Reservations, see the Web site (http://www.fns.usda.gov/fdd/programs/fdpir).

Where to Seek Nutrition Assistance for Clients

Nutrition-assistance programs are usually administered at the local level by the following agencies:

1. Local school food authority: National School Lunch Program, School Breakfast Program, and Special Milk Program.
2. State and local health, social services, education, or agriculture agencies; public or private nonprofit health agencies; and Indian Tribal Organizations or groups recognized by the US Department of the Interior: WIC; Food Distribution Program on Indian Reservations; Summer Food Service Program; Child and Adult Care Food Program; the Emergency Food Assistance Program; Commodity Supplemental Food Program.
3. Local social services, human services, or welfare department: Food Stamp Program.
4. Community or faith-based organizations.

Other Federal Agencies Providing Nutrition Services to Improve Pediatric Health and Well-Being

CDC Nutrition and Physical Activity Program to Prevent Obesity and Other Chronic Diseases

The CDC administers the state-based Nutrition and Physical Activity Program to Prevent Obesity and Other Chronic Diseases. This program is based on a cooperative agreement between the CDC Division of Nutrition and Physical Activity (DNPA) and 28 state health departments. The program was established in fiscal year 1999 to prevent and control obesity and other chronic diseases by supporting states in developing and implementing nutrition and physical activity interventions, particularly through population-based strategies (eg, policy-level changes, environmental supports).

States receive funding from the program to work to prevent and control obesity and other chronic diseases through these strategies: balancing caloric intake and expenditure, increasing physical activity, increasing consumption of fruits and vegetables, decreasing television-viewing and other screen time, and increasing breastfeeding. The program also helps states work to reduce soft-drink consumption and decrease portion size. States funded by the program partner with stakeholders in government, academia, industry, and other areas to create statewide health plans—one of the most important ways to help guide state efforts. State plans promote working with a variety of partners and using all available resources to prevent and control obesity and other chronic diseases. For more information on DNPA programs and campaigns, research reports, surveillance data, training modules, nutrition education, and related resources, see the Web site (http://www.cdc.gov/nccdphp/dnpa).

Department of Health and Human Services Maternal and Child Health Services

The Title V MCH block grant program provides states with federal funds that support a wide variety of health services, including nutrition services. Title V seeks to improve the health of all mothers and children (including children with special health care needs) by assessing needs, setting priorities, and providing programs and services. On the basis of a comprehensive 5-year needs assessment, state Title V MCH programs identify their priority needs and develop a program plan and state performance measures (SPMs) to address these needs, to the extent that they are not addressed by the program's 18 national performance measures (NPMs). Each state is unique in the type of services they provide under their Title V MCH block grant. The conceptual framework for the services of the Title V MCH block grant

V

is a pyramid, which includes 4 tiers of services (ie, direct health care services, enabling services (such as coordination with Medicaid and WIC services), population-based services, and infrastructure building services. The MCH block grant program is the only federal program that provides services at all 4 levels, including state population-based capacity and infrastructure-building services and which targets the entire population and not only the low-income population.

In 2006, the Health Resources and Services Administration's Maternal and Child Health Bureau (MCHB) included a new NPM that addresses the "percentage of children, ages 2 to 5 years, receiving WIC services with a body mass index at or above the 85th percentile." Another NPM, which had previously focused on the "percentage of mothers who breastfeed their infants at hospital discharge," was revised to reflect the "percent of mothers who breastfeed their infants at 6 months of age."

The Title V Information System electronically captures data reported in the annual Title V MCH block grant applications and reports on 59 states, territories, and jurisdictions. State-reported financial data, program data, and information on key measures and indicators of MCH in the United States are posted on the Title V Information System Web site (https://perfdata.hrsa .gov/mchb/mchreports/Search/search.asp).

In addition to the formula block grants to states, Title V supports activities under the Special Projects of Regional and National Significance (SPRANS) grants and the Community Integrated Service Systems grants. Activities supported under Special Projects of Regional and National Significance include MCH research, training, breastfeeding promotion and support, nutrition services, and a broad range of other MCH initiatives and grant projects. The Community Integrated Service Systems program seeks to improve the health of mothers and children by funding projects for the development and expansion of integrated health, education, and social services at the community level. Additional information on MCHB-funded programs is available on the MCHB Web site (www.mchb.hrsa.gov).

The EPSDT program is the child health component of Medicaid. The EPSDT program is required in every state and is designed to improve the health of low-income children by financing appropriate and necessary pediatric services. State Title V agencies can play an important role in fulfilling the potential of EPSDT services. Federal rules encourage partnerships between state Medicaid and Title V agencies to ensure better access to and receipt of the full range of screening, diagnostic, and treatment services.

Bright Futures, initiated in 1990, is a longstanding, major effort of the MCHB and its partners to improve the quality of health promotion and prevention for infants, children, and adolescents and their families. Over the years, Bright Futures has evolved to encompass a vision, a philosophy, and a set of expert guidelines, tools, and other resources to implement a practical developmental approach to providing health supervision for children of all ages, from birth through adolescence.

Recognizing the need for more in-depth materials in certain areas to complement the guidelines, the MCHB launched the Building Bright Futures Project to foster the implementation of the Bright Futures health supervision guidelines by publishing practical tools and materials and by providing technical assistance and training. Using *Bright Futures: Guidelines for Health Supervision of Infants, Children, and Adolescents* as a cornerstone document, a series of implementation guides have been developed. Included in the *Bright Futures* series are the first, second, and upcoming third editions of *Bright Futures in Practice: Nutrition*[16] and the first edition of *Bright Futures: Physical Activity*.[17] Through a cooperative agreement between MCHB and the AAP, the third edition of the *Bright Futures: Guidelines for Health Supervision of Infants, Children, and Adolescents*[18] is available.

Conclusion

As the key provider of child health care, the pediatrician has a major role in ensuring that nutrition services for children include assessment of their nutritional status and provision of a safe food supply adequate in quality and quantity, nutrition counseling, and nutrition education for children and parents. As the primary expert on health in the community and as a concerned citizen, the pediatrician, in coordination with other members of the health care team, including the nutritionist or dietitian and nurse, can provide meaningful leadership in the formulation of sound nutrition policy and the education of legislators, administrators, and others who influence the response of the community to the nutritional needs of its children.

References

1. Eagan MC, Oglesby AC. Nutrition services in the maternal and child health program: a historical perspective. In: Sharbaugh CO, Egan MC, eds. *Call to Action: Better Nutrition for Mothers, Children, and Families.* Washington, DC: National Center for Education in Maternal and Child Health; 1991:73–92

2. US Department of Health and Human Services. *Healthy People 2010. With Understanding and Improving Health and Objectives for Improving Health.* 2 vols. 2nd ed. Washington, DC: US Government Printing Office; 2000

3. McCall M, Keir B. *Survey of the Public Health Nutrition Workforce 1999–2000.* Alexandria, VA: US Department of Agriculture; 2003

4. Institute of Medicine. *The Future of the Public's Health in the 21st Century.* Washington, DC: National Academies Press; 2003

5. Edelstein S. *Nutrition in Public Health: Handbook for Developing Programs and Services.* 2nd ed. Sudbury, MA: Jones and Bartlett Publishers; 2005

6. American Dietetic Association. Position of the American Dietetic Association: cost-effectiveness of medical nutrition therapy. *J Am Diet Assoc.* 1995;95:88–91

7. An Act Further Regulating Insurance Coverage for Certain Inherited Diseases. Massachusetts Session Law. Chapter 384 §1–11 (1993). Available at: http://archives.lib.state.ma.us/actsResolves/1993/1993acts0384.pdf. Accessed November 2, 2007

8. Bayerl CT, Ries J, Bettencourt MF, Fisher P. Nutritional issues of children in early intervention programs: primary care team approach. *Semin Pediatr Gastrointest Nutr.* 1993;4:11–15

9. Owen AY, Splett PL, Owen GM, Frankle RT. *Nutrition in the Community. The Art and Science of Delivering Services.* 4th ed. Boston, MA: McGraw-Hill; 1999

10. *Facts About the Food Stamp Program.* Alexandria, VA: Food and Nutrition Service, US Department of Agriculture; 2007. Available at: http://www.fns.usda.gov/fsp/applicant_recipients/facts.htm. Accessed November 2, 2007

11. US General Accounting Office. *Early Intervention: Federal Investments Like WIC Can Produce Savings: Report to Congressional Requesters.* Washington, DC: US General Accounting Office; 1992. Publication No. GAO/HRD-92-18

12. Mathematica Policy Research Inc. *The Savings in Medicaid Costs for Newborns and Their Mothers From Prenatal Participation in the WIC Program.* Alexandria, VA: Food and Nutrition Service, US Department of Agriculture; 1991

13. Bitler MP, Currie J. Does WIC work? The effects of WIC on pregnancy and birth outcomes. *J Policy Anal Manage.* 2005;24:73–91

14. Henchy W. *WIC in the States: Thirty-One Years of Building a Healthier America.* Washington, DC: Food Research and Action Center; 2005. Available at: http://www.frac.org/WIC/2004_Report/Full_Report.pdf. Accessed November 2, 2007

15. Institute of Medicine. *WIC Food Packages: Time for a Change.* Washington, DC: The National Academies Press; 2006

16. Story M, Holt K, Sofka D. *Bright Futures in Practice: Nutrition.* 2nd ed. Arlington, VA: National Center for Education in Maternal and Child Health; 2002

17. Patrick K. *Bright Futures in Practice: Physical Activity.* Arlington, VA: National Center for Education in Maternal and Child Health; 2001

18. American Academy of Pediatrics, Bright Futures Steering Committee. *Bright Futures: Guidelines for Health Supervision of Infants, Children, and Adolescents.* Hagan JF Jr, Shaw JS, Duncan P, eds. Elk Grove Village, IL: American Academy of Pediatrics; 2008

50 Food Labeling

In 1990, the Nutrition Labeling and Education Act (Pub L No. 101-535) was enacted, mandating numerous changes in food labeling. Before that time, nutrition labeling on food products was voluntary, except for those that contained added nutrients or carried nutrition claims. As Americans became more interested in nutrition, food label regulations were revised to provide nutrition information that would help consumers make food choices to meet national dietary recommendations.

Under the Nutrition Labeling and Education Act, labels of most packaged foods were required to feature the new "Nutrition Facts" panel by 1994.[1] Labeling is voluntary for fresh fruits and vegetables and raw meat, poultry, and seafood. For these raw foods, nutrition information may be printed on the package or on pamphlets or posters displayed near the food in the supermarket. Food labeling of meat and poultry products is regulated by the US Department of Agriculture (USDA), and labeling for the remainder of foods is regulated by the US Food and Drug Administration (FDA).

Ingredient Labeling

Ingredient labeling is an important source of information for consumers about the composition of packaged foods. Both FDA and USDA regulations require that food products with 2 or more ingredients provide a listing of ingredients in descending order of their prominence by weight by their common, specific names.[2-4] The source of some ingredients must be stated by name to help people with specific food needs because of religious or health reasons. These include protein hydrolysates and caseinate as a milk derivative in foods that claim to be nondairy. Certified color additives must also be listed by name (eg, FD&C Blue No. 1 or FD&C Yellow No. 5).

For families with food allergies, it is essential to read the ingredient listings on food labels to determine the presence of the 8 major allergens (milk, egg, wheat, soy, peanuts, tree nuts, fish, and crustaceans). Because food and beverage manufacturers are continually making ingredient changes, food-allergic individuals and their caregivers should read the ingredient declaration or "Contains…" statement on the food label of every product purchased, each time it is purchased and consumed (or served).

In January 2006, food allergen labeling requirements of the Food Allergen Labeling and Consumer Protection Act (Pub L No. 108-282) became effective on FDA-regulated food and beverage products.[5] The act defined the 8 major food allergens and 1 of 2 options for ingredient labeling of food products as follows:

1. Immediately after the ingredient declaration, the label states "Contains" followed by the name of the food source from which the major food allergen is derived (eg, "Contains milk, egg, walnuts"). In the case of tree nuts, fish, or shellfish, each specific food in these classes that is an ingredient in the food must be declared (ie, salmon, cod, crab, pecan, hazelnut) rather than the group listing (see examples).

2. Within the ingredient declaration, in parentheses after the common or usual name of the allergenic ingredient, the label presents the name of the food source from which the major food allergen is derived—for example, "…whey (milk)" (see examples).

Example of ingredient declaration with Food Allergen Labeling and Consumer Protection Act provision using "Contains…" statement:

Ingredients: Flounder, crabmeat, egg, mayonnaise (soybean oil, water, eggs, vinegar, natural flavor [egg, soy]), cracker meal (wheat flour, partially hydrogenated soybean oil, salt, sodium bicarbonate, yeast, malted barley flour, enzymes), green pepper, pimiento, celery, dry mustard, hydrolyzed soy protein, Worcestershire sauce (water, vinegar, molasses, high-fructose corn syrup, anchovies, garlic, shallots, natural flavor [soy], spice), salt, spice, color. Contains flounder, crab, egg, soy, wheat, anchovies.

Example of ingredient declaration with Food Allergen Labeling and Consumer Protection Act provisions within ingredient statement:

Ingredients: Flounder, crabmeat, egg, mayonnaise (soybean oil, water, eggs, vinegar, natural flavor [egg, soy]), cracker meal (wheat flour, partially hydrogenated soybean oil, salt, sodium bicarbonate, yeast, malted barley flour, enzymes), green pepper, pimiento, celery, dry mustard, hydrolyzed soy protein, Worcestershire sauce (water, vinegar, molasses, high-fructose corn syrup, anchovies, garlic, shallots, natural flavor [soy], spice), salt, spice, color.

The Nutrition Facts Panel

The food label carries a variety of nutrition information (Fig 50.1–50.3). It is primarily presented within the Nutrition Facts panel, which indicates the amount of target macronutrients and micronutrients. Simplified or shortened formats may be used for products that contain insignificant amounts (amount declarable as 0 in labeling; generally less than 0.5 g) of certain mandatory label nutrients. Package size constraints may also dictate different formats.

Fig 50.1

Sample Nutrition Facts label for foods for children 4 years and older.

Nutrition Facts

Serving Size 1 cup (228g)
Servings Per Container 2

Amount Per Serving

Calories 260	Calories from Fat 120

	% Daily Value*
Total Fat 13g	**20%**
Saturated Fat 5g	**25%**
Trans Fat 2g	
Cholesterol 30mg	**10%**
Sodium 660mg	**28%**
Total Carbohydrate 31g	**10%**
Dietary Fiber 0g	**0%**
Sugars 5g	
Protein 5g	

Vitamin A 4%	•	Vitamin C 2%
Calcium 15%	•	Iron 4%

* Percent Daily Values are based on a 2,000 calorie diet. Your Daily Values may be higher or lower depending on your calorie needs:

	Calories:	2,000	2,500
Total Fat	Less than	65g	80g
Sat Fat	Less than	20g	25g
Cholesterol	Less than	300mg	300mg
Sodium	Less than	2,400mg	2,400mg
Total Carbohydrate		300g	375g
Dietary Fiber		25g	30g

Calories per gram:

Fat 9 • Carbohydrate 4 • Protein 4

Fig 50.2

Nutrition Facts panel for infant food (for infants and children younger than 2 years).

Nutrition Label Format,
Food for Children under 2

Nutrition Facts

Serving Size 1 jar (140g)

Amount Per Serving

Calories 120	
Total Fat	1g
Trans Fat	0g
Sodium	10mg
Total Carbohydrate	27g
Dietary Fiber	4g
Sugars	18g
Protein	0g

% Daily Value

Protein 0%	•	Vitamin A 6%
Vitamin C 45%	•	Calcium 2%
Iron 2%		

Fig 50.3

Nutrition Facts panel for toddler food (for children younger than 4 years).

Nutrition Label Format,
Food for Children under 4

Nutrition Facts

Serving Size 1 jar (140g)

Amount Per Serving

Calories 110	Calories from Fat 0

Total Fat	0g
Saturated Fat	0g
Trans Fat	0g
Cholesterol	0mg
Sodium	10mg
Total Carbohydrate	27g
Dietary Fiber	4g
Sugars	18g
Protein	0g

% Daily Value

Protein 0%	•	Vitamin A 6%
Vitamin C 45%	•	Calcium 2%
Iron 2%		

The following provides more details about the various features of the Nutrition Facts panel for foods for children and adults older than 4 years:

1. *Serving size.* Serving sizes are standardized for different food categories on the basis of the average amount of food eaten at one time, using data from national food consumption surveys. Sizes do not always match serving sizes specified in MyPyramid (www.mypyramid.gov). Two measurements are provided: common household and metric measures.

2. *Calories.* Total calories in 1 serving are identified. In addition, calories from fat per serving are included. To calculate the total percentage of calories from fat in a diet, however, the fat grams in all food choices must be added. Dietary guidelines emphasize eating 30% or less of calories from fat over a few days, not in 1 food or 1 meal.

3. *Nutrients.* Information about the content of nutrients most related to today's health concerns must be listed. These nutrients include fat, saturated fat, trans fat, cholesterol, sodium, total carbohydrate, fiber, sugars, protein, vitamins A and C, calcium, and iron. Other nutrients are listed voluntarily, and if foods contain insignificant amounts of a required nutrient, that nutrient may be omitted from the label. Information about other nutrients is required in 2 cases: (1) if a claim is made about the nutrients on the label; or (2) if the nutrients are added to the food, as in the case of fortified foods. Nutrient amounts are listed in 1 of 2 ways: in the metric amount or as a percentage of the Daily Value (DV). Percent DV only is used for vitamins and minerals except for sodium and potassium.

4. *Daily Values.* The "% DV" characterizes how the amount of a nutrient in a food or beverage contributes to a moderate, varied, and balanced diet. The term "Daily Value" is an umbrella term for 2 sets of reference values: daily reference values (DRVs) and reference daily intakes (RDIs). The DRVs are set for total fat, saturated fat, cholesterol, total carbohydrate, dietary fiber, sodium, potassium, and protein. They are established for adults and children 4 years or older and are based on current nutrition recommendations. The DRVs for cholesterol, sodium, and potassium are set at a constant level for all calorie levels. The DRVs for total fat, saturated fat, total carbohydrate, dietary fiber, and protein are based on a 2000-kcal reference diet (Table 50.1). Current RDIs are listed in Appendix J.

5. *Label footnotes.* A reference chart for a 2000- and a 2500-kcal diet also appears on the bottom of some Nutrition Facts panels. It suggests the amounts of fat, saturated fat, cholesterol, and sodium not to exceed and the amounts of carbohydrate and dietary fiber to consume. Some labels

also show the number of calories supplied by 1 g of fat, carbohydrate, and protein.

Table 50.1
Daily Values Used to Calculate Percentage Daily Value for Nutrition Panel*

Food	Daily Value for Adults and Children Older Than 4 Years
Total fat	65 g[†]
Saturated fat	20 g[†]
Cholesterol	300 mg
Sodium	2400 mg
Potassium	3500 mg
Total carbohydrate	300 g[†]
Dietary fiber	25 g[‡]
Protein	50 g[†]

* Based on a 2000-kcal diet for adults and children older than 4 years.

[†] Daily value based on a 2000-kcal reference diet.

[‡] Daily value based on 11.5 g/1000 kcal.

Food Labels for Infants Younger Than 2 Years and Children Younger Than 4 Years
Food labels on products designed for infants younger than 2 years and children younger than 4 years are different from food labels on adult products. Specifically, infant food labels (for children younger than 2 years) differ in the listing of calories from fat, saturated fat, and cholesterol as well as DVs and serving sizes. Fat information is not detailed because of the concern that adults may mistakenly apply this information to controlling the calories provided by fat for their infants.

The DVs for fat, cholesterol, sodium, potassium, carbohydrates, and fiber are not listed, because the reference values have not been established for infants and children younger than 4 years. Protein is listed in grams per serving and as a percentage of the DV on foods for infants and children younger than 4 years. The DVs used to calculate the nutrient percentages are calculated based on the RDIs for each population.

Serving sizes of foods for infants and children younger than 4 years are based on government reference amounts and are smaller than typical adult servings.

Table 50.2
Nutrition Claims

Food Component	Definition, per Serving
Calories	
Calorie free	<5 kcal
Low calorie	≤40 kcal
Reduced or fewer calories	At least 25% fewer kcal*
Light or lite	One third fewer kcal or 50% less fat*
Sugar	
Sugar free	<0.5 g
Reduced sugar or less sugar	At least 25% less sugars
No added sugar; without added sugar; no sugar added	No sugars added during processing or packaging, including ingredients that contain sugars, such as juice or dry fruit
Fat	
Fat free	<0.5 g
Low fat	≤3 g
Reduced or less fat	At least 25% less fat*
Light or lite	One third fewer kcal or 50% less fat*

Saturated fat
  Saturated fat free
  Low saturated fat
	<0.5 g
	≤1 g saturated fat and no more than 15% of calories from saturated fat

Reduced or less saturated fat	At least 25% less saturated fat*
Cholesterol	
Cholesterol free	<2 mg cholesterol and <2 g fat
Low cholesterol	≤20 mg cholesterol and <2 g saturated fat
Reduced or less cholesterol	At least 25% less cholesterol* and <2 g saturated fat
Sodium	
Sodium free	<5 mg
Very low sodium	≤35 mg
Low sodium	≤140 mg
Reduced or less sodium	At least 25% less sodium*
Light in sodium	50% less sodium*
Fiber	
High fiber	≤5 g†
Good source of fiber	2.5 to 4.9 g
More or added fiber	At least 2.5 g more or added*

Table 50.2 *(Continued)*
Nutrition Claims

Food Component	Definition, per Serving
Other Claims	
High, rich in, excellent source of (name of nutrient)	≤20% of daily value*
Good source of, contains, provides (name of nutrient)	10% to 19% of daily value*
More, enriched, fortified, added (name of nutrient)	≥10% or more of daily value more or added*
Lean†	<10 g fat, 4.5 g saturated fat, and <95 mg cholesterol
Extra lean†	<5 g fat, 2 g saturated fat, and <95 mg cholesterol
Healthy	Meets standards for "low" fat and saturated fat; contains ≤480 mg sodium, ≤60 mg cholesterol, and at least 10% daily value for vitamin A, vitamin C, calcium, iron, protein, or fiber

* Compared with a standard serving size of the traditional food.

† Must also meet the definition for low fat, or the level of fat must appear next to the high-fiber claim.

‡ On meat, poultry, seafood, and game meats.

Nutrition Claims

Nutrient content claims are those that characterize the amount of a nutrient in a food, using terms such as free, low, reduced, less, more, added, good source, and high. Using these terms in connection with a specific nutrient is strictly defined (Table 50.2).

Infant food labels may carry claims for vitamins and minerals. Claims about protein, fat, and sodium or the content of certain nutritional ingredients (ie, salt and sugar) are not allowed on products intended for infants and children younger than 2 years.

Claims about nonnutrient ingredients (eg, preservatives), the identification of ingredients (eg, made with apples), and taste (eg, unsweetened) are allowed.

Health Claims

In addition to nutrient content claims, a food label may bear claims about the health benefits of the food or a component of the food. Products must meet strict nutrition requirements before they can carry these claims associating foods, nutrients, or substances and reduced risk of a disease or condition.

Health claims are not allowed on the food labels of products intended for infants and children younger than 2 years.

To date, the FDA, on the basis of scientific evidence, has authorized 12 health claims.[6] Although the wording on packages may differ, the following summarizes the claims that link:

1. Calcium and osteoporosis: Physical activity and a calcium-rich diet may reduce the risk of osteoporosis, a condition in which the bones become soft or brittle.
2. Fat and cancer: A diet low in total fat may reduce the risk of some cancers.
3. Saturated fat and cholesterol and heart disease: A diet low in saturated fat and cholesterol may reduce the risk of heart disease.
4. Fiber-containing grain products, fruits, and vegetables and cancer: A low-fat diet rich in fiber-containing grain products, fruits, and vegetables may reduce the risk of some cancers.
5. Fruits, vegetables, and grain products that contain fiber and heart disease: A diet low in saturated fat and cholesterol and rich in fruits, vegetables, and grain products that contain some types of dietary fiber may reduce the risk of heart disease.
6. Sodium and high blood pressure: A low-sodium diet may reduce the risk of high blood pressure, which is a risk factor for heart attacks and strokes.
7. Fruits and vegetables and some cancers: A low-fat diet rich in fruits and vegetables (foods that are low in fat and may contain dietary fiber, vitamin A, or vitamin C) may reduce the risk of some cancers.
8. Folic acid and neural tube birth defects: Women who consume 0.4 mg of folic acid daily may reduce their risk of giving birth to a child affected with a neural tube defect.
9. Noncariogenic carbohydrate sweeteners (sugar alcohols and sucralose) and dental caries: Frequent eating of foods high in sugars and starches as between-meal snacks can promote tooth decay. The [name of sugar alcohol or sucralose] used to sweeten this food may reduce the risk of dental caries.
10. Soluble fiber from certain foods and risk of coronary heart disease: Soluble fiber from [name of food (eg, oat bran, psyllium, or barley fiber)], as part of a diet low in saturated fat and cholesterol, may reduce the risk of heart disease.
11. Soy protein and risk of coronary heart disease: Diets low in saturated fat and cholesterol that include 25 g of soy protein a day may reduce the

risk of heart disease. One serving of [name of food] provides [x] g of soy protein.

12. Plant sterol or stanol esters and risk of coronary heart disease: Diets low in saturated fat and cholesterol that include 2 servings of foods that provide a daily total of at least 1.3 g of vegetable oil sterol esters in 2 meals may reduce the risk of heart disease. A serving of [name of the food] supplies [x] g of vegetable oil sterol esters. Diets low in saturated fat and cholesterol that include 2 servings of foods that provide a daily total of at least 3.4 g of vegetable oil stanol esters in 2 meals may reduce the risk of heart disease. A serving of [name of the food] supplies [x] g of vegetable oil stanol esters.

To bear a health claim, each food must not exceed (unless exempted by the FDA) specified levels of fat, saturated fat, cholesterol, and sodium.

In addition to the above health claims, the FDA Modernization Act of 1997 (Pub L No. 105-115) established an additional route to establish health claims. The act includes procedures that allow a health claim to be made if it is based on a published authoritative statement, currently in effect, about the relationship between a nutrient and a disease or health-related condition to which the claim refers, issued by a scientific body of the US government with official responsibility for public health protection or research directly relating to human nutrition (eg, Dietary Guidelines for Americans from the USDA and DHHS; Dietary Reference Intake reports from the Institute of Medicine).

In July 1999, the first such health claim was established related to whole-grain foods and reduced risk of heart disease and cancer. The health claim states: Diets rich in whole-grain foods and other plant foods and low in total fat, saturated fat, and cholesterol may help reduce the risk of heart disease and certain cancers. To qualify for the claim, a food must contain 51% or more whole-grain ingredients per serving, be low in fat, and meet other general criteria for health claims.

In October 2000, a second health claim was established related to potassium-containing foods and reduced risk of high blood pressure and stroke. The health claim states: Diets containing foods that are good sources of potassium and low in sodium may reduce the risk of high blood pressure and stroke. To qualify for the claim, a food must be a good source of potassium and be low in sodium, total fat, saturated fat, and cholesterol (see nutrition claims).

In December 2003, a third health claim was established related to whole-grain foods with moderate fat content and reduced risk of heart disease. The health claim states: Diets rich in whole-grain foods and other plant foods may help reduced the risk of heart disease. To qualify for the claim, a food must contain 51% or more grain ingredients as whole grain and must meet other FDA-specified criteria. These foods do not have to be low fat (<3 g per serving) but must contain <6 g of fat per serving; must meet other criteria for saturated fat, cholesterol, and sodium; and must have <0.5 g of trans fat per serving.

Juice Labeling

Since 1994, the percentage of juice must be specified on the food label if a beverage claims to contain fruit or vegetable juice.[7] Label statements must be declared using the language, "Contains [x] percent [name of fruit or veg-etable] juice," "[x] percent juice," or similar phrase (eg, Contains 50% apple juice."). If a beverage contains minor amounts of juice for flavoring, the product may use the term "flavor," "flavored," or "flavoring" with a fruit or vegetable name, as long as the product does not bear the term "juice" (other than in the ingredient declaration) and does not visually depict the fruit or vegetable from which the flavor is derived. If the beverage contains no juice, but appears to contain juice, the label must state, "Contains no [name of fruit or vegetable] juice," or similar statements. These percentage juice state-ments appear near the top of the information panel of the beverage label.

Package Dating

Package dating provides a measure of a product's freshness. *Open dates* are stated alphanumerically (eg, Oct 15) or numerically (eg, 10–15 or 1015). An open date might be featured as:

1. Pull or "sell by" date: This is the last day that the manufacturer recom-mends sale of the product. Usually the date allows for additional storage and use time at home.
2. Freshness or quality assurance date: This date suggests how long the manufacturer believes the food will remain at peak quality. The label might read, "Best if used by October 2007." However, the product may be used after this date. A "freshness date" has a different meaning than the word "fresh" printed on the label, which often suggests that a food is raw or unprocessed.
3. Pack date: The date when the food was packaged or processed.
4. Expiration date: The last day the product should be eaten. State govern-ments regulate these dates for perishable foods, such as milk and eggs. The FDA requires expiration dates on infant formula.

Although the FDA does not regulate most package dating, FDA food labeling law and regulations require that such information is truthful and nonmisleading.

Conclusion

Food labeling helps consumers and parents make food choices to meet dietary recommendations by providing specific information about the content of certain nutrients in the product. This information may be used to compare foods, to choose foods that help provide a balance of recommended nutrients, and to build meals and a total diet that is moderate, varied, and balanced. In addition, ingredient declarations are useful for consumers to make food choices on the basis of religious, cultural, health, or food allergy concerns.

References

1. US Food and Drug Administration. Focus on food labeling. *FDA Consum.* May 1993;27(special issue):1–63. Available at: http://www.fda.gov/fdac/special/foodlabel/food_toc.html. Accessed November 2, 2007

2. US Food and Drug Administration. Food: Designation of Ingredients. 21 CFR §104.1 (2007)

3. US Department of Agriculture, Food Safety and Inspection Service. Labels: definitions; required features; 9 CFR §317.2, 9 (2007)

4. US Department of Agriculture, Food Safety and Inspection Service. Ingredients statement; CFR §381.118 (2007)

5. Food Allergen Labeling and Consumer Protection Act. Pub L No. 108-282 (2004)

6. US Food and Drug Administration. Health claims. 21 CFR §101.72–§101. 83 (2007)

7. US Food and Drug Administration. Percentage juice declaration for foods purporting to be beverages that contain fruit or vegetable juice. 21 CFR §101.30 (2007)

51 Current Legislation and Regulations for Infant Formulas

Infant formula is a food that purports to be or is represented for special dietary use solely as a food for infants by reason of its simulation of human milk or its suitability as a complete or partial substitute for human milk. Infant formula that is marketed in the United States is subject to the federal Food, Drug, and Cosmetic Act (FDCA [21 USC 301])[1] and the implementing regulations of the US Food and Drug Administration (FDA).[2] Generally, the FDCA provides specific regulatory controls for the production and the nutrient composition of standard and generic infant formulas (see Appendix E for listing of nutrient specifications).

The purpose of the infant formula provisions of the FDCA is to protect the health of infants consuming infant formula products. In 1978, a major manufacturer of infant formula reformulated 2 of its soy products by discontinuing the addition of salt. This reformulation resulted in infant formula products that contained an inadequate amount of chloride, an essential nutrient for growth and development in infants. By mid-1979, a disorder associated with chloride deficiency, hypochloremic metabolic alkalosis, was diagnosed in a substantial number of infants. Development of this disorder was associated with prolonged exclusive use of chloride-deficient soy formulas. This incident resulted in the passage of the Infant Formula Act of 1980 (Pub L No. 96-359), which amended the FDCA to ensure the adequacy of the nutrient composition of infant formulas. The statutory requirements for infant formula under the FDCA were revised in 1985 to give the FDA broader regulatory authority over infant formulas.[3]

The FDCA, as amended in 1986, provides specific requirements for the nutrient content and nutrient quantity of infant formula, nutrient quality control procedures, record keeping (including records on product testing) and recall procedures for the removal of unsafe infant formula from the marketplace. In addition, the FDCA requires manufacturers of infant formula to register and submit information to the FDA before marketing any new infant formula, including any infant formula that has had a major change in its formulation or processing. The FDA has a responsibility under the FDCA to review the new infant formula submission to ensure that a safe product will be produced. If the information in the submission meets the requirements of the FDCA, the FDA will not object to the marketing of the formula. Although the FDA does not have the authority to approve infant

V

formulas before they are marketed, it has compliance authority if an infant formula is marketed over its objection.

Information in such an infant formula submission must include the quantitative formulation—a listing, with amounts, of all ingredients in the formula. Only food ingredients that have been shown by the manufacturer to be safe and suitable under the applicable food safety provisions of the Act may be used in infant formulas. Some ingredients may qualify for the designation "Generally Regarded as Safe" after appropriate documentation has been submitted and considered by the FDA. In the submission, a manufacturer must provide assurances that the infant formula meets the nutrient content and quantity specifications and the nutrient quality standards in the FDCA.

The FDCA specifies the minimum nutrient amounts and, in some cases, the maximum nutrient amounts that infant formula products must contain. These specifications for the nutrient composition of commercial infant formulas are based in part on recommendations of the American Academy of Pediatrics. Infant formula manufacturers must demonstrate that a required nutrient is present and available in the formula and that the formula maintains appropriate nutrient contents throughout the shelf-life of the product. In addition, manufacturers must demonstrate that no other substance in the formula, such as a contaminant or a required nutrient present in a concentration that exceeds the maximum amount allowed by FDA regulations, will make the formula unsafe or adulterated.

In certain cases, exemptions from the nutrient specifications are allowed. Exempt infant formulas are specialty formulas for use by infants with special medical and dietary needs, such as those for children with inborn errors of metabolism or low birth weight. The exemption allows these infant formulas to be specifically formulated to meet the distinctive nutritional needs of infants with specific medical disorders.

Nutrient quality relates to the bioavailability of a nutrient. Infant formulas must not only contain all of the nutrients required to support normal growth and development as the sole source of nutrition but also provide those nutrients in a bioavailable form. Ordinarily, manufacturers submit documentation from clinical studies showing that the infant formula promotes normal infant growth and development and is suitable as the sole source of nutrients for young infants. Clinical studies are generally conducted in accordance with recommendations specific for infant populations by the American Academy of Pediatrics, together with general recommendations for rigorous clinical trial design, conduct, and analysis.

An infant formula submission also must include assurance that the infant formula complies with the FDCA and is manufactured in a way that is designed to prevent adulteration, for which there are necessary guidelines and regulations. For example, the FDA has guidelines to prevent microbiologic contamination of infant formula during manufacture and market distribution.

The labels of infant formulas must include directions for use, including pictorial instructions, a warning statement informing consumers of the consequences of improper preparation or use of the infant formula, and a statement cautioning consumers to use infant formula as directed by a physician. In addition, the product label of an infant formula must bear a "use by" date that ensures that if the formula is consumed by that date, the infant will receive not less than the quantity of nutrients stated on the product label. Many infant formula labels also contain claims. Although claims must be truthful and not misleading under the FDCA, no requirement exists that label claims for infant formula be approved by the FDA.

References

1. Federal Food, Drug and Cosmetic Act. 21 USC §321 (2000)
2. Infant Formula Quality Control Procedures and Infant Formula. *Fed Regist.* 1996;61(132):36153–36219
3. Federal Food, Drug and Cosmetic Act Amendment relating to infant formula. 99th Cong. 2nd Sess. *Congressional Record.* 1986;132(130):S14042–S14047

V

Introduction

In the United States, an estimated 76 million cases of foodborne illness occur every year, resulting in approximately 5000 deaths and 325 000 hospitalizations.[1] More than 200 infectious and noninfectious agents have been associated with foodborne and waterborne illness with a wide range of clinical manifestations; these agents include bacteria, viruses, parasites and their toxins, marine organisms and their toxins, and chemical contaminants including heavy metals.[2-7] Depending on the agent, infants, children, pregnant women, the elderly, and immunocompromised people are particularly vulnerable to more severe forms of disease.[8,9]

In January 2000, the US Department of Health and Human Services launched Healthy People 2010, a comprehensive, nationwide health promotion campaign that includes national health objective goals for food safety.[10] For instance, Healthy People 2010 aims to reduce of the national incidence of infections with *Salmonella* species, *Escherichia coli* O157:H7, *Campylobacter* species, and *Listeria* species to 50% of their incidence in 1997. Achieving this goal will require concerted public health interventions. As more people live with immunocompromising conditions, the risks of infection and severe illness from foodborne pathogens may increase. Furthermore, identification of new pathogens and established pathogens in unexpected food vehicles will likely occur. Increased importation of food and international travel increases the potential for exposure to novel or rare pathogens.[11] Because general practitioners are often the first to be contacted by people with foodborne illness, an understanding of the possible causes, spectrum of illness, diagnostic methods, and public health importance of foodborne infections is crucial not only for initial patient treatment but also to ensure timely reports to public health authorities for accurate surveillance. Understanding the diversity and nature of foodborne pathogens and associated vehicles of transmission is crucial to recognize, control, and prevent foodborne disease outbreaks. This chapter focuses on (1) the epidemiology of foodborne disease; (2) the signs, symptoms, and diagnosis of foodborne illness; (3) foodborne disease surveillance; (4) control and prevention of foodborne illness; and (5) resource materials available.

Epidemiology of Foodborne Disease

Infectious and noninfectious agents of foodborne disease can be acquired from a variety of sources, with some linked more frequently with specific foods. For instance, *Salmonella* serotype Enteritidis is commonly associated with poultry products or eggs. Table 52.1 lists examples of recent foodborne disease outbreaks in the United States by location, vehicle, and etiology,[12-32] indicating the diversity in vehicles and causes. Of the 2392 outbreaks of foodborne illness reported to the Centers for Disease Control and Prevention (CDC) in 2003–2004, 928 (38%) were of confirmed etiology, of which bacteria accounted for 44%, viruses accounted for 32%, chemical agents accounted for 11%, and parasites accounted for 1% (Table 52.2).[33] Among outbreaks with a known etiology, norovirus (previously known as Norwalk-like virus) was the most common pathogen, causing 32% of outbreaks. *Salmonella* species were the most common bacterial pathogens, causing 25% of outbreaks. Because the etiology was not determined in most outbreaks (61%), increased stool collection and enhanced epidemiologic and laboratory investigations are needed.[4]

Table 52.1
Examples of Recent Foodborne Outbreaks in the United States by Location, Vehicle, and Cause

Pathogen	Food Vehicle	Where	No. of Cases	Reference
Clostridium botulinum	Chili	Texas	15	12
Clostridium botulinum	Beached whale	Alaska	8	14
Staphylococcus aureus	Shredded pork barbeque and coleslaw	Tennessee	3	15
Shiga toxin-producing *Escherichia coli* (O111; H8)	Water or salad	Texas	58	16
Shiga toxin-producing *E coli*	Ground beef	Multistate	18	17
Enterobacter sakazakii	Powdered infant formula	Tennessee	1	13
Enterotoxigenic *E coli*	Cole slaw	Tennessee	36	18
Cryptosporidium species	Food handler	District of Columbia	92	19
Campylobacter species	Tuna salad	Wisconsin	79	20
Shigella flexneri	Tomatoes	New York	116	21

Table 52.1 *(Continued)*
Examples of Recent Foodborne Outbreaks in the United States by Location, Vehicle, and Cause

Pathogen	Food Vehicle	Where	No. of Cases	Reference
Yersinia enterocolitica	Chitterlings	Illinois	9	22
Hepatitis A	Green onions	Pennsylvania	555	24
Hepatitis A	Unknown	Massachusetts	46	23
Vibrio parahaemolyticus	Raw oysters	Alaska	62	25
V parahaemolyticus	Raw oysters and clams	Multistate	23	26
Cyclospora	Uncooked snow peas	Pennsylvania	96	27
Salmonella serotype Typhimurium	Ground beef	Multistate	31	62
Salmonella serotype Braenderup and Javiana	Tomatoes	Multistate	18	29
Norovirus	Food handler	Michigan	23	63
Norovirus	Deli meat	Texas	125	64
Listeria monocytogenes	Deli turkey meat	Multistate	30	31
Rotavirus	Deli sandwich	District of Columbia	85	30
Clostridium perfringens	Corned beef	Ohio and Virginia	156	32

Table 52.2
Foodborne Outbreak Data from 2003–2004, Collected by the Foodborne Outbreak Reporting System, CDC

Etiology	Total Number of Outbreaks	
	2003	2004
Bacterial		
Bacillus species	2	6
Campylobacter species	15	9
Clostridium species	15	23
Escherichia coli	23	22
Plesiomonas species	0	1
Listeria species	2	0

Table 52.2 *(Continued)*
Foodborne Outbreak Data from 2003–2004, Collected by the Foodborne Outbreak Reporting System, CDC

Etiology	Total Number of Outbreaks	
	2003	2004
Salmonella species	108	122
Shigella species	12	9
Staphylococcus species	15	10
Vibrio species	3	4
Yersinia species	1	2
TOTAL	196	208
Chemical		
Ciguatoxin	16	10
Histamine	4	4
Mushroom toxins	0	2
Other chemical	3	1
Paralytic shellfish poison	1	2
Rhaphides-calcium oxalate	1	0
Scombroid toxin	29	28
TOTAL	54	47
Viral		
Hepatitis	9	2
Norovirus	140	249
TOTAL	149	251
Parasitic		
Cryptosporidium species	2	0
Trichinella species	1	0
Cyclospora species	0	2
Giardia species	0	6
TOTAL	3	8
Multiple Etiologies	7	5
Unknown Etiologies	664	800
TOTAL	1073	1319

In the last 10 years, several pathogens have been recognized as frequent or severe causes of foodborne disease. For instance, the proportion of confirmed foodborne disease outbreaks reported to the CDC caused by noroviruses increased from 2 in 1991 to 164 in 2000 (Fig 52.1). This increase is, in large part, attributable to widespread application of molecular diagnostic assays. These viruses are now estimated to be the most common single infectious cause of foodborne disease outbreaks, and because many outbreaks of unknown etiology are likely due to noroviruses, a total of 30% to 50% of all foodborne outbreaks may be attributable to these agents.[34,35] Norovirus infections have been commonly associated with consumption of a variety ready-to-eat food items contaminated at point of service.[36] Several outbreaks of norovirus gastroenteritis have been associated with imported frozen raspberries presumed contaminated in the fields by irrigation waters or human hands.[37,38] As norovirus detection capacity becomes increasingly available, it is likely that additional outbreaks caused by other foods contaminated before distribution will be identified.

Fig 52.1

Confirmed norovirus foodborne outbreaks reported to the Foodborne Outbreak Reporting System, CDC, United States, 1991–2000.*

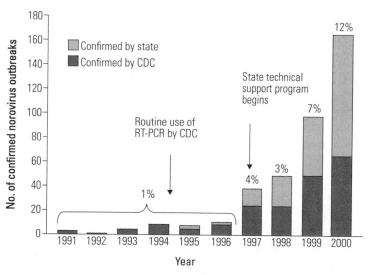

RT-PCR indicates reverse transcriptase-polymerase chain reaction.

*Percentage value above bars represents proportion of all foodborne outbreaks reported to the CDC that were laboratory confirmed to be attributable to norovirus by the Respiratory and Enteric Virus Branch at CDC or by a state public health laboratory.

Enterobacter sakazakii has emerged as a serious cause of foodborne illness in recent years. Although rare, infections in infants younger than 1 month can cause life-threatening meningitis, septicemia, and necrotizing enterocolitis[39-41]; case-fatality rates are as high as 33%.[42] The pathogen can also cause bacteremia and osteomyelitis in adults, albeit rarely.[43] Clusters of *E sakazakii* infections have been reported in a variety of locations over the past several years among infants fed milk-based powdered infant formula products from various manufacturers.[13,39-41,43-46] One study found that *E sakazakii* could be recovered from 14% of samples of milk-based powdered infant formula products,[47] but how contamination occurs is not known.[34]

Important clues for investigating and determining the etiology of an outbreak of foodborne illness include obtaining information about the incubation period, duration of illness, and clinical signs and symptoms. If a foodborne disease outbreak is suspected, appropriate clinical specimens should be submitted for laboratory testing, and local health authorities should be notified.

Clinical Manifestations, Diagnosis, and Treatment

Table 52.3 describes 5 clinicoepidemiologic profiles into which illnesses caused by most foodborne agents can be categorized. These profiles were derived from national data on foodborne outbreaks, including incubation period, duration of illness, percentage of affected people with vomiting or fever, and vomiting-to-fever ratio.[48] These syndromes include vomiting-toxin syndrome, diarrhea-toxin syndrome, diarrheogenic *E coli* syndrome, norovirus syndrome, and *Salmonella*-like syndrome. Most foodborne infections result in gastrointestinal symptoms, such as vomiting, diarrhea, and abdominal cramps.[2,5] Neurologic manifestations are less common but may include paresthesias (fish, shellfish, and monosodium glutamate), hypotonia and descending muscle weakness (*Clostridium botulinum*), and a variety of other signs and symptoms (fish, shellfish, mushrooms). Systemic manifestations are varied and are associated with a variety of infectious agents including *Listeria*, *Brucella*, *Trichinella*, *Toxoplasma*, and *Vibrio* species and hepatitis A virus.

Because the presenting symptoms are common to many causes, many infectious and noninfectious agents must be considered in people suspected of having foodborne illness, and establishing an etiologic diagnosis may be difficult on clinical grounds alone. Testing clinical specimens is often the only way to establish a diagnosis; however, frequently specimens are unavailable for laboratory testing. For individual cases of illness, collecting specimens for

Table 52.3
Distinct Foodborne Pathogen Syndromes[48]

Syndrome	Incubation Period (h)	Duration (h)	Vomiting (%)	Fever (%)	Vomiting-to-Fever Ratio*	Main Causative Agents
Vomiting-toxin	1.5–9.5	6.3–24	50–100	0–28	0–4.3	Chemical, *Bacillus cereus*, *Staphylococcus aureus*, *Salmonella* species, *Clostridium perfringens*, *Escherichia coli* (enterohemorrhagic)
Diarrhea-toxin	10–13.0	12–24	3.6–20	2.3–10	0.40–1.3	*B cereus*, *C perfringens*
Diarrheogenic *E coli*	48–120	104–185	3.1–37	13–25.3	0.25–1.1	*Campylobacter* species, *E coli*, *Salmonella* species, *Shigella* species
Norovirus-like	34.5–38.5	33–47	54–70.2	37–63	0.70–1.7	Norovirus, *Salmonella* species
Salmonella-like	18.0–88.5	63–144	8.9–51	31–81	0.20–1.0	*Campylobacter* species, Norovirus, *Salmonella* species, *Shigella* species

* Ratio of proportion with vomiting to proportion with fever.

laboratory diagnosis should be considered for the following circumstances: (1) patient populations including infants, children, the elderly, pregnant women, and immunocompromised hosts; (2) presence of specific signs and symptoms including bloody diarrhea; severe abdominal pain or fever; sudden onset of nausea, vomiting, or diarrhea, dehydration associated with diarrhea; or neurologic involvement including paresthesias, motor weakness, and cranial nerve palsies; (3) presence of underlying gastrointestinal tract disease, including inflammatory bowel disease, malignancy, gastrointestinal tract surgery or radiation, certain medications; malabsorption syndromes; or other structural or functional conditions; and (4) association of illness with other factors such as travel, hospitalization, occupation, contact with other ill people, and child care or nursing home attendance. The occurrence of neurologic signs and symptoms are particularly worrisome because of the potential for life-threatening complications. For suspected outbreaks of foodborne disease involving gastrointestinal symptoms, stools should always be collected for laboratory testing when possible.

Collaboration and communication with clinical microbiology laboratory personnel and local public health officials will help optimize laboratory testing. Laboratory testing may include at least one of the following: stool cultures for bacteria, polymerase chain reaction assays of stool for viruses, microscopic examination of stool for parasites, and direct antigen detection tests of stool culture broths and blood cultures. More detailed information on laboratory procedures for detection of foodborne pathogens can be obtained from clinical and microbiology specialists and from microbiology and local or state public health personnel. As yet, there is no commercial laboratory test available for diagnosis of norovirus infection, but almost all state public health laboratories and the CDC routinely test stools by polymerase chain reaction assays.

Enteric infections generally are self-limited conditions that require fluid and electrolyte therapy (see also Chapter 28—Oral Therapy for Acute Diarrhea). In some instances, specific antimicrobial therapy may eradicate fecal shedding of the causative organism, prevent transmission of the enteropathogen, abbreviate clinical symptoms, or prevent future complications. However, antibiotic treatment for *E coli* O157:H7 infection has been identified as a risk factor for progression to hemolytic-uremic syndrome.[49] Antibiotic treatment may also disrupt the normal gut flora and may exacerbate the diarrhea, particularly because several pathogens have developed resistance to certain antibiotic agents. Therefore, careful consideration of the illness etiology is important before treatment. A primer on foodborne diseases developed by the American Medical Association, the CDC, the Food and Drug Administration (FDA), and the US Department of Agriculture contains information about causes, clinical considerations, and patient scenarios as well as patient handout materials and resources.[2]

Surveillance for Foodborne Diseases

The CDC collects foodborne disease outbreak information through the Electronic Foodborne Disease Outbreak Reporting System (eFORS). This surveillance system is passive in that it relies on state health departments reporting outbreaks to CDC. The data collected help monitor foodborne disease outbreak etiologies, vehicles, and contributing factors (eg, factors that resulted in contamination of a food vehicle). Data from this surveillance system need to be interpreted with caution, because most people with foodborne illness do not have stool or blood specimen collected and tested uniformly for all agents. For instance, a recent study showed that outbreaks with patients with viral-like symptoms (vomiting, diarrhea) were less likely to be reported than outbreaks with patients with more severe symptoms. The eFORS surveillance system is important for monitoring trends in foodborne disease outbreaks, describing the various types of foodborne pathogens, determining the risk of exposure attributable to different types of foods, and summarizing factors that contributed to the outbreaks.[35]

Another recent development in foodborne disease outbreak detection is PulseNet USA, the national molecular subtyping network system for foodborne disease surveillance.[50] Sixty-four public health and food regulatory laboratories, including all state health departments, participate in PulseNet USA and routinely perform pulsed-field gel electrophoresis (PFGE) of *Campylobacter* species, *E coli* O157, *Shigella* species, *Listeria* species, and *Salmonella* species using standard methods. As a result, public health laboratories can rapidly compare the PFGE patterns of bacteria isolated from ill people and determine whether they are likely to be part of the same outbreak or attributable to the same exposure. Laboratory professionals perform regular searches on their local PFGE databases, looking for clusters of isolates that are indistinguishable by PFGE. The results are reported to CDC, state epidemiologists, and the electronic database. PulseNet USA has been useful in the detection of foodborne disease outbreaks, including *Salmonella* species and *E coli* O157 in ground beef by quickly compiling information on genetic profiles of bacterial isolates from ill people and food specimens.[28,51] The real-time acquisition of PFGE patterns from PulseNet USA as well as eFORS allow for more thorough outbreak detection and control. Because of the extensive food distribution system in the United States, contaminated foods may be distributed to people in many locations.

Surveillance for norovirus and other enteric viruses historically has been performed by the CDC on receipt of specimens from presumed norovirus outbreaks.[52] However, in recent years through technology transfer, most state public health laboratories in the have established the capacity to routinely detect norovirus in specimens collected from people involved in outbreaks, and most foodborne outbreaks of norovirus are now confirmed locally and reported to the CDC via eFORS. Of note, however, because clinical laboratories do not test for norovirus, widespread outbreaks of foodborne illness presenting as dispersed sporadic illnesses may remain undetected.

In 1996, the CDC's Emerging Infection Program (EIP), in collaboration with participating sites, the US Department of Agriculture, and the FDA, initiated the Foodborne Diseases Active Surveillance Network (FoodNet).[53] The rationale of this system was to better define population-based incidence trends in rates of key bacterial foodborne infection as regulatory bodies implemented specific control measures. FoodNet conducts population-based, active laboratory surveillance for 9 foodborne pathogens, including the bacterial pathogens *Salmonella* species, *Shigella* species, *Campylobacter* species, Shiga toxin-producing *Escherichia coli* (STEC), *Listeria monocytogenes*, *Yersinia enterocolitica*, *Vibrio* species, and the parasitic organisms *Cryptosporidium* species and *Cyclospora* species. FoodNet encompasses a surveillance population of 44 million people (15% of the population) and consists of more than 650 clinical laboratories that test specimens in the FoodNet sites. In addition to collecting information on laboratory-diagnosed cases of foodborne pathogens, investigators at FoodNet sites began active surveillance for hemolytic-uremic syndrome, a serious complication of STEC infection.

Table 52.4 shows the incidence by age group, total number of cases, and death rate among people infected with specific pathogens under surveillance in 2004. Bacterial agents including *Campylobacter*, *Salmonella*, and *Shigella* species are the most frequently identified causes of laboratory-confirmed illness in FoodNet.[54] The most severe infections are caused by *Listeria* and *Vibrio* species and *E coli* O157:H7. Children younger than 9 years are at a greater risk than adults for *Campylobacter* species, *Cryptosporidium* species, *E coli* O157:H7, *Salmonella* species, *Shigella* species, and *Yersinia* species infection. Since 1996, various preventive measures have resulted in a decrease in foodborne illness attributable to some of the 9 most common pathogens in the CDC's FoodNet program.[54] Fig 52.2 shows trends in incidence of infection by selected FoodNet pathogens in 2004 compared with the 1996–1998 baseline. Rates of *Campylobacter* species, *E coli* O157:H7, *Listeria* species, and *Salmonella* species infections are declining compared to the incidence reported from 1996–1998. Active surveillance methods used by FoodNet are critical to evaluating the effectiveness of prevention programs, for monitoring emerging foodborne pathogens, and for identifying novel interventions.

Table 52.4

Incidence of Infection by Age Group, Total Cases, and Deaths, FoodNet 2004

| Organism | Age Group and Cases per 100 000 Population in FoodNet | | | | | | No. of Total Cases (Rate*) | No. of Deaths (Rate†) |
	<1 y	1–9 y	10–19 y	20–39 y	40–59 y	>60 y		
Campylobacter species	25.6	15.7	8.3	12.7	13.1	11.4	5684 (12.8)	9 (0.2)
Cryptosporidium species	0.8	2.5	1.2	1.6	1.0	0.8	637 (1.4)	5 (0.9)
Cyclospora species	0.00	0.00	0.04	0.04	0.03	0.04	15 (0.03)	0 0.0
Escherichia coli O157	1.3	2.8	1.2	0. 5	0.5	0.6	402 (0.9)	4 (1.0)
Listeria species	0.3	0.0	0.0	0.1	0.2	0.9	119 (0.3)	19 (16.1)
Salmonella species	113.4	30. 6	10. 7	10.4	9.7	11.6	6498 (14.6)	38 (0.7)
Shigella species	7.6	21.0	2.7	4.1	2.3	1.1	2248 (5.1)	3 (0.2)
Vibrio species	0.0	0.1	0.1	0.3	0.3	0.4	123 (0.3)	5 (5.3)
Yersinia species	8.3	0.6	0.2	0.2	0.2	0.4	176 (0.4)	1 (0.7)

* Cases per 100 000 population for FoodNet areas.
† Deaths per 100 cases with known outcome.

Prevention

From 1993 through 1997, the most commonly reported food preparation practices that contributed to foodborne disease were improper holding temperatures of food and poor personal hygiene of preparers of food.[55] Since these findings, both general and specific measures have been established to improve foodborne disease prevention. The FDA Food Code was originally

Fig 52.2
Trends in selected pathogens in FoodNet sites.

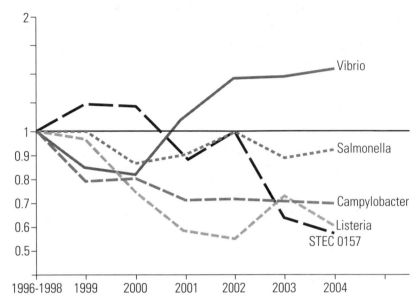

Relative rates compared with 1996–1998 baseline period of laboratory-diagnosed cases of infection with *Campylobacter* species, STEC O157, *Listeria* species, *Salmonella* species, and *Vibrio* species, by year.[54]

created in 1997 but was updated in 2005 and is a model that assists food control jurisdictions by providing them with official, scientifically rigorous guidelines for regulating the retail and foodservice segment of the industry (restaurants and grocery stores and institutions such as nursing homes).[56] The revised Food Code reflects the growing recognition of the frequency of norovirus infection by now stating that food handlers with gastroenteritis should remain away from work for 24 hours after recovery to reduce the risk of transmission of noroviruses, which are usually shed for several days to weeks after resolution of symptoms.[57] Additional measures have been enacted that are specific for defined food products and have changed the incidence of foodborne infections.[58] These measures have included FDA prevention programs for seafood, increased attention to good agriculture practices aimed at fresh fruit and vegetables, new rules on egg and juice safety, increased regulation of imported foods, food safety education, irradiation of meat, and introduction of the Hazard Analysis Critical Control Point regulations for meat and poultry in processing plants.[59] Information about these and other measures enacted to reduce foodborne disease can be found at various Web sites shown in the directory of resources (Table 52.5). One aim of FoodNet surveillance has been to monitor changes in these bacterial and parasitic infection rates that may correspond to efforts to implement measures to control foodborne disease, such as the Hazard Analysis Critical Control Point. Lastly, since the Bioterrorism Act of 2002 (Pub L No. 107-188), regulatory agencies such as the FDA have acted to better protect consumers from food that may have been deliberately contaminated. Measures include improved record keeping for tracing foods, powers to detain suspect foods, improved registration of food facilities, and requirements for previous notice of importation of certain foods in to the United States.

Table 52.5
Directory of Online Resources Regarding Prevention of Foodborne Illness

Food Safety Information and Prevention
• http://www.cdc.gov/foodsafety/about.htm
• http://www.cdc.gov/ounceofprevention
• http://www.cfsan.fda.gov/~mow/chap3.html
• http://www.who.int/foodsafety/fs_management/No_06_GSS_Oct05_en.pdf
• http://www.fao.org/docrep/meeting/008/ae172e/ae172e00.htm
• http://www.paho.org/English/sha/be_v23n1-casedef.htm
• http://www.westchestergov.com/labsresearch/publichealth/microlab/service/service1.htm
• http://www.cdc.gov/foodsafety/
• http://www.cfsan.fda.gov/~dms/fsibroch.html
• http://www.osha.gov/SLTC/foodbornedisease/control.html

Powdered Infant Formula Information and Reconstitution Guidelines
• http://www.ifm.net/issues/esakazakii_position.htm
• http://www.who.int/foodsafety/publications/micro/en/qa2.pdf
• http://peaches.nal.usda.gov/foodborne/fbindex/Outbreak.asp
• http://www.cdc.gov/foodsafety/outbreaks.htm
• http://www.oregon.gov/DHS/ph/acd/reporting/foodrpt.shtml
• http://www.foodsafety.gov/

Clinical Management of Suspected Foodborne Illness
• http://www.cdc.gov/mmwr/preview/mmwrhtml/rr5002a1.htm
• http://www.maine.gov/dhhs/boh/ddc/Feb_06_epigram.htm
• http://www.medscape.com/pages/editorial/public/pguidelines/index-infectiousdiseases
• http://www.ama-assn.org/ama1/pub/upload/mm/36/2004_food_table_bact.pdf

Table 52.5 *(Continued)*
Directory of Online Resources Regarding Prevention of Foodborne Illness

Hazard Analysis and Critical Control Point, FDA FoodCode
• http://www.cfsan.fda.gov/~lrd/haccp.html
• http://www.fao.org/DOCREP/005/Y1579E/y1579e03.htm
• http://www.saferpak.com/haccp.htm
• http://www.fsis.usda.gov/Science/hazard_analysis_&_pathogen_reduction/index.asp
• http://www.mda.state.mn.us/licensing/meategg/haccpssop.htm
• http://www.cfsan.fda.gov/~dms/fc05-toc.html

These measures are especially relevant for specific high-risk segments of the population, including infants, children, the elderly, immunocompromised people, and pregnant women.[9] These high-risk populations should avoid eating or drinking raw (unpasteurized) milk or raw milk products, raw or partially cooked eggs or raw egg products, raw or undercooked meat and poultry, raw or undercooked fish or shellfish, unpasteurized juices, and raw sprouts. Furthermore, certain deli meats and frankfurters should only be eaten once they have been reheated to steaming hot. Raw or unpasteurized honey should be avoided and infants younger than 12 months should not be given honey from any source. Physicians and parents should be aware that powdered infant formulas, although heat-treated during processing, are not sterile, in contrast to liquid formulas.[60] "Transition" infant formulas that are generally used after hospital discharge for infants born preterm or with low birth weight are available in both nonsterile powder form and commercially sterile liquid form. Because of the risk of *E sakazakii* infection, the FDA recommends that powdered infant formulas not be used in neonatal intensive care settings unless no alternative is available.[60]

General measures that can be used to prevent foodborne illness include emphasis on safe food handling practices, with education targeted toward consumers in preparation, cooking, and storage of food, and use of technology including irradiation and food processing methodologies.[61] Major areas of concern with regard to food safety include caution when buying fresh food, handling of ready-to-eat foods, hand washing and surface cleaning, prevention of cross contamination, cooking of food at proper temperatures, and prompt and appropriate refrigeration of food before and after cooking or preparation (see Cooking Guidelines, Table 52.6).

Table 52.6
Cooking Guidelines From the CDC

Eggs
• Cook eggs until they are firm and not runny.
• Do not eat raw or partially cooked eggs.
• Avoid eating other foods that include raw or partially cooked eggs.
Poultry
• Cook poultry until it has an internal temperature of 180°F.
• It is done when the juices run clear and it is white in the middle.
• Never eat rare poultry.
Fish
• Cook fish until it is opaque or white and flaky.
• Cook ground meat to 160°F.
Meat
• It is done when it is brown inside. This is especially critical with hamburger meat.

Personal hygiene and cleaning of surfaces are critical in the prevention of foodborne disease. Cross contamination from one food item to another is a major problem when handling raw meat, poultry, seafood, and eggs. Microorganisms can be transmitted in the kitchen via hands, cutting boards, utensils, and countertops. Hands should be washed before and after handling food and after using the bathroom, changing diapers, or handling pets. Potential vehicles for transmission of organisms, such as cutting boards, dishes, utensils, and countertops, should be washed after preparing each food item. Anyone who prepares food should be familiar with food safety practices, available on the CDC Web site (Table 52.5). Contamination of foods with viruses is particularly easy when preparing food. Any contact of bare, contaminated hands with food subsequently eaten without heating has the potential to transmit virus and cause infection. In addition, food preparation surfaces can become contaminated with viruses; this contamination can be unapparent and may resist disinfection with common products. If viral contamination of the food preparation area is suspected, a 1 in 50 (1000 ppm) solution of domestic bleach in water should be used to clean the area and thoroughly rinsed off. See the Food Code[56] for more details on disinfectants.

Normal cooking of foods will kill most pathogens that cause foodborne illness. Eggs should be cooked until they are firm; poultry should be cooked until it has an internal temperature of 180°F, until the meat is white in the middle and until juices are clear; fish should be cooked until it is opaque and flakes easily with a fork; meat, especially hamburger meat, should be cooked to 160°F, until it is brown inside, and until the juices are clear. Because bacteria grow at room temperature, hot foods should be maintained at 140°F or higher and cold foods at 40°F or lower. Perishables, prepared foods, and leftovers should be refrigerated or frozen within 2 hours of preparation with minimal handling. Foods should be defrosted in the refrigerator, under cold running water, or in a microwave, and foods should be marinated in the refrigerator.

Four major tips can be used to prevent contamination of food (see CDC Food Safety Web site, Table 52.5):

1. Use caution when buying food.

   - Buy perishable food such as meat, eggs, and milk last.

   - Avoid raw or unpasteurized milk.

   - Because eggs, meat, seafood, and poultry are most likely to contain bacteria, do not allow their juices to drip on other food.

   - Shop for groceries when there is time to take food home right away so that it does not spoil in a hot car.

2. Store food properly.

   - Store eggs, raw meat, poultry, and seafood in the refrigerator.

   - Use containers to prevent contaminating other foods or kitchen surfaces.

   - Set refrigerator temperature at 40°F.

   - Set freezer temperature at 0°F.

   - Regularly clean and disinfect the refrigerator and freezer.

3. Use special precautions when preparing and cooking food.

   - Wash hands and clean and disinfect kitchen surfaces before, during, and after handling, cooking, and serving food.

   - Wash raw fruits and vegetables before eating them.

   - Defrost frozen food on a plate either in the refrigerator or in a microwave but not on the counter.

- Cook food immediately after defrosting.

- Use different dishes and utensils for raw foods than for cooked foods.

4. Cool and promptly store leftovers after food has been served.

- Because harmful bacteria grow at room temperature, keep hot food hot at 140°F or higher, and keep cold food cold at 40°F or cooler (this is especially important during picnics and buffets).

- Do not leave perishable foods out for more than 2 hours.

- Promptly refrigerate or freeze leftovers in shallow containers or wrapped tightly in bags.

References

1. Mead PS, Slutsker L, Dietz V, et al. Food-related illness and death in the United States. *Emerg Infect Dis*. 1999;5:607–625

2. Centers for Disease Control and Prevention. Diagnosis and management of foodborne illnesses: a primer for physicians and other health care professionals. *MMWR Recomm Rep*. 2004;53(RR-4):1–33

3. Centers for Disease Control and Prevention. Surveillance for waterborne-disease outbreaks associated with drinking water—United States, 2001–2002. *MMWR Surveill Summ*. 2004;53:23–45

4. Centers for Disease Control and Prevention. Surveillance for foodborne disease outbreaks—United States, 1993–1997. *MMWR CDC Surveill Summ*. 2000;49(SS-1):1–62

5. Guerrant RL, Van Gilder TJ, Steiner TS, et al. Practice guidelines for the management of infectious diarrhea. *Clin Infect Dis*. 2001;32:331–351

6. Pickering LK. Approach to diagnosis and management of gastrointestinal tract infections. In: Long SS, Pickering LK, Prober CG, eds. *Principles and Practice of Pediatric Infectious Diseases*. 2nd ed. Philadelphia, PA: Churchill Livingstone; 2003:362–368

7. Swaminathan B, Gerner-Smidt P, Barrett T. Foodborne disease trends and reports. *Foodborne Pathog Dis*. 2005;2:190–191

8. Koehler KM, Lasky R, Fein SB, et al. Population-based incidence of infection with selected bacterial enteric pathogens in children younger than five years of age, 1996–1998. *Pediatr Infect Dis J*. 2006;25:129–134

9. Gerba CP, Rose JB, Haas CN. Sensitive populations: who is at the greatest risk? *Int J Food Microbiol*. 1996;30:113–123

10. United States Department of Health and Human Services. Healthy People 2010. Washington, DC: United States Department of Health and Human Services; 2000. Available at: http://www.cdc.gov/nchs/about/otheract/hpdata2010/abouthp.htm. Accessed October 29, 2007

11. Tauxe RV. Emerging foodborne pathogens. *Int J Food Microbiol*. 2002;78:31–41

12. Kalluri P, Crowe C, Reller ME, et al. An outbreak of foodborne botulisms associated with food sold at a salvage store in Texas. *Clin Infect Dis.* 2003;37:1490–1495

13. Centers for Disease Control and Prevention. *Enterobacter sakazakii* infections associated with the use of powdered infant formula—Tennessee, 2001. *MMWR Morb Mortal Wkly Rep.* 2002;51:298–300

14. Centers for Disease Control and Prevention. Outbreak of botulism type E associated with eating a beached whale—Western Alaska, July 2002. *MMWR Morb Mortal Wkly Rep.* 2003;52:24–26

15. Jones TF, Kellum ME, Porter SS, Bell M, Schaffner W. An outbreak of community-acquired foodborne illness caused by methicillin-resistant *Staphylocccus aureus. Emerg Infect Dis.* 2002;8:82–84

16. Centers for Disease Control and Prevention. *Escherichia coli* O111:H8 outbreak among teenage campers—Texas, 1999. *MMWR Morb Mortal Wkly Rep.* 2000;49:321–324

17. Centers for Disease Control and Prevention. Multistate outbreak of *Escherichia coli* O157:H7 infections associated with eating ground beef—United States, June–July 2002. *MMWR Morb Mortal Wkly Rep.* 2002;51:637–639

18. Devasia R, Jones T, Ward J, et al. Endemically acquired foodborne outbreak of enterotoxin-producing *Escherichia coli* serotype O169:H41. *Am J Med.* 2006;119:168.e7–168.e10

19. Quiroz ES, Bern C, MacArthur JR, et al. An outbreak of cryptosporidiosis linked to a foodhandler. *J Infect Dis.* 2000;181:695–700

20. Roels TH, Wickus B, Bostrom HH, et al. A foodborne outbreak of *Campylobacter jejuni* (O:33) infection associated with tuna salad: a rare strain in an unusual vehicle. *Epidemiol Infect.* 1998;121:281–287

21. Reller ME, Nelson JM, Molbak K, et al. A large, multiple-restaurant outbreak of infection with *Shigella flexneri* serotype 2a traced to tomatoes. *Clin Infect Dis.* 2006;42:163–169

22. Centers for Disease Control and Prevention. Yersinia enterocolitica gastroenteritis among infants exposed to chitterlings—Chicago, Illinois, 2002. *MMWR Morb Mortal Wkly Rep.* 2003;52:956–958

23. Centers for Disease Control and Prevention. Foodborne transmission of hepatitis A—Massachusetts, 2001. *MMWR Morb Mortal Wkly Rep.* 2003;52:565–567

24. Wheeler C, Vogt TM, Armstrong GL, et al. An outbreak of hepatitis A associated with green onions. *New Engl J Med.* 2005;353:890–897

25. McLaughlin JB, DePaola A, Bopp CA, et al. Outbreak of *Vibrio parahaemolyticus* gastroenteritis associated with Alaskan oysters. *N Engl J Med.* 2005;353:1463–1470

26. Centers for Disease Control and Prevention. Outbreak of *Vibrio parahaemolyticus* infection associated with eating raw oysters and clams harvested from Long Island Sound—Connecticut, New Jersey, and New York, 1998. *MMWR Morb Mortal Wkly Rep.* 1999;48:48–51

27. Centers for Disease Control and Prevention. Outbreak of cyclosporiasis associated with snow peas—Pennsylvania, 2004. *MMWR Morb Mortal Wkly Rep.* 2004;53:876–878

28. Centers for Disease Control and Prevention. Multistate outbreak of *Salmonella* typhimurium infections associated with eating ground beef—United States, 2004. *MMWR Morb Mortal Wkly Rep.* 2006;55:180–182

29. Centers for Disease Control and Prevention. Outbreaks of *Salmonella* infections associated with eating Roma tomatoes—United States and Canada, 2004. *MMWR Morb Mortal Wkly Rep.* 2005;54:325–328

30. Centers for Disease Control and Prevention. Foodborne outbreak of group A rotavirus gastroenteritis among college students—District of Columbia, March–April 2000. *MMWR Morb Mortal Wkly Rep.* 2000;49:1131–1133

31. Olsen SJ, Patrick M, Hunter SB, et al. Multistate outbreak of *Listeria monocytogenes* infection linked to delicatessen turkey meat. *Clin Infect Dis.* 2005;40:962–967

32. Centers for Disease Control and Prevention. *Clostridium perfringens* gastroenteritis associated with corned beef served at St. Patrick's day meals—Ohio and Virginia, 1993. *MMWR Morb Mortal Wkly Rep.* 1994;43:137, 143–144

33. Centers for Disease Control and Prevention. 2004 Foodborne Outbreak Response and Surveillance Unit Summary Statistics. Available at: http://www.cdc.gov/foodborneoutbreaks/outbreak_data.htm. Accessed October 29, 2007

34. Turcios RM, Widdowson MA, Sulka AC, Mead PS, Glass RI. Reevaluation of epidemiological criteria for identifying outbreaks of acute gastroenteritis due to norovirus: United States 1998–2000. *Clin Infect Dis.* 2006;42:964–969

35. Widdowson MA, Sulka A, Bulens SN, et al. Norovirus and foodborne disease, United States, 1991–2000. *Emerg Infect Dis.* 2005;11:95–102

36. Widdowson MA, Monroe SS, Glass RI. Are noroviruses emerging? *Emerg Infect Dis.* 2005;11:735–737

37. Maunula L, Kalso S, Von Bonsdorff CH, Ponka A. Wading pool water contaminated with both noroviruses and astroviruses as the source of a gastroenteritis outbreak. *Epidemiol Infect.* 2004;132:737–743

38. Gaulin CD, Ramsay D, Cardinal P, D'Halevyn MA. [Epidemic of gastroenteritis of viral origin associated with eating imported raspberries.] [Article in French.] *Can J Public Health.* 1999;90:37–40

39. van Acker J, de Smet F, Muyldermans G, Bougatef A, Naessens A, Lauwers S. Outbreak of necrotizing enterocolitis associated with *Enterobacter sakazakii* in powdered milk formula. *J Clin Microbiol.* 2001;39:293–297

40. Biering G, Karlsson S, Clark NC, et al. Three cases of neonatal meningitis caused by *Enterobacter sakazakii* in powdered milk. *J Clin Microbiol.* 1989;27:2054–2056

41. Simmons BP, Gelfand MS, Haas M, Metts L, erguson J. *Enterobacter sakazakii* infections in neonates associated with intrinsic contamination of a powdered infant formula. *Infect Control Hosp Epidemiol.* 1989;10:398–401

42. Lehner A, Stephan R. Microbiological, epidemiological, and food safety aspects of *Enterobacter sakazakii*. *J Food Prot.* 2004;67:2850–2857

43. Lai KK. *Enterobacter sakazakii* infections among neonates, infants, children, and adults. Case reports and a review of the literature. *Medicine (Baltimore).* 2001;80:113–122

44. Clark NC, Hill BC, O'Hara CM, Steinrimsson O, Cooksey RC. Epidemiologic typing of *Enterobacter sakazakii* in two neonatal nosocomial outbreaks. *Diagn Microbiol Infect Dis.* 1990;13:467–472

45. Nazarowec-White M, Farber JM. Phenotypic and genotypic typing of food and clinical isolates of *Enterobacter sakazakii. J Med Microbiol.* 1999;48:559–567

46. Weir E. Powdered infant formula and fatal infection with *Enterobacter sakazakii. CMAJ.* 2002;166:1570–

47. Muytjens HL, Roelofs-Willemse H, Jaspar GH. Quality of powdered substitutes for breast milk with regard to members of the family Enterobacteriaceae. *J Clin Microbiol.* 1988;26:743–746

48. Hall JA, Goulding JS, Bean NH, Tauxe RV, Hedberg CW. Epidemiologic profiling: evaluating foodborne outbreaks for which no pathogen was isolated by routine laboratory testing: United States, 1982–9. *Epidemiol Infect.* 2001;127:381–387

49. Wong CS, Jelacic S, Habeeb RL, Watkins L, Tarr PI. The risk of hemolytic-uremic syndrome after antibiotic treatment of *Escherichia coli* O157:H7 infections. *N Engl J Med.* 2000;342:1930–1936

50. Swaminathan B, Barrett TJ, Hunter SB, Tauxe RV, CDC PulseNet Task Force. PulseNet: the molecular subtyping network for foodborne bacterial disease surveillance, United States. *Emerg Infect Dis.* 2001;7:382–389

51. Gerner-Smidt P, Kincaid J, Kubota K, et al. Molecular surveillance of Shiga toxigenic *Escherichia coli* O157 by PulseNet USA. *J Food Prot.* 2005;68:1926–1931

52. Blanton LH, Adams SM, Beard RS, et al. Molecular and epidemiologic trends of caliciviruses associated with outbreaks of acute gastroenteritis in the United States, 2000–2004. *J Infect Dis.* 2006;193:413–421

53. Centers for Disease Control and Prevention. Foodborne disease active surveillance network, 1996. *MMWR Morb Mortal Wkly Rep.* 1997;46:258–261

54. Centers for Disease Control and Prevention. Preliminary FoodNet data on the incidence of infection with pathogens transmitted commonly through food—10 sites, United States, 2004. *MMWR Morb Mortal Wkly Rep.* 2005;54:352–356

55. Bryan FL, Guzewich JJ, Todd ECD. Surveillance of foodborne disease III. Summary and presentation of data on vehicles and contributory factors; their value and limitations. *J Food Prot.* 1997;60:701–714

56. Federal Drug Administration. *Food Code.* College Park, MD: US Department of Health and Human Services; 2005. Available at: http://www.cfsan.fda.gov/~dms/fc05-toc.html. Accessed November 2, 2007

57. Rockx B, de Wit M, Vennema H, et al. Natural history of human calicivirus infection: a prospective cohort study. *Clin Infect Dis.* 2002;35:246–253

58. Centers for Disease Control and Prevention. Achievements in public health, 1990–1999: safer and healthier foods. *MMWR Morb Mortal Wkly Rep.* 1999;48:905–913

59. Billy TJ, Wachsmuth IK. Hazard analysis and critical control point systems in the United States Department of Agriculture regulatory policy. *Rev Sci Tech.* 1997;16:342–348

60. US Food and Drug Administration. Health Professionals Letter on *Enterobacter sakazakii* Infections Associated With Use of Powdered (Dry) Infant Formulas in Neonatal Intensive Care Units. Rockville, MD: US Food and Drug Administration; 2005. Available at: http://www.cfsan.fda.gov/~dms/inf-ltr3.html. Accessed October 29, 2007

61. Tauxe RV. Food safety and irradiation: protecting the public from foodborne infections. *Emerg Infect Dis*. 2001;7:516–521

62. Centers for Disease Control and Prevention. Multistate outbreak of *Salmonella* Typhimurium infections associated with eating ground beef—United States, 2004. *MMWR Morb Mortal Wkly Rep*. 2006;55:180–182

63. Centers for Disease Control and Prevention. Multisite outbreak of norovirus associated with a franchise restaurant—Kent County, Michigan, May 2005. *MMWR Morb Mortal Wkly Rep*. 2006;55:395–397

64. Daniels NA, Bergmire-Sweat DA, Schwab KJ, et al. A foodborne outbreak of gastroenteritis associated with Norwalk-like viruses: first molecular traceback to deli sandwiches contaminated during preparation. *J Infect Dis*. 2000;181:1467–1470

V

53 Food Safety: Pesticides, Industrial Chemicals, Toxins, Antimicrobial Preservatives and Irradiation, and Indirect Food Additives

Introduction

Foods available in the United States are among the safest found in the world.[1] Nonetheless, there are a wide variety of nonnutritive chemical substances found in the food supply that may have health and safety implications for infants and children.

In contrast with the usually defined illnesses associated with microbial contamination of foods, the safety issues related to nonmicrobial substances in foods are less understood and more difficult to document. As a result, related health issues are less often recognized and less easily diagnosed. Acute toxicity does occur, especially with the organophosphate insecticides, but it is not common and usually not recognized. The chronic effects of these substances are generally more significant for the fetus and young child because of potential neurotoxic and developmental effects, but these effects are even less recognized clinically as related to food than are the acute effects. For the chronic effects, prevention of exposure is more significant than are most treatments.

The primary responsibility for food safety in the United States resides with the US Food and Drug Administration (FDA), which was founded in 1906. Its function was expanded and clarified in 1938 by the Federal Food, Drug and Cosmetic Act (21 USC §301). Within the FDA, now part of the Department of Health and Human Services, most food issues are covered by the Center for Food Safety and Applied Nutrition, which was established in the 1970s and reorganized in 1993. Other agencies also play a supporting role.[1] Additional food safety issues are under the jurisdiction of the US Department of Agriculture (USDA)'s Food Safety and Inspection Service, which is responsible for the safety inspections of meat, poultry, and egg products. The Environmental Protection Agency (EPA) also plays a role in food safety, as it is responsible for setting limits (tolerances) on pesticide residues in food. The Centers for Disease Control and Prevention investigates, conducts surveillance on, and responds to outbreaks of foodborne and waterborne illnesses and monitors emerging pathogens and antimicrobial resistance patterns.

The major legislation that regulates pesticide-related food safety issues for infants and children is the Food Quality and Protection Act of 1996

(Pub L No. 104-170 [see text box]). Up until the passage of this act, the allowable amounts of pesticide residues in food were intended to protect adult health. Concerns for the special vulnerability of infants and children led to the 1993 report from the National Academy of Sciences, "Pesticides in the Diets of Infants and Children,"[2] which preceded the act.

Food Quality and Protection Act of 1996

Actions generated by the act, modifying the Federal Insecticide, Fungicide and Rodenticide Act and the Federal Food, Drug and Cosmetic Act:

- Established a single health-based standard for all pesticides in food.
- Benefits, in general, cannot override the health-based standard.
- Prenatal and postnatal effects are to be considered.
- In the absence of data confirming the safety to infants and children, because of their special sensitivities and exposures, an additional uncertainty factor of up to 10 times can be added to the safety values.
- Aggregate risk, the sum of all exposures to the chemical, must be considered in establishing safe amounts.
- Cumulative risk, the sum of all exposures to chemicals with similar mechanisms of action, must be considered in establishing safe amounts.
- Endocrine disrupters are to be included in the evaluation of safety.
- All existing pesticide registrations were to be reviewed by 2006.
- Expedited review is possible for safer pesticides.
- Risks are to be determined for both 1 year and lifetime exposure.

A major result of that act has been the regulatory recognition that infants and children are potentially more sensitive than adults to environmental chemicals for a number of reasons. Increased susceptibility may result from the greater intake of foods per unit of body weight. This is especially true for foods that are a part of the diet of most infants and young children. The immaturity of developing organ systems is another potential hazard, especially for the nervous, immune, and endocrine systems, and particularly during sensitive periods of development, when relatively brief insults may result in later long-term effects.[3] Altered pharmacokinetics are also of concern because of the immaturity of organs such as the liver and kidney and the changes in the amounts of body fat and extracellular water. Because children have a longer lifespan ahead of them than adults do, the likelihood of long-term effects, such as cancer, is increased.[4]

Sources of Concern for Chemical Food Safety

Chemical substances that are potentially toxic may occur in foods as a deliberate application during agricultural practices (pesticides), through industrial practices (dioxins, metals, flame retardants, and perchlorates), as naturally occurring toxins, or through nonnutritional additives (food contactants or food processing by-products or contaminants from the home environment). For additional information beyond what is in this chapter, see the *Handbook of Pediatric Environmental Health*, published by the American Academy of Pediatrics (AAP) in 2003.[5]

Agricultural Practices

Pesticides

Of the approximately 900 pesticide active ingredients registered with the EPA and more than 9000 preparations licensed for use in the United States, approximately 360 are routinely examined in food products in the United States.[6] They are used primarily on fruits, vegetables, and grains. Pesticides include insecticides, herbicides, fungicides, rodenticides, and fumigants. Although these products can increase both yield and quality of produce, they may be toxic, especially to handlers, but also as residues in the foods we eat. The residues an individual ingests from various foods are determined by the amount of pesticide applied to the crop; the time between application and harvesting, processing, or storage; the type of processing; the treatment of the food in the home; and the amount of the food ingested. The EPA regulates all these processes except what happens in the home. Tolerances are established for each pesticide in related foods and these represent the maximum amount of the pesticide allowed by the EPA. When the tolerance is exceeded, appropriate federal action occurs to remedy the situation.

Residues of pesticides above the allowable amounts in domestic foods were found in 2.4% of the 2344 foods tested in 2003. In foods imported from 99 countries, amounts above those legally allowed vary from year to year but were found in 6% of the 4890 foods tested in 2003. Of special interest was the finding that none of the infant formula and baby food samples that were tested had residues that violated the upper tolerable limits.[7]

The regulations governing these actions are contained in the Federal Insecticide, Fungicide and Rodenticide Act (Pub L No. 108-38 [2003]) and the Federal Food, Drug and Cosmetic Act, as amended by the Food Quality and Protection Act. As a result of regulations and voluntary withdrawals stemming from the Food Quality and Protection Act, several high-use pesticides have been, or are likely to be, significantly reduced in their use. Because the organophosphates are increasingly recognized as potentially toxic to infants and small children, their use, beginning with chlorpyriphos, is being increasingly restricted by the EPA.[8]

There is a significant problem in regulation, because the sampling process can never account for more than a small fraction of the food supply. Moreover, although the same rules about pesticide usage apply to use in home gardens, there is no monitoring or enforcement to ensure proper use. Excessive applications or too short a time between application and harvesting can result in greater residue amounts than are tolerated in commercially produced foods. For detailed information on pesticides in foods, see the EPA report "Pesticides and Food."[9]

Although pesticides in the food chain are not the major source of acute pesticide exposure in infants and children, such events do occur. It also seems clear that chronic toxicity is related to the total exposure to the pesticides, including exposures that occur in the home and outdoor environments as well as in foods. Thus, exposure from consuming foods containing pesticide residues is only one of the significant sources of exposure in infants and children.[2]

Of the pesticides in common use, the insecticides are most likely to cause acute illness. Although pyrethroids are increasing in use because of their lower toxicity, the commonly used insecticides belong to 1 of 2 major groups of compounds: organophosphates and carbamates, both of which are acetylcholinesterase inhibitors. Their acute effects are the direct result of that inhibition. Acute symptoms and signs occur from muscarinic and nicotinic stimuli and usually occur within hours of exposure. These include nausea, vomiting, salivation, lacrimation, blurred vision, miosis, abnormal cardiac rhythm, fasciculations, convulsions, and rarely, death. Treatment, when needed, is atropine initially, and this suffices for most acute situations. In severe cases of organophosphate poisoning, pralidoxime may be required.[10]

The effects of long-term exposures by various routes have been demonstrated in experimental animals, but chronic effects from food sources in human subjects have not been established. Effects that have been postulated, but not validated, on the basis of various epidemiologic studies and animal experiments include a range of neurodevelopmental disorders ranging from mental retardation to attention-deficit/hyperactivity disorder.[11] Undoubtedly, any chronic effects that might occur from exposure through foods would depend on the age of the infant or child at the time exposure begins, the degree of exposure, and the duration. In general, one can assume that exposure in utero and early in infancy would be more harmful to the developing nervous system than would exposure later in childhood. Because infants and children are exposed to many compounds that could have similar effects and exposures may come from a variety of routes, it will likely be a long time before definitive effects of chronic exposure to pesticides in foods can be substantiated.

Reducing Pesticide Exposure From Foods

Although pesticide exposures from use in the home, gardens, lawns, child care centers, and schools may be a greater hazard to children than exposure from foods, reducing exposure from foods can certainly benefit the child.[9] Measures that can be recommended to parents include[12]:

- Thorough washing of foods with cold or warm tap water and scrubbing fruits and vegetables with a brush before consumption.

- After washing, peeling fruits and vegetables when possible.

- Discarding the outer leaves of leafy vegetables, such as lettuce and cabbage.

- Trimming the fat from meats and the skin and fat from poultry and fish.

- Avoidance of pesticide use on home-grown fruits and vegetables.

- Avoidance of fruits and vegetables from nonregulated sources using conventional pesticides, such as other home gardens, country vegetable stands, and local produce markets.

- Limiting produce from other countries to those that can be peeled.

- When and where available, select certified organic foods (although the overall benefits to health from organically grown foods remain to be established).*

_____

* On the basis of the Organic Food Production Act of 1990, the USDA, in October 2002, set definitions for organically grown foods that specify that such foods are grown and processed using no synthetic fertilizers or pesticides. Since that time, producers and handlers must be certified by a USDA-accredited certifying agent to sell, label, or represent their product as "100% organic" or "organic" (at least 95% organic). These activities are part of the National Organic Program and are under the direction of the Agricultural Marketing Service, which is part of the USDA.[13] These standards are not yet applicable to fish or seafood. It should also be noted that there are no standards for the use of the term "natural." In 2005, it is estimated that almost two thirds of consumers purchased some organic foods.[14,15]

Industrial Chemicals

Another source of contaminants in the food supply are products from industrial processes that enter the food chain through contamination of the environment. These include precipitation from the atmosphere into water, onto soil or directly onto food crops, and direct contamination of underground or surface waters that may, in turn, affect the water supply for irrigation or consumption. Industrial chemicals that contaminate food during processing are termed indirect food additives and are covered in a separate section of this chapter.

The most ubiquitous group of compounds resulting from industrial production are the dioxin-like chemicals, which include polychlorinated biphenyls, dibenzofurans, and dibenzodioxins (PCBs, PCDFs, PCDDs, and TCDD, a particularly potent dioxin). These pollutants are part of a larger group of compounds termed persistent organic pollutants (POPs), which also includes the pesticide dichloro-diphenyl-trichloroethane (DDT) and its breakdown products as well as aldrin, dieldrin, chlordane, endrin, heptachlor, hexachlorobenzene, mirex, and toxaphene.[16] Although the continued use of these toxic products has been extensively curtailed by international treaty, they persist in the environment and have accumulated in produce grown in contaminated soils and bioaccumulate in the fat tissue of many animal-based foods, including beef, poultry, dairy products, and fish—both saltwater and freshwater varieties. A major hazard is that the chronic ingestion of small amounts of these toxins ingested with foods may then accumulate in human fat. Persistent organic pollutants can be transferred to the fetus from maternal stores and appear in human milk, because they are fat-soluble and are not significantly metabolized.

No acute exposures from food sources other than some widely publicized accidental exposures have been reported, but chronic effects are a potential problem.[11] Most chronic exposures that have been reported reflect effects on the developing fetus. These include a variety of central nervous system findings, including mental retardation and developmental delay. Endocrine function disruption and immune system disorders have been demonstrated in animals, and possible similar effects on children are under study. The carcinogenic potential of the dioxins has also been recognized by the EPA, and TCDD has been upgraded from a "probable carcinogen" to a "human carcinogen."[17]

No specific treatments are known, and the prevention of excessive intake is the only therapeutic approach. Reducing the ingestion of the fats found in animals, dairy products, and fish are the basis of the recommendations currently proposed. Because the dioxin-like chemicals are minimally metabolized and excreted, intakes are cumulative over years. Fish vary in their fat content by species, and the level of contamination varies with species, location, body size, and the type of feeding, especially in farmed fish.[18] Because of the variation in the contamination in freshwater fish, states in which contaminated fish may be found publish fish advisories about where such fish may exist, along with recommendations on their consumption by pregnant women, lactating mothers, and young children. Recommendations to reduce the intake of dioxin-like compounds in the diet, especially for children, young women, women who may become pregnant, and lactating mothers include:

- Choose lean cuts of meat and trim all visible fat before cooking.

- Choose fish with lower fat content and lower levels of contamination and remove visible fat and skin before cooking.

- Use low-fat dairy products routinely.

- Cook meats and fish by broiling, grilling, or other methods that allow fat to be drained away. Do not save or reuse rendered fats.[19]

Metal Compounds

The next most hazardous chemicals arising from industrial processes are the heavy metals, especially lead and mercury. Exposure to lead is rarely from food sources in the United States. One type of food exposure known to occur in some situations is lead-containing ceramic ware, in which acidic fluids, such as orange juice, may leach lead from the container. In 1995, some types of candy imported from other countries, primarily Mexican-style candy, and powdered snack mix were found to be contaminated with lead. This led to lowering the standard for lead content in candy from 0.5 ppm to 0.1 ppm in 2005. The new standards now apply to sugar-based candy, chocolate candy, and all other candy products that may be ingested by small children.[20]

Mercury is released into the environment by natural and industrial processes. Since the industrial revolution, the majority of environmental mercury comes from manmade sources, such as mining, the burning of fossil fuels, and the incineration of medical waste. Coal-burning power plants remain the largest single source of mercury emissions in the United States. Once released, mercury-containing rains go into lakes, rivers, and oceans, where the mercury is biotransformed by bacteria to methylmercury.

Methylmercury, a potent neurodevelopmental toxicant, is bioconcentrated up the aquatic food chain, and fish consumption is the source of most human mercury exposure in the United States. Chronic effects of methylmercury ingestion have been noted in the offspring of mothers who had elevated concentrations in their bodies. The EPA has determined a reference dose for methylmercury at 0.1 µg/kg per day on the basis of protecting the fetal brain from damage. This amount of intake corresponds roughly to a blood concentration of 5.8 ppb. Approximately 8% of women will have concentrations at or exceeding this amount, and as many as 16% may have concentrations that would lead to fetal exposures above the reference dose.[21] Mercury concentrations in many ocean fish and shellfish have been evaluated.[22] Highly contaminated saltwater fish, including shark, swordfish, king mackerel, and tilefish, should be completely avoided by children and women of childbearing age. A variety of recommendations have been promulgated regarding safe fish consumption for less-contaminated saltwater fish. For example, intake of fresh or frozen tuna and canned albacore should be limited in children and women of childbearing age. Mercury concentrations in freshwater fish vary by location, and many are also highly contaminated. Most states have fish consumption advisories regarding local fish. Often, such advisories include data on mercury as well as PCBs, with guidance on which fish to limit and which to avoid either because of mercury and/or PCBs and other POPs (see text box on next page).

Other metals that may have toxic effects on infants include manganese, which is an essential trace element in human metabolism. Elevated blood manganese concentrations have been tentatively associated with neurologic problems in children, such as hyperactivity and learning disabilities,[27] although these associations are controversial and remain to be validated. Soy products are enriched in aluminum and manganese. For example, soy-based formulas contain manganese at 200–300 µg/L compared with other formulas that contain 77–100 µg/L (see also Chapter 3: Formula Feeding of Term Infants). It should be emphasized, however, that no examples of neurotoxicity have been associated with the ingestion of soy formulas. Cadmium is another metal found to have potential neurotoxicity and is found in foods such as leafy vegetables, grains, and shellfish.

Toxins

There are a wide variety of "endogenous" toxins found in various foods. Seafood may be toxic because of the accumulation of chemical toxicants from the water (PCBs and mercury), because the fish itself is toxic (tetrodotoxin

The Fish Dilemma

Marine and freshwater fish and shellfish can be important components of a balanced healthy diet. Fish is high in protein, is low in saturated fat, and contains essential vitamins, minerals, and long-chain omega-3 fatty acids (see also Chapter 16: Fats and Fatty Acids). Unfortunately, fish are vulnerable to contamination by toxic industrial pollutants, such as mercury, as well as lipophilic chemicals, such as PCBs, dioxins, flame retardants, and others. These pollutants accumulate in fish flesh (as in the case of methylmercury) or fatty tissue (as in the case of PCBs), exposing people who eat them. Mothers can pass on these pollutants to their children both in utero and via human milk, and children may also be exposed to these harmful chemicals directly through diet during critical windows of development. Finding the balance between acquiring the nutritional benefits from adequate fish consumption and avoiding the toxicity from consumption of polluted fish is a challenge uniquely complex for the most vulnerable populations: girls and women of childbearing age, pregnant and lactating mothers, and small children.

A variety of consumption guidelines have been developed; some dealing only with mercury contamination, some dealing with both mercury and lipophilic contaminants. These guidelines often are discordant on the specifics but tend to have consensus on several major points. Women of childbearing age and all children should (1) avoid varieties of fish known to be highly contaminated; (2) know and follow local and federal fish consumption guidelines; (3) eat a wide variety of the least contaminated fish; and (4) limit weekly fish meals depending on which varieties are chosen. In general, leaner, smaller, and younger wild fish are least likely to be heavily polluted. Consumers should ask about the source and time since harvest of fish purchased in grocery stores and restaurants.

A listing of national and state fish advisories can be found.[23] Other consumption guides have been developed by non-profit organizations.[24–26]

Recently, the March of Dimes has revised its recommendations regarding fish consumption by pregnant women. According to the March of Dimes, the 3 categories of fish, on the basis of mercury content, are:

- **Do Not Eat** (high mercury content): swordfish, shark, king mackerel, and tilefish

- **Risky Fish** (varying amounts of mercury): tuna (all forms), halibut, sea bass, grouper, snapper, monkfish

- **Okay to Eat** (low mercury content): canned salmon, sardines, shrimp, pollock.

Advice from the March of Dimes to pregnant women or women actively trying to get pregnant: Fish is a good source of nutrition, and a pregnant woman or a woman actively trying to become pregnant can eat a total of 12 oz of fish per week; however, to reduce risk, it is best if a woman does not eat fish from the "risky" category. If a woman wants to eat a "risky" fish, the March of Dimes recommends eating 6 oz or less per week (http://www.marchofdimes.com/pnhec/pnhec.asp).

V

from puffer fish) or from the ingestion by fish of toxin-producing algae. The most significant algae are the dinoflagellates like Gymnodinium breve, which produces a severe neurotoxin and is the cause of the red tide, Gambierdiscus, which produces the most common fish toxin, ciguatera, and a large number of others that produce toxins affecting shellfish[28,29] (see Table 53.1).

Table 53.1
Toxins in Seafood[28,29]

Organism Producing Toxin	Toxin	Seafood Affected	Health Effects
Gambierdiscus	Ciguatera	Barracudas, groupers, snappers, jacks, mackerel, triggerfish	Acute symptoms of the gastro-intestinal, central nervous, and cardiovascular systems; self-limited; usually subsides in several days
Many dinoflagellates	Saxitoxin derivatives	Mussels, clams, cockles, scallops	Paralytic shellfish poisoning
	Polyethers	Mussels, oysters, scallops	Diarrheic shellfish poisoning
	Brevetoxins	Shellfish from the Florida coast	Neurotoxic shellfish poisoning
	Domoic acid	Mussels	Amnesic shellfish poisoning
Various bacteria	Histamine, also called scombrotoxin	Tuna, mahi mahi, bluefish, sardines, mackerel, amber-jack, abalone (note: may also be in Swiss cheese)	Burning mouth, upper body rash, hypotension, headache, pruritus, vomiting, and diarrhea

Naturally occurring toxins found in other foods include the mushroom toxins, which are classified in 4 groups: protoplasmic poisons, neurotoxins, gastrointestinal irritants, and disulfiram toxins. They are found in a wide variety of mushrooms, which are not easily distinguished from nontoxic varieties. They are not inactivated by cooking. Pyrrolizidine alkaloids are usually associated with home remedies that are derived from legumes and other plants. Phytohemagglutinins are found primarily in red kidney beans that are raw or only partially cooked, as in slow cookers and in salads. Grayanotoxin is found in honey that comes from rhododendrons. Like most others in this group, the symptoms are usually acute. Aflatoxins are fungal in origin and may affect corn, nuts, and milk. They may have long-term carcinogenic effects.[28,29] The frequency of illness reported to result from these toxins is low, but no specific data are available. The rarity of case reports may be related to lack of recognition of specific toxidromes.[28]

Two fungal toxins, patulin and fumonisin, are more widespread and are now under regulation by the EPA. Patulin can be found in apple juice and apple juice products if they are made from rotten or partially rotted apples. At the maximum recommended amount for patulin in juice (50 µg/kg), it is possible for infants and small children to exceed the allowable limit of 0.43 µg/kg of body weight. There are only chronic effects of patulin ingestion, and these occur with long-term consumption. Toxicologic studies in animals indicate premature death, embryotoxic and fetotoxic effects, and possible immunologic effects.[30] Studies in humans have not been performed, but consumption of apple juice should be limited to 4 to 6 oz/day for children 1 to 6 years of age and 8 to 12 oz/day for older children (see also Chapter 6: Feeding the Child).

Fumonisin is a mycotoxin. More than 10 types have been found world-wide[31] in corn and corn products, such as corn flour, corn meal, and grits. They have been found to be at very low concentrations in ready-to-eat breakfast cereals. They are not found in corn syrup. Low amounts are found in corn chips and tortillas as well as in popcorn. The toxicity of the fumonisins in animals includes leukoencephalomalacia in horses, pulmonary edema in pigs, and liver, kidney, cardiac, and atherogenic effects in experimental animals. Rats and mice have been shown to develop liver cancers in chronic feeding experiments.[31] Possible carcinogenic effects in humans are some-what inconclusive. However, because of the extensive nature of effects in animals, fumonisin action levels in corn products are now established.[32]

At this time, there is little material available on how to protect children from the toxins listed here. The EPA is increasing its evaluation of these substances, and regulations are gradually being put into place regarding the most prevalent and serious of these materials. In the interim, there are several things families can do. In relation to seafood, the following suggestions are made:

- Do not use any seafood (fish or shellfish) that looks, smells, or tastes odd.

- Buy seafood from reputable sources.

- Buy only fresh seafood that is refrigerated or properly iced.

- Do not buy cooked seafood if displayed in the same case as raw fish.

- Do not buy frozen seafood with torn, open, or crushed package edges.

- Keep seafood refrigerated immediately after buying it.

Antimicrobial Preservatives

Among the approaches used in achieving food preservation by inhibiting growth of undesirable microorganisms is the use of chemical agents exhibiting antimicrobial activity. These chemicals may be either synthetic compounds intentionally added to foods or naturally occurring, biologically derived substances (ie, "naturally occurring antimicrobials").[33] Most of these substances are classified as "generally regarded as safe." They include traditional substances, such as salt, sugar, or smoke. Other materials may be found naturally in some foods or may be naturally occurring substances that are found in the food as it exists or are added to other foods. The most common of these compounds are the organic acids or their salts or derivatives; sorbic acid and benzoic acid are the most common, but others include propionic, citric, acetic, lactic, and more than a half dozen other acids. Additionally, lipid materials, such as monoacylglycerols (from partially hydrolyzed fat); phenols; lytic enzymes, such as egg white lysozyme; peroxidases and oxidases, such as glucose oxidase; bacteriocins, such as nisin; and hydrogen peroxide, may be added to foods for their preservative function. No specific toxicity to any of these substances is known.

Food Irradiation

Introduction

Food irradiation is a process by which food is exposed to a controlled source of ionizing radiation to prolong shelf life and reduce food losses, to improve microbiologic safety, and/or to reduce the use of chemical fumigants and additives. The dose of the ionizing radiation determines the effects of the process on foods. Food is generally irradiated at levels from 50 Gy to 10 kGy (1 kGy = 1000 Gy), depending on the goals of the process. Low-dose irradiation (up to 1 kGy) is used primarily to delay ripening of produce or kill or render sterile insects and other higher organisms that may infest fresh food. Medium-dose irradiation (1–10 kGy) reduces the number of pathogens and other microbes on food and prolongs shelf life. High-dose irradiation (>10 kGy) sterilizes food.

Food irradiation is regulated by the FDA as a food additive. The USDA also has regulatory responsibilities for some types of foods irradiated for defined purposes. All petitioners for FDA approval of food irradiation must complete a process that ensures that food irradiated for a specific purpose under precise conditions will remain radiologically, toxicologically, and microbiologically safe and nutritionally adequate.[34]

All irradiated food sold in the United States must be labeled with the international sign of irradiation, the Radura (Fig 53.1). Current labeling rules do not require that the dose of the irradiation or the purpose of the irradiation be specified. Thus, it is not possible for consumers to know whether food has been treated to reduce pathogen loads or merely to prolong shelf life. Furthermore, current rules to not require food services to identify irradiated foods they serve.

Fig 53.1
International sign of radiation, the Radura.

Radiological Safety
Neither the food nor the packaging materials become radioactive as a result of food irradiation.[35,36] The sources of radiation approved for use in food irradiation are limited to those producing energy too low to induce subatomic particles or cause chain reactions.

Toxicologic Safety
Radiation absorbed by food causes a host of chemical reactions proportional to the dose of radiation applied. The desired reactions involve disrupting the DNA of spoilage and disease-causing microbes and pests. Undesired reactions could involve creation of toxic compounds. A number of approaches involving hundreds of studies have been used over decades to determine whether such toxic compounds are created during irradiation, and if created, whether they are unique to the irradiation process (versus canning, freezing, drying, etc) or created in amounts large enough to cause harm. With improved analytic techniques, a class of compounds apparently

unique to irradiation has been identified and proposed as a marker of food irradiation. These compounds, known as 2-alkylcyclobutanones, are derived from irradiation of fatty acids in food in a dose-dependent manner. Little is known about their toxicity, but there is evidence that some of these chemicals could be tumor promoters.[37,38] Nonetheless, multigenerational animal feeding studies and analytic chemical modeling studies have failed to identify any unusual toxicity associated with consumption of irradiated foods.[35,39,40] In fact, irradiated food often contains fewer changed molecules (also called radiolytic products) than does food processed in conventional ways. For example, heat-processed foods can contain 50 to 500 times more changed-products molecules than irradiated foods.[41]

Microbiologic Safety

Irradiation kills microbes primarily by fragmenting DNA. The sensitivity of organisms increases with the complexity of the organism. Thus, viruses are most resistant to destruction by irradiation, and insects and parasites are most sensitive. Spores, cysts, toxins, and prions are quite resistant to the effects of irradiation, because they are in highly stable resting states or are not living organisms. The conditions under which irradiation takes place (ie, temperature, humidity, and atmospheric content) can affect the dose required to achieve the food-processing goal. Regardless, the quality of the food to be irradiated must be high, without heavy microbial contamination, for irradiation to achieve food-processing goals at any level.

When irradiation is used at nonsterilizing doses, the possibility of persistent pathogens is always present. Although it is true that pathogen loads can be substantially reduced using this technique, it is always possible for foods to become recontaminated. Irradiation does not obviate the need for strict application of safe food-handling techniques, including adequate storage, hygienic preparation, and complete cooking, particularly of high-risk foods such as foods of animal origin, precooked processed foods, or imported foods.[42]

Nutritional Value

As with any food-processing technique, irradiation can have a negative effect on some nutrients. It does not significantly damage carbohydrates or proteins and does not change the bioavailability or quantity of minerals or trace elements in foods. A slight loss of essential polyunsaturated fatty acids does occur with irradiation, but fats and oils that are major dietary sources of these nutrients tend to become rancid when irradiated and are not good candidates for this kind of treatment.[35]

Vitamin loss is the largest nutritional concern when foods are irradiated. Vitamin losses are most dramatic when studied in pure solutions. Whole foods exert a protective effect on vitamins, because most of the radiation dose is absorbed by macromolecules (proteins, carbohydrates, and fats). Losses can be minimized by irradiating at low temperatures, at low doses, and by excluding oxygen and light.[43] When studied in pure solution, the water-soluble vitamins most sensitive to irradiation are thiamin (vitamin B$_1$), pyridoxine (vitamin B$_6$), and riboflavin (vitamin B$_2$). Vitamin C is converted by irradiation to dehydroascorbic acid, which behaves like ascorbic acid in humans, preserving nearly normal vitamin C activity after irradiation. Vitamins B$_{12}$, niacin, and pantothenic and folic acids are resistant to irradiation. Of the fat-soluble vitamins, vitamins E and A are sensitive. Plant carotenes are relatively resistant, and vitamins D and K are quite resistant to irradiation.[41]

Thiamine loss can be 50% or more under some conditions in some foods. Loss is enhanced with increased irradiation doses, increased storage time after irradiation, and cooking after irradiation. Thiamine is found in meats, milk, whole grains, and legumes. If all sources of thiamine come from irradiated products, a deficiency condition could develop, but this is unlikely in the United States. Irradiation losses of pyridoxine (found in meat, whole grains, corn, and soybeans) are not as severe as with thiamine, and deficiency states are less likely to develop. The biologic availability of riboflavin (found in meat, milk, eggs, green vegetables, whole grains, and legumes) can be paradoxically increased after irradiation by shortening required cooking time. For example, dried legumes irradiated at high dose require less than a quarter of the cooking time of untreated legumes, and measured riboflavin is higher in irradiated versus nonirradiated cooked samples.[41]

Vitamin E loss can be significant. A study of effects of radiation plus heat shows that nonirradiated rolled oats lost 17% of their vitamin E after 10 minutes of cooking and 40% after 30 minutes, whereas rolled oats treated with 1 kGy lost 17% of their vitamin E after irradiation, 27.5% after cooking for 10 minutes, and 57% after cooking for 30 minutes.[41] Many of the sources of vitamin E—cereal grains, seed oils, peanuts, soybeans, milk fat, and turnip greens—are unlikely to be treated with radiation and should provide for adequate alternative sources in a balanced and varied diet. Preformed vitamin A is found primarily in milk fat (vitamin A-fortified milk) and eggs. Thus far, only eggs are approved for irradiation. Furthermore, plant carotenes found in dark green and yellow vegetables are converted by the body into vitamin A and are relatively resistant to irradiation.

Although a few vitamins are significantly affected by irradiation, in general, irradiated food is quite nutritious. As long as a diet is balanced and food choices are varied, deficiency states are unlikely to develop.

Palatability

Taste, texture, color, and smell are all components of palatable foods. Some foods, particularly foods with high fat content, suffer unacceptable changes in these qualities when irradiated. Modified conditions, such as excluding oxygen from the atmosphere, lowering the temperature, excluding light, reducing water content, or lowering the radiation dose, can minimize or eliminate these changes. A welcome consequence of modifying irradiation conditions to preserve palatability is that the same modifications can also minimize vitamin loss.

Table 53.2
Rules From US FDA for Food Irradiation

Food	Purpose of Irradiation	Dose Permitted, kGy	Date of Rule
Spices, dry vegetable seasoning	Decontamination/disinfest insects	30 (maximum)	07/15/63
Wheat, wheat powder	Disinfest insects	0.2–0.5	08/21/63
White potatoes	Extend shelf life	0.05–0.15	11/01/65
Dry or dehydrated enzyme preparations	Control insects and microorganisms	10 (maximum)	06/10/85
Pork carcasses or fresh noncut processed cuts	Control Trichinella spiralis	0.3 (minimum)–1.0 (maximum)	07/22/85
Fresh fruit	Delay maturation	1	04/18/86
Dry or dehydrated enzyme preparations	Decontamination	10	04/18/86
Dry or dehydrated aromatic vegetable substances	Decontamination	30	04/18/86
Poultry	Control pathogens	3	05/02/90
Red meat	Control pathogens and prolong shelf life	4.5 (fresh)–7 (frozen)	12/03/97
Fresh shell eggs	Control Salmonella species	3.0	07/12/00

Conclusion

Irradiation is increasingly suggested as an important adjunct to improving food safety and availability.[44,45] Current rules by the FDA for food irradiation are listed in Table 53.2. In a reversal of previous policy and amid great public controversy, the USDA began allowing the option of using irradiated ground beef by school lunch programs beginning in January 2004.[46] This move has rekindled heated public debate about this technology. Irradiated food is safe and nutritious and produces no toxicity as long as best management practices are followed. It can be safely used as part of a balanced and varied diet. It is important to remember, however, that irradiation of food does not substitute for careful food handling from farm to fork. Widespread use of food irradiation would necessitate construction of irradiation facilities in the United States and other countries. The benefits of expanding this technology and the risks involved must be thoroughly debated. Pediatricians should participate in the dialogue. As with any technology, unforeseen consequences are possible; therefore, careful monitoring and continuous evaluation of this and all food-processing techniques are prudent precautions. (For more information, see the AAP technical report on food irradiation[34] and the AAP *Handbook of Pediatric Environmental Health.*[5])

Nonnutritive Additives

Indirect Food Additives

Indirect food additives are substances used in food-contact materials, including adhesives, dyes, coatings, paper, paperboard, and polymers (plastics), that may come into contact with food as part of packaging or processing equipment but are not intended to be added directly to food.[47] They confer no nutritional value to food. Although direct food additives undergo toxicologic testing before approval on the basis of structure-activity relationships as well as anticipated human exposure levels,[48] testing of indirect food additives is performed primarily on the basis of anticipated exposure levels. Exposures considered "virtually nil" (<0.05 ppm) or "insignificant" (0.05–1.0 ppm) receive subchronic testing (90 days or approximately 12% of postweaning lifetime of test animals) unless "indicated by available data or information."[49] Petitioners for new indirect additive approvals may apply for an exemption from regulation if they can satisfy the agency that exposures will not exceed the regulatory threshold of 0.5 ppb or are at or less than 1% of the acceptable dietary intake.[50] This regulatory approach is based on the concept that "the dose makes the poison," and adverse human health effects are unlikely for most substances when exposure levels are very small. The exposure level is calculated from laboratory-generated migration data of the chemical into food simulants and estimates of the percentage of total daily food intake that would contain the substance for an adult.[51] Additional calculations to estimate daily intake of indirect food additives of infants, children, or adolescents are not routinely performed as part of the approval process.

Many common packaging materials were approved for use before the 1958 Food Additives Amendment to the Food, Drug and Cosmetics Act and, thus, "grandfathered in" for continued use as "prior approved" substances.[52] Some of these substances have since been found to be hormonally active in laboratory animals, raising specific concerns about potential adverse effects on fetuses, infants, children, and adolescents. Examples are plasticizers like the phthalate esters (used in polyvinyl chloride plastics, inks, dyes, and adhesives in food packaging), nonyl phenol (used in polyvinyl chloride, juice boxes, and lid gaskets), and bisphenol A (found in some baby bottles, water bottles, and can liner enamels). There remains considerable scientific uncertainty about the significance of the endocrine-disrupting capacity of these chemicals to humans, the exposure levels at which toxicity might occur, and the extent of real-world human exposures.[53] A recent analysis of infant formulas, baby food, and canned vegetables in the Washington, DC, area found amounts of these chemicals in foods measuring in the low parts per billion.[54] This analysis reinforced earlier reports showing decreasing trends of contamination of infant food with phthalates over the past decade.[55] These decreases correlate with the food industry's move to eliminate many uses of these chemicals in packaging of foods intended for small children.

Nonetheless, chemicals can and will migrate from processing equipment, packaging materials, and storage containers into foods. It is not feasible to subject all possible chemical contaminants to exhaustive toxicology testing. A reasonable approach, therefore, is to develop food-preparation and storage practices that will minimize exposures. The following suggestions should help minimize unnecessary exposure to indirect food contaminants.

- Avoid routine use of single-serving packaging. Such packaging maximizes contact between food and the packaging materials.

- When possible, buy fresh food to minimize contact with packaging materials.

- Use heat-safe glass or crockery when cooking or reheating food in the microwave. Heat increases migration of many contaminants into food, particularly foods containing fats.

- Make sure a generous air space separates the surface of stored food from cling wraps used to seal containers. Avoid using cling wraps when microwaving foods.

Finally, pediatricians are in an ideal position to provide important input and continued encouragement to regulatory agencies to ensure that the special exposures and vulnerabilities of children to toxic exposures remain under consideration as food-related materials and processes are developed, reviewed, and revised.

Chemical By-Products From Food Processing

Food-processing technologies include many processes, such as drying, salting, fermentation, acidification, freeze-drying, freezing, irradiation, pasteurization, canning, pulsed electric field, ohmic heating, high-hydrostatic pressure treatment, and others. All of these approaches are used to increase safety while maintaining palatability and nutrient value. All of these approaches also have the capacity to create chemical changes in the food that may be detrimental. As analytical technology has improved, so has the ability to identify more chemical by-products in processed foods. Thoughtful approaches to assessing the safety or risk from these by-products need to be developed.[56]

Acrylamide, a know neurotoxicant and possible human carcinogen and reproductive toxicant, is one such food processing chemical by-product currently undergoing intensive scrutiny.[57] Once thought to be only of significance in the occupational setting, acrylamide has recently been found in carbohydrate-containing foods treated with high heat, such as butter, crackers, graham crackers, some cereals, French fries, potato chips, corn chips, and vegetable chips.[58] Furans are another group of chemicals recently found to form during traditional processing like canning and have been measured in commercially available foods, such as soups, sauces, beans, pasta meals, and baby foods.[59] The risk posed by dietary exposure to these possible human carcinogens is not yet well understood.

As is the case with indirect food additives, these chemical by-products of processing create unknown risks to children. A precautionary approach would be to use a wide variety of healthy foods in children's diets and to use fresh ingredients as much as is feasible.

V

References

1. US Food and Drug Administration, Center for Food Safety and Applied Nutrition. Food Safety: A Team Approach. Available at: http://www.cfsan.fda.gov/~lrd/foodteam.html. Accessed October 30, 2007

2. Institute of Medicine, National Research Council. *Pesticides in the Diets of Infants and Children.* Washington, DC: National Academies Press; 1993

3. Rice D, Barone S Jr. Critical periods of vulnerability for the developing nervous system: evidence from human and animal models. *Environ Health Perspect.* 2000;108 (Suppl 3):511–533

4. Bearer CF. How are children different from adults? *Environ Health Perspect.* 1995;103 (Suppl 6):7–12

5. American Academy of Pediatrics, Committee on Environmental Health. *Handbook of Pediatric Environmental Health.* Etzel RA, Balk SJ, eds. 2nd ed. Elk Grove Village, IL: American Academy of Pediatrics; 2003

6. US Environmental Protection Agency, Office of Pesticide Programs. *Taking Care of Business: Protecting Public Health and the Environment. EPA's Pesticide Program FY 2004 Annual Report.* Washington, DC: US Environmental Protection Agency; 2004. Publication No. 735-R-05-001. Available at: http://www.epa.gov/oppfead1/annual/2004annualreport.pdf. Accessed October 30, 2007

7. US Food and Drug Administration, Center for Food Safety and Applied Nutrition. Pesticide Program, Residue Monitoring 2003. Available at: http://www.cfsan.fda.gov/~dms/pes03rep .html#program. Accessed October 30, 2007

8. US Environmental Protection Agency. Report on FQPA Tolerance Reassessment Program and Risk Management Decision for Chlorpyrifos Methyl. Available at: http://www.epa.gov/ oppsrrd1/REDs/cpm_tred.pdf. Accessed October 30, 2007

9. US Environmental Protection Agency. Pesticides and Food: Healthy, Sensible Food Practices. Available at: http://www.epa.gov/pesticides/food/tips.htm. Accessed October 30, 2007

10. Reigart JR, Roberts JR. *Recognition and Management of Pesticide Poisonings.* 5th ed. Washington, DC: US Environmental Protection Agency; 1999

11. US Environmental Protection Agency. America's Children and the Environment (ACE)— Measure D7. Available at: http://www.epa.gpv/envirohealth/children/child_illness/ d7-graph.htm. Accessed October 30, 2007

12. Shea KM. *Reducing Low-Dose Pesticide Exposures in Infants and Children.* Washington, DC: Physicians for Social Responsibility; 2006. Available at: http://www.psr.org/site/DocServer/ Reducing_Low-Dose_Pesticide_Exposures.pdf?docID=663. Accessed October 30, 2007

13. US Department of Agriculture, Agricultural Marketing Service. The National Organic Program. Backgrounder. Available at: http://www.ams.usda.gov/nop/FactSheets/ Backgrounder.html. Accessed October 30, 2007

14. Consumer Reports. When it pays to buy organic. Available at: http://www.consumerreports. org/cro/food/diet-nutrition/organic-products/organic-products-206/overview/. Accessed October 30, 2007

15. Lu C, Toepel K, Irish R, Fenske RA, Barr DB, Bravo R. Organic diets significantly lower children's dietary exposure to organophosphorus pesticides. *Environ Health Perspect.* 2006;114:260–263

16. Shafer KS, Kegley SE, Patton S. *Nowhere to Hide: Persistent Toxic Chemicals in the US Food Supply.* San Francisco, CA: Pesticides Action Network; 2001. Available at: http://www.panna.org/resources/documents/nowhereToHideAvail.dv.html. Accessed November 1, 2007

17. US Environmental Protection Agency. Dioxin Reassessment, NAS Review Draft 2004. Available at: http://cfpub.epa.gov/ncea/cfm/recordisplay.cfm?deid=87843. Accessed October 30, 2007

18. Institute of Medicine. *Dioxins and Dioxin-like Compounds in the Food Supply: Strategies to Decrease Exposure.* Washington, DC: National Academies Press; 2003. Available at: http://books.nap.edu/catalog/10763.html. Accessed October 30, 2007

19. US Food and Drug Administration. Questions and Answers about Dioxins. 2004. Available at: http://vm.cfsan.fda.gov/~lrd/dioxinqa.html. Accessed October 30, 2007

20. Document for Recommended Maximum Level for Lead in Candy Likely to be Consumed Frequently by Small Children, December 2005. http://www.cfsan.fda.gov/~dms/pbcandy.html. Accessed October 30, 2007

21. Mahaffey KR, Clickner RP, Bodurow CC. Blood organic mercury and dietary mercury intake: National Health and Nutrition Examination Survey 1999–2000. *Environ Health Perspect.* 2004;112:562–570

22. US Department of Health and Human Services, US Environmental Protection Agency. Mercury Levels in Commercial Fish and Shellfish. 2006. Available at: http://www.cfsan.fda.gov/~frf/sea-mehg.html. Accessed October 30, 2007

23. US Environmental Protection Agency. Fish Advisories. Available at: http://www.epa.gov/waterscience/fish/. Accessed October 30, 2007

24. Physicians for Social Responsibility Web site. Available at: http://www.psr.org. Accessed October 30, 2007

25. Environmental Defense Web site. Available at: http://www.oceansalive.org/eat.cfm?subnav=healthalerts. Accessed October 30, 2007

26. Institute for Agriculture Trade and Policy Web site. Available at: http://www.iatp.org/foodandhealth/fishcalculator. Accessed October 30, 2007

27. Aschner JL, Aschner M. Nutritional aspects of manganese homeostasis. *Mol Aspects Med.* 2005;26:353–362

28. US Food and Drug Administration, Center for Food Safety and Applied Nutrition. *Foodborne Pathogenic Microorganisms and Natural Toxins Handbook (The "Bad Bug Book").* College Park, MD: US Food and Drug Administration; 2000. http://www.cfsan.fda.gov/~mow/intro.htm. Accessed October 30, 2007

29. American Medical Association. *Diagnosis and Management of Foodborne Illnesses: A Primer for Physicians.* Chicago, IL: American Medical Association; 2001

30. US Food and Drug Administration, Center for Food Safety and Applied Nutrition. *Patulin in Apple Juice, Apple Juice Concentrates and Apple Juice Products.* Rockville, MD: US Food and Drug Administration; 2001. Available at: http://www.cfsan.fda.gov/~dms/patubck2.html. Accessed October 30, 2007

31. US Food and Drug Administration Center for Food Safety and Applied Nutrition. Background Paper in Support of Fumonisin Levels in Corn and Corn Products Intended for Human Consumption. College Park, MD: US Food and Drug Administration; 2001. Available at: http://www.cfsan.fda.gov/~dms/fumonbg3.html. Accessed October 30, 2007

32. US Food and Drug Administration. Chapter 7: Mycotoxins in domestic and imported food. In: Compliance Program Guidance Manual. College Park, MD: US Food and Drug Administration; 2004. http://www.cfsan.fda.gov/~acrobat/cp07001.pdf. Accessed October 30, 2007

33. Sofos JN, Beuchat LR, Davidson PM, Johnson EA. *Naturally Occurring Antimicrobials in Food.* Ames, IA: Council for Agricultural Science and Technology; 1998

34. Shea KM, American Academy of Pediatrics, Committee on Environmental Health. Technical report: irradiation of food. *Pediatrics.* 2000;106:1505–1510

35. World Health Organization. *Safety and Nutritional Adequacy of Irradiated Food.* Geneva, Switzerland: World Health Organization; 1994

36. Urbain WM. Ionizing radiation. In: Urbain WM, ed. *Food Irradiation.* Orlando, FL: Academic Press Inc; 1986:1–22

37. Raul F, Gosse F, Delincee H, et al. Food-borne radiolytic compounds (2-alkylcyclobutanones) may promote experimental colon carcinogenesis. *Nutr Cancer.* 2002;44:189–191

38. Rao CV. Do irradiated foods cause or promote colon cancer? *Nutr Cancer.* 2003;46:107–109

39. US Food and Drug Administration. Irradiation in the production, processing, and handling of food. *Fed Regist.* 1986;51(75):13376–13399

40. World Health Organization. *High-Dose Irradiation: Wholesomeness of Food Irradiated With Doses Above 10 kGy.* Geneva, Switzerland: World Health Organization; 1999. WHO Technical Report Series No. 890. Available at: http://www.who.int/foodsafety/publications/fs_management/en/irrad.pdf. Accessed November 1, 2007

41. Diehl JF. *Safety of Irradiated Foods.* 2nd ed. New York, NY: Marcel Dekker; 1995

42. World Health Organization. *Prevention of Foodborne Disease: Five Keys to Safer Food.* Available at: http://www.who.int/foodsafety/consumer/5keys/en/index.html. Accessed October 30, 2007

43. Murano EA, Hayes DJ, eds. *Food Irradiation: A Source Book.* Ames, IA: Iowa State University Press; 1995

44. Osterholm MT, Norgan AP. The role of food irradiation in food safety. *N Engl J Med.* 2004;350:1898–1901

45. Thayer DW. Irradiation of food—helping to ensure food safety. *N Engl J Med.* 2004;350:1811–1812

46. US Department of Agriculture. USDA releases specifications for the purchase of irradiated ground beef in the National School Lunch Program [press release]. Washington, DC: US Department of Agriculture; May 29, 2003. Available at: http://www.fns.usda.gov/cga/PressReleases/2003/PR-0172.htm. Accessed October 30, 2007

47. US Food and Drug Administration, Center for Food Safety and Applied Nutrition. List of "Indirect" Food Additives used in Food Contact Substances. Available at: http://vm.cfsan.fda.gov/~dms/opa-indt.html. Accessed October 30, 2007

48. US Food and Drug Administration, Center for Food Safety and Applied Nutrition. Toxicological Principles for the Safety of Food Ingredients. Redbook 2000. College Park, MD: US Food and Drug Administration; 2007. Available at: http://vm.cfsan.fda.gov/~redbook/red-toca.html. October 30, 2007

49. US Food and Drug Administration, Center for Food Safety and Applied Nutrition, Office of Premarket Approval, Toxicology Review Branch. *Toxicological Testing of Food Additives*. College Park, MD: US Food and Drug Administration; 2007. Available at: http://vm.cfsan.fda .gov/~dms/opa-tg1.html. Accessed October 30, 2007

50. US Food and Drug Administration, Center for Food Safety and Applied Nutrition, Office of Premarket Approval. Guidance for submitting requests under 21 CFR 170.39. Threshold of Regulation for Substances Used in Food-Contact Articles. Available at: http://www.cfsan .fda.gov/~dms/torguid.html. Accessed October 30, 2007

51. US Food and Drug Administration, Center for Food Safety and Applied Nutrition, Office of Premarket Approval, Chemistry Review Branch. *Recommendations for Chemistry Data for Indirect Food Additives Petitions*. Available at: http://vm.cfsan.fda.gov/~dms/opa-cg5.html. Accessed October 30, 2007

52. Frank JF, Barnhart HM. Food and dairy sanitation. In: Last JM, Wallace RB, eds. *Public Health & Preventive Medicine*. 13th ed. Norwalk, CT: Appleton & Lange: 1992:589–618

53. Kaiser J. Endocrine disruptors. Panel cautiously confirms low-dose effects. *Science*. 2000;290:695–697

54. McNeal TP, Biles JE, Begley TH, Craun JC, Hopper ML, Sack CA. Determination of suspected endocrine disruptors in foods and food packaging. In: Keith LH, Jones-Lepp TL, Needham LL, eds. Analysis of Environmental Endocrine Disruptors. American Chemical Society Symposium Series 747. Washington, DC: American Chemical Society; 2000:33–52

55. Koo JW, Parham F, Kohn MC, et al. The association between biomarker-based exposure estimates for phthalates and demographic factors in a human reference population. *Environ Health Perspect*. 2002;110:405–410

56. Tritscher AM. Human health risk assessment of processing-related compounds in food. *Toxicol Lett*. 2004:149:177–186

57. National Toxicology Program, Center for the Evaluation of Risks to Human Reproduction. Monograph on the Potential Human Reproductive and Developmental Effects of Acrylamide. February 2005. Available at: http://cerhr.niehs.nih.gov/chemicals/acrylamide/Acrylamide _Monograph.pdf. Accessed October 30, 2007

58. US Food and Drug Administration. Exploratory Data on Acrylamide in Food. Available at: http://www.cfsan.fda.gov/~dms/acrydata.html#1004. Accessed October 30, 2007

59. US Food and Drug Administration. FDA Action Plan on Furan in Food. Available at: http:// www.cfsan.fda.gov/~dms/furanap.html. Accessed October 30, 2007

V

Appendices APP

Appendix A

Table A-1
Exchange Lists for Diabetic Diets*

Groups/Lists	Carbohydrate, g	Protein, g	Fat, g	kcal
Carbohydrate Group				
Starch	15	3	0–1	80
Fruit	15	...	...	60
Milk				
Skim	12	8	0–3	90
Low-fat	12	8	5	120
Whole	12	8	8	150
Other carbohydrates	15	Varies	Varies	Varies
Vegetables	5	2	...	25
Meat and Meat Substitute Group				
Very lean	...	7	0–1	35
Lean	...	7	3	55
Medium-fat	...	7	5	75
High-fat	...	7	8	100
Fat Group	...	...	5	45

*From the American Diabetes Association, Alexandria, VA (http://store.diabetes.org or 1-800-232-6733) and the American Dietetic Association, Chicago, IL (www.eatright.org or 1-800-366-1655) *Exchange Lists for Meal Planning*, 2003.

Table A-2
Food Exchange Lists

Starch List
Cereals, grains, pastas, breads, crackers, snacks, starchy vegetables, and cooked beans, peas, and lentils are starches. In general, 1 starch is: • 1/2 cup of cooked cereal, grain, or starchy vegetable or 1/3 cup of cooked rice or pasta • 1 oz of a bread product, such as 1 slice of bread • 3/4 to 1 oz of most snack foods (some snack foods may also have added fat)

Nutrition Tips

1. Most starch choices are good sources of B vitamins
2. Foods made from whole grains are good sources of fiber
   • A serving from the bread list, on average, has 1 g of fiber
   • A serving from the cereals and grains list or the crackers and snacks list, on average, has 2 g of fiber
   • A serving from the starchy vegetables list, on average, has 3 g of fiber
3. Beans, peas, and lentils are good sources of protein and fiber
   • A serving from this food group, on average, has 6 g of fiber

Selection Tips
1. Choose starches made with little fat as often as you can. 2. Starchy vegetables prepared with fat count as 1 starch and 1 fat. 3. For many starchy foods (eg, bagels, muffins, dinner rolls, buns), a general rule of thumb is 1 oz equals 1 carbohydrate serving. However, bagels or muffins range widely in size. Check the size you eat. Also, use the Nutrition Facts on food labels when available. 4. Beans, peas, and lentils are also found on the meat and meat substitutes list. 5. A waffle or pancake is about the size of a compact disc (CD) and approximately 1/4 in thick. 6. Because starches often swell during cooking, a small amount of uncooked starch will become a much larger amount of cooked food. 7. Most of the serving sizes are measured or weighed after cooking. 8. For specific information, check Nutrition Facts on the food label.

Starch List
One starch exchange equals: 15 g of carbohydrate, 3 g of protein, 0–1 g of fat, and 80 kcal

Bread	
Bagel, 4 oz	1/4 (1 oz)
Bread, reduced-calorie	2 slices (1 1/2 oz)
Bread, white, whole-wheat, pumpernickel, rye	1 slice (1 oz)
Bread sticks, crisp, 4 in × 1/2 in	4 (2/3 oz)
English muffin	1/2
Hot dog bun or hamburger bun	1/2 (1 oz)
Naan, 8 × 2 in	1/4
Pancake, 4 in across, 1/4 in thick	1

Table A-2 *(Continued)*
Food Exchange Lists

Pita, 6 in across	1/2
Roll, plain, small	1 (1 oz)
Raisin bread, unfrosted	1 slice (1 oz)
Tortilla, corn, 6 in across	1
Tortilla, flour, 6 in across	1
Tortilla, flour, 10 in across	1/3
Waffle, 4-in square or across, reduced-fat	1
Cereals and Grains	
Bran cereals	1/2 cup
Bulgur	1/2 cup
Cereals, cooked	1/2 cup
Cereals, unsweetened, ready-to-eat	3/4 cup
Cornmeal (dry)	3 tbsp
Couscous	1/3 cup
Flour (dry)	3 tbsp
Granola, low-fat	1/4 cup
Grape-Nuts (Kraft Foods, Northfield, IL)	1/4 cup
Grits	1/2 cup
Kasha	1/2 cup
Millet	1/3 cup
Muesli	1/4 cup
Oats	1/2 cup
Pasta	1/3 cup
Puffed cereal	1 1/2 cups
Rice, white or brown	1/3 cup
Shredded wheat	1/2 cup
Sugar-frosted cereal	1/2 cup
Wheat germ	3 tbsp
Starchy Vegetables	
Baked beans	1/3 cup
Corn	1/2 cup
Corn on cob, large	1/2 cob (5 oz)

Table A-2 *(Continued)*
Food Exchange Lists

Mixed vegetables with corn, peas, or pasta	1 cup
Peas, green	1/2 cup
Plantain	1/2 cup
Potato, boiled	1/2 cup or 1/2 medium (3 oz)
Potato, baked with skin	1/4 large (3 oz)
Potato, mashed	1/2 cup
Squash, winter (acorn, butternut, pumpkin)	1 cup
Yam, sweet potato, plain	1/2 cup
Crackers and Snacks	
Animal crackers	8
Graham cracker, 2 1/2-in square	3
Matzoh	3/4 oz
Melba toast	4 slices
Oyster crackers	24
Popcorn (popped, no fat added, or low-fat microwave)	3 cups
Pretzels	3/4 oz
Rice cakes, 4 in across	2
Saltine-type crackers	6
Snack chips, fat-free or baked (tortilla, potato)	15–20 (3/4 oz)
Whole-wheat crackers, no fat added	2–5 (3/4 oz)
Beans, Peas, and Lentils (count as 1 starch exchange, plus 1 very lean meat exchange)	
Beans and peas (garbanzo, pinto, kidney, white, split, black-eyed)	1/2 cup
Lima beans	2/3 cup
Lentils	1/2 cup
Miso†	3 tbsp
Common Measurements	
3 tsp = 1 tbsp	4 oz = 1/2 cup
4 tbsp = 1/4 cup	8 oz = 1 cup
5 1/3 tbsp = 1/3 cup	1 cup = 1/2 pt
Starchy Foods Prepared With Fat (count as 1 starch exchange, plus 1 fat exchange)	
Biscuit, 2 1/2 in across	1

Table A-2 *(Continued)*
Food Exchange Lists

Chow mein noodles	1/2 cup
Corn bread, 2 in cube	1 (2 oz)
Crackers, round butter type	6
Croutons	1 cup
French-fried potatoes (oven-baked) (see also the fast foods list)	3 oz
Granola	1/4 cup
Hummus	1/3 cup
Muffin, 5 oz	1/5 (1 oz)
Popcorn, microwaved	3 cups
Sandwich crackers, cheese or peanut butter filling	3
Snack chips (potato, tortilla)	9–13 (3/4 oz)
Stuffing, bread (prepared)	1/3 cup
Taco shell, 6 in across	2
Waffle, 4-in square or across	1
Whole-wheat crackers, fat added	4–7 (1 oz)

Fruit List

Fresh, frozen, canned, and dried fruits and fruit juices are on this list. In general, 1 fruit exchange is:

- 1 small fresh fruit (4 oz)
- 1/2 cup of canned or fresh fruit or unsweetened fruit juice
- 1/4 cup of dried fruit

Nutrition Tips

1. Fresh, frozen, and dried fruits have approximately 2 g of fiber per choice. Fruit juices contain very little fiber.
2. Citrus fruits, berries, and melons are good sources of vitamin C.

Selection Tips

1. Count 1/2 cup cranberries or rhubarb sweetened with sugar substitutes as free foods.
2. Read the Nutrition Facts on the food label. If 1 serving has more than 15 g of carbohydrate, you will need to adjust the size of the serving you eat or drink.
3. Portion sizes for canned fruits are for the fruit and a small amount of juice.
4. Whole fruit is more filling than fruit juice and may be a better choice.
5. Food labels for fruits may contain the words "no sugar added" or "unsweetened." This means that no sucrose (table sugar) has been added.
6. Generally, fruit canned in extra light syrup has the same amount of carbohydrate per serving as the "no sugar added" or the juice pack. All canned fruits on the fruit list are based on one of these 3 types of pack.

APP

Table A-2 *(Continued)*
Food Exchange Lists

Fruit	
Apple, unpeeled, small	1 (4 oz)
Applesauce, unsweetened	1/2 cup
Apples, dried	4 rings
Apricots, fresh	4 whole (5 1/2 oz)
Apricots, dried	8 halves
Apricots, canned	1/2 cup
Banana, small	1 (4 oz)
Blackberries	3/4 cup
Blueberries	3/4 cup
Cantaloupe, small	1/3 melon (11 oz) or 1 cup cubes
Cherries, sweet, fresh	12 (3 oz)
Cherries, sweet, canned	1/2 cup
Dates	3
Figs, fresh	1 1/2 large or 2 medium (3 1/2 oz)
Figs, dried	1 1/2
Fruit cocktail	1/2 cup
Grapefruit, large	1/2 (11 oz)
Grapefruit sections, canned	3/4 cup
Grapes, small	17 (3 oz)
Honeydew melon	1 slice (10 oz) or 1 cup cubes
Kiwi	1 (3 1/2 oz)
Mandarin oranges, canned	3/4 cup
Mango, small	1/2 fruit (5 1/2 oz) or 1/2 cup
Nectarine, small	1 (5 oz)
Orange, small	1 (6 1/2 oz)
Papaya	1/2 fruit (8 oz) or 1 cup cubes
Peach, medium, fresh	1 (4 oz)
Peaches, canned	1/2 cup
Pear, large, fresh	1/2 (4 oz)
Pears, canned	1/2 cup
Pineapple, fresh	3/4 cup

Table A-2 *(Continued)*
Food Exchange Lists

Pineapple, canned	1/2 cup
Plums, small	2 (5 oz)
Plums, canned	1/2 cup
Plums, dried (prunes)	3
Raisins	2 tbsp
Raspberries	1 cup
Strawberries	1 1/4 cups whole berries
Tangerines, small	2 (8 oz)
Watermelon	1 slice (13 1/2 oz) or 1 1/4 cups cubes
Fruit Juice, Unsweetened	
Apple juice/cider	1/2 cup
Cranberry juice cocktail	1/3 cup
Cranberry juice cocktail, reduced-calorie	1 cup
Fruit juice blends, 100% juice	1/3 cup
Grape juice	1/3 cup
Grapefruit juice	1/2 cup
Orange juice	1/2 cup
Pineapple juice	1/2 cup
Prune juice	1/3 cup

Milk List

Different types of milk and milk products are on this list. Cheeses are on the meat and meat substitutes list, and cream and other dairy fats are on the fat list. On the basis of the amount of fat they contain, milks are divided into fat-free/low-fat milk, reduced-fat milk, and whole milk. One choice of these includes:

	Carbohydrate (g)	Protein (g)	Fat (g)	kcal
Fat-free/low-fat (1/2% or 1%)	12	8	0–3	90
Reduced-fat (2%)	12	8	5	120
Whole	12	8	8	150

Nutrition Tips

1. Milk and yogurt are good sources of calcium and protein. Check the Nutrition Facts on the food label.
2. The higher the fat content of milk and yogurt, the greater the amount of saturated fat and cholesterol. Choose lower-fat varieties.
3. For those who are lactose intolerant, look for lactose-reduced or lactose-free varieties of milk. Check the food label for total amount of carbohydrate per serving.

APP

Table A-2 *(Continued)*
Food Exchange Lists

Selection Tips
1. 1 cup equals 8 fluid oz or 1/2 pt.
2. Look for chocolate milk, rice milk, frozen yogurt, and ice cream on the sweets, desserts, and other carbohydrates list.
3. Nondairy creamers are on the free foods list.

Fat-Free and Low-Fat Milk (0–3 g of fat per serving)	
Fat-free milk	1 cup
1/2% milk	1 cup
1% milk	1 cup
Buttermilk, low-fat or fat-free	1 cup
Evaporated fat-free milk	1/2 cup
Fat-free dry milk	1/3 cup dry
Soy milk, low-fat or fat-free	1 cup
Yogurt, fat-free, flavored, sweetened with nonnutritive sweetener and fructose	(6 oz)
Yogurt, plain fat-free	(6 oz)

Reduced-Fat (5 g of fat per serving)	
2% milk	1 cup
Soy milk	1 cup
Sweet acidophilus milk	1 cup
Yogurt, plain low-fat	6 oz

Whole Milk (8 g of fat per serving)	
Whole milk	1 cup
Evaporated whole milk	1/2 cup
Goat milk	1 cup
Kefir	1 cup
Yogurt, plain (made from whole milk)	8 oz

Sweets, Desserts, and Other Carbohydrates List
You can substitute food choices from this list for a starch, fruit, or milk choice on your meal plan. Some choices will also count as 1 or more fat choices.

Table A-2 *(Continued)*
Food Exchange Lists

Nutrition Tips

1. These foods can be substituted for other carbohydrate-containing foods in your meal plan, even though they contain added sugars or fat. However, they do not contain as many important vitamins and minerals as the choices on the starch, fruit, or milk list.
2. When choosing these foods, include foods from the other lists to eat balanced meals.

Selection Tips

1. Because many of these foods are concentrated sources of carbohydrate and fat, saturated fat, and trans fatty acids, the portion sizes are often very small.
2. Look for the words "hydrogenated" or "partially hydrogenated" on the ingredient label. The lower down on the list these words appear, the fewer trans fatty acids there are.
3. Be sure to check the Nutrition Facts on the food label. It will be your most accurate source of information.
4. Many fat-free or reduced-fat products made with fat replacers contain carbohydrate. When eaten in large amounts, they may need to be counted. Talk with your dietitian to determine how to count these in your meal plan.
5. Look for fat-free salad dressings in smaller amounts on the free foods list.

Food Serving	Size	Exchanges per Serving
Angel food cake, unfrosted	1/12th cake (about 2 oz)	2 carbohydrates
Brownie, small unfrosted	2-in square (about 1 oz)	1 carbohydrate, 1 fat
Cake, unfrosted	2-in square (about 1 oz)	1 carbohydrate, 1 fat
Cake, frosted	2-in square (about 2 oz)	2 carbohydrates, 1 fat
Cookie or sandwich cookie with crème filling	2 small (about 2/3 oz)	1 carbohydrate, 1 fat
Cookies, sugar-free	3 small or 1 large (3/4–1 oz)	1 carbohydrate, 1–2 fats
Cranberry sauce, jellied	1/4 cup	1 1/2 carbohydrates
Cupcake, frosted	1 small (about 2 oz)	2 carbohydrates, 1 fat
Doughnut, plain cake	1 medium (1 1/2 oz)	1 1/2 carbohydrates, 2 fats
Doughnut, glazed	3 3/4 inch across (2 oz)	2 carbohydrates, 2 fats
Energy, sport, or breakfast bar	1 bar (1 1/3 oz)	1 1/2 carbohydrates, 0–1 fat
Energy, sport, or breakfast bar	1 bar (2 oz)	2 carbohydrates, 1 fat
Fruit cobbler	1/2 cup (3 1/2 oz)	3 carbohydrates, 1 fat
Fruit juice bars, frozen, 100% juice	1 bar (3 oz)	1 carbohydrate
Fruit snacks, chewy (pureed fruit concentrate)	1 roll (3/4 oz)	1 carbohydrate

APP

Table A-2 *(Continued)*
Food Exchange Lists

Fruit spreads, 100% fruit	1 1/2 tbsp	1 carbohydrate
Gelatin, regular	1/2 cup	1 carbohydrate
Gingersnaps	3	1 carbohydrate
Granola or snack bar, regular or low-fat	1 bar (1 oz)	1 1/2 carbohydrates
Honey	1 tbsp	1 carbohydrate
Ice cream	1/2 cup	1 carbohydrate, 2 fats
Ice cream, light	1/2 cup	1 carbohydrate, 1 fat
Ice cream, low-fat	1/2 cup	1 1/2 carbohydrates
Ice cream, fat-free, no sugar added	1/2 cup	1 carbohydrate
Jam or jelly, regular	1 tbsp	1 carbohydrate
Milk, chocolate, whole	1 cup	2 carbohydrates, 1 fat
Pie, fruit, 2 crusts	1/6 of 8-inch commercially prepared pie	3 carbohydrates, 2 fats
Pie, pumpkin or custard	1/8 of 8-inch commercially prepared pie	2 carbohydrates, 2 fats
Pudding, regular (made with reduced-fat milk)	1/2 cup	2 carbohydrates
Pudding, sugar-free or sugar-free and fat-free (made with fat-free milk)	1/2 cup	1 carbohydrate
Reduced-calorie meal replacement (shake)	1 can (10–11 oz)	1 1/2 carbohydrates, 0–1 fat
Rice milk, low-fat or fat-free, plain	1 cup	1 carbohydrate
Rice milk, low-fat, flavored	1 cup	1 1/2 carbohydrates
Salad dressing, fat-free†	1/4 cup	1 carbohydrate
Sherbet, sorbet	1/2 cup	2 carbohydrates
Spaghetti sauce or pasta sauce, canned†	1/2 cup	1 carbohydrate, 1 fat
Sports drinks	8 oz (1 cup)	1 carbohydrate
Sugar	1 tbsp	1 carbohydrate
Sweet roll or Danish	1 (2 1/2 oz)	2 1/2 carbohydrates, 2 fats
Syrup, light	2 tbsp	1 carbohydrate
Syrup, regular	1 tbsp	1 carbohydrate
Syrup, regular	1/4 cup	4 carbohydrates
Vanilla wafers	5	1 carbohydrate, 1 fat
Yogurt, frozen, fat-free	1/3 cup	1 carbohydrate

Table A-2 *(Continued)*
Food Exchange Lists

Yogurt, low-fat with fruit	1 cup	3 carbohydrates, 0–1 fat

Nonstarchy Vegetable List

Vegetables that contain small amounts of carbohydrate and calories are on this list. Vegetables contain important nutrients. Try to eat at least 2 or 3 vegetable choices each day. In general, 1 vegetable exchange is:

- 1/2 cup of cooked vegetables or vegetable juice
- 1 cup of raw vegetables

If you eat 3 cups or more of raw vegetables or 1 1/2 cups of cooked vegetables at 1 meal, count them as 1 carbohydrate choice.

Nutrition Tips

1. Fresh and frozen vegetables have less added salt than canned vegetables. Drain and rinse canned vegetables if you want to remove some salt.
2. Choose more dark green and dark yellow vegetables, such as spinach, broccoli, romaine, carrots, chilies, and peppers.
3. Broccoli, Brussels sprouts, cauliflower, greens, peppers, spinach, and tomatoes are good sources of vitamin C.
4. Vegetables contain 1 to 4 g of fiber per serving.

Selection Tips

1. A 1-cup portion of broccoli is a portion about the size of a light bulb.
2. Tomato sauce is different from spaghetti sauce, which is on the sweets, desserts, and other carbohydrates list.
3. Canned vegetables and juices are available without added salt.
4. Starchy vegetables such as corn, peas, winter squash, and potatoes, which contain larger amounts of calories and carbohydrates, are on the starch list.

Nonstarchy Vegetable List

One vegetable exchange (1/2 cup cooked or 1 cup raw) equals: 5 g of carbohydrate, 2 g of protein, 0 g of fat, and 25 kcal

Artichoke
Artichoke hearts
Artichoke hearts
Asparagus
Beans (green, wax, Italian)
Bean sprout
Beets
Broccoli
Brussels sprouts
Cabbage
Carrots

Table A-2 *(Continued)*
Food Exchange Lists

Cauliflower
Celery
Cucumber
Eggplant
Green onions or scallions
Kohlrabi
Leeks
Mixed vegetables (without corn, peas, or pasta)
Mushrooms
Okra
Onions
Pea pods
Peppers (all varieties)
Radishes
Salad greens (endive, escarole, lettuce, romaine, spinach)
Sauerkraut†
Spinach
Summer squash
Tomato
Tomatoes, canned
Tomato sauce†
Tomato/vegetable juice†
Turnips
Water chestnuts
Watercress
Zucchini
Meat and Meat Substitutes List

Meat and meat substitutes that contain both protein and fat are on this list. In general, 1 meat exchange is:

- 1 oz of meat, fish, poultry, or cheese
- 1/2 cup of beans, peas, or lentils

Based on the amount of fat they contain, meats are divided into very lean, lean, medium-fat, and high-fat lists. This is done so you can see which ones contain the least amount of fat. One ounce (1 exchange) of each of these includes:

Table A-2 (Continued)
Food Exchange Lists

	Carbohydrate (g)	Protein (g)	Fat (g)	kcal
Very lean	0	7	0–1	35
Lean	0	7	3	55
Medium-fat	0	7	5	75
High-fat	0	7	8	100

Nutrition Tips

1. Choose very lean and lean meat choices whenever possible. Items from the high-fat group are high in saturated fat, cholesterol, and calories and can raise blood cholesterol concentrations.
2. Beans, peas, and lentils are good sources of fiber, approximately 3 g per serving.
3. Some processed meats, seafood, and soy products may contain carbohydrates when consumed in large amounts. Check the Nutrition Facts on the label to see if the amount is close to 15 g. If so, count it as a carbohydrate choice as well as a meat choice.

Selection Tips

1. Weigh meat after cooking and removing bones and fat. Four ounces of raw meat is equal to 3 oz of cooked meat. Some examples of meat portions are:
   - 1 oz cheese = 1 meat choice and is about the size of a 1-inch cube or 4 cubes the size of dice
   - 2 oz meat = 2 meat choices, such as:
     1 small chicken leg or thigh
     1/2 cup cottage cheese or tuna
   - 3 oz meat = 3 meat choices and is about the size of a deck of cards, such as:
     1 medium pork chop
     1 small hamburger
     1/2 of a whole chicken breast
     1 unbreaded fish fillet
2. Limit your choices from the high-fat group to 3 times per week or less.
3. Most grocery stores stock Select and Choice grades of meat. The Select grades of meat are the leanest. The Choice grades contain a moderate amount of fat, and Prime cuts of meat have the highest amount of fat.
4. "Hamburger" may contain added seasoning and fat, but ground beef does not.
5. Read labels to find products that are low in fat and cholesterol (5 g of fat or less per serving).
6. Dried beans, peas, and lentils are also found on the starch list.
7. Peanut butter, in smaller amounts, is also found on the fat list.
8. Bacon, in smaller amounts, is also found on the fat list.
9. Do not be fooled by ground beef packages that state a percentage of lean (eg, 90% lean). This is the percentage of fat by weight, NOT the percentage of calories from fat. A 3.5-oz patty of this raw ground beef has about half of its calories from fat.
10. Meatless burgers are in the combination foods list (3 oz of soy-based burger = 1/2 carbohydrate + 2 very lean meats; 3 oz of vegetable and starch-based burger = 1 carbohydrate + 1 lean meat).

APP

Table A-2 *(Continued)*
Food Exchange Lists

Very Lean Meat and Substitutes List	
One very lean meat exchange is equal to any one of the following items:	
Poultry: chicken or turkey (white meat, no skin), Cornish hen (no skin)	1 oz
Fish: fresh or frozen cod, flounder, haddock, halibut, trout, lox (smoked salmon)†; tuna fresh or canned in water	1 oz
Shellfish: clams, crab, lobster, scallops, shrimp, imitation shellfish	1 oz
Game: duck or pheasant (no skin), venison, buffalo, ostrich	1 oz
Cheese with 1 g of fat or less per ounce: fat-free or low-fat cottage cheese	1/4 cup
Fat-free cheese	1 oz
Other: Processed sandwich meats with 1 g of fat or less per oz, such as deli-thin, shaved meats, chipped beef†, turkey ham	1 oz
Egg whites	2
Egg substitutes, plain	1/4 cup
Hot dogs with 1 g of fat or less per oz†	1 oz
Kidney (high in cholesterol)	1 oz
Sausage with 1 g of fat or less per oz	1 oz
Count the following items as 1 very lean meat and one starch exchange:	
Beans, peas, lentils (cooked)	1/2 cup
Meal Planning Tips	

1. Bake, roast, broil, grill, poach, steam, or boil meat and fish rather than frying.
2. Place meat on a rack so the fat will drain off during cooking.
3. Use a nonstick spray and a nonstick pan to brown or fry foods.
4. Trim off visible fat or skin before or after cooking.
5. If you add flour, bread crumbs, coating mixes, fat, or marinades when cooking, ask your dietitian how to count it in your meal plan.

One lean meat exchange is equal to any 1 of the following items:	
Beef: USDA Select or Choice grades of lean beef trimmed of fat, such as round, sirloin, and flank steak; tenderloin; roast (rib, chuck, rump); steak (T-bone, porterhouse, cubed); ground round	1 oz
Pork: Lean pork, such as fresh ham; canned, cured, or boiled ham; Canadian bacon†; tenderloin, center loin chop	1 oz
Lamb: Roast, chop, or leg	1 oz
Veal: Lean chop, roast	1 oz
Poultry: Chicken, turkey (dark meat, no skin), chicken (white meat, with skin), domestic duck or goose (well-drained off fat, no skin)	1 oz

Table A-2 *(Continued)*
Food Exchange Lists

Fish: Herring (uncreamed or smoked)	1 oz
Oysters	6 medium
Salmon (fresh or canned), catfish	1 oz
Sardines (canned)	2 medium
Tuna (canned in oil, drained)	1 oz
Game: Goose (no skin), rabbit	1 oz
Cheese: 4.5%-fat cottage cheese	1/4 cup
Grated Parmesan	2 tbsp
Cheeses with 3 g of fat or less per oz	1 oz
Other: Hot dogs with 3 g of fat or less per oz†	1 1/2 oz
Processed sandwich meat with 3 g of fat or less per ounce, such as turkey pastrami or kielbasa	1 oz
Liver, heart (high in cholesterol)	1 oz

Medium-Fat Meat and Substitutes List

One medium-fat meat exchange is equal to any one of the following items:	
Beef: Most beef products fall into this category (ground beef, meatloaf, corned beef, short ribs, Prime grades of meat trimmed of fat, such as prime rib)	1 oz
Pork: Top loin, chop, Boston butt, cutlet	1 oz
Lamb: Rib roast, ground	1 oz
Veal: Cutlet (ground or cubed, unbreaded)	1 oz
Poultry: Chicken (dark meat, with skin), ground turkey or ground chicken, fried chicken (with skin)	1 oz
Fish: Any fried fish product	1 oz
Cheese with 5 g or less fat per oz: Feta	1 oz
Mozzarella	1 oz
Ricotta	1/4 cup (2 oz)
Other: Egg (high in cholesterol, limit to 3 per wk)	1
Sausage with 5 g of fat or less per oz	1 oz
Tempeh	1/4 cup
Tofu	4 oz or 1/2 cup

High-Fat Meat and Substitutes List

Remember these items are high in saturated fat, cholesterol, and calories and may raise blood cholesterol concentrations if eaten on a regular basis.	
One high-fat meat exchange is equal to any one of the following items:	
Pork: Spareribs, ground pork, pork sausage	1 oz
Cheese: All regular cheeses, such as American†, cheddar, Monterey Jack, Swiss	1 oz

APP

Table A-2 *(Continued)*
Food Exchange Lists

Other:	Processed sandwich meats with 8 g of fat or less peroz, such as bologna, pimento loaf, salami	1 oz
	Sausage, such as bratwurst, Italian, knockwurst, Polish, smoked	1 oz
	Hot dog (turkey or chicken)†	1 (10/lb)
	Bacon	3 slices (20 slices/lb)
	Peanut butter (contains unsaturated fat)	1 tbsp

Count the following items as 1 high-fat meat plus 1 fat exchange:

Hot dog (beef, pork, or combination)†	1 (10/lb)

Fat List

Fats are divided into 3 groups on the basis of the main type of fat they contain: monounsaturated, polyunsaturated, and saturated. Monounsaturated and polyunsaturated fats in the foods we eat are linked with good health benefits. Saturated fats and fats called trans fatty acids (or trans unsaturated fatty acids) are linked with heart disease. In general, 1 fat exchange is:

- 1 tsp of regular margarine or vegetable oil
- 1 tbsp of regular salad dressing

Nutrition Tips

1. All fats are high in calories. Limit serving sizes for good nutrition and health.
2. Nuts and seeds contain small amounts of fiber, protein, and magnesium.
3. If blood pressure is a concern, choose fats in the unsalted form to help lower sodium intake, such as unsalted peanuts.

Selection Tips

1. Check the Nutrition Facts on food labels for serving sizes. One fat exchange is based on a serving size containing 5 g of fat.
2. The Nutrition Facts on food labels usually list total fat grams and saturated fat grams per serving. When most of the calories come from saturated fat, the food fits into the saturated fats list.
3. Occasionally, the Nutrition Facts on food labels will list monounsaturated and/or polyunsaturated fats in addition to total and saturated fats. If more than half the total fat is monounsaturated, the food fits into the monounsaturated fats list; if more than half is polyunsaturated, the food fits into the polyunsaturated fats list.
4. When selecting fats to use with your meal plan, consider replacing saturated fats with monounsaturated fats.
5. When selecting regular margarine, choose those with liquid vegetable oil as the first ingredient. Soft margarines are not as saturated as stick margarines and are healthier choices.
6. Avoid foods on the fat list (such as margarines) listing hydrogenated or partially hydrogenated fat as the first ingredient because these foods will contain higher amounts of trans fatty acids.
7. When selecting reduced-fat or lower-fat margarines, look for liquid vegetable oil as the second ingredient. Water is usually the first ingredient.
8. When used in smaller amounts, bacon and peanut butter are counted as fat choices. When used in larger amounts, they are counted as high-fat meat choices.
9. Fat-free salad dressings are on the sweets, desserts, and other carbohydrates list and the free foods list.
10. See the free foods list for nondairy coffee creamers, whipped topping, and fat-free products, such as margarines, salad dressings, mayonnaise, sour cream, cream cheese, and nonstick cooking spray.

Table A-2 *(Continued)*
Food Exchange Lists

Monounsaturated Fats List	
Avocado, medium	2 tbsp (1 oz)
Oil (canola, olive, peanut)	1 tsp
Olives: ripe (black)	8 large
green, stuffed[†]	10 large
Nuts: almonds, cashews	6 nuts
mixed (50% peanuts)	6 nuts
peanuts	10 nuts
pecans	4 halves
Peanut butter, smooth or crunchy	1/2 tbsp
Sesame seeds	2 tsp
Tahini or sesame paste	2 tsp
Polyunsaturated Fats List	
Margarine: stick, tub, or squeeze	1 tsp
lower-fat spread (30% to 50% vegetable oil)	1 tbsp
Mayonnaise: regular	1 tsp
reduced-fat	1 tbsp
Nuts: walnuts, English	4 halves
Oil (corn, safflower, soybean)	1 tsp
Salad dressing: regular[†]	1 tbsp
reduced-fat	2 tbsp
Miracle Whip Salad Dressing (Kraft Foods, Northfield, IL):	
regular	2 tsp
reduced-fat	1 tbsp
Seeds: pumpkin, sunflower	1 tbsp
Saturated Fats List	
Bacon, cooked	1 slice (20 slices/lb)
Bacon, grease	1 tsp
Butter: stick	1 tsp
whipped	2 tsp
reduced-fat	1 tbsp
Chitterlings, boiled	2 tbsp (1/2 oz)
Coconut, sweetened, shredded	2 tbsp
Coconut milk	1 tbsp
Cream, half and half	2 tbsp
Cream cheese: regular	1 tbsp (1/2 oz)
reduced-fat	1 1/2 tbsp (3/4 oz)

Table A-2 *(Continued)*
Food Exchange Lists

Fatback or salt pork[†] (see below[‡])	
Shortening or lard	1 tsp
Sour cream: regular	2 tbsp
reduced-fat	3 tbsp

‡Use a piece 1 in × 1 in × 1/4 in if you plan to eat the fatback cooked with vegetables.
Use a piece 2 in × 1 in × 1/2 in when eating only the vegetables with the fatback removed.

Free Foods List

A free food is any food or drink that contains less than 20 kcal or less than or equal to 5 g of carbohydrate per serving. Foods with a serving size listed should be limited to 3 servings per day. Be sure to spread them out throughout the day. If you eat all 3 servings at one time, it could raise your blood glucose concentration. Foods listed without a serving size can be eaten whenever you like.

Fat-Free or Reduced-Fat Foods	
Cream cheese, fat-free	1 tbsp (1/2 oz)
Creamers, nondairy, liquid	1 tbsp
Creamers, nondairy, powdered	2 tsp
Mayonnaise, fat-free	1 tbsp
Mayonnaise, reduced-fat	1 tsp
Margarine spread, fat-free	4 tbsp
Margarine spread, reduced-fat	1 tsp
Miracle Whip, fat-free	1 tbsp
Miracle Whip, reduced-fat	1 tsp
Nonstick cooking spray	
Salad dressing, fat-free or low-fat	1 tbsp
Salad dressing, fat-free, Italian	2 tbsp
Sour cream, fat-free, reduced-fat	1 tbsp
Whipped topping, regular	1 tbsp
Whipped topping, light or fat-free	2 tbsp
Sugar-Free Foods	
Candy, hard, sugar-free	1 candy
Gelatin dessert, sugar-free	
Gelatin, unflavored	
Gum, sugar-free	
Jam or jelly, light	2 tsp

Table A-2 *(Continued)*
Food Exchange Lists

Sugar substitutes*	
Syrup, sugar-free	2 tbsp

*Sugar substitutes, alternatives, or replacements that are approved by the Food and Drug Administration are safe to use. Common brand names include:
  Equal (aspartame; Merisant Company, Chicago, IL)
  Splenda (sucralose; McNeil Nutritionals, Fort Washington, PA)
  Sweet One (acesulfame K; Stadt Holdings Corp, Brooklyn, NY)
  Sugar Twin (saccharin; Alberto-Culver Company, Melrose Park, IL)
  Sweet 'N Low (saccharin; Cumberland Packing Corp, Brooklyn, NY)

Drinks	
Bouillon, broth, consommé†	
Bouillon or broth, low-sodium	
Carbonated or mineral water	
Club soda	
Cocoa powder, unsweetened	1 tbsp
Coffee	
Diet soft drinks, sugar-free	
Drink mixes, sugar-free	
Tea	
Tonic water, sugar-free	

Condiments	
Catsup	1 tbsp
Horseradish	
Lemon juice	
Lime juice	
Mustard	
Pickle relish	1 tbsp
Pickles, dill†	1 1/2 medium
Pickles, sweet (bread and butter)	2 slices
Pickles, sweet (gherkin)	3/4 oz
Salsa	1/4 cup
Soy sauce, regular or light†	1 tbsp
Taco sauce	1 tbsp
Vinegar	

APP

Table A-2 *(Continued)*
Food Exchange Lists

Yogurt	2 tbsp

Seasonings

Flavoring extracts
Garlic
Herbs, fresh or dried
Pimento
Spices
Tabasco (McIlhenny Co, Avery Island, LA) or hot pepper sauce
Wine, used in cooking
Worcestershire sauce
Be careful with seasonings that contain sodium or are salts, such as garlic or celery salt and lemon pepper.

Combination Foods List

Many of the foods we eat are mixed together in various combinations. These combination foods do not fit into any one exchange list. Often, it is hard to tell what is in a casserole dish or prepared food item. This is a list of exchanges for some typical combination foods. This list will help you fit these foods into your meal plan. Ask your dietitian for information about any other combination foods you would like to eat.

Food	Serving Size	Exchanges per Serving
Entrees		
Tuna noodle casserole, lasagna, spaghetti with meatballs, chili with beans, macaroni and cheese†	1 cup (8 oz)	2 carbohydrates, 2 medium-fat meats
Chow mein (without noodles or rice)†	2 cups (16 oz)	1 carbohydrate, 2 lean meats
Tuna or chicken salad	1/2 cup (3 1/2 oz)	1/2 carbohydrate, 2 lean meats, 1 fat
Frozen Entrees and Meals		
Dinner-type meal	Generally 14–17 oz	3 carbohydrates, 3 medium-fat meats, 3 fats
Meatless burger, soy based	3 oz	1/2 carbohydrate, 2 lean meats
Meatless burger, vegetable and starch based	3 oz	1 carbohydrate, 1 lean meat
Pizza, cheese, thin crust†	1/4 of 12 in (6 oz)	2 carbohydrates, 2 medium-fat meats,

Table A-2 *(Continued)*
Food Exchange Lists

Pizza, meat topping, thin crust†	1/4 of 12 in (6 oz)	2 carbohydrates, 2 medium-fat meats, 1 1/2 fats
Pot pie†	1 (7 oz)	
Entree or meal with less than 340 kcal†	Approx 8–11 oz	2–3 carbohydrates, 1–2 lean meats

Soups		
Bean†	1 cup	1 carbohydrate, 1 very lean meat
Cream (made with water)	1 cup (8 oz)	1 carbohydrate, 1 fat
Instant†	6 oz prepared	1 carbohydrate
Instant with beans/lentils†	8 oz prepared	2 1/2 carbohydrates, 1 very lean meat
Split pea (made with water)†	1/2 cup (4 oz)	1 carbohydrate
Tomato (made with water)†	1 cup (8 oz)	1 carbohydrate
Vegetable beef, chicken noodle, or other broth-type†	1 cup (8 oz)	1 carbohydrate

Fast Foods* List		
Food	**Serving Size**	**Exchange per Serving**
Burrito with beef†	1 (5–7 oz)	3 carbohydrates, 1 medium-fat meat, 1 fat
Chicken nuggets†	6	1 carbohydrate, 2 medium-fat meats, 1 fat
Chicken breast and wing, breaded and fried†	1	1 carbohydrate, 4 medium-fat meats, 2 fats
Chicken sandwich, grilled†	1	2 carbohydrates, 3 very lean meats
Chicken wings, hot†	6 (5 oz)	1 carbohydrate, 3 medium fat meats, 4 fats
Fish sandwich/tartar sauce†	1	3 carbohydrates, 1 medium-fat meat, 3 fats
French fries†	1 medium serving (5 oz)	4 carbohydrates, 4 fats

APP

Table A-2 *(Continued)*
Food Exchange Lists

Hamburger, regular	1	2 carbohydrates, 2 medium-fat meats
Hamburger, large[†]	1	2 carbohydrates, 3 medium-fat meats 1 fat
Hot dog with bun[†]	1	1 carbohydrate, 1 high-fat meat, 1 fat
Individual pan pizza[†]	1	5 carbohydrates, 3 medium-fat meats, 3 fats
Pizza, cheese, thin crust[†]	1/4 12 inch (about 6 oz)	2 1/2 carbohydrates, 2 medium-fat meats 1 1/2 fats
Pizza, meat, thin crust[†]	1/4 12 inch (about 6 oz)	2 1/2 carbohydrates 2 medium-fat meats, 2 fats
Soft-serve ice cream cone	1 small (5 oz)	2 1/2 carbohydrates, 1 fat
Submarine sandwich[†] (regular)	1 sub (6 inch)	3 1/2 carbohydrates, 2 medium-fat meats, 1 fat
Submarine sandwich[†] (less than 6 g fat)	1 sub (6 inch)	3 carbohydrates, 2 very lean meats
Taco, hard or soft shell[†]	1 (3–3 1/2 oz)	1 carbohydrate, 1 medium-fat meat, 1 fat

* Ask at the fast-food restaurant for nutrition information about your favorite fast foods or check Web sites.

† 400 mg or more of sodium per exchange.

Appendix B

Table B-1

Conversions from Conventional Units to Systeme International (SI) Units

	Specimen	Traditional Reference Intervals	Traditional Units	Conversion Factor Multiply→ ←Divide	SI Reference Intervals	SI Units
Acetaminophen (therapeutic)	Serum, plasma	10–30	µg/mL	6.62	70–200	µmol/L
Acetoacetic acid	Serum, plasma	<1	mg/dL	0.098	<0.1	mmol/L
Acetone	Serum, plasma	<2.0	mg/dL	0.172	<0.34	mmol/L
Acetylcholinesterase	Red blood cells	30–40	U/g of Hb	0.0645	2.13–2.63	MU/mol of Hb
Activated partial thromboplastin time (APTT)	Whole blood	25–40	s	1	25–40	s
Adenosine deaminase[†]	Serum	11.5–25.0	U/L	0.017	0.20–0.43	µkat/L
Adrenocorticotropic hormone (ACTH) (see Corticotropin)						
Alanine*	Serum	1.87–5.89	mg/dL	112.2	210–661	µmol/L
Alanine aminotransferase (ALT, SGPT)*	Serum	10–40	U/L	1	10–40	U/L
Albumin*	Serum	3.5–5.0	g/dL	10	35–50	g/L
Alcohol (see Ethanol, Isopropanol, Methanol)						
Alcohol dehydrogenase[†]	Serum	<2.8	U/L	0.017	<0.05	µkat/L
Aldolase*[†]	Serum	1.0–7.5	U/L	0.017	0.02–0.13	µkat/L
Aldosterone*	Serum, plasma	7–30	ng/dL	0.0277	0.19–0.83	nmol/L
Aldosterone	Urine	3–20	µg/24 h	2.77	8–55	nmol/d
Alkaline phosphatase*	Serum	50–120	U/L	1	50–120	U/L
Alprazolam (therapeutic)	Serum, plasma	10–50	ng/mL	3.24	32–162	nmol/L
Aluminum	Serum	0–6	ng/mL	37.06	0.0–222.4	nmol/L

APP

Table B-1 *(Continued)*
Conversions from Conventional Units to Systeme International (SI) Units

	Specimen	Traditional Reference Intervals	Traditional Units	Conversion Factor Multiply → ← Divide	SI Reference Intervals	SI Units
Amikacin (therapeutic, peak)	Serum, plasma	20–30	µg/mL	1.71	34–52	µmol/L
Amino acid fractionation						
Alanine*	Serum	1.87–5.89	mg/dL	112.2	210–661	µmol/L
α-Aminobutyric acid*	Plasma	0.08–0.36	mg/dL	97	8–35	µmol/L
Arginine*	Plasma	0.37–2.40	mg/dL	57.4	21–138	µmol/L
Asparagine*	Plasma	0.40–0.91	mg/dL	75.7	30–69	µmol/L
Aspartic acid*	Plasma	<0.3	mg/dL	75.1	<25	µmol/L
Citrulline*	Plasma	0.2–1.0	mg/dL	57.1	12–55	µmol/L
Cystine*	Plasma	0.40–1.40	mg/dL	83.3	33–117	µmol/L
Glutamic acid*	Plasma	0.2–2.8	mg/dL	67.97	15–190	µmol/L
Glutamine*	Plasma	6.1–10.2	mg/dL	68.42	420–700	µmol/L
Glycine*	Plasma	0.9–4.2	mg/dL	133.3	120–560	µmol/L
Histidine*	Plasma	0.5–1.7	mg/dL	64.5	32–110	µmol/L
Hydroxyproline*	Plasma	<0.55	mg/dL	76.3	<42	µmol/L
Isoleucine*	Plasma	0.5–1.3	mg/dL	76.24	40–100	µmol/L
Leucine*	Plasma	1.0–2.3	mg/dL	76.3	75–175	µmol/L
Lysine*	Plasma	1.2–3.5	mg/dL	68.5	80–240	µmol/L
Methionine*	Plasma	0.1–0.6	mg/dL	67.1	6–40	µmol/L
Ornithine*	Plasma	0.4–1.4	mg/dL	75.8	30–106	µmol/L

Table B-1 *(Continued)*
Conversions from Conventional Units to Systeme International (SI) Units

	Specimen	Traditional Reference Intervals	Traditional Units	Conversion Factor Multiply → ← Divide	SI Reference Intervals	SI Units
Phenylalanine*	Plasma	0.6–1.5	mg/dL	60.5	35–90	µmol/L
Proline*	Plasma	1.2–3.9	mg/dL	86.9	104–340	µmol/L
Serine*	Plasma	0.7–2.0	mg/dL	95.2	65–193	µmol/L
Taurine*	Plasma	0.3–2.1	mg/dL	80	24–168	µmol/L
Threonine*	Plasma	0.9–2.5	mg/dL	84	75–210	µmol/L
Tryptophan*	Plasma	0.5–1.5	mg/dL	48.97	25–73	µmol/L
Tyrosine*	Plasma	0.4–1.6	mg/dL	55.19	20–90	µmol/L
Valine*	Plasma	1.7–3.7	mg/dL	85.5	145–315	µmol/L
α-Aminobutyric acid*	Plasma	0.08–0.36	mg/dL	97	8–35	µmol/L
Amiodarone (therapeutic)	Serum, plasma	0.5–2.5	µg/mL	1.55	0.8–3.9	µmol/L
δ–Aminolevulinic acid	Urine	1.0–7.0	mg/24 h	7.626	8–53	µmol/d
Amitriptyline (therapeutic)	Serum, plasma	80–250	ng/mL	3.61	289–903	nmol/L
Ammonia (as NH3)*	Plasma	19–60	µg/dL	0.587	11–35	µmol/L
Amobarbital (therapeutic)	Serum	1–5	µg/mL	4.42	4–22	µmol/L
Amoxapine (therapeutic)	Plasma	200–600	ng/mL	1	200–600	µg/L
Amylase*†	Serum	27–130	U/L	0.017	0.46–2.21	µkat/L
Androstenedione*, male	Serum	75–205	ng/dL	0.0349	2.6–7.2	nmol/L
Androstenedione*, female	Serum	85–275	ng/dL	0.0349	3.0–9.6	nmol/L
Angiotensin I	Plasma	<25	pg/mL	1	<25	ng/L

APP

Table B-1 *(Continued)*
Conversions from Conventional Units to Systeme International (SI) Units

	Specimen	Traditional Reference Intervals	Traditional Units	Conversion Factor Multiply → ← Divide	SI Reference Intervals	SI Units
Angiotensin II	Plasma	10–60	pg/mL	1	10–60	ng/L
Angiotensin-converting enzyme (ACE)*†	Serum	8–52	U/L	0.017	0.14–0.88	μkat/L
Anion gap (Na+) –(Cl– + HCO3–)	Serum, plasma	8–16	mEq/L	1	8–16	nmol/L
Antidiuretic hormone (ADH, vasopressin) (varies with osmolality: 285–290 mOsm/kg)	Plasma	1–5	pg/mL	0.926	0.9–4.6	pmol/L
α₂-Antiplasmin	Plasma	80–130	%	0.01	0.80–1.3	Fraction of 1.0
Antithrombin III	Plasma	21–30	mg/dL	10	210–300	mg/L
Antithrombin III activity	Plasma	80–130	%	0.01	0.8–1.3	Fraction of 1.0
α₁-Antitrypsin	Serum	126–226	mg/dL	0.01	1.26–2.26	g/L
Apolipoprotein A*						
Male	Serum	80–151	mg/dL	0.01	0.8–1.5	g/L
Female	Serum	80–170	mg/dL	0.01	0.8–1.7	g/L
Apolipoprotein B*						
Male	Serum, plasma	50–123	mg/dL	0.01	0.5–1.2	g/L
Female	Serum, plasma	25–120	mg/dL	0.01	0.25–1.20	g/L
Arginine*	Plasma	0.37–2.40	mg/dL	57.4	21–138	μmol/L
Arsenic (As)	Whole blood	<23	μg/L	0.0133	<0.31	μmol/L
Arsenic (As), acute poisoning	Whole blood	600–9300	μg/L	0.0133	7.98–123.7	μmol/L
Ascorbate, ascorbic acid (see Vitamin C)						

Table B-1 *(Continued)*
Conversions from Conventional Units to Systeme International (SI) Units

	Specimen	Traditional Reference Intervals	Traditional Units	Conversion Factor Multiply → ← Divide	SI Reference Intervals	SI Units
Asparagine*	Plasma	0.40–0.91	mg/dL	75.7	30–69	µmol/L
Aspartate amino transferase (AST, SGOT)*†	Serum	20–48	U/L	0.017	0.34–0.82	µkat/L
Aspartic acid*	Plasma	<0.3	mg/dL	75.1	<25	µmol/L
Atrial natriuretic hormone	Plasma	20–77	pg/mL	1	20–77	ng/L
Barbiturates (see individual drugs; Pentobarbital, Phenobarbital, Thiopental)						
Basophils (see Complete blood cell count, White blood cell count)						
Benzodiazepines (see individual drugs; Alprazolam, Chlordiazepoxide, Diazepam, Lorazepam)						
Bicarbonate	Plasma	21–28	mEq/L	1	21–28	mmol/L
Bile acids (total)	Serum	0.3–2.3	µg/mL	2.448	0.73–5.63	µmol/L
Bilirubin						
Total*	Serum	0.3–1.2	mg/dL	17.1	2–18	µmol/L
Direct (conjugated)	Serum	<0.2	mg/dL	17.1	<3.4	µmol/L
Biotin	Whole blood, serum	200–500	pg/mL	0.0041	0.82–2.05	nmol/L
Bismuth	Whole blood	1–12	µg/L	4.785	4.8–57.4	nmol/L
Blood gases						
Pco₂	Arterial blood	35–45	mm Hg	1	35–45	mm Hg
pH	Arterial blood	7.35–7.45	…	1	7.35–7.45	…
Po₂	Arterial blood	80–100	mm Hg	1	80–100	mm Hg

APP

Table B-1 (Continued)
Conversions from Conventional Units to Systeme International (SI) Units

	Specimen	Traditional Reference Intervals	Traditional Units	Conversion Factor Multiply → ← Divide	SI Reference Intervals	SI Units
Blood urea nitrogen (BUN, see Urea nitrogen)						
C1 esterase inhibitor	Serum	12–30	mg/dL	0.01	0.12–0.30	g/L
C3 complement*	Serum	1200–1500	µg/mL	0.001	1.2–1.5	g/L
C4 complement*	Serum	350–600	µg/mL	0.001	0.35–0.60	g/L
Cadmium (nonsmoker)	Whole blood	0.3–1.2	µg/L	8.897	2.7–10.7	nmol/L
Caffeine (therapeutic, infants)	Serum, plasma	8–20	µg/mL	5.15	41–103	µmol/L
Calciferol (see Vitamin D)						
Calcitonin	Serum, plasma	<19	pg/mL	1	<19	ng/L
Calcium, ionized	Serum	4.60–5.08	mg/dL	0.25	1.15–1.27	mmol/L
Calcium, total	Serum	8.2–10.2	mg/dL	0.25	2.05–2.55	mmol/L
Calcium, normal diet	Urine	<250	mg/24 h	0.025	<6.2	mmol/d
Carbamazepine (therapeutic)	Serum, plasma	8–12	µg/mL	4.23	34–51	µmol/L
Carbon dioxide	Serum, plasma, venous blood	22–28	mEq/L	1	22–28	mmol/L
Carboxyhemoglobin (carbon monoxide), as fraction of hemoglobin saturation						
Nonsmoker	Whole blood	<2.0	%	0.01	<0.02	Fraction of 1.0
Toxic	Whole blood	>20	%	0.01	>0.2	Fraction of 1.0
β-Carotene	Serum	10–85	µg/dL	0.0186	0.2–1.6	µmol/L
Catecholamines, total (see Norepinephrine)						
Ceruloplasmin*	Serum	20–40	mg/dL	10	200–400	mg/L

Table B-1 *(Continued)*
Conversions from Conventional Units to Systeme International (SI) Units

	Specimen	Traditional Reference Intervals	Traditional Units	Conversion Factor Multiply — Divide	SI Reference Intervals	SI Units
Chloramphenicol (therapeutic)	Serum	10–25	μg/mL	3.1	31–77	μmol/L
Chlordiazepoxide (therapeutic)	Serum, plasma	0.7–1.0	μg/mL	3.34	2.3–3.3	μmol/L
Chloride	Serum, plasma	96–106	mEq/L	1	96–106	mmol/L
Chloride	CSF	118–132	mEq/L	1	118–132	mmol/L
Chlorpromazine (therapeutic, adult)	Plasma	50–300	ng/mL	3.14	157–942	nmol/L
Chlorpromazine (therapeutic, child)	Plasma	40–80	ng/mL	3.14	126–251	nmol/L
Chlorpropamide (therapeutic)	Plasma	75–250	mg/L	3.61	270–900	μmol/L
Cholesterol, high-density lipoprotein (HDL)						
Male	Plasma	35–65	mg/dL	0.02586	0.91–1.68	mmol/L
Female	Plasma	35–80	mg/dL	0.02586	0.91–2.07	mmol/L
Cholesterol, low-density lipoprotein (LDL)*	Plasma	60–130	mg/dL	0.02586	1.55–3.37	mmol/L
Cholesterol (total), adult						
Desirable	Serum	<200	mg/dL	0.02586	<5.17	mmol/L
Borderline high	Serum	200–239	mg/dL	0.02586	5.17–6.18	mmol/L
High	Serum	>240	mg/dL	0.02586	>6.21	mmol/L
Cholesterol (total), children						
Desirable	Serum	<170	mg/dL	0.02586	4.40	mmol/L
Borderline high	Serum	170–199	mg/dL	0.02586	4.40–5.15	mmol/L
High	Serum	>200	mg/dL	0.02586	>5.18	mmol/L

Table B-1 *(Continued)*
Conversions from Conventional Units to Systeme International (SI) Units

	Specimen	Traditional Reference Intervals	Traditional Units	Conversion Factor Multiply → ← Divide	SI Reference Intervals	SI Units
Cholesterol esters (as % of total cholesterol)	Plasma	60–75	%	0.01	0.60–0.75	Fraction of 1.0
Chromium	Whole blood	0.7–28.0	µg/L	19.2	13.4–538.6	nmol/L
Citrate	Serum	1.2–3.0	mg/dL	52.05	60–160	µmol/L
Citrulline*	Plasma	0.2–1.0	mg/dL	57.1	12–55	µmol/L
Clonazepam (therapeutic)	Serum	15–60	ng/mL	3.17	48–190	nmol/L
Coagulation factor I (fibrinogen)	Plasma	150–400	mg/dL	0.01	1.5–4.0	g/L
Coagulation factor II (prothrombin)	Plasma	60–140	%	0.01	0.60–1.40	Fraction of 1.0
Coagulation factor V	Plasma	60–140	%	0.01	0.60–1.40	Fraction of 1.0
Coagulation factor VII	Plasma	60–140	%	0.01	0.60–1.40	Fraction of 1.0
Coagulation factor VIII	Plasma	50–200	%	0.01	0.50–2.00	Fraction of 1.0
Coagulation factor IX	Plasma	60–140	%	0.01	0.60–1.40	Fraction of 1.0
Coagulation factor X	Plasma	60–140	%	0.01	0.60–1.40	Fraction of 1.0
Coagulation factor XI	Plasma	60–140	%	0.01	0.60–1.40	Fraction of 1.0
Coagulation factor XII	Plasma	60–140	%	0.01	0.60–1.40	Fraction of 1.0
Cobalt	Serum	4.0–10.0	µg/L	16.97	67.9–169.7	nmol/L
Codeine (therapeutic)	Serum	10–100	ng/mL	3.34	33–334	nmol/L
Complete blood cell (CBC) count						
Hematocrit*						

Table B-1 *(Continued)*
Conversions from Conventional Units to Systeme International (SI) Units

	Specimen	Traditional Reference Intervals	Traditional Units	Conversion Factor Multiply→ ←Divide	SI Reference Intervals	SI Units
Male	Whole blood	41–50	%	0.01	0.41–0.50	Fraction of 1.0
Female	Whole blood	35–45	%	0.01	0.35–0.45	Fraction of 1.0
Hemoglobin (mass concentration)*						
Male	Whole blood	13.5–17.5	g/dL	10	135–175	g/L
Female	Whole blood	12.0–15.5	g/dL	10	120–155	g/L
Hemoglobin (substance concentration, Hb [Fe])						
Male	Whole blood	13.6–17.2	g/dL	0.6206	8.44–10.65	mmol/L
Female	Whole blood	12.0–15.0	g/dL	0.6206	7.45–9.30	mmol/L
Mean corpuscular hemoglobin (MCH), mass concentration*	Whole blood	27–33	pg/cell	1	27–33	pg/cell
Mean corpuscular hemoglobin (MCH), substance concentration, Hb [Fe]	Whole blood	27–33	pg/cell	0.06206	1.70–2.05	fmol
Mean corpuscular hemoglobin concentration (MCHC), mass concentration	Whole blood	33–37	g Hb/dL Ercs	10	330–370	g Hb/L Ercs
Mean corpuscular hemoglobin concentration (MCHC), substance concentration, Hb [Fe]	Whole blood	33–37	g Hb/dL Ercs	0.6206	20–23	mmol/L
Mean cell volume (MCV)*	Whole blood	80–100	μm^3	1	80–100	fl
Platelet count	Whole blood	150–450	$10^3/\mu L$	1	150–450	$10^9/L$
Red blood cell count						

APP

Table B-1 *(Continued)*

Conversions from Conventional Units to Systeme International (SI) Units

	Specimen	Traditional Reference Intervals	Traditional Units	Conversion Factor Multiply → ← Divide	SI Reference Intervals	SI Units
Female	Whole blood	3.9–5.5	$10^6/\mu L$	1	3.9–5.5	$10^{12}/L$
Male	Whole blood	4.6–6.0	$10^6/\mu L$	1	4.6–6.0	$10^{12}/L$
Reticulocyte count*	Whole blood	25–75	$10^3/\mu L$	1	25–75	$10^9/L$
Reticulocyte count* (fraction)	Whole blood	0.5–1.5	% of RBCs	0.01	0.005–0.015	Fraction of RBCs
White blood cell count*	Whole blood	4.5–11.0	$10^3/\mu L$	1	4.5–11.0	$10^9/L$
Differential count* (absolute)						
Neutrophils	Whole blood	1800–7800	$/\mu L$	1	1.8–7.8	$10^9/L$
Bands	Whole blood	0–700	$/\mu L$	1	0.00–0.70	$10^9/L$
Lymphocytes	Whole blood	1000–4800	$/\mu L$	1	1.0–4.8	$10^9/L$
Monocytes	Whole blood	0–800	$/\mu L$	1	0.00–0.80	$10^9/L$
Eosinophils	Whole blood	0–450	$/\mu L$	1	0.00–0.45	$10^9/L$
Basophils	Whole blood	0–200	$/\mu L$	1	0.00–0.20	$10^9/L$
Differential count* (number fraction)						
Neutrophils	Whole blood	56	%	0.01	0.56	Fraction of 1.0
Bands	Whole blood	3	%	0.01	0.03	Fraction of 1.0
Lymphocytes	Whole blood	34	%	0.01	0.34	Fraction of 1.0
Monocytes	Whole blood	4	%	0.01	0.04	Fraction of 1.0
Eosinophils	Whole blood	2.7	%	0.01	0.027	Fraction of 1.0
Basophils	Whole blood	0.3	%	0.01	0.003	Fraction of 1.0

Table B-1 *(Continued)*
Conversions from Conventional Units to Systeme International (SI) Units

	Specimen	Traditional Reference Intervals	Traditional Units	Conversion Factor Multiply → ← Divide	SI Reference Intervals	SI Units
Copper*	Serum	70–140	µg/dL	0.1574	11.0–22.0	µmol/L
Coproporphyrin	Urine	<200	µg/24 h	1.527	<300	nmol/d
Corticotropin*	Plasma	<120	pg/mL	0.22	<26	pmol/L
Cortisol, total*						
Fasting, 8 AM–noon	Plasma	5–25	µg/dL	27.6	138–690	nmol/L
Noon–8 PM	Plasma	5–15	µg/dL	27.6	138–414	nmol/L
8 PM–8 AM	Plasma	0–10	µg/dL	27.6	0–276	nmol/L
Cortisol, free*	Urine	30–100	µg/24 h	2.759	80–280	nmol/d
Cotinine (smoker)	Plasma	16–145	ng/mL	5.68	91–823	nmol/L
C-peptide	Serum	0.5–2.5	ng/mL	0.333	0.17–0.83	nmol/L
Creatine, male	Serum	0.2–0.7	mg/dL	76.3	15.3–53.3	µmol/L
Creatine, female	Serum	0.3–0.9	mg/dL	76.3	22.9–68.6	µmol/L
Creatine kinase (CK)†	Serum	50–200	U/L	0.017	0.85–3.40	µkat/L
Creatine kinase-MB fraction	Serum	<6	%	0.01	<0.06	Fraction of 1.0
Creatinine*	Serum, plasma	0.6–1.2	mg/dL	88.4	53–106	µmol/L
Creatinine	Urine	1–2	g/24 h	8.84	8.8–17.7	mmol/d
Creatinine clearance	Serum, urine	75–125	mL/min	0.01667	1.24–2.08	mL/s
Cyanide (toxic)	Whole blood	>1.0	µg/mL	38.4	>38.4	µmol/L
Cyanocobalamin (see Vitamin B₁₂)						

APP

Table B-1 (Continued)
Conversions from Conventional Units to Systeme International (SI) Units

	Specimen	Traditional Reference Intervals	Traditional Units	Conversion Factor Multiply → ← Divide	SI Reference Intervals	SI Units
Cyclic adenosine monophosphate (cAMP)	Plasma	4.6–8.6	ng/mL	3.04	14–26	nmol/L
Cyclosporine (toxic)	Whole blood	>400	ng/mL	0.832	>333	nmol/L
Cystine*	Plasma	0.40–1.40	mg/dL	83.3	33–117	μmol/L
D-dimer	Plasma	Negative (<500)	ng/mL	1	Negative (<500)	ng/mL
Dehydroepiandrosterone (DHEA) (unconjugated, male)*	Plasma, serum	180–1250	ng/dL	0.0347	6.2–43.3	nmol/L
Dehydroepiandrosterone sulfate (DHEA-S) (male)*	Plasma, serum	10–619	μg/dL	0.027	0.3–16.7	μmol/L
Desipramine (therapeutic)	Plasma, serum	50–200	ng/mL	3.75	170–700	nmol/L
Diazepam (therapeutic)	Plasma, serum	100–1000	ng/mL	0.00351	0.35–3.51	μmol/L
Digoxin (therapeutic)	Plasma	0.5–2.0	ng/mL	1.281	0.6–2.6	nmol/L
Disopyramide (therapeutic)	Plasma, serum	2.8–7.0	mg/L	2.95	8–21	μmol/L
Doxepin (therapeutic)	Plasma, serum	150–250	ng/mL	3.58	540–890	nmol/L
Electrolytes						
Chloride	Serum, plasma	96–106	mEq/L	1	96–106	mmol/L
Carbon dioxide (CO_2)	Serum, plasma, venous blood	22–28	mEq/L	1	22–28	mmol/L
Potassium	Plasma	3.5–5.0	mEq/L	1	3.5–5.0	mmol/L
Sodium*	Plasma	136–142	mEq/L	1	136–142	mmol/L

Table B-1 *(Continued)*
Conversions from Conventional Units to Systeme International (SI) Units

	Specimen	Traditional Reference Intervals	Traditional Units	Conversion Factor Multiply→ ←Divide	SI Reference Intervals	SI Units
Eosinophils (see Complete blood cell count, White blood cell count)						
Epinephrine	Plasma	<60	pg/mL	5.46	<330	pmol/L
Epinephrine*	Urine	<20	µg/24 h	5.46	<109	nmol/d
Erythrocyte count (see Complete blood cell count, Red blood cell count)						
Erythrocyte sedimentation rate (ESR)*	Whole blood	0–20	mm/h	1	0–20	mm/h
Erythropoietin	Serum	5–36	mU/mL	1	5–36	IU/L
Estradiol (E_2, unconjugated)*, female						
Follicular phase	Serum	20–350	pg/mL	3.67	73–1285	pmol/L
Mid-cycle peak	Serum	150–750	pg/mL	3.67	551–2753	pmol/L
Luteal phase	Serum	30–450	pg/mL	3.67	110–1652	pmol/L
Postmenopausal	Serum	<59	pg/mL	3.67	<218	pmol/L
Estradiol (unconjugated)*, male	Serum	<20	pg/mL	3.67	<184	pmol/L
Estriol (E_3, unconjugated), varies with length of gestation	Serum	5–40	ng/mL	3.47	17.4–138.8	nmol/L
Estrogens (total)*, female						
Follicular phase	Serum	60–200	pg/mL	1	60–200	ng/L
Luteal phase	Serum	160–400	pg/mL	1	160–400	ng/L
Postmenopausal	Serum	<130	pg/mL	1	<130	ng/L
Estrogens (total)*, male	Serum	20–80	pg/mL	1	20–80	ng/L

APP

Table B-1 *(Continued)*
Conversions from Conventional Units to Systeme International (SI) Units

	Specimen	Traditional Reference Intervals	Traditional Units	Conversion Factor Multiply → Divide ←	SI Reference Intervals	SI Units
Estrone (E₁)*, female						
Follicular phase	Plasma, serum	1.5–25	pg/mL	37	55–925	pmol/L
Luteal phase	Plasma, serum	1.5–20	pg/mL	37	55–740	pmol/L
Postmenopausal	Plasma, serum	1.5–5.5	pg/mL	37	55–204	pmol/L
Estrone (E₁)*, male	Plasma, serum	1.5–6.5	pg/mL	37	55–240	pmol/L
Ethanol (ethyl alcohol), toxic	Serum, whole blood	>100	mg/dL	0.2171	>21.7	mmol/L
Ethosuximide	Plasma, serum	40–100	µg/mL	7.08	283–708	µmol/L
Ethylene glycol (toxic)	Plasma, serum	>30	mg/dL	0.1611	>5	mmol/L
Fatty acids (nonesterified)	Plasma	8–25	mg/dL	0.0354	0.28–0.89	mmol/L
Fecal fat (as stearic acid)	Stool	2.0–6.0	g/d	1	2–6	g/d
Ferritin*	Plasma	15–200	ng/mL	1	15–200	µg/L
α₁-Fetoprotein*	Serum	<10	ng/mL	1	<10	µg/L
Fibrinogen	Plasma	150–400	mg/dL	0.01	1.5–4.0	g/L
Fibrin breakdown products (fibrin split products)	Serum	<10	µg/mL	1	<10	mg/L
Folate (folic acid)	Red blood cells	166–640	ng/mL	2.266	376–1450	nmol/L
Folate (folic acid)	Serum	5–25	ng/mL	2.266	11–57	nmol/L
Follicle-stimulating hormone (FSH, follitropin)*, female						
Follicular phase	Serum	1.37–9.9	mIU/mL	1	1.37–9.9	IU/L

Table B-1 *(Continued)*
Conversions from Conventional Units to Systeme International (SI) Units

	Specimen	Traditional Reference Intervals	Traditional Units	Conversion Factor Multiply → ← Divide	SI Reference Intervals	SI Units
Ovulatory phase	Serum	6.17–17.2	mIU/mL	1	6.17–17.2	IU/L
Luteal phase	Serum	1.09–9.2	mIU/mL	1	1.09–9.2	IU/L
Postmenopausal	Serum	19.3–100.6	mIU/mL	1	19.3–100.6	IU/L
Follicle-stimulating hormone (FSH, follitropin)*, male	Serum	1.42–15.4	mIU/mL	1	1.42–15.4	IU/L
Follicle-stimulating hormone (FSH, follitropin)*, female	Urine	2–15	IU/24 h	1	2–15	IU/d
Follicle-stimulating hormone (FSH, follitropin)*, male	Urine	3–12	IU/24 h	1	3–11	IU/d
Fructosamine*	Serum	1.5–2.7	mmol/L	1	1.5–2.7	mmol/L
Fructose	Serum	1–6	mg/dL	55.5	55.5–333	µmol/L
Galactose	Plasma, serum	<20	mg/dL	0.0555	<1.10	mmol/L
Gastrin (fasting)	Serum	<100	pg/mL	1	<100	ng/L
Gentamicin (therapeutic, peak)	Serum	6–10	µg/mL	2.1	12–21	µmol/L
Glucagon*	Plasma	20–100	pg/mL	1	20–100	ng/L
Glucose*	Serum, plasma	70–110	mg/dL	0.05551	3.9–6.1	mmol/L
Glucose	Cerebrospinal fluid	50–80	mg/dL	0.05551	2.8–4.4	mmol/L
Glucose-6-phosphate dehydrogenase	Red blood cells	10–14	U/g of Hb	0.0645	0.65–0.90	MU/mol of Hb
Glutamic acid*	Plasma	0.2–2.8	mg/dL	67.97	15–190	µmol/L
Glutamine	Plasma	6.1–10.2	mg/dL	68.42	420–700	µmol/L

APP

Table B-1 *(Continued)*
Conversions from Conventional Units to Systeme International (SI) Units

	Specimen	Traditional Reference Intervals	Traditional Units	Conversion Factor Multiply → ← Divide	SI Reference Intervals	SI Units
γ-Glutamyltransferase (GGT; γ-glutamyl transpeptidase)†	Serum	0–30	U/L	0.017	0–0.51	μkat/L
Glycerol (free)*	Serum	<1.5	mg/dL	0.1086	<0.16	mmol/L
Glycine*	Plasma	0.9–4.2	mg/dL	133.3	120–560	μmol/L
Glycosylated hemoglobin (glycated hemoglobin; hemoglobin A1, A1c)	Whole blood	4–7	% of total Hb	0.01	0.04–0.07	Fraction of total Hb
Gold (therapeutic)	Serum	100–200	μg/dL	0.05077	5.1–10.2	μmol/L
Growth hormone, adult (GH, somatotropin)*	Plasma, serum	<20	ng/mL	1	<20	μg/L
Haloperidol (therapeutic)	Serum, plasma	5–20	ng/mL	2.6	13–52	nmol/L
Haptoglobin*	Serum	40–180	mg/dL	0.01	0.4–1.8	g/L
Hematocrit (see Complete blood cell count)						
Hemoglobin (see Complete blood cell count)						
Hemoglobin A1c (see Glycosylated hemoglobin)						
Hemoglobin A2*	Whole blood	2.0–3.0	%	0.01	0.02–0.03	Fraction of 1.0
Hemoglobin F* (fetal hemoglobin in adult)	Whole blood	<2	%	0.01	<0.02	Fraction of 1.0
High-density lipoprotein cholesterol (HDL)						
Male	Plasma	35–65	mg/dL	0.02586	0.91–1.68	mmol/L
Female	Plasma	35–80	mg/dL	0.02586	0.91–2.07	mmol/L
Histidine*	Plasma	0.5–1.7	mg/dL	64.5	32–110	μmol/L

Table B-1 *(Continued)*
Conversions from Conventional Units to Systeme International (SI) Units

	Specimen	Traditional Reference Intervals	Traditional Units	Conversion Factor Multiply → ← Divide	SI Reference Intervals	SI Units
Homocysteine (total)	Plasma, serum	4–12	μmol/L	1	4–12	μmol/L
Homovanillic acid*	Urine	<8	mg/24 h	5.489	<45	μmol/d
Human chorionic gonadotropin (HCG) (nonpregnant adult female)	Serum	<3	mIU/mL	1	<3	IU/L
β-Hydroxybutyric acid	Serum	0.21–2.81	mg/dL	96.05	20–270	μmol/L
5-Hydroxyindoleacetic acid (5-HIAA)	Urine	<25	mg/24 h	5.23	<131	μmol/d
17 α-Hydroxyprogesterone*, female						
Follicular phase	Serum	15–70	ng/dL	0.03	0.4–2.1	nmol/L
Luteal phase	Serum	35–290	ng/dL	0.03	1.0–8.7	nmol/L
Postmenopausal	Serum	<70	ng/dL	0.03	<2.1	nmol/L
17 α-Hydroxyprogesterone*, male	Serum	27–199	ng/dL	0.03	0.8–6.0	nmol/L
Hydroxyproline	Plasma	<0.55	mg/dL	76.3	<42	μmol/L
5-Hydroxytryptamine (see Serotonin)						
Ibuprofen (therapeutic)	Plasma, serum	10–50	μg/mL	4.85	49–243	μmol/L
Imipramine (therapeutic)	Plasma	150–250	ng/mL	3.57	536–893	nmol/L
Immunoglobulin A (IgA)*	Serum	50–350	mg/dL	0.01	0.5–3.5	g/L
Immunoglobulin D (IgD)	Serum	0.5–3.0	mg/dL	10	5–30	mg/L
Immunoglobulin E (IgE)	Serum	10–179	IU/mL	2.4	24–430	μg/L
Immunoglobulin G (IgG)*	Serum	650–1600	mg/dL	0.01	6.5–16.0	g/L
Immunoglobulin M (IgM)*	Serum	54–222	mg/dL	0.01	0.5–2.2	g/L

Table B-1 (Continued)
Conversions from Conventional Units to Systeme International (SI) Units

	Specimen	Traditional Reference Intervals	Traditional Units	Conversion Factor Multiply → ← Divide	SI Reference Intervals	SI Units
Insulin	Plasma	5–20	µU/mL	6.945	34.7–138.9	pmol/L
Insulin C-peptide (see C-peptide)						
Insulin-like growth factor*	Plasma	130–450	ng/mL	1	130–450	µg/L
Ionized calcium (see Calcium)						
Iron (total)*	Serum	60–150	µg/dL	0.179	10.7–26.9	µmol/L
Iron-binding capacity	Serum	250–400	µg/dL	0.179	44.8–71.6	µmol/L
Isoleucine*	Plasma	0.5–1.3	mg/dL	76.24	40–100	µmol/L
Isoniazid (therapeutic)	Plasma	1–7	µg/mL	7.29	7–51	µmol/L
Isopropanol (toxic)	Plasma, serum	>400	mg/L	0.0166	>6.64	mmol/L
Lactate (lactic acid)	Arterial blood	3–11.3	mg/dL	0.111	0.3–1.3	mmol/L
Lactate (lactic acid)	Venous blood	4.5–19.8	mg/dL	0.111	0.5–2.2	mmol/L
Lactate dehydrogenase (LDH)	Serum	50–200	U/L	1	50–200	U/L
Lactate dehydrogenase isoenzymes						
LD1	Serum	17–27	%	0.01	0.17–0.27	Fraction of 1.0
LD2	Serum	27–37	%	0.01	0.27–0.37	Fraction of 1.0
LD3	Serum	18–25	%	0.01	0.18–0.25	Fraction of 1.0
LD4	Serum	8–16	%	0.01	0.08–0.16	Fraction of 1.0
LD5	Serum	6–16	%	0.01	0.06–0.16	Fraction of 1.0
Lead	Whole blood	<25	µg/dL	0.0483	<1.21	µmol/L
Leucine*	Plasma	1.0–2.3	mg/dL	76.3	75–175	µmol/L

Table B-1 *(Continued)*
Conversions from Conventional Units to Systeme International (SI) Units

	Specimen	Traditional Reference Intervals	Traditional Units	Conversion Factor Multiply → ← Divide	SI Reference Intervals	SI Units
Leukocyte count (see Complete blood cell count, White blood cell count)						
Lidocaine (therapeutic)	Serum, plasma	1.5–6.0	µg/mL	4.27	6.4–25.6	µmol/L
Lipase†	Serum	0–160	U/L	0.017	0–2.72	µkat/L
Lipoprotein(a) [Lp(a)]	Serum, plasma	10–30	mg/dL	0.01	0.1–0.3	g/L
Lithium (therapeutic)	Serum	0.6–1.2	mEq/L	1	0.6–1.2	mmol/L
Lorazepam (therapeutic)	Serum, plasma	50–240	ng/mL	3.11	156–746	nmol/L
Low-density lipoprotein cholesterol (LDL)*	Plasma	60–130	mg/dL	0.02586	1.55–3.37	mmol/L
Luteinizing hormone (LH)*, female						
Follicular phase	Serum	2.0–15.0	mIU/L	1	2.0–15.0	IU/L
Ovulatory peak	Serum	22.0–105.0	mIU/L	1	22.0–105.0	IU/L
Luteal phase	Serum	0.6–19.0	mIU/L	1	0.6–19.0	IU/L
Postmenopausal	Serum	16.0–64.0	mIU/L	1	16.0–64.0	IU/L
Luteinizing hormone (LH)*, male	Serum	2.0–12.0	mIU/L	1	2.0–12.0	IU/L
Lymphocytes (see Complete blood cell count, White blood cell count)						
Lysine*	Plasma	1.2–3.5	mg/dL	68.5	80–240	µmol/L
Lysozyme (muramidase)	Serum	4–13	mg/L	1	4–13	mg/L
Magnesium*	Serum	1.5–2.5	mg/dL	0.4114	0.62–1.03	mmol/L
Magnesium*	Serum	1.3–2.1	mEq/L	0.5	0.65–1.05	mmol/L
Manganese	Whole blood	10–12	µg/L	18.2	182–218	nmol/L

Table B-1 *(Continued)*
Conversions from Conventional Units to Systeme International (SI) Units

	Specimen	Traditional Reference Intervals	Traditional Units	Conversion Factor Multiply→ ←Divide	SI Reference Intervals	SI Units
Maprotiline (therapeutic)	Plasma	200–600	ng/mL	1	200–600	µg/L
Mean corpuscular hemoglobin (see Complete blood cell count)						
Mean corpuscular hemoglobin concentration (see Complete blood cell count)						
Meperidine (therapeutic)	Serum, plasma	0.4–0.7	µg/mL	4.04	1.6–2.8	µmol/L
Mercury	Whole blood	0.6–59.0	µg/L	4.99	3.0–294.4	nmol/L
Metanephrines (total)*	Urine	<1.0	mg/24 h	5.07	<5	µmol/d
Methadone (therapeutic)	Serum, plasma	100–400	ng/mL	0.00323	0.32–1.29	µmol/L
Methanol	Whole blood, serum	<1.5	mg/L	0.0312	<0.05	mmol/L
Methemoglobin	Whole blood	<0.24	g/dL	155	<37.2	µmol/L
Methemoglobin	Whole blood	<1.0	% of total Hb	0.01	<0.01	Fraction of total Hb
Methionine*	Plasma	0.1–0.6	mg/dL	67.1	6–40	µmol/L
Methsuximide (therapeutic)	Serum	10–40	µg/mL	5.29	53–212	µmol/L
Methyldopa (therapeutic)	Serum, plasma	1–5	µg/mL	4.73	5–24	µmol/L
Metoprolol (therapeutic)	Serum, plasma	75–200	ng/mL	3.74	281–748	nmol/L
β_2-Microglobulin	Serum	<2	µg/mL	85	<170	nmol/L
Monocytes (see Complete blood cell count, White blood cell count)						
Morphine (therapeutic)	Serum, plasma	10–80	ng/mL	3.5	35–280	nmol/L
Muramidase (see Lysozyme)						

Table B-1 (Continued)
Conversions from Conventional Units to Systeme International (SI) Units

	Specimen	Traditional Reference Intervals	Traditional Units	Conversion Factor Multiply→ ←Divide	SI Reference Intervals	SI Units
Myoglobin	Serum	19–92	µg/L	1	19–92	µg/L
Naproxen (therapeutic trough)	Plasma, serum	>50	µg/mL	4.34	>217	µmol/L
Neutrophils (see Complete blood cell count, White blood cell count)						
Niacin (nicotinic acid)	Urine	2.4–6.4	mg/24 h	7.3	17.5–46.7	µmol/d
Nickel	Whole blood	1.0–28.0	µg/L	17	17–476	nmol/L
Nicotine (smoker)	Plasma	0.01–0.05	mg/L	6.16	0.062–0.308	µmol/L
Nitrogen (nonprotein)	Serum	20–35	mg/dL	0.714	14.3–25.0	mmol/L
Norepinephrine*	Plasma	110–410	pg/mL	5.91	650–2423	nmol/L
Norepinephrine*	Urine	15–80	µg/24 h	5.91	89–473	nmol/d
Nortriptyline (therapeutic)	Serum, plasma	50–150	ng/mL	3.8	190–570	nmol/L
Ornithine*	Plasma	0.4–1.4	mg/dL	75.8	30–106	µmol/L
Osmolality*	Serum	275–295	mOsm/kg H₂O	1	275–295	mmol/kg H₂O
Osmolality	Urine	250–900	mOsm/kg H₂O	1	250–900	mmol/kg H₂O
Osteocalcin*	Serum	3.0–13.0	ng/mL	1	3.0–13.0	µg/L
Oxalate	Serum	1.0–2.4	mg/L	11.4	11–27	µmol/L
Oxazepam (therapeutic)	Serum, plasma	0.2–1.4	µg/mL	3.49	0.7–4.9	µmol/L
Oxycodone (therapeutic)	Plasma, serum	10–100	ng/mL	3.17	32–317	nmol/L
Oxygen, partial pressure (Po₂)	Arterial blood	80–100	mm Hg	1	80–100	mm Hg
Pantothenic acid (see Vitamin B₅)						

APP

Table B-1 (Continued)
Conversions from Conventional Units to Systeme International (SI) Units

	Specimen	Traditional Reference Intervals	Traditional Units	Conversion Factor Multiply → Divide	SI Reference Intervals	SI Units
Parathyroid hormone						
Intact*	Serum	10–50	pg/mL	1	10–50	ng/L
N-terminal specific*	Serum	8–24	pg/mL	1	8–24	ng/L
C-terminal (mid-molecule)	Serum	0–340	pg/mL	1	0–340	ng/L
Pentobarbital (therapeutic)	Serum, plasma	1–5	µg/mL	4.42	4.0–22	µmol/L
Pepsinogen I	Serum	28–100	ng/mL	1	28–100	µg/L
pH (see Blood gases)						
Phenobarbital (therapeutic)	Serum, plasma	15–40	µg/mL	4.31	65–172	µmol/L
Phenylalanine*	Plasma	0.6–1.5	mg/dL	60.5	35–90	µmol/L
Phenytoin (therapeutic)	Serum, plasma	10–20	µg/mL	3.96	40–79	µmol/L
Phosphorus (inorganic)*	Serum	2.3–4.7	mg/dL	0.3229	0.74–1.52	mmol/L
Phosphorus (inorganic)*	Urine	0.4–1.3	g/24 h	32.29	12.9–42.0	mmol/d
Phospholipid phosphorus (total)	Serum	8.0–11.0	mg/dL	0.3229	2.58–3.55	mmol/L
Placental lactogen (5 to 38 wks' gestation)	Serum	0.5–11	µg/mL	46.3	23–509	nmol/L
Plasminogen	Plasma	8.4–14.0	mg/dL	10	84–140	mg/L
Plasminogen	Plasma	80–120	%	0.01	0.80–1.20	Fraction of 1.0
Plasminogen activator inhibitor	Plasma	<15	IU/mL	1	<15	kIU/L
Platelet count (see Complete blood cell count, platelet count)						
Porphobilinogen deaminase	Red blood cells	>7.0	nmol/s/L	1	>7.0	nmol/(s·L)

Table B-1 *(Continued)*
Conversions from Conventional Units to Systeme International (SI) Units

	Specimen	Traditional Reference Intervals	Traditional Units	Conversion Factor Multiply→ ←Divide	SI Reference Intervals	SI Units
Porphyrins (total)	Urine	<320	nmol/L	1	<320	nmol/L
Potassium	Plasma	3.5–5.0	mEq/L	1	3.5–5.0	mmol/L
Pregnanediol*, female						
Follicular phase	Urine	<2.6	mg/24 h	3.12	<8	μmol/d
Luteal phase	Urine	2.3–10.6	mg/24 h	3.12	8–33	μmol/d
Pregnanediol*, male	Urine	0–1.9	mg/24 h	3.12	0–5.9	μmol/d
Pregnanetriol*	Urine	<2.5	mg/24 h	2.97	<7.5	μmol/d
Primidone (therapeutic)	Plasma	5–12	μg/mL	4.58	23–55	μmol/L
Procainamide (therapeutic)	Serum, plasma	4–10	μg/mL	4.23	17–42	μmol/L
Progesterone*, female						
Follicular phase	Serum	0.15–0.7	ng/mL	3.18	0.5–2.2	nmol/L
Luteal phase	Serum	2.0–25.0	ng/mL	3.18	6.4–79.5	nmol/L
Progesterone*, male	Serum	0.13–0.97	ng/mL	3.18	0.4–3.1	nmol/L
Prolactin (nonlactating subject)	Serum	1–25	ng/mL	1	1–25	μg/L
Proline*	Plasma	1.2–3.9	mg/dL	86.9	104–340	μmol/L
Propoxyphene (therapeutic)	Serum	0.1–0.4	μg/mL	2.946	0.3–1.2	μmol/L
Propranolol (therapeutic)	Serum	50–100	ng/mL	3.86	190–386	nmol/L
Protein (total)*	Serum	6.0–8.0	g/dL	10	60–80	g/L
Protein C	Plasma	70–140	%	0.01	0.70–1.40	Fraction of 1.0

APP

6TH EDITION

Table B-1 *(Continued)*
Conversions from Conventional Units to Systeme International (SI) Units

	Specimen	Traditional Reference Intervals	Traditional Units	Conversion Factor Multiply → ← Divide	SI Reference Intervals	SI Units
Protein electrophoresis (SPEP), fraction of total protein						
Albumin	Serum	52–65	%	0.01	0.52–0.65	Fraction of 1.0
α₁-Globulin	Serum	2.5–5.0	%	0.01	0.025–0.05	Fraction of 1.0
α₂-Globulin	Serum	7.0–13.0	%	0.01	0.07–0.13	Fraction of 1.0
β-Globulin	Serum	8.0–14.0	%	0.01	0.08–0.14	Fraction of 1.0
γ-Globulin	Serum	12.0–22.0	%	0.01	0.12–0.22	Fraction of 1.0
Protein electrophoresis (SPEP), concentration						
Albumin	Serum	3.2–5.6	g/dL	10	32–56	g/L
α₁-Globulin	Serum	0.1–0.4	g/dL	10	1–10	g/L
α₂-Globulin	Serum	0.4–1.2	g/dL	10	4–12	g/L
β-Globulin	Serum	0.5–1.1	g/dL	10	5–11	g/L
γ-Globulin	Serum	0.5–1.6	g/dL	10	5–16	g/L
Protein S (activity)	Plasma	70–140	%	0.01	0.70–1.40	Fraction of 1.0
Prothrombin time (PT)	Plasma	10–13	s	1	10–13	s
Protoporphyrin	Red blood cells	15–50	µg/dL	0.0177	0.27–0.89	µmol/L
Pyridoxine (see Vitamin B₆)						
Pyruvate (as pyruvic acid)	Whole blood	0.3–0.9	mg/dL	113.6	34–102	µmol/L
Quinidine (therapeutic)	Serum	2.0–5.0	µg/mL	3.08	6.2–15.4	µmol/L
Red blood cell count (See Complete blood cell count)						

Table B-1 *(Continued)*
Conversions from Conventional Units to Systeme International (SI) Units

	Specimen	Traditional Reference Intervals	Traditional Units	Conversion Factor Multiply→ ←Divide	SI Reference Intervals	SI Units
Red cell folate (see Folate)						
Renin (normal sodium diet)*	Plasma	1.1–4.1	ng/mL/h	1	1.1–4.1	ng/(mL · h)
Reticulocyte count*	Whole blood	25–75	10³/μL	1	25–75	10⁹/L
Reticulocyte count* (fraction)	Whole blood	0.5–1.5	% of RBCs	0.01	0.005–0.015	Fraction of RBCs
Retinol (see Vitamin A)						
Rheumatoid factor	Serum	<30	IU/mL	1	<30	kIU/L
Riboflavin (see Vitamin B₂)						
Salicylates (therapeutic)	Serum, plasma	15–30	mg/dL	0.0724	1.08–2.17	mmol/L
Sedimentation rate (see Erythrocyte sedimentation rate)						
Selenium	Whole blood	58–234	μg/L	0.0127	0.74–2.97	μmol/L
Serine*	Plasma	0.7–2.0	mg/dL	95.2	65–193	μmol/L
Serotonin (5-hydroxytryptamine)	Whole blood	50–200	ng/mL	0.00568	0.28–1.14	μmol/L
Serum protein electrophoresis (SPEP, see Protein electrophoresis)						
Sex hormone-binding globulin*	Serum	0.5–1.5	μg/dL	34.7	17.4–52.1	nmol/L
Sodium*	Plasma	136–142	mEq/L	1	136–142	mmol/L
Somatostatin	Plasma	<25	pg/mL	1	<25	ng/L
Somatomedin C (see Insulin-like growth factor)						
Strychnine (toxic)	Whole blood	>0.5	mg/L	2.99	>1.5	μmol/L
Substance P	Plasma	<240	pg/mL	1	<240	ng/L

APP

Table B-1 (Continued)
Conversions from Conventional Units to Systeme International (SI) Units

	Specimen	Traditional Reference Intervals	Traditional Units	Conversion Factor Multiply → ← Divide	SI Reference Intervals	SI Units
Sulfhemoglobin	Whole blood	<1.0	% of total Hb	0.01	<0.010	Fraction of total Hb
Taurine*	Plasma	0.3–2.1	mg/dL	80	24–168	µmol/L
Testosterone*, male	Plasma, serum	300–1200	ng/dL	0.0347	10.4–41.6	nmol/L
Testosterone*, female	Plasma, serum	<85	ng/dL	0.0347	2.95	nmol/L
Theophylline (therapeutic)	Plasma, serum	10–20	µg/mL	5.55	56–111	µmol/L
Thiamine (see Vitamin B$_1$)						
Thiocyanate (nonsmoker)	Plasma, serum	1–4	mg/L	17.2	17–69	µmol/L
Thiopental (therapeutic)	Plasma, serum	1–5	µg/mL	4.13	4–21	µmol/L
Thioridazine (therapeutic)	Plasma, serum	1.0–1.5	µg/mL	2.7	2.7–4.1	µmol/L
Thrombin time	Plasma	16–24	s	1.0	16–24	s
Threonine*	Plasma	0.9–2.5	mg/dL	84	75–210	µmol/L
Thyroglobulin*	Serum	3–42	ng/mL	1	3–42	µg/L
Thyrotropin (thyroid-stimulating hormone, TSH)*	Serum	0.5–5.0	µIU/mL	1	0.5–5.0	mU/L
Thyroxine, free (FT$_4$)*	Serum	0.9–2.3	ng/dL	12.87	12–30	pmol/L
Thyroxine, total (T$_4$)*	Serum	5.5–12.5	µg/dL	12.87	71–160	nmol/L
Thyroxine-binding globulin (TBG)*, as T$_4$-binding capacity	Serum	10–26	µg/dL	12.9	129–335	nmol/L
Tissue plasminogen activator	Plasma	<0.04	IU/mL	1000	<40	IU/L

Table B-1 *(Continued)*
Conversions from Conventional Units to Systeme International (SI) Units

	Specimen	Traditional Reference Intervals	Traditional Units	Conversion Factor Multiply → ← Divide	SI Reference Intervals	SI Units
Tobramycin (therapeutic, peak)	Plasma, serum	5–10	µg/mL	2.14	10–21	µmol/L
Tocainide (therapeutic)	Plasma, serum	4–10	µg/mL	5.2	21–52	µmol/L
α-Tocopherol (see Vitamin E)						
Transferrin (siderophilin)*	Serum	200–380	mg/dL	0.01	2.0–3.8	g/L
Triglycerides*	Plasma, serum	10–190	mg/dL	0.01129	0.11–2.15	mmol/L
Triiodothyronine, free (FT₃)*	Serum	260–480	pg/dL	0.0154	4.0–7.4	pmol/L
Triiodothyronine, resin uptake*	Serum	25–35	%	0.01	0.25–0.35	Fraction of 1.0
Triiodothyronine, total (T₃)*	Serum	70–200	ng/dL	0.0154	1.08–3.14	nmol/L
Troponin I (cardiac)	Serum	0–0.4	ng/mL	1	0–0.4	µg/L
Troponin T (cardiac)	Serum	0–0.1	ng/mL	1	0–0.1	µg/L
Tryptophan*	Plasma	0.5–1.5	mg/dL	48.97	25–73	µmol/L
Tyrosine*	Plasma	0.4–1.6	mg/dL	55.19	20–90	µmol/L
Urea nitrogen (BUN)*	Serum	8–23	mg/dL	0.357	2.9–8.2	mmol/L
Uric acid*	Serum	4.0–8.5	mg/dL	0.0595	0.24–0.51	mmol/L
Urobilinogen*	Urine	0.05–2.5	mg/24 h	1.693	0.1–4.2	µmol/d
Valine*	Plasma	1.7–3.7	mg/dL	85.5	145–315	µmol/L
Valproic acid (therapeutic)	Plasma, serum	50–150	µg/mL	6.93	346–1040	µmol/L
Vancomycin (therapeutic, peak)	Plasma, serum	18–26	µg/mL	0.69	12–18	µmol/L
Vanillylmandelic acid (VMA)*	Urine	2.1–7.6	mg/24 h	5.046	11–38	µmol/d

APP

Table B-1 *(Continued)*
Conversions from Conventional Units to Systeme International (SI) Units

	Specimen	Traditional Reference Intervals	Traditional Units	Conversion Factor Multiply → — Divide	SI Reference Intervals	SI Units
Vasoactive intestinal polypeptide	Plasma	<50	pg/mL	1	<50	ng/L
Verapamil (therapeutic)	Plasma, serum	100–500	ng/mL	2.2	220–1100	nmol/L
Vitamin A (retinol)*	Serum	30–80	μg/dL	0.0349	1.05–2.80	μmol/L
Vitamin B_1 (thiamine)	Whole blood	2.5–7.5	μg/dL	29.6	74–222	nmol/L
Vitamin B_2 (riboflavin)	Plasma, serum	4–24	μg/dL	26.6	106–638	nmol/L
Vitamin B_5 (pantothenic acid)	Whole blood	0.2–1.8	μg/mL	4.56	0.9–8.2	μmol/L
Vitamin B_6 (pyridoxine)	Plasma	5–30	ng/mL	4.046	20–121	nmol/L
Vitamin B_{12} (cyanocobalamin)*	Serum	160–950	pg/mL	0.7378	118–701	pmol/L
Vitamin C (ascorbic acid)	Plasma, serum	0.4–1.5	mg/dL	56.78	23–85	μmol/L
Vitamin D 1,25-dihydroxyvitamin D	Plasma, serum	16–65	pg/mL	2.6	42–169	pmol/L
Vitamin D 25-hydroxyvitamin D	Plasma, serum	14–60	ng/mL	2.496	35–150	nmol/L
Vitamin E (α-tocopherol)*	Plasma, serum	0.5–1.8	mg/dL	23.22	12–42	μmol/L
Vitamin K	Plasma, serum	0.13–1.19	ng/mL	2.22	0.29–2.64	nmol/L
von Willebrand factor (ranges vary according to blood type)	Plasma	70–140	%	0.01	0.70–1.40	Fraction of 1.0
Warfarin (therapeutic)	Plasma, serum	1.0–10	μg/mL	3.24	3.2–32.4	μmol/L
White blood cell count*	Whole blood	4.5–11.0	10^3/μL	1	4.5–11.0	10^9/L
White blood cell, differential count (see Complete blood cell count)						
Xylose absorption test (25-g dose)*	Whole blood	>25 mg/dL	mg/dL	0.06661	>1.7	mmol/L

Table B-1 *(Continued)*
Conversions from Conventional Units to Systeme International (SI) Units

Specimen	Traditional Reference Intervals	Traditional Units	Conversion Factor Multiply→ ←Divide	SI Reference Intervals	SI Units
Zidovudine (therapeutic)	Plasma, serum	0.15–0.27	µg/mL	3.74	0.56–1.01	µmol/L
Zinc	Serum	50–150	µg/dL	0.153	7.7–23.0	µmol/L

The normal ranges listed here are included as a helpful guide and are by no means comprehensive. The listed reference, unless noted, pertains to adults. Laboratory results are method dependent and can have intralaboratory variation. Conversion factors are not affected by age-related differences. The information in this table is from the following sources: (1) Tietz NW, ed. Clinical Guide to Laboratory Tests. 3rd ed. Philadelphia, PA: WB Saunders Co; 1995; (2) Laposata M. SI Unit Conversion Guide. Boston, MA: NEJM Books; 1992; (3) American Medical Association Manual of Style: A Guide for Authors and Editors. 9th ed. Chicago, IL: American Medical Association; 1998; (4) Jacobs DS, Demott WR, Oxley DK, eds. Jacobs & DeMott Laboratory Test Handbook with Key Word Index. 5th ed. Hudson, OH: Lexi-Comp Inc; 2001; (5) Henry JB, ed. Clinical Diagnosis and Management by Laboratory Methods. 20th ed. Philadelphia, PA: WB Saunders Co; 2001; and (6) Kratz A, Ferraro M, Sluss PM, Lewandrowski KB. Case records of the Massachusetts General Hospital. Weekly clinicopathological exercises. Laboratory reference values. N Engl J Med. 2006;351:1548–1563.

* For this analyte, there is age dependence for the reference range. There may be several different normal ranges for different pediatric age ranges. Consult your clinical laboratory for the local institution age-specific reference range. Pediatric reference values may also be found in Soldin SJ, Brugnara C, Wong EC, eds. *Pediatric References Intervals.* 5th ed. Washington, DC: American Association for Clinical Chemistry Press; 2005.

† The SI unit katal is the amount of enzyme generating 1 mol of product per second. Although provisionally recommended as the SI unit for enzymatic activity, it has not been universally accepted. It is suitable to maintain use of U/L in these circumstances (conversion factor 1.0).

APP

Appendix C

Table C-1
Representative Values for Constituents of Human Milk*

Constituent (Per L)†	Early Milk	Mature Milk
Energy (kcal)		650–700
Carbohydrate		
Lactose (g)	20–30	67
Glucose (g)	0.2–1.0	0.2–0.3
Oligosaccharides (g)	22–24	12–14
Total nitrogen (g)	3.0	1.9
Nonrotein nitrogen (g)	0.5	0.45
Protein nitrogen (g)	2.5	1.45
Total protein (g)	16	9
Casein (g)	3.8	5.7
β-Casein (g)	2.6	4.4
κ-Casein (g)	1.2	1.3
α-Lactalbumin (g)	3.62	3.26
Lactoferrin (g)	3.53	1.94
Albumin (g)	0.39	0.41
sIgA (g)	2.0	1.0
IgM (g)	0.12	0.2
IgG (g)	0.34	0.05
Total lipids (%)	2	3.5
Triglyceride (% total lipid)	97–98	97–98
Cholesterol‡ (% total lipids)	0.7–1.3	0.4–0.5
Phospholipids (% total lipids)	1.1	0.6–0.8
Fatty acids (weight %)	88	88
Total saturated fatty acids (%)	43–44	44–45
Palmitic acid (C16:0)		20
Monounsaturated fatty acids (%)		40
Oleic acid (C18:1 ω9)	32	31
Polyunsaturated fatty acids (%)	13	14–15
Total ω3 fatty acids (%)	1.5	1.5
Linolenic acid (C18:3 ω3)	0.7	0.9

Table C-1 **1201**

APP

Table C-1 *(Continued)*
Representative Values for Constituents of Human Milk*

Constituent (Per L)†	Early Milk	Mature Milk
Carbohydrate (continued)		
Eicosapentaenoic acid (C22:5 ω3)	0.2	0.1
Docosahexaenoic acid (C22:6 ω3)	0.5	0.2
Total ω6 fatty acids (%)	11.6	13.06
Linoleic acid (C18:2 ω6)	8.9	11.3
Arachidonic acid (C20:4 ω6)	0.7	0.5
Water-soluble vitamins		
Ascorbic acid (mg)		100
Thiamin (μg)	20	200
Riboflavin (μg)		400–600
Niacin (mg)	0.5	1.8–6.0
Vitamin B$_6$ (mg)		0.09–0.31
Folate (μg)		80–140
Vitamin B$_{12}$ (μg)		0.5–1.0
Pantothenic acid (mg)		2–2.5
Biotin (μg)		5–9
Fat-soluble vitamins		
Retinol (mg)	2	0.3–0.6
Carotenoids (mg)	2	0.2–0.6
Vitamin K (μg)	2–5	2–3
Vitamin D (μg)		0.33
Vitamin E (mg)	8–12	3–8
Minerals		
Calcium (mg)	250	200–250
Magnesium (mg)	30–35	30–35
Phosphorus (mg)	120–160	120–140
Sodium (mg)	300–400	120–250
Potassium (mg)	600–700	400–550
Chloride (mg)	600–800	400–450
Iron (mg)	0.5–1.0	0.3–0.9
Zinc (mg)	8–12	1–3

Table C-1 (Continued)
Representative Values for Constituents of Human Milk*

Constituent (Per L)†	Early Milk	Mature Milk
Copper (mg)	0.5–0.8	0.2–0.4
Manganese (µg)	5–6	3
Selenium (µg)	40	7–33
Iodine (µg)		150
Fluoride (µg)		4–15

sIgA indicates secretory immunoglobulin A; IgM, immunoglobulin M; IgG, immunoglobulin G.

* Adapted from Picciano MF. Representative values for constituents of human milk. *Pediatr Clin North Am.* 2001;48:263–272

† All values are expressed per L of milk with the exception of lipids that are expressed as a percentage on the basis of milk volume or weight of total lipids.

‡ The cholesterol content of human milk ranges from 100 to 200 mg/L in most samples of human milk after day 21 of lactation.

APP

Table C-1 **1203**

Appendix D

Appendix D-1
Set I

Birth to 36 months: Boys
Length-for-age and Weight-for-age percentiles

NAME _____

RECORD # _____

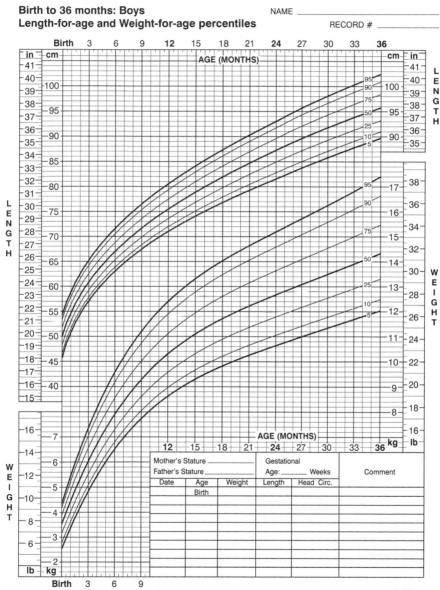

Published May 30, 2000 (modified 4/20/01).
SOURCE: Developed by the National Center for Health Statistics in collaboration with
the National Center for Chronic Disease Prevention and Health Promotion (2000).
http://www.cdc.gov/growthcharts

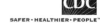

SAFER·HEALTHIER·PEOPLE™

Birth to 36 months: Boys
Head circumference-for-age and
Weight-for-length percentiles

NAME _____

RECORD # _____

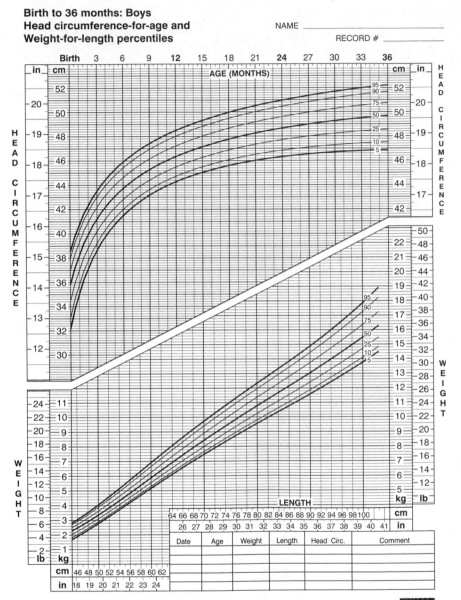

Published May 30, 2000 (modified 10/16/00).
SOURCE: Developed by the National Center for Health Statistics in collaboration with
the National Center for Chronic Disease Prevention and Health Promotion (2000).
http://www.cdc.gov/growthcharts

SAFER·HEALTHIER·PEOPLE™

Birth to 36 months: Girls
Length-for-age and Weight-for-age percentiles

NAME _____

RECORD # _____

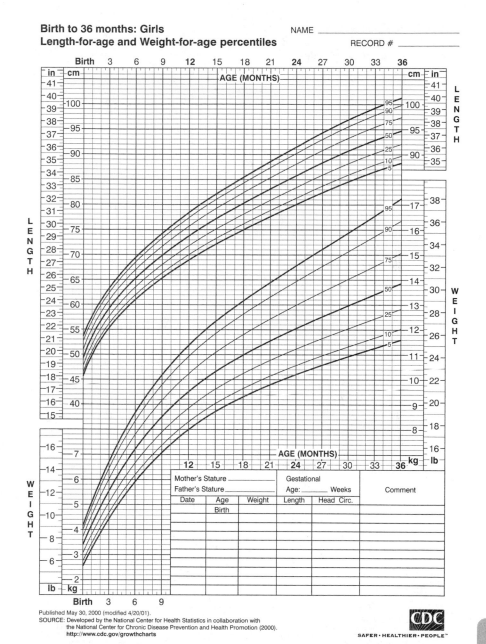

Published May 30, 2000 (modified 4/20/01).
SOURCE: Developed by the National Center for Health Statistics in collaboration with
the National Center for Chronic Disease Prevention and Health Promotion (2000).
http://www.cdc.gov/growthcharts

CDC
SAFER·HEALTHIER·PEOPLE™

APP

**Birth to 36 months: Girls
Head circumference-for-age and
Weight-for-length percentiles**

NAME _____

RECORD # _____

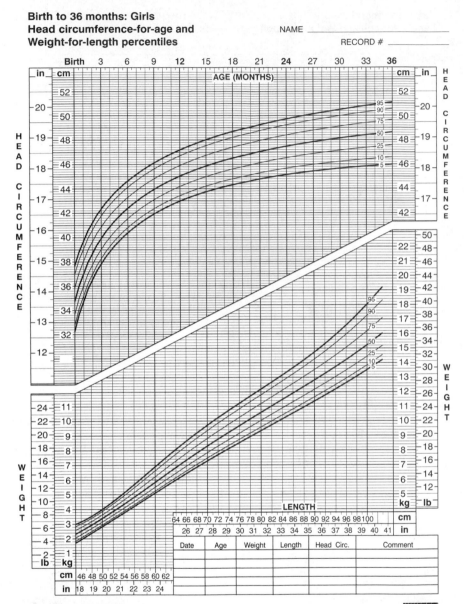

Published May 30, 2000 (modified 10/16/00).
SOURCE: Developed by the National Center for Health Statistics in collaboration with
the National Center for Chronic Disease Prevention and Health Promotion (2000).
http://www.cdc.gov/growthcharts

SAFER · HEALTHIER · PEOPLE™

2 to 20 years: Boys
Stature-for-age and Weight-for-age percentiles

NAME _____

RECORD # _____

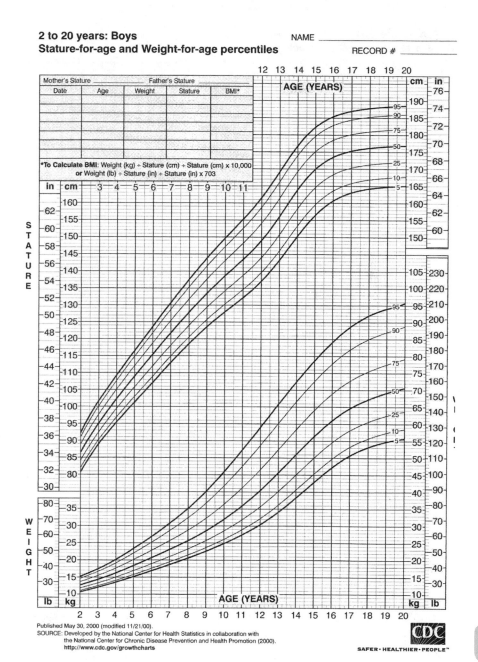

Published May 30, 2000 (modified 11/21/00).
SOURCE: Developed by the National Center for Health Statistics in collaboration with
the National Center for Chronic Disease Prevention and Health Promotion (2000).
http://www.cdc.gov/growthcharts

CDC

SAFER·HEALTHIER·PEOPLE™

2 to 20 years: Boys
Body mass index-for-age percentiles

NAME _____

RECORD # _____

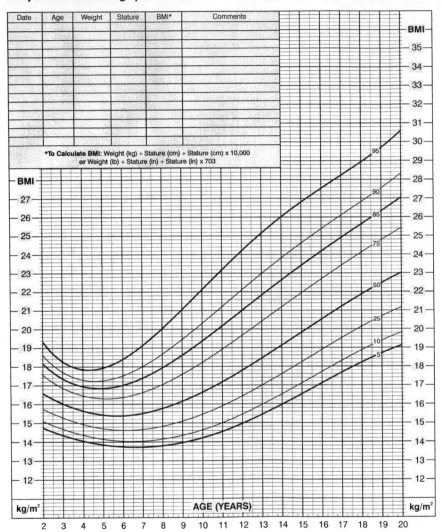

Date	Age	Weight	Stature	BMI*	Comments

*To Calculate BMI: Weight (kg) ÷ Stature (cm) ÷ Stature (cm) x 10,000
or Weight (lb) ÷ Stature (in) ÷ Stature (in) x 703

AGE (YEARS)

kg/m²

SOURCE: Developed by the National Center for Health Statistics in collaboration with
the National Center for Chronic Disease Prevention and Health Promotion (2000).
http://www.cdc.gov/growthcharts

2 to 20 years: Girls
Stature-for-age and Weight-for-age percentiles

NAME _____

RECORD # _____

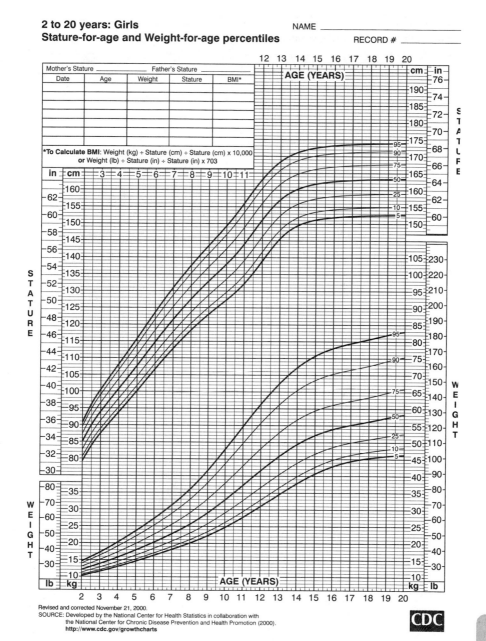

Mother's Stature _____ Father's Stature _____

Date	Age	Weight	Stature	BMI*

*To Calculate BMI: Weight (kg) ÷ Stature (cm) ÷ Stature (cm) x 10,000
or Weight (lb) ÷ Stature (in) ÷ Stature (in) x 703

Revised and corrected November 21, 2000.
SOURCE: Developed by the National Center for Health Statistics in collaboration with
the National Center for Chronic Disease Prevention and Health Promotion (2000).
http://www.cdc.gov/growthcharts

CDC

2 to 20 years: Girls
Body mass index-for-age percentiles

NAME _____

RECORD # _____

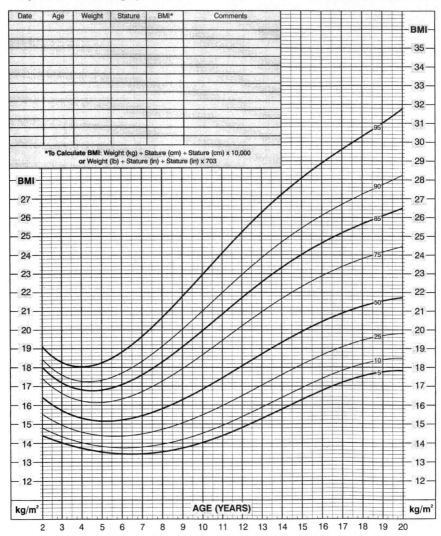

Date	Age	Weight	Stature	BMI*	Comments

*To Calculate BMI: Weight (kg) ÷ Stature (cm) ÷ Stature (cm) x 10,000
or Weight (lb) ÷ Stature (in) ÷ Stature (in) x 703

AGE (YEARS)

SOURCE: Developed by the National Center for Health Statistics in collaboration with
the National Center for Chronic Disease Prevention and Health Promotion (2000).
http://www.cdc.gov/growthcharts

Weight-for-stature percentiles: Boys

NAME _____

RECORD # _____

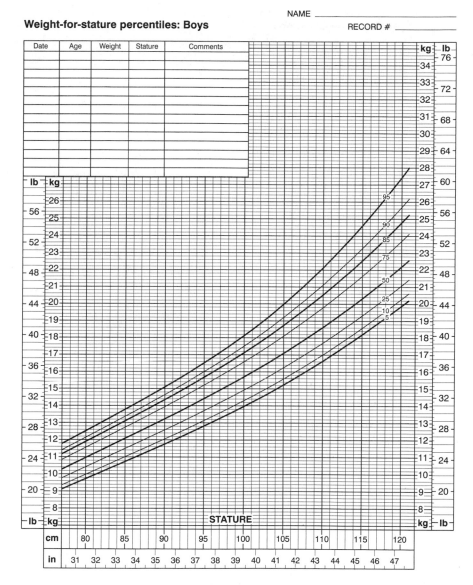

Date	Age	Weight	Stature	Comments

STATURE

SOURCE: Developed by the National Center for Health Statistics in collaboration with
the National Center for Chronic Disease Prevention and Health Promotion (2000).
http://www.cdc.gov/growthcharts

Weight-for-stature percentiles: Girls

NAME _____

RECORD # _____

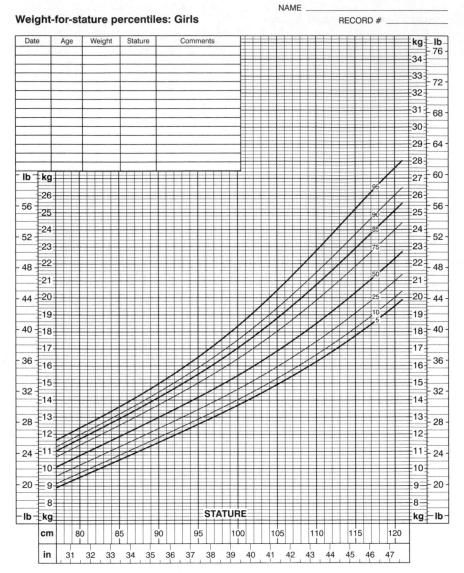

Date	Age	Weight	Stature	Comments

STATURE

SOURCE: Developed by the National Center for Health Statistics in collaboration with
the National Center for Chronic Disease Prevention and Health Promotion (2000).
http://www.cdc.gov/growthcharts

Appendix D-1
Set II

Birth to 36 months: Boys
Length-for-age and Weight-for-age percentiles

NAME _____

RECORD # _____

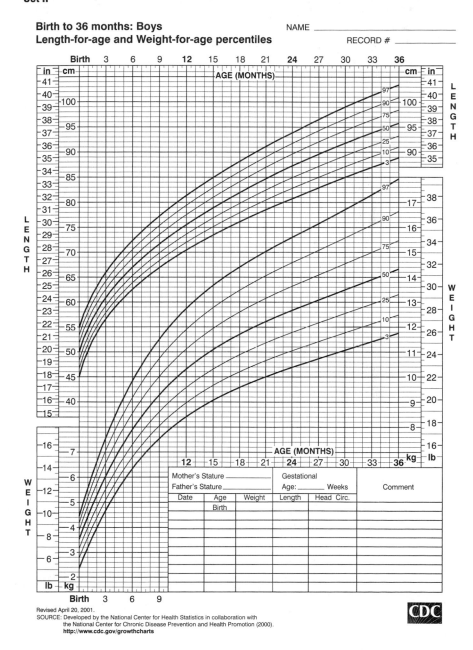

Revised April 20, 2001.
SOURCE: Developed by the National Center for Health Statistics in collaboration with
the National Center for Chronic Disease Prevention and Health Promotion (2000).
http://www.cdc.gov/growthcharts

Birth to 36 months: Boys
Head circumference-for-age and
Weight-for-length percentiles

NAME _____

RECORD # _____

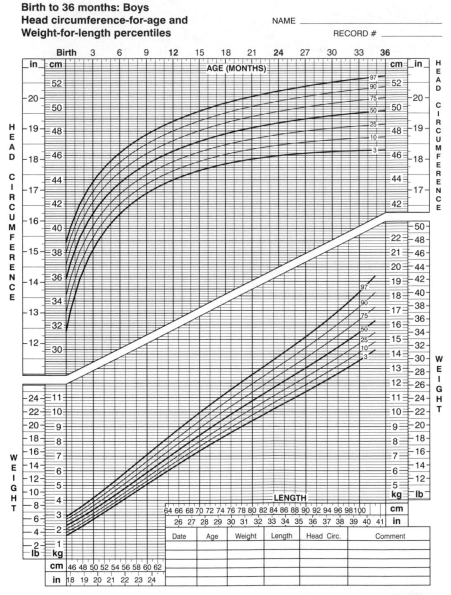

SOURCE: Developed by the National Center for Health Statistics in collaboration with
the National Center for Chronic Disease Prevention and Health Promotion (2000).
http://www.cdc.gov/growthcharts

Birth to 36 months: Girls
Length-for-age and Weight-for-age percentiles

NAME _____

RECORD # _____

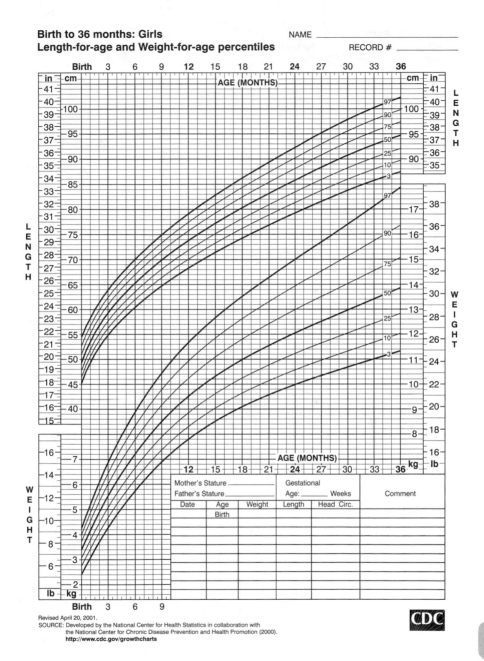

Revised April 20, 2001.
SOURCE: Developed by the National Center for Health Statistics in collaboration with
the National Center for Chronic Disease Prevention and Health Promotion (2000).
http://www.cdc.gov/growthcharts

CDC

APP

Birth to 36 months: Girls
Head circumference-for-age and
Weight-for-length percentiles

NAME _____

RECORD # _____

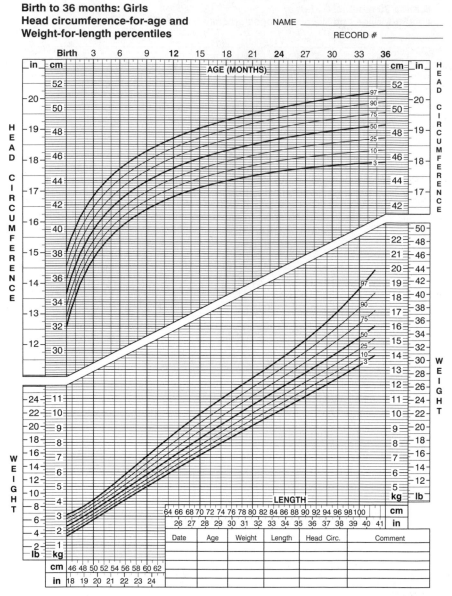

Date	Age	Weight	Length	Head Circ.	Comment

SOURCE: Developed by the National Center for Health Statistics in collaboration with
the National Center for Chronic Disease Prevention and Health Promotion (2000).
http://www.cdc.gov/growthcharts

2 to 20 years: Boys
Stature-for-age and Weight-for-age percentiles

NAME _____

RECORD # _____

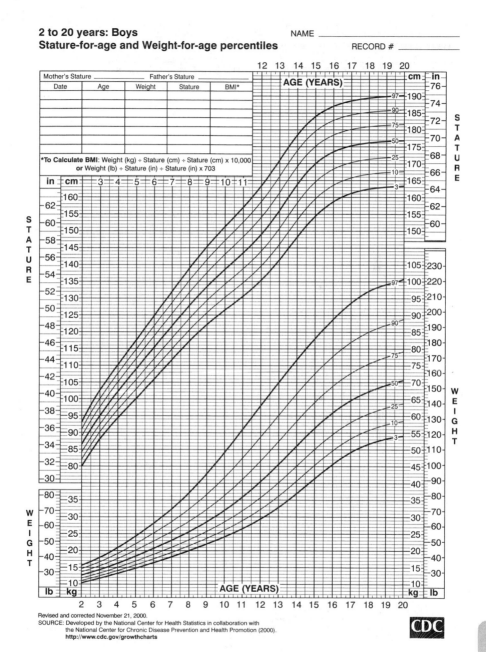

Revised and corrected November 21, 2000.
SOURCE: Developed by the National Center for Health Statistics in collaboration with
the National Center for Chronic Disease Prevention and Health Promotion (2000).
http://www.cdc.gov/growthcharts

CDC

APP

2 to 20 years: Boys
Body mass index-for-age percentiles

NAME _____

RECORD # _____

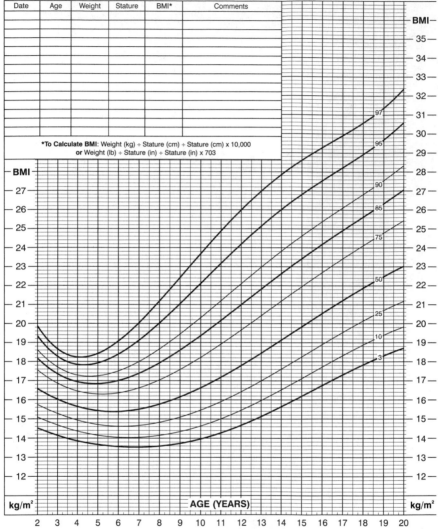

Date	Age	Weight	Stature	BMI*	Comments

*To Calculate BMI: Weight (kg) ÷ Stature (cm) ÷ Stature (cm) x 10,000
or Weight (lb) ÷ Stature (in) ÷ Stature (in) x 703

AGE (YEARS)

SOURCE: Developed by the National Center for Health Statistics in collaboration with
the National Center for Chronic Disease Prevention and Health Promotion (2000).
http://www.cdc.gov/growthcharts

2 to 20 years: Girls
Stature-for-age and Weight-for-age percentiles

NAME _____

RECORD # _____

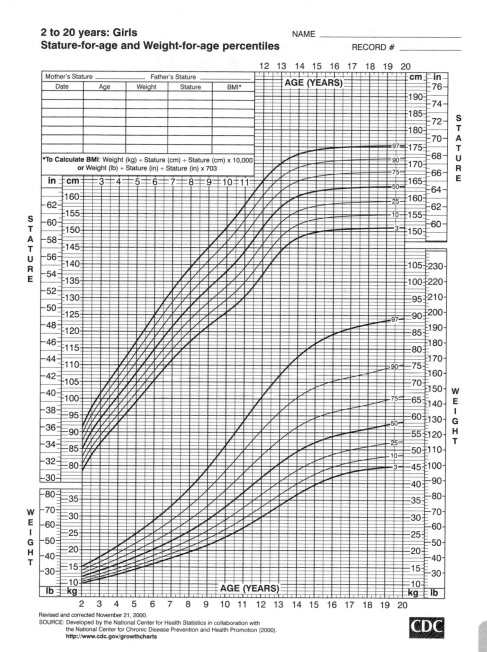

Mother's Stature _____ Father's Stature _____

Date	Age	Weight	Stature	BMI*

*To Calculate BMI: Weight (kg) ÷ Stature (cm) ÷ Stature (cm) x 10,000
or Weight (lb) ÷ Stature (in) ÷ Stature (in) x 703

AGE (YEARS)

Revised and corrected November 21, 2000.
SOURCE: Developed by the National Center for Health Statistics in collaboration with
the National Center for Chronic Disease Prevention and Health Promotion (2000).
http://www.cdc.gov/growthcharts

CDC

APP

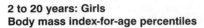

2 to 20 years: Girls
Body mass index-for-age percentiles

NAME _____

RECORD # _____

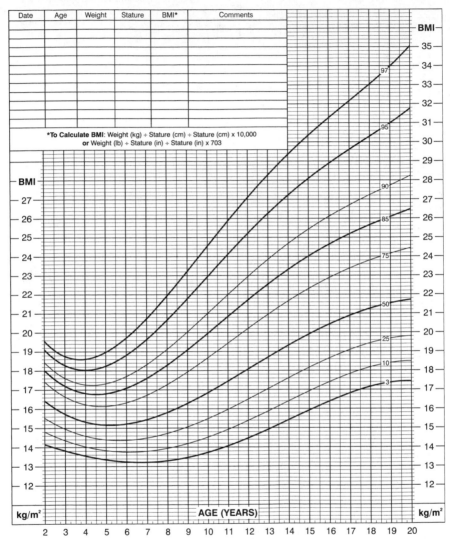

*To Calculate BMI: Weight (kg) ÷ Stature (cm) ÷ Stature (cm) x 10,000
or Weight (lb) ÷ Stature (in) ÷ Stature (in) x 703

AGE (YEARS)

SOURCE: Developed by the National Center for Health Statistics in collaboration with
the National Center for Chronic Disease Prevention and Health Promotion (2000).
http://www.cdc.gov/growthcharts

Appendix D-2

Fig. D-2.1
WHO length-for-age percentiles for boys from birth to 24 months

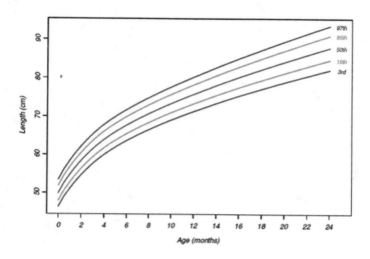

Fig. D-2.2
WHO length-for-age percentiles for girls from birth to 24 months

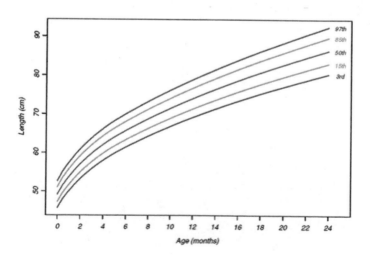

Fig. D-2.3
WHO height-for-age percentiles for boys from 24 months to 60 months

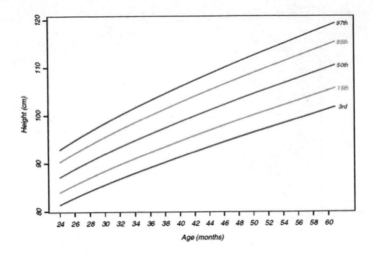

Fig. D-2.4
WHO height-for-age percentiles for girls from 24 months to 60 months

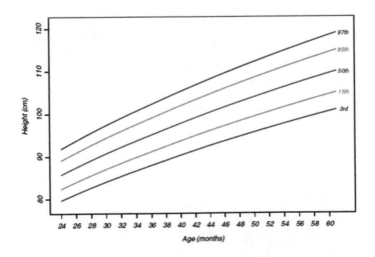

Fig. D-2.5
WHO weight-for-age percentiles for boys from birth to 60 months

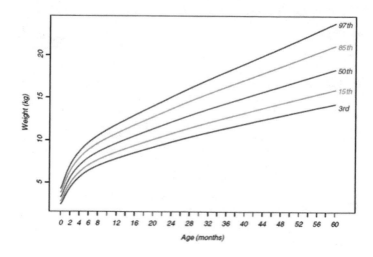

Fig. D-2.6
WHO weight-for-age percentiles for girls from birth to 60 months

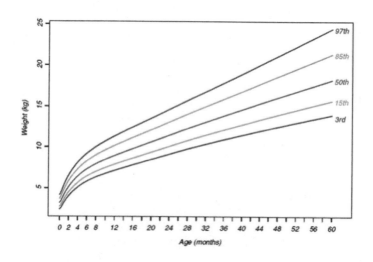

Appendix D-3

Fig. D-3.A
Low Birth Weight Growth Charts

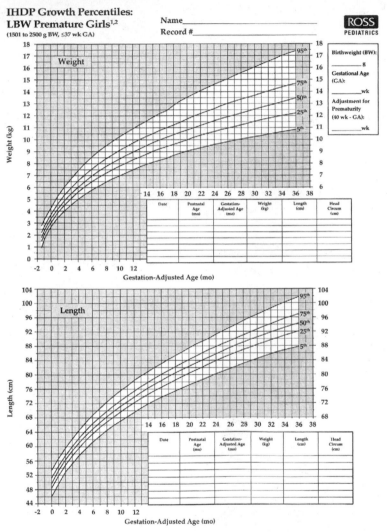

IHDP Growth Percentiles:
LBW Premature Girls[1,2]
(1501 to 2500 g BW, ≤37 wk GA)

Name_____

Record #_____

ROSS
PEDIATRICS

Birthweight (BW):
_____ g
Gestational Age
(GA):
_____ wk
Adjustment for
Prematurity
(40 wk - GA):
_____ wk

IHDP Growth Percentiles: LBW Premature Girls[1,2]

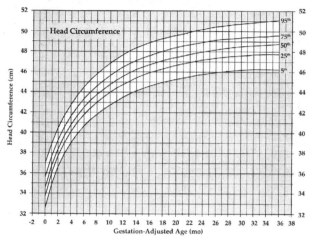

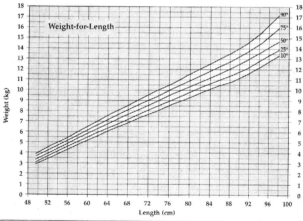

References

1. Guo SS, Roche AF, Chumlea WC, et al: Growth in weight, recumbent length, and head circumference for preterm low-birthweight infants during the first three years of life using gestation-adjusted ages. *Early Hum Dev* 1997;47:305-325.

2. Guo SS, Wholihan K, Roche AF, et al: Weight-for-length reference data for preterm, low-birth-weight infants. *Arch Pediatr Adolesc Med* 1996;150:964-970. Copyright 1996, American Medical Association.

Acknowledgment

IHDP studies were supported by grants from the Robert Wood Johnson Foundation, Pew Charitable Trusts, and the Bureau of Maternal and Child Health, US Department of Health and Human Services. The IHDP growth percentile graphs were prepared by S.S. Guo and A.F. Roche, Wright State University, Yellow Springs, Ohio. IHDP, its sponsors and the investigators do not endorse specific products.

© 1999 Abbott
A7223/MARCH 1999
LITHO IN USA

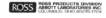
ROSS PRODUCTS DIVISION
ABBOTT LABORATORIES INC.
COLUMBUS, OHIO 43215-1724

Provided as a service of
Similac NeoSure™
Infant Formula With Iron

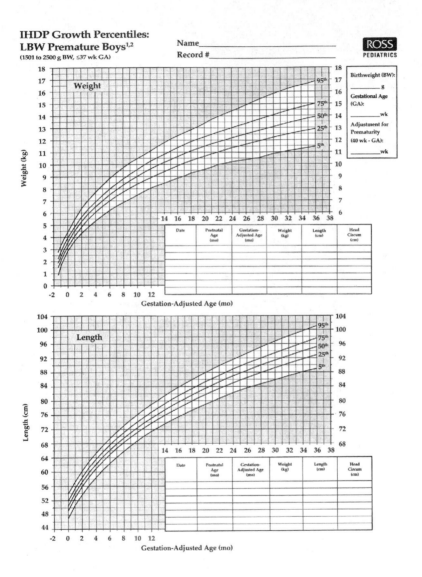

IHDP Growth Percentiles:
LBW Premature Boys[1,2]
(1501 to 2500 g BW, ≤37 wk GA)

Name_____

Record #_____

ROSS
PEDIATRICS

Birthweight (BW):
_____g

Gestational Age
(GA):
_____wk

Adjustment for
Prematurity
(40 wk - GA):
_____wk

Weight

95th
75th
50th
25th
5th

Weight (kg)

Gestation-Adjusted Age (mo)

Date	Postnatal Age (mo)	Gestation-Adjusted Age (mo)	Weight (kg)	Length (cm)	Head Circum (cm)

Length

95th
75th
50th
25th
5th

Length (cm)

Gestation-Adjusted Age (mo)

Date	Postnatal Age (mo)	Gestation-Adjusted Age (mo)	Weight (kg)	Length (cm)	Head Circum (cm)

IHDP Growth Percentiles: LBW Premature Boys[1,2]

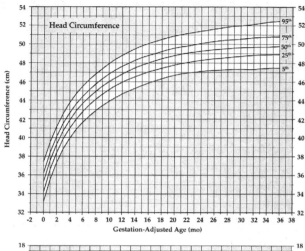

Head Circumference

95th
75th
50th
25th
5th

Head Circumference (cm)

Gestation-Adjusted Age (mo)

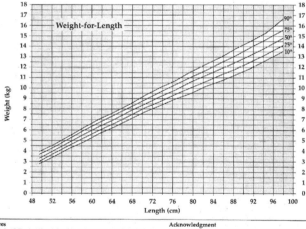

Weight-for-Length

90th
75th
50th
25th
10th

Weight (kg)

Length (cm)

References

1. Guo SS, Roche AF, Chumlea WC, et al: Growth in weight, recumbent length, and head circumference for preterm low-birthweight infants during the first three years of life using gestation-adjusted ages. *Early Hum Dev* 1997;47:305-325.

2. Guo SS, Wholihan K, Roche AF, et al: Weight-for-length reference data for preterm, low-birth-weight infants. *Arch Pediatr Adolesc Med* 1996;150:964-970. Copyright: 1996, American Medical Association.

Acknowledgment

IHDP studies were supported by grants from the Robert Wood Johnson Foundation, Pew Charitable Trusts, and the Bureau of Maternal and Child Health, US Department of Health and Human Services. The IHDP growth percentile graphs were prepared by S.S. Guo and A.F. Roche, Wright State University, Yellow Springs, Ohio. IHDP, its sponsors and the investigators do not endorse specific products.

APP

Fig. D-3.B
Very Low Birth Weight Growth Charts

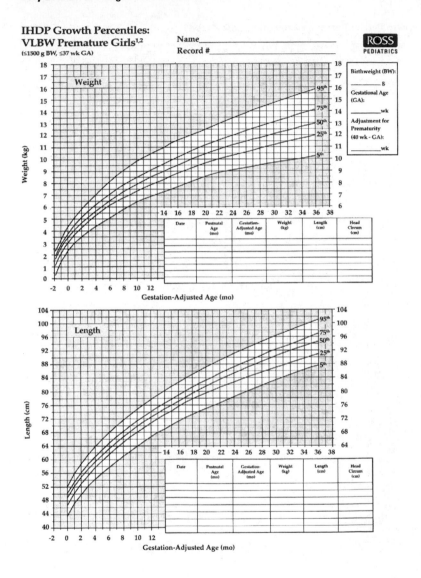

IHDP Growth Percentiles:
VLBW Premature Girls[1,2]
(≤1500 g BW, ≤37 wk GA)

Name_____

Record #_____

ROSS
PEDIATRICS

IHDP Growth Percentiles: VLBW Premature Girls[1,2]

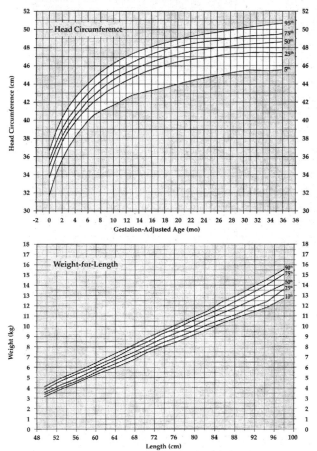

References

1. Guo SS, Roche AF, Chumlea WC, et al: Growth in weight, recumbent length, and head circumference for preterm low-birthweight infants during the first three years of life using gestation-adjusted ages. *Early Hum Dev* 1997;47:305-325.

2. Guo SS, Wholihan K, Roche AF, et al: Weight-for-length reference data for preterm, low-birth-weight infants. *Arch Pediatr Adolesc Med* 1996;150:964-970. Copyright: 1996, American Medical Association.

© 1999 Abbott
A7220/MARCH 1999
LITHO IN USA

Acknowledgment

IHDP studies were supported by grants from the Robert Wood Johnson Foundation, Pew Charitable Trusts, and the Bureau of Maternal and Child Health, US Department of Health and Human Services. The IHDP growth percentile graphs were prepared by S.S. Guo and A.F. Roche, Wright State University, Yellow Springs, Ohio. IHDP, its sponsors and the investigators do not endorse specific products.

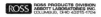

ROSS PRODUCTS DIVISION
ABBOTT LABORATORIES INC.
COLUMBUS, OHIO 43215-1704

Provided as a service of
Similac NeoSure™
Infant Formula With Iron

APP

IHDP Growth Percentiles:
VLBW Premature Boys[1,2]
(≤1500 g BW, ≤37 wk GA)

Name_____

Record #_____

ROSS
PEDIATRICS

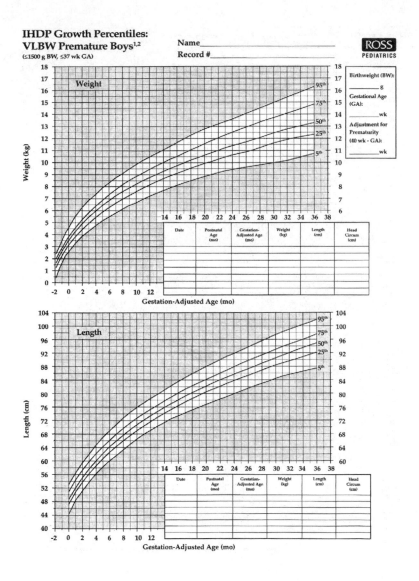

Birthweight (BW):

_____ g

Gestational Age
(GA):

_____ wk

Adjustment for
Prematurity
(40 wk - GA):

_____ wk

IHDP Growth Percentiles: VLBW Premature Boys[1,2]

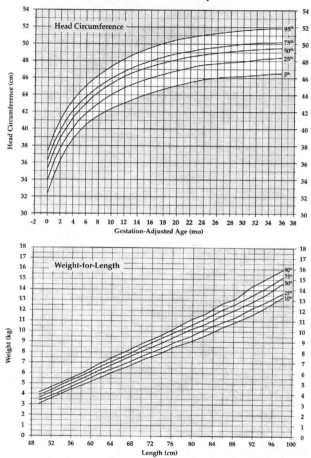

References

1. Guo SS, Roche AF, Chumlea WC, et al: Growth in weight, recumbent length, and head circumference for preterm low-birthweight infants during the first three years of life using gestation-adjusted ages. *Early Hum Dev* 1997;47:305-325.

2. Guo SS, Wholihan K, Roche AF, et al: Weight-for-length reference data for preterm, low-birth-weight infants. *Arch Pediatr Adolesc Med* 1996;150:964-970. Copyright: 1996, American Medical Association.

Acknowledgment

IHDP studies were supported by grants from the Robert Wood Johnson Foundation, Pew Charitable Trusts, and the Bureau of Maternal and Child Health, US Department of Health and Human Services. The IHDP growth percentile graphs were prepared by S.S. Guo and A.F. Roche, Wright State University, Yellow Springs, Ohio. IHDP, its sponsors and the investigators do not endorse specific products.

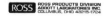
Provided as a service of
Similac NeoSure™
Infant Formula With Iron

Fig. D-3.C
Intrauterine Growth Charts
Canadian male singletons, crude curves

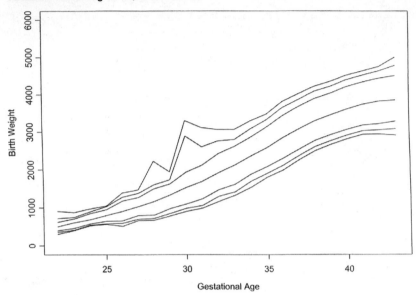

Fig. D-3.D
Intrauterine Growth Charts
Canadian female singletons, crude curves

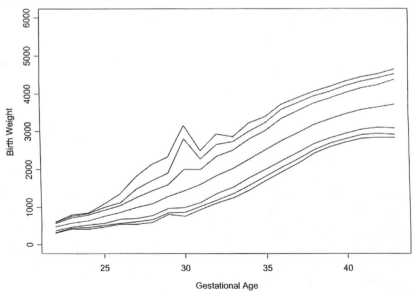

Fig. D-3.E
Intrauterine Growth Charts
Canadian male singletons, corrected and smooth curves

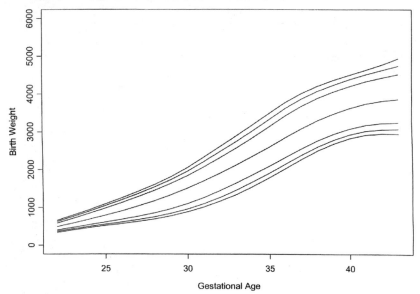

Fig. D-3.F
Intrauterine Growth Charts
Canadian female singletons, corrected and smooth curves

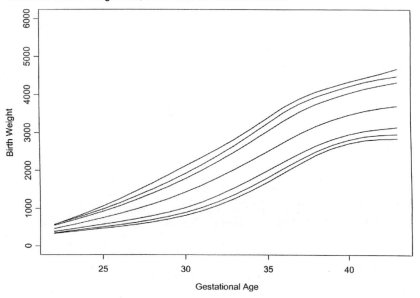

Appendix D-4

Arm circumference-for-age BOYS

3 months to 5 years (percentiles)

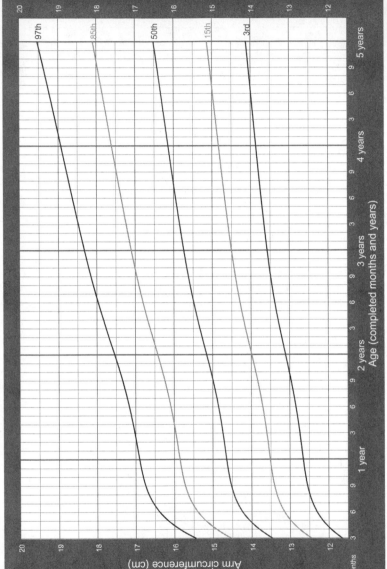

WHO Child Growth Standards

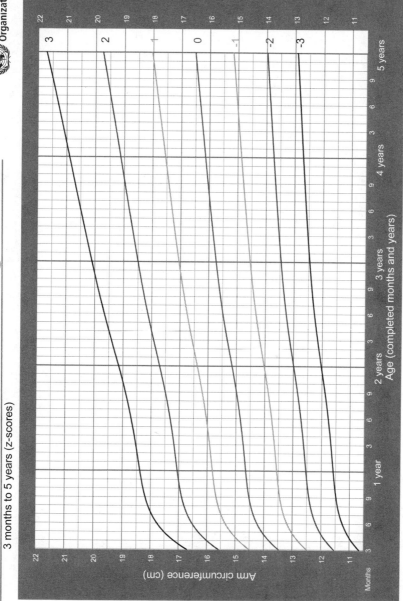

World Health Organization

Arm circumference-for-age BOYS
3 months to 5 years (z-scores)

WHO Child Growth Standards

APP

Arm circumference-for-age GIRLS

3 months to 5 years (percentiles)

World Health
Organization

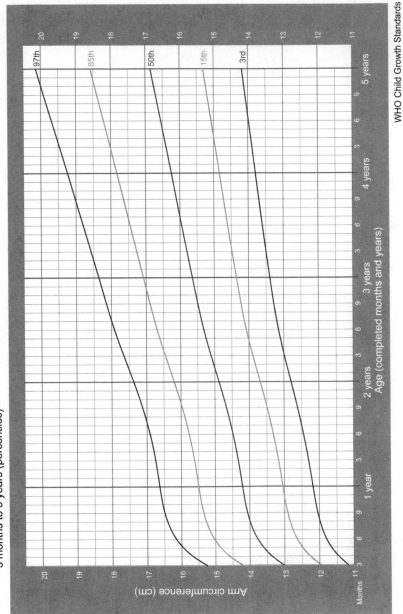

WHO Child Growth Standards

Arm circumference-for-age GIRLS
3 months to 5 years (z-scores)

World Health Organization

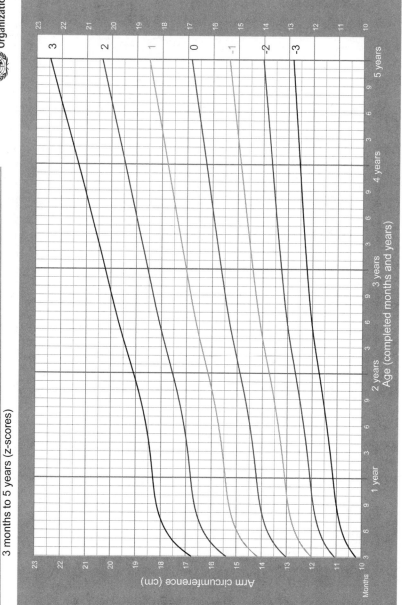

WHO Child Growth Standards

APP

Appendix E

Table E-1

Recommended Nutrient Levels of Infant Formulas (per 100 kcal) (From the US Infant Formula Act of 1980 [Pub L No. 96-359], Amended 1986 [Pub L No. 99-570])

Nutrient	Range	
	Minimum	Maximum
Protein, g	1.8*	4.5*
Fat, g	3.3 (30% of kcal)	6.0 (54% of kcal)
Linoleic acid (18:2 ω6), mg	300 (2.7% of kcal)	
Vitamins		
A, IU	250 (75 µg)†	750 (225 µg)†
D, IU	40 (1 µg)‡	100 (2.5 µg)‡
K, µg§	4	...
E, IU	0.7 (0.5 mg)‖ at least 0.7 IU (0.5 mg)/g linoleic acid	...
C (ascorbic acid), mg	8	...
B₁ (thiamine), µg	40	
B₂ (riboflavin), µg	60	...
B₆ (pyridoxine), µg	35¶	...
B₁₂, µg	0.15	...
Niacin, µg	250 (or 0.8 mg niacin equivalents)	...
Folic acid, µg	4	...
Pantothenic acid, µg	300	...
Biotin, µg	1.5#	...
Choline, mg	7#	...
Inositol, mg	4#	...
Minerals		
Calcium, mg	60**	...
Phosphorus, mg	30**	...
Magnesium, mg	6	...
Iron, mg††	0.15	3.0
Iodine, µg	5	75
Zinc, mg	0.5	...
Copper, µg	60	...
Manganese, µg	5	...
Sodium, mg	20 (0.9 mEq)	60 (2.6 mEq)

APP

Table E-1 *(Continued)*
Recommended Nutrient Levels of Infant Formulas (per 100 kcal) (From the US Infant Formula Act of 1980 [Pub L No. 96-359], Amended 1986 [Pub L No. 99-570]

Nutrient	Range	
	Minimum	Maximum
Potassium, mg	80 (2.1 mEq)	200 (5.1 mEq)
Chloride, mg	55 (1.6 mEq)	150 (4.2 mEq)

* Biologically equivalent to or better than casein. If protein of lower quality used, minimum is increased in proportion. In no case, protein with biological value <70%.
† Retinol equivalents.
‡ Cholecalciferol.
§ Any vitamin K added shall be in the form of phylloquinone.
‖ all-*rac*-α-tocopherol equivalents.
¶ At least 15 µg for each g protein in excess of 18 g/100 kcal.
⁑ Naturally present in cow milk-based formulas; addition required only non-cow milk-based formulas.
** Calcium-to-phosphorus ratio should be no less than 1.1 and no more than 2.
†† If contains ≥1 mg/100 kcal, must be labeled as formula "with iron."

Appendix F

Table F-1
Increasing the Caloric Density of Infant Formula
Using Concentrated Liquid

Caloric Density	Water	Concentrated Liquid	Approximate Yield
20 kcal/fl oz	13 fl oz	13 fl oz (1 can)	26 fl oz
22 kcal/fl oz	11 fl oz	13 fl oz (1 can)	24 fl oz
24 kcal/fl oz	9 fl oz	13 fl oz (1 can)	22 fl oz
27 kcal/fl oz	6 fl oz	13 fl oz (1 can)	19 fl oz
30 kcal/fl oz	4.5 fl oz	13 fl oz (1 can)	17.5 fl oz

Using Powder

Because of the variability of scoop sizes for different formulas from different manufacturers and the variability of household measures, no single set of recipes can be provided that is safe for all products. Some manufacturers provide recipes for their specific products on their Web sites. In the absence of such information, contact the manufacturer directly.

Increasing Caloric Density Using Other Additives

- Medium-chain triglyceride oil provides 7.7 kcal/mL; 1 teaspoon provides 38 kcal.
- Vegetable oils provide 40 kcal/teaspoon.
- Polycose powder (Abbott Nutrition, Columbus, OH) contains 8 kcal/teaspoon.

Note that increasing caloric density using fat and/or carbohydrate should be done with caution, because the additional energy (kcal) effectively decreases the density (amount per 100 kcal) of all other nutrients.

Table F-2, Part 1 of 3
Cow Milk-Based Infant Formulas: Label Claim Nutrient Contents (per L at 20 kcal/oz)

Contents	Enfamil LIPIL*‡ (Mead Johnson, Evansville, IN)	Enfamil Gentlease LIPIL (Mead Johnson, Evansville, IN)	Enfamil LactoFree LIPIL*† (Mead Johnson, Evansville, IN)	Enfamil A.R. LIPIL* (Mead Johnson, Evansville, IN)	Nestlé Good Start*† (Nestlé, Glendale, CA)	Nestlé Good Start DHA & ARA*† (Mead Johnson, Evansville, IN)	Nestlé Good Start DHA & ARA Natural Cultures† (powder only) (Nestlé, Glendale, CA)
Energy, kcal	680	680	680	680	670	670	670
Protein, g	14.2	15.6	14.2	16.9	15	15	15
Casein, % of total protein	40	40‡	80	80	0	0	0
Whey, % of total protein	60	60‡	20	20	100‡	100‡	100‡
Fat, g	36	36	36	34	34	34	34
Polyunsaturated, %	20	20	20	20	22	22	22
Monounsaturated, %	37	37	37	37	33	33	33
Saturated, %	43	43	43	43	45	45	45
Source	Palm olein, soy, coconut, high-oleic sunflower, DHA and ARA§	Palm olein, soy, coconut, high-oleic sunflower, DHA and ARA§	Palm olein, soy, coconut, high-oleic sunflower, DHA and ARA§	Palm olein, soy, coconut, high-oleic sunflower, DHA and ARA§	Palm olein, soy, coconut, high-oleic safflower/ sunflower	Palm olein, soy, coconut, high-oleic safflower/sun- flower, DHA and ARA§	Palm olein, soy, coconut, high-oleic safflower/sun- flower, DHA and ARA§
Carbohydrate, g	74	73	74	74	75	75	75
Source	Lactose	Corn-syrup solids, lactose	Corn-syrup solids	Lactose, rice starch, and maltodextrin	Lactose, corn maltodextrin	Lactose, corn maltodextrin	Lactose, corn maltodextrin
Osmolality, mOsm/kg	300	220	200	230‖/240¶	260	260	260
Minerals							
Calcium, mg	530	550	550	530	449	449	449

Table F-2, Part 1 of 3 *(Continued)*
Cow Milk-Based Infant Formulas: Label Claim Nutrient Contents (per L at 20 kcal/oz)

Contents	Enfamil LIPIL*‡ (Mead Johnson, Evansville, IN)	Enfamil Gentlease LIPIL (Mead Johnson, Evansville, IN)	Enfamil LactoFree LIPIL*† (Mead Johnson, Evansville, IN)	Enfamil A.R. LIPIL* (Mead Johnson, Evansville, IN)	Nestlé Good Start*† (Nestlé, Glendale, CA)	Nestlé Good Start DHA & ARA*† (Mead Johnson, Evansville, IN)	Nestlé Good Start DHA & ARA Natural Cultures† (powder only) (Nestlé, Glendale, CA)
Phosphorus, mg	290	310	310	360	255	255	255
Magnesium, mg	54	54	54	54	47	47	47
Iron, mg	12.2	12.2	12.2	12.2	10	10	10
Zinc, mg	6.8	6.8	6.8	6.8	5	5	5
Manganese, µg	101	101	101	101	101	101	101
Copper, µg	510	510	510	510	536	536	536
Iodine, µg	68	68	101	68	80	80	80
Sodium, mEq	8	9.6	8.7	11.7	8	8	8
Potassium, mEq	18.7	18.7	18.9	18.7	19	19	19
Chloride, mEq	12.1	12.1	12.7	14.4	12	12	12
Vitamins							
A, IU	2000	2000	2000	2000	2010	2010	2010
D, IU	410	410	410	410	402	402	402
E, IU	13.5	13.5	13.5	13.5	13	13	13
K, µg	54	54	54	54	54	54	54
Thiamine (B_1), µg	540	540	540	540	670	670	670
Riboflavin (B_2), µg	950	950	950	950	938	938	938

Table F-2, Part 1 of 3 *(Continued)*
Cow Milk-Based Infant Formulas: Label Claim Nutrient Contents (per L at 20 kcal/oz)

Contents	Enfamil LIPIL*‡ (Mead Johnson, Evansville, IN)	Enfamil Gentlease LIPIL (Mead Johnson, Evansville, IN)	Enfamil LactoFree LIPIL*‡ (Mead Johnson, Evansville, IN)	Enfamil A.R. LIPIL* (Mead Johnson, Evansville, IN)	Nestlé Good Start**‡ Nestlé, Glendale, CA)	Nestlé Good Start DHA & ARA*‡ (Mead Johnson, Evansville, IN)	Nestlé Good Start DHA & ARA Natural Cultures‡ (powder only) (Nestlé, Glendale, CA)
Pyridoxine, μg	410	410	410	410	503	503	503
B$_{12}$, μg	2	2	2	2	2	2	2
Niacin, mg	6.8	6.8	6.8	6.8	7	7	7
Folic acid, μg	108	108	108	108	101	101	101
Pantothenic acid, mg	3.4	3.4	3.4	3.4	3	3	3
Biotin, μg	20	20	20	20	29	29	29
C (ascorbic acid), mg	81	81	81	81	60	60	60
Choline, mg	162	162	162	81	161	161	161
Inositol, mg	41	41	41	41	40	40	40

LCPUFA indicates long-chain polyunsaturated fatty acids; DHA, docosahexaenoic acid; ARA, arachidonic acid.

* Liquid and powder.
† With nucleotides.
‡ Partially hydrolyzed.
§ From single-cell oils *Crypthecodinium cohnii* and *Mortierella alpina*, respectively.
‖ Powder form.
¶ Liquid form.
# Organic ingredients.
** Low iron.

Table F-2, Part 2 of 3
Cow Milk–Based Infant Formulas: Label Claim Nutrient Contents (per L at 20 Kcal/oz)

Contents	Similac with Iron*† (Abbott Nutrition, Columbus, OH)	Similac Advance*† (Abbott Nutrition, Columbus, OH)	Similac Organic*† (Abbott Nutrition, Columbus, OH)	Similac PM 60/40 (powder only) (Abbott Nutrition, Columbus, OH)	Similac Sensitive*† (Abbott Nutrition, Columbus, OH)
Energy, kcal	676	676	676	676	676
Protein, g	14	14	14.0‡	15	14.47
Casein, % of total protein	52	52	82	40	18
Whey, % of total protein	48	48	18	60	82
Fat, g	36.5	36.5	37.1	37.9	36.5
Polyunsaturated, %	26	27	21	26	27
Monounsaturated, %	40	40	44	40	40
Saturated, %	34	33	35	34	33
Source	High-oleic safflower, soy, coconut	High-oleic safflower, soy, coconut, DHA and ARA§	High-oleic,‖ sunflower,‖ soy,‖ coconut,‖ DHA and ARA§	High-oleic safflower, soy, coconut	High-oleic safflower, soy, coconut, DHA and ARA§
Carbohydrate, g	73	73	71.4	69	72.4
	Lactose	Lactose	Corn maltodextrin,‖ lactose,‖ sucrose‖	Lactose	Corn maltodextrin, sucrose
Osmolality, mOsm/kg	300	300	225	280	200
Minerals					
Calcium, mg	528	528	528	379	568
Phosphorus, mg	284	284	284	189	379
Magnesium, mg	41	41	41	40.6	40.6
Iron, mg	12.2	12	12.2	4.7**	12.2

APP

Table F-2, Part 2 of 3 (*Continued*)
Cow Milk-Based Infant Formulas: Label Claim Nutrient Contents (per L at 20 Kcal/oz)

Contents	Similac with Iron*† (Abbott Nutrition, Columbus, OH)	Similac Advance*† (Abbott Nutrition, Columbus, OH)	Similac Organic*† (Abbott Nutrition, Columbus, OH)	Similac PM 60/40 (powder only) (Abbott Nutrition, Columbus, OH)	Similac Sensitive*† (Abbott Nutrition, Columbus, OH)
Zinc, mg	5.1	5.1	5.1	5.1	5.1
Manganese, µg	34	34	34	34	34
Copper, µg	609	609	609	609	609
Iodine, µg	41	41	41	41	61
Sodium, mEq	7.1	7.1	7.1	7.1	8.8
Potassium, mEq	18.2	18.2	18.1	13.8	18.5
Chloride, mEq	12.4	12.4	12.4	11.3	12.4
Vitamins					
A, IU	2029	2029	2029	2029	2029
D, IU	406	406	406	406	406
E, IU	10.1	10.1	10.1	10.1	20.3
K, µg	54	54	54	54	54
Thiamine (B$_1$), µg	676	676	676	676	676
Riboflavin (B$_2$), µg	1014	1014	1014	1014	1014
Pyridoxine, µg	406	406	406	406	406
B$_{12}$, µg	1.7	1.7	1.69	1.7	1.7
Niacin, mg	7.1	7.1	7.1	7.1	7.1
Folic acid, µg	101	101	101	101	101

Table F-2, Part 2 of 3 (*Continued*)

Cow Milk-Based Infant Formulas: Label Claim Nutrient Contents (per L at 20 Kcal/oz)

Contents	Similac with Iron*† (Abbott Nutrition, Columbus, OH)	Similac Advance*† (Abbott Nutrition, Columbus, OH)	Similac Organic*† (Abbott Nutrition, Columbus, OH)	Similac PM 60/40 (powder only) (Abbott Nutrition, Columbus, OH)	Similac Sensitive*† (Abbott Nutrition, Columbus, OH)
Pantothenic acid, mg	3.04	3.04	3.04	3.04	3.04
Biotin, µg	29.8	29.8	29.8	30.4	29.8
C (ascorbic acid), mg	61	61	61	61	61
Choline, mg	108	108	108	81	108
Inositol, mg	31.8	32	31.8	162	29.1

LCPUFA indicates long-chain polyunsaturated fatty acids; DHA, docosahexaenoic acid; ARA, arachidonic acid.

* Liquid and powder.
† With nucleotides.
‡ Partially hydrolyzed.
§ From single-cell oils *Crypthecodinium cohnii* and *Mortierella alpina*, respectively.
‖ Powder form.
¶ Liquid form.
\# Organic ingredients.
** Low iron.

APP

Table F-2, Part 3 of 3
Cow Milk-Based Infant Formulas: Label Claim Nutrient Contents (per L at 20 kcal/oz)

Contents	Store Brand Milk-Based Formula With Iron† (powder only) (PBM Nutritionals, Georgia, VT)	Store Brand Milk-Based Formula With LCPUFA*† (PBM Nutritionals, Georgia, VT)	Store Brand Milk-Based Lactose-Free Formula With LCPUFA† (powder only) (PBM Nutritionals, Georgia, VT)	Store Brand Milk-Based Partially Hydro-lyzed Formula With LCPUFA† (powder only) (PBM Nutritionals, Georgia, VT)	Store Brand Milk-Based A.R. Formula With LCPUFA (powder only) (PBM Nutritionals, Georgia, VT)	Store Brand Organic Milk-Based Formula With LCPUFA† (powder only) (PBM Nutritionals, Georgia, VT)
Energy, kcal	672	668	672	672	666	672
Protein, g	15	14	15	15	17	15ᵈ
Casein, % of total protein	40	40	40	40	80	40
Whey, % of total protein	60	60	60	60ᵃ	20	60
Fat, g Polyunsaturated, % Monounsaturated, % Saturated, %	36	36	36	36	34	36
Source	Palm olein, soy, coconut, high-oleic safflower or sunflower	Palm olein, soy, coconut, high-oleic safflower/ sunflower, DHA and ARA§	Palm olein, soy, coconut, high-oleic safflower/ sunflower, DHA and ARA§	Palm olein, soy, coconut, high-oleic safflower/sunflower, DHA and ARA§	Palm olein, soy, coconut, high-oleic safflower/ sunflower, DHA and ARA§	Palm or palm olein,ᵉ soy,ᵉ coconut,ᵉ soy,ᵉ high-oleic safflower/ sunflowerᵉ DHA and ARA§
Carbohydrate, g	72 Lactose	72 Lactose	72 Corn-syrup solids	72 Corn-syrup solids	73 Lactose, malto-dextrin, rice starch	72 Lactoseᵉ
Osmolality, mOsm/kg	281	293	207	182		274
Minerals						
Calcium, mg	420	520	550	547	520	420
Phosphorus, mg	280	287	366	307	353	280

Table F-2, Part 3 of 3 (Continued)
Cow Milk-Based Infant Formulas: Label Claim Nutrient Contents (per L at 20 kcal/oz)

Contents	Store Brand Milk-Based Formula With Iron† (powder only) (PBM Nutritionals, Georgia, VT)	Store Brand Milk-Based Formula With LCPUFA*† (PBM Nutritionals, Georgia, VT)	Store Brand Milk-Based Lactose-Free Formula With LCPUFA† (powder only) (PBM Nutritionals, Georgia, VT)	Store Brand Milk-Based Partially Hydro-lyzed Formula With LCPUFA† (powder only) (PBM Nutritionals, Georgia, VT)	Store Brand Milk-Based A.R. Formula With LCPUFA (powder only) (PBM Nutritionals, Georgia, VT)	Store Brand Organic Milk-Based Formula With LCPUFA† (powder only) (PBM Nutritionals, Georgia, VT)
Magnesium, mg	45	53	45	53	53	45
Iron, mg	12	12	12	12	12	12
Zinc, mg	5	6.7	5	6.7	6.7	5
Manganese, µg	100	100	100	100	100	100
Copper, µg	470	500	470	500	500	470
Iodine, µg	60	67	60	67	67	60
Sodium, mEq	6.52	7.83	6.52	9.26	11.6	6.52
Potassium, mEq	14.34	18.72	14.34	18.43	18.43	14.34
Chloride, mEq	10.72	11.85	11.44	12.01	14.3	11.44
Vitamins						
A, IU	2000	2000	2000	2000	2000	2000
D, IU	400	400	400	400	400	400
E, IU	9.5	13	13	13	13	13
K, µg	55	53	55	53	53	55
Thiamine (B_1), µg	670	533	670	533	533	670
Riboflavin (B_2), µg	1000	933	1000	933	933	1000

APP

Table F-2, Part 3 of 3 (Continued)
Cow Milk-Based Infant Formulas: Label Claim Nutrient Contents (per L at 20 kcal/oz)

Contents	Store Brand Milk-Based Formula With Iron† (powder only) (PBM Nutritionals, Georgia, VT)	Store Brand Milk-Based Formula With LCPUFA*† (PBM Nutritionals, Georgia, VT)	Store Brand Milk-Based Lactose-Free Formula With LCPUFA† (powder only) (PBM Nutritionals, Georgia, VT)	Store Brand Milk-Based Partially Hydrolyzed Formula With LCPUFA‡ (powder only) (PBM Nutritionals, Georgia, VT)	Store Brand Milk-Based A.R. Formula With LCPUFA (powder only) (PBM Nutritionals, Georgia, VT)	Store Brand Organic Milk-Based Formula With LCPUFA¶ (powder only) (PBM Nutritionals, Georgia, VT)
Pyridoxine, μg	420	400	420	400	400	420
B_{12}, μg	1.3	2	1.3	2	2	1.3
Niacin, mg	5	6.7	5	6.7	6.7	5
Folic acid, μg	50	107	100	107	107	50
Pantothenic acid, mg	2.1	3.3	2.1	3.3	3.3	2.1
Biotin, μg	15	20	15	20	20	15
C (ascorbic acid), mg	55	80	55	80	80	60
Choline, mg	100	160	100	160	160	100
Inositol, mg	27	40	114	40	40	27

LCPUFA indicates long-chain polyunsaturated fatty acids; DHA, docosahexaenoic acid; ARA, arachidonic acid.
* Liquid and powder.
† With nucleotides.
‡ Partially hydrolyzed.
§ From single-cell oils Crypthecodinium cohnii and Mortierella alpina, respectively.
‖ Powder form.
¶ Liquid form.
# Organic ingredients.
** Low iron.

Table F-3, Part 1 of 2

Soy-Based Infant Formulas: Label Claim Nutrient Contents (per L at 20 kcal/oz)

Contents	Nestlé Good Start Soy DHA & ARA* (Nestlé, Glendale, CA)	Enfamil ProSobee LIPIL* (Mead Johnson, Evansville, IN)	Similac Isomil* (Abbott Nutrition Columbus, OH)	Similac Isomil Advance* (Abbott Nutrition, Columbus, OH)	Similac Isomil DF (liquid only) (Abbott Nutrition, Columbus, OH)
Energy, kcal	670	680	676	676	676
Protein, g	17	16.9	16.55	16.57	17.99
Source	Soy protein† isolate and L-methionine	Soy protein isolate and L-methionine	Soy protein isolate and L-methionine	Soy protein isolate and L-methionine	Soy protein isolate and L-methionine
Fat, g	34	36	36.9	36.9	36.9
Polyunsaturated, %	23	20	27	27	39
Monounsaturated, %	32	37	40	40	17
Saturated, %	45	43	33	33	44
Sources	Palm olein, soy, coconut, high-oleic safflower/sunflower, DHA and ARA‡	Palm olein, soy, coconut, high-oleic sunflower, DHA and ARA‡	High-oleic safflower, soy, coconut	High-oleic safflower, soy, coconut, DHA and ARA‡	Soy, coconut
Carbohydrate, g	74	72	69.6	69.7	68.3
	Corn maltodextrins, sucrose (+ cornstarch in liquids)	Corn-syrup solids	Corn-syrup solids and sucrose	Corn-syrup solids and sucrose	Corn-syrup solids and sucrose
Osmolality, mOsm/kg	185	170	200	200	240
Minerals					
Calcium, mg	704	710	710	710	710
Phosphorus, mg	422	470	507	507	507
Magnesium, mg	74	74	50.7	50.7	50.7
Iron, mg	12	12.2	12.2	12.2	12.2

APP

Table F-3, Part 1 of 2 *(Continued)*
Soy-Based Infant Formulas: Label Claim Nutrient Contents (per L at 20 kcal/oz)

Contents	Nestlé Good Start Soy DHA & ARA* (Nestlé, Glendale, CA)	Enfamil ProSobee LIPIL* (Mead Johnson, Evansville, IN)	Similac Isomil* (Abbott Nutrition Columbus, OH)	Similac Isomil Advance* (Abbott Nutrition, Columbus, OH)	Similac Isomil DF (liquid only) (Abbott Nutrition, Columbus, OH)
Zinc, mg	6	8.1	5.07	5.07	5.07
Manganese, µg	168	169	169	169	169
Copper, µg	536	510	507	507	507
Iodine, µg	101	101	101	101	101
Sodium, mEq	12	10.4	12.9	12.9	12.9
Potassium, mEq	20	21	18.7	18.7	18.7
Chloride, mEq	13	15.2	11.8	11.8	11.8
Vitamins					
A, IU	2010	2000	2029	2029	2029
D, IU	402	410	406	406	406
E, IU	20	13.5	10.1	10.1	10.1
K, µg	60	54	74	74	74
Thiamine (B_1), µg	402	540	406	406	406
Riboflavin (B_2), µg	630	610	609	609	609
Pyridoxine, µg	402	410	406	406	406
B_{12}, µg	2	2	3.04	3.04	3.04
Niacin, mg	9	6.8	9.13	9.13	9.13

Table F-3, Part 1 of 2 *(Continued)*
Soy-Based Infant Formulas: Label Claim Nutrient Contents (per L at 20 kcal/oz)

Contents	Nestlé Good Start Soy DHA & ARA* (Nestlé, Glendale, CA)	Enfamil ProSobee LIPIL* (Mead Johnson, Evansville, IN)	Similac Isomil* (Abbott Nutrition, Columbus, OH)	Similac Isomil Advance* (Abbott Nutrition, Columbus, OH)	Similac Isomil DF (liquid only) (Abbott Nutrition, Columbus, OH)
Folic acid, µg	107	108	101	101	101
Pantothenic acid, mg	3	3.4	5.1	5.1	5.1
Biotin, µg	34	20	30.4	30.4	30.4
C (ascorbic acid), mg	80	81	61	61	61
Choline, mg	161	162	81	81	81
Inositol, mg	40	41	33.8	33.8	33.8

* Liquid and powder.
† Partially hydrolyzed.
‡ From single-cell oils Crypthecodinium cohnii and Mortierella alpina, respectively.
§ Organic ingredients.

Table F-3, Part 2 of 2
Soy-Based Infant Formulas: Label Claim Nutrient Contents (per L at 20 kcal/oz)

Contents	Store Brand Soy Infant Formula With Iron (powder only) (PBM Nutritionals, Georgia, VT)	Store Brand Soy Infant Formula With LCPUFA* (PBM Nutritionals, Georgia, VT)	Store Brand Soy Organic, Kosher, Vegetarian and Halal-Certified Infant Formula With LCPUFA (powder only) (PBM Nutritionals, Georgia, VT)
Energy, kcal	672	667	664
Protein, g	18	16.7	16.7
Source	Soy protein isolate and L-methionine	Soy protein isolate and L-methionine	Soy protein isolate and L-methionine
Fat, g Polyunsaturated, % Monounsaturated, % Saturated, %	36	35.3	35.3
Source	Palm olein, coconut, soy, high-oleic safflower/sunflower	Palm olein, coconut, soy, high-oleic safflower/sunflower, DHA and ARA‡	Palm olein,§ coconut,§ soy,§ high-oleic safflower/sunflower,§ DHA and ARA‡
Carbohydrate, g	69	70.7	70
	Corn-syrup solids, sucrose	Corn-syrup solids	Corn-syrup solids§
Osmolality, mOsm/kg	217	162	178
Minerals			
Calcium, mg	600	700	700
Phosphorus, mg	420	553	460
Magnesium, mg	67	73	73
Iron, mg	12	12	12
Zinc, mg	5	8	8

Table F-3, Part 2 of 2 *(Continued)*
Soy-Based Infant Formulas: Label Claim Nutrient Contents (per L at 20 kcal/oz)

Contents	Store Brand Soy Infant Formula With Iron (powder only) (PBM Nutritionals, Georgia, VT)	Store Brand Soy Infant Formula With LCPUFA* (PBM Nutritionals, Georgia, VT)	Store Brand Soy Organic, Kosher, Vegetarian and Halal-Certified Infant Formula With LCPUFA (powder only) (PBM Nutritionals, Georgia, VT)
Manganese, µg	200	167	167
Copper, µg	470	500	500
Iodine, µg	60	100	100
Sodium, mEq	8.7	10.4	10.4
Potassium, mEq	17.9	20.5	20.5
Chloride, mEq	10.7	15.2	15.2
Vitamins			
A, IU	2000	2000	2000
D, IU	400	400	400
E, IU	9.5	13	13
K, µg	55	53	53
Thiamine (B₁), µg	670	533	533
Riboflavin (B₂), µg	1000	600	600
Pyridoxine, µg	420	400	400
B₁₂, µg	2	2	2
Niacin, mg	5	6.7	6.7
Folic acid, µg	50	107	107

APP

Table F-3, Part 2 of 2 *(Continued)*
Soy-Based Infant Formulas: Label Claim Nutrient Contents (per L at 20 kcal/oz)

Contents	Store Brand Soy Infant Formula With Iron (powder only) (PBM Nutritionals, Georgia, VT)	Store Brand Soy Infant Formula With LCPUFA* (PBM Nutritionals, Georgia, VT)	Store Brand Soy Organic, Kosher, Vegetarian and Halal-Certified Infant Formula With LCPUFA (powder only) (PBM Nutritionals, Georgia, VT)
Pantothenic acid, mg	3.0	3.3	3.3
Biotin, µg	35	20	20
C (ascorbic acid), mg	55	80	80
Choline, mg	85	80	160
Inositol, mg	27	40	40

* Liquid and powder.
† Partially hydrolyzed.
‡ From single-cell oils *Crypthecodinium cohnii* and *Mortierella alpina*, respectively.
§ Organic ingredients.

Table F-4
Selected Nutrients in Human Milk, Various Forms of Cow Milk, and Goat Milk (Values are per 100 g, approximately 100 mL)

	Energy, kcal	Protein, g	Fat, g	Carbohydrate, g	Calcium, mg	Phosphorus, mg	Sodium, mg (mEq)*	Potassium, mg (mEq)*	Iron, mg	Zinc, mg
Human milk	64–80†	1.03	4.38	6.89	32	14	17 (0.74)	51 (1.30)	0.03	0.2
Cow milk, whole	64	3.28	3.66	4.65	119	93	49 (2.13)	151 (3.86)	0.05	0.4
Cow milk, 2%	50	3.33	1.92	4.80	122	95	50 (2.17)	154 (3.94)	0.05	0.4
Cow milk, 1%	42	3.29	1.06	4.78	123	96	51 (2.22)	156 (3.99)	0.05	0.4
Cow milk, skim	35	3.41	0.18	4.85	123	101	52 (2.26)	166 (4.25)	0.04	0.4
Cow milk, evaporated	134	6.81	7.56	10.04	261	203	106 (4.61)	303 (7.75)	0.19	0.8
Goat milk	69	3.56	4.14	4.45	134	111	50 (2.17)	204 (5.22)	0.05	0.3

Source: US Department of Agriculture. Nutrient Database for Standard Reference. Beltsville, MD: US Department of Agriculture, Agricultural Research Service, Human Nutrition Research Center; 2001 (except for energy in human milk).

* mEq data calculated from US Department of Agriculture data using atomic weights of 23.0 for sodium and 39.1 for potassium.
† Values from Lucas A, Ewing G, Roberts SB, Coward WA. How much energy does the breast fed infant consume and expend? *BMJ.* 1987;295:75–77

Comments

Human Milk: Energy content is variable. Commonly used value is 67 kcal/dL. Protein has variable whey-to-casein ratio during lactation (90:10 in early lactation, 60:40 in mature lactation, 50:50 in late lactation). Carbohydrate is predominantly lactose, with approximately 10% as oligosaccharides.

Cow Milk: Whey-to-casein ratio is 18:82. Carbohydrate is lactose. Fat is poorly digested relative to human milk and infant formula. Low-fat versions are hypocaloric. All forms are very low in iron. No form of cow milk is recommended for feeding during the first year of life. Evaporated milk can be diluted with water and additional carbohydrate to produce a formula, but trace elements and vitamins will be inadequate if unsupplemented.

Goat Milk: Whey-to-casein ratio is 18:82. Protein cross-reacts immunologically with cow milk protein. Fat more readily digested than cow milk. Not suitable for feeding during the first year of life. Contains very low concentrations of folic acid and low concentrations of other nutrients similar to cow milk.

Appendix G

Table G-1

Extensively Hydrolyzed Protein-Based and Amino Acid-Based Formulas for Infants: Label Claim Nutrient Contents (per L at 20/kcal/oz)

	EleCare Unflavored and Vanilla (Abbott Nutrition, Columbus, OH)	Pregestimil LIPIL (Mead Johnson, Evansville, IN)	Neocate Infant (Nutricia North America, Rockville, MD)	Neocate Infant with DHA and ARA (Nutricia North America, Rockville, MD)	Nutramigen LIPIL (Mead Johnson, Evansville, IN)	Similac Alimentum Advance (Abbott Nutrition, Columbus, OH)
Form	Powder	Liquid/powder unflavored	Powder unflavored	Powder unflavored	Liquid/powder unflavored	Liquid/powder unflavored
Energy, kcal	676	680	670	670	680	676
Protein, Equivalent g	20.6	18.9	20.7	20.7	18.9	18.6
Protein source	Free L-amino acids	Casein hydrolysate and L-amino acids	Free L-amino acids	Free L-amino acids	Casein hydrolysate and L-amino acids	Casein hydrolysate and L-amino acids
Carbohydrate, g	72.4	69	78.5	78.5	70	69
Fat, g	32.7	38	30.4	30.4	36	37.5
Linoleic acid, mg	5680	6400	4536	4536	5800	12,850
Energy Distribution						
Protein	15%	11%	12%	12%	11%	11%
Fat	42%	48%	41%	41%	48%	48%
LCT	67%	45%	95%	95%	100%	67%
MCT	33%	55%	5%	5%	0%	33%
% Total energy from EFA	7.6	9.58/9.36*	7.7	7.7	8.5	17.1
LCPUFA	DHA and ARA†	DHA and ARA†		DHA and ARA†	DHA and ARA†	DHA and ARA†
Carbohydrate	43%	41%	47%	47%	41%	41%
Osmolality, mOsm/kg	350	290/320*	375	375	320/300*	370

APP

Table G-1 *(Continued)*
Extensively Hydrolyzed Protein-Based and Amino Acid-Based Formulas for Infants: Label Claim Nutrient Contents (per L at 20/kcal/oz)

	EleCare Unflavored and Vanilla (Abbott Nutrition, Columbus, OH)	Pregestimil LIPIL (Mead Johnson, Evansville, IN)	Neocate Infant (Nutricia North America, Rockville, MD)	Neocate Infant with DHA and ARA (Nutricia North America, Rockville, MD)	Nutramigen LIPIL (Mead Johnson, Evansville, IN)	Similac Alimentum Advance (Abbott Nutrition, Columbus, OH)
Minerals						
Calcium, mg	781	640	831	831	640	710
Phosphorus, mg	568	350	624	624	350	507
Magnesium, mg	56.8	74	83	83	74	50.7
Iron, mg	9.9	12.2	12.5	12.5	12.2	12.2
Zinc, mg	5.7	6.8	11.14	11.14	6.8	5.07
Manganese, μg	568	169	60	60	169	54
Copper, μg	710	510	828	828	510	507
Iodine, μg	57	101	103	103	101	101
Sodium, mEq	13.3	13.9	11	11	13.9	12.9
Potassium, mEq	26	18.9	26	26	18.9	20.3
Chloride, mEq	11.4	16.3	15	15	16.3	15.5
Vitamins						
A, IU	1846	2600	2738	2738	2000	2029
D, IU	284	340	401	401	340	304
E, IU	14.2	27	7.6	7.6	13.5	20.3

Table G-1 (Continued)

Extensively Hydrolyzed Protein-Based and Amino Acid-Based Formulas for Infants: Label Claim Nutrient Contents (per L at 20/kcal/oz)

	EleCare Unflavored and Vanilla (Abbott Nutrition, Columbus, OH)	Pregestimil LIPIL (Mead Johnson, Evansville, IN)	Neocate Infant (Nutricia North America, Rockville, MD)	Neocate Infant with DHA and ARA (Nutricia North America, Rockville, MD)	Nutramigen LIPIL (Mead Johnson, Evansville, IN)	Similac Alimentum Advance (Abbott Nutrition, Columbus, OH)
K, µg	40.5	81	59	59	54	101
Thiamine (B_1), µg	1420	540	620	620	540	406
Riboflavin (B_2), µg	710	610	923	923	610	609
Pyridoxine, µg	568	410	827	827	410	406
B_{12}, µg	2.84	2	1.75	1.75	2	3.04
Niacin, mg	11.4	6.8	10.3	10.3	6.8	9.13
Folic acid, µg	199	108	68.41	68.41	108	101
Pantothenic acid, mg	2.8	3.4	4.2	4.2	3.4	5.07
Biotin, µg	28.4	20	20.68	20.68	20	30.4
C (ascorbic acid), mg	61	81	62.05	62.05	81	61
Choline, mg	64	162	87.5	87.5	162	81
Inositol, mg	34	115	156	156	115	33.8

* Values for 20 kcal/oz liquid and powder, respectively.
† From single-cell oils Crypthecodinium cohnii and Mortierella alpina, respectively.

APP

Appendix H

Table H-1

Milk-Based Follow-up Infant Formulas: Label Claim Nutrient Contents (per L at 20 kcal/oz)

Contents	Enfamil NEXT STEP LIPIL* (Mead Johnson, Evansville, IN)	Nestlé Good Start 2 DHA and ARA (powder only) (Nestlé, Glendale, CA)	Nestlé Good Start 2 DHA and ARA Natural Cultures (powder only) (Nestlé, Glendale, CA)	Similac Go & Grow Milk-Based Formula (powder only) (Abbott Nutrition, Columbus, OH)	Store Brand Formula for Older Infants With LCPUFA (unflavored or vanilla flavored) (powder only) (PBM Nutritionals, Georgia, VT)	Store Brand Formula for Older Infants With LCPUFA and FOS† (powder only) (PBM Nutritionals, Georgia, VT)
Energy, kcal	680	670	670	676	681	681
Protein	17.6	15	15	14.0	18	18
Casein, % of total calories	80	0	0	52	50	50
Whey, %	20	100‡	100‡	48	50	50
Fat, g	36	34	34	37	37	36
Polyunsaturated, %	20	23	23	27		
Monounsaturated, %	37	32	32	40		
Saturated, %	43	45	45	33		
Source	Palm olein, soy, coconut, high-oleic sunflower, DHA & ARA§	Palm olein, soy,coconut & high-oleic saf-flower/sunflower, DHA & ARA§	Palm olein, soy,coconut & high-oleic saf-flower/sunflower, DHA & ARA§	High-oleic saf-flower, coconut, soy, DHA & ARA§	Palm or palm olein, coconut, soy, high-oleic (saf-flower/sunflower) DHA & ARA§	Palm olein, coconut, soy, high-oleic (saf-flower/sunflower) DHA & ARA§
Carbohydrate, g	71	75	75	71.4	69	71.5
	Lactose and corn syrup solids	Lactose, corn maltodextrin	Lactose, corn maltodextrin	Lactose	Lactose and corn syrup solids	Lactose and corn syrup solids
Osmolality, mOsm/kg	270	255	265	300	279/274‖	274

APP

Table H-1 (Continued)
Milk-Based Follow-up Infant Formulas: Label Claim Nutrient Contents (per L at 20 kcal/oz)

Contents	Enfamil NEXT STEP LIPIL* (Mead Johnson, Evansville, IN)	Nestlé Good Start 2 DHA and ARA (powder only) (Nestlé, Glendale, CA)	Nestlé Good Start 2 DHA and ARA Natural Cultures (powder only) (Nestlé, Glendale, CA)	Similac Go & Grow Milk-Based Formula (powder only) (Abbott Nutrition, Columbus, OH)	Store Brand Formula for Older Infants With LCPUFA (unflavored or vanilla flavored) (powder only) (PBM Nutritionals, Georgia, VT)	Store Brand Formula for Older Infants With LCPUFA and FOS† (powder only) (PBM Nutritionals, Georgia, VT)
Minerals						
Calcium, mg	1320	1273	1273	1014	816	1330
Phosphorus, mg	880	710	710	548	579	885
Magnesium, mg	54	47	47	40.6	68	55
Iron, mg	13.5	13	13	13.5	12	14
Zinc, mg	6.8	5	5	5.1	6.0	6.8
Manganese, μg	101	101	101	34	40	102
Copper, μg	510	536	536	609	580	511
Iodine, μg	68	80	80	41	69	68
Sodium, mEq	10.4	8	8	7.1	9.6	9.6
Potassium, mEq	23	19	19	18.2	21.8	21.8
Chloride, mEq	15.2	12	12	12.4	15.6	15.6

Table H-1 (Continued)

Milk-Based Follow-up Infant Formulas: Label Claim Nutrient Contents (per L at 20 kcal/oz)

Contents	Enfamil NEXT STEP LIPIL* (Mead Johnson, Evansville, IN)	Nestlé Good Start 2 DHA and ARA (powder only) (Nestlé, Glendale, CA)	Nestlé Good Start 2 DHA and ARA Natural Cultures (powder only) (Nestlé, Glendale, CA)	Similac Go & Grow Milk-Based Formula (powder only) (Abbott Nutrition, Columbus, OH)	Store Brand Formula for Older Infants With LCPUFA (unflavored or vanilla flavored) (powder only) (PBM Nutritionals, Georgia, VT)	Store Brand Formula for Older Infants With LCPUFA and FOS† (powder only) (PBM Nutritionals, Georgia, VT)
Vitamins						
A, IU	2000	2010	2010	2029	2520	2049
D, IU	410	402	402	406	440	410
E, IU	13.5	13	13	20.3	14	13.6
K, µg	54	54	54	54	67	54.5
Thiamine (B$_1$), µg	540	670	670	676	1022	545
Riboflavin (B$_2$), µg	950	938	938	1014	1500	955
Pyridoxine, µg	410	503	503	406	613	410
B$_{12}$, µg	2	2	2	1.7	2	2
Niacin, mg	6.8	7	7	7.1	6.9	6.83
Folic acid, µg	108	101	101	101	102	110

Table H-1 *(Continued)*
Milk-Based Follow-up Infant Formulas: Label Claim Nutrient Contents (per L at 20 kcal/oz)

Contents	Enfamil NEXT STEP LIPIL* (Mead Johnson, Evansville, IN)	Nestlé Good Start 2 DHA and ARA (powder only) (Nestlé, Glendale, CA)	Nestlé Good Start 2 DHA and ARA Natural Cultures (powder only) (Nestlé, Glendale, CA)	Similac Go & Grow Milk-Based Formula (powder only) (Abbott Nutrition, Columbus, OH)	Store Brand Formula for Older Infants With LCPUFA (unflavored or vanilla flavored) (powder only) (PBM Nutritionals, Georgia, VT)	Store Brand Formula for Older Infants With LCPUFA and FOS† (powder only) (PBM Nutritionals, Georgia, VT)
Pantothenic acid, mg	3.4	3	3	3.04	3	3.42
Biotin, μg	20	29	29	29.8	20	20
C (ascorbic acid), mg	81	80	80	81	90	82
Choline, mg	162	161	161	108	100	164
Inositol, mg	41	40	40	31.8	27	41

* Liquid and powder.
† Fructo-oligosaccharides.
‡ Partially hydrolyzed.
§ From single-cell oils *Crypthecodinium cohnii* and *Mortierella alpina*, respectively.
‖ Unflavored/flavored.

Table H-2
Soy Follow-up Infant Formulas: Label Claim Nutrient Contents (per L at 20 kcal/oz)

	Enfamil NEXT STEP ProSobee LIPIL (powder only) (Mead Johnson, Evansville, IN)	Nestlé Good Start 2 Supreme Soy DHA and ARA (powder only) (Nestlé, Glendale, CA)	Similac Go & Grow Soy-Based Formula (powder only) (Abbott Nutrition, Columbus, OH)
Energy, kcal	680	670	676
Protein	22	19	16.6
	Soy protein isolate and L-methionine	Soy protein isolate* and L-methionine	Soy protein isolate and L-methionine
Fat, g			
Polyunsaturated, %	30	34	36.9
Monounsaturated, %	20	23	27
Saturated, %	37	32	40
	43	45	33
Source	Palm olein, soy, coconut, high-oleic sunflower, DHA and ARA†	Palm olein, soy, coconut, high-oleic safflower/sunflower, DHA and ARA†	High-oleic safflower, soy, coconut, DHA and ARA†
Carbohydrate, g	80	73	69.6
	Corn-syrup solids	Corn maltodextrin, sucrose	Corn-syrup solids, sucrose
Osmolality, mOsm/kg	230	185	200
Minerals			
Calcium, mg	1320	1273	1014
Phosphorus, mg	880	710	676
Magnesium, mg	74	74	50.7
Iron, mg	13.5	13	13.5
Zinc, mg	8.1	6	5.1
Manganese, µg	340	335	169
Copper, µg	510	503	507

APP

Table H-2 *(Continued)*
Soy Follow-up Infant Formulas: Label Claim Nutrient Contents (per L at 20 kcal/oz)

	Enfamil NEXT STEP ProSobee LIPIL (powder only) (Mead Johnson, Evansville, IN)	Nestlé Good Start 2 Supreme Soy DHA and ARA (powder only) (Nestle, Glendale, CA)	Similac Go & Grow Soy-Based Formula (powder only) (Abbott Nutrition, Columbus, OH)
Iodine, µg	101	101	101
Sodium, mEq	10.4	12	12.9
Potassium, mEq	21	20	18.7
Chloride, mEq	15.2	13	11.8
Vitamins			
A, IU	2000	2010	2029
D, IU	410	402	406
E, IU	13.5	20	10.1
K, µg	54	60	74
Thiamine (B$_1$), µg	540	402	406
Riboflavin (B$_2$), µg	610	630	609
Pyridoxine, µg	410	402	406
B$_{12}$, µg	2	2	3
Niacin, mg	6.8	9	9.1
Folic acid, µg	108	107	101
Pantothenic acid, mg	3.4	3	5.1
Biotin, µg	20	34	30

Table H-2 *(Continued)*
Soy Follow-up Infant Formulas: Label Claim Nutrient Contents (per L at 20 kcal/oz)

	Enfamil NEXT STEP ProSobee LIPIL (powder only) (Mead Johnson, Evansville, IN)	Nestlé Good Start 2 Supreme Soy DHA and ARA (powder only) (Nestlé, Glendale, CA)	Similac Go & Grow Soy-Based Formula (powder only) (Abbott Nutrition, Columbus, OH)
C (ascorbic acid), mg	81	80	81
Choline, mg	162	161	81
Inositol, mg	41	40	33.8

* Partially hydrolyzed.

† From single-cell oils: *Crypthecodinium cohnii* and *Mortierella alpina*, respectively.

Appendix I

Table I-1
Formulas for Infants With Low Birth Weight and Preterm Infants (per L)

	Similac Special Care Advance 24 cal* Liquid (Abbott Nutrition, Columbus, OH)	Enfamil Premature LIPIL 24 cal* Iron Fortified Liquid (Mead Johnson, Evansville, IN)	Similac Neosure Advance 22 cal* Liquid (Abbott Nutrition, Columbus, OH)	Enfamil Enfacare LIPIL 22 cal* Liquid (Mead Johnson, Evansville, IN)	Similac Special Care 30 cal† Liquid (Abbott Nutrition, Columbus, OH)
Energy, kcal	810	810	746	740	1000
Protein, g	24	24	21	21	30
Fat, g	44.1‡	41§	41	39	67.1
Polyunsaturated, g	8.3	10.3	—	—	
Monounsaturated, g	3.5	4.5	—	—	
Saturated, g	32	26.2‖	—	—	
Linoleic acid, g	5.7	8.5	5.6	7.1	
Carbohydrate, g	84¶	90#	76.9	79	78¶
Mineral					
Calcium, mg	1460	1340	784	890	1830
Phosphorus, mg	810	670	463	490	1010
Magnesium, mg	97	55	67.2	59	122
Iron, mg	14.6	14.4	13.4	13.3	18.3
Zinc, mg	12.2	12.2	9.0	9.	15.2
Manganese, μg	100	51	75	111	120
Copper, μg	2030	1010	896	890	2540
Iodine, μg	50	200	112	111	60

Table I-1 1285

Table I-1 *(Continued)*
Formulas for Infants With Low Birth Weight and Preterm Infants (per L)

	Similac Special Care Advance 24 cal* Liquid (Abbott Nutrition, Columbus, OH)	Enfamil Premature LIPIL 24 cal* Iron Fortified Liquid (Mead Johnson, Evansville, IN)	Similac Neosure Advance 22 cal* Liquid (Abbott Nutrition, Columbus, OH)	Enfamil Enfacare LIPIL 22 cal* Liquid (Mead Johnson, Evansville, IN)	Similac Special Care 30 cal† Liquid (Abbott Nutrition, Columbus, OH)
Sodium, mEq	15	13.9	10.7	11.3	19.0
Potassium, mEq	27	21	27.1	20.2	34
Chloride, mEq	19	19.4	15.8	16.5	23
Vitamin					
A, USP Units	10 140	10 100	3433	3330	12 680
D, USP Units	1220	2200	522	590	1520
E, USP Units	32	51	27	30	41
K, µg	97	65	82	59	122
Thiamine (B$_1$), µg	2003	1620	1642	1480	2540
Riboflavin (B$_2$), µg	5030	2400	1119	1480	6290
Pyridoxine, µg	2030	1220	746	740	2540
B$_{12}$, µg	4.5	2	3.0	2.2	5.6
Niacin, mg	40.6	32	14.5	14.8	50.7
Folic acid, µg	300	280	187	192	375
Pantothenic acid, mg	15.4	9.7	6.0	6.3	19.3

Table I-1 *(Continued)*

Formulas for Infants With Low Birth Weight and Preterm Infants (per L)

	Similac Special Care Advance 24 cal* Liquid (Abbott Nutrition, Columbus, OH)	Enfamil Premature LIPIL 24 cal* Iron Fortified Liquid (Mead Johnson, Evansville, IN)	Similac Neosure Advance 22 cal* Liquid (Abbott Nutrition, Columbus, OH)	Enfamil Enfacare LIPIL 22 cal* Liquid (Mead Johnson, Evansville, IN)	Similac Special Care 30 cal† Liquid (Abbott Nutrition, Columbus, OH)
Biotin, µg	300	32	67	44	375
C (ascorbic acid), mg	300	162	112	118	380
Choline, mg	80	97	119	111	100
Inositol, mg	320	138	45	220	410

* Kcal/oz.

† To be mixed with Similac Special Care Advance 24 to increase caloric content of formula as well as other nutrients.

‡ Nonfat milk, whey protein concentrate.

‖ Included 17.4 g of MCT oils.

‡ Medium-chain triglyceride (MCT) oil, 50%; soy oil, 30%; coconut oil, 20%.

¶ Lactose, 50%; glucose polymers, 50%.

§ MCT oil, 40%; soy oil, 40%; coconut oil, 20%.

Glucose polymers, 60%; lactose, 40%.

APP

Table I-1 **1287**

Table I-2
Nutrients Provided by Human Milk Fortifiers for Preterm Infants Fed Human Milk

Nutrient	Enfamil Human Milk Fortifier (Powder, 4 packets)* (Mead Johnson, Evansville, IN)	Similac Human Milk Fortifier (4 packets) (Abbott Nutrition, Columbus, OH)	Similac Natural Care Fortifier (Liquid, 100 mL)† (Abbott Nutrition, Columbus, OH)
Energy, kcal	14	14	81.2
Protein, g	1.1	1.0	2.4
Fat, g	1	0.36	4.4
Linoleic acid, mg	140	0	568
α-Linolenic acid, mg	17	0	
Carbohydrate, g	<0.40	1.8	8.36
Vitamins			
Vitamin A, IU	950	620	1014
Vitamin D, IU	150	120	122
Vitamin E, IU	4.6	3.2	3.2
Vitamin K, µg	4.4	8.3	9.7
Vitamin C (ascorbic acid), mg	12	25	30
Thiamin, µg	150	233	203
Riboflavin, µg	220	417	503
Pyridoxine, µg	115	211	203
Niacin, mg	3	3.57	4
Pantothenic acid, mg	0.73	1.5	1.5
Biotin, µg	2.7	26	30

Table I-2 (Continued)
Nutrients Provided by Human Milk Fortifiers for Preterm Infants Fed Human Milk

Nutrient	Enfamil Human Milk Fortifier (Powder, 4 packets)* (Mead Johnson, Evansville, IN)	Similac Human Milk Fortifier (4 packets) (Abbott Nutrition, Columbus, OH)	Similac Natural Care Fortifier (Liquid, 100 mL)† (Abbott Nutrition, Columbus, OH)
Folic acid, µg	25	23	30
Vitamin B$_{12}$, µg	0.18	0.64	0.44
Minerals			
Calcium, mg	90	117	170
Phosphorus, mg	50	67	94
Magnesium, mg	1	7	9.7
Iron, mg	1.44	0.35	0.30
Zinc, mg	0.72	1	1.2
Manganese, µg	10	7.0	9.7
Copper, µg	44	170	202
Sodium, mEq	0.7	0.65	1.5
Potassium, mEq	0.74	1.6	2.7
Chloride, mEq	0.37	1.1	1.9

* Four packets of Enfamil Human Milk Fortifier is usually added to 100 mL of human milk.
† Similac Natural Care is to be diluted 1:1 with human milk.

Table I-2   1289

APP

Appendix J

The Standing Committee on the Scientific Evaluation of Dietary Reference Intakes of the Food and Nutrition Board, Institute of Medicine, National Academy of Sciences, has undertaken a comprehensive expansion of the periodic reports called Recommended Dietary Allowances (RDAs) into a set of 4 nutrient-based values known as Dietary Reference Intakes (DRIs). These reference values include the Estimated Average Requirement (EAR), Recommended Dietary Allowance (RDA), Adequate Intake (AI), and the Tolerable Upper Intake Level (UL). If sufficient scientific evidence is not available to calculate an RDA, a reference intake called an Adequate Intake (AI) is provided instead. RDAs and AIs are levels of intake recommended for individuals. They should reduce the risk of developing a condition that is associated with the nutrient in question that has a negative functional outcome. The DRIs apply to the apparently healthy general population. They are based on nutrient balance studies, the nutrient intakes of breastfed infants and healthy adults, biochemical measurement of tissue saturation or molecular function, and extrapolation from animal models. Unfortunately, only limited data are available on vitamin requirements in infants and children because of ethical, cost, and time concerns. Meeting the recommended intakes for the nutrients would not necessarily provide enough for individuals who are already malnourished, nor would they be adequate for certain disease states marked by increased nutritional requirements.

Table J-1
Dietary Reference Intakes: Recommended Intakes for Individuals, Food and Nutrition Board, Institute of Medicine

	Infants 0–6 mo	Infants 7–12 mo	Children 1–3 y	Children 4–8 y	Males 9–13 y	Males 14–18 y	Females 9–13 y	Females 14–18 y	Pregnancy ≤18 y	Lactation ≤18 y
Carbohydrate (g/day)	60*	95*	130	130	130	130	130	130	175	210
Total Fiber (g/day)	ND	ND	19*	24*	31*	38*	26*	26*	28*	29*
Fat (g/day)	31*	30*	ND	ND	ND	ND	ND	ND	ND	ND
n-6 Polyunsaturated Fatty Acids (g/day) (Linoleic Acid)	4.4*	4.6*	7*	10*	12*	16*	10*	11*	13*	13*
n-3 Polyunsaturated Fatty Acids (g/day) (α-Linolenic Acid)	0.5*	0.5*	0.7*	0.9*	1.2*	1.6*	1.0*	1.1*	1.4*	1.3*
Protein (g/kg/day)	1.52*	1.05*	0.95*	0.95*	0.95*	0.85*	0.95*	0.85*	1.1*	1.3*
Vitamin A μg/day†	400*	500*	300	400	600	900	600	700	750	1200
Vitamin C mg/day	40*	50*	15	25	45	75	45	65	80	115
Vitamin D μg/day†§	5*	5*	5*	5*	5*	5*	5*	5*	5*	5*
Vitamin E mg/day‖	4*	5*	6	7	11	15	11	15	15	19
Vitamin K μg/day	2.0*	2.5*	30*	55*	60*	75*	60*	75*	75*	75*
Thiamin (mg/day)	0.2*	0.3*	0.5	0.6	0.9	1.2	0.9	1.0	1.4	1.4
Riboflavin (mg/day)	0.3*	0.4*	0.5	0.6	0.9	1.3	0.9	1.0	1.4	1.6
Niacin (mg/day)¶	2*	4*	6	8	12	16	12	14	18	17
Vitamin B$_6$ (mg/day)	0.1*	0.3*	0.5	0.6	1.0	1.3	1.0	1.2	1.9	2.0
Folate (μg/day)#	65*	80*	150	200	300	400	300	400**	600††	500

Table J-1 *(Continued)*
Dietary Reference Intakes: Recommended Intakes for Individuals, Food and Nutrition Board, Institute of Medicine

	Infants 0–6 mo	Infants 7–12 mo	Children 1–3 y	Children 4–8 y	Males 9–13 y	Males 14–18 y	Females 9–13 y	Females 14–18 y	Pregnancy ≤18 y	Lactation ≤18 y
Vitamin B_{12} (mg/day)	0.4*	0.5*	0.9	1.2	1.8	2.4	1.8	2.4	2.6	2.8
Pantothenic Acid (mg/day)	1.7*	1.8*	2*	3*	4*	5*	4*	5*	6*	7*
Biotin (μg/day)	5*	6*	8*	12*	20*	25*	20*	25*	30*	35*
Calcium (mg/day)	210*	270*	500*	800*	1300*	1300*	1300*	1300*	1300*	1300*
Choline‡‡ (mg/day)	125*	150*	200*	250*	375*	550*	375*	400*	450*	550*
Chromium (μg/day)	0.2*	5.5*	11*	15*	25*	35*	21*	24*	29*	44
Copper (μg/day)	200*	220*	340	440	700	890	700	890	1000	1300
Fluoride (mg/day)	0.01*	0.5*	0.7*	1*	2*	3*	2*	2*	3*	3*
Iodine (μg/day)	110*	130*	90	90	120	150	120	150	220	290
Iron (mg/day)	0.27*	11	7	10	8	11	8	15	27	10
Magnesium (mg/day)	30*	75*	80	130	240	410	240	360	400	360
Manganese (mg/day)	0.003*	0.6*	1.2*	1.5*	1.9*	2.2*	1.6*	1.6*	2.0*	2.6*
Molybdenum (μg/day)	2*	3*	17	22	34	43	34	43	50	50
Phosphorus (mg/day)	100*	275*	460	500	1250	1250	1250	1250	1250	1250
Selenium (μg/day)	15*	20*	20	30	40	55	40	55	60	70
Zinc (mg/day)	2*	3	3	5	8	11	8	9	13	14
Potassium (g/day)	0.4*	0.7*	3.0*	3.8*	4.5*	4.7*	4.5*	4.7*	4.7*	5.1*
Sodium (g/day)	0.12*	0.37*	1.0*	1.2*	1.5*	1.5*	1.5*	1.5*	1.5*	1.5*
Chloride (g/day)	0.18*	0.57*	1.5*	1.9*	2.3*	2.3*	2.3*	2.3*	2.3*	2.3*

APP

Table J-1 (Continued)
Dietary Reference Intakes: Recommended Intakes for Individuals, Food and Nutrition Board, Institute of Medicine

This table (taken from the DRI reports; see http://www.iom.edu/CMS/3788/21370.aspx) presents Recommended Dietary Allowances (RDAs) in **bold type**, and Adequate Intakes (AIs) are in ordinary type followed by the symbol (*). ND indicates not determined.

* RDAs and AIs may both be used as goals for individual intake. RDAs are set to meet the needs of almost all (97%–98%) individuals in a group. For healthy breastfed infants, the AI is the mean intake. The AI for other life stage and gender groups is believed to cover needs of all individuals in the group, but lack of data or uncertainty in the data prevent being able to specify with confidence the percentage of individuals covered by this intake.

† As retinol activity equivalents (RAEs). 1 RAE = 1 μg retinol, 12 μg β-carotene, 24 μg α-carotene, or 24 μg β-cryptoxanthin in foods. The RAE for dietary provitamin A carotenoids is twofold greater than retinol equivalents (RE), whereas the RAE for preformed vitamin A is the same as RE.

‡ As cholecalciferol. 1 μg cholecalciferol = 40 IU vitamin D.

§ In the absence of adequate exposure to sunlight.

‖ As α-tocopherol. α-Tocopherol includes RRR-α-tocopherol, the only form of α-tocopherol that occurs naturally in foods, and the 2R-stereoisomeric forms of α-tocopherol (RRR-, RSR-, RRS-, and RSS-α-tocopherol) that occur in fortified foods and supplements. It does not include the 2S-stereoisomeric forms of α-tocopherol (SRR-, SSR-, SRS-, and SSS-α-tocopherol), also found in fortified foods and supplements.

¶ As niacin equivalents (NEs). 1 mg of niacin = 60 mg of tryptophan; 0–6 mo = preformed niacin (not NEs).

As dietary folate equivalents (DFEs). 1 DFE = 1 μg food folate = 0.6 μg of folic acid from fortified food or as a supplement consumed with food = 0.5 μg of a supplement taken on an empty stomach.

** In view of evidence linking folate intake with neural tube defects in the fetus, it is recommended that all women capable of becoming pregnant consume 400 μg from supplements or fortified foods in addition to intake of food folate from the diet.

†† It is assumed that women will continue consuming 400 μg from supplements or fortified food until their pregnancy is confirmed and they enter prenatal care, which ordinarily occurs after the end of the periconceptional period—the critical time for formation of the neural tube.

‡‡ Although AIs have been set for choline, there are few data to assess whether a dietary supply of choline is needed at all stages of the life cycle, and it may be that the choline requirement can be met by endogenous synthesis at some of these stages. 2004.

Table J-2
Dietary Reference Intakes (DRIs): Tolerable Upper Intake Levels (UL*), Food and Nutrition Board, Institute of Medicine

	Infants 0–6 mo	Infants 7–12 mo	Children 1–3 y	Children 4–8 y	Males/Females 9–13 y	Males/Females 14–18 y	Pregnancy ≤18 y	Lactation ≤18y
Vitamin A (µg/day)†	600	600	600	900	1700	2800	2800	2800
Vitamin C (mg/day)	ND‡	ND	400	650	1200	1800	1800	1800
Vitamin D (µg/day)	25	25	50	50	50	50	50	50
Vitamin E (mg/day)§‖	ND	ND	200	300	600	800	800	800
Vitamin K (µg/day)	ND	ND	ND	ND	ND	ND	ND	ND
Thiamin (mg/day)	ND	ND	ND	ND	ND	ND	ND	ND
Riboflavin (mg/day)	ND	ND	ND	ND	ND	ND	ND	ND
Niacin (mg/day)‖	ND	ND	10	15	20	30	30	30
Vitamin B$_6$ (mg/day)	ND	ND	30	40	60	80	80	80
Folate (µg/day)‖	ND	ND	300	400	600	800	800	800
Vitamin B$_{12}$ (mg/day)	ND	ND	ND	ND	ND	ND	ND	ND
Pantothenic acid (mg/day)	ND	ND	ND	ND	ND	ND	ND	ND
Biotin (µg/day)	ND	ND	ND	ND	ND	ND	ND	ND
Choline (mg/day)	ND	ND	1.0	1.0	2.0	3.0	3.0	3.0
Carotenoids¶	ND	ND	ND	ND	ND	ND	ND	ND
Arsenic†	ND‡	ND	ND	ND	ND	ND	ND	ND
Boron (mg/day)	ND	ND	3	6	11	17	17	17
Calcium (mg/day)	ND	ND	2.5	2.5	2.5	2.5	2.5	2.5

APP

Table J-2 *(Continued)*
Dietary Reference Intakes (DRIs): Tolerable Upper Intake Levels (UL*), Food and Nutrition Board, Institute of Medicine

	Infants 0–6 mo	Infants 7–12 mo	Children 1–3 y	Children 4–8 y	Males/Females 9–13 y	Males/Females 14–18 y	Pregnancy ≤18 y	Lactation ≤18 y
Chromium	ND	ND	ND	ND	ND	ND	ND	ND
Copper (µg/day)	ND	ND	1000	3000	5000	8000	8000	8000
Fluoride (mg/day)	0.7	0.9	1.3	2.2	10	10	10	10
Iodine (µg/day)	ND	ND	200	300	600	900	900	900
Iron (mg/day)	40	40	40	40	40	45	45	45
Magnesium (mg/day)§	ND	ND	65	110	350	350	350	350
Manganese (mg/day)	ND	ND	2	3	6	9	9	9
Molybdenum (µg/day)	ND	ND	300	600	1100	1700	1700	1700
Nickel (mg/day)	ND	ND	0.2	0.3	0.6	1.0	1.0	1.0
Phosphorus (mg/day)	ND	ND	3	3	4	4	3.5	4
Potassium	ND	ND	ND	ND	ND	ND	ND	ND
Selenium (µg/day)	45	60	90	150	280	400	400	400
Silicon‖	ND	ND	ND	ND	ND	ND	ND	ND
Sulfate	ND	ND	ND	ND	ND	ND	ND	ND
Vanadium (mg/day)§	ND	ND	ND	ND	ND	ND	ND	ND
Zinc (mg/day)	4	5	7	12	23	34	34	34
Sodium (g/day)	ND	ND	1.5	1.9	2.2	2.3	2.3	2.3
Chloride (g/day)	ND	ND	2.3	2.9	3.4	3.6	3.6	3.6

Table J-2 (Continued)
Dietary Reference Intakes (DRIs): Tolerable Upper Intake Levels (UL*), Food and Nutrition Board, Institute of Medicine

This table taken from the DRI reports; see http://www.iom.edu/CMS/3788/21370.aspx.

*UL indicates the maximum level of daily nutrient intake that is likely to pose no risk of adverse effects. Unless otherwise specified, the UL represents total intake from food, water, and supplements. Because of a lack of suitable data, ULs could not be established for vitamin K, thiamin, riboflavin, vitamin B_{12}, pantothenic acid, biotin, or carotenoids. In the absences of ULs, extra caution may be warranted in consuming amounts above recommended intakes.

† As preformed vitamin A only.

‡ ND = Not determinable because of a lack of data on adverse effects in this age group and concern with regard to lack of ability to handle excess amounts.

§ As α-tocopherol; applies to any form of supplemental α-tocopherol.

‖ The ULs for vitamin E, niacin, and folate apply to synthetic forms obtained from supplements, fortified foods, or a combination of the two.

¶ β-Carotene supplements are advised only to serve as a provitamin A source for individuals at risk of vitamin A deficiency.

APP

Table J-3
Nutrition During Pregnancy

Dietary Reference Intakes (DRIs) During Pregnancy					
	Females			Pregnancy		
Life Stage Group	14–18 y	19–30 y	31–50 y	≤18 y	19–30 y	31–50 y
Vitamin A (µg/day)*	700	700	700	750	770	770
Vitamin C (mg/day)	65	75	75	80	85	85
Vitamin D (µg/day)†‡	5§	5§	5§	5§	5§	5§
Vitamin E‖ (mg/day)	15	15	15	15	15	15
Vitamin K (µg/day)	15§	15§	15§	15§	15§	15§
Thiamin (mg/day)	1.1	1.1	1.1	1.4	1.4	1.4
Riboflavin (mg/day)	1.0	1.1	1.1	1.4	1.4	1.4
Niacin (mg/day)¶	14	14	14	18	18	18
Vitamin B₆ (mg/day)	1.2	1.3	1.3	1.9	1.9	1.9
Folate (µg/day)#	400**	400**	400**	600††	600††	600††
Vitamin B₁₂ (µg/day)	2.4	2.4	2.4	2.6	2.6	2.6
Pantothenic acid (mg/day)	5§	5§	5§	6§	6§	6§
Biotin (µg/day)	25§	30§	30§	30§	30§	30§
Choline‡‡ (mg/day)	400§	425§	425§	450§	450§	450§
Calcium (mg/day)	1300§	1000§	1000§	1300§	1000§	1000§
Chromium (µg/day)	24§	25§	25§	29§	30§	30§
Copper (µg/day)	890	900	900	1000	1000	1000
Fluoride (mg/day)	3§	3§	3§	3§	3§	3§
Iodine (µg/day)	150	150	150	220	220	220
Iron (mg/day)	15	18	18	27	27	27
Magnesium (mg/day)	360	310	320	400	350	360
Manganese (mg/day)	1.6§	1.8§	1.8§	2.0§	2.0§	2.0§
Molybdenum (µg/day)	43	45	45	50	50	50
Phosphorus (mg/day)	1250	700	700	1250	700	700
Selenium (µg/day)	55	55	55	60	60	60
Zinc (mg/day)	9	8	8	12	11	11
Potassium (mg/day)	4.7§	4.7§	4.7§	4.7§	4.7§	4.7§
Sodium (mg/day)	1.5§	1.5§	1.5§	1.5§	1.5§	1.5§
Chloride (mg/day)	2.3§	2.3§	2.3§	2.3§	2.3§	2.3§

Table J-3 *(Continued)*
Nutrition During Pregnancy

Note: This table (taken from the DRI reports; see http://www.iom.edu/CMS/3788/21370.aspx) presents Recommended Dietary Allowances (RDAs) in **bold type** and Adequate Intakes (AIs) in ordinary type followed by the symbol (§).

* As retinol activity equivalents (RAEs). 1 RAE = 1 μg retinol, 12 μg β-carotene, 24 μg α-carotene, or 24 μg β-cryptoxanthin in foods. The RAE for dietary provitamin A carotenoids is twofold greater than retinol equivalents (REs), whereas the RAE for preformed vitamin A is the same as the RE.

† As cholecalciferol. 1 μg cholecalciferol = 40 IU vitamin D.

‡ In the absence of adequate exposure to sunlight.

§ RDAs and AIs may both be used as goals for individual intake. RDAs are set to meet the needs of almost all individuals in a group (97%–98%). For healthy breastfed infants, the AI is the mean intake. The AI for other life stage and gender groups is believed to cover needs of all individuals in the group, but lack of data or uncertainty in the data prevent being able to specify with confidence the percentage of individuals covered by this intake.

‖ As α-tocopherol. α-Tocopherol includes RRR-α-tocopherol, the only form of α-tocopherol that occurs naturally in foods, and the 2R-stereoisomeric forms of α-tocopherol (RRR-, RSR-, RRS-, and RSS-α-tocopherol) that occur in fortified foods and supplements. It does not include the 2S-stereoisomeric forms of α-tocopherol (SRR-, SSR-, SRS-, and SSS-α-tocopherol), also found in fortified foods and supplements.

¶ As niacin equivalents (NEs). 1 mg of niacin = 60 mg of tryptophan; 0–6 mo = preformed niacin (not NEs).

As dietary folate equivalents (DFEs). 1 DFE = 1 μg food folate = 0.6 μg of folic acid from fortified food or as a supplement consumed with food = 0.5 μg of a supplement taken on an empty stomach.

** In view of evidence linking folate intake with neural tube defects in the fetus, it is recommended that all women capable of becoming pregnant consume 400 μg from supplements or fortified foods in addition to intake of food folate from the diet.

†† It is assumed that women will continue consuming 400 μg from supplements or fortified food until their pregnancy is confirmed and they enter prenatal care, which ordinarily occurs after the end of the periconceptional period—the critical time for formation of the neural tube.

‡‡ Although AIs have been set for choline, there are few data to assess whether a dietary supply of choline is needed at all stages of the life cycle, and it may be that the choline requirement can be met by endogenous synthesis at some of these stages.

APP

Appendix K

Fig. K-1

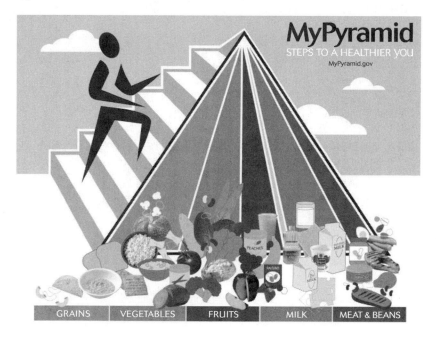

Illustration of mini-poster from the US Department of Agriculture's MyPyramid, which provides food-based guidance for professionals and the public to help implement the recommendations of the Dietary Guidelines for Americans for people 2 years and older (for Web version of poster, see http://www.mypyramid.gov/downloads/MiniPoster.pdf).

APP

Fig. K-2.A
Simplified version.

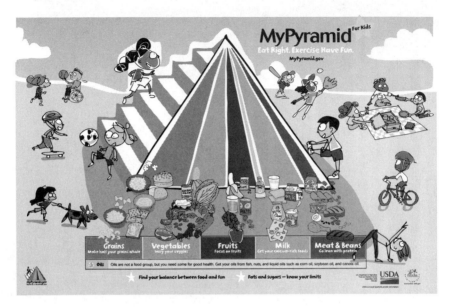

Fig. K-2.A and Fig. K-2.B Illustration of posters from the US Department of Agriculture's MyPyramid for Kids, which provides age-appropriate information for children 6 to 11 years of age about the 2005 Dietary Guidelines for Americans and MyPyramid (for Web version, see http://teamnutrition.usda.gov/Resources/mpk_poster.pdf for simplified version or http://teamnutrition.usda.gov/Resources/mpk_poster2.pdf for advanced version).

Fig. K-2.B
Advanced version.

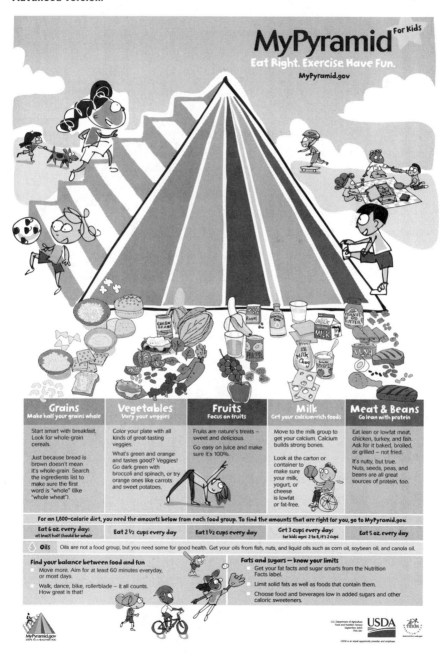

Fig. K-3

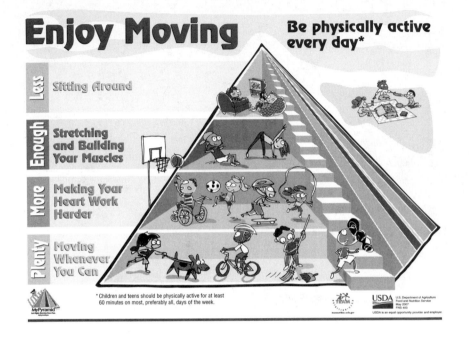

Appendix L

Table L-1
Beverages and Alcoholic Drinks: Calories and Selected Electrolytes (per fl oz)*

Beverage	Energy, kcal	Sodium, mg	Potassium, mg	Phosphorous, mg
Regular Soft Drinks				
Cola or "pepper"	11	1	1	3
Decaffeinated cola or "pepper"	13	1	1	3
Lemon-lime (clear)	13	3	0	0
Orange	15	4	1	0
Root beer	13	4	0	0
Ginger ale	10	2	0	0
Tonic water	10	4	0	0
Diet Soft Drinks				
Diet cola or "pepper"	1	2	2	3
Decaffeinated diet cola or "pepper"	0	1	2	3
Diet lemon-lime	0	2	0	1
Diet root beer	0	5	3	1
Other Beverages				
Club soda, seltzer, sparkling water	0	6	1	0
Apricot nectar, canned	18	1	36	3
Apple juice, unsweetened	15	1	37	2
Cranberry juice cocktail, bottled	17	1	4	0
Grape juice, canned, unsweetened	19	1	4	3
Grapefruit juice, canned, unsweetened	12	0	47	3
Orange juice, raw	14	0	62	5
Pear nectar, canned	17	2	12	2
Pineapple juice, canned, unsweetened	17	1	41	3
Tomato juice, canned, without salt added	5	3	70	5

Table L **1311**

Table L-1 *(Continued)*
Beverages and Alcoholic Drinks: Calories and Selected Electrolytes (per fl oz)*

Beverage	Energy, kcal	Sodium, mg	Potassium, mg	Phosphorous, mg
Alcoholic Beverages				
Beer	13	1	8	4
Gin, rum, vodka, whiskey (80 proof)	64	0	1	1
Dessert wine (sweet)	47	3	27	3
Table wine (red)	25	1	37	7

*Based on data from US Department of Agriculture, Agricultural Research Service. 2005. USDA Nutrient Database for Standard Reference, Release 18. Nutrient Data Available at: http://www.ars.usda.gov/ba/bhnrc/ndl.

Nutrition Data System for Research software version 2005. Minneapolis, MN: Nutrition Coordinating Center (NCC), University of Minnesota; 2005.

Appendix M

Table M-1
Carbohydrate Content of Juices

Fruit or Juice	Fructose	Glucose	Sucrose	Sorbitol
Prune	14.0	23.0	0.6	12.7
Pear	6.6	1.7	1.7	2.1
Sweet cherry	7.0	7.8	0.2	1.4
Peach	1.1	1.0	6.0	0.9
Apple	6.0	2.3	2.5	0.5
Grape	6.5	6.7	0.6	Trace
Strawberry	2.2	2.3	0.9	0.0
Raspberry	2.0	1.9	1.9	0.0
Blackberry	3.4	3.2	0.2	0.0
Pineapple	1.4	2.3	7.9	0.0
Orange	2.4	2.4	4.7	0.0

Source: American Academy of Pediatrics. The use of fruit juice in the diets of young children. *AAP News.* 1991;7:11

Appendix N

Food-Drug Interactions

Food-drug interactions occur when an ingested food or nutrient alters the effects of a medication. Food components can enhance, delay, or decrease drug absorption. Some foods or nutrients in the foods can alter drug metabolism and, thereby, alter the therapeutic effect of the medication. Certain medications should be administered with food to minimize gastrointestinal distress or to maximize the drug's effect. There are many food-drug interactions reported in the literature of varying clinical significance.

In recent years, there has been increased awareness of the potential for medications to interact with grapefruit juice. Drugs that interact with grapefruit and/or grapefruit juice undergo cytochrome p450 oxidative metabolism in the intestinal wall or liver. Grapefruit juice contains substances that have been demonstrated to affect the cytochrome p450 (CYP) system by binding to the isoenzyme as a substrate and impairing first-pass metabolism by direct inactivation or inhibition of the enzyme. This seems to result in a selective down-regulation of CYP3A4 in the small intestine. For certain drugs that are known to be metabolized this way, less drug is metabolized before absorption, so greater amounts reach the systemic circulation, leading to higher blood levels and potential increases in therapeutic and/or toxic effects. If patients are accustomed to ingesting grapefruit juice while on chronic medications, it is best that they avoid significant increases or decreases in the amount of grapefruit juice they are ingesting.

A drug-nutrient interaction is the effect a medication has on the bioavailability or metabolism of a nutrient in food. Some well-known drug-nutrient interactions include monoamine oxidase (MAO) inhibitors with tyramine containing foods, such as red wine and aged cheese, and warfarin with green, leafy vegetables and other foods high in vitamin K. In addition, drugs can affect the metabolism or disposition of minerals and vitamins. Examples of this include low folate levels in patients on chronic anticonvulsant therapy and diuretics causing potassium depletion. Laxatives can decrease the absorption of many vitamins and minerals.

The following tables provide information about some specific food-drug interactions and issues related to administration of medications. Please be advised that the information in this list is not a substitute for clinical judgment. Readers are also advised to consult current references, because formulation of some of these medications may have changed since the publication of this handbook.

Table N-1
Drugs for Which Absorption Is Increased by Food

Atovaquone (administer with a high-fat meal)
Cefpodoxime
Cefuroxime
Erythromycin
Griseofulvin (administer with a high-fat meal)
Morphine sulfate (oral solution)
Nitrofurantoin
Theophylline sustained release (food may induce sudden release of sustained-release preparation)

APP

Table N-2
Drugs for Which Absorption May Be Delayed by Food or Milk

Medication Name	Comments
Acetaminophen	Rate may decreased by high carbohydrate load
Amitriptyline	Increased fiber may decrease effect
Ampicillin	Food decreases rate and extent of absorption
Cefaclor	Delays and decreases peak concentration
Cephalexin	Food may delay absorption
Cimetidine	Limit xanthine-containing food and beverages
Ciprofloxacin	Dairy products/minerals decrease concentration
Digoxin	Increased fiber or pectin may decrease absorption
Diltiazem	Food may increase absorption from sustained-release product
Fluoxetine	Food may delay absorption
Furosemide	Avoid acidic solutions
Glipizide	Rate of absorption, not extent, delayed by food
Lansoprazole	Food decreases bioavailability by 40%
Metronidazole	
Omeprazole	Administering with food decreases level by 50%
Penicillin	
Trazodone	Rate of absorption, not extent, delayed by food
Valproic acid	Rate of absorption, not extent, delayed by food
Zafirlukast	Food decreases absorption by 40%
Zalcitabine	

(Drugs in this category should either be administered on an empty stomach or taken consistently with regard to food.)

Table N-3
Drugs That Should Be Administered on an Empty Stomach

Medication Name	Comments
Ampicillin	
Amprenavir	Avoid antacids and high-fat meals
Captopril	
Ceftibuten	
Cloxacillin	
Dicloxacillin	
Didanosine	
Diltiazem	
Efavirenz	
Erythromycin base	
Indinavir	
Iron	Avoid milk and antacids
Isoniazid	
Itraconazole oral solution	
Ketoconazole	Administer 2 h before antacids; may administer with food to decrease gastrointestinal distress
Lansoprazole	
Levofloxacin oral solution	
Loracarbef	
Mycophenolate	
Nifedipine	
Omeprazole	
Rifampin	May administer with food to decrease gastrointestinal distress
Tacrolimus	Separate antacids by at least 2 hours
Tetracycline	
Zafirlukast	

APP

Table N-4
Miscellaneous Food-Nutrient Effects

Drug or Class	Nutrient	Comment
Albuterol	Glucose	May cause hyperglycemia
	Potassium	May cause hypokalemia
Amiloride	Potassium	May cause hyperkalemia
Amphotericin	Magnesium	Causes electrolyte wasting
	Potassium	
	Sodium	
Aspirin	Folate	May cause folate deficiency
	Vitamin C	May increase vitamin C excretion
	Iron	May cause iron-deficiency anemia
Captopril	Potassium	May cause small increases in serum potassium
	Zinc	May cause zinc deficiency (long-term)
Ciprofloxacin	Enteral feeds	Enteral feeds may interfere with absorption
	Caffeine	May increase caffeine concentration
Cisplatin	Magnesium	Causes magnesium depletion
Cholestyramine	Fat-soluble vitamins	May result in deficiency
Corticosteroids	Glucose	May cause hyperglycemia
Digoxin	Calcium	May cause arrhythmias as a result of inotropic effect
	Antacids, fiber	May decrease digoxin effects
	Licorice	Avoid natural licorice
Ethambutol	Aluminum salts	May decrease absorption of ethambutol
Furosemide	Calcium	May cause electrolyte depletion
	Magnesium	
	Potassium	
	Sodium	
Gabapentin	Glucose	May cause fluctuations in glucose and weight gain
Glipizide, glyburide	Alcohol	Disulfuram-like reaction with alcohol
Insulin	Concentrated sugar	Can increase insulin requirement
Isoniazid	Pyridoxine	Isoniazid is a B_6 antagonist
Isotretinoin	Vitamin A	May result in increased toxicity

Table N-4 *(Continued)*
Miscellaneous Food-Nutrient Effects

Drug or Class	Nutrient	Comment
Lithium	Sodium	Maintain constant sodium intake
	Caffeine	Caffeine may decrease lithium effects to avoid toxicity
MAOIs	Tyramine	Dietary tyramine can cause hypertensive crisis
Methotrexate	Folic acid	Folic acid may decrease effects
Metronidazole	Alcohol	Causes disulfuram-like reaction
Mineral oil	Fat-soluble vitamins	May decrease absorption of fat-soluble vitamins
NSAIDs	Potassium	May cause hyperkalemia in patients with renal impairment or on supplements or potassium-sparing diuretics
Omeprazole, Lansoprozole	Acid	Acid-labile drug, administer with beads intact
Pancreatic enzymes	Calcium carbonate	May increase drug effect
	Magnesium hydroxide	
Phenobarbital	Protein	Be consistent with protein intake
	Vitamin C	Displaces drug from binding sites
	Vitamin D	Deficiency may result from malabsorption
Phenytoin	Enteral feeds	May interfere with phenytoin absorption
	Folate	High-dose folic acid may reverse drug effects
	Calcium	Phenytoin decreases absorption
	Vitamin D	May interfere with phenytoin metabolism
	Vitamin C	Displaces drug from binding sites
	Glucose	May cause hypoglycemia
Primidone	Folic acid	Megaloblastic anemia attributable to folate deficiency may occur
Propranolol	Protein-rich foods	May result in increased propranolol effects
Spironolactone	Potassium	May cause hyperkalemia; avoid supplements
Sulfasalazine	Folic acid	May inhibit absorption of folate
Terbutaline	Glucose, potassium	May cause hyperglycemia, hypokalemia
Theophylline	Caffeine	May cause increased theophylline toxicity

Table N-4 *(Continued)*
Miscellaneous Food-Nutrient Effects

Drug or Class	Nutrient	Comment
Thiazide diuretics	Magnesium	May cause electrolyte depletion
	Sodium	
	Potassium	
Trimethoprim	Folate	May cause folate depletion
Valproic acid	Carbonated beverages	Avoid carbonated beverages with syrup
	Carnitine	May cause carnitine deficiency with Hyperammonemia
Warfarin	Vitamin K	May inhibit response to warfarin
	Vitamins A, C, E	May alter prothrombin time
Zidovudine	Folate, B_{12}	Deficiency may increase myelosuppression

MAOI indicates monoamine oxidase inhibitors; NSAID, nonsteroidal anti-inflammatory drug.

Table N-5
Drug-Grapefruit Juice Interactions

Drug	Effect of Grapefruit Juice on Drug Concentration	Clinical Significance	Onset
Amlodipine	Increases	Minor	Delayed
Atorvastatin	Increases	Moderate	Rapid
Buspirone	Increases	Moderate	Rapid
Carbamazepine	Increases	Moderate	Rapid
Cisapride	Increases	Major	Rapid
Clomipramine	Increases	Moderate	Delayed
Cyclosprine	Increases	Moderate	Delayed
Diazepam	Increases	Moderate	Rapid
Felodipine	Increases	Moderate	Rapid
Indinavir	Decreases	No dose changes needed per manufacturer	Not applicable
Itraconazole	Decreases	Moderate	Rapid
Lovastatin	Increases	Moderate	Rapid
Methylprednisolone	Increases	Unknown	Unknown
Midazolam	Increases	Moderate	Rapid

Table N-5 *(Continued)*
Drug-Grapefruit Juice Interactions

Drug	Effect of Grapefruit Juice on Drug Concentration	Clinical Significance	Onset
Nifedipine	Increases	Moderate	Rapid
Nimodipine	Increases	Moderate	Rapid
Nisoldipine	Increases	Moderate	Rapid
Omeprazole	Decreases	Minor	Rapid
Pimozide	Increases	Major	Rapid
Pravastatin	Increases	None	Unknown
Quinidine	Unknown	Moderate	Rapid
Saquinavir	Increases	Moderate	Rapid
Sertraline	Increases	Moderate	Delayed
Simvastatin	Increases	Moderate	Rapid
Sirolimus	Increases	Moderate	Delayed
Tacrolimus	Increases	Moderate	Delayed
Triazolam	Increases	Minor	Rapid

Sources:

Bland SE. Drug-food interactions. *J Pharm Soc Wisc.* 1998;Nov/Dec:28–35

Elbe D. Drug commentary: grapefruit juice-drug interactions. *BC Pharm.* 1998;7:18–19

Kane G, Lipsky J. Drug-grapefruit juice interactions. *Mayo Clin Proc.* 2000;75(9):933–942

Kirk J. Significant drug-nutrient interactions. *Am Fam Physician.* 1995;51:1175–1182

Lacy C, ed. *Drug Information Handbook.* 7th ed. Hudson, OH: Lexi-Comp Inc; 2006

Maka D, Murphy L. Drug-nutrient interactions: a review. *Adv Pract Acute Crit Care.* 2000;11:580–588

Beers MH, Berkow R, Bogin RM, Fletcher AJ, eds. *Merck Manual of Diagnosis and Therapy.* Whitehouse Station, NJ: Merck Inc; 1999

Thomson Micromedex. *Micromedex Healthcare Series.* Greenwood Village, CO: Thomson. Available at: http://www.micromedex.com/products/hcs/. Accessed August 6, 2007

APP

Appendix O

Table O-1

Review of Fad Diets and Other Popular Weight-Loss Diets

Diet	Premise	Positive Aspects	Negative Aspects
Fad Diets: None Are Recommended for Children or Adolescents			
Acid Alkaline Diet			
The Acid Alkaline Diet for Optimum Health: Restore Your Health by Creating Balance in Your Diet—Christopher Vasey, ND; Healing Arts Press, 2003	The body needs equal amounts of acid and alkaline to achieve balance.	Does not give quick solutions for weight loss or health. Recommends increasing intake of omega-3 fatty acids, avoiding trans-fatty acids, and consuming plenty of fiber-rich foods and green, leafy vegetables.	Little research available to support theories. Uses scientific words and concepts that are difficult to understand. Recommends organic foods that are expensive and do not provide a health benefit. Recommends doses of many vitamins and minerals well above recommendations.
The Acid Alkaline Balance Diet: An Innovative Program for Ridding Your Body of Acidic Wastes—Felicia Drury Kliment; Contemporary Books/McGraw Hill Companies, 2002			
Atkins Diet			
Dr. Atkins' New Diet Revolution—Robert C. Atkins, MD; Avon, 2002	Very low carbohydrate to induce ketosis.	Weight loss.	Serious ketoacidosis has been reported. Low-carbohydrate, high-fat diets are not more efficacious in long-term weight loss than low-energy or low-fat diets. Long-term effects of high-fat diets and ketosis are unknown. Deficient in vitamins, minerals, and dietary fiber. Allows high intakes of fat without specific type recommendations.
Dr. Atkins' New Diet Revolution, New and Revised—Robert C. Atkins, MD; Collins, 2002			
The Atkins Essentials: A Two-Week Program to Jump-Start Your Low Carb Lifestyle—Atkins Health & Medical Information; Avon, 2004			

Table O-1 *(Continued)*
Review of Fad Diets and Other Popular Weight-Loss Diets

Diet	Premise	Positive Aspects	Negative Aspects
The Carbohydrate Addict's Diet: The Lifelong Solution to Yo-Yo Dieting—Rachael F. Heller, Richard F. Heller; Signet, 1993	By stopping carbohydrate addiction, the amount of insulin produced decreases and people lose weight and reduce the risk of "carbohydrate-addicted" diseases.	As with all low-carbohydrate, low-energy diets, weight loss will ensue.	Faulty premise—there is no scientific support for a carbohydrate addiction. Complicated diet schedules and confusing advice (eg, high-fiber, low-carbohydrate foods). Not recommended for pregnant or nursing women or those with diabetes, hypoglycemia, a history of heart disease, or kidney or liver disorders because of specialized diet plans.
Carbohydrate Addicted Kids—Harper Collins, 1997			
The Carbohydrate Addict's 7-Day Plan: Start Fresh on Your Low-Carb Diet!—Rachael F. Heller, Richard F. Heller; Signet, 2004			
The Carbohydrate Addict's Lifespan Program: A Personalized Plan for Becoming Slim, Fit and Healthy in Your 40s, 50s, 60s and Beyond—Rachael F. Heller, Richard F. Heller; Plume, 1998			
The Complete Scarsdale Medical Diet—Herman Tarnower, MD; Bantam Doubleday Dell, 1980	Low-energy, low-carbohydrate. Ketosis.		Does not meet vitamin and mineral requirements. Very rapid weight loss, but because compliance is difficult, this is usually temporary. Limited food choices and does not promote a balanced diet. Not recommended for diabetics, pregnant women, or alcoholics. Scientific support is unavailable.

Table O-1 *(Continued)*
Review of Fad Diets and Other Popular Weight-Loss Diets

Diet	Premise	Positive Aspects	Negative Aspects
The Detox Diet: The How-To & When-To Guide for Cleansing the Body—Elson M. Haas, MD; Celestial Arts Publishing, 1996	Not specifically for weight loss, but rather "eliminates toxins from the body."	Promotes the intake of fruits, vegetables, and fiber.	Prolonged fasting and use of enemas may have unnecessary risks. Many herbal supplements are included in this diet and have possible adverse effects. Foods that are considered "toxic" contain important nutrients. Relies on testimonials.
The New Detox Diet: The Complete Guide for Lifelong Vitality with Recipes, Menus, and Detox Plans—Elson M. Haas, MD, Daniella Chace; Celestial Arts Publishing, 2004			
Dr. Kushner's Personality Type Diet—Robert Kushner and Nancy Kushner; St Martin's Press, 2003	Recognizing and controlling behavior patterns that guide food choices.	Does not promote rapid weight loss. Does not limit intake of any foods or food groups.	There is no scientific support that "specific personalities" are related to nutrient needs or specific recommendations for diet. Recommends high fiber but does not give guidelines on how to gradually incorporate this into the diet. Does not discuss sodium when talking about reading food labels. Does not stress maintenance of weight loss.
Eat Right 4 Your Type: The Individualized Diet Solution to Staying Healthy, Living Longer, & Achieving Your Ideal Weight—Peter J. D'Adamo, ND; JP Putnam & Sons, 1996	Your blood type reflects your unique internal chemistry and determines your susceptibility to illness, the foods you should eat, and ways to avoid health problems.		No scientific support. Eliminates whole food groups and restricts nutritious foods from every food group. Relies heavily on case histories and anecdotes. Implies quick, unintentional weight loss. Author has little credibility.

APP

Table 0-1 *(Continued)*
Review of Fad Diets and Other Popular Weight-Loss Diets

Diet	Premise	Positive Aspects	Negative Aspects
The False Fat Diet—Elson M. Haas, MD, Cameron Stauth; Ballantine, 2000	Excess weight is a result of food "reactions."		No scientific support. Use of "personalized diets." Elimination diets can be especially risky for children.
The Food Revolution: How Your Diet Can Help Save Your Life and Our World—John Robbins; Conari Press, 2001		Promotes high intake of fruits, vegetables, and whole grains as well as low intake of refined and processed foods. High-energy, high-fat foods are discouraged.	Author has no credentials as a health expert. Restricts intake of all animal products, which may lead to nutrient deficiencies. Pregnant and lactating women should exercise caution if following this diet.
The G-Index Diet: The Missing Link that Makes Permanent Weight Loss Possible—Richard N. Podell, Johanna C. Burani, William Proctor; Warner Books Inc, 1993	Low–glycemic-index diet.	Written with recipes and menus by a registered dietitian with an advanced degree. Does not restrict foods or food groups. Physical activity is encouraged.	Evidence lacking that diets based on the glycemic index promote permanent weight loss.
How I Gave Up My Low-Fat Diet and Lost 40 Pounds...And How You Can Too!—Dana Carpender; Fair Winds Press, 2003	Low carbohydrate.		Relies on testimonials. Low carbohydrate.
The Insulin Resistance Diet: How to Turn Off Your Body's Fat-Making Machine—Cheryle R. Hart, MD, Mary Kay Grossman, RD; McGraw-Hill, 2001	Balancing carbohydrate and protein foods to reduce insulin spiking.	Recommends a permanent lifestyle change rather than a "quick fix" for weight loss. Promotes use of mono- and polyunsaturated fats.	Unproven scientific premise. Complicated regimen for eating carbohydrate and protein foods. Diet is not appropriate for people with renal disease. No guidelines for sodium or energy intake.

Table O-1 *(Continued)*
Review of Fad Diets and Other Popular Weight-Loss Diets

Diet	Premise	Positive Aspects	Negative Aspects
Living Low Carb: The Complete Guide to Long-Term Low-Carb Dieting—Fran McCullough; Little, Brown & Co, 2000	Low carbohydrate.		No indication that long-term weight loss results from this diet. Author is not a qualified expert in the medical or nutrition fields. Recommends low/no carbohydrates, which could lead to dangerous ketosis. Restricts everything white. Advises not to worry about fat intake. Not sufficient for people with kidney disease or women who are pregnant or nursing. Promotes rapid weight loss.
The Metabolic Typing Diet—William L. Wolcott, Trish Fahey; Doubleday, 2000	Diet based on "homeostatic controls."		There is no scientific premise for this diet; simplistic conclusions to a complex problem. Recommendations for specific products, brands, and supplements are inappropriate. Raw or minimally cooked foods are encouraged and are not appropriate for everyone. States chronic health problems (eg, AIDS) are the result of inadequate nutrition. Diet should not be used for those with kidney disease, diabetes, gout, or heart disease.
The Omega Diet: The Lifesaving Nutritional Program Based on the Diet of the Island of Crete—Artemis P. Simopoulos, MD, Jo Robinson; Harper Collins, 1999	Fat is essential: 35% kcal from fat.	Recommends intake of omega-3 fatty acids and monounsaturated fats as well as avoidance of saturated and trans-fats. Recommendations are supported by scientific research.	Modest increases in low-density lipoprotein cholesterol. Mercury levels in fish.

APP

Table O-1 (Continued)
Review of Fad Diets and Other Popular Weight-Loss Diets

Diet	Premise	Positive Aspects	Negative Aspects
The Paleo Diet: Lose Weight and Get Healthy by Eating the Foods You Were Designed to Eat—Loren Cordain, PhD; Wiley, 2001	Low carbohydrate- High protein.		No scientific evidence. Eliminates dairy, grains, and legumes. Confusing guidelines for macronutrient intakes. Claims that food can change body chemistry. Makes unrealistic and incorrect claims (eg, cure for Crohn disease). Recommends buying certain products.
The New Sugar Busters!—H. Leighton Steward, Morrison C. Bethea, MD, Sam S. Andrews, MD, Luis A. Balart, MD; Ballantine Books, 2002	Manipulates insulin and glucagon secretion through food choices.	Weight loss attributable to low overall energy in the diet. Does not eliminate whole food groups but uses the glycemic index to limit carbohydrate choices. Restricts refined sugars.	Restricts some fruits and vegetables that could contribute vitamins and minerals to the diet. Compliance is difficult because some foods are restricted and timing of eating some foods is dictated.
The Rotation Diet—Martin Katahn, PhD; Bantam Books, 1987	Rotating low energy intake for weight loss.	Very low-calorie diet, promotes rapid weight loss. Katahn developed the Vanderbilt University weight loss program.	No indication that this diet supports long-term weight loss. Unproven claims. Contains elements of sacrifice. Should be avoided by diabetics, children, adolescents, pregnant or lactating women, and highly active people.
The South Beach Diet: The Delicious, Doctor-Designed, Foolproof Plan for Fast and Healthy Weight Loss—Arthur Agatston, MD; Rodale, 2003	Emphasizes carbohydrates and fat type as part of healthy, balanced diet.	Encourages eating a variety of healthy foods and snacks on a regular basis (after phase 1). Developed by medical professional.	Promises immediate weight loss. Temporarily eliminates certain foods from the diet (phase 1). Does not recommend physical activity.

Table O-1 *(Continued)*
Review of Fad Diets and Other Popular Weight-Loss Diets

Diet	Premise	Positive Aspects	Negative Aspects
The Starch Blocker Diet: The Safe, New Way to Eat the Foods You love And Lose Weight—Steven Rosenblatt, MD, PhD, Cameron Stauth; Harper Collins, 2003	Use of a starch blocker pill to neutralize calories from starch.	Developed by medical professional.	Conflicting evidence as to whether "starch blockers" block digestion of starch and result in weight loss. Relies on an over-the-counter pill. Should not be used by pregnant or lactating women, children, or diabetics.
Your Last Diet! The Sugar Addict's Weight-Loss Plan—Kathleen DesMaisons, PhD; Ballantine Books, 2002	Eliminating white foods from the diet to "detoxify" body to lose weight.	Recommends keeping a food journal.	Not supported in scientific literature. Designed for people who are "sugar sensitive." Uses testimonials. Recommends digestive enzymes and supplements (flaxseed, fish oil, vitamin C).
Suzanne Somers' Eat, Cheat, and Melt the Fat Away—Suzanne Somers; Three Rivers Press, 2003	Low carbohydrate, high protein.	Promotes complex carbohydrate, high fiber consumption. Encourages lifestyle modification. Does not exclude whole food groups.	No scientific evidence to backup claims. Author has no credibility in nutrition. Uses testimonials. Promotes certain products.
What Color is Your Diet?—David Heber, MD, PhD, Susan Bowerman, MS, RD; Harper Collins, 2002	Intake a variety of nutrients to maximize health and longevity.	Developed by medical and nutrition professionals. Promotes lifelong dietary changes. Does not offer a quick fix. Recommends intake of a variety of fruits and vegetables. Does not restrict food groups—although some foods are restricted.	Recommends soy, which may not be for everyone. People taking potassium-sparing diuretics may need to consult a doctor before beginning this diet.

APP

Table O-1 *(Continued)*
Review of Fad Diets and Other Popular Weight-Loss Diets

Diet	Premise	Positive Aspects	Negative Aspects
The Zone			
A Week in the Zone: A Quick Course in the Healthiest Diet for You—Barry Sears, PhD, Deborah Kotz; Harper Collins, 2000	Low carbohydrate, high protein to maintain hormones within zones from meal to meal.	Immediate weight loss in adults.	Low carbohydrate—restricts fruit, vegetables, and grains—suggesting vitamin supplementation is needed. Expensive. Confusing and complicated to follow. Limited scientific support. Athletes should not follow this diet. Not backed by any professional organizations or scientific evidence.
Enter The Zone: The Dietary Road Map To Lose Weight Permanently, Reset Your Genetic Code, Prevent Disease, Achieve Maximum Physical Performance—Barry Sears, PhD, Bill Lawren; Harper Collins, 1995			
Mastering The Zone: The Next Step in Achieving Superhealth and Permanent Fat Loss—Barry Sears, PhD; Harper Collins, 1997			
The Sonoma Diet: Trimmer Waist, Better Health in Just 10 Days!—Connie Guttersen, PhD, RD; Meredith Books, 2005	Lose weight by following the Mediterranean diet.	Does not eliminate food groups. Encourages physical activity. Emphasizes food enjoyment, portion control, food label reading, and trans fat elimination.	May be too idealistic for people to follow long-term. Relies heavily on cooking. Eliminates fruit and restricts calories in wave 1.

Table O-1 *(Continued)*
Review of Fad Diets and Other Popular Weight-Loss Diets

Diet	Premise	Positive Aspects	Negative Aspects
Other Types of Diets or Lifestyle Changes: Although Some Represent Healthy Lifestyles, These Diets Are Not Recommended for Most Children or Adolescents			
Dieting for Dummies—Jane Kirby, RD, American Dietetic Association; For Dummies, 2003	Overall health/wellness.	Supported by the American Dietetic Association. Focuses on consuming a wide variety of foods and no food group is excluded. Promotes a healthy lifestyle with which compliance is easy, rather than a quick fix or a magic food. Recommends daily physical activity.	
Dr. Shapiro's Picture Perfect Weight Loss: The Visual Program for Permanent Weight Loss—Howard M. Shapiro, DO; Rodale, 2000	Lifestyle change involving becoming aware of food and its nutritional aspects, as well as taking control of your food choices.	Provides an overview of basic nutrition. Pictures provide examples of food choices and portion sizes. No foods are eliminated; instead, a variety of alternatives to high-fat foods are offered. No quick, unhealthy, unrealistic weight loss claims.	Vague when explaining specific energy goals; relies on individual hunger cues rather than calorie counting. Soy is recommended instead of milk. Sodium intake is not addressed. It may be difficult to equate pictures to real food and serving sizes.

Table O-1 (Continued)
Review of Fad Diets and Other Popular Weight-Loss Diets

Diet	Premise	Positive Aspects	Negative Aspects
Eat, Drink, and Be Healthy: The Harvard Medical School Guide to Healthy Eating—Walter C. Willett, MD; Free Press, 2001	Healthy lifestyle through better food choices and exercise.	Recommendations are based on scientific evidence and aimed at optimal health Not a weight-loss diet.	Includes alcohol, which may encourage people to drink, which could have negative health and social consequences. Encourages calcium antacids as a cheaper and sometimes better way to consume calcium than dairy products.
Eat More, Weigh Less: Dr. Dean Ornish's Life Choice Program for Losing Weight Safely While Eating Abundantly—Dean Ornish, MD; Harper Collins, 2000	Lifestyle modification to lower cholesterol and reduce risk of heart disease.	Weight loss. Reduces atherosclerotic plaque.	Vegetarian based, very low fat (10% of energy). Diet may be deficient in zinc and vitamin B_{12}. No portion sizes are listed in the sample menu or on the recipes. High-fiber intake may cause gastrointestinal distress. Compliance is difficult.

Appendix P

PEDIATRIC NUTRITION HANDBOOK

Table P-1
Sources of Dietary Fiber

Food	Fiber (g/100g)	Fiber (g/serving)	Food	Fiber (g/100g)	Fiber (g/serving)
Fruits			**Uncooked Vegetables**		
Apple (without skin)	2.1	2.9/1 medium-sized apple	Bean sprout, soy	2.6	2.6/1 cup
Apple (with skin)	2.5	3.5/1 medium-sized apple	Celery, diced	1.5	3.7/1 large stalk
Apricot (fresh)	1.7	1.8/3 apricots	Cucumber	0.8	0.2/6–8 slices with skin
Apricot (dried)	8.1	10.5/1 cup	Lettuce, sliced	1.5	20/1 wedge iceberg
Banana	2.1	2.5/1 banana	Mushrooms, sliced	2.5	0.8/half cup (sliced)
Blueberries	2.7	3.9/1 cup	Onions, sliced	1.3	1.3/1 cup
Cantaloupe	1.0	2.7/half edible portion	Peppers, green, sliced	1.3	1.0/1 pod
Cherries, sweet	1.2	1.2/15 cherries	Tomato	1.5	1.8/1 tomato
Dates	7.6	13.5/1 cup (chopped)	Spinach	4.0	8.0/1 cup (chopped)
Grapefruit	1.3	1.6/half edible portion	**Legumes**		
Grapes	1.3	2.6/10 grapes	Baked beans, Tomato sauce	7.3	18.6/1 cup
Oranges	2.0	2.6/1 orange	Dried peas, cooked	4.7	4.7/half cup (cooked)
Peach (with skin)	2.1	2.1/1 peach	Kidney beans, cooked	7.9	7.4/half cup (cooked)
Peach (without skin)	1.4	1.4/1 peach	Lima beans, cooked/canned	5.4	2.6/half cup (cooked)
Pear (with skin)	2.8	4.6/1 pear	Lentils, cooked	3.7	1.9/half cup (cooked)
Pear (without skin)	2.3	3.8/1 pear	Navy beans, cooked	6.3	3.1/half cup (cooked)
Pineapple	1.4	2.2/1 cup (diced)			

Table P-1 (Continued)
Sources of Dietary Fiber

Food	Fiber (g/100g)	Fiber (g/serving)	Food	Fiber (g/100g)	Fiber (g/serving)
Plums, damsons	1.7	1.7/3 plums	Breads, Pastas, and Flours		
Prunes	11.9	11.9/11 dried prunes			
Raisins	8.7	2.2/packet	Bagels	1.1	1.1/half bagel
Raspberries	5.1	6.3/1 cup	Bran muffins	6.3	6.3/muffin
Strawberries	2.0	3.0/1 cup	Cracked wheat	4.1	4.1/slice
Watermelon	0.3	1.3/4 × 8-inch wedge	Crisp bread, rye	14.9	
Juices			Crisp bread, wheat	12.9	
			French bread	2.0	0.67/slice
Apple	0.3	0.74/1 cup	Italian bread	1.0	0.33/slice
Grapefruit	0.4	1.0/1 cup	Mixed grains	3.7	
Grape	0.5	1.3/1 cup	Oatmeal	2.2	5.3/1 cup
Orange	0.4	1.0/1 cup	Pita bread (5 in)	0.9	
Papaya	0.6	1.5/1 cup	Pumpernickel bread	3.2	1.0/slice
Vegetables Cooked			Raisin bread	2.2	0.55/slice
			White bread	2.2	0.55/slice
Asparagus, cut	1.5	1.5/7 spears	Whole-wheat bread	5.7	1.66/slice
Beans, string green	2.6	3.4/1 cup	Pasta and Rice Cooked		
Broccoli	2.8	5.0/1 stalk			

Table P-1 (Continued)
Sources of Dietary Fiber

Food	Fiber (g/100g)	Fiber (g/serving)	Food	Fiber (g/100g)	Fiber (g/serving)
Brussel sprouts	3.0	4.6/7–8 sprouts	Macaroni	0.8	1.0/1 cup (cooked)
Cabbage, red	2.0	2.9/1 cup (cooked)	Rice, brown	1.2	2.4/1 cup (cooked)
Cabbage, white	2.0	2.9/1 cup (cooked)	Rice, polished	0.3	0.6/1 cup (cooked)
Carrots	3.0	4.6/1 cup	Spaghetti (regular)	0.8	1.0/1 cup (cooked)
Cauliflower	1.7	2.1/1 cup	Spaghetti (whole wheat)	2.8	3.0/1 cup (cooked)
Corn, canned	2.8	4.5/1 cup	Flours and Grains		
Kale leaves	2.6	2.9/1 cup (cooked)			
Parsnip	3.5	5.4/1 cup (cooked)	Bran, corn	62.2	18.7/oz
Peas	4.5	7.2/1 cup (cooked)	Bran, oat	27.8	8.3/oz
Potato (without skin)	1.0	1.4/1 boiled	Bran, wheat	41.2	12.4/oz
Potato (with skin)	1.7	2.3/1 boiled	Rolled oats	5.7	13.7/1 cup (cooked)
Spinach	2.3	4.1/1 cup (raw)	Rye flour (72%)	4.5	5.2/1 cup
Squash, summer	1.6	3.4/1 cup (cooked, diced)	Rye flour (100%)	12.8	15.4/1 cup
Sweet potatoes	2.4	2.7/1 baked (5x2 inches)	Wheat flour		
Turnip	2.2	3.4/1 cup (cooked, diced)	Whole meal (100%)	8.9	10.6/1 cup
Zucchini	2.0	4.2/1 cup (cooked, diced)	Brown (85%)	7.3	8.8 1 cup
			White (72%)	2.9	2.9/1 cup

APP

Table P-1 *(Continued)*
Sources of Dietary Fiber

Food	Fiber (g/100g)	Fiber (g/serving)	Food	Fiber (g/100g)	Fiber (g/serving)
				Nuts	
			Almonds	7.2	3.6/half cup (slivered)
			Peanuts	8.1	11.7/1 cup
			Filberts	6.0	2.8/half cup

Table P-2
Available Over-the-Counter Preparations of Fiber

Brand	Form	Fiber Source	Fluid Required?
Benefiber*	Caplets	Guar gum Microcrystalline cellulose	No
	Tablets	Guar gum	No
	Powder	Guar gum	4 oz/tbsp
Citrucel[†]	Caplets	Methylcellulose	8 oz/dose
	Powder	Methylcellulose	8 oz/tbsp
Fiber Choice[‡]	Tablets	Inulin	No
Fibercon[§]	Caplets	Calcium polycarbophil	8 oz/dose
Metamucil[‖]	Capsules	Psyllium husk	8 oz/dose
	Powder	Psyllium husk	8 oz/dose
	Wafers	Psyllium husk	8 oz/dose
Senokot[¶]	Powder	Fructose, wheat bran, sucrose, gum, no senna	8 oz/dose
Ultra Fiber[#]	Caplets	Chicory fiber, citrus fiber, microcrystalline cellulose, oat bran fiber, prune fiber, apple fiber, psyllium fiber	8 oz/dose

* Novartis, Freemont, MI.

[†] GlaxoSmithKline, Philadelphia, PA.

[‡] GlaxoSmithKline, Philadelphia, PA.

[§] Wyeth Consumer Healthcare, Richmond, VA.

[‖] Procter & Gamble, Mason, OH.

[¶] Purdue Products LP, Stamford, CT.

[#] Alva-Amco Pharmacal Companies Inc, Niles, IL.

APP

Appendix Q

Table Q-1

Approximate Calcium Contents of 1 Serving of Some Common Foods That Are Good Sources of Calcium

Food	Serving Size	Calcium Content, mg	No. of Servings to Equal Calcium Content in 1 Cup of Low-Fat Milk
Dairy Foods			
Whole milk	1 cup (244 g)	246	1.0
Low-fat (1%) milk	1 cup (244 g)	264	—
Nonfat milk	1 cup (245 g)	223	1.2
Yogurt, nonfat, fruit variety	6 oz (170 g)	258	1.0
Frozen yogurt, vanilla, soft serve	1/2 cup (72 g)	103	2.6
Cheese	1 1-oz slice (28 g)	202	1.3
Cheese, pasteurized, processed	1 3/4-oz slice (21 g)	144	1.8
Cheese, ricotta, part skim milk	1/2 cup (124 g)	337	0.7
Nondairy Foods			
Salmon, sockeye canned, drained, with bones	3 oz (85 g)	203	1.3
Tofu, firm, prepared with calcium sulfate and magnesium chloride	1/2 cup (126 g)	204	1.3
White beans, cooked, boiled	1 cup (179 g)	161	1.6
Broccoli, cooked	1 cup, chopped (156 g)	62	4.3
Collards, cooked, boiled, drained	1 cup, chopped (190 g)	266	1.0
Baked beans, canned	1 cup (253 g)	127	2.1
Tomatoes, canned, stewed	1 cup (255 g)	87	3.0
Foods Fortified with Calcium			
Calcium-fortified orange juice	1 cup (240 mL)	300	0.9
Selected fortified breakfast cereals	3/4–1 cup (30 g)	100	2.6

APP

Table Q-1 *(Continued)*
Approximate Calcium Contents of 1 Serving of Some Common Foods That Are Good Sources of Calcium

Food	Serving Size	Calcium Content, mg	No. of Servings to Equal Calcium Content in 1 Cup of Low-Fat Milk
Instant oatmeal, fortified, plain, prepared with water	1/2 cup (117 g)	65	4.1
English muffin, plain, enriched, with calcium propionate	1 muffin (57 g)	99	2.7
Calcium-fortified soy milk*	1 cup (240 mL)	200–500	0.5–1.3

Reprinted from Greer FR, Krebs NF, American Academy of Pediatrics, Committee on Nutrition. Optimizing bone health and calcium intakes of infants, children, and adolescents. *Pediatrics*. 2006;117:578–585.

Source: US Department of Agriculture, Agriculture Research Service. US Department of Agriculture Nutrient Data Laboratory. Available at: www.ars.usda.gov/main/site_main.htm?modecode=12354500. Accessed December 21, 2005.

* Native soy milk contains 10 mg of calcium per cup (240 mL).

Table Q-2
Calcium Content of Foods (mg/Serving)*

100	150	200	250
1 cup cooked kale (94)	1 cup ice cream (184)	3.5 oz almonds (246)	1 cup milk (352)
3 tbsp light (reg) molasses (41)	1/2 cup cooked rhubarb (174)	6 medium stalks broccoli (328)	1/2 cup cooked ricotta cheese (337)
5 oz sunflower seeds (81)	3 oz canned salmon with bones (188)	1/2 cup soybean curd (Tofu) (212)	1 cup of cooked collards (266)
9 oz oysters (41)		1 oz cheddar or Muenster cheese (204)	
1/2 cup maple syrup (108)		1 oz Swiss or Parmesan cheese (224)	
16 Brazil nuts (112)		1 cup cooked spinach (245)	
1 cup cooked navy beans (126)			
1 oz feta or mozzarella cheese (140)			
1 cup cottage cheese, regular or low fat (138)			
1 cup beet greens (44)			
1 cup of dandelion greens (148)			
2 sardines with bones (92)			
1 tbsp blackstrap molasses (145)			

Source: US Department of Agriculture, Agricultural Research Service. USDA Nutrient Database for Standard Reference, Release 18. 2005. Available at: http://www.ars.usda.gov/ba/bhnrc/ndl. Accessed August 22, 2007

* Column value categorizations are approximate.

APP

Appendix R

Table R-1
Iron Content of Selected Foods

Food	Portion	Iron, mg
Apricots, raw	3 medium	0.41
Avocado, California	1 medium	1.11
Banana, raw	1 medium	0.31
Black-eyed peas, boiled	1/2 cup	2.1
Bread, white	1 slice	0.75
Bread, whole wheat	1 slice	0.92
Broccoli, boiled	1/2 cup	0.52
Brussels sprouts	1/2 cup	0.94
Butter	1 tsp	0.00
Cheddar cheese	1 oz	0.19
Chicken, light and dark, without skin, roasted	3.5 oz	1.19
Chocolate, bittersweet	1 oz	0.89
Chocolate, sweet	1 oz	1.13
Clams, raw	3 oz	11.88
Cream of wheat, instant, cooked	3/4 cup	8.98
Egg, white	1 large	0.03
Egg, whole	1 large	0.92
Egg, yolk	1 large	0.46
Frankfurter, beef	1 frank, 8/lb	0.86
Frankfurter, turkey	1 frank, 8/lb	0.83
Garbanzos, canned	1/2 cup	1.62
Grape juice, from frozen concentrate	8 oz	0.78
Grapes, adherent skin	1 cup	0.55
Halibut, cooked	3 oz	0.71
Ham, 11% fat	1 oz	0.38
Hamburger, extra lean, broiled, medium	3.5 oz	2.00
Lettuce, iceberg	1 leaf	0.06
Lettuce, romaine, shredded	1/2 cup	0.46
Liver (beef)	3 1/2 oz	4.90
Liver (pork)	3 1/2 oz	19.82
Milk, 2%	8 oz	0.15

APP

Table R-1 *(Continued)*
Iron Content of Selected Foods

Food	Portion	Iron, mg
Molasses, blackstrap	1 T	0.30
Navy beans, canned	1/2 cup	2.42
Oatmeal, cooked	3/4 cup	1.19
Orange juice, from frozen concentrate	8 oz	0.99
Oysters, raw	6 medium	4.86
Papaya nectar	8 oz	0.85
Peanut butter, smooth	1 T	0.60
Potato, baked with skin, medium	6 1/2 oz	1.87
Prune juice	1/2 cup	1.51
Prunes, dried, cooked	1/2 cup	2.32
Raisins, seedless	2/3 cup	1.80
Rice, brown, cooked	1 cup	0.82
Rice, white, enriched	1 cup	0.38
Soybeans, green, boiled	1/2 cup	2.25
Spinach, boiled	1/2 cup	3.21
Tomato juice	1/2 cup	0.52
Tortilla, corn, enriched	1 (1 oz)	0.66
Yeast, brewers	1 oz	1.99
Yogurt, low-fat	8 oz	0.18

Source: US Department of Agriculture, Agricultural Research Service. USDA Nutrient Database for Standard Reference, Release 18. Washington, DC: US Department of Agriculture; 2005. Available at: http://www.ars.usda.gov/ba/bhnrc/ndl.

Appendix S

Table S-1
Zinc Content of Common Household Portions of Selected Foods

Food	Portion	Zinc, mg
Fish (flounder)	3 oz	0.54
Oysters, eastern, wild, raw	3 oz	77.28
Crab, blue, cooked	3 oz	3.51
Chicken Dark meat Light meat	 3.5 oz 3.5 oz	 2.78 1.22
Turkey Dark meat Light meat	 3.5 oz 3.5 oz	 4.42 2.02
Beef, tenderloin	3.5 oz	4.75
Pork, loin	3 oz	2.51
Bologna	1 oz	0.65
Liver (beef)	3 oz	4.5
Whole egg	1 large	0.53
Lentils	1 cup	2.51
Milk, whole	1 cup	0.98
Cheese (cheddar)	1 oz	0.88
Bread White Whole wheat	 1 oz 1 oz	 0.21 0.55
Rice White Brown	 1/2 cup 1/2 cup	 0.29 0.61
Cornmeal, dry	1/2 cup	0.50
Oatmeal, cooked	1/2 cup	0.57
Bran flakes	1 oz	1.42
Corn flakes	1 oz	0.14

Source: US Department of Agriculture, Agricultural Research Service. USDA Nutrient Database for Standard Reference, Release 18. 2005. Available at: http://www.ars.usda.gov/ba/bhnrc/ndl.

Appendix T

Table T-1
Commercially Available Parenteral Nutrition Solutions

Contents	Solutions Designed for Infants					Solutions Designed for Individuals ≥1 Year		
	Aminosyn PF 10%*	TrophAmine 10%†	Premasol 10%†	Aminosyn 3.5%*	Aminosyn II 3.5%*	FreAmine III 10%†	Novamine*	Travasol 10%‡
Essential Amino Acids (g/100 mL)								
Isoleucine	0.760	0.820	0.820	0.252	0.231	0.690	0.570	0.600
Leucine	1.200	1.400	1.400	0.329	0.350	0.910	0.790	0.730
Lysine	0.677	0.820	0.820	0.252	0.368	0.730	0.900	0.580
Methionine	0.180	0.340	0.340	0.140	0.060	0.530	0.570	0.400
Phenylalanine	0.427	0.48	0.480	0.154	0.104	0.560	0.790	0.560
Threonine	0.512	0.420	0.420	0.182	0.140	0.400	0.570	0.420
Tryptophan	0.180	0.200	0.200	0.056	0.070	0.150	0.190	0.180
Valine	0.673	0.780	0.780	0.280	0.175	0.660	0.730	0.580
Nonessential Amino Acids (g/100 mL)								
Alanine	0.698	0.540	0.540	0.448	0.348	0.710	1.650	2.070
Arginine	1.227	1.200	1.200	0.343	0.356	0.950	1.120	1.150
Histidine§	0.312	0.480	0.480	0.105	0.105	0.280	0.680	0.480
Proline	0.812	0.680	0.680	0.300	0.253	1.120	0.680	0.680
Serine	0.495	0.380	0.380	0.147	0.186	0.590	0.450	0.500
Taurine	0.070	0.025	0.025	—	—	—	—	—
Tyrosine	0.044	0.240	0.240	0.031	0.095	—	0.030	0.040

Table T-1 (Continued)
Commercially Available Parenteral Nutrition Solutions

Contents	Solutions Designed for Infants			Solutions Designed for Individuals ≥1 Year				
	Aminosyn PF 10%*	TrophAmine 10%†	Premasol 10%‡	Aminosyn 3.5%*	Aminosyn II 3.5%*	FreAmine III 10%†	Novamine*	Travasol 10%‡
Glycine	0.385	0.360	0.360	0.448	0.175	1.400	0.790	1.030
Glutamic acid	0.820	0.500	0.500	—	0.258	—	0.570	—
Aspartic acid	0.527	0.320	0.320	—	0.245	—	0.330	—
Cysteine	—	<0.016	<0.016	—	—	—	—	—
N-ac-L-tyrosine	0.044	0.240	0.240	—	—	—	—	—
Nitrogen (g/100 mL)	1.52	1.55	1.55	0.55	0.54	1.53	1.8	1.65

* Hospira, Lake Forest, IL.

† B. Braun Medical Inc, Bethlehem, PA.

‡ Baxter, Deerfield, IL.

§ Histidine is considered an essential amino acid in infants and in renal failure.

Appendix U

Table U-1
Selected Enteral Products for Special Indications

Product	Energy, kcal/L	Protein Source	Protein g/L	Carbohydrate Source	Carbohydrate g/L	Fat Source	Fat g/L	Fiber g/L	Purpose
Additions*	526/100g	Na caseinate, whey protein isolate	31.6/100 g	Corn-syrup solids	47.4/100 g	Canola oil, soy lecithin	26.3/100 g		Neutral-flavored powdered blend of protein, carbohydrate, and fat used to supplement regular food
Beneprotein*	25/7g (1 scoop)	Whey protein isolates	6	None	0	None	0		Protein powder supplement
Boost*	1010	Milk protein concentrate	42	Corn-syrup solids, sucrose	180	Canola, high-oleic sunflower, and corn oils	17	13	Nutritionally complete liquid food, lactose-free, with fiber and fructo-oligosaccharides
Boost High Protein*	1010	Milk protein concentrate, Na and Ca caseinate	61	Corn-syrup solids, sucrose	139	Canola, high-oleic sunflower, and corn oils	23		High-protein, nutritionally complete oral supplement
Boost Plus*	1520	Na and Ca caseinate, milk protein concentrate	59	Corn-syrup solids, sucrose	190	Canola, high-oleic sunflower and corn oils	58		High-calorie, nutritionally complete oral supplement
Boost Diabetic*	1060	Sodium and calcium caseinates (milk), L-arginine	58.2	Tapioca dextrin, fructose, corn-syrup solids	84	Canola oil	49.4	14.8	Specifically formulated for use in the dietary management of diabetes mellitus

APP

Table U-1 (Continued)
Selected Enteral Products for Special Indications

Product	Energy, kcal/L	Protein Source	g/L	Carbohydrate Source	g/L	Fat Source	g/L	Fiber g/L	Purpose
Carnation Instant Breakfast*	1000	Ca caseinate	35	Corn-syrup solids, sucrose	132.4	Canola and corn oils, soy lecithin	36.8		Oral supplement, lactose free, gluten free
Carnation Instant Breakfast Plus*	1500	Ca caseinate	52.4	Corn-syrup solids, sucrose	176.4	Canola and corn oils, soy lecithin	64.8		High-calorie, lactose-free, oral supplement
Compleat*	1070	Chicken, Na caseinate, pea puree	48	Corn-syrup, maltodextrin, fruits, vegetables,	128	Canola oil, chicken	40	6.0	Blenderized tube feed formulated from traditional foods
Compleat Pediatric*	1000	Chicken, Na caseinate, pea puree	38	Hydrolyzed cornstarch, fruits, vegetables, apple juice Corn-syrup solids, fruits, vegetables, cranberry juice	130	High-oleic sunflower, soybean, MCT (18%) oils, canola oil, chicken	39	6.8	Intact protein, formulated from traditional foods including meats, vegetables, and fruits
Crucial*	1500	Hydrolyzed casein, L-arginine	94	Maltodextrin	134	MCT oil (50%), deodorized fish oil, soy oil, soy lecithin	68		High-calorie and protein peptide-based formula designed for critically ill patients

Table U-1 (Continued)
Selected Enteral Products for Special Indications

Product	Energy, kcal/L	Protein Source	g/L	Carbohydrate Source	g/L	Fat Source	g/L	Fiber g/L	Purpose
Diabeti-source*	1200	Soy protein, L-arginine	60	Corn-syrup, fructose, tapioca dextrin, vegetables, fruits	100	Oil, menhaden oil	59	15	Traditional food ingredients, designed for abnormal glucose tolerance and stress-induced hypoglycemia
EleCare†	1000	Free L-amino acids	30	Corn-syrup solids	107	High-oleic safflower, MCT (33%) oil, and soy oils	48		Nutritionally complete elemental formula specifically indicated for children who need an amino acid-based medical food or who cannot tolerate intact protein
Duocal‡	490/100 g		0	Hydrolyzed cornstarch	73	Corn, coconut, MCT (35%) oils	22		Powdered carbohydrate and fat supplement
Enlive†	1234	Whey protein isolate	41	Corn maltodextrin, sucrose	267		0		High-calorie, fat-free, clear liquid oral supplement
Ensure Fiber†	1060	Na and Ca caseinate, soy protein isolate	38	Maltodextrin, sucrose, soy fiber, oat fiber, fructo-oligosaccharides	177	High-oleic safflower, canola, and corn oils	26	11.8	Complete or supplemental nutrition with fiber and fructo-oligosaccharides

APP

Table U-1 (Continued)
Selected Enteral Products for Special Indications

Product	Energy, kcal/L	Protein Source	Protein g/L	Carbohydrate Source	Carbohydrate g/L	Fat Source	Fat g/L	Fiber g/L	Purpose
Ensure†	1060	Ca caseinate, soy protein isolate, whey protein concentrate	38	Corn-syrup, sucrose, maltodextrin	167	Corn, high-oleic safflower, and canola oils	25		Nutritionally complete oral supplement
Ensure High Calcium†	950	Ca and Na caseinates, soy protein isolate	51	Sucrose, maltodextrin	129	High-oleic safflower, canola, and soy oils	0		Supplemental high-protein oral nutrition with 1667 mg Ca/L
Ensure High Protein†	950	Ca and Na caseinates, soy protein isolate	51	Sucrose, maltodextrin	128	High-oleic safflower, canola, and soy oils	0		High-protein, complete oral nutritional supplement
Ensure Plus†	1500	Na and Ca caseinate, soy protein isolate	55	Corn-syrup, maltodextrin, sucrose	211	High-oleic safflower, canola, and corn oils	0		High-calorie, complete oral supplement
Ensure Plus HN†	1500	Na and Ca caseinate, soy protein isolate	62	Maltodextrin, sucrose	200	Corn oil	50		High-calorie, high-protein, nutritionally complete liquid for oral supplementation or tube feeding
FAA*	1000	Free amino acids	50	Maltodextrin, cornstarch	176	Soybean and MCT (25%) oils	11.2		Low-fat elemental diet with 20% of calories from free amino acids

Table U-1 *(Continued)*
Selected Enteral Products for Special Indications

Product	Energy, kcal/L	Protein Source	g/L	Carbohydrate Source	g/L	Fat Source	g/L	Fiber g/L	Purpose
Fibersource Standard*	1200	Soy concentrate, soy isolate	43	Corn-syrup, Maltodextrin	170	Canola and MCT (20%) oils	39	10	Higher calories, contains soluble and insoluble fiber
Fibersource HN*	1200	Soy isolate, soy concentrate	53	Corn-syrup, Maltodextrin	160	Canola and MCT (20%) oils	39	10	Higher calories and protein, contains soluble and insoluble fiber
Glucerna†	1000	Na and Ca caseinate	41.8	Maltodextrin, fructose, soy fiber	95.6	High-oleic safflower and canola oils, soy lecithin	54.4	14.1	Supplemental or complete tube feeding or oral nutrition for patients with abnormal glucose tolerance
Glytrol*	1000	Ca and K caseinate	45	Maltodextrin, corn starch, fructose, gum arabic, pectin, soy polysaccharides	100	Canola, high-oleic safflower and MCT (20%) oils, soy lecithin	47.5	15	Fiber, fat, and carbohydrate containing, designed for better glucose control
Hepatic-Aid§	1176	L-amino acids	44	Maltodextrin, sucrose	169	Partially hydrogenated soybean oil, lecithin, mono- and diglycerides	36		High-branched-chain amino acid and high-calorie supplement for patients with chronic liver disease; contains no vitamins or minerals

Table U-1 *(Continued)*
Selected Enteral Products for Special Indications

Product	Energy, kcal/L	Protein Source	Protein g/L	Carbohydrate Source	Carbohydrate g/L	Fat Source	Fat g/L	Fiber g/L	Purpose
Immun-Aid[5]	1000	Lactalbumin, supplemental amino acids	80	Maltodextrin	120	MCT (50%) and canola oils	22		High-nitrogen, nutritionally complete feeding for immunocompromised patients
Impact with fiber*	1000	Na and Ca caseinate, L-arginine	56	Maltodextrin	140	Palm kernel and sunflower oil, menhaden oil	28	10	Designed for critically ill patients who have fiber needs but not high energy needs
Impact Glutamine*	1300	Wheat protein hydrolysate, free amino acids, sodium caseinate	78	Maltodextrin	150	Palm kernel, menhaden, and sunflower oils	43		High-glutamine (15 g/L), immune-enhancing enteral formula for critically ill patients
Impact 1.5*	1500	Na and Ca caseinate, L-arginine	84	Maltodextrin	140	Palm kernel and sunflower oil, menhaden and MCT (55%) oil	69		High calorie and high protein designed for critically ill patients
Isocal*	1060	Ca and Na caseinate, soy protein isolate	34	Maltodextrin	135	Soy and MCT (20%) oils	44		Nutritionally complete, isotonic, tube-feeding formula

Table U-1 *(Continued)*
Selected Enteral Products for Special Indications

Product	Energy, kcal/L	Protein Source	g/L	Carbohydrate Source	g/L	Fat Source	g/L	Fiber g/L	Purpose
Isocal HN*	1060	Na and Ca caseinate, soy protein isolate	44	Maltodextrin	124	Soy and MCT (40%) oils	45		Moderately high-nitrogen, isotonic, nutritionally complete tube feeding
Isosource*	1200	Soy isolate	43	Corn-syrup, maltodextrin	170	Canola and MCT (20%) oils	39		High-calorie soy protein formula
Isosource 1.5 Cal*	1500	Na and Ca caseinate	68	Sugar Maltodextrin	170	Canola, MCT (30%), and soybean oils	65	8	High calorie, high nitrogen, contains soluble and insoluble soy fiber
Isosource HN*	1200	Soy isolate	53	Corn-syrup, maltodextrin	160	Canola and MCT (20%) oils	39		High-nitrogen, high-calorie soy protein formula
Isosource VHN*	1000	Na and Ca caseinate	62	Maltodextrin	130	Canola and MCT (50%) oils	29	10	High nitrogen, isotonic, contains soluble and insoluble fiber
Jevity 1 cal†	1060	Na and Ca caseinate	44.3	Maltodextrin, soy fiber, Corn-syrup	154.7	High-oleic safflower, canola, and MCT (20%) oils	34.7	14.4	Isotonic, fiber-containing, nutritionally complete tube-feeding formula
Jevity 1.2 cal†	1200	Na and Ca caseinate, soy protein isolate	55.5	Corn-syrup, maltodextrin, fructo-oligosaccharide, fiber blend	171.5	High-oleic safflower, canola, and MCT (19%) oils	39.3	12	Higher-calorie, high-protein, fiber-containing tube feeding

APP

Table U-3 **1373**

Table U-1 *(Continued)*
Selected Enteral Products for Special Indications

Product	Energy, kcal/L	Protein Source	g/L	Carbohydrate Source	g/L	Fat Source	g/L	Fiber g/L	Purpose
Kindercal with fiber‖	1060	Milk protein concentrate	30	Maltodextrin, sucrose, (gum Arabic, soy fiber)	135	Canola, high-oleic sunflower, corn, and MCT (20%) oils	44	6.3	Nutritionally complete, lactose-free oral beverage for children 1–10 y of age
Kindercal TF with fiber‖	1060	Milk protein concentrate	30	Sugar, maltodextrin, (gum Arabic, soy fiber)	135	Canola, high-oleic sunflower, MCT (20%), and corn oils	44	6.3	Nutritionally complete, isotonic, lactose-free tube feeding for children 1–10 y of age
MCT oil*	115 kcal/tbsp 8.3 kcal/g	None	0	None	0	Coconut oil	14 g/tbsp		Fat supplement or substitute for patients with long-chain fatty acid malabsorption—directly absorbed into portal vein
Microlipid*	68 kcal/tbsp	None	0	None	0	Safflower oil	7.5 g/tbsp		50% Fat emulsion for special dietary use in oral or tube-feeding formulas
Modulen IBD*	1000	Acid casein	36	Glucose syrup, sucrose	110	Milk fat, MCT (25%) and corn oils	47		Oral intact protein formula designed for people with Crohn disease

Table U-1 (Continued)
Selected Enteral Products for Special Indications

Product	Energy, kcal/L	Protein Source	g/L	Carbohydrate Source	g/L	Fat Source	g/L	Fiber g/L	Purpose
Neocate Jr‡	1000	Free amino acids	30	Corn-syrup solids	104	MCT (35%), canola, high-oleic safflower, and coconut oils	50		Nutritionally complete elemental formula for children >1 y of age with severe gastrointestinal impairment; more vitamins and minerals than Neocate 1+
Neocate 1+‡	1000	Free amino acids	25	Corn-syrup solids	146	MCT (35%), canola, high-oleic safflower and coconut oils	35		Elemental diet suitable for children >1 y of age with protein hypersensitivity or allergy
Nepro†	2000	Ca, Mg, and Na caseinate, milk protein isolate	70	Corn-syrup, sucrose, fructo-oligosaccharides	222.7	High-oleic safflower and canola oils	95.6		Very high-calorie, complete oral or tube feeding designed for dialysis patients
NovaSource Pulmonary*	1500	Na and Ca caseinates	75	Corn-syrup, sugar	150	Canola and MCT (20%) oils	68	8	High-calorie and high-nitrogen formula, designed for pulmonary patients

Table U-1 (Continued)
Selected Enteral Products for Special Indications

Product	Energy. kcal/L	Protein		Carbohydrate		Fat		Fiber g/L	Purpose
		Source	g/L	Source	g/L	Source	g/L		
NovaSource Renal*	2000	Na and Ca caseinate, l-arginine	74	Corn-syrup, fructose	200	High-oleic sun-flower, corn, and MCT (14%) oils	100		Very high calorie, vi-tamin, and mineral profile specifically formulated for dialysis patients in a Tetra Pak (Pully/Lausanne, Switzerland)
NovaSource 2.0*	2000	Ca and Na caseinate	90	Corn-syrup, sucrose, maltodextrin	220	Canola and MCT (20%) oils	88		Very high calorie, high nitrogen, reduced level of sodium in a Tetra Pak
Nutren 1.0 With fiber*	1000	Ca and K caseinate	40	Maltodextrin, corn-syrup solids (soy polysaccharides)	127	Canola, MCT (25%), and corn oils, soy lecithin	38	14	Complete liquid nutrition, fiber for management of diarrhea or consti-pation
Nutren 1.5*	1500	Ca and K caseinate	60	Maltodextrin	169	MCT (50%), canola, and corn oils, soy lecithin	67.6		High calorie for fluid restriction, 50% MCT oil
Nutren 2.0*	2000	Ca and K caseinate	80	Corn-syrup solids, maltodextrin, sucrose	196	MCT (75%), canola, and corn oils, soy lecithin	104		Very high calorie, severe fluid restric-tion, 75% MCT oil

Table U-1 *(Continued)*

Selected Enteral Products for Special Indications

Product	Energy, kcal/L	Protein Source	g/L	Carbohydrate Source	g/L	Fat Source	g/L	Fiber g/L	Purpose
Nutren Jr With fiber*	1000	Casein, whey	30	Maltodextrin, sucrose (soy polysaccharides)	110	MCT (25%), canola, and soybean oils, soy lecithin	49.6	6	Balanced formula designed to meet needs of children 1–10 y of age
Nutren Pulmonary*	1500	Ca and K caseinate	68	Maltodextrin	100	Canola, MCT (40%), and corn oils, soy lecithin	94.8		High fat content, designed to reduce carbon dioxide production
Nutren Replete with fiber*	1000	Ca and K caseinate	62.4	Maltodextrin, corn-syrup solids (soy polysaccharides)	113.2	Canola and MCT (25%) oils, soy lecithin	34	14	High protein, vita-min, and mineral profile designed for wound healing
NutriHep*	1500	L-amino acids, whey protein (50% BCAA)	40	Maltodextrin, modified corn starch	290	MCT (70%), canola, and corn oils, soy lecithin	21.2		High branched-chain amino acids, low aromatic and ammonogenic amino acids
NutriRenal*	2000	Ca and K caseinate	70	Corn-syrup solids, maltodextrin, sucrose	205	MCT (50%), canola, and corn oils	104		High calorie, high biological protein, designed for the patient on dialysis

Table U-1 *(Continued)*
Selected Enteral Products for Special Indications

Product	Energy, kcal/L	Protein Source	g/L	Carbohydrate Source	g/L	Fat Source	g/L	Fiber g/L	Purpose
Optimental†	1000	Soy protein hydrolysate, partially hydrolyzed Na caseinate, free arginine	51.3	Maltodextrin, sucrose, fructo-oligosaccharides	138.5	Sardine oil/MCT structured lipid, canola, and soybean oils	28.4		Complete elemental oral or tube-feeding formula designed for patients with malabsorptive conditions
Osmolite†	1060	Na and Ca caseinates, soy protein isolate	37.1	Maltodextrin	151.1	High-oleic safflower, canola, and MCT (20%) oils	34.7		Isotonic, low-residue, complete nutrition for oral or tube-feeding use
Osmolite 1 cal†	1060	Na and Ca caseinates, soy protein isolate	44.3	Maltodextrin	143.9	High-oleic safflower, canola, and MCT (20%) oils	34.7		Isotonic, nutritionally complete, high-nitrogen, mild-flavored liquid for oral or tube feeding
Osmolite 1.2 cal†	1200	Na and Ca caseinates	55.5	Maltodextrin	157.5	High-oleic safflower, canola, and MCT (19%) oils	39.3		High-calorie, high-nitrogen complete oral or tube feeding
Oxepa†	1500	Na and Ca caseinates	62.7	Sucrose, maltodextrin	105.3	Canola, MCT (25%), and borage and refined, deodorized sardine oils	93.8		High-calorie complete tube feeding formula for patients with lung injury

Table U-1 *(Continued)*
Selected Enteral Products for Special Indications

Product	Energy, kcal/L	Protein Source	g/L	Carbohydrate Source	g/L	Fat Source	g/L	Fiber g/L	Purpose
Pediasure and Pediasure Enteral with fiber†	1000	Na caseinate, whey protein concentrate	30	Maltodextrin, sucrose	138	High-oleic safflower, soy, and MCT (20%) oils	40	8	Complete oral or tube feeding designed for patients 1–10 y of age
Pediatric E028‡	1000	Free amino acids	25	Maltodextrin, sucrose	146	MCT (33%), canola, and high-oleic safflower oils	35		Ready-to-feed, flavored elemental liquid for children >1 y of age with severe gastrointestinal impairment
Pediatric Peptinex DT*	1000	Casein hydrolysate, free amino acids	30	Maltodextrin, food starch modified—corn	138	MCT (50%), soybean oil (50%)	39		Nutritionally complete semi-elemental tube feeding for children 1 to 12 y of age
Pepdite One+ (banana flavored)‡	1000	Soy and pork hydrolysates, free amino acids	31	Corn-syrup solids (sucrose, aspartame)	106	MCT (35%), canola, and safflower oils	50		Semi-elemental formula for children >1 y of age with severe gastrointestinal impairment
Peptamen Oral*	1000	Enzymatically hydrolyzed whey	40	Maltodextrin, corn starch (sucrose)	127	MCT (70%) and soybean oils	37		Peptide-based, isotonic, designed for general malabsorption

APP

Table U-3   **1379**

Table U-1 *(Continued)*
Selected Enteral Products for Special Indications

Product	Energy, kcal/L	Protein Source	g/L	Carbohydrate Source	g/L	Fat Source	g/L	Fiber g/L	Purpose
Peptamen 1.5 oral*	1500	Enzymatically hydrolyzed whey	67.6	Maltodextrin, corn starch (sucrose)	188	MCT (70%) and soybean oils, soy lecithin	56		High-calorie, peptide-based, high-percentage MCT oil designed for malabsorption
Peptamen VHP oral*	1000	Enzymatically hydrolyzed whey	62.5	Maltodextrin, (sucrose) potato starch	104.5	MCT (70%) and soybean oils, soy lecithin	39.2		High-protein, peptide-based, high-percentage MCT oil designed for general malabsorption
Peptamen, Jr oral*	1000	Enzymatically hydrolyzed whey	30	Maltodextrin, cornstarch (sucrose)	137.6	MCT (60%), soybean, and canola oils, soy lecithin	38.5		Designed for children 1–10 y of age, peptide based, 60% of fat from MCT oil
Perative†	1300	Partially hydrolyzed Na caseinate, lactalbumin hydrolysate, L-arginine	66.6	Maltodextrin	180.3	Canola, MCT (40%), and corn oils	37.4		Higher calorie, 40% of fat from MCT oil, designed for metabolically stressed patients
Polycose†	380/100 g powder, 2000/L liquid	None	0	Glucose polymers from cornstarch	94/100 g, 500/L	None	0		Carbohydrate calorie supplement, available in powder or liquid

Table U-1 (Continued)
Selected Enteral Products for Special Indications

Product	Energy, kcal/L	Protein g/L	Protein Source	Carbohydrate g/L	Carbohydrate Source	Fat g/L	Fat Source	Fiber g/L	Purpose
ProBalance*	1200	54	Ca and K caseinate	156	Maltodextrin, corn-syrup solids, polysaccharides, gum arabic	40.8	Canola, MCT (20%), and corn oils, soy lecithin	10	Higher calorie, fiber for the mature adult
Promote with fiber†	1000	62.5	Sodium and calcium caseinate, soy protein isolate	138	Maltodextrin, sucrose (oat and soy fiber)	28	High-oleic safflower, canola, and MCT (19%) oils, soy lecithin	14.4	High-protein complete oral or tube feeding
Pulmocare†	1500	62.6	Na and Ca Caseinates	106	Sucrose, maltodextrin	93.3	Canola, MCT (20%), high-oleic safflower, and corn oils		High-fat, low-carbohydrate complete oral or tube feeding designed for pulmonary patients
Renalcal Diet*	2000	34.4	Essential and select nonessential amino acids, whey protein	290.4	Maltodextrin, modified corn starch	82.4	MCT (70%), canola, and corn oils, soy lecithin		Very high calorie, low protein designed to maintain positive nitrogen balance, added histidine for renal failure, negligible electrolytes
ReSource Diabetic*	1060	64	Na and Ca caseinate, soy protein isolates	95	Corn-syrup solids, soy protein isolate	47	High-oleic sunflower and soybean oils	13	Fiber containing, designed for diabetics, in a Tetra Pak

APP

Table U-1 *(Continued)*
Selected Enteral Products for Special Indications

Product	Energy, kcal/L	Protein		Carbohydrate		Fat		Fiber g/L	Purpose
		Source	g/L	Source	g/L	Source	g/L		
Resource Breeze*	1060	Whey protein isolate	38	Sugar, Corn-syrup	230	None	0		Fat-free, clear liquid nutritional supplement
ReSource Just For Kids with fiber*	1000	Na and Ca caseinate, whey protein concentrate	30	Sucrose, maltodextrins	110	High-oleic sun-flower, soybean, and MCT (20%) oils	50	6	Complete formula designed for chil-dren 1-10 y of age, available with fiber, in a Tetra Pak
ReSource 2.0*	2000	Ca and Na caseinates	9	Corn-syrup; sucrose, maltodextrin	215	Canola and MCT (20%) oils	89		Very high calorie, designed for medi-cation pass supple-ment programs, in a pouch pack
Suplena†	2000	Na and Ca caseinates	30	Maltodextrin, sucrose	255.2	High-oleic saf-flower and soy oils	95.6		Very high-calorie, low-protein, com-plete formula for renal failure
Tolerex*	1000	Free amino acids	21	Maltodextrin, modi-fied corn starch	230	Safflower oil	1.5		Nutritionally com-plete, truly elemen-tal diet, low fat
TraumaCal*	1500	Na and Ca caseinate	82	Corn-syrup, sucrose	144	Soy and MCT (30%) oils	68		High calorie, high nitrogen for meta-bolically stressed patients

Table U-1 *(Continued)*
Selected Enteral Products for Special Indications

Product	Energy, kcal/L	Protein Source	g/L	Carbohydrate Source	g/L	Fat Source	g/L	Fiber g/L	Purpose
TwoCal HN†	2000	Na and Ca caseinates	83.5	Maltodextrin, sucrose, fructo-oligosaccharides	218.5	High oleic safflower, MCT (19%), and canola oils	90.5		Complete, very high-calorie feeding with fructo-oligosaccharides
Vital High Nitrogen†	1000	Partially hydrolyzed whey, meat, soy, free essential amino acids	41.7	Maltodextrin, sucrose	185	Safflower and MCT (45%) oils	10.8		Nutritionally complete, peptide-based formula for patients with impaired gastrointestinal function
Vivonex T.E.N.*	1000	Free amino acids	38	Maltodextrin, modified corn starch	210	Safflower oil	2.8		Free amino acids plus additional glutamine, designed for gastrointestinal impairment
Vivonex Plus*	1000	Free amino acids	45	Maltodextrin, modified corn starch	190	Soybean oil	6.7		High-nitrogen, very low-fat elemental diet; additional glutamine, arginine, and branched-chain amino acids

APP

Table U-1 **1383**

Table U-1 *(Continued)*
Selected Enteral Products for Special Indications

Product	Energy, kcal/L	Protein Source	Protein g/L	Carbohydrate Source	Carbohydrate g/L	Fat Source	Fat g/L	Fiber g/L	Purpose
Vivonex Pediatric*	800	Free amino acids	24	Maltodextrin, modified starch	130	MCT (68%) and soybean oils	24		Nutritionally complete, elemental formula for children, can be flavored with Vivonex Flavor Packets
Vivonex RTF*	1000	Free amino acids	50	Maltodextrin, modified cornstarch	175	Soybean and MCT (40%) oils	12		Ready-to-use, high-nitrogen, low-fat elemental diet for use in stressed, catabolic patients

Na indicates sodium; Ca, calcium; MCT, medium-chain triglycerides.

* Nestlé Nutrition, Glendale, CA.

† Abbott Nutrition, Columbus, OH.

‡ Nutricia North America, Gaithersburg, MD

§ B. Braun Medical Inc, Irvine, CA.

‖ Mead Johnson Nutritionals, Evansville, IN.

Table U-2
Enteral Products Grouped by Usage Indication

Standard adult oral	Boost,* Ensure,† Ensure High Calcium,† Ensure Fiber,† Carnation Instant Breakfast*
Standard adult tube feeding	FiberSource Standard,* Isocal,* Isosource,* Jevity 1 cal,† Nutren 1.0,* Osmolite†
High-protein oral feeding	Boost High Protein,* Ensure High Protein,† Ensure Plus HN†
High-protein tube feeding	FiberSource HN,* Isocal HN,* Isosource HN,* Jevity 1.2 cal,† Osmolite 1 cal,† Osmolite 1.2 cal,† ProBalance,* Promote†
1.5 kcal/mL	Boost Plus,* Ensure Plus,† Carnation Instant Breakfast Plus,* Nutren 1.5*
2.0 kcal/mL	NovaSource 2.0,* Carnation Instant Breakfast VHC,* Nutren 2.0,* ReSource 2.0,* TwoCal HN†
Standard pediatric (>1 y of age)	Kindercal,‡ Kindercal TF,‡ Nutren Jr,* Pediasure,† ReSource Just For Kids*
Blenderized	Compleat,* Compleat Pediatric*
Clear fortified liquid	Enlive,† Resource Breeze*
Peptide-based adult	Peptamen,* Peptamen 1.5,* Peptamen VHP,* Perative,† Vital High Nitrogen†
Peptide-based pediatric	Pepdite One+,§ Peptamen Jr*
Free amino acid adult	Tolerex,* Vivonex T.E.N.,* Vivonex Plus,* Vivonex RTF*
Free amino acid pediatric (>1 y of age)	EleCare,† Neocate Junior,§ Neocate One+,§ Pediatric EO28,§ Vivonex Pediatric,* FAA*
Immune enhancing	Immun-Aid,‖ Impact,* Impact 1.5,* Impact Glutamine*
Wound healing	Crucial,* Isosource VHN,* Replete,* TraumaCal*
Diabetes	Boost Diabetic,* Diabeti-source,* Glucerna,† Glytrol,* ReSource Diabetic*
Kidney disease	Nepro,† NovaSource Renal,* NutriRenal,* Renalcal Diet,* Suplena†
Liver disease	Hepatic-Aid,‖ NutriHep*
Pulmonary disease	Isosource 1.5,* NovaSource Pulmonary,* Nutren Pulmonary,* Oxepa,† Pulmocare†

APP

Table U-2 (Continued)
Enteral Products Grouped by Usage Indication

Inflammatory bowel disease	Modulen,* Optimental[†]
Carbohydrate modular	Polycose[†]
Protein modular	Beneprotein*
Calorie enhancers	Additions,* Duocal[§]
Fat modulars	MCT oil,* Microlipid*

* Nestlé Nutrition, Glendale, CA.

[†] Abbott Nutrition, Columbus, OH.

[‡] Mead Johnson, Evansville, IN.

[§] Nutricia North America, Gaithersburg, MD.

[||] B. Braun Medical Inc, Irvine, CA.

Table U-3
Sources of Medical Food Modules for Treatment of Inborn Errors of Metabolism

Company	Medical Protein Module	Low-Protein Substitute Modules
Applied Nutrition 10 Saddle Road Cedar Knolls, NJ 07927 Tel: (800) 605-0410 Fax: (973) 734-0029 E-mail: info@medicalfood.com Web site: www.medicalfood.com	Beverage powders, bars	Cereals, snacks, sweets
Cambrooke Foods 2 Central Street Framingham, MA 01701 Tel: (866) 456-9776 Fax: (978) 443-1318 E-mail: info@cambrookefoods.com Web site: www.cambrookefoods.com		Bagels, breads, cheese, meat alternatives, pastas, mixes, rice, seasonings, snacks, sweets
Canbrands Specialty Foods 15 Connie Crescent Concord, ON Canada L4K 1L3 Tel: (905) 761-5008 Fax: (905) 761-5009 E-mail: info@canbrands.ca Web site: www.canbrands.ca		Breads, cookies, egg substitute, mixes
Dietary Specialties 10 Leslie Court Whippany, NJ 07981 Tel: (888) 640-2800 Fax: (973) 884-5907 E-mail: info@dietspec.com Web site: www.dietspec.com		Breads, cheese, cookies, dessert mixes, meat alternatives, mixes, pastas, pizza, rice, sauce mixes, snacks
Ener-G Foods 5960 First Avenue South P.O. Box 84487 Seattle, WA 98124-5787 Tel: (800) 331-5222 Fax: (206) 764-3398 E-mail: customerservice@ener-g.com Web site: www.ener-g.com		Breads, cheese, cookies, crackers, egg substitute, milk substitutes, mixes, pastas, soup mix, snacks, sweets
Glutino 2055 Dagenais West Laval, Quebec Canada H7L 5V1 Tel: (800) 363-3438 Fax: (450) 629-4781 E-mail: info@glutino.com Web site: www.glutino.com		Cookies, crackers, mixes, pastas, rice

Table U-3 *(Continued)*
Sources of Medical Food Modules for Treatment of Inborn Errors of Metabolism

Company	Medical Protein Module	Low-Protein Substitute Modules
Liv-N-Well Distributors 7900 River Road Unit #1 Richmond, British Columbia Canada V6X 1X7 Tel: (877) 270-8479 Fax: (604) 270-8477 E-mail: info@liv-n-well.com Web site: www.liv-n-well.com		Breads, cookies, mixes, pastas
Mead Johnson 2400 West Lloyd Expressway Evansville, IN 47721-0001 Tel: (812) 429-6399 Fax: (812) 429-7189 Web site: www.meadjohnson.com	Beverage powders	
Med-Diet 3600 Holly Lane, Suite 80 Plymouth, MN 55447 Tel: (800) 633-3438 Fax: (763) 550-2022 E-mail: meddiet@med-diet.com Web site: www.med-diet.com		Breads, cookies, crackers, desserts, mixes, pastas, rice, sauces, soups
Nutricia North America P.O. Box 117 Gaithersburg, MD 20884 Tel: (800) 365-7354 Fax: (301) 795-2301 E-mail: nutritionservices@shsna.com Web site: www.shsna.com	Bars, beverage powders, capsules, drink boxes	Cereal, cookies, crackers, milk substitute, mixes, pastas, snacks
PKU Chippery 1021 Hahman Drive Santa Rosa, CA 95405 Tel: (707) 579-2447 E-mail: info@pkuchips.com Web site: www.pkuchips.com		Snacks
PKU Perspectives PO Box 696 Pleasant Grove, UT 84062 Tel: (866) 758-3663 Fax: (801) 785-0952 E-mail: sales@pkuperspectives.com Web site: www.pkuperspectives.com		Cheese, desserts, egg substitute, meat alternative, milk substitute, mixes, pasta, soups, sweets

Table U-3 *(Continued)*
Sources of Medical Food Modules for Treatment of Inborn Errors of Metabolism

Company	Medical Protein Module	Low-Protein Substitute Modules
Ross Products/Abbott Laboratories Metabolic Division 3300 Stelzer Road Columbus, OH 43219-3034 Tel: (800) 551-5838 Web site: www.ross.com/product Handbook/metabolic.asp	Beverage powders, chews	
Taste Connections 612 Meyer Lane #13 Redondo Beach, CA 90278 Tel: (310) 371-8861 Fax: (310) 371-8861 E-mail: lopro@webuniverse.net Web site: www.tasteconnections.com		Cookies, mixes, snacks
Vitaflo 123 East Neck Road Huntington, NY 11743 Tel: (888) 848-2356 Fax: (631) 367-2868 E-mail: vitaflo@vitaflo.co.uk Web site: www.vitaflousa.com	Beverage powders, drink boxes, gel	Sweets

Appendix V

Table V-1
Sports/Nutrition Bars

Product (Weight, g) (Manufacturer)	Calories	Protein	Fat (Saturated Fat)	Fiber	Sodium	Calcium (% DV)	Iron (% DV)
Apex Fit (55 g)	210	13 g	5 g (3.5 g)	>1 g	100 mg	15%	20%
Apex Fix Crisp Bars (40 g)	150	9 g	3.5 g (2 g)	3 g	120 mg	10%	10%
Atkins' Advantage (60 g) (ANI, New York, NY)	240	19 g	12 g (6 g)	10 g	180 mg	30%	15%
Balance (50 g) (The Balance Bar Co, Tarrytown, NY)	210	15 g	7 g (2.5)	3 g	230 mg	25%	15%
Balance Outdoor (50 g)	200	15 g	6 g (1 g)	2 g	140 mg	8%	15%
Burn Bar (50 g) (Unipro, Jamul, CA)	200	15 g	6 g (2.5 g)	2 g	160 mg	25%	6%
Clif (68 g) (Clif Bar Inc, Berkeley, CA)	230	10 g	3 g (0.5 g)	5 g	125 mg	25%	25%
Clif's Luna Bar (48 g)	190	9 g	6 g (3 g)	4 g	125 mg	35%	35%
Clif Mojo (45 g)	200	10 g	8 g (1 g)	3 g	160 mg	0%	8%
GeniSoy (61.5 g) (GeniSoy Food Co, Tulsa, OK)	240	14 g	4.5 g (2.5 g)	1 g	250 mg	25%	25%
Kashi GoLean (78 g) (Kashi Co, La Jolla, CA)	280	13 g	5 g (4 g)	6 g	85 mg	10%	8%
Kashi TLC (35 g)	140	5 g	5 g (0.5 g)	4 g	115 mg	0%	8%
Met-Rx (100 g) (Met-Rx USA, Bohemia, NY)	340	27 g	4 g (0.5 g)	0	135 mg	70%	40%
Nature's Path Organic Optimum Energy (56 g) (Nature's Path Foods, Richmond, British Columbia, Canada)	200	7 g	3 g (1 g)	7 g	125 mg	4%	10%
Odwalla (62 g) (Odwalla, Half Moon Bay, CA)	240	8 g	7 g (1.5 g)	3 g	210 mg	25%	8%
PowerBar (65 g) (Nestlé, Glendale, CA)	234	10 g	2 g (0.5 g)	3 g	90 mg	33%	38%
PowerBar Harvest (65 g)	240	10 g	4 g (0.5 g)	5 g	140 mg	40%	25%
PowerBar Pria (28 g)	188	5.3 g	30 g (1.7 g)	0	25 mg	25%	0%

Table V-1 **1393**

APP

Table V-1 (Continued)
Sports/Nutrition Bars

Product (Weight, g) (Manufacturer)	Calories	Protein	Fat (Saturated Fat)	Fiber	Sodium	Calcium (% DV)	Iron (% DV)
PowerBar Protein Plus (65 g)	258	18 g	5.6 g (3.8 g)	1 g	102 mg	45%	57%
Pro 42 (105 g) (ISS Research, Charlotte, NC)	390	42 g	11 g (6 g)	2 g	125 mg	35%	110%
Probar (85 g) (Probar LLC, Heber City, UT)	380	9 g	18 g (4.5 g)	6 g	45 mg	0%	0%
Promax (68 g) (Promax Nutrition, Concord, CA)	280	20 g	6 g (3 g)	2 g	170 mg	25%	25%
PureFit (58 g) (PureFit Inc, Irvine, CA)	240	18 g	6 g (1 g)	2 g	240 mg	5%	2%
Solo (50 g) (Solo GI Nutrition, Edmonton, Alberta, Canada)	200	11 g	6 g (2.5 g)	3 g	125 mg	20%	4%
Steel Bar (65 g) (American Body Building, Aurora, IL)	250	16 g	4 g (2.5 g)	1 g	250 mg	10%	10%
Think Energy (35 g) (Think Products, San Francisco, CA)	140	6 g	5 g (2 g)	2 g	35 mg	15%	25%
Tigers Milk (35 g) (Schiff Nutrition Group, Salt Lake City, UT)	145	7 g	5 g (1 g)	1 g	70 mg	30%	15%
Usana (41 g) (Usana Health Sciences, Salt Lake City, UT)	150	12 g	4 g (2 g)	1 g	95 mg	0%	0%
Worldwide Sport Nutrition Bar (78 g) (Worldwide Sport Nutrition, Bohemia, NY)	260	32 g	6 g (3.5 g)	1 g	95 mg	50%	50%
Zone Perfect (50 g) (Abbott Nutrition, Columbus, OH)	190	16 g	7 g (1.5 g)	<1 g	280 mg	2%	8%

DV indicates daily value.

Appendix W

Table W-1
Arm Measurements

Length/Height (cm)	Boys			Combined Sexes			Girls			Length/Height* (cm)
	Median	−2 SD	−3 SD	Median	−2 SD	−3 SD	Median	−2 SD	−3 SD	
65.0	14.6	12.7	11.7	14.0	12.4	11.5	14.0	12.1	11.2	65.0
65.5	14.7	12.7	11.8	14.4	12.5	11.5	14.1	12.2	11.2	65.5
68.0	14.7	12.8	11.8	14.5	12.5	11.6	14.2	12.3	11.3	66.0
68.5	14.8	12.8	11.8	14.5	12.6	11.6	14.3	12.3	11.3	66.5
67.0	14.8	12.9	11.9	14.6	12.6	11.6	14.4	12.4	11.4	67.0
67.5	14.9	12.8	11.9	14.7	12.7	11.7	14.4	12.4	11.4	67.5
68.0	15.0	12.0	11.0	14.7	12.7	11.7	14.5	12.5	11.5	68.0
68.5	15.0	13.0	12.0	14.8	12.8	11.7	14.6	12.6	11.5	68.5
60.0	10.1	13.0	12.0	14.8	12.8	11.8	14.7	12.8	11.6	69.0
69.5	15.1	13.0	12.0	14.9	12.8	11.8	14.7	12.7	11.6	69.5
70.0	15.1	13.1	12.0	15.0	12.9	11.8	14.8	12.7	11.7	70.0
70.5	15.2	13.1	12.0	15.0	12.9	11.9	14.8	12.8	11.7	70.5
71.0	15.2	13.1	12.1	15.1	13.0	11.9	14.9	12.8	11.7	71.0
71.5	15.3	13.1	12.1	15.1	13.0	11.9	15.0	12.8	11.8	71.5
72.0	15.3	13.2	12.1	15.2	13.0	11.8	15.0	12.9	11.8	72.0
72.5	15.3	13.2	12.1	15.2	13.1	12.0	15.1	12.9	11.8	72.5
73.0	15.4	13.2	12.1	15.2	13.1	12.0	15.1	13.0	11.9	73.0

APP

Table W-1 (Continued)
Arm Measurements

Length/Height* (cm)	Mid-Upper-Arm-Circumference (MUAC) for Length or Height Reference Data									Length/Height* (cm)
	Boys			Combined Sexes			Girls			
	Median	−2 SD	−3 SD	Median	−2 SD	−3 SD	Median	−2 SD	−3 SD	
73.5	15.4	13.2	12.2	15.3	13.1	12.0	15.2	13.0	11.9	73.5
74.0	15.4	13.3	12.2	15.3	13.1	12.1	15.2	13.0	11.9	74.0
74.5	15.5	13.3	12.2	15.4	13.2	12.1	15.2	13.1	12.0	74.5
75.0	15.5	13.3	12.2	15.4	13.2	12.1	15.3	13.1	12.0	75.0
75.5	15.5	13.3	12.2	15.4	13.2	12.1	15.3	13.1	12.0	75.5
76.0	15.6	13.4	12.2	15.5	13.3	12.2	15.4	13.2	12.1	76.0
76.5	15.6	13.4	12.3	15.5	13.3	12.2	15.4	13.2	12.1	76.5
77.0	15.6	13.4	12.3	15.5	13.3	12.2	15.4	13.2	12.1	77.0
77.5	15.6	13.4	12.3	15.6	13.3	12.2	15.5	13.3	12.1	77.5
78.0	15.7	13.4	12.3	15.6	13.4	12.2	15.5	13.3	12.2	78.0
78.5	15.7	13.4	12.3	15.6	13.4	12.3	15.6	13.3	12.2	78.5
79.0	15.7	13.5	12.3	15.6	13.4	12.3	15.6	13.3	12.2	79.0
79.5	15.7	13.5	12.4	15.7	13.4	12.3	15.6	13.4	12.2	79.5
80.0	15.8	13.5	12.4	15.7	13.4	12.3	15.6	13.4	12.3	80.0
80.5	15.8	13.5	12.4	15.7	13.5	12.3	15.7	13.4	12.3	80.5
81.0	15.8	13.6	12.4	15.8	13.5	12.4	15.7	13.5	12.3	81.0
81.5	15.8	13.6	12.4	15.8	13.5	12.4	15.7	13.5	12.3	81.5

Table W-1 *(Continued)*
Arm Measurements

Mid–Upper-Arm-Circumference (MUAC) for Length or Height Reference Data

Length/Height (cm)	Boys			Combined Sexes			Girls			Length/Height* (cm)
	Median	–2 SD	–3 SD	Median	–2 SD	–3 SD	Median	–2 SD	–3 SD	
82.0	15.9	13.6	12.4	15.8	13.5	12.4	15.8	13.5	12.3	82.0
82.5	15.9	13.6	12.5	15.8	13.6	12.4	15.8	13.5	12.4	82.5
83.0	15.9	13.6	12.5	15.9	13.6	12.4	15.8	13.5	12.4	83.0
83.5	15.9	13.6	12.5	15.9	13.6	12.5	15.8	13.6	12.4	83.5
84.0	15.9	13.7	12.5	15.9	13.6	12.5	15.9	13.6	12.4	84.0
84.5	16.0	13.7	12.5	15.9	13.6	12.5	15.9	13.6	12.5	84.5
85.0	16.0	13.7	12.5	15.9	13.6	12.5	15.9	13.6	12.5	85.0
85.5	16.0	13.7	12.6	16.0	13.7	12.5	15.9	13.6	12.5	85.5
86.0	16.0	13.7	12.6	16.0	13.7	12.5	15.9	13.6	12.5	86.0
86.5	16.0	13.7	12.6	16.0	13.7	12.6	16.0	13.7	12.5	86.5
87.0	16.1	13.8	12.6	16.0	13.7	12.6	16.0	13.7	12.6	87.0
87.5	16.1	13.8	12.6	16.0	13.7	12.6	16.0	13.7	12.6	87.5
88.0	16.1	13.8	12.6	16.1	13.8	12.6	16.0	13.7	12.6	88.0
88.5	16.1	13.8	12.7	16.1	13.8	12.6	16.1	13.8	12.6	88.5
89.0	16.1	13.8	12.7	16.1	13.8	12.7	16.1	13.8	12.6	89.0
89.5	16.2	13.9	12.7	16.1	13.8	12.7	16.1	13.8	12.7	89.5
90.0	16.2	13.9	12.7	16.2	13.9	12.7	16.1	13.8	12.7	90.0

APP

Table W-1 *(Continued)*
Arm Measurements

Mid-Upper-Arm-Circumference (MUAC) for Length or Height Reference Data

Length/Height* (cm)	Boys			Combined Sexes			Girls			Length/Height* (cm)
	Median	−2 SD	−3 SD	Median	−2 SD	−3 SD	Median	−2 SD	−3 SD	
90.5	16.2	13.9	12.8	16.2	13.9	12.7	16.2	13.8	12.7	90.5
91.0	16.2	13.9	12.8	16.2	13.9	12.7	16.2	13.9	12.7	91.0
91.5	16.3	14.0	12.8	16.2	13.9	12.8	16.2	13.9	12.7	91.5
92.0	16.3	14.0	12.8	16.3	13.9	12.8	16.2	13.9	12.8	92.0
92.5	16.3	14.0	12.9	16.3	14.0	12.8	16.2	13.9	12.8	92.5
93.0	16.3	14.0	12.9	16.3	14.0	12.8	16.3	14.0	12.8	93.0
93.5	16.4	14.1	12.9	16.3	14.0	12.9	16.3	14.0	12.8	93.5
94.0	16.4	14.1	12.9	16.4	14.0	12.9	16.3	14.0	12.8	94.0
94.5	16.4	14.1	13.0	16.4	14.1	12.9	16.3	14.0	12.9	94.5
95.0	16.4	14.1	13.0	16.4	14.1	12.9	16.4	14.1	12.9	95.0
95.5	16.5	14.2	13.0	16.4	14.1	13.0	16.4	14.1	12.9	95.5
96.0	16.5	14.2	13.0	16.5	14.1	13.0	16.4	14.1	12.9	96.0
96.5	16.5	14.2	13.1	16.5	14.2	13.0	16.4	14.1	13.0	96.5
97.0	16.5	14.2	13.1	16.5	14.2	13.0	16.5	14.1	13.0	97.0
97.5	16.6	14.3	13.1	16.5	14.2	13.1	16.5	14.2	13.0	97.5
98.0	16.6	14.3	13.1	16.6	14.2	13.1	16.5	14.2	13.0	98.0
98.5	16.6	14.3	13.2	16.6	14.3	13.1	16.5	14.2	13.1	98.5

Table W-1 *(Continued)*
Arm Measurements

Length/Height (cm)	Mid-Upper-Arm-Circumference (MUAC) for Length or Height Reference Data									Length/Height* (cm)
	Boys			Combined Sexes			Girls			
	Median	−2 SD	−3 SD	Median	−2 SD	−3 SD	Median	−2 SD	−3 SD	
99.0	16.7	14.3	13.2	16.6	14.3	13.1	16.6	14.3	13.1	99.0
99.5	16.7	14.4	13.2	16.6	14.3	13.2	16.6	14.3	13.1	99.5
100.0	16.7	14.4	13.2	16.7	14.4	13.2	16.6	14.3	13.1	100.0
100.5	16.8	14.4	13.3	16.7	14.4	13.2	16.7	14.3	13.2	100.5
101.0	16.8	14.5	13.3	16.7	14.4	13.2	16.7	14.4	13.2	101.0
101.5	16.8	14.5	13.3	16.8	14.5	13.3	16.7	14.4	13.2	101.5
102.0	16.9	14.5	13.4	16.8	14.5	13.3	16.7	14.4	13.2	102.0
102.5	16.9	14.6	13.4	16.8	14.5	13.3	16.8	14.4	13.3	102.5
103.0	16.9	14.6	13.4	16.9	14.6	13.4	16.8	14.5	13.3	103.0
103.5	16.9	14.6	13.4	16.9	14.6	13.4	16.8	14.5	13.3	103.5
104.0	17.0	14.6	13.5	16.9	14.6	13.4	16.9	14.5	13.4	104.0
104.5	17.0	14.7	13.5	17.0	14.6	13.4	16.9	14.6	13.4	104.5
105.0	17.0	14.7	13.5	17.0	14.6	13.5	16.9	14.6	13.4	105.0
105.5	17.1	14.7	13.6	17.0	14.7	13.5	17.0	14.6	13.4	105.5
106.0	17.1	14.8	13.6	17.1	14.7	13.5	17.0	14.6	13.5	106.0
106.5	17.1	14.8	13.6	17.1	14.7	13.6	17.0	14.7	13.5	106.5
107.0	17.2	14.8	13.6	17.1	14.8	13.6	17.1	14.7	13.6	107.0

Table W-1 (Continued)
Arm Measurements

Mid-Upper-Arm-Circumference (MUAC) for Length or Height Reference Data

Length/Height* (cm)	Boys			Combined Sexes			Girls			Length/Height* (cm)
	Median	–2 SD	–3 SD	Median	–2 SD	–3 SD	Median	–2 SD	–3 SD	
107.5	17.2	14.8	13.7	17.2	14.8	13.6	17.1	14.7	13.6	107.5
108.0	17.3	14.9	13.7	17.2	14.8	13.6	17.1	14.8	13.6	108.0
108.5	17.3	14.9	13.7	17.2	14.9	13.7	17.2	14.8	13.6	108.5
109.0	17.3	14.9	13.7	17.3	14.9	13.7	17.2	14.8	13.6	109.0
109.5	17.4	15.0	13.8	17.3	14.9	13.7	17.2	14.9	13.7	109.5
110.0	17.4	15.0	13.8	17.4	15.0	13.8	17.3	14.9	13.7	110.0
110.5	17.4	15.0	13.8	17.4	15.0	13.8	17.3	14.9	13.7	110.5
111.0	17.5	15.1	13.9	17.4	15.0	13.8	17.4	15.0	13.8	111.0
111.5	17.5	15.1	13.9	17.5	15.1	13.9	17.4	14.0	13.8	111.5
112.0	17.5	15.1	13.9	17.5	15.1	13.9	17.5	15.0	13.8	112.0
112.5	17.6	15.1	13.9	17.6	15.1	13.9	17.5	15.1	13.9	112.5
113.0	17.6	15.2	14.0	17.6	15.2	13.9	17.6	15.1	13.9	113.0
113.5	17.7	15.2	14.0	17.6	15.2	14.0	17.6	15.2	13.9	113.5
114.0	17.7	15.2	14.0	17.7	15.2	14.0	17.7	15.2	14.0	114.0
114.5	17.7	15.3	14.0	17.7	15.3	14.0	17.7	15.2	14.0	114.5
115.0	17.8	15.3	14.0	17.8	15.3	14.0	17.8	15.3	14.0	115.0
115.5	17.8	15.3	14.1	17.8	15.3	14.1	17.8	15.3	14.1	115.5

Table W-1 *(Continued)*
Arm Measurements

Length/Height* (cm)	Mid-Upper-Arm-Circumference (MUAC) for Length or Height Reference Data									Length/Height* (cm)
	Boys			Combined Sexes			Girls			
	Median	−2 SD	−3 SD	Median	−2 SD	−3 SD	Median	−2 SD	−3 SD	
116.0	17.9	15.4	14.1	17.9	15.3	14.1	17.9	15.3	14.1	116.0
116.5	17.9	15.4	14.1	17.9	15.4	14.1	17.9	15.4	14.1	116.5
117.0	18.0	15.4	14.1	18.0	15.4	14.1	18.0	15.4	14.1	117.0
117.5	18.0	15.4	14.2	18.0	15.4	14.2	18.0	15.5	14.2	117.5
118.0	18.0	15.5	14.2	18.1	15.5	14.2	18.1	15.5	14.2	118.0
118.5	18.1	15.5	14.2	18.1	15.5	14.2	18.1	15.5	14.2	118.5
119.0	18.1	15.5	14.2	18.2	15.6	14.3	18.2	15.6	14.3	119.0
119.5	18.2	15.6	14.2	18.2	15.6	14.3	18.2	15.6	14.3	119.5
120.0	18.2	15.6	14.3	18.3	15.7	14.3	18.3	15.7	14.3	120.0
120.5	18.3	15.6	14.3	18.3	15.7	14.3	18.4	15.7	14.4	120.5
121.0	18.3	15.6	14.3	18.4	15.7	14.4	18.4	15.7	14.4	121.0
121.5	18.4	15.7	14.0	18.4	15.8	14.4	18.5	15.8	14.4	121.5
122.0	18.4	15.7	14.3	18.5	15.8	14.4	18.5	15.8	14.5	122.0
122.5	18.5	15.7	14.4	18.6	15.8	14.4	18.6	15.9	14.5	122.5
123.0	18.5	15.8	14.4	18.6	15.9	14.5	18.7	15.9	14.5	123.0
123.5	18.6	15.8	14.4	18.6	15.9	14.5	18.7	16.0	14.6	123.5
124.0	18.6	15.8	14.4	18.7	15.9	14.5	18.8	16.0	14.6	124.0

Table W-1 (Continued)
Arm Measurements

Length/Height* (cm)	Mid-Upper-Arm-Circumference (MUAC) for Length or Height Reference Data									Length/Height* (cm)
	Boys			Combined Sexes			Girls			
	Median	−2 SD	−3 SD	Median	−2 SD	−3 SD	Median	−2 SD	−3 SD	
124.5	18.7	15.8	14.4	18.8	15.9	14.5	18.9	16.1	14.6	124.5
125.0	18.7	15.9	14.5	18.8	16.0	14.6	18.9	16.1	14.7	125.0
125.5	18.8	15.9	14.5	18.9	16.0	14.6	19.0	16.1	14.7	125.5
126.0	18.8	15.9	14.5	19.0	16.1	14.6	19.1	16.2	14.7	126.0
126.5	18.9	16.0	14.5	19.0	16.1	14.6	19.2	16.2	14.8	126.5
127.0	18.9	16.0	14.5	19.1	16.1	14.7	19.2	16.3	14.8	127.0
127.5	19.0	16.0	14.5	19.2	16.2	14.7	19.3	16.3	14.8	127.5
128.0	19.1	16.1	14.6	19.2	16.2	14.7	19.4	16.4	14.9	128.0
128.5	19.1	16.1	14.6	19.3	16.3	14.7	19.5	16.4	14.9	128.5
129.0	19.3	16.1	14.6	19.4	16.3	14.8	19.5	16.5	14.9	129.0
129.5	19.3	16.2	14.6	19.4	16.3	14.8	19.6	16.5	14.9	129.5
130.0	19.3	16.2	14.6	19.5	16.4	14.8	19.7	16.6	15.0	130.0
130.5	19.4	16.2	14.6	19.6	16.4	14.9	19.8	16.6	15.1	130.5
131.0	19.5	16.3	14.7	19.7	16.5	14.9	19.9	16.7	15.1	131.0
131.5	19.6	16.3	14.7	19.8	16.5	14.9	20.0	16.7	15.1	131.5
132.0	19.6	16.3	14.7	19.8	16.6	14.9	20.1	16.8	15.2	132.0
132.5	19.7	16.4	14.7	19.9	16.6	15.0	20.2	16.8	15.2	132.5

Table W-1 *(Continued)*
Arm Measurements

Mid-Upper-Arm-Circumference (MUAC) for Length or Height Reference Data

Length/Height* (cm)	Boys			Combined Sexes			Girls			Length/Height* (cm)
	Median	–2 SD	–3 SD	Median	–2 SD	–3 SD	Median	–2 SD	–3 SD	
133.0	19.8	16.4	14.7	20.0	16.7	15.0	20.2	16.9	15.2	133.0
133.5	19.8	16.5	14.8	20.1	16.7	15.0	20.3	17.0	15.3	133.5
134.0	19.9	16.5	14.8	20.2	16.8	15.0	20.4	17.0	15.3	134.0
134.5	20.0	16.5	14.8	20.3	16.8	15.1	20.5	17.1	15.3	134.5
135.0	20.1	16.6	14.8	20.4	16.9	15.1	20.5	17.1	15.4	135.0
135.5	20.2	16.6	14.9	20.5	16.9	15.1	20.7	17.2	15.4	135.5
136.0	20.3	16.7	14.9	20.6	17.0	15.2	20.8	17.2	15.5	136.0
136.5	20.4	16.7	14.9	20.7	17.0	15.2	20.9	17.3	15.5	136.5
137.0	20.5	16.8	14.9	20.8	17.1	15.2	21.1	17.4	15.5	137.0
137.5	20.5	16.8	15.0	20.9	17.1	15.3	21.2	17.4	15.6	137.5
138.0	20.7	16.9	15.0	21.0	17.2	15.3	21.3	17.5	15.6	138.0
138.5	20.8	16.9	15.0	21.1	17.3	15.3	21.4	17.6	15.7	138.5
139.0	20.9	17.0	15.0	21.2	17.3	15.4	21.5	17.6	15.7	139.0
139.5	21.0	17.0	15.1	21.3	17.4	15.4	21.6	17.7	15.7	139.5
140.0	21.1	17.1	15.1	21.4	17.4	15.4	21.7	17.8	15.8	140.0
140.5	21.2	17.2	15.2	21.5	17.5	15.5	21.8	17.9	15.8	140.5
141.0	21.3	17.2	15.2	21.7	17.6	15.5	22.0	17.9	15.9	141.0

APP

Table W-1 (Continued)
Arm Measurements

Length/Height* (cm)	Mid-Upper-Arm-Circumference (MUAC) for Length or Height Reference Data												Length/Height* (cm)
	Boys			Combined Sexes				Girls				
	Median	−2 SD	−3 SD	Median	−2 SD	−3 SD	Median	−2 SD	−3 SD			
141.5	21.5	17.3	15.2	21.8	17.6	15.6	22.1	18.0	15.9			141.5
142.0	21.6	17.4	15.3	21.9	17.7	15.6	22.2	18.0	15.9			142.0
142.5	21.7	17.5	15.3	22.0	17.8	15.7	22.4	18.1	16.0			142.5
143.0	21.9	17.5	15.4	22.2	17.9	15.7	22.5	18.2	16.0			143.0
143.5	22.0	17.6	15.4	22.3	17.9	15.8	22.7	18.3	16.1			143.5
144.0	22.1	17.7	15.5	22.5	18.0	15.8	22.8	18.4	16.1			144.0
144.5	22.3	17.8	15.5	22.6	18.1	15.9	22.9	18.4	16.2			144.5
145.0	22.4	17.9	15.6	22.6	18.2	15.9	23.1	18.5	16.2			145.0

* Length <85 cm, height ≥85 cm.

Reprinted with permission from Mei Z, Grummer-Strawn LM, de Onis M, Yip R. The development of a MUAC-for-height reference, including a comparison to other nutritional status screening indicators. *Bull World Health Organ.* 1997;75:333–341.

Table W-2
Arm Measurements

Age, mo	−4 SD	−3 SD	−2 SD	−1 SD	Mean	+1 SD	+2 SD	+3 SD
			MUAC-for-Age Reference Data for Boys Aged 6–59 Months*					
6	10.3	11.5	12.6	13.8	14.9	16.1	17.3	18.4
7	10.4	11.6	12.7	13.9	15.1	16.3	17.5	18.6
8	10.5	11.7	12.8	14.0	15.2	16.4	17.6	18.8
9	10.5	11.7	12.9	14.2	15.4	16.6	17.8	19.0
10	10.6	11.8	13.0	14.2	15.5	16.7	17.9	19.1
11	10.6	11.9	13.1	14.3	15.6	16.8	18.0	19.3
12	10.7	11.9	13.2	14.4	15.7	16.9	18.1	19.4
13	10.7	12.0	13.2	14.5	15.7	17.0	18.2	19.5
14	10.8	12.0	13.3	14.5	15.8	17.1	18.3	19.6
15	10.8	12.1	13.3	14.6	15.9	17.1	18.4	19.7
16	10.8	12.1	13.4	14.6	15.9	17.2	18.5	19.8
17	10.8	12.1	13.4	14.7	16.0	17.3	18.6	19.8
18	10.8	12.1	13.4	14.7	16.0	17.3	18.6	19.9
19	10.9	12.2	13.5	14.8	16.1	17.4	18.7	20.0
20	10.9	12.2	13.5	14.8	16.1	17.4	18.7	20.0
21	10.9	12.2	13.5	14.8	16.1	17.5	18.8	20.1

Table W-2 (Continued)
Arm Measurements

				MUAC-for-Age Reference Data for Boys Aged 6–59 Months*						
Age, mo	−4 SD	−3 SD	−2 SD	−1 SD	Mean	+1 SD	+2 SD	+3 SD		
22	10.9	12.2	13.5	14.8	16.2	17.5	18.8	20.1		
23	10.9	12.2	13.5	14.8	16.2	17.6	18.9	20.2		
24	10.9	12.3	13.6	14.8	16.2	17.6	18.9	20.2		
25	10.9	12.3	13.6	14.9	16.3	17.6	18.9	20.3		
26	10.9	12.3	13.6	14.9	16.3	17.6	19.0	20.3		
27	10.9	12.3	13.6	15.0	16.3	17.7	19.0	20.4		
28	10.9	12.3	13.6	15.0	16.3	17.7	19.1	20.4		
29	10.9	12.3	13.7	15.0	16.4	17.7	19.1	20.4		
30	10.9	12.3	13.7	15.0	16.4	17.8	19.1	20.5		
31	11.0	12.3	13.7	15.1	16.4	17.8	19.2	20.5		
32	11.0	12.3	13.7	15.1	16.5	17.8	19.2	20.6		
33	11.0	12.4	13.7	15.1	16.5	17.9	19.2	20.6		
34	11.0	12.4	13.8	15.1	16.5	17.9	19.3	20.6		
35	11.0	12.4	13.8	15.2	16.5	17.9	19.3	20.7		
36	11.0	12.4	13.8	15.2	16.6	18.0	19.3	20.7		
37	11.0	12.4	13.8	15.2	16.6	18.0	19.4	20.8		

Table W-2 (Continued)
Arm Measurements

| | | | | MUAC-for-Age Reference Data for Boys Aged 6–59 Months* | | | | |
Age, mo	–4 SD	–3 SD	–2 SD	–1 SD	Mean	+1 SD	+2 SD	+3 SD
38	11.0	12.4	13.8	15.2	16.6	18.0	19.4	20.8
39	11.1	12.5	13.9	15.3	16.7	18.1	19.5	20.9
40	11.1	12.5	13.9	15.3	16.7	18.1	19.5	20.9
41	11.1	12.5	13.9	15.3	16.7	18.1	19.6	21.0
42	11.1	12.5	13.9	15.4	16.8	18.2	19.6	21.0
43	11.1	12.5	14.0	15.4	16.8	18.2	19.7	21.1
44	11.1	12.5	14.0	15.4	16.8	18.3	19.7	21.1
45	11.1	12.6	14.0	15.4	16.9	18.3	19.8	21.2
46	11.1	12.6	14.0	15.5	16.9	18.4	19.8	21.3
47	11.1	12.6	14.0	15.5	17.0	18.4	19.9	21.3
48	11.1	12.6	14.1	15.5	17.0	18.4	19.9	21.4
49	11.1	12.6	14.1	15.6	17.0	18.5	20.0	21.4
50	11.1	12.6	14.1	15.6	17.1	18.5	20.0	21.5
51	11.1	12.6	14.1	15.6	17.1	18.6	20.1	21.6
52	11.1	12.6	14.1	15.6	17.1	18.6	20.1	21.6
53	11.1	12.6	14.1	15.7	17.2	18.7	20.2	21.7

APP

Table W-2 (Continued)
Arm Measurements

MUAC-for-Age Reference Data for Boys Aged 6–59 Months*

Age, mo	−4 SD	−3 SD	−2 SD	−1 SD	Mean	+1 SD	+2 SD	+3 SD
54	11.1	12.6	14.2	15.7	17.2	18.7	20.2	21.8
55	11.1	12.6	14.2	15.7	17.2	18.8	20.3	21.8
56	11.1	12.6	14.2	15.7	17.3	18.8	20.4	21.9
57	11.1	12.6	14.2	15.8	17.3	18.9	20.4	22.0
58	11.1	12.6	14.2	15.9	17.3	18.9	20.5	22.1
59	11.1	12.6	14.2	15.9	17.4	19.0	20.6	22.2

* Reprinted with permission from: de Onis et al. The development of MUAC-for-age reference data recommended by a WHO expert committee. *WHO Bull.* 1997;75:11–18.

Table W-3
Arm Measurements

Age, mo	−4 SD	−3 SD	−2 SD	−1 SD	Mean	+1 SD	+2 SD	+3 SD
6	9.2	10.4	11.5	12.7	13.9	15.0	16.2	17.4
7	9.4	10.6	11.8	13.0	14.1	15.3	16.5	17.7
8	9.6	10.8	12.0	13.2	14.4	15.6	16.8	18.0
9	9.8	11.0	12.2	13.4	14.6	15.8	17.0	18.2
10	9.9	11.1	12.3	13.6	14.8	16.0	17.2	18.4
11	10.0	11.3	12.5	13.7	15.0	16.2	17.4	18.6
12	10.1	11.4	12.6	13.9	15.1	16.4	17.6	18.8
13	10.2	11.5	12.7	14.0	15.2	16.5	17.7	19.0
14	10.3	11.6	12.8	14.1	15.4	16.6	17.9	19.2
15	10.4	11.7	12.9	14.2	15.5	16.7	18.0	19.3
16	10.4	11.7	13.0	14.3	15.6	16.8	18.1	19.4
17	10.5	11.8	13.1	14.4	15.7	16.9	18.2	19.5
18	10.5	11.8	13.1	14.4	15.7	17.0	18.3	19.6
19	10.6	11.9	13.2	14.5	15.8	17.1	18.4	19.7
20	10.6	11.9	13.2	14.5	15.8	17.2	18.5	19.8
21	10.6	11.9	13.3	14.6	15.9	17.2	18.5	19.8

MUAC-for-Age Reference Data for Girls Aged 6–59 Months*

APP

Table W-3 *(Continued)*
Arm Measurements

Age, mo	−4 SD	−3 SD	−2 SD	−1 SD	Mean	+1 SD	+2 SD	+3 SD
22	10.7	12.0	13.3	14.6	15.9	17.3	18.6	19.9
23	10.7	12.0	13.3	14.7	16.0	17.3	18.6	20.0
24	10.7	12.0	13.4	14.7	16.0	17.4	18.7	20.0
25	10.7	12.0	13.4	14.7	16.1	17.4	18.7	20.1
26	10.7	12.1	13.4	14.7	16.1	17.4	18.8	20.1
27	10.7	12.1	13.4	14.8	16.1	17.5	18.8	20.2
28	10.7	12.1	13.4	14.8	16.1	17.5	18.8	20.2
29	10.7	12.1	13.5	14.8	16.2	17.5	18.9	20.3
30	10.8	12.1	13.5	14.8	16.2	17.6	18.9	20.3
31	10.8	12.1	13.5	14.9	16.2	17.6	19.0	20.3
32	10.8	12.1	13.5	14.9	16.3	17.6	19.0	20.4
33	10.8	12.2	13.5	14.9	16.3	17.7	19.0	20.4
34	10.8	12.2	13.6	14.9	16.3	17.7	19.1	20.5
35	10.8	12.2	13.6	15.0	16.3	17.7	19.1	20.5
36	10.8	12.2	13.6	15.0	16.4	17.8	19.2	20.6
37	10.8	12.2	13.6	15.0	16.4	17.8	19.2	20.6

MUAC-for-Age Reference Data for Girls Aged 6–59 Months*

Table W-3 *(Continued)*
Arm Measurements

					MUAC-for-Age Reference Data for Girls Aged 6–59 Months*				
Age, mo	−4 SD	−3 SD	−2 SD	−1 SD	Mean	+1 SD	+2 SD	+3 SD
38	10.9	12.2	13.6	15.0	16.4	17.8	19.2	20.6
39	10.9	12.3	13.7	15.1	16.5	17.9	19.3	20.7
40	10.9	12.3	13.7	15.1	16.6	17.9	19.3	20.7
41	10.9	12.3	13.7	15.1	16.6	18.0	19.4	20.8
42	10.9	12.3	13.8	15.2	16.6	18.0	19.4	20.8
43	10.9	12.4	13.8	15.2	16.6	18.1	19.5	20.9
44	10.9	12.4	13.8	15.2	16.7	18.1	19.5	21.0
45	11.0	12.4	13.8	15.3	16.7	18.1	19.6	21.0
46	11.0	12.4	13.9	15.3	16.7	18.2	19.6	21.1
47	11.0	12.4	13.9	15.3	16.8	18.2	19.7	21.2
48	11.0	12.4	13.9	15.4	16.8	18.3	19.8	21.2
49	11.0	12.5	13.9	15.4	16.9	18.3	19.8	21.3
50	11.0	12.5	14.0	15.4	16.9	18.4	19.9	21.4
51	11.0	12.5	14.0	15.5	17.0	18.4	19.9	21.4
52	11.0	12.5	14.0	15.5	17.0	18.5	20.0	21.5
53	11.0	12.5	14.0	15.5	17.0	18.6	20.1	21.6

APP

Table W-3 (Continued)
Arm Measurements

	MUAC-for-Age Reference Data for Girls Aged 6–59 Months*							
Age, mo	−4 SD	−3 SD	−2 SD	−1 SD	Mean	+1 SD	+2 SD	+3 SD
54	11.0	12.5	14.0	15.6	17.1	18.6	20.1	21.7
55	11.0	12.5	14.1	15.6	17.1	18.7	20.2	21.7
56	11.0	12.5	14.1	15.6	17.2	18.7	20.3	21.8
57	11.0	12.5	14.1	15.7	17.2	18.8	20.3	21.9
58	11.0	12.5	14.1	15.7	17.3	18.8	20.4	22.0
59	11.0	12.5	14.1	15.7	17.3	18.9	20.5	22.1

* Reprinted with permission from: de Onis et al. The development of MUAC-for-age reference data recommended by a WHO expert committee. *WHO Bull.* 1997; 75: 11–18.

Appendix X

Table X-1
Saturated and Polyunsaturated Fat and Cholesterol Content of Common Foods*

Foods	Portion	Saturated Fat, g	Polyunsaturated Fat, g	Cholesterol, mg	kcal
Almonds (roasted, salted, shelled)	1 oz	1.1	3.6	0	169
Bacon (cured, cooked)	2 slices	2.2	0.8	18	87
Beef, lean, chuck blade roast	3 oz	8.5	0.8	88	290
Bread	1 oz	0.2	0.4	0	75
Butter	1 tbsp	7.3	0.4	31	102
Cheese					
Cheddar	1 oz	6.0	0.3	30	114
Cottage, creamed	1/2 cup	3.1	0.2	16	112
Cream or spread	2 tbsp	5.4	0.3	27	88
Chicken (light meat without skin)	3.5 oz	1.3	1.0	84	172
Coconut (dried, sweetened, shredded)	1/4 c	7.3	0.1	0	116
Corn oil	1 tbsp	1.3	6.2	0	124
Cottonseed oil	1 tbsp	3.5	7.1	0	120
Egg					
Whole	1 large	1.6	0.7	212	78
White	1 large	0	0	0	17
Yolk	1 large	1.6	0.7	210	55
Fish (fillet or flounder, sole)	3 oz	0.3	0.5	58	99
Hamburger (80% lean) broiled	3 oz	5.6	0.4	77	231
Ice cream (10% fat) vanilla	1/2 cup	4.9	0.3	32	145

Table X-1 **1417**

Table X-1 (*Continued*)
Saturated and Polyunsaturated Fat and Cholesterol Content of Common Foods*

Foods	Portion	Saturated Fat, g	Polyunsaturated Fat, g	Cholesterol, mg	kcal
Lamb (lean leg)	3.5 oz	5.6	1.0	91	241
Lard and other animal fats	1 tbsp	6.4	1.1	14	126
Liver (beef) braised	3.5 oz	1.7	1.0	393	189
Margarine					
Regular (hydrogenated)	1 tbsp	1.9	2.5	0	101
Liquid oil	1 tbsp	1.5	3.3	0	87
Milk					
Whole	1 cup	4.6	0.5	24	146
2%	1 cup	3.1	0.2	20	122
Skim	1 cup	0.3	0	5	83
Olive oil	1 tbsp	1.9	1.4	0	119
Oysters (Eastern) wild, raw	6 medium	0.6	0.8	45	57
Peanut oil	1 tbsp	2.3	4.3	0	119
Pork (lean) center loin, roasted	3.5 oz	3.5	0.8	83	213
Safflower oil	1 tbsp	0.8	2.0	0	120
Salmon, pink (canned, drained)	3 1/2 oz	0.7	1.2	70	116
Shrimp (canned in wet pack)	3 1/2 oz	0.2	0.7	250	99
Soybean oil	1 tbsp	2	7.9	0	120
Sweetbreads (calf)	3 oz	7.3	4.0	250	271

Table X-1 *(Continued)*
Saturated and Polyunsaturated Fat and Cholesterol Content of Common Foods*

Foods	Portion	Saturated Fat, g	Polyunsaturated Fat, g	Cholesterol, mg	kcal
Tuna fish, white canned in oil	3 oz	1.1	2.5	26	158
Turkey (light meat, without skin, roasted)	3.5 oz	1.0	0.9	68	156

* From U.S. Department of Agriculture, Agricultural Research Service. 2005. USDA Nutrient Database for Standard Reference, Release 18. Nutrient Data Laboratory Home Page, http://www.ars.usda.gov/ba/bhnrc/ndl

A low-cholesterol, low-fat diet should limit cholesterol intake to 300 mg per day, have less than 30% of calories as fat, and no more than 10% of calories as saturated fats. Calories contributed by monounsaturated fats, hence total fat, are not included except under kcal.

Appendix Y

Table Y-1
Sodium Content of Foods*

350–500+ mg	200–350 mg	100–200 mg	50–100 mg	<50 mg
1/4 tsp salt (581 mg sodium)	1/2 cup spinach, beets, celery, kale, seasoned with 1/16 tsp salt	1/2 cup canned carrots, Swiss chard, or seasoned vegetables not listed elsewhere	1/2 cup of the following unsalted vegetables: frozen mixed peas and carrots	1/2 cup of the following fresh, frozen, or canned vegetables, canned without salt:
3/4 tsp monosodium glutamate	1 oz salami	1 oz natural cheddar cheese	3/4 cup milk (6 oz)	1 artichoke (edible base and leaves)
1/2 bouillon cube	1 hard roll	1 tbsp catsup	1/2 cup pasta cooked in salted (1/16 tsp) water	beets, carrots, celery, dandelion greens, kale, mustard greens, peas (black-eyed), spinach, succotash, turnip greens, turnip (white), lima beans, peas
1/2 cup hominy seasoned with 1/8 tsp salt	1/2 cup rice or grits cooked in salted water	5 saltine crackers	1 oz tuna, drained (not rinsed)	
1 average frankfurter (1 1/2 oz)	1/2 cup tomato juice	1/2 cup beet greens		
3 oz canned sardines or salmon	1/2 cup cooked rice, spaghetti, noodles, seasoned with 1/8 tsp salt	1 1/2 oz turkey luncheon meat		
1 grilled cheese sandwich made with 2 slices white bread, 2 oz American cheese, 2 tsp margarine	1/3 cup drained sauerkraut	3 oz shrimp (fresh) cooked in salted water		
1 box 4-ct McDonalds Chicken McNuggets[†]	2 thin slices bacon, crisp and drained	1 oz frozen fish fillets		
1 McDonalds hamburger on bun		1 slice regular bread		
1 McDonalds cheeseburger on bun		1 small order of McDonalds French fries		
1 McDonalds Big Mac[†]				
1 cup Kraft Macaroni & Cheese[‡]				
1 cup Spaghetti O's[§]				

*Based on data from US Department of Agriculture, Agricultural Research Service. USDA Nutrient Database for Standard Reference, Release 18. Available at: http://www.ars.usda.gov/ba/bhnrc/ndl.

† McDonalds Corporation, Oak Brook, IL.

‡ Kraft Foods, Northfield, IL.

§ Campbell Soup, Camden, NJ.

APP

Index

A

G

Gabapentin, food or nutrient interactions with, 1322

Gagging
  in feeding disorders, 579
  in neurologic impairment, 823
  reflex for, 121

Galactomannans, 511

Galactose, absorption of, 11

Galactosemia
  breastfeeding contraindicated in, 39
  screening for, 661–662
  soy formulas for, 72–74
  treatment of, 666, 667

Galanin, in energy homeostasis, 746

Gallbladder, development of, 4

Gamma-linolenic acid, 362

Garlic, 304

Gastric bypass surgery, 766–767

Gastric emptying
  in breastfed infants, 34
  in eating disorders, 869

Gastric lipase, in fat digestion, 8, 9, 359

Gastric tolerance, in sports, 229–230

Gastroenteritis
  diarrhea after, 645–646
  feeding during, 161–162
  lactase deficiency after, 347

Gastroesophageal reflux
  in enteral feeding, 552–553
  in neurologic impairment, 824, 829, 836
  swallowing disorders in, 582, 583

Gastrointestinal disorders. See also Gastroenteritis
  breastfeeding protection against, 36, 127
  in cancer therapy, 928–929
  in congenital heart disease, 983
  enteral feeding for, 543–545
  in food hypersensitivity, 784, 785, 793
  in HIV infection, 878, 880–882

Gastrointestinal function
  in breastfed infants, 34
  development of, 3–28
    carbohydrate processing, 10–12
    disorders of, 4–5
    in embryonic period, 3–5
    fat processing, 7–10
    for human milk utilization, 16–19
    intestinal epithelium, 5–6
    microbiota population, 19–20
    mineral absorption, 16
    nutrient assimilation, 6–7

protein processing, 12–15
    vitamin absorption, 15–16
  in parenteral nutrition, 534–535

Gastrojejunostomy feeding, for neurologic impairment, 836

Gastroplasty, vertical banded, 766–767

Gastroschisis, 5

Gastrostomy tube feeding, 552–554
  for cancer, 934–936
  for congenital heart disease, 995
  for cystic fibrosis, 1008–1009
  for neurologic impairment, 834–836
  of vegetarian diets, 218

Gaucher disease, 670

Genetic factors
  in eating disorders, 859
  in obesity, 740, 749–752

Genetically modified foods. See Biotechnology

Gentamicin, for hepatic encephalopathy, 977

Ghrelin, in energy homeostasis, 746

Giardiasis, 639, 1098

Ginger, 304

Ginkgo, 304

Gitelman syndrome, 913

Glipizide, food or nutrient interactions with, 1320, 1322

Global Strategy for Infant and Young Child Feeding, 50

Globulin, measurement of, in nutritional status assessment, 572, 573

Glomerulonephritis, 915

Glucagon
  in energy homeostasis, 746
  for hypoglycemia, 714, 715

Glucagon-like peptides, in energy homeostasis, 746

Glucoamylase, 343

Gluconeogenesis, 346, 847–848

Glucose
  abnormal. See Hyperglycemia; Hypoglycemia
  absorption of, 10–11
  amino acid conversion to, 13
  in beverages, cariogenic potential of, 1043–1044
  for hypoglycemia, 711–716
  for inborn errors of metabolism, 663
  metabolism of, 344–346, 847–848
  monitoring of, in diabetes mellitus, 674
  in oral rehydration therapy, 651–653
  in parenteral nutrition, 100, 525–526
  requirements of, 257, 345–346

etiology of, 704–706
evaluation of, 706–708
in hyperinsulinism, 709–709
in ketogenic diet, 1033
ketotic, 705, 710
in neonates, 701–709, 711–714
nonketotic, 706, 710–711
pathophysiology of, 701–702
reactive, 707
treatment of, 711–716
unawareness of, 703
unexplained, 708
Hypolactasia, 12
Hypoleptinemia, 747
Hypomagnesemia, 389, 396–397
Hyponatremia
in cystic fibrosis, 1006–1007
in sports, 229
Hypophosphatemic rickets, familial, 667
Hypopituitarism, hypoglycemia in, 708
Hypothalamus, in energy homeostasis,
743–749
Hypothermia, in anorexia nervosa, 862
Hypothyroidism
obesity in, 757
screening for, 661–662
Hypoxemia, in congenital heart disease, 986

I

Idiosyncrasy, food, 784
Illness, feeding during, 161–162
Immunity
human milk and, 18–19, 34–35, 803–806
neonatal intestine function in, 6
nutrient interactions with, 801–819
in deficiencies, 802
early, 802–807
herbal products, 811–812
importance of, 801–802
iron, 808
long-chain polyunsaturated fatty
acids, 810–811
nucleotides, 810
in preterm infants, 807
probiotics, 811
vitamins, 809–810
zinc, 808–809
Immunizations, for failure to thrive, 615
Immunodeficiency, in malnutrition, 612
Immunoglobulin(s), measurement of, in
diarrhea, 640

Immunoglobulin A, in human milk, 17–18,
803–804
Immunoglobulin E, in food hypersensitivity,
790–791
Inborn errors of metabolism, 661–672
community nutrition services for, 1059
definitions of, 661
hypoglycemia in, 706–707
inheritance of, 661
parent education on, 664
screening for, 661–662
signs and symptoms of, 662
treatment of
emergency, 663–664
enzyme replacement in, 670
gene therapy in, 670–671
ketogenic diet in, 1025
organ transplantation in, 670
pharmacologic, 669–670
restrictions in, 666–669
supplements for, 666–669
synthetic medical foods for, 664–665,
1387–1389
Indian reservations, food distribution
programs for, 1066, 1073–1074
Indinavir, food or nutrient interactions with,
1321, 1324
Indirect calorimetry, for energy expenditure
measurement, 321
Individuals with Disabilities Education Act,
1062–1063
Industrial chemicals, safety concerns with,
1122–1123
Infant(s)
breastfeeding of. See Breastfeeding
calcium requirements of, 387, 390–393
carbohydrate requirements of, 345–346
complementary foods for. See
Complementary foods
copper requirements of, 432–434
critical illness in, 843–854
cultural food practices related to,
185–190
cystic fibrosis in, 1001–1003, 1005–1006,
1009–1010, 1013–1015
dental caries in, 1041
diarrhea in, chronic or persistent,
637–649
Dietary Reference Intakes for, 1294–1296
energy requirements of, 321–323
fat digestion in, 359
fat processing in, 7–10
fat requirements of, 359–361